# Medical Radiology

## Diagnostic Imaging



For further volumes:
http://www.springer.com/series/4354

Denis Tack • Mannudeep K. Kalra
Pierre Alain Gevenois
Editors

# Radiation Dose from Multidetector CT

Second Edition

Foreword by
Maximilian F. Reiser

Springer

*Editors*
Prof. Dr. Denis Tack
Department of Radiology
Réseau Hospitalier de Médecine Sociale
Rue Louis Caty 136
7331 Baudour
Belgium

Prof. Dr. Pierre Alain Gevenois
Department of Radiology
Université libre de Bruxelles Hôspital Erasme
Route de Lennik 808
1070 Brussels
Belgium

Asst. Prof. Dr. Mannudeep K. Kalra
Department of Radiology
Harvard Medical School
Massachusetts General Hospital
55 Fruit Street
02114 Boston MA
USA

Additional material to this book can be downloaded from http://extras.springer.com/

ISSN 0942-5373
ISBN 978-3-642-24534-3 ISBN 978-3-642-24535-0 (eBook)
DOI 10.1007/978-3-642-24535-0
Springer Heidelberg New York Dordrecht London

Library of Congress Control Number: 2012934251



Printed on acid-free paper

Springer is part of Springer Science+Business Media (www.springer.com)

# Foreword

The introduction of spiral and multi-detector-row computed tomography has a profound impact on radiological practice. Within one and a half decades we witnessed a breathtaking technological development allowing for high quality imaging data within a very short acquisition time and providing excellent image quality and diagnostic accuracy. Not surprisingly, there was also a considerable increase in radiation exposure to the patients and the population. This resulted in concerns about potential health hazards as well as various initiatives and actions of governmental and non-governmental bodies. At the same time great efforts were made in order to reduce the radiation exposure to patients without compromising image quality and diagnostic efficacy.

The high actuality of this topic is underlined by the fact, that within a short period of time a second edition of the book "Radiation dose in CT" became necessary. It is the great merit of the editors Denis Tack, Mannudeep K. Kalra and Pierre Alain Gevenois and the authors contributing to this book, to compose a second edition which covers many important issues such as CT technology and use, general aspects of CT radiation, practical approaches to dose reduction, radiation risk management in low dose MDCT screening programmes, initiatives for dose reduction and the vendor perspective on CT radiation dose. The editors as well as the authors are internationally distinguished scientists in the field. This book gives a comprehensive overview on all aspects of radiation dose in CT. I would like to express my great appreciation and thanks for this magnificent work which I am confident will be of great use not only for radiologists and CT practitioners but also for those interested in radiation protection as well as for political decision makers.

Prof. Dr. Maximilian F. Reiser
Munich

# Preface

*Radiation dose in CT* is the second edition of our textbook titled *Radiation Dose from Adult and Pediatric Multidetector Computed Tomography*. The second edition of this textbook was necessitated by continued technologic advances in multidetector-row computed tomography (MDCT) since the first edition as well as by development of new and promising radiation dose reduction technologies. Despite these developments, MDCT still poses challenges in radiological protection to the extent that CT radiation dose has been labelled by some as one of the topmost patient safety concerns. Applications and use of MDCT continue to proliferate with emergence of newer clinical indications; requests of clinicians for high diagnostic confidence as provided by MDCT are factors contributing to a continuous increase in the collective radiation dose from diagnostic CT imaging.

The first edition of the textbook dealt with radiation issues with MDCT in two parts. The first part was preceded with detailed discussions on the clinical use and expansion of CT in modern medical practice. In Part I, the book provided a comprehensive approach to perceived and potential risks of low radiation dose, influence of CT technical factors on the radiation dose, and technologic developments for optimization and reduction of the radiation dose per acquisition. In Part II, a comprehensive clinical approach of radiation dose justification, optimization, and reduction was provided, covering the fields of pediatric, head and neck, chest, abdomen, cardiovascular, bone and joint, and interventional MDCT. Finally, a detailed discussion on the balance between the risks and benefits of screening for cancer using low-dose MDCT was presented in the field of lung cancer and colon cancer.

The second edition of the textbook has recent and updated information about the two parts presented in the first edition. Several new chapters from renowned international radiation experts have been added to embellish the second edition, which now boasts seven parts including an online only Interactive Atlas-based teaching part which has four additional chapters for understanding the effect of CT radiation dose on image quality and lesion detection and appearance. In the second edition, Part I deals with technologic advances in MDCT and updates on clinical expansion in use of MDCT. Part II deals with risk issues with CT, and several technical aspects of CT radiation dose management with new chapters on iterative reconstruction techniques, noise reduction filters, hardware developments for dose optimization, tube potential adjustments for dose reduction, and an unbiased perspective on the use of shielding devices in CT. A new chapter on radiation dose recording and auditing has also been added to this part.

Practical and clinical approaches to dose optimization in different radiology subspecialties are presented in Part III of the second edition, which has been enhanced by addition of a chapter based on issues with CT scanning in pregnant patients. Part IV deals with radiation issues and dose reduction strategies for lung and colon cancer screening CT protocols. Part V presents perspectives of several regulatory bodies, organizations, and campaigns on CT radiation dose including the IAEA, FDA, ICRP, Image Gently, and Image Wisely. This part also includes two chapters on software for estimating CT dose and risks, and on discussion of guidelines for appropriate use of CT. Part VI brings entirely new content to the second chapter with four new chapters from major CT vendors outlining their CT radiation dose reduction and optimization technologies.

Several international experts, from Europe and North America, selected for their important contributions to the scientific literature, have contributed to this book with a common objective of providing readers with a comprehensive, up-to-date, practical, clinical, and well-documented approach on radiation dose optimization and reduction, suitable for daily MDCT practice.

Among the three editors, Denis Tack, is a general radiologist subspecialized in MDCT, and Pierre Alain Gevenois is Chest radiologist and Professor of medical imaging at the Faculty of Medicine and the School of Public Health of the University of Brussels, Belgium. Their researches deal with radiation dose reduction with MDCT, and quantification of pulmonary emphysema and pulmonary edema by computed tomography. The new editor, Mannudeep K. Kalra is a Chest and Cardiac radiologist at the Massachusetts General Hospital and an Assistant Professor at Harvard Medical School in Boston with key interest in CT radiation dose research and education.

Denis Tack
Mannudeep K. Kalra
Pierre Alain Gevenois

# Contents

## Part VI Vendor Perspective on CT Radiation Dose

# Contributors

**E. Stephen Amis** Department of Diagnostic Radiology, Yale University School of Medicine, Tomkins East 2-230 789 Howard Avenue, New Haven, CT, 06520-9128, USA; Department of Radiology, Albert Einstein College of Medicine and Montefiore Medical Center Department of Radiology, 111 E 210th St., Bronx, NY 10467-2401, USA

**Shima Aran** Department of Radiology, Harvard Medical School, Massachusetts General Hospital, Boston, MA, USA

**A. A. Bankier** Department of Radiology, Beth Israel Deaconess Medical Center, 330 Brookline Ave, Boston, MA 02215, USA

**Patrick Bellinck** Department of Radiology, Heilig Hart Ziekenhuis, Mechelsestraat 24, 2500 Lier, Belgium

**A. Blum** Guilloz Imaging Department, Hôpital Central, CHU Nancy, 29 avenue du Maréchal de Lattre de Tassigny, 54035, Nancy Cedex, France

**Thierry N. Boellaard** Department of Radiology, Academic Medical Center, University of Amsterdam, P.O. Box 22660, 1100 DD Amsterdam, The Netherlands, e-mail: t.n.boellaard@amc.uva.nl

**William W. Boonn** Hospital of the University of Pennsylvania, Philadelphia, PA, USA

**Sean Boyd** U.S. Department of Health and Human Services, U.S. Food and Drug Administration, Silver Spring, MD, USA

**James A. Brink** Department of Diagnostic Radiology, Yale University School of Medicine, Tomkins East 2-230, 789 Howard Avenue, New Haven, CT, 06520-9128, USA, e-mail: james.brink@yale.edu

**Alan Britten** Department of Physics and Clinical Engineering, St. George's Hospital, ImPACT CT Scanner Evaluation Centre, London, SW170QT, UK

**N. Buls** UZ Brussel, Laarbeeklaan 101, 1090 Brussel, Belgium, e-mail: Nico.Buls@uzbrussel.be

**Michael J. Callahan** Department of Radiology, Children's Hospital, 300 Longwood Ave, Boston, MA 02115-5737, USA

**Kenneth H. Chadwick** 3 Ellerbank, Cowan Head, Kendal, Cumbria, LA8 9HX, UK, e-mail: kennethhchadwick@aol.com

**Kish Chakrabarti** U.S. Department of Health and Human Services, U.S. Food and Drug Administration, Silver Spring, MD, USA

**Olivera Ciraj-Bjelac** International Atomic Energy Agency, Vienna International Centre, 1400 Vienna, Austria; Vinca Institute of Nuclear Sciences, , M.P. Alasa 12-14, Vinca, Belgrade, Serbia,

**Bernard L. Cohen** Department of Physics, University of Pittsburgh, Pittsburgh, PA 15260, USA, e-mail: blc@pitt.edu

**Tessa S. Cook** Hospital of the University of Pennsylvania, Philadelphia, PA, USA, e-mail: tessa.cook@uphs.upenn.edu

**Synho Do** Department of Radiology, Massachusetts General Hospital, Boston, MA, USA

**Sue Edyvean** Department of Physics and Clinical Engineering, St. George's Hospital, ImPACT CT Scanner Evaluation Centre, London, SW170QT, UK, e-mail: sue.edyvean@gmail.com; sue@impactscan.org

**Joel G. Fletcher** Department of Radiology, Mayo Clinic College of Medicine, 200 First Street SW, Rochester, MN 55905, USA

**Thomas Flohr** Siemens Healthcare, Forchheim, Germany; Eberhard Karls University, Tübingen, Germany, e-mail: thomas.flohr@siemens.com

**Donald P. Frush** Division of Pediatric Radiology, Duke University Medical Center, 1905 McGovern Davison Childrens Health Center, Durham, NC 27710-3808, USA

**Jacob Geleijns** Radiology Department, Leiden University Medical Center, Albinusdreef 2, 2333 ZA, Leiden, The Netherlands, e-mail: J.Geleijns@lumc.nl

**A. Gervaise** Guilloz Imaging Department, Hôpital Central, CHU Nancy, 29 avenue du Maréchal de Lattre de Tassigny, 54035, Nancy Cedex, France; Medical Imaging Department, Hôpital d'Instruction des Armées Legouest, 27 avenue de Plantières, BP 90001, 57077 Metz Cedex 3, France, e-mail: alban.gervaise@hotmail.fr

**Pierre Alain Gevenois** Department of Radiology, Clinic of Chest Imaging, Hôpital Erasme, Université Libre de Bruxelles, Brussels, Belgium, e-mail: Pierre.Alain.Gevenois@erasme.ulb.ac.be

**Stephen Golding** Radiology Group, Nuffield Department of Surgical Sciences, University of Oxford, Oxford, UK, e-mail: stephen.golding@surgery.oxford.ac.uk

**Marilyn J. Goske** Department of Radiology, Cincinnati Children's Hospital Medical Center, MLC 5031, 3333 Burnet Ave, Cincinnati, OH 45229-3039, USA, e-mail: Marilyn.Goske@cchmc.org

**Kristie M. Guite** Departments of Radiology, University of Wisconsin, Mail Code 3252, 600 Highland Avenue, Madison, WI 53792, USA

**J. Louis Hinshaw** Departments of Radiology, University of Wisconsin, Mail Code 3252, 600 Highland Avenue, Madison, WI 53792, USA, e-mail: jhinshaw @uwhealth.org

**R. Irwan** CT Business Unit, Toshiba Medical Systems Europe, Zoetermeer, The Netherlands

**Mannudeep K. Kalra** Department of Radiology, Harvard Medical School, Massachusetts General Hospital, 55 Fruit Street, 02114, Boston, MA, USA; Department of Radiology, Emory University School of Medicine, 1364 Clifton Road NE, Atlanta GA 30322, USA; Department of Radiology, Harvard Medical School, Massachusetts General Hospital, Boston, MA 02114, USA, e-mail: mkalra@partners.org; mkalra@emory.edu

**Sue C. Kaste** Radiologic Science Division of Diagnostic Imaging, St Jude Children's Research Hospital, 262 Danny Thomas Place, Memphis, TN 38105-2794, USA

**Caroline Keyzer** Department of Radiology, Hôpital Erasme, Université libre de Bruxelles, Route de Lennik 808, 1070 Brussels, Belgium, e-mail: caroline. keyzer@erasme.ulb.ac.be

**Woojin Kim** Hospital of the University of Pennsylvania, Philadelphia, PA, USA

**Iacovos S. Kyprianou** U.S. Department of Health and Human Services, U.S. Food and Drug Administration, Silver Spring, MD, USA

**S. Lecocq** Guilloz Imaging Department, Hôpital Central, CHU Nancy, 29 avenue du Maréchal de Lattre de Tassigny, 54035, Nancy Cedex, France

**Fred T. Lee** Departments of Radiology, University of Wisconsin, Mail Code 3252, 600 Highland Avenue, Madison, WI 53792, USA

**Hendrik P. Leenhouts** FredBantinglaan 6, 6721 BC, Bennekom, The Netherlands

**Christianne Leidecker** Siemens Medical Solutions, Erlangen, Germany, e-mail: Christianne.Leidecker@siemens.com

**Maria Lewis** Department of Physics and Clinical Engineering, St. George's Hospital, ImPACT CT Scanner Evaluation Centre, London, SW170QT, UK

**D. E. Litmanovich** Department of Radiology, Beth Israel Deaconess Medical Center, 330 Brookline Ave, Boston, MA 02215, USA, e-mail: dlitmano@ bidmc.harvard.edu

**M. Louis** Guilloz Imaging Department, Hôpital Central, CHU Nancy, 29 avenue du Maréchal de Lattre de Tassigny, 54035, Nancy Cedex, France

**Rich Mather** Toshiba Medical Research Institute, 706 N Deerpath Dr, Vernon Hills, IL 60061, USA, e-mail: rmather@tmriusa.com

**Cynthia H. McCollough** Department of Radiology, Mayo Clinic College of Medicine, 200 First Street SW, Rochester, MN 55905, USA

**Stuart Meeson** Radiology Group, Nuffield Department of Surgical Sciences, University of Oxford, Oxford, UK

**Dhruv Mehta** Philips Healthcare, Miner Road 595, Cleveland, OH, USA

**J. de Mey** UZ Brussel, Laarbeeklaan 101, 1090 Brussel, Belgium

**Thalia T. Mills** U.S. Department of Health and Human Services, U.S. Food and Drug Administration, Silver Spring, MD, USA

**Gregory Morrison**, American Society of Radiologic Technologists, 15000 Central Ave SE, Albuquerque, NM 87123-3909, USA

**Krijn van Muiswinkel** Department of Radiology, Meander Medical Center Amersfoort, Utrechtseweg 160, 3800 BM, Amersfoort, The Netherlands

**Tom Mulkens** Department of Radiology, Heilig Hart Ziekenhuis, Mechelsestraat 24, 2500 Lier, Belgium, e-mail: tom.mulkens@scarlet.betom.mulkens@hhzhlier.be

**Roy A. Nilsen** GE Healthcare, Waukesha, WI, USA, e-mail: Roy.Nilsen@med.ge.com

**Rajesh Patel** Radiology Group, Nuffield Department of Surgical Sciences, University of Oxford, Oxford, UK

**Jean François Paul** Department of Radiology, Marie Lannelongue Surgical Centre, Plessis-Robinson, France

**Mathias Prokop** Department of Radiology, Diagnostic Image Analysis Group, University Hospital Nijmegen, St Radboud, 6500 HB, Nijmegen, The Netherlands

**Homer Pien** Department of Radiology, Massachusetts General Hospital, Boston, MA, USA, e-mail: hpien@partners.org

**Cornelia Schaefer-Prokop** Department of Radiology, Meander Medical Center Amersfoort, Utrechtseweg 160, 3800 BM, Amersfoort, The Netherlands; Department of Radiology, Diagnostic Image Analysis Group, University Hospital Nijmegen, St Radboud, 6500 HB, Nijmegen, The Netherlands

**Frank N. Ranallo** Departments of Radiology, University of Wisconsin, Mail Code 3252, 600 Highland Avenue, Madison, WI 53792, USA; Departments of Medical Physics, University of Wisconsin, Madison, WI, USA

**Madan M. Rehani** International Atomic Energy Agency, Vienna International Centre, 1400 Vienna, Austria; Secretary, Protection in Medicine Committee, International Commission on Radiological Protection (ICRP), Ottawa, ON, Canada, e-mail: M.M.Rehani@iaea.org; madan.rehani@gmail.com

**Rodrigo Salgado** Department of Radiology, Universitair Ziekenhuis Antwerpen, Wilrijkstraat 10, 2650 Edegem, Belgium

**Cornelia Schaefer-Prokop** Department of Radiology, Meander Medical Center Amersfoort, Utrechtseweg 160, 3800 BM, Amersfoort, The Netherlands

**Bernhard Schmidt** Siemens Medical Solutions, Erlangen, Germany

**Sarabjeet Singh** Department of Radiology, Harvard Medical School Massachusetts General Hospital, 55 Fruit Street, 02114 Boston, MA, USA; Department of Radiology, Harvard Medical School, Massachusetts General Hospital, Boston, MA, USA; Department of Radiology, Harvard Medical School, Massachusetts General Hospital, Boston, MA 02114, USA

**David C. Spelic** U.S. Department of Health and Human Services, U.S. Food and Drug Administration, Silver Spring, MD, USA

**Georg Stamm** Medizinische Hochschule Hannover, Institut für Diagnostische und Interventionelle Radiologie, Carl-Neuberg-Str. 1, 30625 Hannover, Germany, e-mail: stamm.georg@mh-hannover.de

**Stanley H. Stern** U.S. Department of Health and Human Services, U.S. Food and Drug Administration, Silver Spring, MD, USA, e-mail: Stanley.Stern@fda.hhs.gov

**Jaap Stoker** Department of Radiology, Academic Medical Center, University of Amsterdam, P.O. Box 22660, 1100 DD Amsterdam, The Netherlands

**Enno Stranzinger** Department of Diagnostic, Interventional and Pediatric Radiology, University Hospital, Inselspital, 3010 Bern, Switzerland

**Keith J. Strauss** Department of Radiology, Cincinnati Children's Hospital Medical Center, MLC 5031, 3333 Burnet Ave, Cincinnati, OH 45229-3039, USA

**Denis Tack** Department of Radiology, Clinique Louis Caty, Hôpital RHMS, Rue Louis Caty 136, 7331, Baudour, Belgium; Department of Radiology, RHMS Clinique Louis Caty, Rue Louis Caty 136, 7331, Baudour, Belgium

**P. Teixeira** Guilloz Imaging Department, Hôpital Central, CHU Nancy, 29 avenue du Maréchal de Lattre de Tassigny, 54035 Nancy Cedex, France

**Thomas L. Toth** General Electric Healthcare Technologies, 3000 North Grandview, Boulevard, Waukesha, WI 53188, USA; GE Healthcare, Brookfield, WI, USA, e-mail: Thomas.toth@plexar.com

**F. Vandenbroucke** UZ Brussel, Laarbeeklaan 101, 1090 Brussel, Belgium

**Henk W. Venema** Department of Radiology, Academic Medical Center, University of Amsterdam, P.O. Box 22660, 1100 DD Amsterdam, The Netherlands

**N. Villani** Medical Radiophysics Unit, CRAN UMR 7039 CNRS, Centre Alexis Vautrin, Avenue de Bourgogne, 54511 Vandoeuvre-les-Nancy, France

**Alain Vlassenbroek** Philips Healthcare, Miner Road 595, Cleveland, OH, USA, e-mail: alain.vlassenbroek@philips.com

**Peter Vock** Department of Diagnostic, Interventional and Pediatric Radiology, University Hospital, Inselspital, 3010 Bern, Switzerland, e-mail: peter.vock@insel.ch

**Michelle Williams** University of Edinburgh/British Heart Foundation Centre for Cardiovascular Science, Chancellor's Building, 49, Little France Crescent, EH16SU4, Edinburgh, UK

**Rainer Wolf** Department of Diagnostic, Interventional and Pediatric Radiology, University Hospital, Inselspital, 3010 Bern, Switzerland

**Jeffrey Yanof** Philips Healthcare, Miner Road 595, Cleveland, OH, USA

**Lifeng Yu** Department of Radiology, Mayo Clinic College of Medicine, 200 First Street SW, Rochester, MN 55905, USA, e-mail: yu.lifeng@mayo.edu

# Part I

# CT Technology and Use

# Multi-Detector Row CT–Recent Developments, Radiation Dose and Dose Reduction Technologies

Thomas Flohr

## Contents




**Abstract**

Clinical experience with the most recent 64-slice and 128-slice CT-systems indicates that a further increase of the number of detector rows will not automatically translate into improved clinical performance. Consequently, recent CT developments have focused on solving remaining limitations of multi-detector row CT, such as limited potential to dynamically scan entire organs or insufficient temporal resolution for cardiac imaging. We discuss new CT system concepts such as CT-scanners with area detectors large enough to cover entire organs, or dual-source CT-systems with considerably enhanced temporal resolution below 100 ms and fast volume coverage by means of high pitch scanning. Furthermore, we introduce and explain the basic radiation dose parameters in CT and their measurement. We briefly discuss established and new techniques for radiation dose reduction, such as anatomical X-ray tube current modulation, organ-based tube current modulation, ECG-controlled tube current modulation, adaptation of the X-ray tube voltage to the patient's anatomy and the planned examination type, dynamically adjustable pre-patient collimators and iterative reconstruction.


## 1 Recent Developments in CT

During the last decade, multi-detector row CT (MDCT) has been driven by a fast development from 4-slice scanners to the most recent 64-slice and 128-slice systems. This technical progress has been accompanied by a significant enhancement of the


T. Flohr (✉)
Siemens Healthcare, Forchheim, Germany
e-mail: thomas.flohr@siemens.com

T. Flohr
Eberhard Karls University, Tübingen, Germany



D. Tack et al. (eds.), *Radiation Dose from Multidetector CT*, Medical Radiology. Diagnostic Imaging,
DOI: 10.1007/174_2011_499, © Springer-Verlag Berlin Heidelberg 2012

clinical potential of CT. On the other hand, clinical experience indicates that a level of saturation has meanwhile been reached, and that adding even more detector rows will not by itself translate into increased clinical benefit.

Consequently, recent CT developments have focused on solving remaining limitations of MDCT, such as limited potential to dynamically scan entire organs or insufficient temporal resolution for cardiac CT. As a result, new CT-system concepts have been introduced, such as CT-scanners with large area detectors providing 16 cm volume coverage, or dual-source CT-systems enabling CT imaging at a temporal resolution of up to 75 ms.

In the following sections, we will discuss some of these new developments.

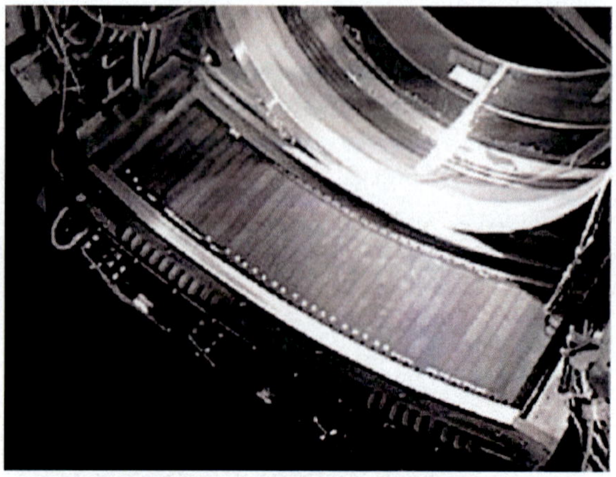

**Fig. 1** Prototype of a CT area detector providing 256 × 0.5 mm collimation (from: Mori et al. (2006))

## 1.1 CT-Systems with Area Detector

One remaining challenge for MDCT is the visualization of dynamic processes in extended anatomical ranges, e.g. to characterize the inflow and outflow of contrast agent in the arterial and venous system in dynamic CT angiographic studies (CTAs), or to determine the enhancement characteristics of the contrast agent in volume perfusion scans. One way to solve this problem is the introduction of area detectors large enough to cover entire organs, such as the heart, the kidneys or the brain, in one axial scan. In 2007, a CT-scanner with 320 × 0.5 mm collimation and 0.35 s gantry rotation time was commercially introduced by one vendor, after a long evaluation phase using prototype systems (see Fig. 1) with 256 × 0.5 mm collimation and 0.5 s gantry rotation time (Mori et al. 2004; Mori et al. 2006a; Funashabi et al. 2005; Mori et al. 2006b; Kido et al. 2007).

CT-scanners with area detectors are optimized for the acquisition of axial (sequential) scan data without table movement. The reconstructed scan field of view (SFOV) is cone-shaped, see Fig. 2. With 320 × 0.5 mm detector collimation, a SFOV of 16 cm z-width is feasible at the iso-center, however, z-coverage reduces to only 11.7 cm at a distance of 160 mm from the iso-center. Larger scan volumes in the z-direction have to be covered by "stitching", i.e. by appending axial scans shifted in the z-direction. With increasing SFOV, more overlap in the z-direction is required for gapless volume coverage.

CT-scanners with area detector show advantages in cardiac scanning and in the acquisition of dynamic CT data.

With the typical MDCT detector z-coverages of 40 mm (and recently up to 80 mm, Weigold 2009), ECG-controlled CT volume imaging of the heart is comprised of several subvolumes acquired during two to four consecutive heart beats (Flohr et al. 2007). These image subvolumes can be blurred or shifted relative to each other as a consequence of insufficient temporal resolution or variations of the heart motion from one cardiac cycle to the next, resulting in stair-step or banding artifacts in multi-planar reformations (MPRs) or volume rendered images (VRTs). The width of an image slab originating from one heart beat is proportional to the detector z-coverage. CT-systems with large area detectors can image the entire heart in one axial scan without table movement, in this way avoiding stair-step artifacts. As a downside, the entire scan will be distorted in case of arrhythmia or ectopic beats during data acquisition. Meanwhile, successful use of the commercially available CT-system with 320 × 0.5 mm detector collimation for coronary CTA has been demonstrated (Rybicki et al. 2008; Hoe and Toh 2009; Steigner et al. 2009; Dewey et al. 2009).

As a second benefit, CT-systems with area detectors can acquire dynamic volume data by repeatedly scanning the same anatomical range without table movement, which is useful in dynamic CT angiographic studies or in volume perfusion studies (see Fig. 3), e.g. to differentiate hepatocellular carcinoma

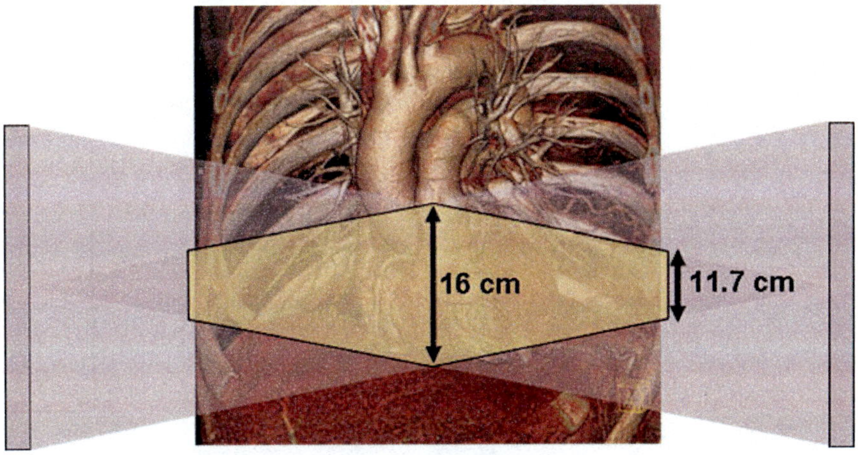


**Fig. 2** The scan volume acquired in an axial scan with an area detector is cone-shaped. To obtain gapless volume coverage, consecutive scans have to overlap in the z-direction

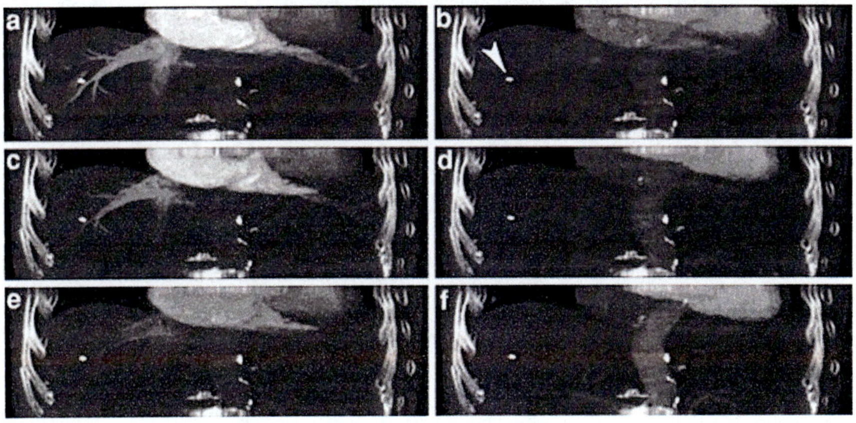


**Fig. 3** Dynamic CT scan of a patient with hepatocellular carcinoma using a CT-system with area detector. Coronal images with maximum intensity projection (MIP) beginning **a** 30 s, **b** 31.0 s, **c** 33.1 s, **d** 34.5 s, **e** 37.4 s, **f** 39.4 s after contrast injection (from Mori et al. (2006c))

(HCC) from normal liver tissue (Mori et al. 2007), or for the evaluation of myocardial perfusion defects.

A challenge of larger detector z-coverage in particular for perfusion scanning is increased X-ray scatter. Scattered radiation may cause hypodense artifacts, may affect CT-number stability, and the scatter-induced noise may reduce the contrast-to-noise ratio (CNR) in the images (Flohr et al. 2009b). The magnitude of scatter artifacts scales linearly with the illuminated z-width of the detector (Engel et al. 2008).

An alternative approach to dynamic CT scanning of a larger volume is the use of a spiral shuttle mode. By periodically moving the patient forward and backward during data acquisition (Fig. 4), a scan range larger than the detector z-width is covered. The scan range can be flexibly adapted to the organ of interest. As a downside, the maximum temporal sampling rate is lower than with a wide detector, and data sampling is temporally equidistant only in the center of the scanned area. The non-equidistant data sampling at different z-positions within the volume has to be considered in the calculation of the perfusion parameters; their accuracy, however, is not compromised (Haberland et al. 2010). Using a spiral shuttle mode with a 4 cm detector, a scan range of about 15 cm can be dynamically covered at an average sampling rate of 1.5 s, which is sufficient for perfusion scanning of the brain and of abdominal organs (Abels et al. 2011).

Figure 5 shows an example for the use of dynamic volume perfusion CT in oncology. Changes of tumor vascularity demonstrated by a change of perfusion parameters might be earlier indicators for response to modern anti-angiogenesis therapy than a change of the tumor size, which is the conventional parameter to assess therapy response.

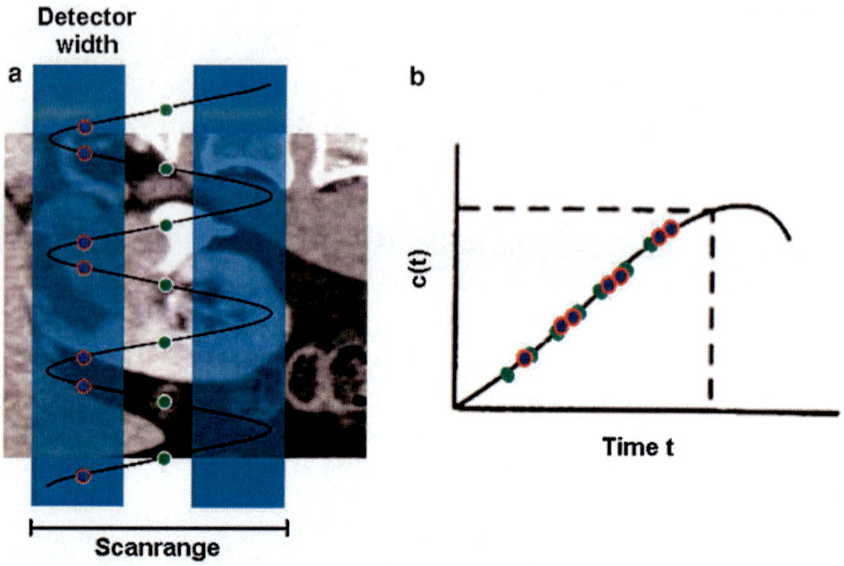


**Fig. 4** **a** Using a spiral shuttle mode to acquire dynamic CT data in an extended scan range. **b** Time attenuation curve with temporal sampling points at different z-positions. Note the temporally non-equidistant sampling outside the center of the scanned area (*blue circles*)

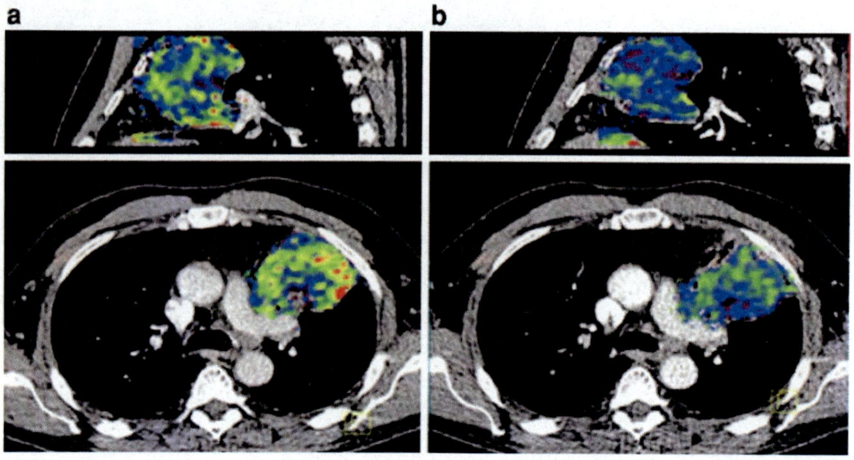


**Fig. 5** Permeability map obtained from a volume perfusion scan of a patient with bronchial carcinoma. Initial scan (**a**) and scan 2 weeks after combined treatment with radiotherapy and a vascular targeting drug (**b**). Although there is no change in tumor size, permeability decreases and indicates therapy response (courtesy of Vicky Goh, King's College London, Great Britain)

## 1.2 Dual-Source CT

Cardiac imaging with CT requires excellent temporal resolution, i.e. very short exposure time of the individual axial slices, and the corresponding dedicated scan and image reconstruction techniques. To improve temporal resolution in a clinically reliable way, the gantry has to rotate faster. Despite gantry rotation times of 0.3 s and less, motion artifacts at higher and irregular heart rates remain a challenge for coronary CTA even with the latest generation of MDCT. An alternative scanner concept that provides considerably enhanced temporal resolution but does not require faster gantry rotation is a CT with multiple tubes and corresponding detectors (Robb and Ritman 1979; Ritman et al. 1980). In 2006, a dual-source CT (DSCT), i.e. a CT scanner with two X-ray tubes and two corresponding detectors offset by 90° (Flohr et al. 2006), was commercially introduced by one vendor, see Fig. 6.

Detector A covers the full SFOV of 50 cm diameter, while detector B is restricted to a central 26 cm FOV. Both detectors provide 64 overlapping 0.6 mm slices with the use of a z-flying focal spot. The shortest gantry rotation time is 0.33 s. Each of the two X-ray tubes can be operated independently with regard to their kV- and mA-settings. This allows the acquisition of dual-energy data, with one tube being operated at e.g. 80 kV while the other is operated at e. g. 140 kV.

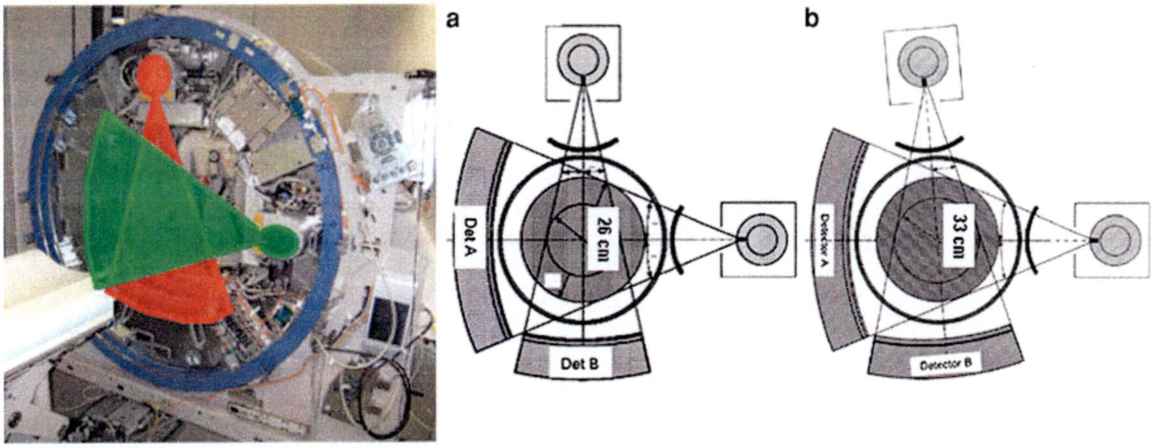


**Fig. 6** Dual-source CT-scanner with two independent measurement systems. **a** First-generation. The measurement systems are at an angle of 90°. **b** Second-generation. To enlarge the SFOV of detector B, the system angle was increased to 95°

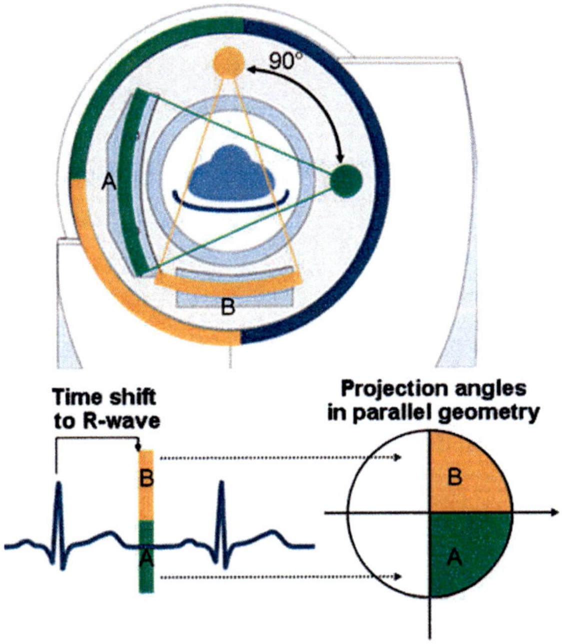


**Fig. 7** Principle of dual-source CT: Two simultaneously acquired quarter-scan sinograms in parallel geometry are put together to the half-scan sinogram needed for image reconstruction. The total data acquisition time is a quarter of the gantry rotation time

In 2009, the second-generation of DSCT-systems was introduced. The angle between the X-ray tubes was increased to 95° to allow for a larger SFOV of 33 cm with detector B (see Fig. 6). The detectors have a larger z-coverage and acquire 128 overlapping 0.6 mm slices. The shortest gantry rotation time is 0.28 s.

The key benefit of DSCT for cardio-thoracic scanning is improved temporal resolution. In parallel geometry, 180° of scan data (a half-scan sinogram) are necessary for image reconstruction. Due to the 90° angle between both X-ray tubes, the half-scan sinogram can be split up into two 90° data segments which are simultaneously acquired by the two acquisition systems in the same phase of the patient's cardiac cycle and at the same anatomical level, see Fig. 7. Therefore, the total data acquisition time per image is a quarter of the gantry rotation time $t_{rot}/4$ in a sufficiently centered region of the SFOV (Flohr et al. 2006). For the first-generation DSCT with $t_{rot} = 0.33$ s, the temporal resolution is $t_{rot}/4 = 83$ ms. For the second-generation DSCT with $t_{rot} = 0.28$ s, it is 75 ms as a consequence of the increased system angle of 95°.

With the dual-source approach, temporal resolution is independent of the patient's heart rate, because data from one cardiac cycle only are used to reconstruct an image. This is a major difference to single-source MDCT-systems, which can provide similar temporal resolution by combining data from several heart cycles to an image in a multi-segment reconstruction. Then, however, temporal resolution strongly depends on the relation of heart rate and gantry rotation time. Meanwhile, several clinical studies have demonstrated the potential of DSCT for coronary CTA with little or no dependence on the patient's heart rate (Achenbach et al. 2006; Johnson et al. 2006; Scheffel et al. 2006; Matt et al. 2007; Leber et al. 2007; Ropers et al. 2007).

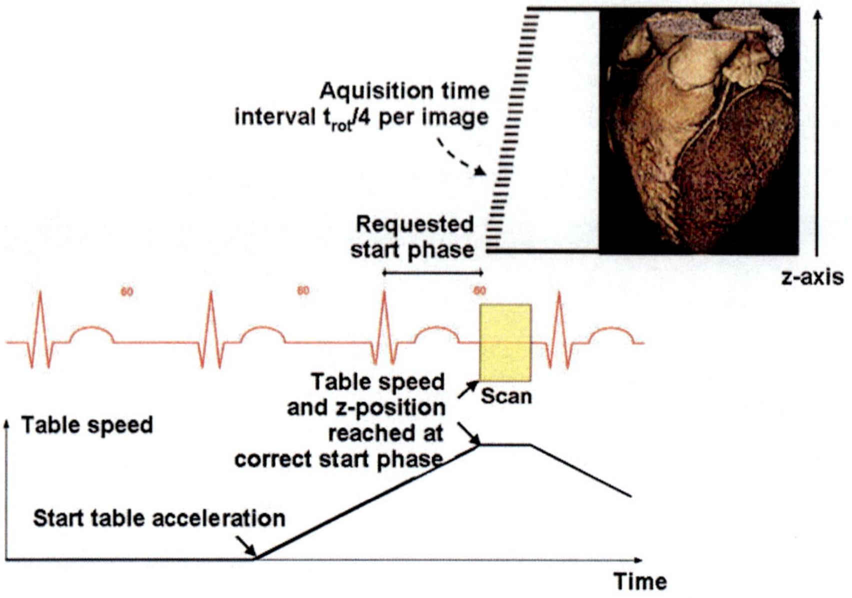


**Fig. 8** ECG-triggered start of table movement and data acquisition for the high-pitch DSCT spiral

DSCT-systems offer an alternative way to scan the heart within one heartbeat. With a single-source CT, the spiral pitch $p$ is limited to $p \leq 1.5$ to ensure gapless volume coverage along the z-axis. $p$ is defined as the table feed per rotation divided by the total detector z-coverage. If the pitch is increased beyond $p = 1.5$, sampling gaps will lead to severe image artifacts. With DSCT-systems, however, data acquired with the second measurement system a quarter rotation later can be used to fill these gaps. In this way, the pitch can be increased up to $p = 3.4$ in a limited SFOV that is covered by both detectors (Petersilka et al. 2008; Flohr et al. 2009a). Because of the high-pitch, no redundant data are acquired, and a quarter rotation of data per measurement system (in parallel geometry) is used for image reconstruction. Therefore, each of the individual axial images has a temporal resolution of $t_{rot}/4$.

At a pitch of 3.4, and with $t_{rot} = 0.28$ s, the table feed with 38.4 mm detector z-coverage (2nd generation DSCT) is 450 mm/s, which is sufficient to cover the heart (12 cm) in about 0.27 s. The patient's ECG is used to trigger both table motion and data acquisition. The patient table is positioned, and table acceleration is started in a way that the table arrives at the prescribed start z-position (e.g., the base or the apex of the heart) at the requested cardiac phase after full table speed has been reached, see Fig. 8. Then data acquisition begins. The scan data for images at adjacent z-positions are acquired at slightly different phases of the cardiac cycle. With a length of the diastolic phase of the heart of about 300 ms for low to medium heart rates (e.g., below 65 bpm), visualization of the coronary arteries without image quality degradation by motion artifacts can be expected. Meanwhile, several clinical studies have demonstrated the successful use of the high-pitch scan technique for coronary CT angiography in patients with sufficiently low and stable heart rate, with the potential to scan the entire heart in one beat at very low radiation dose (Achenbach et al. 2009, 2010; Lell et al. 2009; Leschka et al. 2009).

In a non-ECG-gated version, the high-pitch mode has also frequently been used for the examination of larger anatomical ranges in very short scan times, e.g., when the patient has limited ability to cooperate, such as in pediatric radiology, see Fig. 9.

DSCT-systems show interesting properties for general radiology applications too. Both X-ray tubes can be operated at different kV- and mA-settings, allowing for the acquisition of dual-energy data. While dual-energy CT was evaluated 20 years prior (Kalender et al. 1986; Vetter et al. 1986), technical limitations of the CT-scanners at those times prevented the development of routine clinical applications. With a DSCT-system, dual-energy data can be acquired with subsecond scan times and flexible selection of other scan parameters such as mAs per tube or spiral pitch. The use of dual-energy CT can in

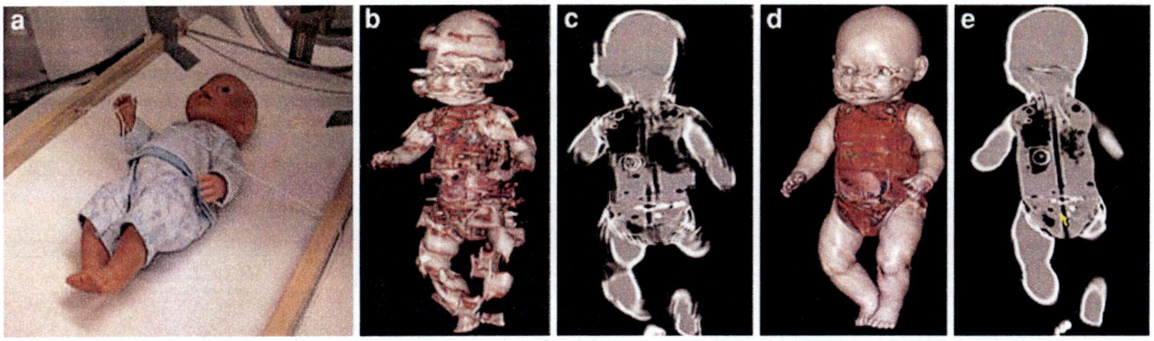


**Fig. 9** CT scans of a moving doll phantom simulating motion of a child without sedation. **a** the moving phantom. **b** and **c** VRTs and MPRs of the phantom scanned with a standard spiral (pitch 1, 0.33 s rotation time) show significant motion artifacts. **d** and **e** Using the DSCT high-pitch spiral (pitch 3.4, 0.33 s rotation time) motion artifacts are significantly reduced because of the very short scan time and the good temporal resolution per image. Courtesy of C. McCollough, Clinical Innovation Center, Mayo Clinic Rochester, MN, USA

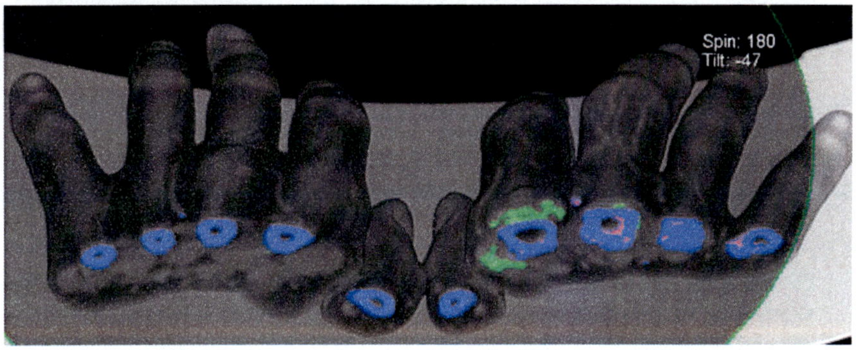


**Fig. 10** Dual-energy scan of a patient's hand. The dual-energy information is used to identify uric acid crystals (*highlighted in green*), which are characteristic for gout. Courtesy of Clinical Innovation Center, Mayo Clinic Rochester, MN, USA

principle add functional information to the morphological information based on X-ray attenuation that is usually obtained in a CT examination. In CT the two relevant interaction mechanisms of X-ray photons with matter are the photo effect and the Compton effect. Both show different dependence on the photon energy $E$ and on the atomic number $Z$ of the investigated materials. A material can therefore be identified by its characteristic change of attenuation when scanned with two different mean X-ray energies, provided by running one X-ray tube at e.g., 80 kV and the other at e.g. 140 kV. Clinical applications of dual-energy CT include tissue characterization, calcium quantification, calculation of pseudo-monochromatic images and quantification of the local blood volume in contrast-enhanced scans (Johnson et al. 2007; Primak et al. 2007; Scheffel et al. 2007; Graser et al. 2008, 2010; Glazebrook et al. 2001). Figure 10 shows an example of dual-energy-based identification of uric acid crystals for the differential diagnosis of gout.

Despite their clinical benefits, DSCT-systems have to address a number of challenges. One major challenge for image reconstruction is cross-scattered radiation, i.e. scattered radiation from X-ray tube (B) detected by detector (A) and vice versa. Cross-scattered radiation can produce artifacts and degrade the contrast-to-noise ratio of the images. The most straightforward correction approach is to directly measure the cross-scattered radiation in detectors (A) and (B) and to subtract it from the signal. This technique is implemented in the second generation DSCT (Petersilka et al. 2010). It requires additional detector elements on each detector outside the direct beam. An alternative to direct measurement is a model-based cross-scatter correction. The primary source of cross-scattered radiation is Compton scatter at the object surface, hence knowledge of the surface is sufficient to predict cross-scatter. The object surface, however, can be readily determined by analyzing the outline of the raw data sinogram. This technique is realized in

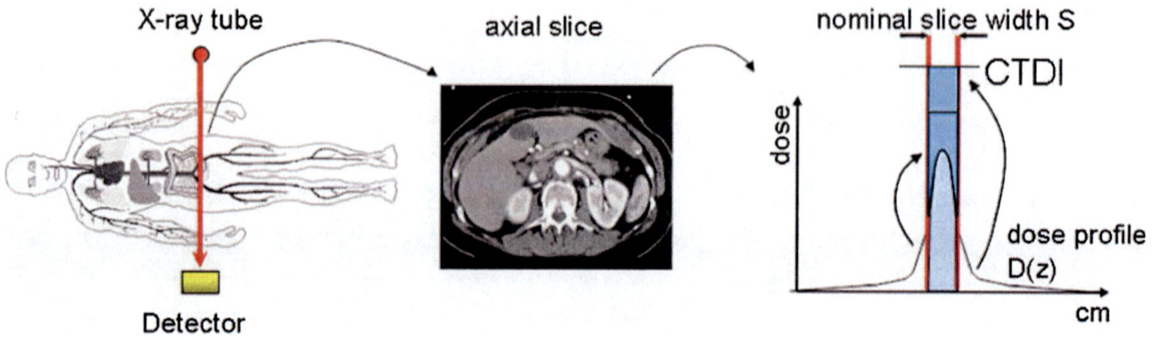


**Fig. 11** Schematic illustration of the definition of the CTDI as a measure for the radiation energy deposited in one axial slice of the patient

the first-generation DSCT. Pre-stored cross-scatter tables for objects with similar surface shape are used for an online correction of the cross-scattered radiation. Scatter correction can efficiently reduce scatter artifacts, however, at the expense of increased image noise.

## 2 Radiation Dose in CT

Radiation exposure of the patient by computed tomography and the resulting potential radiation hazard have gained considerable attention both in the public and in the scientific literature (e.g., Brenner et al. 2007). Typical values for the effective patient doses of selected CT protocols are 1–2 mSv for head, 5–7 mSv for chest and 8–14 mSv for abdomen and pelvis (McCollough 2003; McCollough et al. 2009; Morin et al. 2003). This radiation exposure should be appreciated in the context of the average annual background radiation, which is 2–5 mSv. If medically indicated, the benefits of a properly performed CT examination by far outweigh the potential radiation risks. Nevertheless, it is mandatory to optimize data acquisition modes and scan protocols with regard to radiation exposure in all CT examinations, and to utilize techniques to reduce radiation dose.

In CT the established parameter to describe the average radiation dose in the axial scan plane is the computed tomographic dose index CTDI (Morin et al. 2003; McCollough et al. 2003), which is a measure for the radiation energy deposited both in a slice with nominal slice width S and outside of it (as a consequence of scattered radiation), see Fig. 11. CTDI is measured with ionization chambers in lucite phantoms with a diameter of 16 cm for head and 32 cm for body scans (Fig. 12). Most commonly $CTDI_{100}$ is used, which is defined as

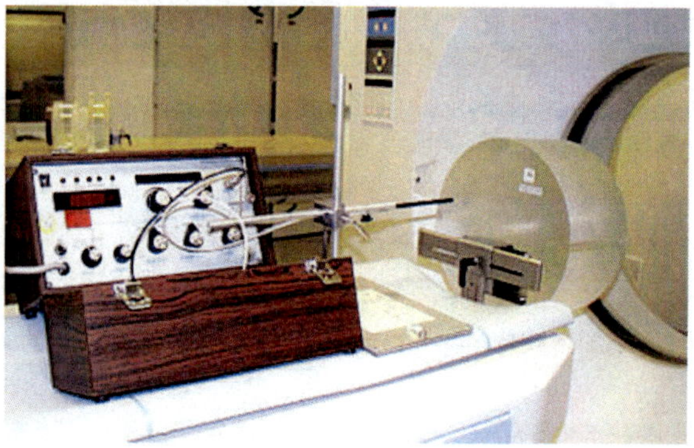

**Fig. 12** Ionization chamber and 32 cm lucite phantom used to measure CTDI

$$CTDI_{100} = \frac{1}{S}\int_{-50\text{mm}}^{50\text{mm}} D(z)\text{d}z$$

D(z) is the dose distribution along the z-axis. The integration range accounts for the typical length of an ionization chamber (100 mm).

Note that $CTDI_{100}$ significantly underestimates the dose for MDCT systems with wider detectors in the z-direction, such as the newer scanners with 8 or 16 cm detector coverage at isocenter.

Dose measurements are performed both in the center (position A) and at the periphery (position B) of the lucite phantoms, resulting in the $CTDI_w$ (weighted CTDI)

$$CTDI_w = \frac{1}{3}CTDI_{100}^A + \frac{2}{3}CTDI_{100}^B.$$

$CTDI_w$ is an indicator for the average patient dose only if the patient's scanned area has about the same diameter as the lucite phantoms used for measurement. $CTDI_w$ will overestimate radiation dose for large patients, and it will underestimate radiation dose for small patients.

Scan protocols for different CT-scanners should always be compared on the basis of $CTDI_w$ and never on the basis of mAs, since different system geometries can lead to significant differences in the radiation dose that is applied at identical mAs. $CTDI_w$ depends on scanner geometry, in particular source-isocenter distance, slice collimation and beam prefiltration as well as on X-ray tube voltage, tube current mA and gantry rotation time $t_{rot}$. To obtain a parameter characteristic for the scanner used, it is helpful to introduce a normalized nCTDI given in mGy/mAs:

$$CTDI_w = mA \cdot t_{rot} \cdot nCTDI_w = mAs \cdot nCTDI_w.$$

To represent the dose in a spiral/helical scan, it is essential to account for gaps or overlaps between the radiation dose profiles from consecutive rotations of the X-ray source (Morin et al. 2003). For this purpose $CTDI_{vol}$, the volume $CTDI_w$, has been introduced

$$CTDI_{vol} = 1/p \cdot CTDI_w$$

$p$ is the pitch of the spiral examination. The factor $1/p$ accounts for the increasing dose accumulation with decreasing spiral pitch due to the increasing spiral overlap. Some manufacturers such as Siemens use an "effective" mAs-concept for spiral/helical MDCT scanning which includes the factor $1/p$ into the mAs-definition:

$$(mAs)_{eff} = mA \cdot t_{rot} \cdot 1/p = mAs \cdot 1/p.$$

The dose of a spiral/helical scan is then equivalent to the dose of a sequential CT acquisition with the same detector collimation and the same mAs, and is simply given by

$$CTDI_{vol} = (mAs)_{eff} \cdot nCTDI_w.$$

Some other manufacturers stay with the conventional mAs-definition, and the user has to perform the $1/p$ correction by himself. When comparing the scan parameters for CT-systems of different manufacturers, the underlying mAs-definition needs to be taken into account.

Radiation dose as given by the CTDI is a local parameter, it does not reflect differences in the total radiation exposure to the patient due to different scanned ranges. The dose-length product DLP, defined as

$$DLP = CTDI_{vol} \cdot L$$

and measured in mGy·cm, accounts for the scan range L of a CT examination. $CTDI_{vol}$ and DLP are physical dose measures, they do not inform about the radiation risk associated with a CT examination. For this purpose the concept of "effective dose" E has been introduced by the International Commission on Radiological Protection (ICRP). The effective dose, measured in mSv, is the weighted sum of the organ doses $D_{org,\ i}$ to all organs i in a CT examination, and includes both direct and scattered radiation. The weighting factors $w_i$ depend on the biological radiation sensitivities of the respective organs

$$E = \Sigma w_i \cdot D_{org,i}.$$

The $w_i$ are estimated and published on a regular basis by the ICRP. As research and measuring technologies advance, these factors may undergo significant changes. The recommendations of the ICRP of 2007 (ICRP Report 103) indicate that gonads are less radiosensitive and the breast is more radiosensitive than assumed in the ICRP report of 1990 (ICRP Report 60).

Effective dose can be measured using whole-body phantoms such as the Alderson-Rando phantom, or derived from computer simulations using Monte Carlo techniques in mathematical models of "standardized patients". Because each individual patient deviates from this idealized mathematical model, effective dose cannot be used to quantify the radiation exposure to an individual patient, but rather the mean radiation exposure to a standard patient group.

For different scan ranges, the effective dose E can be approximated from the DLP by applying a conversion factor

$$E = DLP \cdot f.$$

Examples of $f$ for the different body regions are
*Head*. $f = 0.0021$ mSv/(mGy·cm)
*Neck*. $f = 0.0059$ mSv/(mGy·cm)
*Thorax*. $f = 0.014$ mSv/(mGy·cm)
*Abdomen and Pelvis*. $f = 0.015$ mSv/(mGy·cm)

## 3 Radiation Dose Reduction

Modern CT-scanners are equipped with a variety of different techniques to reduce radiation exposure. Some of them will be explained in this section.

### 3.1 Anatomical Tube Current Modulation

The most effective means to reduce radiation exposure is an adaptation of the dose to the patient's body size and shape (Donelly et al. 2001; Frush et al. 2002; Wildberger et al. 2001).

This can be achieved by an adaptation of the X-ray tube current to the patient's anatomy, either manually by selecting patient-individual mAs-settings or automatically with the use of automatic anatomical tube current modulation (automatic exposure control). This technique modifies the tube output in the through-plane (z-axis) direction to maintain adequate dose when scanning body regions with different attenuation, for instance thorax and abdomen. In addition, angular tube current modulation is performed during each rotation of the gantry to compensate for strongly varying X-ray attenuations in asymmetrical body regions such as the shoulders and pelvis. The variation of the tube output is either predefined by an analysis of the localizer scan (topogram, scout view) or determined online by evaluating the signal of a detector row (Fig. 13). In some approaches, the attenuation of a "standard-sized" patient is stored in the control computer for each body region. The user selects a reference mAs-setting in the standard scan protocol that will be applied if the patient's attenuation matches the stored standard attenuation. If the patient's attenuation deviates, the tube output will be adapted accordingly. Some vendors try to adapt the tube current such as to maintain constant image noise in all examined body parts. Others allow for a weaker increase of the tube current with increasing body size, since radiologists tend to accept noisier images with more obese patients.

With use of anatomical dose modulation approaches, radiation exposure can be significantly reduced. Several authors demonstrated radiation dose reduction by 20–68% depending on the body region without degrading image quality (Mulkens et al. 2005; Greess et al. 2004). It has to be noted, however, that automatic exposure control reaches its limits with larger detector z-coverage because the detector then covers different anatomical regions at the same time which would require different mA-settings, such as the transition from liver to lung or from shoulder to neck.

### 3.2 Organ-Based Tube Current Modulation

Organ-based tube current modulation is a variant of automatic anatomical tube current modulation designed to specifically reduce radiation exposure to selected organs, such as the female breast. For this purpose, bismuth breast shields have so far been used. Their benefit, however, is doubtful, since they result in increased image artifacts and reduced overall image quality. Using organ-based tube current modulation, the X-ray tube current is reduced in a selectable angular range, e.g. when the X-ray tube moves directly in front of the female breast. The tube current has to be correspondingly increased when the X-ray tube is on the opposite side, see Fig. 14.

Organ-based tube current modulation therefore does not lead to an overall radiation dose reduction, but to a different distribution of the radiation dose in the scan plane (Fig. 15). It has been shown that the local radiation dose to the breast or to the thyroid gland can be reduced by 20–35% without loss of image quality (Ketelsen et al. 2011).

### 3.3 ECG-Controlled Tube Current Modulation

The radiation dose in electrocardiogram (ECG)-gated spiral/helical examinations of the heart can be reduced by means of ECG-controlled tube current modulation. This technique is also sometimes called "ECG-pulsing". During scan data acquisition, the X-ray tube current is modulated according to the patient's ECG. It is high (100%) in a user-defined phase of the cardiac cycle, in general the mid- to end-diastolic phase, and reduced to 4–25%, depending on the implementation, during the rest of the cardiac cycle, see Fig. 16.

Clinical studies with 4-slice CT-systems and ECG-controlled modulation of the tube current to 20% of

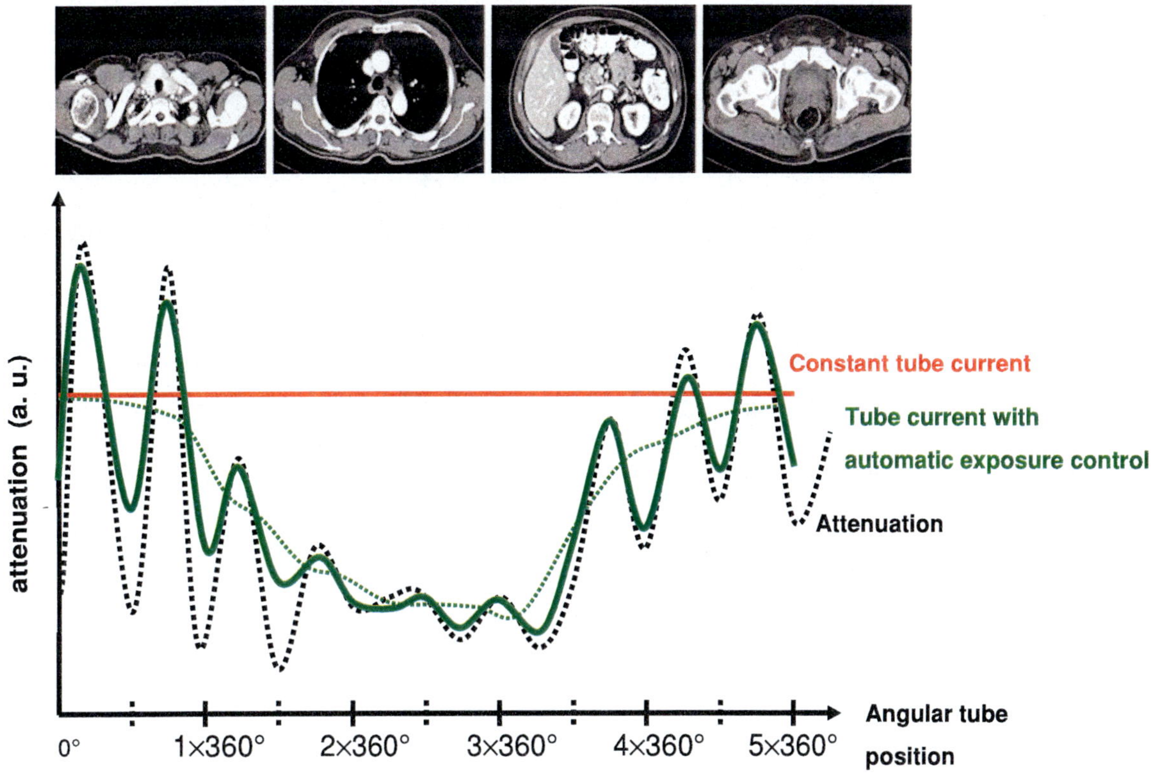


**Fig. 13** Principle of automatic adaptation of the X-ray tube current to patient size and shape (automatic exposure control)

**Fig. 14** Principle of organ-based tube current modulation to reduce the radiation dose to the female breast

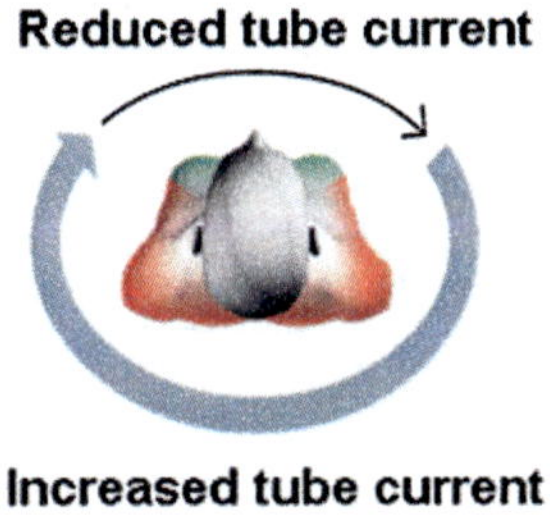


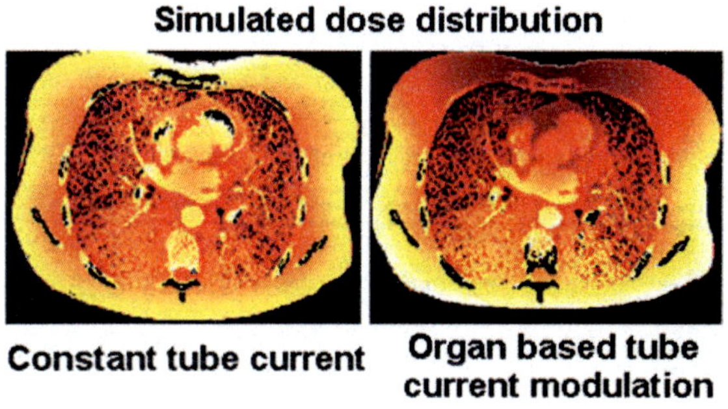


**Fig. 15** Monte Carlo simulation of radiation dose distribution with constant tube current (*left*) and organ-based tube current modulation (*right*). *Red* means lower dose. Note the reduced dose to the female breast with organ-based tube current modulation

its nominal value demonstrated dose reduction by 30–50%, with higher dose savings at lower heart rate (Jakobs et al. 2002). Further reduction of the tube current to 4% of its nominal value outside the targeted heart phase can reduce the radiation dose by another 10–15% (Stolzmann et al. 2008a). ECG-controlled dose modulation needs to reliably predict the patient's next RR-interval length by analyzing the preceding RR-intervals. While the first ECG-controlled dose modulation approaches only worked in patients with stable sinus rhythm, more refined algorithms have now been developed that can also be used in arrhythmic patients.

If the patient's heart rate is not too high and sufficiently stable, ECG-gated spiral/helical scans may be replaced by ECG-triggered axial scans, which lead to a further level of dose reduction. Using modern ECG-triggering approaches, the scan can be automatically repeated at the same table position in case of ectopic beats, and a flexible selection of the width of the data

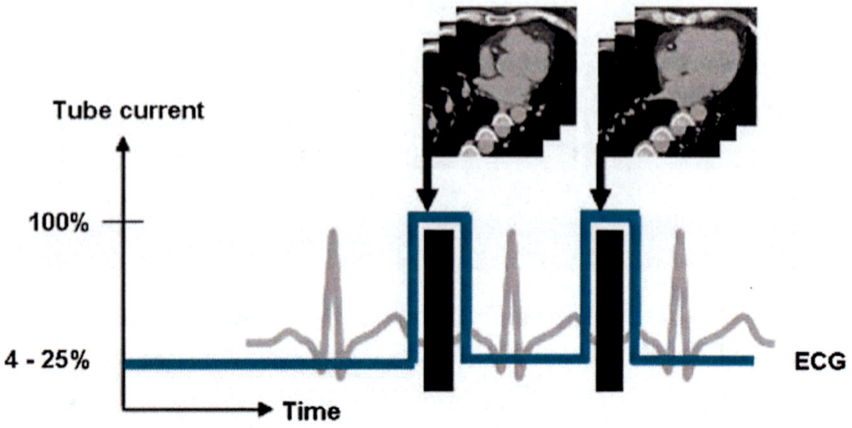


**Fig. 16** Principle of ECG-controlled dose modulation for ECG-gated spiral scans

acquisition window allows for retrospective optimization of the reconstruction phase similar to ECG-gated spiral scanning. Depending on patient size and scan technique, the effective patient dose can be as low as 1.5–3 mSv for ECG-triggered coronary CTA (Earls et al. 2008; Scheffel et al. 2008; Shumann et al. 2008; Stolzmann et al. 2008b; Blankstein et al. 2009).

## 3.4 Adaptation of the X-ray Tube Voltage

Automatic dose modulation approaches modify the X-ray tube current according to the patient's anatomy or the patient's ECG, but they do not change the user-prescribed X-ray tube voltage. Adaptation of the X-ray tube voltage to patient size and to the intended application, however, is another powerful means to reduce radiation exposure, in particular in contrast-enhanced studies such as CT angiographies. In these examinations the contrast-to-noise ratio at equal radiation dose increases with decreasing X-ray tube voltage because the iodine contrast significantly increases at lower kV (McCollough et al. 2009). This effect is most pronounced for small- and medium-sized patients, see Fig. 17.

As a consequence patient dose can be reduced by applying lower kV, if a certain contrast-to-noise ratio is considered adequate for diagnosis. Ideally, contrast-enhanced CT examinations in small- and medium-sized patients should be performed at 80 kV. In reality, however, the maximum X-ray tube current available at 80 kV may not be sufficient to obtain the desired contrast-to-noise ratio.

It is therefore difficult in clinical practice to manually pick the right kV-setting and the correspondingly adapted mAs for a particular patient and a particular scan. Recently, approaches for automatic tube voltage selection (ATVS) have been introduced, such as CARE kV (Siemens Healthcare, Forchheim, Germany). Prior to each scan, the scanner software analyzes the patient's attenuation by evaluating the localizer scan (topogram, scout view), and proposes optimized kV- and mAs-settings according to the planned examination type (e.g., CTA, scan of organ parenchyma, non-enhanced scan) and the system limitations (e.g., maximum tube current available, maximum system load). CARE kV provides different decision criteria for tube voltage selection, depending on the relative importance of iodine enhancement for the particular diagnostic task (more aggressive for CT angiography, less aggressive for scans of organ parenchyma, conservative for unenhanced scans). Compared with the standard 120 kV protocol, Winklehner et al. (Winklehner et al. 2011) demonstrated radiation dose reduction by 25% when using automatic tube voltage selection for thoraco-abdominal CT angiography in a group of 40 patients, see Fig. 18.

## 3.5 Dynamically Adjustable Pre-patient Collimator to Avoid Spiral Over-Ranging

CT-systems face the problem of over-ranging in spiral scans, because scan data beyond the user-defined scan volume in the z-direction (through-plane direction) are required for spiral image reconstruction. Usually,

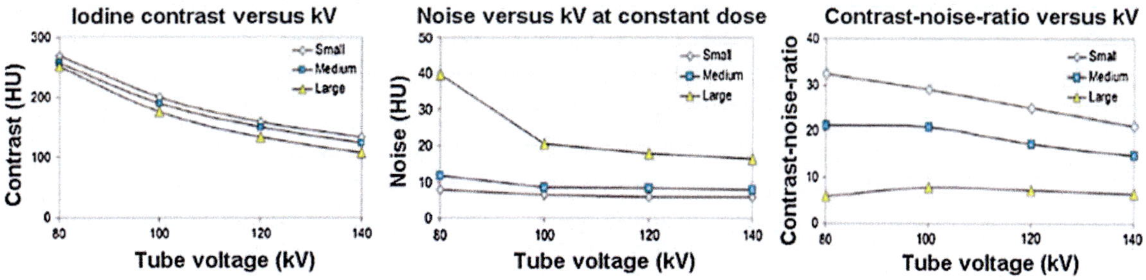


**Fig. 17** Contrast of a 2% iodine solution (*left*), image noise at constant dose (*center*) and contrast-to-noise ratio at constant dose (*right*) for different kV settings and different phantom sizes (small, medium and large). Iodine contrast significantly increases at lower tube potential. For small- and medium-sized patients, image noise at constant dose is independent of the tube potential, as expected. For large patients, image noise at constant dose increases at 80 kV for the evaluated CT-scanner, because of the increased relative contribution of electronic noise. As a consequence, CNR increases at lower tube potential for small- and medium-sized patients (*right*)

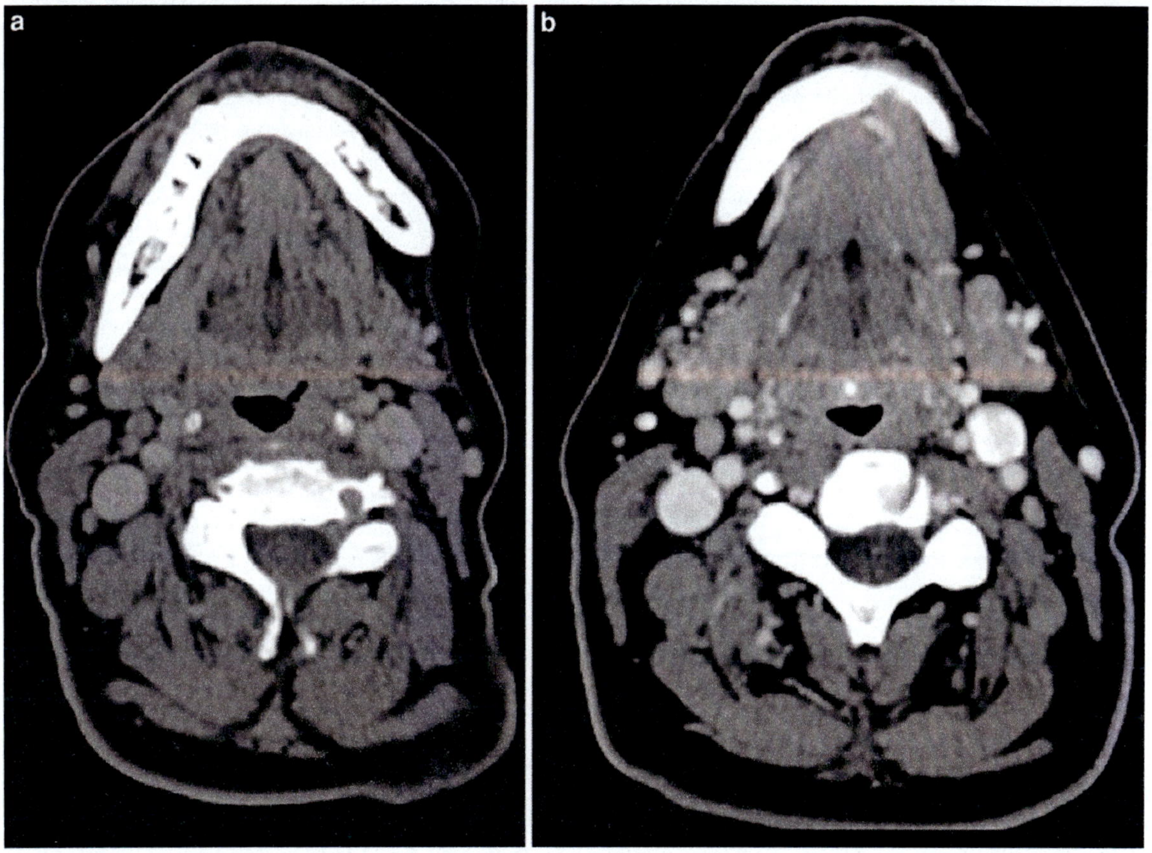


**Fig. 18** Automatic adaptation of the X-ray tube voltage to the patient anatomy and the examination type. **a** Contrast-enhanced scan of the neck with standard parameters: 120 kV, 132 mAs, CTDI = 8.9 mGy. **b** Follow-up scan using automatic tube voltage selection, resulting in modified scan parameters: 70 kV, 403 mAs, CTDI = 4.6 mGy. In this example, dose could be reduced by 50% without degradation of image quality (courtesy of H. Alkadhi, University Hospital of Zurich, Switzerland)

the corresponding pre- and post-spiral scan ranges are fully irradiated by the X-ray tube. The resulting scan data, however, are not fully used for image reconstruction and represent wasted dose (Fig. 19). The relative amount of unused radiation dose increases with increasing z-coverage of the detector.

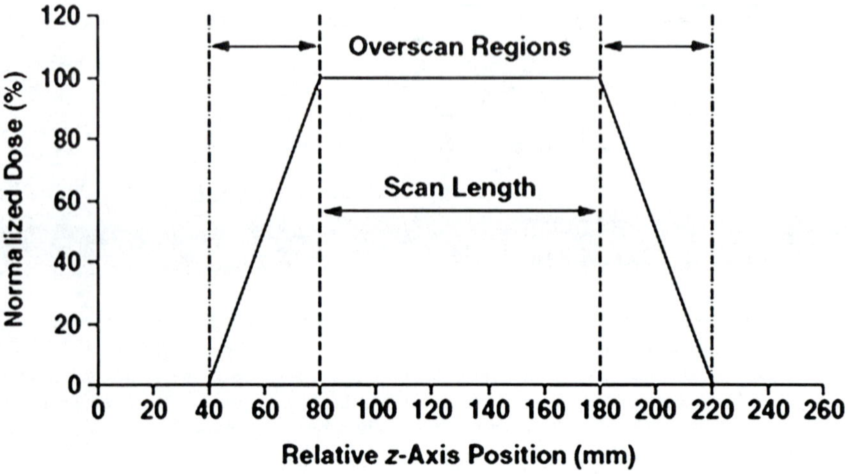


**Fig. 19** Graph illustrating z-axis profiles of over-scanned regions in a spiral scan with 100 mm scan length, using a detector with 40 mm z-coverage at pitch 1 (from Christner 2010)

Meanwhile, some CT-vendors mitigate the problem with dynamically adjustable pre-patient collimators allowing independent control of both tube collimator blades. The collimator blades open and close asymmetrically at the beginning and at the end of each spiral scan, thereby reducing spiral over-ranging. Radiation reduction depends on detector z-coverage, scan range and spiral pitch. For one implementation, estimated reductions in effective dose were 16% for the head, 10% for the chest and liver, 6% for the abdomen and pelvis and 4 and 55% for coronary CT angiography at pitches of 0.2 and 3.4 (Christner et al. 2010).

## 3.6 Iterative Reconstruction

Iterative reconstruction is not a new image reconstruction technique. For many years, it has been a well-established reconstruction method for positron emission tomography (PET) or single photon emission computed tomography (SPECT). Recently, iterative reconstruction was reintroduced to computed tomography (CT) as a method to improve image quality, enhance image resolution and lower image noise (Thibault et al. 2007).

While increased spatial resolution is directly correlated with increased image noise in filtered back projection reconstruction as it is used in all commercially available CT-scanners today, iterative reconstruction to a certain extent allows decoupling of spatial resolution and image noise.

In an iterative reconstruction, a correction loop is introduced in the image reconstruction process. After an image has been reconstructed from the measured projection data, a ray-tracing in the image is performed to calculate synthetic projections that exactly represent the reconstructed image. The deviation between measured and calculated projections is used to reconstruct a correction image and update the original image in an iterative loop. Each time the image is updated, nonlinear image processing algorithms are used to stabilize the solution. They maintain or enhance spatial resolution at higher object contrasts and reduce image noise in low contrast areas. This step, called regularization, is responsible for the image noise reduction properties of an iterative reconstruction. The repeated calculation of correction projections removes image artifacts introduced by the approximate nature of the filtered back projection reconstruction, but does not necessarily reduce image noise. In addition to artifact reduction, image resolution can be increased by carefully modeling the measurement system during forward projection in a so-called model-based iterative reconstruction.

Several iterative reconstruction algorithms have so far been introduced by the different vendors, such as adaptive statistical iterative reconstruction (ASIR), iterative reconstruction in image space (IRIS), sinogram affirmed iterative reconstruction (SAFIRE) or model-based iterative reconstruction (MBIR). The potential of these techniques with regard to radiation dose reduction is discussed in Chapter "Conventional and Newer Reconstruction Techniques in CT".

## References

Abels B, Klotz E, Tomandl BF, Villablanca JP, Kloska SP, Lell MM (2011) CT perfusion in acute ischemic stroke: a comparison of 2-second and 1-second temporal resolution. AJNR Am J Neuroradiol 32(9):1632–1639

Achenbach S, Ropers D, Kuettner A, Flohr T, Ohnesorge B, Bruder H, Theessen H, Karakaya M, Daniel WG, Bautz W, Kalender WA, Anders K (2006) Contrast-enhanced coronary artery visualization by dual-source computed tomography—initial experience. Eur J Radiol 57(3):331–335

Achenbach S, Marwan M, Schepis T, Pflederer T, Bruder H, Allmendinger T, Petersilka M, Anders K, Lell M, Kuettner A, Ropers D, Daniel WG, Flohr T (2009) High-pitch spiral acquisition: a new scan mode for coronary CT angiography. J Cardiovasc Comput Tomogr 3:117–121

Achenbach S, Marwan M, Ropers D, Schepis T, Pflederer T, Anders K, Kuettner A, Daniel WG, Uder M, Lell MM (2010) Coronary computed tomography angiography with a consistent dose below 1 mSv using prospectively electrocardiogram-triggered high-pitch spiral acquisition. Eur Heart J 32(3):340–346

Blankstein R, Shah A, Pale R, Abbara S, Bezerra H, Bolen M, Mamuya WS, Hoffmann U, Brady TJ, Cury RC (2009) Radiation dose and image quality of prospective triggering with dual-source cardiac computed tomography. Am J Cardiol 103(8):1168–1173

Brenner DJ, Hall EJ (2007) Computed tomography–an increasing source of radiation exposure. N Engl J Med 357(22):2277–2284

Christner JA, Zavaletta VA, Eusemann CD, Walz-Flannigan AI, McCollough CH (2010) Dose reduction in helical CT: dynamically adjustable z-axis X-ray beam collimation. Am J Roentgenol 2010(194):W49–W55

Dewey M, Zimmermann E, Deissenrieder F, Laule M, Dübel HP, Schlattmann P, Knebel F, Rutsch W, Hamm B (2009) Noninvasive coronary angiography by 320-row computed tomography with lower radiation exposure and maintained diagnostic accuracy: comparison of results with cardiac catheterization in a head-to-head pilot investigation. Circulation 120(10):867–875

Donelly LF, Emery KH, Brody AS et al (2001) Minimizing radiation dose for pediatric body applications of single-detector helical CT: strategies at a large children's hospital. AJR 2001(176):303–306

Earls JP, Berman EL, Urban BA, Curry CA, Lane JL, Jennings RS, McCulloch CC, Hsieh J, Londt JH (2008) Prospectively gated transverse coronary CT angiography versus retrospectively gated helical technique: improved image quality and reduced radiation dose. Radiology 246(3):742–753

Engel KJ, Herrmann C, Zeitler G (2007) X-ray scattering in single- and dual-soure CT. Med Phys 35(1):318–332

Flohr TG, McCollough CH, Bruder H, Petersilka M, Gruber K, Süß C, Grasruck M, Stierstorfer K, Krauss B, Raupach R, Primak AN, Küttner A, Achenbach S, Becker C, Kopp A, Ohnesorge BM (2006) First performance evaluation of a dual-source CT (DSCT) system. Eur Radiol 16(2):256–268

Flohr T, Schoepf UJ, Ohnesorge B (2007) Chasing the heart-new developments for cardiac CT. J Thorac Imaging 22(1): 4–16

Flohr TG, Leng S, Yu L, Allmendinger T, Bruder H, Petersilka M, Eusemann CD, Stierstorfer K, Schmidt B, McCollough C (2009a) Dual-source spiral CT with pitch up to 3.2 and 75 ms temporal resolution: image reconstruction and assessment of image quality. Med Phys 36(12):5641–5653

Flohr TG, Raupach R, Bruder H (2009b) Cardiac CT: how much can temporal resolution, spatial resolution, and volume coverage be improved? J Cardiovasc Comput Tomogr 3(3): 143–152

Funabashi N, Yoshida K, Tadokoro H, Nakagawa K, Komiyama N, Odaka K, Tsunoo T, Mori S, Tanada S, Endo M, Komuro I (2005) Cardiovascular circulation and hepatic perfusion of pigs in 4-dimensional films evaluated by 256-slice cone-beam computed tomography. Circ J 69(5):585–589

Glazebrook KN, Guimarães LS, Murthy NS, Black DF, Bongartz T, Manek JN, Leng S, Fletcher JG, McCollough CH (2001) Identification of intraarticular and periarticular uric acid crystals with dual-energy CT: initial evaluation. Radiology 261(2): 516–524

Graser A, Johnson TR, Bader M, Staehler M, Haseke N, Nikolaou K, Reiser MF, Stief CG, Becker CR (2008) Dual energy CT characterization of urinary calculi: initial in vitro and clinical experience. Invest Radiol 43(2):112–119

Graser A, Becker CR, Staehler M, Clevert DA, Macari M, Arndt N, Nikolaou K, Sommer W, Stief C, Reiser MF, Johnson TR (2010) Single-phase dual-energy CT allows for characterization of renal masses as benign or malignant. Invest Radiol 45(7):399–405

Greess H, Wolf H, Suess C, Kalender WA, Bautz W, Baum U (2004) Automatic exposure control to reduce the dose in subsecond multislice spiral CT: phantom measurements and clinical results. Röfo Fortschr Geb Rontgenstr Neuen Bildgeb Verfahr 176(6):862–869

Haberland U, Klotz E, Abolmaali N (2010) Performance assessment of dynamic spiral scan modes with variable pitch for quantitative perfusion computed tomography. Invest Radiol 45(7):378–386

Hoe J, Toh KH (2009) First experience with 320-row multi-detector CT coronary angiography scanning with prospective electrocardiogram gating to reduce radiation dose. J Cardiovasc Comput Tomogr 3(4):257–261

Jakobs TF, Becker CR, Ohnesorge B, Flohr T, Suess C, Schoepf UJ, Reiser MF (2002) Multislice helical CT of the heart with retrospective ECG gating: reduction of radiation exposure by ECG-controlled tube current modulation. Eur Radiol 2002(12):1081–1086

Johnson TRC, Nikolaou K, Wintersperger BJ, Leber AW, von Ziegler F, Rist C, Buhmann S, Knez A, Reiser MF, Becker CR (2006) Dual source cardiac CT imaging: initial experience. Eur Radiol 2006(16):1409–1415

Johnson TRC, Krauß B, Sedlmair M, Grasruck M, Bruder H, Morhard D, Fink C, Weckbach S, Lenhard M, Schmidt B, Flohr T, Reiser MF, Becker CR (2007) Material differentiation by dual energy CT: initial experience. Eur Radiol 17(6):1510–1517

Kalender WA, Perman WH, Vetter JR, Klotz E (1986) Evaluation of a prototype dual-energy computed tomographic apparatus. I. Phantom studies. Med Phys 13(3): 334–339

Ketelsen D, Buchgeister M, Fenchel M, Schmidt B, Flohr TG, Syha R, Thomas C, Tsiflikas I, Claussen CD, Heuschmid M

(2011) Automated computed tomography dose-saving algorithm to protect radiosensitive tissues: estimation of radiation exposure and image quality considerations. Invest Radiol 2012 47(2):148–152

Kido T, Kurata A, Higashino H, Sugawara Y, Okayama H, Higaki J, Anno H, Katada K, Mori S, Tanada S, Endo M, Mochizuki T (2007) Cardiac imaging using 256-detector row four-dimensional CT: preliminary clinical report. Radiat Med 25(1):38–44

Leber AW, Johnson T, Becker A, von Ziegler F, Tittus J, Nikolaou K, Reiser M, Steinbeck G, Becker CR, Knez A (2007) Diagnostic accuracy of dual-source multi-slice CT-coronary angiography in patients with an intermediate pretest likelihood for coronary artery disease. Eur Heart J 28(19):2354–2360

Lell M, Marwan M, Schepis T, Pflederer T, Anders K, Flohr T, Allmendinger T, Kalender W, Ertel D, Thierfelder C, Kuettner A, Ropers D, Daniel WG, Achenbach S (2009a) Prospectively ECG-triggered high-pitch spiral acquisition for coronary CT angiography using dual source CT: technique and initial experience. Eur Radiol 19(11):2576–2583

Leschka S, Stolzmann P, Desbiolles L, Baumueller S, Goetti R, Schertler T, Scheffel H, Plass A, Falk V, Feuchtner G, Marincek B, Alkadhi H (2009) Diagnostic accuracy of high-pitch dual-source CT for the assessment of coronary stenoses: first experience. Eur Radiol 19(12):2896–2903

Matt D, Scheffel H, Leschka S, Flohr TG, Marincek B, Kaufmann PA, Alkadhi H (2007) Dual-source CT coronary angiography: image quality, mean heart rate, and heart rate variability. Am J Roentgenol 189(3):567–573

McCollough C (2003) Patient Dose in Cardiac Computed Tomography. Herz 2003(28):1–6

McCollough CH, Primak AN, Braun N, Kofler J, Yu L, Christner J (2009) Strategies for Reducing Radiation Dose in CT. Radiol Clin North Am 47(1):27–40

Mori S, Endo M, Tsunoo T, Kandatsu S, Tanada S, Aradate H et al (2004) Physical performance evaluation of a 256-slice CT-scanner for four-dimensional imaging. Med Phys 31(6):1348–1356

Mori S, Endo M, Obata T, Tsunoo T, Susumu K, Tanada S. (2006a) Properties of the prototype 256-row (cone beam) CT scanner. Eur Radiol 16(9):2100–2108

Mori S, Kondo C, Suzuki N, Hattori A, Kusakabe M, Endo M (2006b) Volumetric coronary angiography using the 256-detector row computed tomography scanner: comparison in vivo and in vitro with porcine models. Acta Radiol 47(2):186–191

Mori S, Endo M, Obata T, Kishimoto R, Kato H, Kandatsu S, Tsujii H, Tanada S (2006c) Noise properties for three weighted Feldkamp algorithms using a 256-detector row CT-scanner: case study for hepatic volumetric cine imaging. Eur J Radiol 59(2):289–294

Mori S, Obata T, Kato H, Kishimoto R, Kandatsu S, Tanada S, Endo M (2007) Preliminary study: color map of hepatocellular carcinoma using dynamic contrast-enhanced 256-detector row CT. Eur J Radiol 62(2):308–310

Morin R, Gerber T, McCollough C (2003) Radiation dose in computed tomography of the heart. Circulation 2003(107): 917–922

Mulkens TH, Bellinck P, Baeyaert M, Ghysen D, Van Dijck X, Mussen E, Venstermans C, Termote JL (2005) Use of an automatic exposure control mechanism for dose optimization in multi–detector row CT examinations: clinical evaluation. Radiology 237:213–223

Petersilka M, Bruder H, Krauss B, Stierstorfer K, Flohr TG (2008) Technical principles of dual source CT. Eur J Radiol 68(3):362–368

Petersilka M, Stierstorfer K, Bruder H, Flohr T (2010) Strategies for scatter correction in dual source CT. Med Phys 37(11):5971–5992

Primak AN, Fletcher JG, Vrtiska TJ, Dzyubak OP, Lieske JC, Jackson ME, Williams JC Jr, McCollough CH (2007) Noninvasive differentiation of uric acid versus non-uric acid kidney stones using dual-energy CT. Acad Radiol 14(12): 1441–1447

Ritman E, Kinsey J, Robb R, Gilbert B, Harris L, Wood E (1980) Three-dimensional imaging of heart, lungs, and circulation. Science 210(4467):273–280

Robb R, Ritman E (1979) High speed synchronous volume computed tomography of the heart. Radiology 133(3 Pt 1): 655–661

Ropers U, Ropers D, Pflederer T, Anders K, Kuettner A, Stilianakis NI, Komatsu S, Kalender W, Bautz W, Daniel WG, Achenbach S (2007) Influence of heart rate on the diagnostic accuracy of dual-source computed tomography coronary angiography. J Am Coll Cardiol 50(25):2393–2398

Rybicki FJ, Otero HJ, Steigner ML, Vorobiof G, Nallamshetty L, Mitsouras D, Ersoy H, Mather RT, Judy PF, Cai T, Coyner K, Schultz K, Whitmore AG, Di Carli MF (2008) Initial evaluation of coronary images from 320-detector row computed tomography. Int J Cardiovasc Imaging 24(5):535–546

Scheffel H, Alkadhi H, Plass A, Vachenauer R, Desbiolles L, Gaemperli O, Schepis T, Frauenfelder T, Schertler T, Husmann L, Grunenfelder J, Genoni M, Kaufmann PA, Marincek B, Leschka S (2006) Accuracy of dual-source CT coronary angiography: first experience in a high pre-test probability population without heart rate control. Eur Radiol 16(12):2739–2747

Scheffel H, Stolzmann P, Frauenfelder T, Schertler T, Desbiolles L, Leschka S, Marincek B, Alkadhi H (2007) Dual-energy contrast-enhanced computed tomography for the detection of urinary stone disease. Invest Radiol 42(12): 823–829

Scheffel H, Alkadhi H, Leschka S, Plass A, Desbiolles L, Guber I, Krauss T, Gruenenfelder J, Genoni M, Luescher TF, Marincek B, Stolzmann P (2008) Low-dose CT coronary angiography in the step-and-shoot mode: diagnostic performance. Heart 94(9):1132–1137

Shuman WP, Branch KR, May JM, Mitsumori LM, Lockhart DW, Dubinsky TJ, Warren BH, Caldwell JH (2008) Prospective versus retrospective ECG gating for 64-detector CT of the coronary arteries: comparison of image quality and patient radiation dose. Radiology 248(2):431–437

Steigner ML, Otero HJ, Cai T, Mitsouras D, Nallamshetty L, Whitmore AG, Ersoy H, Levit NA, Di Carli MF, Rybicki FJ (2009) Narrowing the phase window width in prospectively ECG-gated single heart beat 320-detector row coronary CT angiography. Int J Cardiovasc Imaging 25(1):85–90

Stolzmann P, Scheffel H, Schertler T, Frauenfelder T, Leschka S, Husmann L, Flohr TG, Marincek B, Kaufmann PA, Alkadhi H (2008a) Radiation dose estimates in dual-source computed tomography coronary angiography. Eur Radiol 18(3):592–599

Stolzmann P, Leschka S, Scheffel H, Krauss T, Desbiolles L, Plass A, Genoni M, Flohr TG, Wildermuth S, Marincek B, Alkadhi H (2008b) Dual-source CT in step-and-shoot mode: noninvasive coronary angiography with low radiation dose. Radiology 249(1):71–80

Thibault JB, Sauer KD, Bouman CA, Hsieh J (2007) A three-dimensional statistical approach to improved image quality for multislice helical CT. Med Phys 34:4526–4544

Vetter JR, Perman WH, Kalender WA, Mazess RB, Holden JE (1986) Evaluation of a prototype dual-energy computed tomographic apparatus. II. Determination of vertebral bone mineral content. Med Phys 13(3):340–343

Weigold WG, Olszewski ME, Walker MJ (2009) Low-dose prospectively gated 256-slice coronary computed tomographic angiography. Int J Cardiovasc Imaging 2009 25:217–230

Wildberger JE, Mahnken AH, Schmitz-Rode T, Flohr T, Stargardt A, Haage P, Schaller S, Guenther RW (2001) Individually adapted examination protocols for reduction of radiation exposure in chest CT. Invest Radiol 36(10):604–611

Winklehner A, Goetti R, Baumueller S, Karlo C, Schmidt B, Raupach R, Flohr T, Frauenfelder T, Alkadhi H (2011) Automated attenuation-based tube potential selection for thoracoabdominal computed tomography angiography improved dose effectiveness. Invest Radiol 46(12):767–773

# Clinical Expansion of CT and Radiation Dose

Stuart Meeson, Rajesh Patel, and Stephen Golding

## Contents



S. Meeson · R. Patel · S. Golding (✉)
Radiology Group, Nuffield Department of Surgical Sciences, University of Oxford, Oxford, UK
e-mail: stephen.golding@surgery.oxford.ac.uk

**Abstract**

The principles of protecting the patient undergoing clinical investigation using radiation are clear and well established: it is the responsibility of all radiological services to ensure the information required for the clinical management of the patient is obtained with the lowest practicable exposure to radiation. Within this clear objective, however, medical investigation operates in a constantly changing scenario influenced by increasing knowledge of disease processes and advancing technological development. This syndrome ensures that as time passes differing objectives and concerns come to the fore. With the now widespread adoption of multidetector computed tomography (MDCT), for a broad range of examinations, MDCT continues to be the dominant source of dose from medical X-ray examinations, thereby posing significant challenges in radiological protection to the extent that some now claim that this represents today's greatest single challenge in radiation protection in diagnostic use. This book expounds the challenges posed by MDCT to scientists and physicians and in this chapter we provide an introduction to the main themes which are of concern.

## 1 Introduction

The principles of protecting the patient undergoing clinical investigation using radiation are clear and well established: it is the responsibility of all radiological services to ensure the information required for the clinical management of the patient is obtained

D. Tack et al. (eds.), *Radiation Dose from Multidetector CT*, Medical Radiology. Diagnostic Imaging,
DOI: 10.1007/174_2012_541, © Springer-Verlag Berlin Heidelberg 2012

with the lowest practicable exposure to radiation. Within this clear objective, however, medical investigation operates in a constantly changing scenario influenced by increasing knowledge of disease processes and advancing technological development. This syndrome ensures that as time passes differing objectives and concerns come to the fore. With the now widespread adoption of multidetector computed tomography (MDCT), for a broad range of examinations, MDCT continues to be the dominant source of dose from medical X-ray examinations, thereby posing significant challenges in radiological protection to the extent that some now claim that this represents today's greatest single challenge in radiation protection in diagnostic use. This book expounds the challenges posed by MDCT to scientists and physicians and in this chapter we provide an introduction to the main themes which are of concern.

Since its inception in 1973 (Hounsfield 1973) the development of computed tomography (CT) has been dramatic and the technique continues to mature and expand. Over 30 years ago a typical study consisted of 10 mm sections, a 20 s exposure time and a 60 s image reconstruction time. Technical developments including the development of slip rings, increased X-ray tube heat capacity, advances in multi-detector technology and improvement in computer processing now permit rapid sub-second exposures for acquiring sub-millimeter sections and almost instantaneous image reconstruction along with options of multi-planar reconstruction and three-dimensional (3-D) imaging. These improvements have brought benefits in clinical examination, extending the applications of CT into new areas and facilitating difficult or demanding examinations in all applications. The major development in technology has been MDCT, which has dramatically increased the performance capability of CT. It is now routine to expect modern radiology departments to have systems capable of acquiring 64 or more sections simultaneously have been introduced (Berland and Smith 1998; Hu et al. 2000; Kalender 2000; Prokop 2005). Even greater configurations are now becoming available, with the latest cone beam systems capable of simultaneously acquiring 256 sections (Mori et al. 2006). Beyond this dual energy scanners, for the distinction of bone and vessel structures (Morhard et al. 2009), and iterative reconstruction methods, as a means for dose reduction with controllable noise reduction (Gervaise et al. 2011), are both being trialled clinically. The incorporation of slip ring technology into the design of scanners in the late 1980s removed the need for rigid mechanical linkage between the power cables and the X-ray tube. The ability to rotate the tube continuously in one direction allowed the development of helical CT and re-established CT as a front-line imaging modality. Helical CT allows a volume of tissue rather than individual slices to be scanned as the table supporting the patient also moves continuously while the tube is rotating; the data are reformatted automatically to display the images as axial slices. Furthermore, whereas conventional and spiral scanners use a single row of detectors, MDCT scanners now have multiple active rows of detectors and selectable geometry. The increased number of detectors combined with sub-second tube rotation times have increased the speed and the ability to cover large body areas without anatomical misregistration (Garney and Hanlon 2002). Whole CT examinations may now be carried out within a single breath-hold (e.g. thorax, abdomen and pelvis in a trauma patient in 20 s) (Kalender et al. 1990). As well as increased speed and volume coverage, MDCT offers excellent opportunities for dedicated 2-D and 3-D visualization and post processing. Continuous data acquisition also means lesions can be evaluated during different phases of contrast enhancement and small lesions which may be missed with conventional CT can now be detected (Ichikawa et al. 2006).

Thus, modern CT scanners now offer clinical tools of vast flexibility. However, these benefits have not been without a price and it is arguable that MDCT has become Diagnostic Radiology's major radiation protection challenge.

## 2 Clinical Expansion

The continued development of MDCT means it remains a challenge of patient protection, owing to increased use in established applications and the introduction of a wide range of new applications. Despite efforts to move away from CT in some traditional examination areas, using either ultrasound (US) or magnetic resonance imaging (MRI) as the first imaging modality for patient examination, the further development of new CT technology and associated applications means the volume of patient examinations shows no signs of decreasing yet.

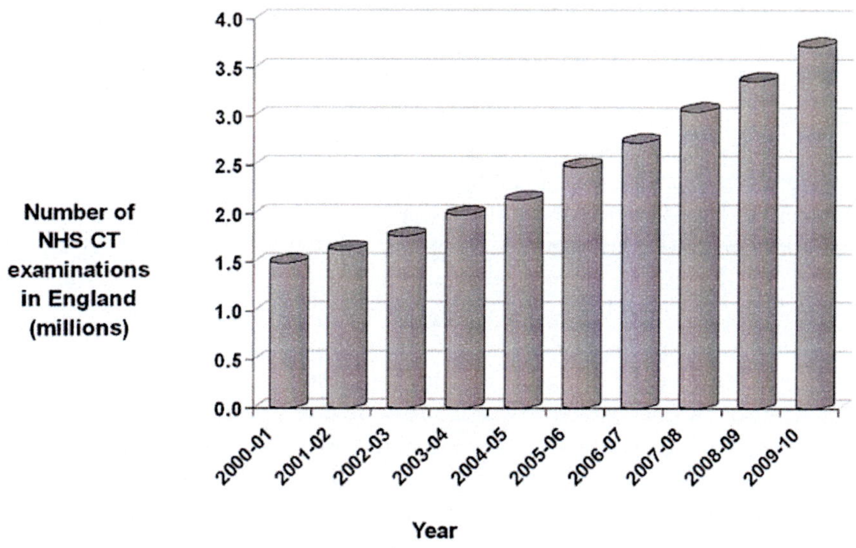


**Fig. 1** Annual numbers of NHS CT examinations in England, showing the growth in frequency of scans since the millennium

Figure 1 shows how in England CT use has continued to grow (Hart et al. 2010) with the National Health Service (NHS) referral frequency increasing year on year since the millennium (Meeson et al. 2011).

MDCT is routinely used for multiphase enhancement studies (Zoetelief and Geleijns 1998) including optimized injection protocols in multiphasic contrast-enhanced MDCT of the liver (Ichikawa et al. 2006). CT angiography continues to expand (Makayama et al. 2001; F or Lederlin et al. 2011), with CT urography (Anderson and Cowan 2004) and CT virtual colonoscopy (VC) (Landeras et al. 2007) contributing to greater use of 3-D imaging and virtual reality (Caramella and Bartolozzi 2002). For example, in the case of a neoplasm of the pancreas, it is possible to outline the primary neoplasm at an optimal phase of enhancement while at the same time gathering images of the liver in different phases of enhancement in order to examine for metastatic disease (Johnson 2001). Where the investigation is justified, completing it in one sitting is clearly of benefit in terms of facilitating treatment planning and for the patient.

It is recognized that the effective dose from CT scans of the head and neck is considerably lower than that from CT examinations of the abdomen or chest. However, head and neck CT examinations for well-established clinical indications (such as sinusitis, unilateral conductive hearing loss and acute stroke) are more common and the collective dose to the population from cranial examinations is therefore higher. Scan parameters for head and neck CT examination protocols are generally chosen to obtain the best image quality and meet the highest diagnostic criteria, but with an associated radiation dose cost. Radiation dose from head CT scans may vary considerably as a result of inherent differences in equipment and because of variations in exposure technique and scanning protocol. Previous studies where systematic changes in scanning parameters were analyzed with respect to resulting image quality have reported dose reductions of 40% or more in CT scans of the head without loss of relevant information or diagnostic image quality (Smith et al. 1998; Cohnen et al. 2000; AC or Kröpil et al. 2010; AD or Abul-Kasim et al. 2011).

The use of CT for the evaluation of cervical spine trauma achieves an end health state of high value compared to just conventional radiography (Theocharopoulos et al. 2009; European Commission 2008). However, our latest cervical spine test phantom and low dose CT studies suggest there is clear latitude for reducing dose while preserving image quality (publication forthcoming).

Well-established clinical indications for CT of the chest include bronchiectasis and the evaluation of interstitial lung disease. Chest CT is also commonly used to detect pulmonary metastases. CT is now the "gold standard" in imaging suspected pulmonary embolism (PE) (European Commission 2008; Henzler et al. 2011) replacing pulmonary scintigraphy or angiography as a first line investigation for PE

(Mayo 1997). While traditional angiography will continue to be used for various treatment options (such as the placement of stents or angioplasty) the diagnostic role of angiography is increasingly being carried out using the non-invasive procedure of CT angiography. A meta-analysis of this technique has demonstrated sensitivities of 53–100% and specificities of 83–100%, wide ranges which are partly explained by technologic improvements over time (Rathburn et al. 2000; Wittram et al. 2004).

MDCT has reduced scan times to a few seconds allowing patients to be scanned with very high resolution. Also, patients with severe pulmonary disease and congestive heart failure can be examined in a single breath-hold. Fast acquisition of narrow slices combined with ECG gating permits scans with greater temporal resolution. The main use of these images is for the visualization of the coronary arteries and calcium scoring for assessment of stenoses. The evaluation of the effect of ECG controlled tube current modulation on radiation exposure in retrospectively ECG-gated multi-slice CT of the heart has been shown to reduce dose by 37% (Poll et al. 2002) or more (Lehmkuhl et al. 2010).

Established indications for CT of the abdomen include detecting causes of sepsis (sensitivity 95% and specificity 91% (Meeson et al. 2009)), and detection of retroperitoneal lymphadenopathy or liver metastases from neoplasms. A relatively new clinical indication is urolithiasis. CT urography (CTU) allows comprehensive evaluation of the urinary tracts and it is now the primary imaging study for the evaluation of adults over 40 years old with hematuria (European Commission 2008). Together with other genitourinary conditions CTU has become an established technique for examining patients with acute renal colic (Kawashima et al. 2004; Wells et al. 1998). The sensitivity and accuracy of non-contrast CT in assessing ureteral calculi has been reported to be as high as 97% (Smith et al. 1996). Both CT angiography and CT urography cover large body areas with several hundred sections. The field of 3-D imaging and virtual reality is too large to cover here but MDCT has made these studies remarkably easy, for example, facilitating the development of CT virtual colonography. The technique of virtual colonoscopy was first introduced in the mid-1990s as a non-invasive technique to image the colon (Vining 1997). Thin axial slices through the abdomen are obtained in supine and prone positions and may be reconstructed into 3-D surface rendered images giving the impression of viewing the large bowel via an endoscope. It has now been suggested that best practices for polyp size measurement with VC include the use of 3-D endoluminal displays, 2-D displays with a window level near −500 HU and automated measurement software (Summers 2010).

A further development has been CT fluoroscopy which enables real-time monitoring for image-guided biopsy procedures. Improved needle manipulation has made previously difficult procedures easier. However, careful use of this technique is essential as there is potential for large skin doses to both patient and operator (Olerud et al. 2002). The use of tube currents as low as 10–30 mA have been shown to give significantly lower patient skin doses while still providing sufficient image quality in order to control the difficult steps of the procedure. In addition, lead protection has been shown to reduce the scattered dose to the operator by more than 90% (Irie et al. 2001).

CT screening is an emerging concept targeting early detection of disease entities such as lung cancer, colon cancer and coronary artery disease. The issue of screening for disease by CT is a difficult area, as clinical benefit has to be demonstrated conclusively to justify irradiation of a large number of normal individuals. Furthermore the impact on patients and health care services also needs to be quantified to determine the physical, psychological and financial costs of false negative impressions and subsequent unnecessary clinical interventions. One American study of the detection of pulmonary nodules found a primary neoplasm rate of only 0.03% (Benjamin et al. 2003).

In situations where the diagnostic yield of CT is expected to be so low, alternative, safer examinations should always be considered. Contrary to the general expectation that, with the advent of magnetic resonance imaging and its widespread use the use of X-ray computed tomography would decline rapidly, MDCT has continued to gain importance (Kalender 2000). However, MRI is an imaging modality that is considerably safer than CT on the basis of a number of factors, of which radiation dose is perhaps the most significant. It therefore provides the main "competition" for MDCT in clinical practice where it is available and applicable. A recent article has shown that screening MRI of the entire body may be more accurate than individual "gold standard" diagnostic investigations of individual organ systems (Lauenstein et al. 2004). There are important differences between MDCT and MRI, including speed, metal object compatibility, availability and cost. However, the present high use of MDCT suggests powerfully that whether MRI can replace CT for various indications should be continuously re-evaluated, perhaps even in circumstances where MDCT may be diagnostically more accurate (Semelka 2005).

The extension of CT into new areas continues. Several studies have already demonstrated that CT is ideally suited to the challenges posed by patients with suspected appendicitis. Raptopoulos et al. (2003) have reported the use of CT for selecting patients for management of acute appendicitis, finding that with increased use of CT there were less severe imaging findings, a significant decrease in surgical–pathologic severity and shortened hospital stay. These would seem to be clinical benefits but the routine use of a high radiation dose in a relatively benign process requires careful study of costs and benefits, especially as most patients with acute appendicitis, of whatever stage, are managed effectively without specialized investigation. In the latest update to the European Guidelines on the use of MDCT (European Commission 2008) US is now recommended as the first modality of imaging in acute abdominal pain, with CT used in clinically equivocal cases.

## 3 The Dose Problem

The fact that CT is a modality giving significant exposure is well known. In the past this was seen as permissible as in areas of its greatest application, such as the investigation of malignancy; its diagnostic value was greater than its inherent risk. However, CT is now used extensively in benign disease and in the young in whom cumulative dose considerations are of the utmost importance.

This issue of radiation dose from CT has received much attention in both the popular media and scientific literature, due in part to the fact that the dose levels from CT typically exceed those from conventional radiography and fluoroscopy, and that the use of CT continues to grow. CT contributes a significant portion of the total collective dose from ionizing radiation delivered to the public from medical procedures. The United Nations Scientific Committee on the Effects of Atomic Radiation (UNSCEAR) has highlighted that medical radiology is the largest artificial source of exposure to ionizing radiation (UNSCEAR 2010) and that in the USA there about 67 million CT examinations performed annually at a rate of about 223 examinations per 1000 persons. UNSCEAR also estimated previously that CT constitutes about 5% of all X-ray examinations worldwide while accounting for about 34% of the resultant collective dose. In the countries that were identified as having the highest levels of healthcare, the corresponding figures were 6 and 41%, respectively (UNSCEAR 2000). In the UK the most recent estimate from the Health Protection Agency (HPA) put the contribution from medical X-ray examinations (including dental) at 90% of the dose from all artificial sources of exposure in the UK.

In a frequently cited study performed by the Federal Bureau on Radiation Protection in Germany, it was found that between 1990 and 1992 only 4% of all X-ray examinations were performed on CT scanners, yet CT accounted for 35% of the collective effective dose (BMU 1996). In the United Kingdom, in 1991 the National Radiological Protection Board (NRPB) pointed out that CT makes a disproportionately large contribution to dose, at that time representing only 2.5% of examinations but constituting 25% of the collective dose to the population from diagnostic use (Shrimpton et al. 1991). Subsequent studies indicate that this proportion has increased; in 1998 Shrimpton and Edyvean (1998) suggested that the cumulative radiation dose was closer to 40%. Mettler et al. (2000) have indicated that in their department CT comprises 11% of examinations and 67% of the collective dose, 11% of these examinations being carried out in children, in whom radiation protection considerations are paramount. These growing trends have continued with population doses from diagnostic X-rays in the UK and USA showing CT remains the dominant source of dose from medical X-ray examinations. In the UK 68% of the population dose comes from CT examinations, while CT represents only 11% of all of the X-ray examinations performed (excluding nuclear medicine) (Hart et al. 2010). Similarly in the USA the percentages are 66 and 18%, respectively (NCRP 2009). In the UK HPA (includes former NRPB) report of 2010, per caput CT dose in the UK was less than five times the equivalent figure in the USA. However, in the UK there were typically 56 CT examinations per 1000 population rising to 223 per 1000 in the USA.

Whereas, there is still a paucity of published data available on the trends in patient doses following the introduction of MDCT, an increased contribution to patient dose may be expected due to reduced geometric efficiency and the more prominent impact of the additional tube rotations necessary before and after data acquisition over the planned scan range. When scanning in helical mode, all CT scanners acquire additional rotations at each end of the scan length in order to obtain sufficient data to reconstruct the full imaged volume. Two studies have reported significant increases in effective dose per patient of 10% and 34% for multislice compared with single slice CT (Brix et al. 2003; Yates et al. 2004a, b). Reconstruction methods on multidetector systems sometimes require a greater number of additional rotations. This together with greater X-ray beam widths used can result in a significant increase in effective dose, particularly for short scan lengths (Nicholson and Fetherston 2002). Published results from the 2003 UK CT dose survey (Shrimpton et al. 2005), a review of CT practice after the introduction of helical CT nationally, show that there has been a reduction in average patient doses from CT examinations since the previous national CT dose survey published in 1991. However, they also show that doses from MDCT are consistently slightly higher than dose levels from single slice CT scanners. The Third UK national CT dose survey of current practice (2010/2011) is currently under way with the aims of updating existing examination-specific national reference doses and providing guidance for some new establishing examinations.

Of particular concern is the fact that many of the new applications are especially applicable to young patients and those with benign disease. However, this challenge is not the only problem facing radiation protection in CT. The short scanning time of MDCT means there is a danger of uncritical use being made of the technique and previous studies have shown that there are large variations in the scanning protocols employed for the use of CT (Lewis and Edyvean 2005). The risk is that the flexibility of MDCT in terms of long scan lengths and use of narrow imaged slices with high mAs values can lead to unnecessarily high doses if diagnostic requirements are not adequately considered (Shrimpton et al. 2005).

Controlling technique variations may be problematic. Recommendations of CT manufacturers vary with regard to clinical protocols and cannot be compared easily because of different scanner makes and models (Scheck et al. 1998). Institutions may also change protocols according to their needs with variations even noted between different departments in the same hospital where equivalent technology is in use. Further, different CT scanners employ specific detector geometry and filtration characteristics. As a result it has been shown that even identical scanning parameters can result in considerable dose differences in the patient (Scheck et al. 1998). Consequently, there is a worrying level of variation in exposure for examinations carried out for identical purposes.

Shrimpton et al. (2005) reported that effective dose could differ by a factor between 10 and 40 in examinations for the same application and Olerud (1997) has reported variations between 8 and 20 times. These differences seem to relate principally to variations in examination technique. In our experience (unpublished data) a 10-fold variation in the number of sections and exposure factors is found across the work of one general department. It is inevitable that some complex cases will require a larger number of CT sections and multiple phases, but the disparity occurring between apparently similar applications is of serious concern.

It is now widely accepted that unoptimized CT examination protocols are a significant contributor of unnecessary radiation dose. There appears to be much scope for dose optimization through use of appropriate protocols (Lewis and Edyvean 2005). Efforts and measures to reduce dose can be initiated by the examiner by critically considering the indication and the choice of scanning protocols and parameters for CT examination.

There may be justifiable reasons for some variability in practice, of which the most important one is the difference in clinical indication. Furthermore, as techniques develop there is a period of learning during which the examination technique should develop to a mature level. This difference is greater if operators and practitioners are insufficiently educated in newly emerging technology. Further, increasing demand in radiology may induce radiologists to use over-intense protocols for CT, for viability to supervise the examination directly while engaged in other work. It is perceived that this is more likely to occur with relatively inexperienced workers and, it is also possible that some examinations are carried out more intensively than needed as a means of clinical risk limitations. These factors indicate strongly against measures to provide effective radiation protection. Low annual referral frequencies for examinations may also lead to unnecessarily high patient exposures where a lack of familiarity with the procedure and a failure to optimize the examination parameters increase the dose cost to the patient. This is particularly the case for centers with low numbers of pediatric referrals.

A further factor is the frequency with which patients may undergo CT in a single illness. Surveys have shown that it is not difficult for a patient with a complex illness to acquire several exposures in a short time (European Commission 2008). In our own study in patients with abdominal sepsis (Meeson et al. 2009)—a non-malignant condition—we found when looking at all CT referrals locally a maximum of 18 examinations for a single patient during one year. The relative percentages of patients with six or more CT in a year were comparable with other institutes taking part in the European survey. It was agreed that the high number of patients receiving more than six CT examinations in a year raised concern about the appropriateness of the repeated CT examinations. This has significant implication for interpreting the impact of population exposure; many population surveys give an average exposure per caput, whereas what is happening in practice is that there are patients who are receiving a large number of exposures over a short period. This makes protection measures even more important in the individual case.

One of the critical questions to ask is to what extent developments in technology should alter examination technique. There is a natural tendency for changes in the examination technique to be driven by advances in technology but the person carrying out the examination has to ask if there is added benefit in intensifying the examination and therefore the radiation exposure. It has to be accepted that clinical demand and workload pressures currently motivate against protection measures and that optimization of practice is one of the greatest challenges facing dose constraint in CT (Golding and Shrimpton 2002).

Unfortunately, despite the development of exposure reducing technology, the evidence base for practice is limited (Kalra et al. 2004). Optimization of scanning protocols involves many parameters including tube voltage, tube current, section thickness, collimation and pitch (McCollough et al. 2006). A dose reduction of 90% has been reported in high resolution CT of the face in patients with orbital trauma (Jackson and Whitehouse 1993), and in CT of the chest minimizing tube current has been reported to reduce the dose by 50%. Starck et al. (1998) reported that in very specialized circumstances a 96% reduction in dose can be achieved and similar levels of reduction may be possible in CT colonography (Iannaccone et al. 2003). Our own studies in this area bear out this experience. These studies related to areas of high natural contrast and high resolution imaging, where large exposure latitude may be expected. However, research is needed in the main areas of application of CT, where detection of low contrast lesions is paramount. It is necessary to establish the minimum exposure threshold that will deliver adequate image quality in each application, preferably expressed in terms of clinical effectiveness (Mini et al. 1995). Dose reductions achieved in studies with test objects also need to be confirmed in clinical trials, demonstrating image suitability, before potential dose savings can be achieved more widely.

## 4 Approaches to the Problem

The answers to the challenges facing the use of MDCT must come both from technological development and from the clinical practice. On the industrial side the significant developments that have already been achieved in dose-constraint technology must continue and must impact on the way that MDCT operates in practice, as described in the following chapters. A harmonization of dose-constraint methods employed by all manufacturers, including the different options for automatic tube current modulation, is also desirable to achieve the best possible image with the lowest dose and to ensure that operators understand both the protocol settings selected and the impact of modifying them. The advances in practice must be based upon a clear perception of the factors important in protecting the patient in MDCT, as outlined below.

## 5 The ALARA Principle

The ALARA principle states that all medicinal exposure for diagnostic purposes shall be kept as low as reasonably achievable. It is based on the radiation assurance recommendations of various international expert committees and organizations and forms the cornerstone of radiation protection. Based on the assumption that there is no lower threshold for carcinogenesis (i.e. there is no dose that can be considered completely safe or harmless), the reduction of radiation exposure to 'ALARA' remains an ongoing challenge.

## 6 The Role of the Referrer: Justification

It is a sine qua nom of investigational medicine that the risk of the procedure is outweighed by the putative benefit to the patient. Although simple in essence, this principle may be difficult to put into practice. In many areas of established use of CT the potential benefit to the patient is clear and its application therefore well justified. However, patients are all individuals and in other areas it may be difficult to quantify accurately the potential benefit to the patient in many instances, it is accepted, clinicians may tend to refer patients for examination in order to give themselves reassurance concerning their intended management regime; in such cases benefit is difficult to demonstrate and dose constraint should be employed here.

The aims of radiation protection—and of effective justification and the ALARA Principle—may best be met by encouraging referring clinicians to adopt a critical appraisal of their own referral practice. The clinician needs to ask, before referring a patient for MDCT, "do I really need this investigation? Will it change what I do?" If the answer to these questions is positive, the next critical question is to ask whether the information that is needed could be obtained without the use of ionizing radiation. In many abdominal and pelvic applications ultrasound and MRI provide acceptable alternatives to MDCT, and MRI is also an effective competitor elsewhere in the body. Even where these two techniques may not be as sensitive as MDCT, there may be a case for employing them first, especially in young patients, on the basis that if they yield the required information then exposure of the patient to radiation may not be required. In our own practice the investigation of some cases of orbital fracture—an application usually regarded as exclusively a requirement for CT—have been successfully achieved using MRI. In such clinical decisions referral guidelines such as those issued by the Royal College of Radiologists in the UK have an established value.

## 7 The Role of the Operator: Optimization

It should be a given principle that all MDCT equipment is operated at optimum technical performance and subject to regular quality assurance. However, the objectives of optimization of the examination go beyond this. As indicated above, there are current technological advances which may be used to constrain exposure and, in appropriate circumstances, image quality can be manipulated to reduce exposure, provided that the resulting examination does not fall below an acceptable threshold of image quality and therefore of sensitivity appropriate to the clinical application. All departments should have in place local guidelines, based on the best evidence to date, to ensure that these objectives are met.

## 8 The Role of Guidelines in MDCT

As indicated above, the evidence base for dose constraint in CT is not strong and in these circumstances practice guidelines may be important. In 1994, the European Commission set up a working group on image quality and dose in CT, resulting in publication in 2000 of the European Guidelines on Quality Criteria for Computed Tomography (European Commission 2000). This group continued its work and produced updates to the guidelines. The second edition of the guidelines (European Commission 2000) surveyed technical and clinical principles in MDCT and made recommendations on good technique in common areas of application, together with the guidelines on dose measurement and audit. Particular attention was also paid to pediatrics, a group of patients who should always be examined using protocols that have been optimized for children and not adults. In 2008, the updates concentrated on MDCT scanners that can acquire data with at least 16 slices simultaneously (European Commission 2008).

One problem that the group has had to face is the variation in the performance of individual CT scanners. Whereas, in the first edition it was possible to make specific recommendations on slice thickness and pitch, only ranges can now be specified. As in the first edition, the guidelines recommend quality criteria that enable examinations to be assessed. However, the key issue of diagnostic effectiveness and exposure still needs to be addressed by robust research studies for both established and emerging applications of MDCT.

## 9 The Role of Evidence: Vigilance

Overall, experience indicates that the dramatic rise in applications of CT has not yet reached a plateau. This is despite the fact that both technically and clinically, MSCT may be used in a way to aid dose constraint (Olerud 1997; Kalendar 2004; Yates et al. 2004a, b). A number of factors actually offer the potential of dose reduction if taken into consideration by clinicians. For example, repeat scans which were frequently required if the patient moved significantly or breathed between single scans, have been practically eliminated by MDCT. Overlapping scans which were often selected for good multiplanar or 3-D displays and led to corresponding increases in dose are no longer a necessity because overlapping images are routinely available in helical CT with no additional exposure. Also, the selection of pitch factors >1 results in a reduction in dose corresponding to the pitch factor (Kalender 2000). Significant reduction of dose can also be obtained through attenuation-dependent tube current modulation which allows constant image quality to be maintained regardless of patient attenuation characteristics and is now widely available on most MSCT systems (Yates et al. 2004a, b).

It is important that all practitioners in CT continue to review emerging evidence and adapt their practice accordingly. For the present dose audit remains mandatory and further surveys of practice are required. Departments must ensure that their justification criteria are soundly applied, and that examinations are carefully targeted to clinical applications and do not exceed the clinical requirements. Where evidence supports the approach, exposure should be adjusted to the lowest threshold that delivers the required clinical sensitivity. It is necessary to follow published guidelines and observe all updates in these. Beyond this, however, new legislation has now been passed in the USA to enforce radiation protection at a patient level. The Governor of California, Arnold Schwarzenegger, has signed a bill into law related to CT dose. SB1237, that was signed into law September 30, 2010, paves the way for the implementation of the first state law aimed at protecting patients from excessive radiation exposure received during CT scans and radiation therapy procedures. The bill will impose strict new procedures and reporting requirements to protect patients from medical radiation overdoses when it becomes effective July 1, 2012. The bill also provides an accreditation mandate for CT scanners that will take effect from January 1, 2013 (American Association of Physicists in Medicine (AAPM) 2011). The bill requires that dose be recorded on the scanned image and in a patient's health records, and that radiation overdoses be reported to patients, physicians, and the state Department of Public Health.

CT manufacturers are constantly reviewing dose optimization and regulation. Five companies that manufacture the majority of the world's CT scanners are cooperating in an initiative to improve patients' safety by including additional radiation dose safeguards on their equipment. Under the Medical Imaging and Technology Alliance (MITA) "dose check" initiative (Computed Tomography Dose Check (NEMA Standards Publication XR 25-2010) 2010), manufacturers of computed tomography equipment have agreed to add an alert feature to notify CT operators when recommended radiation dose levels are exceeded. The AAPM have also issued dose check recommendations regarding notification and alert values for CT scanners (AAPM Dose Check Guidelines 2011).

Overall, the challenge of patient exposure in MDCT will best be served by continuing vigilance; from the manufacturers toward new dose-saving developments and advice to their uses, from clinical referrers to ensure that over-demand is avoided, and from radiology department staff to ensure that the principles of best practice are always applied. This is, therefore, a field in which understanding of the balance between risks and benefits is most likely to be served by effective inter-disciplinary communication, education and vigilance.

## 10 Conclusion: The Professional Responsibility

It is an unfortunate fact of radiation protection in this field that we are not in a position to judge definitely whether the increase in population exposure due to CT will or will not create a future problem in radiation-induced disease, as many claim. All our estimations of risk are based on extrapolation from outside the range of diagnostic exposures. It is not even known if the Linear No Threshold (LNT) model is applicable at this level of exposure. However, in Medicine it is insufficient practice to assume safety; if we do not know for certain that we are safe we have a professional obligation to proceed with caution. The evidence from successive surveys makes it clear that this is not happening.

It is essential that all available guidelines for patient protection and adherence to protection law are applied. Wide variations in exposure for similar indications need to be outlawed, possibly by international action. However, we also need to reverse the climb in exposure. This may be done by replacement of CT wherever practicable but also by department staff taking a proactive approach to introducing the results of protection research as they become available. Diagnostic Radiology staff should also be alert to the number of examinations that patients may have in a single disease episode, together with their total numbers of examinations in any given year, and be prepared to modify examination protocols to limit repeat exposures. While departments carry the legal responsibility for protection, there is much that individual staff can achieve by being sensitive to the perceived challenge in exposure from MDCT and having the aspiration to go further in protecting the patient than required by law. In this sense the issues addressed in this book are as much a matter of individual professional responsibility as the application of science.

## References

AAPM Dose Check Guidelines (2011) Version1.0, 04/27/2011. Available from: http://www.aapm.org/pubs/CTProtocols/documents/NotificationLevelsStatement_2011-04-27.pdf

Abul-Kasim K, Strömbeck A, Sahlstrand-Johnson P (2011) Low-dose computed tomography of the paranasal sinuses: radiation doses and reliability analysis. Am J Otolaryngol 32(1):47–51 [Epub 2009 Oct 12]

American Association of Physicists in Medicine (AAPM) (2011) AAPM Government Affairs. Available from http://www.aapm.org/government_affairs/default.asp

Anderson K, Cowan NC (2004) Multidetector CT urography. Radiol Now 21:4–6

Benjamin MS, Drucker EA, McLoud TC, Shepherd J (2003) Small pulmonary nodules: detection at chest CT and outcome. Radiology 226:489–493

Berland LL, Smith JK (1998) Multidetector-array CT: once again, technology creates new opportunities. Radiology 209: 327–329

BMU (1996) (Bundesministerium fur Umwelt, Naturschutz und Reaktorsicher-heit). Umweltradioaktivitat und Strahlenbelastung im Jahre. Deutscher Bundestag 13. Wahlperiode; Drucksache 13/8630

Brix G, Nagel HD, Stamm G et al (2003) Radiation exposure in multi-slice versus single slice spiral CT: results of a nationwide survey. Eur Radiol 13:1979–1991

Caramella D, Bartolozzi C (eds) (2002) 3D image processing: techniques and applications. Springer, Brelin

Cohnen M, Fischer H, Hamacher J et al (2000) CT of the head by use of reduced current and kilovoltage: relationship between image quality and dose reduction. Am J Neuradiol 21(1654):1660

Computed Tomography Dose Check (NEMA Standards Publication XR 25-2010) (2010) http://www.nema.org/stds/xr25.cfm)

European Commission (2000) European guidelines on quality criteria for computed tomography. EUR 16262EN. EC, Luxembourg

European Commission (2004) MSCT quality criteria. European guidelines for multislice computed tomography. Contract number FIGM-CT2000-20078-CT-TIP. Bongartz G, Golding SJ, Jurik AG, Leonardi M, van Persijn van Meerten E, Rodríguez R, Schneider K, Calzado A, Geleijns J, Jessen KA, Panzer W, Shrimpton PC, Tosi G. Available from http://www.drs.dk/guidelines/ct/quality/index.htm

European commission (2008) Safety and efficacy of computed tomography: a broad perspective (CT safety and efficacy). European commission Euratom research and training programme on nuclear energy (area: radiation protection) report. Contract FI6R-CT2004-002388. Geleijns J (Koos), Kalender W, Krispijn W, Schneider K, Shrimpton P. Available from ftp://ftp.cordis.europa.eu/pub/fp6-euratom/docs/ct_safety_efficacy_projrep_en.pdf

Garney CJ, Hanlon R (2002) Computed tomography in clinical practice. BMJ 324:1077–1080

Gervaise A, Osemont B, Lecocq S, Noel A, Micard E, Felblinger J, Blum A (2011) CT image quality improvement using adaptive iterative dose reduction with wide-volume acquisition on 320-detector CT. Eur Radiol 17 Sep 2011 [Epub ahead of print]

Golding SJ, Shrimpton PC (2002) Radiation dose in CT: are we meeting the challenge? Br J Radiol 75:1–4

Hart D, Wall BF, Hillier MC, Shrimpton PC (2010) Frequency and collective dose for medical and dental X-ray examinations in the UK, 2008. Chilton HPA-CRCE-012, 2010. Available from http://www.hpa.org.uk/radiation/

Henzler T, Barraza JM Jr, Nance JW Jr, Costello P, Krissak R, Fink C, Schoepf UJ (2011) CT imaging of acute pulmonary embolism. J Cardiovasc Comput Tomogr. 5(1):3–11 [Epub 29 Oct 2010]

Hounsfield GN (1973) Computerised transverse axial scanning (tomography). Br J Radiol 46:1016

Hu H, He HD, Foley WD, Fox SH (2000) Four multidetector-row helical CT: image quality and volume coverage speed. Radiology 215:55–62

Iannaccone R, Laghi A, Catalano C et al (2003) Feasibility of ultra-low dose multislice CT colography for the detection of colorectal lesions: preliminary experience. Eur Radiol 13: 1297–1302

Ichikawa T, Erturk SM, Araki T (2006) Multiphasic contrast-enhanced multidetector-row CT of liver: contrast-enhancement theory and practical scan protocol with a combination of fixed injection duration and patients' body-weight-tailored dose of contrast material. Eur J Radiol 58(2): 165–176 [Epub 18 Jan 2006]

Irie T, Kajitani M, Itai Y (2001) CT fluoroscopy-guided intervention: marked reduction of scattered radiation dose to the physicians hand by use of a lead plate and an improved I–I device. J Vasc Interv Radiol 12:1417–1421

Jackson A, Whitehouse RW (1993) Low-dose computed tomographic imaging in orbital trauma. Br J Radiol 66:655–661

Johnson CD (2001) Pancreatic carcinoma: developing a protocol for multidetector row CT. Radiology 220:3–4

Kalendar W (2004) Dose management in multislice spiral computed tomography. Eur Radiol Syllabus 14:40–49

Kalender WA (2000) Computed tomography, Publicis MCD Verlag, Munich

Kalender WA, Seissler W, Klotz E, Vock P (1990) Spiral volumetric CT with single-breath-hold technique, continuous transport, and continuous scanner rotation. Radiology 176:181–183

Kalra KM, Maher M, Toth TL et al (2004) Techniques and applications of automatic tube current modulation. Radiology 233:649–657

Kawashima A, Vrtiska TJ, LeRoy AJ et al (2004) CT urography. RadioGr 24:S35–S54

Kröpil P, Cohnen M, Andersen K, Heinen W, Stegmann V, Mödder U (2010) Image quality in multidetector CT of paranasal sinuses: potential of dose reduction using an adaptive post-processing filter. Rofo 182(11):973–978 [Epub 18 Aug 2010]. German

Landeras LA, Aslam R, Yee J (2007) Virtual colonoscopy: technique and accuracy. Radiol Clin North Am 45(2):333–345

Lauenstein TC, Goehde SC, Herborn CU et al (2004) Whole-body MR imaging: evaluation of patients for metastases. Radiology 233:139–148

Lederlin M, Thambo JB, Latrabe V, Corneloup O, Cochet H, Montaudon M, Laurent F (2011) Coronary imaging techniques with emphasis on CT and MRI. Pediatr Radiol 41(12): 1516–1525 [Epub 30 Nov 2011]

Lehmkuhl L, Gosch D, Nagel HD, Stumpp P, Kahn T, Gutberlet M (2010) Quantification of radiation dose savings in cardiac computed tomography using prospectively triggered mode and ECG pulsing: a phantom study. Eur Radiol 20(9):2116–2125 [Epub 9 Apr 2010]

Lewis MA, Edyvean S (2005) Patient dose reduction in CT. Br J Radiol 78:880–883

Makayama Y, Yamashita Y and Takahahi M (2001) CT of the aorta and its major branches. In: Multislice CT. Reiser M, Takahashi M, Modic M and Bruening R (eds) Multislice CT, Springer, Berlin

Mayo JR (1997) Opinion response to acute pulmonary embolism: the role of computed tomographic imaging. J Thoracic Imaging 12:95–97

Meeson S, Alvey CM, Golding SJ (2009) Justifying multi-detector CT in abdominal sepsis: time for review? Br J Radiol 82:190–197 [Epub 27 Oct 2008]

Meeson S, Shrimpton PC, MacLachlan SA, Golding SJ (2011) Update on radiation exposure from CT: early progress in the third UK CT dose survey. In: (e103) Proceedings of UK radiological congress 2011, BJR Congress Series, pp 55–56

Mettler FA, Wiest PW, Locken JA, Kelsey CA (2000) CT scanning: patterns of use and dose. J Radiol Prot 20:353–359

Mini RL, Vock P, Mury R, Schneeberger PP (1995) Radiation exposure of patients who undergo CT of the Trunk. Radiology 195:557–562

Morhard D, Fink C, Graser A, Reiser MF, Becker C, Johnson TR (2009) Cervical and cranial computed tomographic angiography with automated bone removal: dual energy computed tomography versus standard computed tomography. Invest Radiol 44(5):293–297

Mori S, Endo M, Nishizawa K et al (2006) Comparison of patient doses in 256-slice CT and 16-slice CT scanners. Br J Radiol 79:56–61

McCollough CH, Bruesewitz MR, Kofler JM Jr (2006) CT dose reduction and dose management tools: overview of available options. Radiographics 26:503–512 (review)

NCRP (2009) Ionizing radiation exposure of the population of the United States. NCRP report 160. National Council on Radiation Protection and Measurements, Bethesda

Nicholson R, Fetherston S (2002) Primary radiation outside the imaged volume. Br J Radiol 75:518–522

Olerud HM (1997) Analysis of factors influencing patient doses from CT in Norway. Radiat Prot Dosim 71:123–133

Olerud HM, Obberg S, Widmark A, Hauser M (2002) Physician and patient radiation dose in various CT guided biopsy protocols. In: Sixth European ALARA network on "occupational exposure optimisation in the medical field and radiopharmaceutical industry". Madrid, Spain, 23–25 Oct 2002

Poll LW, Cohnen M, Brachten S, Ewen K, Modder U (2002) Dose reduction in multi-slice CT of the heart by use of ECG-controlled tube current modulation ("ECG pulsing"): phantom measurements. Rofo 174:1500–1505

Prokop (2005) New challenges in MDCT. Eur Radiol 15(suppl 5): E35–E45

Raptopoulos V, Katson G, Rosen P et al (2003) Acute appendicitis: effect of increased use of CT on selecting patients earlier. Radiology 226:521–526

Rathburn SW, Raskob GE, Whitsett TL (2000) Sensitivity and specificity of helical computed tomography in the diagnosis of pulmonary embolism: a systematic review. Ann Int Med 132:227–232

Scheck RJ, Coppenrath EM, Kellner MW et al (1998) Radiation dose and image quality in spiral computed tomography: multicentre evaluation at six institutions. Br J Radiol 71: 734–744

Semelka RC (2005) Radiation risks from CT scans: a call for patient-focused imaging. Medscape Radiol 6(1) http://www.medscape.com/article/496297

Shrimpton PC, Edyvean S (1998) CT scanner dosimetry. Br J Radiol 71:1–3

Shrimpton PC, Hillier MC, Lewis MA, Dunn M (2005) Doses from computed tomography (CT). Examinations in the UK—2003 Review. NRPB-W67

Shrimpton PC, Jones DG, Hillier MC et al (1991) Survey of CT practice in the UK. Part 2: dosimetric aspects. NRPB Report R249. NRPB, Chilton

Smith A, Shah GA, Kron T (1998) Variation of patient dose in head CT. Br J Radiol 71:1296–1301

Smith RC, Verga M, McCarthy S, Rosenfield AT (1996) Diagnosis of acute flank pain: value of unenhanced helical CT. Am J Roentgenol 166:97–101

Starck G, Lonn L, Cederblad A et al (1998) Radiation dose reduction in CT: application to tissue area and volume determination. Radiology 209:397–403

Summers RM (2010) Polyp size measurement at CT colonography: what do we know and what do we need to know? Radiology 255(3):707–720

Theocharopoulos N, Chatzakis G, Damilakis J (2009) Is radiography justified for the evaluation of patients presenting with cervical spine trauma? Med Phys 36(10):4461–4470

United Nations Scientific Committee on the Effects of Atomic Radiation (2000) Sources and effects of ionising radiation, vol 1. UNSCEAR, New York

UNSCEAR (2010) United Nations scientific committee on the effects of atomic radiation 2008 report: sources and effects of ionizing radiation, vol 1. Annex A: Medical radiation exposures. Available from www.unscear.org

Vining DJ (1997) Virtual colonoscopy. Gastrointest Endosc Clin N Amer 7:285–291

Wells ES et al (1998) Use of a clinical model for safe management of patients with suspected pulmonary embolism. Ann Intern Med 129:997–1005

Wittram C, Maher MM, Yoo AJ et al (2004) CT angiography of pulmonary embolism: diagnosis criteria and causes of misdiagnosis. RadioGraphics 24:1219–1238

Yates SJ, Pike LC, Goldstone KE (2004a) Effect of multislice scanners on patient dose from routine CT examinations in East Anglia. Br J Radiol 77:472–478

Yates SJ, Pike LC, Golstone KE (2004b) Effect of multislice scanners on patient dose from routine CT examinations in East Anglia. Br J Radiol 77:472–478

Zoetelief J, Geleijns J (1998) Patient dose in spiral CT. Br J Radiol 71:584–586

# Part II

# General Aspects of CT Radiation

# Risks from Ionising Radiation

Kenneth H. Chadwick and Hendrik P. Leenhouts

## Contents



K. H. Chadwick (✉)
3 Ellerbank, Cowan Head, Kendal,
Cumbria,
LA8 9HX, UK
e-mail: kennethhchadwick@aol.com

H. P. Leenhouts
FredBantinglaan 6, 6721 BC Bennekom,
The Netherlands

**Abstract**

The outline of a quantitative model is presented which can be used to derive the pathway from radiation-induced molecular damage, the DNA double strand break, to cellular effects such as cell killing, chromosomal aberrations and mutations and on to radiation-induced cancer. Evidence is provided to support the links in the chain which relate the different cellular end-points to each other and to cancer. The influence of differing dose rates and types of radiation on dose effect relationships are discussed. The extension to radiation induced cancer is made using a two mutation multi-step model for carcinogenesis and evidence is provided to support the assumption that radiation induced cancer arises from a somatic mutation. The dose response for radiation induced cancer is presented and various implications for radiation risks are outlined. The model is also extended to a consideration of deterministic effects by assuming that these effects arise as a result of multi-cell killing at high acute doses. The implications of the model for medical diagnostic radiology are discussed.

## 1 Introduction

### 1.1 Preamble

Deleterious health effects induced by ionising radiation are conventionally divided into two different categories, deterministic effects and stochastic effects.

Exposures to high acute doses in excess of one or two gray (Gy) or sievert (Sv) cause substantial levels of

D. Tack et al. (eds.), *Radiation Dose from Multidetector CT*, Medical Radiology. Diagnostic Imaging,
DOI: 10.1007/174_2011_400, © Springer-Verlag Berlin Heidelberg 2012

cell killing which is expressed as organ and tissue damage and, soon after exposure, as deleterious clinical effects. These effects are called deterministic and the dose-effect relationships exhibit a long threshold dose with no observable effect after which the effect increases in severity as the radiation dose increases.

At lower doses, deleterious health effects, such as cancer or hereditary disease which may take years to be revealed, can occur as a consequence of molecular damage to the nucleus of a single cell. These effects are called stochastic effects and the probability for their occurrence increases as the dose increases but the severity of the effect is unrelated to the dose.

The radiation doses received by patients undergoing diagnostic radiological examinations using computed tomography (CT) are generally in the order of 1–24 mSv per examination for adults (UNSCEAR 2000) and 2–6.5 mSv for children (Shrimpton et al. 2003). These effective doses can be classified as low even though they are invariably larger than doses from conventional diagnostic radiology. The immediate question which comes to mind is whether these low doses carry any risk for the patient.

Under normal circumstances with doses in the range of 1–24 mSv per examination deterministic health effects, such as radiation sickness or organ and tissue damage, can be excluded. However, there are some diagnostic procedures where skin damage can occur (Buls and de Mey 2007) and the report of a 6 Gy exposure during a brain examination (Smith-Bindman 2010) suggests that the occurrence of deterministic effects cannot be completely excluded. Consequently, although a thorough treatment of deterministic radiation effects is beyond the scope of this chapter, a brief section illustrating the analysis of deterministic effects is presented to draw attention to the potential dangers and implications of larger exposure doses.

The potential for stochastic health effects to occur as a consequence of computed tomography examinations cannot be so easily dismissed because the shape of the dose-effect relationship at low doses is not known. The aim of this chapter is, therefore, to present a model of radiation action at the cellular level which provides a comprehensive understanding of radiation biological effects, defines dose-effect relationships down to zero dose, can be extended to the induction of cancer and identifies the nature of radiation risk at low doses.

## 1.2 Cancer Risk: Threshold or Linear No-Threshold

The estimation of the risk for radiation-induced cancer relies on the analyses of epidemiological data from exposed populations, most notably the atomic bomb survivors. In all the epidemiological data, the cancer inducing effects of low doses are not significantly different from the background levels of cancer in unexposed populations so that the dose-effect relationship at low doses is not well defined. There are essentially two different opinions about the shape of the dose-effect relationship for stochastic effects at low doses. There are those who believe that very low doses of radiation carry no risk so that a threshold dose has to be exceeded before an effect will be induced and there are others who support the concept of radiation risk increasing linearly with dose from zero dose up, i.e. the linear no-threshold (LNT) concept.

The LNT concept of radiation risk has been the subject of much debate (Academie des Sciences 1997; Clarke 1998; Tubiana 1998; Kellerer 2000; Kellerer and Nekolla 2000) and supporters of the "threshold" concept (Bond et al. 1996; Becker 1997; Tubiana 2000) include some who support the idea that low doses can have a beneficial health effect, i.e. "radiation hormesis" (Calabrese 2002; Luckey 1997; Sagan 1992; Kesavan and Sugahara 1992). Others who support the LNT concept include some who claim that the linear no-threshold concept underestimates the risk of low dose radiation (Gofman and Tamplin 1971; Stewart and Kneale 1990; Edwards 1997). However, it is important to note that, following extensive reviews, both the United Nations Scientific Committee on the Effects of Atomic Radiation (UNSCEAR 2000) and the National Council on Radiation Protection and Measurements of the United States of America (NCRP 2001) have concluded that the LNT extrapolation provides the interpretation of low dose radiation effects which is most consistent with current scientific data and developing knowledge. UNSCEAR qualifies this by adding that a strictly linear dose response should not be expected in all circumstances.

Even more important is the fact that the Recommendations of the International Commission on Radiological Protection (ICRP), outlined in its Publication 60 (ICRP 1991), implicitly adopt the LNT concept and ICRP considers that the risks estimated using the concept are probably conservative. The concept has formed the basis for the development of an extremely useful radiological protection philosophy including the valuable As Low As Readily Achievable [ALARA] principle and Collective Dose which is a parameter that, while useful, is also open to abuse. In this context, it is worth noting that there are indications that the ICRP might adopt a different strategy in the future (Clarke 1999; ICRP 2003).

However, the ICRP has, in its current Recommendations which date from 1991, adopted the LNT concept and estimated low dose-rate radiation risk essentially using an interpretation of the data on cancer induction in the atomic bomb survivors. ICRP uses a dose and dose-rate reduction factor (DDREF) of 2 to convert from high dose-rate risk to low dose, low dose-rate risk to take account of the sparing effect of low dose-rate which is commonly found in radiation biology. The ICRP quantified radiation risk in 1991 by adopting a value of 5% for the nominal lifetime excess absolute risk (EAR) per sievert (Sv) for fatal cancer for a general population exposed to low doses. A value of 4% for the nominal lifetime excess absolute risk per sievert for fatal cancer was adopted for a population of working age.

More recently UNSCEAR (2000) has derived a quantification of radiation risk in a somewhat different way. Starting from an assessment of lifetime risk estimates for solid cancer mortality in a population of all ages after an acute dose of 1 Sv (9% for men, 13% for women) UNSCEAR applies a 50% reduction to estimate risk for chronic exposures but suggests that solid cancer incidence risks are about twice those for mortality. Children are thought to have twice the levels of risk compared with adults. The lifetime risk for leukaemia is taken as 1% for both men and women following an acute dose of 1 Sv but the nonlinearity of the acute dose-response is expected to lead to a 20-fold reduction in risk if the acute dose is reduced from 1 to 0.1 Sv.

## 1.3 What the Data Tell

The debate about the LNT concept continues to rage because the extrapolation of epidemiological and experimental radiation biological data measured at higher doses down to zero dose is open to several interpretations and has important economic and policy implications for radiological protection and medical radiology as well as energy production and nuclear decommissioning. The discussion about the different interpretations of the shape of the dose–effect relationship at low doses continues to be unresolved because the statistical and systematic variations inherently associated with the zero dose effect make it impossible to measure a significant increase in the effect at very low doses.

This problem is unavoidable in experimental radiation biology (Pohl-Ruhling et al. 1983, 1986; Lloyd et al. 1988, 1992; Mill et al. 1998) as well as in epidemiology (Brenner et al. 2003). In a multi-laboratory exercise, the lowest dose at which a significant effect of radiation on the induction of dicentric chromosome aberrations in human lymphocytes could be measured was 20 mGy (Lloyd et al. 1992). The lowest dose at which a statistically significant excess of cancer can be detected in the atomic bomb survivors has been estimated to be 50 mSv (Pierce et al. 1996) although others have claimed that the value should be 200 mSv (Heidenreich et al. 1997a, b; Pierce and Preston 1997). The data on the occurrence of leukaemia in children following prenatal exposure to diagnostic X-rays indicates a risk from accumulated doses of a few tens of millisieverts (Stewart et al. 1956, 1958; Bithell and Stiller 1988; Doll and Darby 1991; Wakeford et al. 1997). Other epidemiological data on chronically exposed nuclear workers (Muirhead et al. 1999; Cardis et al. 2005) while being interpreted in terms of a linear dose-effect relationship and showing general agreement with the ICRP risk estimate within the statistical limits of the studies (Wakeford 2005) illustrate the problem of detecting statistically significant effects at low dose and the difficulties of defining the shape of the dose-effect relationship at low doses. This can be seen in Fig. 1 where the data reveal that there is no statistically significant radiation effect in the range of dose from 0 to 100 mSv which is of greatest relevance to computed tomography.

## 1.4 The Way Forward

The unavoidable conclusion is that it will never be possible to determine the real shape of the dose–effect relationship at the low doses relevant to radiological protection and computed tomography using experimental and epidemiological studies. It is clear that the only way that progress will be made to define the real shape of the dose-effect relationship is by understanding the mechanism of radiation action at the

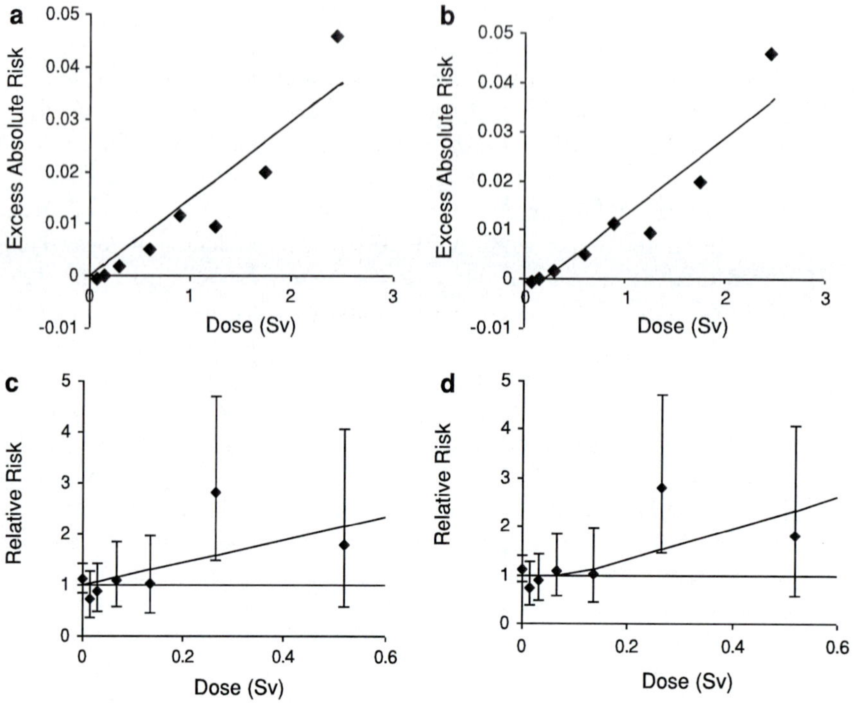


**Fig. 1** Two examples illustrating the difficulty of determining the shape of the dose-effect relationship at low doses. The upper graphs (**a, b**) present the atomic bomb survivor data (Pierce et al. 1996) with a straight line from the origin through the data (**a**) and a straight line from a threshold dose through the data (**b**). The lower graphs (**c, d**) present similar extrapolations through data for the UK nuclear workers (Muirhead et al. 1999)

molecular level and developing a credible model approach which provides a coherent interpretation of the higher dose, statistically significant, experimental and epidemiological data (Brenner et al. 2003; Chadwick et al. 2003). The model must take account of the biophysics of radiation action, induction and repair of molecular damage, occurrence of effects at the cellular level and the influence of cellular effects on the development of cancer.

In the following sections we present the outline of a model which can be used to derive the pathway from radiation-induced molecular damage to radiation-induced cancer and we provide evidence supporting the various links in the chain required to complete the pathway. The model is based on a mechanism of radiation action at the molecular level that results in different cellular end-points and provides a quantifiable description of the dose response for a variety of radiation effects.

## 1.5 Model Development

The pathway from radiation energy deposition through cellular effects to the induction of cancer is described here in two parts. The first part describes a model which provides an explanation of the cellular effects of radiation in terms of a basic lesion and mathematical expressions for the dose-effect relationships. The second part incorporates the cellular effects model into a biologically based cancer model in order to derive the implications that the pathway has for radiation risk at low doses.

The cellular effects model is presented in a series of stages which closely follow its historical development starting from the fitting of dose-effect relationships for cell killing, through the choice of lesion with all its implications, to the inter-relationship of different cellular end-points. The features of the cancer model are discussed in a qualitative way to show how the incorporation of the cellular model can be envisaged and to derive some important conclusions for radiological protection.

We have been using and developing the cellular model for 30 years and have benefitted from the insight into radiation biological effects that the model has given us. All models represent a simplification of reality and the one presented here is but one of many although we are not aware of another radiobiological model which is as far-reaching and comprehensive. We commend it for its straight-forward simplicity but warn that, in some aspects, it contradicts some current radiobiological dogma. It provides a logical explanation of experimental and epidemiological findings and, although the model is supported by fits to cellular and cancer data, it is not yet proven.

## 1.6 Dose-Effect Relationships

The development of the model started when we noticed that different cell survival curves could all be very closely fitted using a linear-quadratic dose-effect relationship of the type:

$$S = \exp[-p(\alpha D + \beta D^2)] \qquad (1)$$

where $S$ is cell survival, $D$ is radiation dose and p$\alpha$ and p$\beta$ are values derived from fitting the data (Chadwick and Leenhouts 1973).

Sinclair (1966) had already found that the linear-quadratic relationship gave the best fit by analysing cell survival data using various possible mathematical functions although he did not have a mechanistic interpretation for the equation. Later Gillespie et al. (1975a, b) showed, in a series of elegant experiments, that the linear-quadratic function fitted cell survival as well as could be statistically expected and Skarsgard et al. (1993) showed, in equally elegant experiments, that the survival of synchronised cells was accurately described by the equation down to low doses.

The equation suggests that cell killing is a result of "things" induced in a single radiation event (p$\alpha$D) and "things" arising from a combination of two radiation events (p$\beta$D$^2$). Our analysis of several sets of cell survival data revealed consistent results and indicated that the equation could provide straightforward explanations for known radiation biological phenomena, such as dose-rate and fractionation effects and radiation quality effects, in terms of changes in the values of the curve fitting coefficients p$\alpha$ and p$\beta$. For example, decreasing the dose-rate of exposure leads to a sparing effect and increased cell survival and this is expressed in the linear-quadratic equation by a decrease in the quadratic coefficient ($p\beta$), which goes to zero at very low dose rates, while the linear coefficient ($p\alpha$) does not change (Wells and Bedford 1983; Metting et al. 1985). This effect is often referred to as the repair of sub-lethal damage.

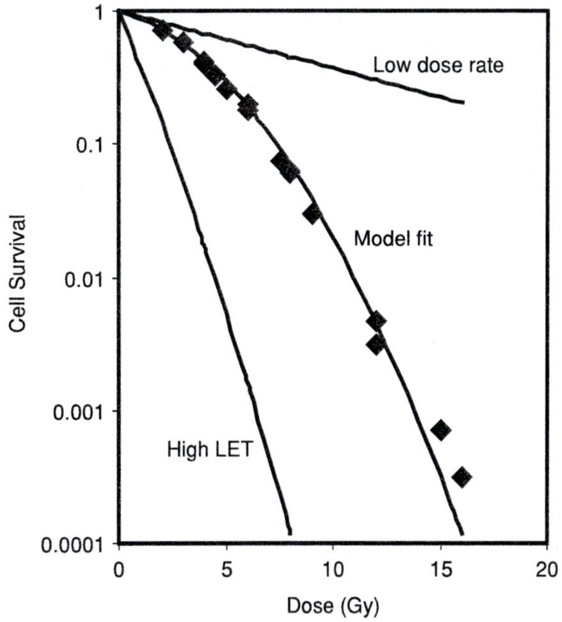


**Fig. 2** An example of the fitting of the linear-quadratic dose-effect Eq. 3 to the survival of stationary CHO cells after acute gamma ray exposure ($\alpha = 0.0992$ Gy$^{-1}$; $\beta = 0.0291$ Gy$^{-2}$). The figure also shows the expected low dose-rate curve when $\beta = 0$ and a typical survival curve after exposure to densely ionising radiation with $\alpha = 0.9$ Gy$^{-1}$; $\beta = 0.029$ Gy$^{-2}$

Another example is the effect of radiation quality which is revealed in a change in the value of the (p$\alpha$) coefficient. In general, (p$\alpha$) increases as the radiation becomes more densely ionising. Alpha particles, for example, which are more densely ionising than gamma radiation, induce a virtually linear survival curve because (p$\alpha$) dominates and is substantially larger than the (p$\alpha$) found following gamma radiation (Barendsen 1964; Todd 1967) (see Fig. 2).

An additional indication of the consistency of the curve fitting was revealed by the analysis of the survival of cells synchronised in different phases of the cell cycle. This showed that the linear-quadratic equation fitted all the different survival curves and, in addition, it was found that the linear and quadratic coefficients varied through the cell cycle in a typical way independent of the type or strain of cell line examined (Chadwick and Leenhouts 1975).

The linear-quadratic equation for cell killing is a first suggestion of the shape of dose-effects at low doses. It is important to note that the quadratic term only starts to influence the response at acutely delivered doses above about 2 Gy and that the linear term, which is dependent on radiation quality but not on dose-rate, is the term defining cell killing at very low doses.

Although comparable effects of dose-rate and radiation quality were known for other end-points, such as the induction of chromosomal aberrations and somatic mutations, and the dose-effect relationship for these end-points had been found to be linear-quadratic, it was only when we decided on the nature of the radiation-induced "thing" responsible for cell killing that we found real insight into radiation effects and a whole panoply of explanations offered themselves.

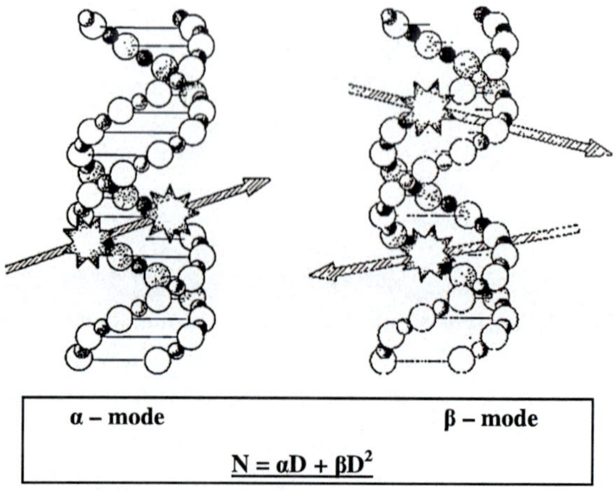


**Fig. 3** A schematic representation of the possible modes of radiation action for the induction of DNA double strand breaks. In the $\alpha$-mode, a single particle track causes two spatially and temporally correlated ionisation events close to the two strands of the DNA helix. In the $\beta$-mode, two separate particle tracks each induce a single strand break in the two strands of the DNA helix. $N$ represents the number of DNA double strand breaks induced by a dose ($D$) of radiation

## 1.7 The Choice of Lesion–DNA Double Strand Breaks

There are several reasons why a DNA double strand break is a suitable choice for the crucial radiation-induced lesion.

- The DNA helix is a large, important, structured target molecule in the nucleus of the cell.
- Cells which are deficient in the repair of double strand breaks are very sensitive to ionising radiation.
- In the unineme concept of chromosome structure, where the chromosome backbone is a single DNA helix, a double strand break is the same as a chromosome break.
- Permanent damage to DNA can cause mutations.
- The error free repair of single strand breaks can be ascribed to sub-lethal damage repair to explain dose-rate and fractionation effects.
- The repair of double strand breaks, which is unlikely to be completely error free, can be ascribed to potentially lethal damage repair to explain changes in survival that occur on post-irradiation storage of non-cycling cells.
- The interaction of radiation with the two strands of the DNA helix offers an explanation for the increased effectiveness of densely ionising radiation.

### 1.7.1 Modes of Radiation Action

The DNA helix can, at least hypothetically, be disrupted in two modes of radiation action as is illustrated in Fig. 3.

The two strands of the helix can be broken in the passage of a single ionising particle if two energy depositions, closely associated in time and space, occur along the particle track close to, or on, the two strands. A double strand break also results if two independent ionising particles induce single strand breaks in each strand of the helix. This leads to the equation for the number ($N$) of DNA double strand breaks induced by a dose ($D$) of radiation as:

$$N = (\alpha D + \beta D^2) \tag{2}$$

so that if $f_p$ is the proportion of unrestituted double strand breaks and if $p_0$ is the probability for an unrestituted double strand break to cause cell killing, then cell survival ($S$) is given by:

$$S = \exp[-pN] = \exp\left[-p(\alpha D + \beta D^2)\right] \tag{3}$$

where $p = p_0 f_p$.

In fuller derivations of this equation (Chadwick and Leenhouts 1973, 1981) the $\alpha$ and $\beta$ coefficients are made up of several parameters which take the effects of radiation quality and repair into account. A parameter ($f_1$) is included in the $\beta$-coefficient to take account of the repair of single strand breaks so that $f_1 = 1$ for acute exposure but decreases to $f_1 = 0$

for chronic exposure where $\beta$ becomes zero. This essentially reflects the probability that a single strand break can be repaired during exposure before a second single strand break converts it to a double strand break and provides a mechanistic explanation for the dose-rate effect and fractionation.

A consideration of the α-mode of double strand break induction should, intuitively, lead to the understanding that more densely ionising particle tracks have a higher probability of causing two energy deposition events close to the two strands of the helix than sparsely ionising particle tracks and should, therefore, be more effective per unit dose. This provides a mechanistic understanding for the effect of radiation quality.

The association of the double strand break with cell killing, chromosome arm breakage and mutations and the knowledge that similar effects of dose-rate and radiation quality had been found in aberration and mutation studies (Lloyd et al. 1984; Iliakis 1984; Vivek Kumar et al. 2006; Leenhouts and Chadwick 1990; Lloyd et al. 1976; Goodhead et al. 1979; Albertini et al. 1997) led us to propose that each of the three cellular end-points derive from the same type of molecular damage, namely, DNA double strand breaks. In this case, the yield of chromosomal aberrations ($Y$) can be described by the equation:

$$Y = cN = c(\alpha D + \beta D^2) \quad (4)$$

where c relates induced double strand breaks to chromosomal aberrations and the mutation frequency per surviving cell ($M$) can be described (to a first approximation) by the equation:

$$M = qN = q(\alpha D + \beta D^2) \quad (5)$$

where $q$ relates induced double strand breaks to mutations. The full equation is given by:

$$M = \{1 - \exp[-q(\alpha D + \beta D^2)]\} \quad (6)$$

and this leads to the equation for mutation frequency per irradiated cell ($M_s$), which is the case for human, animal or organism exposure, as:

$$M_s = \mathrm{M} * \mathrm{S} = \{1 - \exp[-\mathrm{q}(\alpha \mathrm{D} + \beta \mathrm{D}^2)]\} \times \{exp[-\mathrm{p}(\alpha \mathrm{D} + \beta \mathrm{D}^2)]\} \quad (7)$$

This equation is initially linear-quadratic but at increasing doses it flattens to a peak and decreases at higher doses where cell killing starts to dominate. It expresses the fact that a mutated cell must survive to express the mutation.

### 1.7.2 Correlations

Comparison of Eqs. 4 and 5 with Eq. 3 leads to the equations which correlate cell killing with the yield of chromosomal aberrations:

$$\ln S = -(\mathrm{p/c})\mathrm{Y} \quad (8)$$

and cell killing with mutation frequency:

$$\ln S = -(\mathrm{p/q})\mathrm{M} \quad (9)$$

Equations 8 and 9 predict that the logarithm of cell survival should correlate as a linear function of chromosomal aberration yield or mutation frequency when the end-points are measured in the same experiment irrespective of the non-linear shape of the dose-effect relationships. Several examples of these correlations have been measured (Dewey et al. 1970, 1971a, b, 1978; Bhambhani et al. 1973; Franken et al. 1999; Richold and Holt 1974; Thacker and Cox 1975; Thacker et al. 1977; Rao and Hopwood 1982; Iliakis 1984). Examples of these correlations are presented in Figs. 4 and 5.

In accordance with the model, our interpretation of these correlations is not that aberrations or mutations cause cell killing but that each end-point arises from the same type of molecular lesion, the DNA double strand break. In this respect Eq. 3 predicts that the logarithm of cell survival should be linearly related to the number (N) of DNA double strand breaks measured in the same experiment irrespective of the nonlinear shape of the dose-effect relationships. The development of sensitive neutral filter elution techniques to measure DNA double strand breaks in the 1980 s enabled these correlations to be measured (Radford 1985, 1986; Prise et al. 1987; Murray et al. 1989, 1990). An example of this correlation is presented in Fig. 6.

These correlations create a linkage chain between DNA double strand breaks and all three cellular end-points, survival, chromosome aberrations and mutations.

There is one further implied correlation arising from Eq. 7 because, when the type of lesion leading

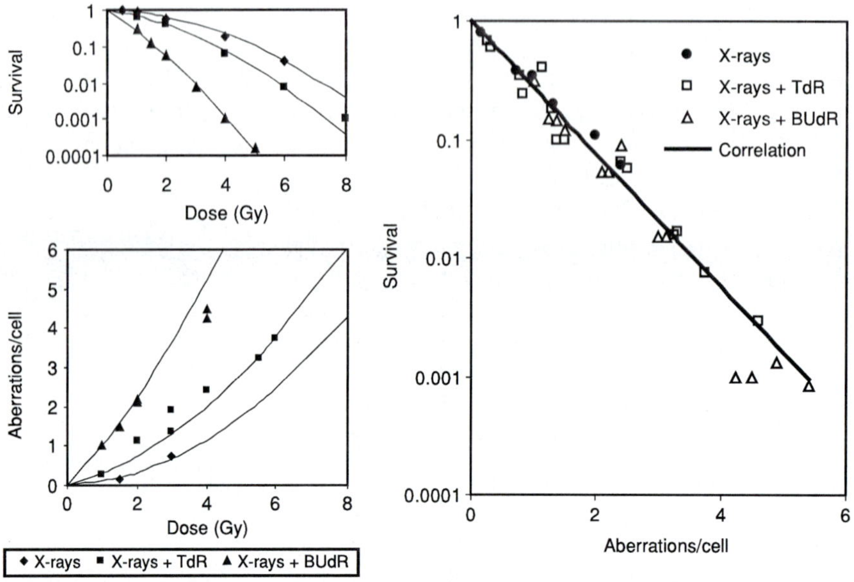


**Fig. 4** The correlation between the induction of chromosomal aberrations and cell survival in accordance with Eq. 8 predicted by the model. The data are taken from Dewey et al. (1970, 1971a, b). The correlation shows data from nine different nonlinear survival and aberration yield dose-effect curves of which three are shown in the graphs on the *left* of the figure

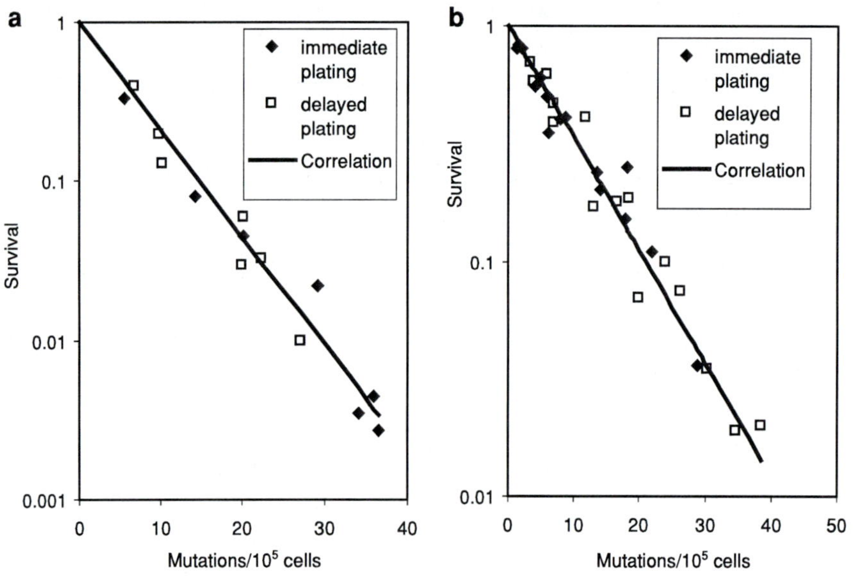


**Fig. 5** Two examples of the correlation between mutation frequency and cell survival in accordance with Eq. 9 predicted by the model. The data are taken from Rao and Hopwood (1982) (**a**) and Iliakis (1984) (**b**)

to mutation is the same as the type of lesion leading to cell killing, then the peak height of the equation depends only on the values of $p$ and $q$ and is independent of the radiation dose kinetics. This feature is revealed in Fig. 7 for the induction of pink mutations in the stamen hairs of Tradescantia. This implied correlation is important as it leads to the association of a somatic mutation and radiation-induced cancer, as will be shown later.

### 1.7.3 Implications for Low Dose Effects

The association of cell killing, chromosomal aberrations and mutations with DNA double strand breaks permits an understanding of the shape of the dose-effect relationships for these end-points down to very low doses. This is not achieved by extrapolating the data to lower and lower doses but by considering the modes of radiation action in the production of double strand breaks. At low doses the α- mode (see Fig. 3) is

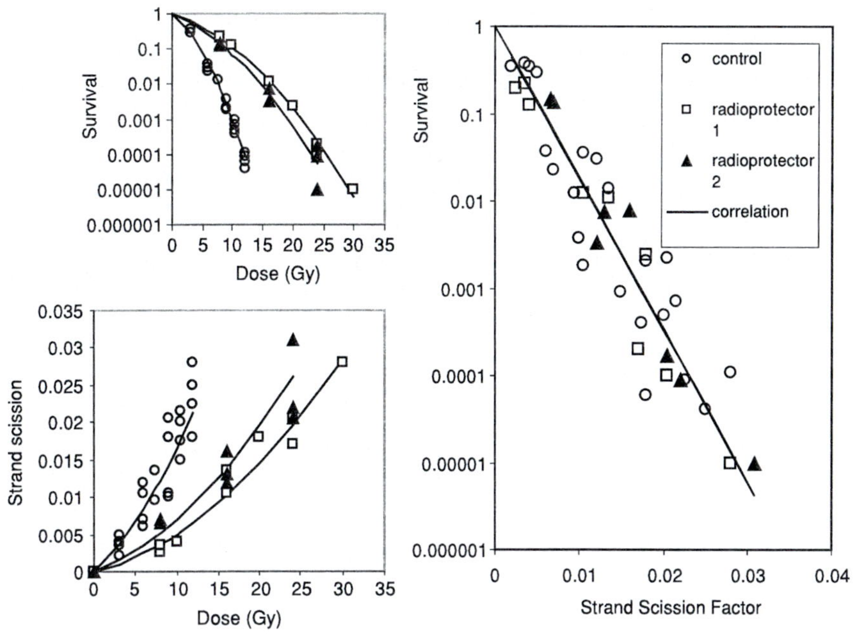


**Fig. 6** An example of the correlation between the induction of DNA double strand breaks and cell survival in accordance with Eq. 3 predicted by the model. The data are taken from Murray et al. (1989)

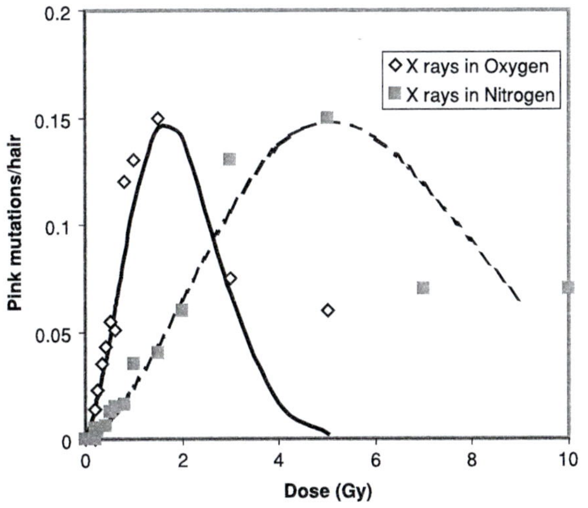


**Fig. 7** The induction of mutations in the stamen hairs of Tradescantia after exposure in oxygen or nitrogen to gamma rays revealing the same peak height in each case. The curves are fitted by eye using Eq. 7. Data from Underbrink et al. 1975)

obviously dominant, even for acute exposure, and the biophysics of radiation energy deposition suggests that two energy depositions close to, or on, each of the DNA strands in one radiation track is needed to cause the double strand break (Brenner and Ward 1992; Nikjoo et al. 1994, 1999; Friedland et al. 1998, 1999). This has been confirmed by experiments which have shown the role of pairs of hydroxyl radicals in the induction of DNA double strand breaks (Prise et al. 1993, 1999; Milligan et al. 1995, 2000). The three-dimensional molecular structure and the 2 nm distance between the two strands of the DNA helix impose the requirement that a single radiation track must have energy deposition events occurring every couple of nanometres along its path in order to induce a double strand break. It is not difficult to understand that the densely ionising tracks produced by α-particles, for example, will have the required ionisation clustering to cause double strand breaks efficiently. Although it is less intuitive, sparsely ionising radiation, such as X-rays, which lose energy by electron scattering, produce electron tracks with a sufficiently high ionisation clustering, especially at the track ends, to induce double strand breaks. Indeed, Goodhead et al. (1979); (Thacker et al. 1986) have shown that 0.3 keV carbon ultrasoft X-rays creating electron tracks of only 7 nm in length have a high efficiency for inducing cell killing, aberrations and mutations. These results put an upper limit on the size of the "target" for the effects and also suggest that each of the cellular end-points arises from the same type of damage.

The important conclusion from this is that all types of ionising radiation from the very sparsely ionising high-energy gamma rays to the most densely ionising energetic heavy particles are able to induce DNA double strand breaks in a single radiation track. And this means that the dose-effect relationship for DNA double strand breaks and for the three cellular endpoints must be linear at low doses from zero dose up. So the risk for hereditary mutations deriving from cellular effects in germ cells must also be linear at low doses from zero dose up.

An important corollary from this is that the low dose effectiveness of different sparsely ionising radiations, in terms of the α-coefficient, will not be the same. This arises because, although gamma rays and X-rays lose energy by electron scattering it is the less energetic electrons at the end of the tracks which have the required, nanometer, clustering of energy deposition events to be effective at inducing the double strand break. Lower energy or softer X-rays deposit a larger proportion of dose in the form of the track end electrons than more energetic gamma rays and X-rays and are therefore more biologically damaging or effective. Thus, we may anticipate that the relative biological effectiveness (RBE) or Radiation Weighting Factor of soft X-rays such as are used in mammography, will be larger than for energetic gamma rays and hard X-rays. There are good experimental data sets (Heyes et al. 2006, 2009; Heyes and Mill 2004; Frankenberg et al. 2002) which suggest that mammography X-rays are possibly four times more biologically damaging per unit dose than conventional 250 kVp X-rays.

The idea that softer X-rays will be more biologically damaging, and thus have a larger radiation risk, than hard X-rays at low doses might appear to be counter intuitive but could have important repercussions on the choice of the optimum X-ray spectra for different imaging procedures in medical radiology.

It should, however, be remembered that for practical radiological protection purposes the ICRP continues to recommend a Radiation Weighting Factor of 1 for all sparsely ionising radiations.

### 1.7.4 The Formation of Chromosomal Aberrations

One major problem which arose in the development of the model was the clash that it created with the Classical and Exchange Theories for the formation of chromosomal aberration(Sax 1940; Lea and Catcheside 1942; Lea 1946; Revell 1963, 1974). Briefly, both of these theories generate linear-quadratic equations for the yield of aberrations. The Classical Theory assumes that radiation induces chromosome arm breaks in proportion with dose so that exchange aberrations, requiring two breaks, have a linear-quadratic yield with dose while deletions are linear with dose. The Exchange Theory assumes that primary events, not breaks, in chromosome arms are induced in proportion with dose and that two primary events interact to produce both exchange aberrations and deletions.

The major difference between the Classical and Exchange Theories and the model presented here is that we propose that the chromosome arm break, which is a DNA double strand break, is induced by radiation with linear-quadratic dose kinetics. Thus, while our model predicts linear-quadratic dose-effect relationships for all types of chromosomal aberrations, except complex aberrations, we are left to explain the origin of the second break which is so clearly evident in exchange aberrations, such as dicentrics or reciprocal exchanges.

The explanation that we have proposed derives from the work of Resnick (1976) who devised a model for the repair of DNA double strand breaks via a recombinational exchange process. In this process, the broken DNA helix pairs with a homologous undamaged DNA helix, DNA strands are exchanged which allows copying of the homologous DNA at the site of the break, a Holliday junction is formed which can be resolved to give either perfect repair or misrepair involving the reciprocal exchange of DNA strands (see Fig. 8). In terms of the unineme concept of chromosome structure, the reciprocal exchange of DNA strands represents the reciprocal exchange of chromosome arms (see Fig. 8). In other words, the second break, so clearly visible in exchange chromosome aberrations, is not radiation-induced but arises as a consequence of the repair of the radiation-induced double strand break.

We expanded on the proposals of Resnick by suggesting that complete homology between the broken and unbroken helixes might not be needed and that the recombination repair process would also occur in regions of short-range homology on either side of the double strand break. In this case, the short-range homologous association at the break can be developed between the broken DNA and the undamaged DNA from any other chromosome, not just the homologous chromosome. The large proportion of repetitive and closely homologous DNA sequences in

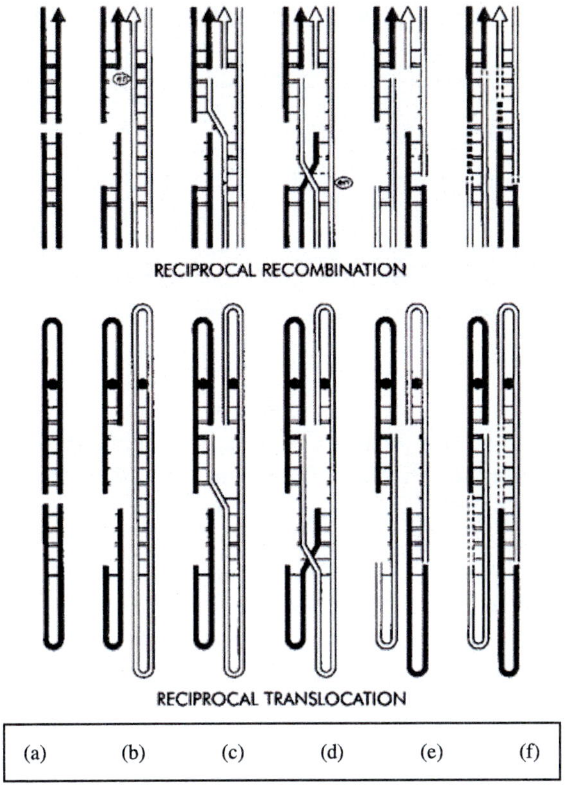


**Fig. 8** A schematic representation of how homologous recombinational repair of a DNA double strand break can lead to the formation of a chromosomal aberration. The upper part of the drawing presents the repair of the DNA while the lower part presents the same repair at the level of the chromosome. The broken ends of the helix (**a**) are trimmed by endonuclease and an undamaged stretch of homologous DNA aligns with the break (**b**). Strand exchange (**c**) leads to the formation of a Holliday junction (**d**) which can be resolved to give either perfect repair (not shown) or the complete exchange of the DNA helices (**e**) and (**f**). The misrepair of the DNA double strand break leads to the exchange of chromosome arms and the formation of exchange aberrations. A reciprocal translocation is illustrated

eukaryotic chromosomes provides a multitude of regions on all the chromosomes for the short-range, homologous association to occur. This, in turn, means that the recombinational repair of a radiation-induced DNA double strand break can lead to the exchange of chromosome arms between different chromosomes as well as regions on the same chromosome with the result that all the different chromosomal aberration configurations can be derived in this way (Chadwick and Leenhouts 1978, 1981).

Our proposals for the formation of chromosome aberrations from one radiation- induced chromosome arm break were in contradiction with the accepted conventional cytological wisdom and there were no experimental data which could be interpreted to resolve this contradiction. There are now some experiments which appear to suggest that we may be right.

The experiments of Goodhead and his colleagues using the ultrasoft X-rays with radiation tracks of only a few nanometers were expected to induce chromosome aberration with an almost completely quadratic dose-effect relationship according to traditional cytological theory. Such short tracks were not expected to break more than one chromosome arm so that there would be no alpha-mode of radiation action. In fact, several workers (Virsik et al. 1980; Goodhead et al. 1980; Thacker et al. 1986; Simpson and Savage 1996; Griffin et al. 1996, 1998) found that the ultrasoft X-rays with tracks as short as 7 nm induced chromosomal aberrations efficiently with a yield that was closely linear with dose i.e. a strong alpha-mode of radiation action.

Another piece of evidence in favour of the model comes from the experiments of Aten and his colleagues (Ludwików et al. 2002) who were able to induce double strand breaks in one chromosome and show that exchange chromosome aberrations were formed between the damaged chromosome and other undamaged chromosomes in the cells. The double strand breaks could be induced in only one chromosome because it was unusually late replicating so that, by adding iodine-125 labelled iodo-deoxyuridine (IUdR) to the medium after the other chromosomes had replicated, only the late replicating chromosome carried the iodine-125 which emits very short-range Auger-electrons. This experiment provides an extremely clear indication of the formation of exchange aberrations by the interaction of the damaged chromosome with the other undamaged chromosomes.

Further support for the interaction of damaged and undamaged chromosomes to create exchange aberrations comes from experiments studying aberrations formed after the fusion of irradiated and un-irradiated cells. The first experiment of this type appeared not to show interaction between the irradiated and unirradiated chromosomes (Cornforth 1990) but more recent work contradicts this (Darroudi et al. 2001).

In addition, the molecular biology, biochemistry and genetics of DNA double strand break repair has advanced considerably in recent years and a gene

(*RAD54*) controlling homologous recombinational repair (HR) in mammalian cells has been identified and cells deficient in this repair process are sensitive to ionising radiation (Essers et al. 1997).

We remain confident that the problem of the mechanisms involved in the formation of chromosomal aberrations will be resolved in the near future.

### 1.7.5 The $\beta$-mode of Radiation Action

Another problem which has dogged the development of the model is the $\beta$-mode of radiation action where the model proposes that two independently induced DNA single strand breaks can combine to produce a double strand break. It is a particularly attractive process because it is known that the repair of single strand breaks is correct, thus error free, and because the repair process explains very straight forwardly the dose-rate and fractionation effects which also appear to be error free.

The problem arises because calculations based purely on the physics of energy deposition predict that two, independently induced, single strand breaks will only occur close enough together to produce a double strand break at much larger doses than those at which the quadratic component of dose-effect relationships becomes apparent. We assume that what happens in the cell is not just physics but that chemistry and biology must also be involved and we believe that there are certain extenuating circumstances which need to be taken into account but we acknowledge that our arguments are more conjectural than established.

The first point to be made is that the $\beta$-coefficient measured for cell survival in synchronous cells is maximum at the start of the S-phase when the DNA starts to replicate and is at a minimum, often close to zero, in the $G_2$-phase and in mitosis. In other words, when the DNA and chromosomes are tightly bound in mitosis the cell may be behaving more or less in accordance with the physics. However, there are indications that the DNA 'relaxes' and unwinds as it enters replication and it might even form regions or 'microbubbles' of single stranded DNA (Gaudette and Benbow 1986; Benbow et al. 1985; Chadwick and Leenhouts 1994). These extended regions of single stranded DNA would increase the distance along DNA over which two single strand breaks could combine to form a double strand break.

In addition, it has been shown that the sensitivity of DNA to hydroxyl attack increases by some 100-fold as the proteins surrounding cellular DNA are stripped away (Ljungman 1991; Ljungman et al. 1991; Nygren et al. 1995). If a first single strand break led to an uncoiling of the DNA helix, as a result of the relaxation of the strain normally experienced by the helix, and the DNA spiralled away from the histones, which coil it into the chromosomes, this region of single stranded DNA might be more susceptible to the induction of a second single strand break by hydroxyl radical attack.

We have also made calculations which show that, in the $\alpha$-mode the two breaks are induced by radicals induced within about 0.5 nm of the helix. In the $\beta$-mode, if the first single strand break is caused by hydroxyl radical attack from within about 0.5 nm of the helix, then the second independently induced break would need to be caused by radical attack from within about 5 nm of the second strand to comply with the values found for the $\beta$-coefficient in radiation biology (Leenhouts and Chadwick 1976; Chadwick and Leenhouts 1981). The radical scavenging experiments of Chapman et al. (1975) support our conclusion that the radiation chemistry of the $\alpha$-mode and $\beta$-mode should be different.

One other completely different piece of evidence which, we think, supports our ideas on the combination of two single strand breaks to form a double strand break comes from the fact that we were able to extend our model to describe the cell- killing effects of UV light as well as cytotoxic chemicals (Chadwick and Leenhouts 1983; Leenhouts and Chadwick 1984). A photon of UV light cannot interact with both strands of the DNA helix but can induce a pyrimidine dimer on one strand. Mono-functional cytotoxic chemicals only interact with a single strand of the DNA. In both cases, the extension of our model predicted a purely quadratic cell survival curve, i.e. no $\alpha$-mode action, in good agreement with experimental data. We were also able to derive a mathematical expression to describe the synergistic interaction of cytotoxic chemicals or UV light with ionising radiation based on the combination of a radiation-induced single strand break with single strand damage induced by the chemical or UV (Leenhouts and Chadwick 1978).

Thus, although there is no definite proof for our interpretation of the $\beta$-mode of radiation action, there is enough conjectural evidence in support of this interpretation for us to continue with our approach and maintain the implications we derive from it.

### 1.8 Conclusions from the Cellular Model

At this stage we conclude that:

- the linear-quadratic equation provides an accurate description of the dose-effect relationships of cellular end-points,
- the DNA double strand break is the crucial radiation-induced lesion causing each of the end-points,
- the $\alpha$-mode of radiation action is responsible for low dose effects, even after an acute exposure,
- all ionising radiation is capable of inducing a DNA double strand break in the $\alpha$-mode,
- not all DNA double strand breaks will be repaired perfectly,
- the induction of DNA double strand breaks and, consequently, of chromosomal aberrations, mutations and cell killing, will be initially linear with radiation dose from zero dose up.

In other words, cellular end-points, including hereditary mutations, will be induced at low doses in direct proportion with radiation dose, in accordance with the LNT concept.

## 2 Radiation-Induced Cancer

Insight can be gained into the induction of cancer by radiation and the shape of the dose-effect relationship at low doses by incorporating the cellular model into a multi-step model of carcinogenesis. A 'two-mutation step with clonal expansion of intermediate cells' model for cancer was derived by Moolgavkar and Knudson (1981). The cancer model has a firm biological basis because it was developed from conclusions drawn by Knudson from a study of the occurrence of retinoblastoma in children (Knudson 1971, 1985, 1991). The conclusions have been subsequently confirmed by molecular biological analysis.

Evidence that supports the association of a radiation-induced somatic mutation and radiation-induced cancer is found in the many studies of the dose-effect relationships for cancer in animals which reveal the same peak height under different radiation conditions (Chadwick and Leenhouts 2011). The dose-effect relationships increase with dose, flattening to a peak and decreasing at higher doses and can be closely described by an equation with the same form as Eq. 7. The same peak height in cancer incidence implies that the same type of lesion is involved in both the induction of cancer and the cell killing which causes the decrease in cancer at higher doses and cell killing has been correlated with mutations, aberrations and DNA double strand breaks. An example of the same peak height occurring in radiation-induced cancer is presented in Fig. 9.

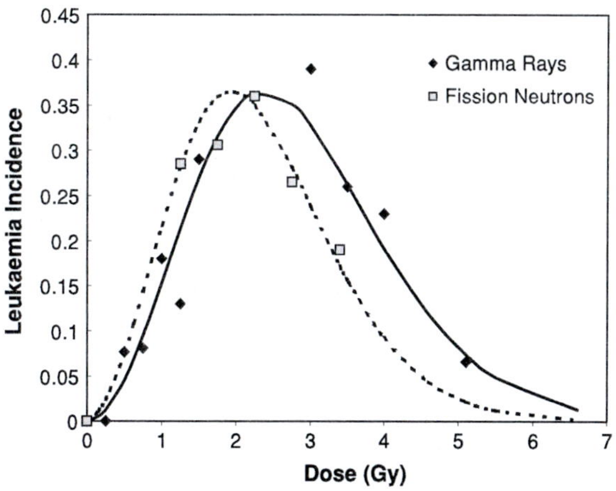


**Fig. 9** The induction of leukaemia in mice after gamma and fast neutron irradiation showing the same peak height. Data from Upton et al. (1964)

### 2.1 A Multi-Step Cancer Model

Figure 10 presents, schematically, a two-mutation model for carcinogenesis.

A population of normal stem cells in an organ is at risk of a mutation ($\mu_1$), 'initiation', to an intermediate state. A cell in the intermediate state can divide and undergo clonal expansion ($\varepsilon$), 'promotion', to form, as time passes, an increasing population of cells at risk of a second mutation ($\mu_2$), 'conversion', that creates a malignant cell. The malignant cell divides, 'progression', and produces a detectable tumour after a certain lag time ($t_0$).

There have been some criticisms levelled at the model because mutational and cytological analyses of tumour cells appear to show more than two-mutational changes but there may be several explanations for this. Firstly, many of these changes might

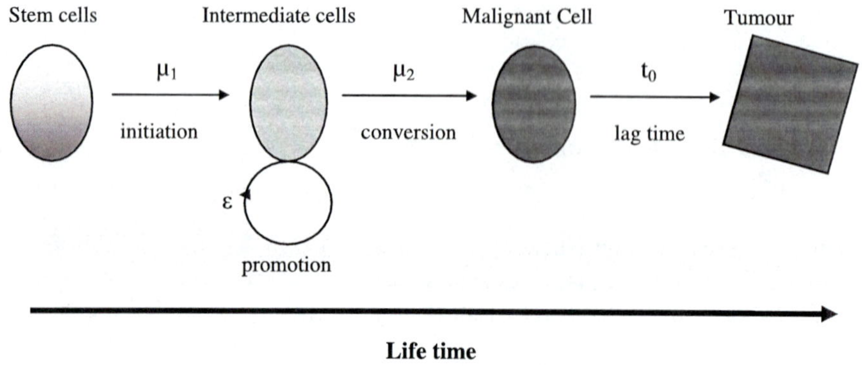


**Fig. 10** A schematic representation of the two-mutation cancer model showing the development from normal stem cells via an intermediate state to the malignant cell which can grow out to form a detectable tumour. The intermediate cell population expands exponentially in time. Note the important role that time plays in the model

occur during the progression of the malignant cells to tumour formation. Then, the recent findings that only certain cells in a tumour are able to divide continuously and act as "cancer stem cells" (Beachy et al. 2004) seem to suggest that not all cells in a tumour will be informative for the malignant process. Alternatively, the two mutations may be rate limiting for the process, i.e. other steps occur quickly and do not affect the mathematics of the model.

We have used a slightly modified version of the Moolgavkar model which allows us to calculate, simultaneously, the age-dependent increase in cancer incidence and the dose-effect relationships and we have been able to apply the modified version of the model to the analysis of animal radiation biological data and epidemiological data from exposed human populations (Leenhouts and Chadwick 1994a, b; Leenhouts 1999; Leenhouts and Brugmans 2000, 2001; Leenhouts et al. 2000).

It is not necessary to go into the complicated mathematics associated with the model but it is useful to form a basic understanding of how the model functions especially because the model has some important implications for the shape of the dose-effect relationship at low doses and for levels of radiation risk.

### 2.1.1 Spontaneous Cancers

Consider first the case of spontaneous cancer which, according to the model, must arise as a consequence of spontaneous mutations ($\mu_{b1}$, $\mu_{b2}$). The probability that one of the normal organ stem cells mutates to an intermediate cell increases proportionally with time as long as the spontaneous mutation rate ($\mu_{b1}$) remains approximately constant. The intermediate cell divides and by population doubling at each division, produces an exponentially increasing population of intermediate cells which are all targets for a second spontaneous mutation ($\mu_{b2}$) to create a malignant cell. Time, a significant part of lifetime, plays a major role in the model and it is important to realise that while the mutation probabilities are proportional with time the cellular expansion of the intermediate cells is exponential in time. The model has been shown to describe the rapidly increasing incidence of several spontaneous cancers at later age (Moolgavkar and Venzon 1979) (see Fig. 11a).

### 2.1.2 Cancers Induced by an Acute Exposure

If we now consider an acute exposure to radiation, the mutations it causes can only be taken into account in the model together with the spontaneous mutations. In this case, there are two possibilities, either the radiation affects the first mutational step, e.g., if the person exposed is young and has none or very few intermediate cells, ($\mu_1 \rightarrow \{\mu_b + f(\mathrm{D})\}_1$) and an intermediate cell derived from a radiation-induced mutation will need a spontaneous mutation ($\mu_{b2}$) to convert it to malignancy (Fig. 11b), or, if the person exposed is older and already has many intermediate cells, radiation is more likely to affect the second mutation ($\mu_2 \rightarrow \{\mu_b + f(\mathrm{D})\}_2$) and convert an intermediate cell deriving from a spontaneous mutation ($\mu_{b1}$) to a malignant state (Fig. 11b). $f(D)$ is a function of dose ($D$), normally linear-quadratic, which represents the contribution of the acute exposure to the mutations in the initiation step or the conversion step, although $f(\mathrm{D})_1$ is not necessarily the same as $f(D)_2$.

In each case, the radiation-induced mutation in one step relies on a spontaneous mutation in the other step to complete the path from a normal to a malignant state and radiation may be seen to be a co-factor in the induction of cancer.

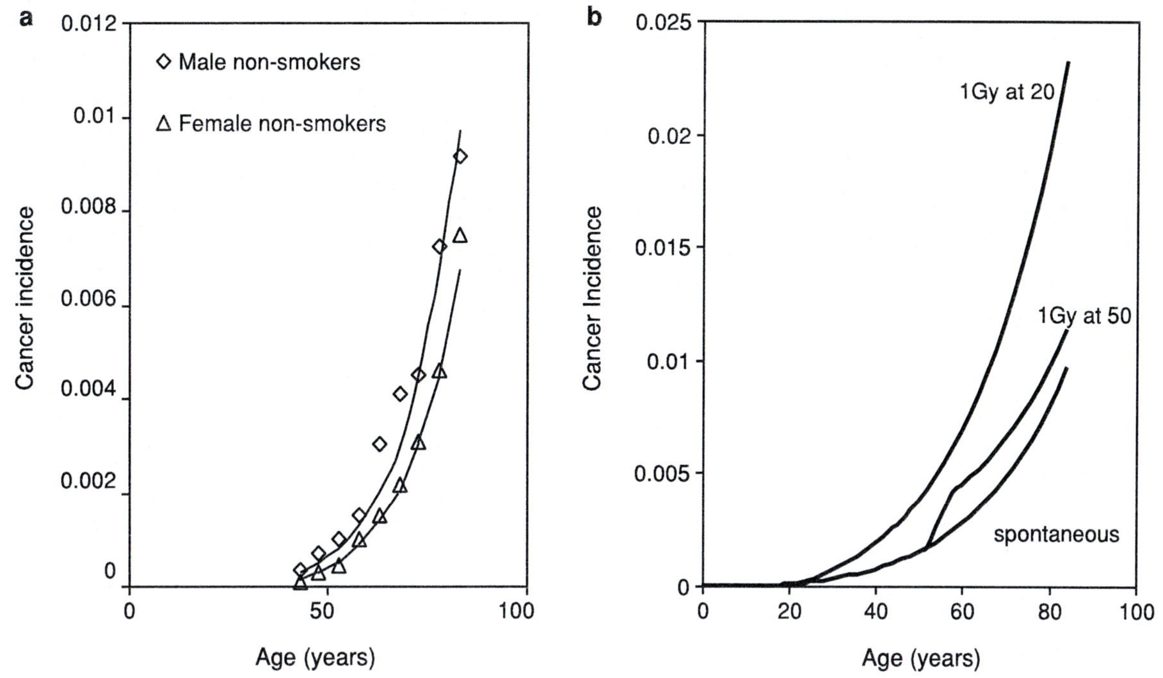


**Fig. 11** **a** The fitting of the model to the occurrence of lung cancers in non-smoking males and females as a function of age (Data from Hammond 1966). The fitting of the model to spontaneous cancers is used to define values for the basic parameters, e.g. $\mu_{b1}$, $\mu_{b2}$, $\varepsilon$, $t_0$. **b** A model simulation showing the effect of 1 Gy at 20 and 50 on the increasing incidence of cancer as a function of age after exposure

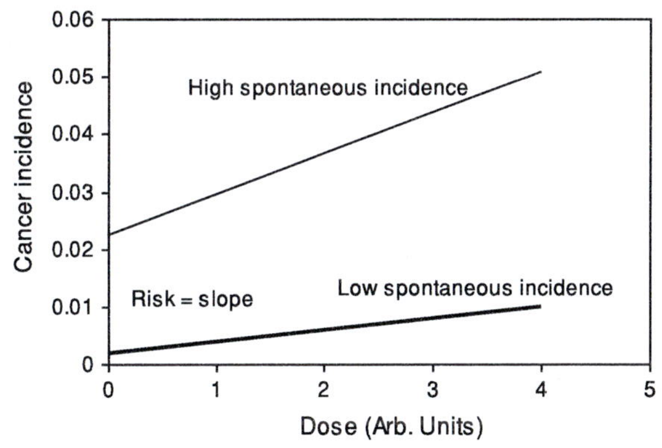


**Fig. 12** A model simulation showing the effect of spontaneous cancer incidence on the radiation risk, the slope of the line, even when the cellular radiation sensitivities are held constant

### 2.1.3 Implications and Consequences

Several important implications derive from the fact that the radiation-induced mutations cannot be treated separately from the spontaneous mutations, namely:

- The spontaneous mutation rates in the stem and intermediate cells define the spontaneous incidence of a specific cancer and, in general, the higher the spontaneous mutation rates the higher the spontaneous incidence of the cancer,
- The effect of radiation is irrevocably inter-woven with the spontaneous mutations and consequently, with the spontaneous cancer incidence,
- The effect of radiation on cancer incidence, i.e. the radiation risk, depends on the level of the spontaneous mutation rates and will be different for different cancers,
- In general, the effect of radiation, or radiation risk, will be greater for cancers with higher specific incidence levels (see Fig. 12),
- The shape of the dose-effect relationship for cancer is defined by the dose-effect relationship for cellular mutation frequency, or aberration yield, so that at low to moderate doses $f(D)$ can be approximated to $f(D) = k(\alpha D + \beta D^2)$ which is linear with dose at very low doses.
- All of this means:
- Each specific cancer will have its own level of radiation risk dependent upon its spontaneous incidence,
- The radiation risk for a specific cancer in populations with different spontaneous incidences of that

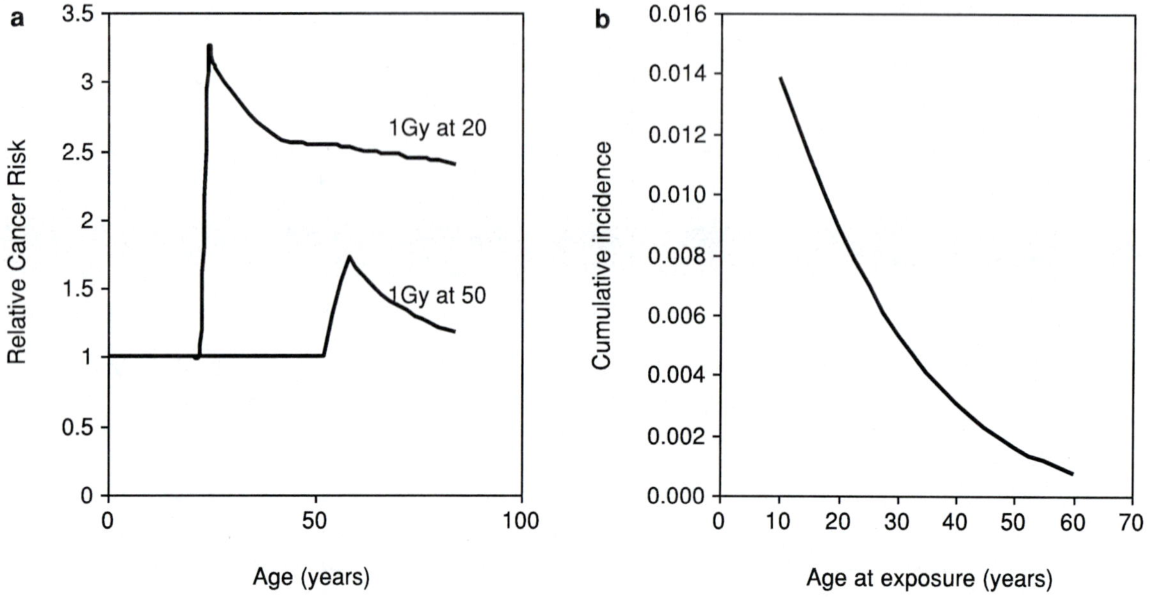


**Fig. 13** **a** A model simulation of the relative cancer risk after exposure at 20 and 50 years of age as a function of time after exposure. **b** A model simulation of the cumulative cancer incidence as a function of age-at-exposure showing an increasing risk following exposure at younger ages

cancer (cf. Japanese atomic bomb survivors with a European population) will not be the same although the model offers a way of extrapolating risk across populations,

- The shape of the dose-effect curve for radiation-induced cancer in animals or man will resemble the shape of the dose-effect curve for cellular mutation and show, at least qualitatively, the same dose-rate and radiation quality effects.
- At very low doses, the shape of the dose-effect curve is linear,
- The slope of the linear dose-effect curve, which defines radiation risk for a specific cancer, is dependent on the cellular sensitivity (k$\alpha$) and the spontaneous mutation rates $\mu_b$.

### 2.1.4 Age-Dependent Risk

Using the modified cancer model to calculate the age-dependent increase in cancer incidence for spontaneous cancers and cancers after exposure at different ages (see Fig. 11) has allowed a simulation of the dependence of risk in adults on age-at-exposure, although the model has not been used to consider the case of babies and infants. Briefly, the pattern of the relative risk, the induced cancer incidence divided by the spontaneous cancer incidence, is similar for an adult acutely exposed at age 20 to that for an adult exposed at age 50 (Fig. 13a). The relative risk increases rapidly after the lag period, peaks and drops gradually over time. At the same exposure level, and using the same cellular radiation sensitivity, the increase is larger following exposure at the younger age but it should be born in mind that the rapid increase in relative risk results because a small induced effect is divided by a very small spontaneous incidence that is much smaller at age 20 than at age 50. Figure 13b presents the cumulative risk as a function of age-at-exposure and reveals that the risk is higher in those exposed at younger ages. This, to some extent, reflects the 'amplification' resulting from a longer period for the exponential clonal expansion of intermediate cells. We think it prudent to assume that the risk in babies and children would be greater than that in young adults although the model has not been used to simulate these risks.

## 2.2 Some Additional Considerations

Some additional points need to be made even though they are of lesser relevance to the dose levels and practices associated with computed tomography.

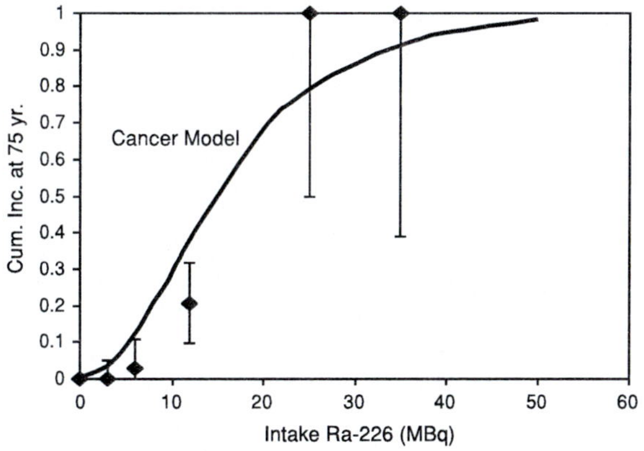


**Fig. 14** The model fitting to the cumulative bone cancer incidence at 75 years in radium dial painters illustrating the strongly curved risk resulting from a combination of the very low spontaneous incidence of bone cancer and the radiation-induced mutations in both steps of the cancer pathway. The incidence has been interpreted as indicating a threshold but the model provides an alternative explanation

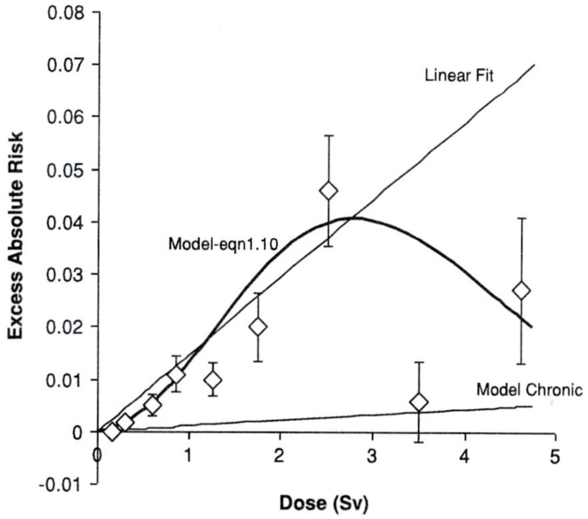


**Fig. 15** An illustration of how a linear-quadratic model (Eq. 10) might be fitted to the data (shown in Fig. 1 but including higher dose data) for the acute exposure of the atomic bomb survivors compared with a linear interpretation. The lower straight line shows the risk that would be predicted by the model for chronic exposure

### 2.2.1 Protracted Exposure

The complementation of a radiation-induced mutation in one step by a spontaneous mutation in the other step, which is rather intuitive for an acute exposure, also applies for the case of an exposure protracted over a major part of lifetime as long as the spontaneous mutation rate is comparable with the radiation-induced mutation rate. One interesting exception to this rule occurs when the spontaneous mutation rates are very low and, consequently, the spontaneous cancer incidence is very low. In this case, a long-term radiation exposure may induce mutations in both steps of the pathway and the radiation risk curve becomes much more quadratic with accumulated dose. An example of this is to be found in the bone cancers occurring in the Radium Dial painters who ingested high levels of the bone seeking alpha-particle emitters radium-226 and radium-228 (Rowland 1994). Primary bone cancer has a very low spontaneous incidence and the bone cancer incidence in the dial painters appears to show a threshold dose type of response (Fig. 14). However, the model offers an explanation based on the induction of both mutations by the alpha-particle radiation and suggests that the incidence is more likely to be closely quadratic. Even so, there will be a very small low dose linear component because the spontaneous bone cancer incidence and thus, the spontaneous mutation rate, is low but not completely zero (Leenhouts and Brugmans 2000).

### 2.2.2 The Role of Cell Killing

At high acute doses the effect of cell killing has to be taken into account because a mutated cell which fails to survive cannot express the mutation. Cellular studies score mutations per surviving cell but, in an organ, the mutations expressed are per irradiated cell. This means that the approximate function $f(\mathrm{D})$, which is accurate enough for low doses, must be modified by a term for survival and:

$$f(D) \rightarrow [1 - \exp(-k(\alpha D + \beta D^2))] \exp(-p(\alpha D + \beta D^2)) \qquad (10)$$

This equation, which is analogous to Eq. 7, is linear-quadratic at lower doses, flattens to a peak and decreases at high doses where cell killing dominates. This is illustrated in Fig. 15 which also shows how the data for leukaemia in the atomic bomb survivors presented in Fig. 1a, but including data at higher doses showing a decreasing risk, might be described by the equation.

The multi-step cancer model incorporating a function equivalent to Eq. 10 offers an alternative analysis of the epidemiological data from the Atom

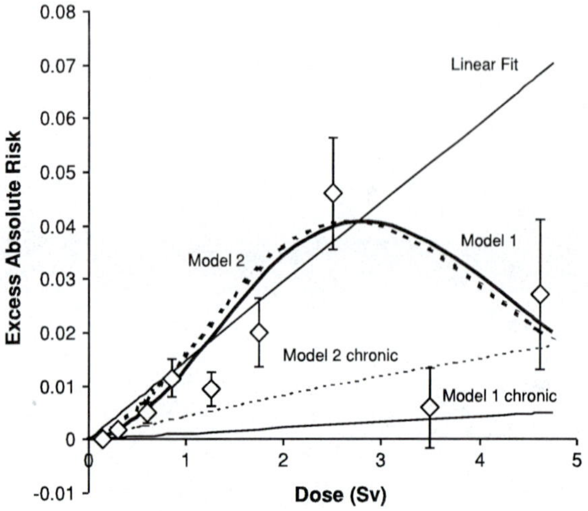


**Fig. 16** Two acute curves drawn using Eq. 10 with the same parameters as shown in Fig. 15 (*Model 1*) but with the α coefficient larger by a factor 4 (*Model 2*). The chronic curves have $\beta = 0$

Bomb survivors to the linear analysis used by ICRP to derive low dose radiation risk. However, further consideration of Fig. 15 reveals that the curve is almost totally dominated by the quadratic component of radiation action and the linear component in the fitting shown is very small as is indicated by the slope of the chronic model curve. This dominant role of the quadratic term is further illustrated by Fig. 16 which shows the same data with two curves drawn through the data which have the same value for the quadratic term but the dotted curve (Model 2) has a linear term which is four times bigger than the solid line curve (Model 1). The difference between the two curves is clearly very small because the linear component plays such an insignificant role and the implication for the determination of low dose risk is that the data from the Atomic bomb survivors is unlikely to give a good determination of the linear component of radiation action irrespective of how it is analysed (Leenhouts and Chadwick 2011). The epidemiological study of chronically exposed populations is needed to reveal low dose radiation risk (cf. Model 1 chronic and Model 2 chronic).

### 2.2.3 Different Mutations to the Same Cancer

The schematic diagram of the multi-step cancer model suggests that there is one mutation ($\mu_{b1}$) which changes an organ stem cell into an intermediate cell and one mutation ($\mu_{b2}$) which changes an intermediate cell into a malignant cell which divides to produce a tumour. This is a simplified way of looking at the cancer process and we are convinced that there are several different mutations which can change an organ stem cell into an intermediate cell and several other different mutations which can change an intermediate cell into a malignant cell, even though the tumours eventually formed are classified pathologically in the same type. However, with different mutagenic pathways leading to the same pathological tumour it is reasonable to expect that the tumours would express different molecular signatures and possibly express different levels of virulence. In spite of these considerations, the model calculations and simulations remain useful as the mutation rates used ($\mu_1$, $\mu_2$) will represent average values for the spectrum of mutations involved in each step of the pathway to a specifically classified tumour.

The situation is different when different types of tumours are considered because the stem cells of one organ, for example, the kidney, need not necessarily have the same radiation sensitivity to cellular mutation as the stem cells of, for example, the brain, and the rate of cell expansion (ε) of the intermediate cells and the lag time ($t_0$) might differ from one organ to the next. This means that, especially in the case of acute exposure when the dose-effect curve is likely to be nonlinear, each type of tumour needs to be analysed individually so that the grouping of all solid tumours arising in the atomic bomb survivors (Pierce et al. 1996) is unlikely to provide much useful information about the dose-effect relationship or radiation risk for radiation-induced cancer. This situation is probably less critical for populations exposed to low acute or to protracted irradiation when the dose-effect curve will be linear.

## 2.3 Conclusions from the Cancer Model

By combining the cellular model of radiation action with the two-mutation model of cancer we can predict the following:

- radiation-induced cancer arises from a radiation-induced somatic mutation,
- the radiation-induced mutation will almost always be complemented by a spontaneous mutation on the

path from a normal to a malignant state, which implies that radiation is a co-factor in the induction of cancer,

- the dose-effect relationship for acute sparsely ionising radiation will increase as a linear-quadratic fuction from zero dose, pass through a maximum and decrease at higher doses,
- the dose-effect relationship at low doses will be linear from zero dose up,
- the risk will vary from one cancer to the other and be related to the spontaneous incidence of the cancer,
- those exposed at a young age will be at a greater risk.

In other words, the radiation-induced cancer will be induced at low doses in direct proportion to the exposure dose from zero dose up.

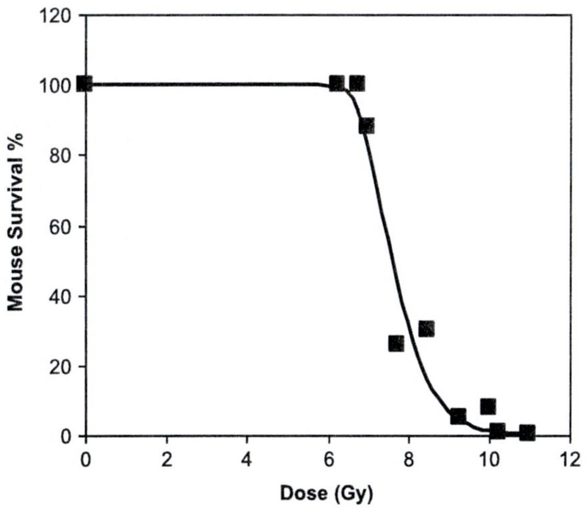


**Fig. 17** A typical dose-effect relationship for a deterministic effect, in this case mouse survival at 30 days after a total body exposure to acute gamma rays. Data from Traynor and Still (1968). The curve is drawn according to Eq. 11

## 3 Deterministic Effects

An acute exposure to substantial doses of radiation leads to observable deleterious biological effects within a relatively short period of time, such as, a few days to some weeks. These deleterious effects, which are called deterministic effects, arise as a result of gross damage to the exposed organ caused by significant cell killing and unlike stochastic radiation effects, such as cancer induction, the severity of deterministic effects increases as the dose increases. If the amount of damage, which is dependent on the magnitude of the dose, does not cause the complete malfunction of the organ, cell renewal over time may lead to recovery and a continued functioning of the organ. Consequently, these effects are not easily studied but in the case of a total body exposure of, for example, a small animal, when death may be the resultant effect, studies have shown that the dose-effect relationship for these deterministic effects exhibits a long threshold, where no effect is apparent, followed by a steep decrease where the severity of the observed effect i.e. the number of animals dying, increases with the increasing dose of radiation. Figure 17 presents a typical example of the dose-effect relationship for a deterministic effect, in this case mouse lethality following a total body exposure to acute gamma rays (Traynor and Still 1968).

In extending our cellular effects model to deterministic effects (Leenhouts and Chadwick 1989) we assume that the majority, if not all, of these effects arise as a consequence of multi-cell killing when a substantial proportion of cells in an organ die so that the surviving stem cells for that organ are unable to repopulate the organ in time to prevent its malfunction. Using this assumption, an equation can be derived for organ survival ($L$):

$$L = 1 - \{1 - \exp[-p(\alpha D + \beta D^2)]\}^n \qquad (11)$$

where $n$ is related to the proportion of the stem cell population needed for organ repopulation such that when an average proportion of less than $1/n$ of the original stem cell population survives, organ function is impaired. For example, if n = 200, the organ fails when less than 0.5% of the stem cells survive.

Figure 18a illustrates organ survival according to Eq. 11 in a direct comparison with Fig. 17 and Fig. 18b presents the same curve together with the equivalent single cell survival curve (Eq. 3) (note the logarithmic scale for both cell and organ survival in Fig. 18b.

The important message that we wish to convey with these figures is that, even when there is apparently no observable deterministic effect in the threshold dose region, there is a considerable amount of cell killing and, consequently, some tissue or organ damage. It is therefore crucial that the radiologist is aware of this cell killing so that any potential deterministic effects are avoided or at least minimised wherever possible in all diagnostic examinations.

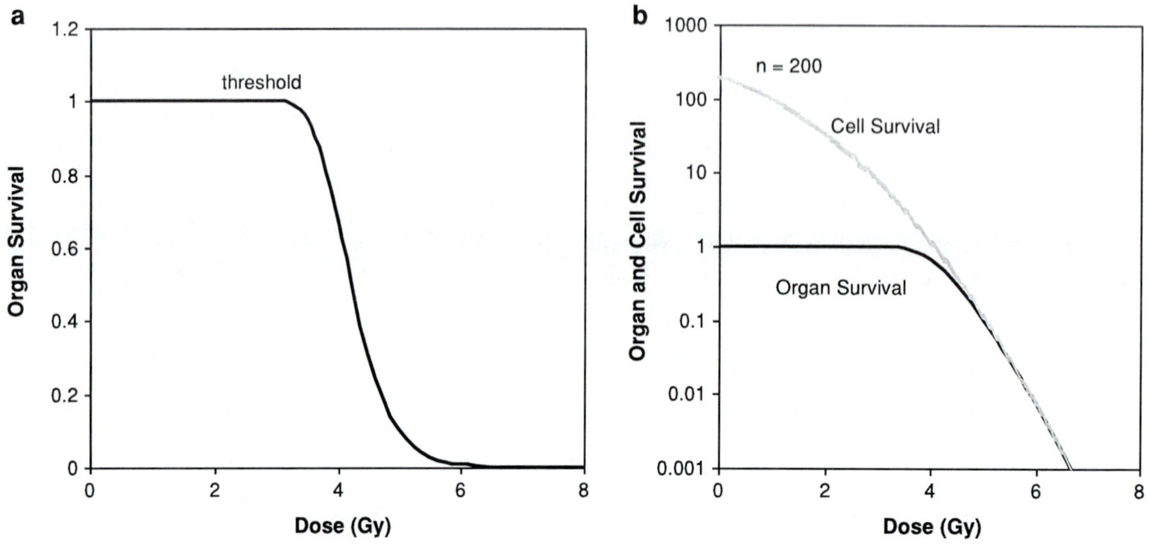


**Fig. 18** a The normal representation of a deterministic dose-effect relationship drawn according to Eq. 11 with $n = 200$ and b the same curve drawn to show the relationship between the deterministic effect, organ survival, (Eq. 11) and single cell survival (Eq. 3) using a logarithmic scale for survival

On the basis of the changes in the alpha and beta coefficients determined in cellular experiments it is possible, using Eq. 11, to make the following predictions about deterministic effects with respect to protraction of exposure and of radiation quality:

- an acute exposure of sparsely ionising radiation will exhibit a shorter (lower) threshold dose than a chronic (over hours or days) exposure,
- densely ionising radiation will exhibit a shorter threshold dose than sparsely ionising radiation.

These predictions are supported by the analysis of experimental data (Leenhouts and Chadwick 1989).

In computer tomography, where exposures are in general acute, the exposure will be localised to the organ being investigated and the nature of any deterministic effect will depend on the exposed organ. Exposure of the bone marrow could eventually lead to signs of anaemia, exposure of the stomach could lead to intestinal disturbance and exposure of the brain could lead to memory problems. For some diagnostic examinations the effects are especially related to exposure of the skin which may be locally exposed to a relatively high dose. In these cases the effects may range from skin erythema to dermal atrophy (Buls and de Mey 2007). It should be realised that even below the threshold dose considerable cell killing and organ or tissue damage may occur dependent on the exposure dose.

## 4 Discussion and Conclusions

We have established a link from a radiation-induced molecular lesion in the nucleus of the cell to the development of cancer. The molecular lesion, the DNA double strand break, is known to be a critical lesion which cannot always be perfectly repaired and which is strongly associated with sensitivity to ionising radiation. The cellular model provides a link from the molecular lesion to chromosomal aberrations, mutations and cell killing and evidence has been presented supporting these links and associations. The biophysics of energy deposition clearly reveals that all forms of ionising radiation are able to induce DNA double strand breaks directly in proportion with radiation dose and that this mode of radiation action will dominate at low doses down to zero dose. This means the dose–effect relationship for cellular effects must be linear at low doses down to zero dose. Biophysics also reveals that the induction of double strand breaks by a single particle traversal of the DNA helix will depend on radiation quality so that different energy X-rays will have different efficiencies for the production of the breaks and the relative effectiveness for sparsely ionising radiation will not always be the same.

The multi-step cancer model allows the radiation biology of cellular effects to be applied to the induction of cancer and suggests that, in general, radiation will only affect one of the mutational steps on the pathway to cancer. Spontaneous mutations, responsible for spontaneous cancers, will be needed to complement the radiation-induced mutation and produce a malignant cell. This means that the dose-effect relationship for the induction of cancer is linear at low doses from zero dose up and that the slope of that straight line, the radiation risk, depends on the spontaneous incidence of the cancer and will be larger for cancers with a high spontaneous incidence. This argument is valid even if more than two-mutational steps are involved in cancer development.

In conclusion, if we accept that the DNA double strand break is the critical radiation-induced lesion which can, ultimately, lead to cancer, we must accept that the dose-effect relationship for radiation-induced cancer, the main radiation risk, is linear with dose from zero dose up because:

- The lowest dose imaginable is a single electron track through one of a population of cells,
- The track has a small positive probability of causing a DNA double strand break in the nucleus of that cell,
- The double strand break has a small positive probability of causing a mutation,
- The mutation has a small positive probability of being involved in a pathway to cancer.

The potential risk of radiation exposures incurred in computed tomography and indeed in all diagnostic radiology is a small increase in the probability of developing cancer which will be in direct proportion with the size of the total accumulated exposure dose.

The arguments presented here are based on a mechanism of radiation action at the level of the DNA in the nucleus of the cell. The conclusions are in accordance with a Linear No-Threshold concept of radiation risk at low acute or protracted exposures although we stress that our approach to the LNT concept is different from that applied by ICRP. The modelling does not provide any value of the slope of the dose effect relationship which quantifies the radiation risk but does imply that it will vary from cancer type to cancer type. Further analysis of epidemiological data using the model is required to obtain quantified estimates of risk.

A LNT concept of radiation risk implies that each increment of dose carries a concomitant increase in radiation risk so the ALARA principle remains valid and the development of improvements in computed tomography which lead to a reduction of the dose to the patient continues to be worthwhile.

Deterministic effects of radiation (organ damage, skin burn), which exhibit a long dose threshold followed by a steep decline where the severity of the effect increases as the dose increases, can also be traced back to DNA damage on the assumption that the effects arise as a result of multicell killing. It is important to realise that, even in the region of the threshold dose where no apparent organ damage is observable, substantial cell killing is occurring together with a more than proportional (linear-quadratic) increase in the risk of developing cancer. In diagnostic radiology every effort should be made to avoid exposures which might cause the onset of deterministic effects. .

## References


Académie des Sciences (1997) Problems associated with the effects of low doses of ionising radiations. Académie des Sciences, Rapport N° 38 (Technique and Documentation, Paris)

Albertini RJ, Clark LS, Nicklas JA et al (1997) Radiation quality affects the efficiency of induction and the molecular spectrum of *HPRT* mutations in human T cells. Radiat Res 148(Suppl):S76–S86

Barendsen GW (1964) Impairment of the proliferative capacity of human cells in culture by α-particles with different linear energy transfer. Int J Radiat Biol 8:453–466

Beachy PA, Karhadkar SS, Berman DM (2004) Tissue repair and stem cell renewal in carcinogenesis. Nature 432: 324–331

Becker K (1997) Threshold or no threshold, that is the question. Radiat Prot Dosim 71:3–5

Benbow RM, Gaudette MF, Hines PJ et al (1985) Initiation of DNA replication in eukaryotes. In: Boynton AL, Leffert HL (eds) Control of Animal Cell Proliferation Vol 1. Academic Press, New York, pp 449–483

Bhambhani R, Kuspira J, Giblak RE (1973) A comparison of cell survival and chromosomal damage using CHO cells synchronised with and without colcemid. Can J Genet Cytol 15:605–618

Bithell JF, Stiller CA (1988) A new calculation of the carcinogenic risk of obstetric X-raying. Stat Med 7:857–864

Bond VP, Wielopolski L, Shani G (1996) Current misinterpretations of the linear no-threshold hypothesis. Health Phys 70:877–882

Brenner DJ, Ward JF (1992) Constraints on energy deposition and target size of multiply damaged sites associated with DNA double-strand breaks. Int J Radiat Biol 61:737–748

Brenner DJ, Doll R, Goodhead DT et al (2003) Cancer risks attributable to low doses of ionizing radiation: Assessing what we really know. Proc Natl Acad Sci 100:13761–13766

Buls N, de Mey J (2007) Dose reduction in CT fluotoscopy. In: Tack D, Genevois PA (eds) Radiation Dose from Adult and Pediatric Multidetector Computed Tomography. Diagnostic Imaging. Medical Radiology. Springer, Berlin, pp 195–222

Calabrese EJ (2002) Hormesis: changing view of the dose-response, a personal account of the history and current status. Mutat Res 511:181–189

Cardis E, Vrijheid M, Blettner M et al (2005) Risk of cancer after low doses of ionising radiation: retrospective cohort study in 15 countries. Br Med J 331:77–83

Chadwick KH, Leenhouts HP (1973) A molecular theory of cell survival. Phys Med Biol 18:78–87

Chadwick KH, Leenhouts HP (1975) The effect of an asynchronous population of cells on the initial slope of dose–effect curves. In: Alper T (ed) Cell survival after low doses of radiation: Theoretical and clinical implications. The Institute of Physics and John Wiley and Sons, London, pp 57–63

Chadwick KH, Leenhouts HP (1978) The rejoining of DNA double-strand breaks and a model for the formation of chromosomal rearrangements. Int J Radiat Biol 33:517–529

Chadwick KH, Leenhouts HP (1981) The molecular theory of radiation biology. Springer, Berlin

Chadwick KH, Leenhouts HP (1983) A quantitative analysis of UV-induced cell killing. Phys Med Biol 28:1369–1383

Chadwick KH, Leenhouts HP (1994) DNA double strand breaks from two single strand breaks and cell cycle radiation sensitivity. Radiat Prot Dosim 52:363–366

Chadwick KH, Leenhouts HP (2011) Radiation induced cancer arises from a somatic mutation. J Radiol Prot 31:41–48

Chadwick KH, Leenhouts HP, Brugmans MJP (2003) A contribution to the linear no-threshold discussion. J Radiol Prot 23:53–78

Chapman JD, Gillespie CJ, Reuvers AP et al (1975) The inactivation of Chinese hamster cells by X-rays: the effects of chemical modifiers on single- and double-events. Radiat Res 64:365–375

Clarke R (1998) Conflicting scientific views on the health risks of low-level ionising radiation. J Radiol Prot 18:159–160

Clarke R (1999) Control of low-level radiation exposure: time for a change? J Radiol Prot 19:107–115

Cornforth MN (1990) Testing the notion of the one-hit exchange. Radiat Res 121:21–27

Darroudi F, Natarajan AT, Savage JRK et al (2001) Induction of chromosomal aberrations by low and high LET radiations: mechanisms and spectra. In: Proceedings European Radiation Research, Dresden 2001 (ISBN 3-00-007790-1)

Dewey WC, Furman SC, Miller HH (1970) Comparison of lethality and chromosomal damage induced by X-rays in synchronised Chinese hamster cell in vitro. Radiat Res 43:561–581

Dewey WC, Stone LE, Miller HH et al (1971a) Radiosensitization with 5-bromodeoxyuridine of Chinese hamster cells irradiated during different phases of the cell cycle. Radiat Res 47:672–688

Dewey WC, Miller HH, Leeper DB (1971b) Chromosomal aberrations and mortality of X-irradiated mammalian cells: emphasis on repair. Proc Natl Acad Sci U S A 68:667–671

Dewey WC, Saparetto SA, Betten DA (1978) Hyperthermic radiosensitization of synchronised Chinese hamster cells: relationship between lethality and chromosomal aberrations. Radiat Res 76:48–59

Doll R, Darby S (1991) Leukaemia: some unsolved problems. Brit Inst Radiol Rep 22:1–6

Edwards R (1997) Radiation roulette. New Sci. (11 October), pp 36–40

Essers J, Hendriks RW, Swagemakers SMA et al (1997) Disruption of mouse RAD54 reduces ionizing radiation resistance and homologous recombination. Cell 89:195–204

Franken NA P, Ruurs P, Ludwikow G et al (1999) Correlation between cell reproductive death and chromosome aberrations assessed by FISH for low and high doses of radiation and sensitization by iodo-deoxyuridine in human SW-1573 cells. Int J Radiat Biol 75:293–299

Frankenberg D, Kelnhofer K, Bar K et al (2002) Enhanced neoplastic transformation by mammography X-rays relative to 200 kVp X-rays: indication for a strong dependence on photon energy of the $RBE_M$ for various end points. Radiat Res 157:99–105

Friedland W, Jacob P, Paretzke HG et al (1998) Monte Carlo simulation of the production of short DNA fragments by low-linear energy transfer radiation using high-order DNA models. Radiat Res 150:170–182

Friedland W, Jacob P, Paretzke HG et al (1999) Simulation of DNA-fragment distribution after irradiation with photons. Radiat Environ Biophys 38:39–47

Gaudette MF, Benbow RM (1986) Replication forks are under-represented in chromosomal DNA of *Xenopus laevis* embryos. Proc Natl Acad Sci USA 83:5953–5957

Gillespie CJ, Chapman JD, Reuvers AP et al (1975a) The inactivation of Chinese hamster cells by X-rays: synchronized and exponential cell populations. Radiat Res 64:353–364

Gillespie CJ, Chapman JD, Reuvers AP et al (1975b) Survival of X-irradiated hamster cells: analysis in terms of the Chadwick–Leenhouts model. In: Alper T (ed) Cell survival after low doses of radiation: Theoretical and clinical implications. The Institute of Physics and John Wiley and Sons, London, pp 25–31

Gofman JW, Tamplin AR (1971) The question of safe radiation thresholds for alpha-emitting bone seekers in man. Health Phys 21:47–51

Goodhead DT, Thacker J, Cox R (1979) Effectiveness of 0.3 keV carbon ultrasoft X-rays for the inactivation and mutation of cultured mammalian cells. Int J Radiat Biol 36:101–114

Goodhead DT, Virsik RP, Harder D et al (1980) Ultrasoft X-rays as a tool to investigate radiation-induced dicentric chromosome aberrations. In: Booz J, Ebert HG, Hartfield HD (eds) Proceedings of the seventh symposium on microdosimetry EUR 7147. Harewood Academic Press, London, pp 1275–1285

Griffin CS, Stevens DL, Savage JRK (1996) Ultrasoft 1.5 keV aluminium X-rays are efficient producers of complex chromosome exchange aberrations revealed by fluorescence in situ hybridization. Radiat Res 146:144–150

Griffin CS, Hill MA, Papworth DG et al (1998) Effectiveness of 0.28 keV carbon K ultrasoft X-rays at producing simple and complex chromosome exchanges in human fibroblasts in vitro detected using FISH. Int J Radiat Biol 73:591–598

Hammond EC (1966) Smoking in relation to the death rates of one million men and women. In: Epidemiological study of cancer and other chronic diseases. National Cancer Institute Monograph 19, pp 127—204

Heidenreich WF, Paretzke HG, Jacob P (1997a) No evidence for increased tumor rates below 200 mSv in the atomic bomb survivors data. Radiat Environ Biophys 36:205–207

Heidenreich WF, Paretzke HG, Jacob P (1997b) Reply to the 'Commentary' by D. A. Pierce and D. L. Preston. Radiat Environ Biophys 36:211–212

Heyes GJ, Mill AJ (2004) The neoplastic transformation potential of mammography X-rays and atomic bomb radiation. Radiat Res 162:120–127

Heyes GJ, Mill AJ, Charles MW (2006) Enhanced biological effectiveness of low energy X-rays and implications for the UK breast screening programme. Brit J Radiol 79:195–200

Heyes GJ, Mill AJ, Charles MW (2009) Mammography—oncogenicity at low doses. J Radiol Prot 29:A123–A132

ICRP 1991 (1990) Recommendations of the International Commission on Radiological Protection. ICRP Publication 60. Annals of the ICRP 21:1–3

ICRP (2003) The evolution of the current system of radiological protection: the justification for new ICRP recommendations (a memorandum from the International Commission on Radiological Protection). J Radiol Prot 23:129–142

Iliakis G (1984) The influence of conditions affecting repair and fixation of potentially lethal damage on the induction of 6-thioguanine resistance after exposure of mammalian cells to X-rays. Mutat Res 126:215–225

Kellerer AM (2000) Risk estimates for radiation-induced cancer—the epidemiological evidence. Radiat Environ Biophys 39:17–24

Kellerer AM, Nekolla EA (2000) The LNT-controversy and the concept of "Controllable Dose". Health Phys 74:412–418

Kesavan PC, Sugahara T (1992) Perspectives in mechanistic considerations of biological effects of low dose radiations. In: Sugahara T, Sagan L, Aoyama T (eds) Low dose irradiation and biological defence mechanisms. Excerpta Medica International Congress Series 1013. Elsevier, Amsterdam, pp 439–443

Knudson AG (1971) Mutation and cancer: statistical study of retinoblastoma gene. Proc Natl Acad Sci USA 68:620–623

Knudson AG (1985) Hereditary cancer, oncogenes and antioncogenes. Cancer Res 45:1437–1443

Knudson AG (1991) Overview: genes that predispose to cancer. Mutat Res 247:185–190

Lea DE (1946) Actions of radiations on living cells. University Press, Cambridge

Lea DE, Catcheside DG (1942) The mechanism of induction by radiation of chromosome aberrations in *Tradescantia*. J Genet 44:216–245

Leenhouts HP (1999) Radon-induced lung cancer in smokers and non-smokers: risk implications using a two mutation carcinogenesis model. Radiat Environ Biophys 38:57–71

Leenhouts HP, Brugmans MJP (2000) An analysis of bone and head sinus cancers in radium dial painters using a two-mutation carcinogenesis model. J Radiol Prot 20:169–188

Leenhouts HP, Brugmans MJP (2001) Calculation of the 1995 lung cancer incidence in the Netherlands and Sweden caused by smoking and radon: risk implications for radon. Radiat Environ Biophys 40:11–21

Leenhouts HP, Chadwick KH (1976) Stopping power and the radiobiological effects of electrons, gamma rays and ions. In: Booz J, Ebert HG, Smith BGR (eds) Fifth Symposium on Microdosimetry. Commission of the European Communities EUR 5452, Luxembourg, pp 289–308

Leenhouts HP, Chadwick KH (1978) An analysis of synergistic sensitization. Br J Cancer 37:198–201

Leenhouts HP, Chadwick KH (1984) A quantitative analysis of the cytotoxic action of chemical mutagens. Mutat Res 129:345–357

Leenhouts HP, Chadwick KH (1989) The molecular basis of stochastic and nonstochastic effects. Health Phys 57(Suppl. 1): 343–348

Leenhouts HP, Chadwick KH (1990) The influence of dose rate on the dose–effect relationship. J Radiat Prot 10:95–102

Leenhouts HP, Chadwick KH (1994a) A two-mutation model of radiation carcinogenesis: applications to lung tumours in rodents and implications for risk evaluations. J Radiol Prot 14:115–130

Leenhouts HP, Chadwick KH (1994b) Analysis of radiation induced carcinogenesis using a two stage carcinogenesis model: Implications for dose-effect relationships. Radiat Protect Dosim 52:465–469

Leenhouts HP, Chadwick KH (2011) Dose-effect relationships, epidemiological analysis and the derivation of low dose risk. J Radiol Prot 31:95–105

Leenhouts HP, Brugmans MJP, Chadwick KH (2000) Analysis of thyroid cancer data from the Ukraine after 'Chernobyl' using a two-mutation carcinogenesis model. Radiat Environ Biophys 39:89–98

Ljungman M (1991) The influence of chromatin structure on the frequency of radiation-induced DNA breaks: a study using nuclear and nucleoid monolayers. Radiat Res 126: 58–64

Ljungman M, Nyberg S, Nygren J et al (1991) DNA-bound proteins contribute much more than soluble intracellular compounds to the intrinsic protection against radiation-induced DNA strand breaks in human cells. Radiat Res 127:171–176

Lloyd DC, Purrott RJ, Dolphin GW et al (1976) Chromosome aberrations induced in human lymphocytes by neutron irradiation. Int J Radiat Biol 29:169–182

Lloyd DC, Edwards AA, Prosser JS et al (1984) The dose response relationship obtained at constant irradiation times for the induction of chromosome aberrations in human lymphocytes by cobalt-60 gamma rays. Radiat Environ Biophys 23:179–189

Lloyd DC, Edwards AA, Leonard A et al (1988) Frequencies of chromosomal aberrations induced in human blood lymphocytes by low doses of X-rays. Int J Radiat Biol 53:49–55

Lloyd DC, Edwards AA, Leonard A et al (1992) Chromosomal aberrations in human lymphocytes induced in vitro by very low doses of X-rays. Int J Radiat Biol 61:335–343

Luckey TD (1997) Low-dose irradiation reduces cancer deaths. Radiat Prot Manag 14 (6): pp 58–64

Ludwików G, Xiao Y, Hoebe RA et al (2002) Induction of chromosome aberrations in unirradiated chromatin after partial irradiation of a cell nucleus. Int J Radiat Biol 78:239–247

Metting NF, Braby LA, Roesch WC et al (1985) Dose-rate evidence for two kinds of radiation damage in stationary-phase mammalian cells. Radiat Res 103:204–212

Mill AJ, Frankenberg D, Bettega D et al (1998) Transformation of C3H 10T1/2 cells by low doses of ionising radiation: a collaborative study by six European laboratories strongly supporting a linear dose -response relationship. J Radiol Prot 18:79–100

Milligan JR, Ng JY-Y, Wu CCL et al (1995) DNA repair by thiols in air shows two radicals make a double-strand break. Radiat Res 143:273–280

Milligan JR, Aguilera JA, Nguyen T-TD et al (2000) DNA strand-break yields after post-irradiation incubation with base excision repair endonucleases implicate hydroxyl radical pairs in double-strand break formation. Int J Radiat Biol 76:1475–1483

Moolgavkar SH, Knudson AG (1981) Mutation and cancer: a model for human carcinogenesis. J Natl Cancer Inst 68:1037–1052

Moolgavkar SH, Venzon D (1979) Two-event models for carcinogenesis. Incidence curves for childhood and adult tumors. Math Biosci 47:55–77

Muirhead CR, Goodill AA, Haylock RGE et al (1999) Occupational radiation exposure and mortality: second analysis of the National Registry for Radiation Workers. J Radiol Prot 19:3–26

Murray D, Prager A, Milas L (1989) Radioprotection of cultured mammalian cells by amniothiols WR-1065 and WR-255591: correlation between protection against DNA double-strand breaks and cell killing after $\gamma$-radiation. Radiat Res 120:154–163

Murray D, Prager A, Vanankeren SC (1990) Comparative effect of the thiols dithiothreitol, cysteamine and WR-151326 on survival and on the induction of DNA damage in cultured Chinese hamster ovary cells exposed to $\gamma$-radiation. Int J Radiat Biol 58:71–91

NCRP (2001) Evaluation of the linear-nonthreshold dose-response model for ionizing radiation. NCRP Report No. 136. National Council on Radiation Protection and Measurements, Washington

Nikjoo H, O'Neill P, Terrisol M et al (1994) Modelling of radiation-induced DNA damage: the early physical and chemical events. Int J Radiat Biol 66:453–457

Nikjoo H, O'Neill P, Terrissol M et al (1999) Quantitative modelling of DNA damage using Monte Carlo track structure method. Radiat Environ Biophys 37:1–8

Nygren J, Ljungman L, Ahnstrom G (1995) Chromatin structure and radiation-induced DNA strand breaks in human cells: soluble scavengers and DNA-bound proteins offer a better protection against single- than double-strand breaks. Int J Radiat Biol 68:11–18

Pierce DA, Preston DL (1997) On 'No evidence for increased tumor rates below 200 mSv in the atomic bomb survivors data'. Radiat Environ Biophys 36:209–210

Pierce DA, Shimuzu Y, Preston DL et al (1996) Studies of the mortality of atomic bomb survivors. Report 12, Part I. Cancer: 1950–1990. Radiat Res 146:1–27

Pohl-Ruhling J, Fischer P, Haas O et al (1983) Effects of low-dose acute X-irradiation on the frequencies of chromosomal aberrations in human peripheral lymphocytes in vitro. Mutat Res 110:71–82

Pohl-Ruling J, Fischer P, Lloyd DC et al (1986) Chromosomal damage induced in human lymphocytes by low doses of D-T neutrons. Mutat Res 173:267–272

Prise KM, Davies S, Michael BD (1987) The relationship between radiation-induced DNA double-strand breaks and cell kill in hamster V79 fibroblasts irradiated with 250-kVp X-rays, 2.3 MeV neutrons or $^{238}$Pu $\alpha$-particles. Int J Radiat Biol 52:893–902

Prise KM, Davies S, Michael BD (1993) Evidence for induction of DNA double-strand breaks at paired radical sites. Radiat Res 134:102–106

Prise KM, Gillies NE, Michael BD (1999) Further evidence for double-strand breaks originating from a paired radical precursor from studies of oxygen fixation processes. Radiat Res 151:635–641

Radford IR (1985) The level of induced DNA double-strand breakage correlates with cell killing after X-irradiation. Int J Radiat Biol 48:45–54

Radford IR (1986) Evidence for a general relationship between the induced level of DNA double-strand breakage and cell killing after X-irradiation of mammalian cells. Int J Radiat Biol 49:611–620

Rao BS, Hopwood LE (1982) Modification of mutation frequency in plateau Chinese hamster ovary cells exposed to gamma radiation during recovery from potentially lethal damage. Int J Radiat Biol 42:501–508

Resnick MA (1976) The repair of double-strand breaks in DNA: a model involving recombination. J Theor Biol 59:97–106

Revell SH (1963) Chromatid aberrations—the general theory. In: Wolff S (ed) Radiation induced chromosome aberrations. Columbia University Press, New York, pp 41–72

Revell SH (1974) The breakage-and-reunion theory and the exchange theory for chromosomal aberrations induced by ionizing radiation: a short history. Adv Radiat Biol 4: 367–416

Richold M, Holt PD (1974) The effect of differing neutron energies on mutagenesis in cultured Chinese hamster cells. In: Biological Effects of Neutron Irradiation (IAEA, Vienna) pp 237–244

Rowland RE (1994) Radium in humans: a review of US studies. US Department of Commerce. Technology Administration, National Technical Information Service, Springfield

Sagan L (1992) It's time to re-think the radiation paradigm. In: Sugahara T, Sagan L, Aoyama T (eds) Low dose irradiation and biological defence mechanisms. Excerpta Medica International Congress Series 1013. Elsevier, Amsterdam pp 3–12

Sax K (1940) X-ray-induced chromosomal aberrations in *Tradescantia*. Genetics 25:41–68

Shrimpton PC, Hillier MC, Lewis MA et al (2003) Data from computed tomography (CT) examinations in the UK—2003 Review. NRPB—67, National Radiological Protection Board, Chilton

Simpson P, Savage JRK (1996) Dose-response curves for simple and complex chromosome aberrations induced by X-rays and detected using fluorescence in situ hybridization. Int J Radiat Biol 69:429–436

Sinclair WK (1966) The shape of radiation survival curves of mammalian cells cultured in vitro. In: Biophysical aspects of radiation quality, Techn Rep Ser 58. International Atomic Energy Agency, Vienna, pp 21–43

Skarsgard LD, Wilson DJ, Durrand RE (1993) Survival at low dose in asynchronous and partially synchronized Chinese hamster V79–171 cells. Radiat Res 133:102–107

Smith-Bindman R (2010) Is computed tomography safe? New eng. J Med 363:1–4

Stewart AM, Kneale GW (1990) A-bomb radiation and evidence of late effects other than cancer. Health Phys 58:729–735

Stewart AM, Webb J, Giles D et al (1956) Malignant disease in childhood and diagnostic radiation in utero. Lancet 2:p 447

Stewart AM, Webb J, Hewitt D (1958) A survey of childhood malignancies. Br Med J 1:1495–1508

Thacker J, Cox R (1975) Mutation induction and inactivation in mammalian cells exposed to ionizing radiation. Nature 258:429–431

Thacker J, Stretch A, Stephens MA (1977) The induction of thioguanine-resistant mutants of Chinese hamster cells by $\gamma$-rays. Mutat Res 42:313–326

Thacker J, Wilkinson RE, Goodhead DT (1986) The induction of chromosome exchange aberrations by carbon ultrasoft X-rays in V79 hamster cells. Int J Radiat Biol 49:645–656

Todd P (1967) Heavy-ion irradiation of cultured human cells. Radiat Res Suppl 7:196–207

Traynor JE, Still ET (1968) Dose rate effect on LD50/30 in mice exposed to cobalt-60 gamma irradiation. Brooks Air Force Base, TX:USAF School of Aerospace Medicine; Rep. SAM-TR-68-97

Tubiana M (1998) The report of the French Academy of Science: problems associated with the effects of low doses of ionising radiations. J Radiat Prot 18:243–248

Tubiana M (2000) Radiation risks in perspective: radiation-induced cancer among cancer risks. Radiat Environ Biophys 39:3–16

Underbrink AG, Sparrow AH, Sautkulis D, Mills RE (1975) Oxygen enhancement ratios (OERs) for somatic mutations in Tradescantia stamen hairs. Radiat Bot 15: 161–168

UNSCEAR (2000) Sources and effects of ionizing radiation. United Nations Scientific Committee on the Effects of Atomic Radiation Report to the General Assembly, New York

Upton AC, Jenkins VK, Conklin JW (1964) Myeloid leukemia in the mouse. Ann N Y Acad Sci 114:189–202

Virsik RP, Schafer CH, Harder D et al (1980) Chromosome aberrations induced in human lymphocytes by ultrasoft Al-K and Cu X-rays. Int J Radiat Biol 38:545–557

Vivek Kumar PR, Mohankumar MN, Zareena Hamza V et al (2006) Dose-rate effect on the induction of *HPRT* mutants in Human $G_0$ lymphocytes exposed in vitro to gamma radiation. Radiat Res 165:43–50

Wakeford R (2005) Cancer risk among nuclear workers. J Radiat Prot 25:225–228

Wakeford R, Doll R, Bithell JF (1997) Childhood cancer and intrauterine irradiation, In: Health effects of low dose radiation: challenges of the 21st century. British Nuclear Energy Society, London, pp 114–119

Wells RL, Bedford JS (1983) Dose-rate effects in mammalian cells IV: repairable and non-repairable damage in non-cycling C3H 10T1/2 cells. Radiat Res 94:105–134

# The Cancer Risk from Low Level Radiation

Bernard L. Cohen

## Contents



**Abstract**

We present a wide variety of experimental data indicating that linear no-threshold theory (LNT) greatly exaggerates the cancer risk from low level radiation. LNT is based on cancer initiating hits on DNA molecules, but many other factors affect the progression from DNA damage to a fatal tumor, such as availability of DNA repair enzymes, immune response, and cell suicide. Data are presented to show that these are generally stimulated by low level radiation (LLR) and suppressed by high doses that serve as calibrations for LNT. Since the great majority of cancers are caused by natural chemical processes, the protection against these provided by LLR may make LLR beneficial rather than harmful. Genes turned on and turned off by LLR are often different from those affected by high doses. Direct studies of cancer risk vs dose are reviewed: animal experiments generally indicate that LNT exaggerates the risk of low level radiation, and the same is true of most data on humans except possibly where dose rates are very high. Data show that the time delay between receipt of dose and cancer death increases with decreasing dose, which means that, with low level radiation, death from natural causes will often occur first. This implies an effective threshold. Responses to this type of information by various official and prestigious groups charged with estimating cancer risks from radiation are reviewed.

B. L. Cohen (✉)
Department of Physics, University of Pittsburgh,
Pittsburgh, PA 15260, USA
e-mail: blc@pitt.edu

D. Tack et al. (eds.), *Radiation Dose from Multidetector CT*, Medical Radiology. Diagnostic Imaging,
DOI: 10.1007/174_2011_401, © Springer-Verlag Berlin Heidelberg 2012

## 1 Introduction

It is commonly stated that "any radiation dose, no matter how small, can cause cancer". The basis for that statement is the linear no-threshold theory (LNT) of radiation carcinogenesis. According to LNT, if 1 Gy (100 rads) of exposure gives a cancer risk *R*, the risk from 0.01 Gy (1 rad) of exposure is *R*/100, the risk from 0.00 001 Gy (1 millirad) is *R*/100 000, and so on. Thus the cancer risk is not zero regardless of how small the exposure.

However, over the past several years, a strong sentiment has developed in the community of radiation health scientists to regard risk estimates in the low-dose region based on LNT as being grossly exaggerated or completely negligible. For example, the 6000 member Health Physics Society, the principal organization for radiation protection scientists, issued a position paper (HPS 1996) stating "Below 10 rad …risks of health effects are either too small to be observed or are non-existent". A similar position statement was issued by American Nuclear Society. When the Health Physics Society Newsletter asked for submission of comments on validity of LNT, there were about 20 negative comments submitted and only a single comment supportive of LNT. In a worldwide poll conducted by the principal on-line discussion group of radiation protection professionals (RADSAFE), the vote was 118 to 12 against LNT A 2001 Report by the French Academy of Medicine concluded that LNT is "without any scientific validity, and an elaborate joint study by the French Academy of Medicine and the French Academy of Sciences (Aurengo et al. 2005) strongly condemned the use of LNT. While U.S. official agencies have been slower to accept this position, the U.S, National Council on Radiation Protection and Measurements (NCRP) stated in NCRP Publication No. 121 (NCRP 1995) "Few experimental studies and essentially no human data can be said to prove or even provide direct support for the [LNT] concept", and in NCRP Publication No.136 (NCRP-2001) stated "It is important to note that the rates of cancer in most populations exposed to low level radiation have not been found to be detectably increased, and in most cases the rates appear to be decreased". A group of scientists opposing use of LNT (Radiation Science and Health) submitted several hundred papers supporting their position to National Research Council. A recent Workshop on health risks from low level radiation (Feinendegen et al. 2011; Brooks 2011; Morgan 2011) provided much support for that position.

Beyond failure of LNT, there is substantial evidence that low level radiation may be protective against cancer; a view known as "hormesis". There is an International Hormesis Society which sponsors an annual International Scientific Conference and publishes a peer reviewed scientific journal and a regular newsletter. A recent issue of that journal was devoted to radiation hormesis (Scott 2010).

The purpose of this chapter is to review the basis for LNT and to present some of the mostly recent information that has caused this strong shift in sentiment. Other recent reviews have been published with somewhat different approaches to similar objectives (Feinendegen 2005a, b, 2011; Tubiana 2005).

## 2 Problems with the Basis for Linear No-Threshold Theory

The original basis for linear no-threshold theory (LNT), as that theory emerged in the mid-twentieth century, was theoretical and very simple. A single particle of radiation hitting a single DNA molecule in a single cell nucleus of the human body can initiate a cancer. The probability of such a cancer initiation is therefore proportional to the number of such hits, which is proportional to the number of particles of radiation, which is proportional to the dose. Thus the risk is proportional to the dose—this is LNT.

An important problem with this simple argument is that factors other than initiating events affect the cancer risk. Human bodies have biological defense mechanisms which prevent the vast majority of initiating events from developing into a fatal cancer (Pollycove and Feinendagen 2001). A list of some of the most important examples including how they are affected by low level radiation follows (Feinendegen 2005b):

- Our bodies produce repair enzymes which repair DNA damage with high efficiency, and low level radiation stimulates production of these repair enzymes.
- Apoptosis, a process by which damaged cells "commit suicide" to avoid extending the effects of

the damage, is stimulated by low level radiation. A similar effect is achieved by premature differentiation and maturation to senescence.

- The immune system is important for preventing mutations from developing into a cancer; there is abundant evidence that low level radiation stimulates the immune system, but high radiation levels depress it.
- The overwhelmingly most important cause of DNA damage is corrosive chemicals (reactive oxygen species—ROS); there are processes for scavenging these out of cells, and low level radiation stimulates these scavenging processes (Kondo 1993). Elevated ROS levels have been shown to initiate a broad array of biochemical reactions that are stress responses, leading to the conclusion that "the best protection against stress is stress itself"(Finkel and Holbrook 2000).
- Radiation can alter cell cycle timing. This can extend the time before the next cell division (mitosis). Damage repair is most effective before the next mitosis, so changing this available time can be important (Elkind M, personal communication). Altered cell timing can also affect DNA repair processes in many ways by changing chemical processes (Boothman et al. 1996).
- Various other effects of low level radiation on cell survival have been observed and are referred to as "low dose hypersensitivity", "increased radiation radioresistance", and "death inducing effects" (Bonner 2004).

It is now recognized that development of cancer is a much more complex process than was originally envisioned. The role of "bystander effects", signaling between neighboring cells relevant to their radiation experiences, is now recognized to be an important, albeit poorly understood factor In fact it seems that tissue response, and even whole organ response, rather than just cellular response, must be considered (Aurengo et al. 2005).

There is also apparently obvious evidence for the failure of the original simple model. For example, the number of initiating events is roughly proportional to the mass of the animal—more DNA targets mean more hits. Thus, the simple theory predicts that the cancer risk should be approximately proportional to the mass of the animal. But the cancer risk in a given radiation field is similar for a 30 g mouse and a 70,000 g human. As another example, our very definition of dose, based on the energy absorbed per unit mass of tissue, which is proportional to the number of radiation hits per unit target mass, would be misleading if only the total number of hits (which is proportional to the number of initiating events) were relevant regardless of the target mass.

A detailed theoretical approach to evaluating the validity of LNT is based on the commonly accepted idea that double strand breaks (DSB) in DNA molecules are the principal initiating event in causing cancer. But DSBs are also caused by endogenous corrosive chemicals, reactive oxygen species (ROS). In fact the DNA damage caused by radiation is mostly due to the production of ROS by the ionizing effects of the radiation on omnipresent water. It is estimated that endogenous ROS causes about 0.1 DSB per cell per day, whereas 100 mSv (10 rem) of radiation, which is close to the upper limit of what is normally called low level radiation, causes about 4 DSB per cell (Feinendegen 2005a). Assuming that the number of cancers is proportional to the number of DSB, a 100 mSv dose of radiation would increase the lifetime (28,000 days × 0.1 DSB/day) risk of cancer by only about (4/2800 =) 0.14%, whereas LNT predicts an increase of 1%. From this it is concluded that the underlying assumption of LNT that, cancer initiating events are the controlling factors in determining the dose–response relationship for radiation is a serious over-simplification.

## 3 Direct Experimental Challenges to the Basis for LNT

A direct demonstration of the failure of the basis for LNT derives from microarray studies determining what genes are up regulated and down regulated by radiation. It is found that generally different sets of genes are affected by low level radiation than by a high level dose. For example, in one study of mouse brain (Yin et al. 2005), 191 genes were affected by a dose of 0.1 Sv but not by a dose of 2.0 Sv, 213 genes were affected by 2.0 Sv but not by 0.1 Sv, while 299 genes were affected by both doses. The 0.1 Sv dose-induced expression of genes involved in protective and repair functions while down-modulating genes involved in unrelated processes.

A similar study with even lower doses on human fibroblast cells (Golder-Novoselsky et al. 2002) found that a dose of 0.02 Sv caused more than 100 genes to change their expression, and these were generally different than the genes affected by 0.5 Sv. The former group was heavily weighted by stress response genes.

Several other microarray studies have shown that high radiation doses which serve as the calibration for application of LNT, are not equivalent to an accumulation of low radiation doses (Tubiana and Aurengo 2005).

Sophisticated experimental techniques have been developed for observing the effects of a single alpha particle hitting a single cell. It was found (Miller et al. 1999) that the probability for transformation to malignancy from N particle hits on a cell is much greater than N times the probability for transformation to malignancy from a single hit. This is a direct violation of LNT, indicating that the estimated effects based on extrapolating the risk from high exposure, represented by N hits, greatly exaggerate the risk from low level exposure as represented by a single hit.

A very clear demonstration of a threshold response, in contrast to LNT, was found in tumor induction by irradiation throughout life of mouse skin (Tanooka 2001). For irradiation rates of 1.5, 2.2, and 3 Gy/week, the percentage of mice that developed tumors was 0, 35, and 100% respectively.

## 4 Effects of Low Level Radiation on Biological Defense Mechanisms

### 4.1 Adaptive Response

An important type of biological defense mechanism is known as "adaptive response" (UNSCEAR 1994)—exposing a cell to a stress like radiation stimulates the natural defense against such stresses and hence protects against subsequent further stresses. On an experimental basis, this is most easily studied by exposing cells to a low dose to prime the adaptive response and then later exposing it to a high radiation "challenge dose"; the adaptive response is observed as the reduced effect of the challenge dose in comparison with a similar challenge exposure without the priming dose.

The most widely studied examples have involved observations on chromosome aberrations, perhaps the simplest tool for detecting genetic damage. It has long been recognized that radiation increases the number of these aberrations. However, an in vitro study on human lymphocyte cells (Shadley and Dai 1992) shows, in Table 1, how that process is affected if the high dose is preceded a few hours before by a low dose. We see that the number of chromosome aberrations caused by the high dose is substantially reduced. This is an example of adaptive response.

**Table 1** Effects of pre-exposure to 5 cGy on two types of chromosome aberrations in human lymphocyte cells, induced by 400 cGy of X-rays 6 h later (Shadley and Dai 1992)

| Dicentrics & Rings | | | Deletions | |
|---|---|---|---|---|
| Donor | 400 cGy | (5 + 400) cGy | 400 cGy | (5 + 400) cGy |
| 1 | 136 | 92 | 52 | 51 |
| 2 | 178 | 120 | 62 | 46 |
| 3 | 79 | 50 | 39 | 15 |
| 4 | 172 | 42 | 46 | 34 |
| 5 | 134 | 106 | 58 | 41 |

As an example of an in vivo experiment (Cai and Liu 1990), it was found that exposure of mouse cells to 65 cGy (65 rad) caused chromosome aberrations in 38% of bone marrow cells and in 12.6% of spermatocytes, but if these exposures are preceded 3 h earlier by an exposure to 0.2 cGy, these percentages are reduced to 19.5 and 8.4% respectively. There are many other examples of such experiments, both in vitro and in vivo (UNSCEAR 1994), and the results are usually explained as stimulated production of repair enzymes by low level radiation.

The effects of adaptive response in protecting against chromosome aberrations were observed for in vivo human exposures in comparing residents of a high background radiation area (1 cGY/year) and a normal background radiation area (0.1 cGy/year) in Iran (Ghiassi-nejad et al. 2002). When lymphocytes from these groups were exposed to 1.5 Gy (150 rad), the mean frequency of chromosome aberrations per cell was 0.098 ± 0.012 for the high background area versus 0.176 ± 0.017 for the low background area, a four standard deviation difference. Presumably, adaptive response induced by radiation in the high background area protected its citizens against chromosome aberrations induced by the 1.5 Gy dose.

A microarray study on human lymphoblastoid cells (Coleman et al. 2005), was carried out to investigate the processes involved in adaptive response. A 0.05 Sv priming dose was followed by a 2.0 Sv challenge dose, and adaptive response was measured by the reduction of chromosome aberrations; the goal was to identify genes involved in adaptive response and determine how their states of activation were affected by the priming dose. It reported that 145 genes were affected by the priming dose, generally up regulated for protein synthesis—a key element in DNA repair—and down regulated for metabolic and signal transduction, perhaps as a means to conserve resources for devotion to DNA repair. Many genes associated with DNA repair, stress response, cell cycle control, and apoptosis were strongly affected by the priming dose. The specifics of the process were found to be highly complex and sometimes pointing in different directions; for example, the TP53 gene, which can act as either a tumor promoter or a tumor suppressor, plays an important but not clearly defined role.

Apart from studies using chromosome aberrations, another type of experiment that reveals effects of "adaptive response" involves detection of genetic mutations. As an example of an in vitro experiment (Kelsey et al. 1991), it was found that an X-ray exposure of 300 cGy to human lymphocytes induced a frequency of mutations at the *hprt locus* of 15.5 x $10^{-6}$, but if this large exposure was preceded 16 h earlier by an exposure of 1 cGy, this frequency was reduced to 5.2 x $10^{-6}$.

As an in vivo example (Fritz-Niggli and Schaeppi-Buechi 1991), it was found that the percentage of dominant lethal mutations in offspring resulting from exposures of female drosophila to 200 cGy of X-rays before mating was substantially reduced by preceding this high dose with an exposure to 2 cGy; for different strains of drosophila and different oocyte maturities these percentages were reduced from 42 to 27%, from 11 to 4.5%, from 40 to 36%, from 32 to 12.5%, from 42 to 30%, and from 51 to 22%.

An alternative for studying chromosome aberrations directly is to observe micronuclei from unrepaired double strand breaks after mitosis (Mitchel 2007); this allows consideration of DNA repair and other natural biological processes. This was used in studying mice exposed near Chernobyl, and showed clear effects of adaptive response (Rodgers and Holmes 2008).

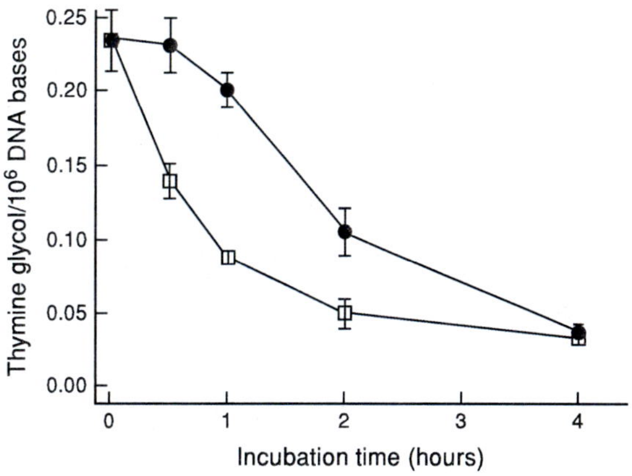


**Fig. 1** Comparison of removal of thymine glycol by A549 cells after 2 Gy irradiation, with (*open squares*) or without (*shaded circles*) a 0.25 Gy priming dose given 4 h before (Le et al. 1998)

A technique has been developed for directly observing repair of DNA base damage (Le et al. 1998). It was found that preceding an exposure to 2 Gy of gamma radiation with 0.25 Gy 4 h before reduced the time for 50% DNA lesion removal from 100 to 50 min. The progression of the repair vs time is shown in Fig. 1 with and without the 0.25 Gy priming dose.

From the types of data discussed above, one might consider the possibility that adaptive response is only effective in protecting against damage caused by subsequent large doses of radiation. But there are data on its effectiveness against spontaneous transformation to malignancy on cells with a predisposition to such transformation. This was shown (Azzam et al. 1996) for exposures of C3H 10T1/2 mouse cells where one day after exposure to low doses of radiation the rate of spontaneous neoplastic transformation was reduced by 78%. In a similar experiment (Redpath and Antoniono 1998) with human HeLa x skin fibroblast cells, the reduction was by 55%. The dependence on dose for this cell type is shown in Fig. 2 (Redpath et al. 2003) with error bars indicating 95% confidence intervals. We see there that the effect is statistically indisputable even at very low doses, below 1 cGy.

The question has been raised as to how long adaptive response persists following a priming dose. In one in vivo experiment (Zaichkina et al. 2003) measuring chromosome damage in bone marrow cells of mice, both spontaneously and by a challenge dose, adaptive response was found after 1, 3, 6, 9, and 12

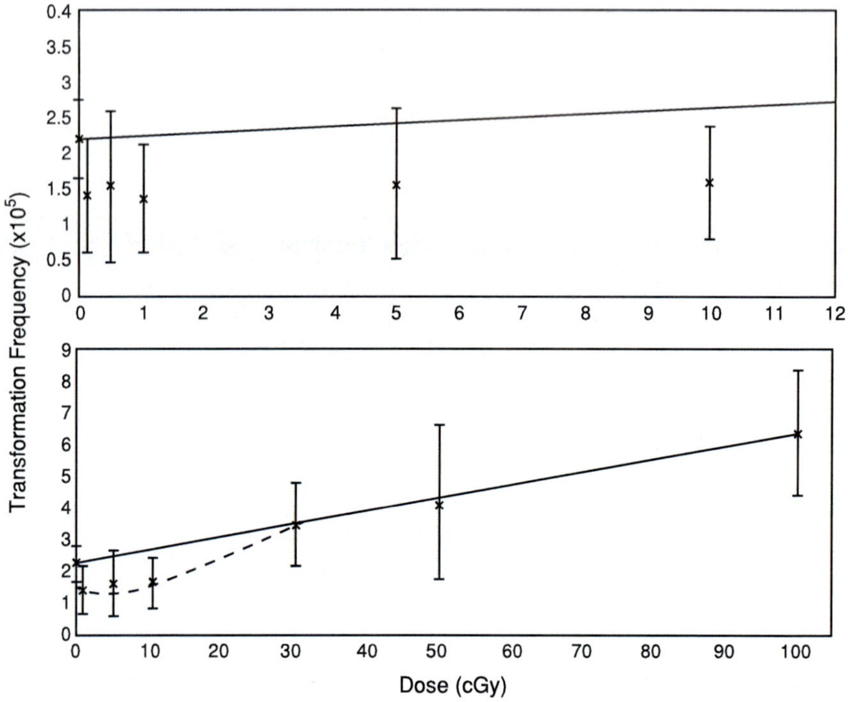


**Fig. 2** Transformations per surviving cell as a function of dose for HeLa X skin fibroblast human hybrid cells irradiated with gamma rays (Redpath et al. 2003). Upper plot is of same data on an expanded scale. Error bars represent 95% confidence limits

months following priming doses of 0.1 and 0.2 Gy, and the protection against spontaneous damage persisted to the end of life (20 months).

This adaptive response protection against spontaneous development of cancer may be understood from effects of radiation on corrosive chemicals (ROS). Since ROS is the dominant cause of spontaneous cancers through initiating DNA damage, reducing the amount of ROS and increasing the amount of antioxidants that scavenge them out of cells is protective against development of spontaneous cancers. The results of a study of these on rat cells (Yamaoka 1991) are shown in Fig. 3. We see there that 50 cGy of X-ray exposure decreases the amount of the oxidant lipid peroxide by about 20%, and increases the amount of the antioxidant SOD by about 25%, and that these beneficial effects are appreciable over the entire dose range up to above 100 cGy. Many other studies with similar results have been summarized and extended (Yukawa et al. 2005).

It is interesting to point out that adaptive response to protect against harmful effects of radiation, such as that provided by previous low level radiation, can also be provided by other stresses such as heat or chemical exposures (Mitchel 2006). This adaptive response has

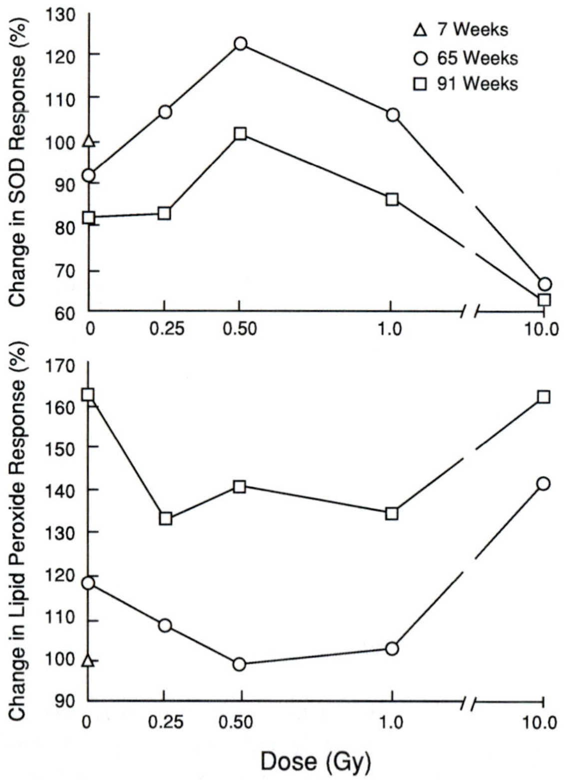


**Fig. 3** Antioxidant SOD and lipid peroxide response to age and radiation of rat brain cortex (Yamaoka 1991)

**Table 2** Effects of radiation on immune response.

| Test | 2.5 cGy | 5 cGy | 7.5 cGy |
|---|---|---|---|
| PFC Reaction | 110 | 143 | 174 |
| MLC Reaction | 109 | 133 | 122 |
| Reaction to Con A | 191 | 155 | 530 |
| NK activity | 112 | 109 | 119 |
| ADCC Activity | 109 | 128 | 132 |

Different columns are percent of response to various tests in unexposed mice, to response in mice exposed as indicated (Liu 1992). *PFC* plaque forming cell, *MLC* mixed lymphocyte culture, used as test of T-cell function, *Con A* concanavalin-A, lectin that stimulates T-lymphocytes, *NK* natural killer cells which recognize and kill tumor cells, *ADCC* anti body dependent cell mediated cytotoxicity, which assists NK activity

been found in all forms of life, from single cell eukaryotes to mammals.

There has been recent interest in "bystander effect", effects of radiation on cells not directly struck by radiation due to inter cell signaling. This might increase the harmful effects of radiation on these cells, except for the fact that it provides them protection through adaptive response (Michel 2010).

In radiation therapy for tumors, effectiveness is limited by damage to surrounding tissue. This damage can be reduced by low level radiation pre-exposure of this tissue (Blankenbecker 2010); this procedure has worked successfully on dogs.

### 4.2 Stimulation of the Immune System

Since the immune system destroys cells with persistent DNA damage and is thus important in protecting against the development of cancer, the effects of low level radiation on it are relevant here. Such effects on several different measures of the immune response (Liu 1992) are listed in Table 2. We see that by each of these measures, the immune response is increased by low level radiation, and increasingly so at least up to 7.5 cSv.

The results of one study of this effect over a wide range of radiation doses (Makinodan and James 1990) is shown in Fig. 4. We see there increases in immune response by 80% in vitro and by 40% in vivo at about 20 cGy followed by a rapid decrease to well below the unirradiated level at doses above 50 cGy.

In a review (Liu 2003) of extensive mouse studies utilizing about 10 levels of whole body radiation exposure, effects on 52 immunologic parameters were analyzed to determine dose–response curves for two categories of these The first category included 20 parameters which would lead to decreased immune activity, for which the results are shown in the upper part of Fig. 5, and the second category included the remaining 32 parameters that would lead to increased immune activity for which the results are shown in the lower part of Fig. 5. We see from Fig. 5 that low doses down regulate the parameters indicative of decreased immune activity, and that these low doses up regulate parameters indicative of increased immune activity. In both cases, these effects are reversed for high level radiation exposure. The conclusion is that low level radiation increases immune activity and high level exposures reduce immune activity, in agreement with what was seen in Fig. 4.

Contrary to expectations from the basic assumption of LNT that the cancer risk depends only on total dose, effects on the immune system are very different for the same total dose given at low dose rate versus high dose rate. In a study of effects on various indicators of immune response in several wild type mouse strains (Ina and Sakai 2005), continuous whole body irradiation at 1.2 mGy per hour stimulated immune response as shown for a few example indicators in Fig. 6, but the same doses given at a high rate had the opposite effect.

Further information on the dose rate dependence was reported in a mouse study of thymic lymphomas (Ina et al. 2005). Acute challenge doses totaling 7.2 Gy induced tumors in 90% of the mice, but if the mice were previously exposed at a rate of 1.2 mGy per hour for 258 days (a total of 7.2 Gy) prior to the 7.2 Gy challenging dose, only 43% developed such tumors—this may seem like an extreme case of adaptive response although the priming dose is equal to the challenge dose and doubling the total dose resulted in fewer tumors. But most significantly for the present discussion, the low dose rate exposure, even extended to 450 days for a total exposure of 12.6 Gy, resulted in no tumors without a challenge dose. Various indicators of immune response were significantly increased by the continuous whole body radiation, and the authors attribute their observations to stimulation of the immune system by this radiation.

Several studies have shown that the immune system provides resistance to metastasis of tumors; one example is shown in Fig. 7. When tumor cells are transplanted into the groins of mice, the rate of their metastasis into the lung is cut about in half by total

**Fig. 4** Immune system response to radiation. Mouse splenic cells primed with antigenic sheep red blood cells (Makinodan and James 1990)

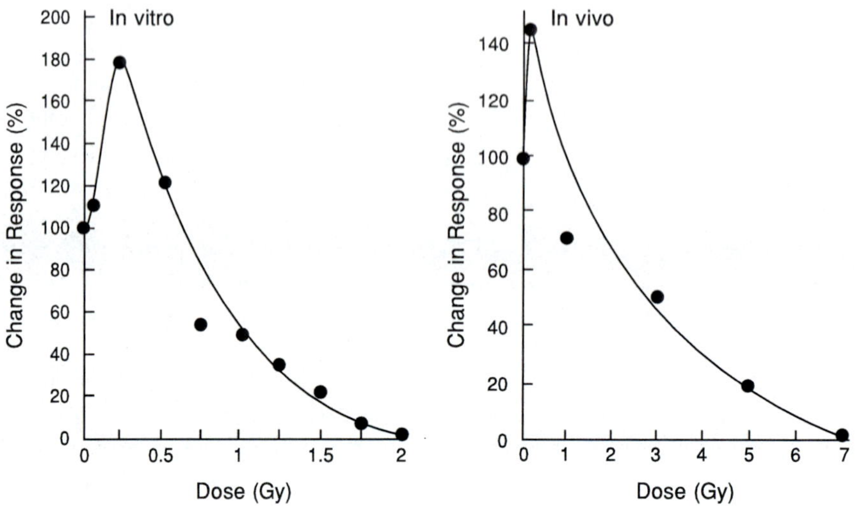


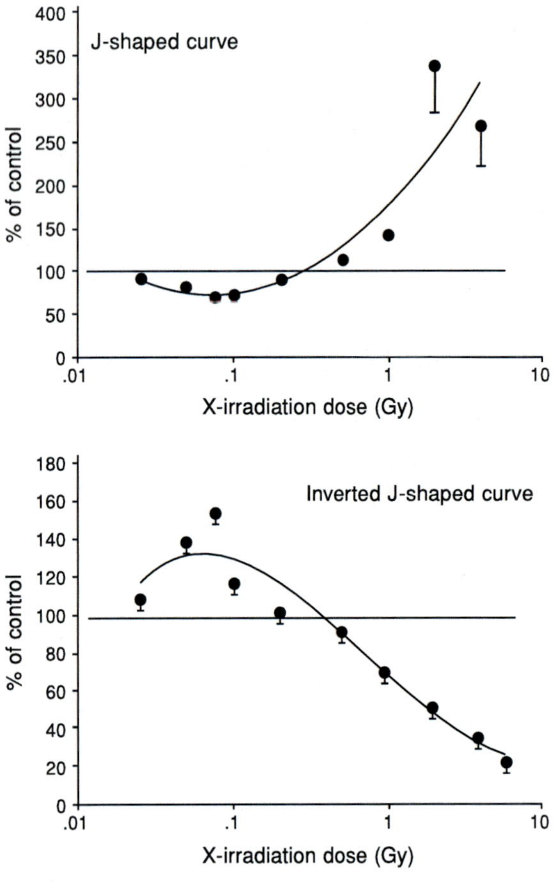


**Fig. 5** Dose–response curves constructed from multiple parameters of the immune system following whole body irradiation of C57BL/6 and Kunming mice (Liu 2003). Upper figure is for 20 parameters that lead to decreased immune activity, and lower figure is for 32 parameters that lead to increased immune activity

body irradiation with 15–30 cGy 12 days after the transplantation (Sakamoto et al. 1997). Doses above 50 cGy on the other hand, reduce the immune response, leading to increased rates of metastasis. A study in rats (Hashimoto et al. 1999) showed that total body irradiation—but not tumor irradiation—with low level radiation reduces the rate of metastasis and increases infiltration into the tumor of immune system agents (Makinodan and James 1990).

Studies on naturally cancer-prone mice (Mitchel et al. 2003) showed that, while low level radiation exposure does not prevent eventual development of cancer, it delays the process substantially. Total body irradiation with low level radiation has also been shown to reduce tumor size (Makinodan 1992; Anderson 1992). The only reasonable explanation for such effects of total body low level radiation would seem to be stimulation of the body's immune system.

## 5 Cancer Risk Versus Dose in Animal Experiments

There have been numerous direct studies of cancer risk vs dose, testing the validity of LNT, with animals exposed to various radiation doses. An example was a series of external gamma ray exposure studies at Oak Ridge National Laboratory, of which one result (Ullrich and Storer 1979) is shown in Fig. 8; we see there clear evidence for the failure of LNT in the low dose region. In those experiments, exposed animals lived considerably longer (up to 40%) than their controls. Another example

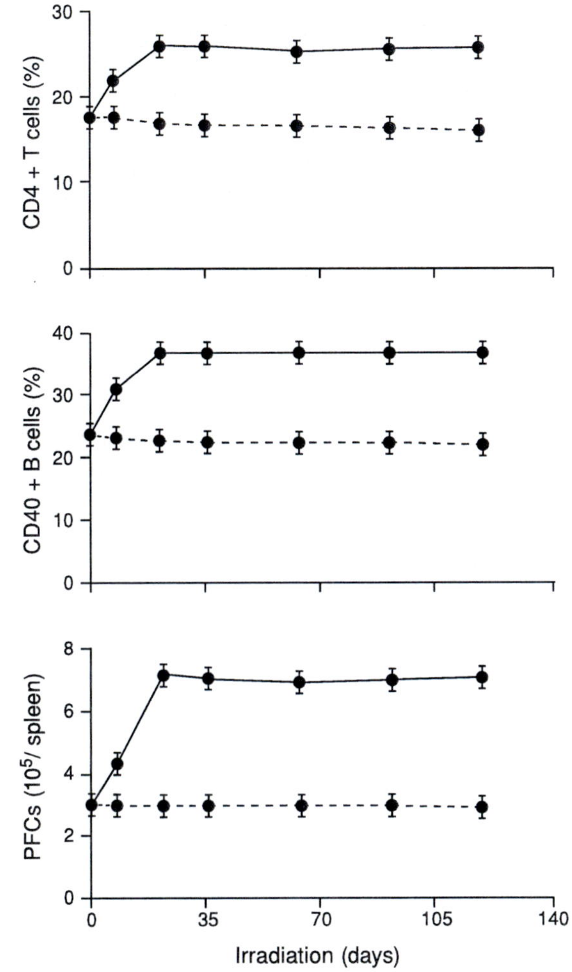


**Fig. 6** Solid lines show activation by continuous low-dose rate $\gamma$ irradiation at 1.2 mGy hour$^{-1}$ from 5 weeks of age, of three different immune cell populations in the spleens of C57BL/6 mice challenged intraperitoneally by SRBC; data are plotted as a function of irradiation time. Dashed lines are the same for unirradiated control mice (Ina and Sakai 2005)

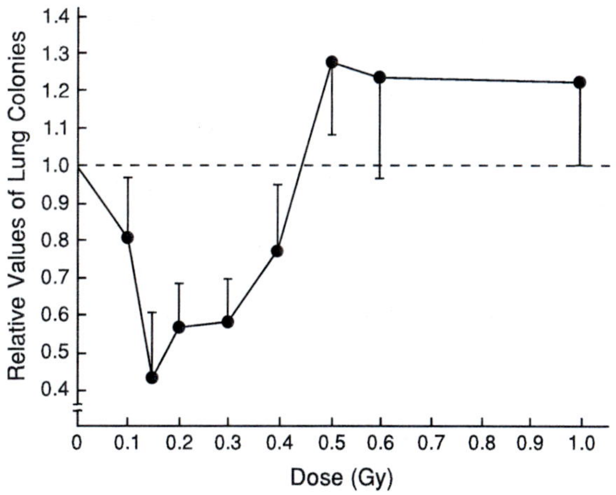


**Fig. 7** Spontaneous lung metasteses after total body irradiation of mice, given 12 days after tumor transplantation into groin (Sakamoto et al. 1997)

was a series of animal studies at Argonne National Laboratory in the 1950s and 1960s with injection of radioactive materials; these are reviewed by Finkel and Biskis (1962, 1969). The results of one of these studies, for bone cancers in mice injected with radioactive isotopes of calcium and strontium (Finkel and Biskis 1968), is shown in Fig. 9. Nearly all of these studies indicate, with high statistical significance, that LNT over-estimates the cancer risk from low level radiation, generally suggesting a threshold.

A review of over 100 such experiments (Duport 2001) involved a total of 85,000 exposed animals with their 45,000 corresponding controls, with a total of 60,000 and 12,000 cancers in exposed and control animals respectively. In cases where cancers were observed in control animals, either no effect or an apparent reduction in cancer risk was observed in 40% of the data sets for neutron exposure, 50% of the data sets for X-rays, 53% of the data sets for gamma rays, and 61% of the data sets for alpha particles.

## 6 Cancer Risk Versus Dose: Data from Human Exposures

### 6.1 Data Supportive of LNT

The principal data that have been cited by those in influential positions to support LNT are those for solid tumors (all cancers except leukemia) among the Japanese A-bomb survivors. The data up to 1990 (Pierce et al. 1996) are shown in Fig. 10, where the error bars represent 95% confidence limits (2 standard deviations). If error bars are ignored, the points do indeed suggest a linear relationship with intercept near zero dose.

But the data themselves give no statistically significant indication of excess cancers for doses below about 25 cSv. This conclusion applies to the incidence data as well as to the mortality data (Heidenreich et al. 1997). In fact, it was shown (Cohen 1998) that considering the three lowest dose points alone (i.e. up to 20 cSv), the slope of the dose–response curve has a

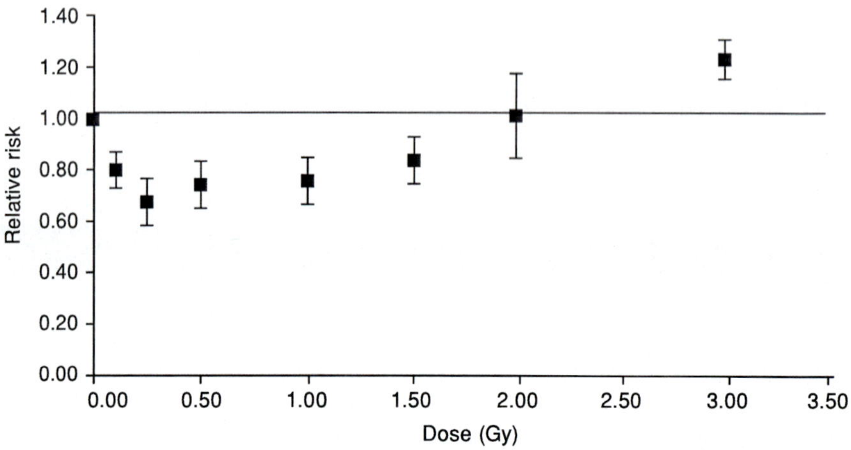


**Fig. 8** Relative risk of lung cancer in mice following gamma ray exposure (Ullrich and Storer 1979)

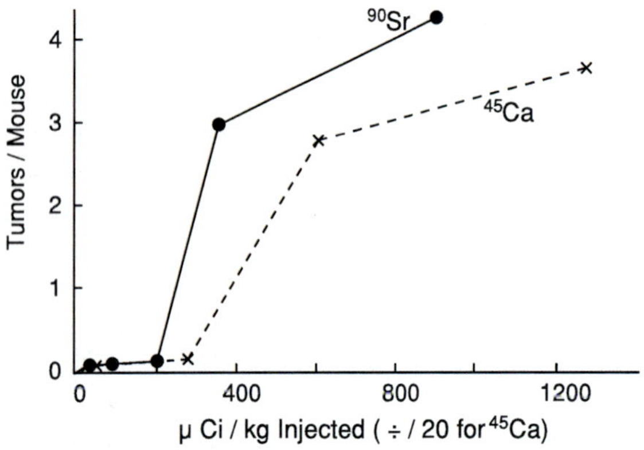


**Fig. 9** Osteogenic sarcomas produced in CF1 female mice by injection of Sr-90 and Ca-45 at age 70 days (Finkel and Biskis 1968). Sr-90 experiments used 810 mice and 150 controls; results for 1.3, 4.5, and 20 microcuries/kg, not shown on the plot, had ordinate values zero

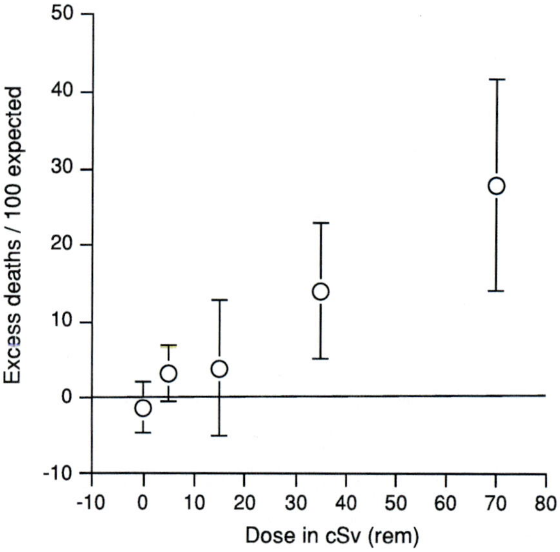


**Fig. 10** Excess deaths from solid tumors per 100 "expected" among Japanese A-bomb survivors (1950–1990) versus their dose (Pierce et al. 1996). Error bars are 95% confidence limits

20% probability of being negative (risk decreasing with increasing dose). A more recent update (Preston et al. 2004) of the data on A-bomb survivors has been published but with insufficient detail to repeat the above analysis. A crude preliminary analysis indicates that the above conclusions will not be appreciably changed.

It has also been pointed out (Kaminski 2011) that non-radiation causes of carcinogenesis, such as thermal burns, non-radioactive toxins from the explosion and fires, malnutrition, and psychosocial factors, may play a prominent role in the data for cancers among the A-bomb survivors with low radiation exposures.

The data on leukemia among A-bomb survivors (Pierce et al. 1996) are shown in Fig. 11, with error bars indicating 95% confidence limits. These data strongly suggest a threshold above 20 cSv, and this difference from LNT expectations is recognized by the authors and in all widely recognized reviews.

The other principal evidence that has been widely cited as supporting LNT is the International Association for Research on Cancer(IARC) studies of monitored radiation workers. The first and most fully reported (Cardis et al. 1995) was a study of 95,673 monitored radiation workers in the U.S., U.K., and Canada. For all cancers except leukemia, there were 3,830 deaths but no excess over the number expected.

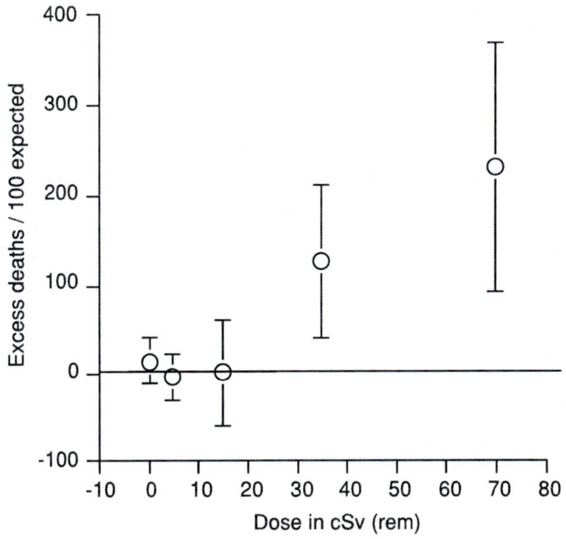


**Fig. 11** Excess deaths from leukemia per 100 "expected" among Japanese A-bomb survivors (1950–1990) versus their dose (Pierce et al. 1996). Error bars are 95% confidence limits

The risk is reported as −0.07/Sv with 90% confidence limits (−04, +0.3). There is surely no support for LNT here.

However, for the 146 leukemia deaths, they did report a positive risk versus dose relationship and vociferously claimed that this supports LNT. Their data are listed in Table 3. It is obvious from those data that there is no indication of any excess risk below 40 cSv (even the excess for >40 cSv is by only 1.4 standard deviations). The conclusion by the authors that this supports LNT is based on an analysis which arbitrarily discards the data in Table 3 for which o/e (observed/expected) is less than unity. They thus arbitrarily discard three of the seven data points.

A follow-up study (Cardis et al. 2007) by the same leader involved over 400,000 monitored workers in 154 facilities spread through 15 countries, and reported some confirmation for LNT, but several objections to this interpretation have been raised. For example, no information on smoking status, an important risk factor for cancer, was collected. There was no consideration given to non-occupational exposure; the average occupational exposure was 2 cSv and 90% were below 5 cSv, whereas the average person is exposed throughout life to about 25 cSv of non-occupational radiation with large variations, typically at least 10 cSv, depending on geography and medical treatment. Over and above

**Table 3** Leukemia deaths from International Association for Research on Cancer (IARC) Study (Cardis 1995). The final column is the ratio of observed to expected *O/E*

| Dose (cSv) | Observed | Expected | O/E |
|---|---|---|---|
| 0–1 | 72 | 75.7 | 0.95 |
| 1–2 | 23 | 21.2 | 1.08 |
| 2–5 | 20 | 21.8 | 0.92 |
| 5–10 | 12 | 11.3 | 1.06 |
| 10–20 | 9 | 7.8 | 1.15 |
| 20–40 | 4 | 5.5 | 0.73 |
| >40 | 6 | 2.6 | 2.3 |

these limitations, more sophisticated analysis of their data (Fornalski 2010) lead to the contrary conclusion, that LNT is not valid in the low dose region.

Many other studies have been reported on cancer risk vs dose for such normal occupational exposures. In response to heavy media coverage of some non-scientific reporting, a $10 million study (Matanoski 1991, 2008) was carried out by the U.S. Center for Disease Control and Prevention of workers in eight U.S. Navy shipyards involved in servicing nuclear-propelled ships. The study included 28,000 exposed workers and 33,000 age- and job-matched controls who worked on non-nuclear ships. The former group all had exposures above 0.5 cSv and average exposures of 5 cSv. The cancer mortality rate for the exposed was only 85% of that for the unexposed, a difference of nearly two standard deviations. Hiring procedures, medical surveillance, job type, and other factors were the same for both groups, so the often used explanation of "healthy worker effect" does not apply here—the study was specifically designed to eliminate that factor. The issue of non-occupational exposure was not addressed, but there was a high degree of homogeneity among the different worker groups being compared.

More discussion of "healthy worker effect" may be appropriate here (Fornalski 2010). In studies comparing mortality rates among employed workers with those of the general population, it is invariably found that employed workers have lower mortality, and it is widely understood that this results from the fact that unemployed persons may be unemployed because of health problems which lead to their earlier demise. However it has been pointed out (Monson 1986) that healthy worker effect should not apply to cancers occurring long after their initial employment because health problems leading to such cancers would not be apparent in a pre-employment medical exam. A direct test of this in Sweden (Gridley et al. 1999) comparing 545,000 employed women with 1,600,000 unemployed women found that the standardized cancer incidence rate for employed women was 1.05 (1.04–1.06) times higher than for the unemployed women. This would seem to eliminate healthy worker effects for cancer. Several other studies of cancer rates among people whose employment involves radiation exposure have been published:

- Studies of British radiologists compared with other British medical practitioners (Berrington et al. 2001) found that radiologists who began work in earlier years, when radiation exposure restrictions were much looser than recent standards, did experience excess cancers. But among the most recent cohort, radiologists who began work between 1955 and 1979, cancer mortality was only 0.71 (95% confidence limits, 0.49–1.00) times that for other medical practitioners who presumably had considerably lower radiation exposures.
- A study of medical X-ray workers in China (Wang et al. 2002) used cancer incidence rather than mortality, and a comparison group of workers in the same hospitals who were not involved with X-rays. The relative risks for earlier workers whose average exposure was 55 cGy were 2.4 for leukemias and 1.2 for solid cancers, while for the more recent workers whose average exposure was only 8.2 cGy, these risks were 1.73 for leukemias (based on 11 cases) and 1.06 (based on 232 cases) for solid cancers. For the recent workers, the differences from 1.0 are not statistically significant.
- A U.S. study of 146,000 radiologic technologists (Mohan et al. 2003) used only the total U.S. population as a comparison group and reported an SMR of 0.82 for all cancers, but a statistically significant increase among those first employed before 1940 as compared with those who began work after 1960.
- A review of studies of eight cohorts of radiologists and radiological technologists in various countries, comprising 270,000 monitored radiation workers (Yoshinaga et al. 2004), concluded that there was good evidence for excess cancers among the early workers, but no such evidence among more recent workers.
- A study of 22,000 monitored workers in the French nuclear power industry (Rogel et al. 2005) found that the cancer mortality rate was only 0.58 (90% confidence interval 0.49–0.68) times that of the general population of France. The authors attribute this to healthy worker effect, but such an explanation seems like an extreme "stretch" for explaining such a large effect. There was no evidence for increased cancer as a function of increasing radiation exposure.

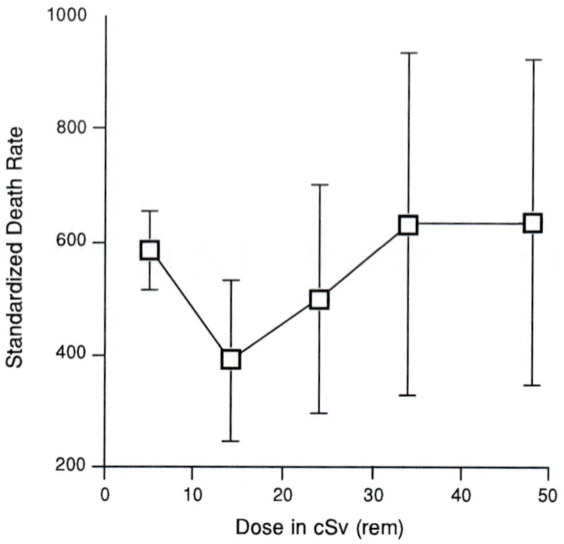


**Fig. 12** Standardized death rates per million person-years from breast cancer among Canadian women after irradiation in fluoroscopic examinations versus their radiation dose (Miller et al. 1989). Error bars are 95% confidence limits

Perhaps the most reasonable conclusion from studies of normally exposed radiation workers is that they give no conclusive information on effects of low level radiation. There is as much information suggesting zero or negative risk as information indicating the increased risk claimed by the IARC study. In any case, the fact that the monitored radiation received by the subjects was much lower than their non-occupational unmonitored exposures, make these data inherently of marginal significance.

## 6.2 Data Contradictory to LNT

There are substantial statistically robust human data contradictory to LNT. One example is for breast cancer among Canadian women exposed to frequent X-ray fluoroscopic examinations in a tuberculosis sanitorium (Miller et al. 1989); the data are shown in Fig. 12. While the statistical uncertainties are

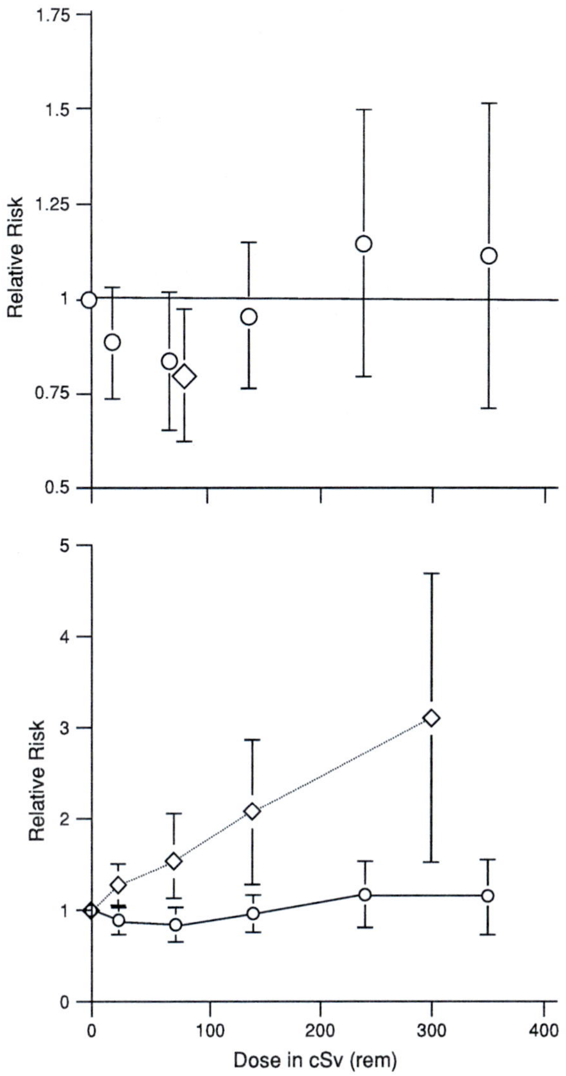


**Fig. 13** Relative risk of mortality from lung cancer versus dose to lung, with 95% confidence limits. In upper figure with expanded vertical scale, circles are from (Howe 1995) and diamond is from (Davis 1989). In lower figure (Howe 1995), solid line connects data from Canadian fluoroscopy patients, and dashed line connects data from A-bomb survivors

substantial, there seems to be a decrease in risk with increasing dose at least up to about 25 cSv.

The data on lung cancer among these Canadian women (Howe 1995), and also a one point study of 10,000 individuals in Massachusetts (Davis et al. 1989) are shown in Fig. 13. Here again we see a decrease in the low dose region, in this case extending at least up to 100 cSv. In Fig. 13, these data are compared with lung cancer data for the Japanese A-bomb survivors, and we see there a difference between the two data sets that is clearly statistically significant; the A-bomb survivor data gives a much higher risk at all doses. This is probably explained by the difference between the very high dose rate to the A-bomb survivors and the low dose rate from protracted fluoroscopic exams extending over many weeks. In any case, Fig. 13 must give one pause before accepting the widely practiced approach of using A-bomb survivor data to predict risks from low dose rate low-level radiation. Other arguments confirming the importance of dose rate, rather than only of total dose, have been expounded elsewhere (Tubiana and Aurengo 2005; Brooks 2011).

In 1957, there was an explosion in an incredibly mismanaged radioactive waste storage facility at the U.S.S.R. Mayak nuclear weapons complex in the Eastern Urals of Siberia, causing large radiation exposures to people in nearby villages. A follow-up on 7852 of these villagers (Kostyuchenko and Krestina 1994) found that the rate of subsequent cancer mortality was much lower among these than among unexposed villagers in the same area. The ratio for exposed to unexposed was $0.73 \pm 0.07$ for 4 cGy, $0.61 \pm 0.07$ for 12 cGy, and $0.72 \pm 0.12$ for 50 cGy (here, $\pm$indicate one standard deviation).

Studies are underway on the workers at this Mayak complex (Koshurnikova et al. 2002), among whom there have been many excess cancers, but exposures were generally quite high and the data reported give little information on the dose–response relationship in the low dose region.

Stimulation of the immune system by low level radiation is being used on an experimental basis for medical treatment of non-Hodgkin's lymphoma with total body and half body (trunk only) irradiation. This radiation was administered to one group of patients ("irradiated" group), but not to an otherwise similar "control" group, before both groups were given similar other standard treatments such as chemotherapy with or without accompanying high radiation doses to tumors. In one such study (Sakamoto et al. 1997), after nine years, 50% of the control group, but only 16% of the irradiated group had died. In a 25 year old study (Chaffey et al. 1976) with different standard treatments, 4-year survival was 70% for the irradiated group versus 40% for the controls. In another slightly later study (Choi et al. 1979) with a more advanced chemotherapy, 4-year survival was 74% for the irradiated group versus 52% for the control group. The information in the scientific literature is very supportive of using whole body or half body low level radiation to stimulate the immune system. The U.S. physicians have not utilized it but further applications are underway in Japan. The scientific basis for this treatment was reviewed by Liu (2007).

Potentially very significant human data on low level radiation is still in the preliminary research stage, but the results (Chen et al. 2004; Hwang et al. 2008) seem to be extremely interesting. In Taipai and other nearby areas of Taiwan, 1700 apartment units were built using steel contaminated with Cobalt-60, exposing 10,000 occupants for up to 20 years to an average of 40 cSv in total. From national Taiwan statistics, 232 cancer deaths would be expected from natural sources, and according to LNT, there should have been 70 additional cancer deaths due to this radiation. However, a total of only seven cancers have occurred among these people. Differences in the age distribution of the affected people as compared with the general population have not been carefully investigated, but preliminary estimates are that this might reduce the expected number of cancers by about 20%, a relatively insignificant change. It would seem to be very important to do a full epidemiological study of this situation, but the funding agencies have not been cooperative, despite heavy pressures from some segments of the scientific community.

Another source of information in the study of those affected by the Chernobyl accident (Jaworowski 2010). In comparison with the general population of Russia, a 15–30% deficit of solid cancer mortality was found among the Russian emergency clean up workers, and a 5% deficit solid cancer incidence among the population of most contaminated areas. The only positive effect was an increase in thyroid cancers among children, but this evidence has been questioned as to whether it was the consequence of increased screening.

The above described data deal with radiation by X-rays and gamma rays (and some neutrons for the A-bomb survivors). There are also impressive relevant data from radiation with alpha particles. One such study is of bone and head cancers among watch dial painters, chemists, and others occupationally exposed to ingested radium (Evans 1974). There were no tumors among those with exposures below 1,000 cGy, but for dose ranges centered about 1800, 3500, 7500 and 20,000 cGy, 25–38% in each category developed tumors. Elaborate analyses of these data show that a Linear no-threshold fit is statistically unsupportable and a threshold behavior is strongly suggested.

Several studies have reported that workers who inhaled plutonium, resulting in sizable radiation exposures to their lungs, have equal or lower lung cancer mortality rates than those not so exposed (Tokarskaya et al. 1997; Voelz et al. 1983; Gilbert et al. 1989).

Very strong evidence against LNT is provided by a very extensive study of lung cancer mortality rates, m, versus average radon exposure in homes for 1,729 U.S. counties—more than half of all U.S. counties, and including 90% of the U.S. population (Cohen 1995, 2006). Plots of age-adjusted rates are shown in Fig. 14a, c where, rather than showing individual points for each county, these are grouped into intervals of radon exposure (shown on the base-line along with the number of counties in each group) and plotted as the mean value of m for each group, its standard deviation indicated by the error bars, and the first and third quartiles of the distribution. Figures 14b, d shows these data corrected for prevalence of cigarette smoking. Note that when there are a large number of counties in an interval, the standard deviation of the mean is quite small. We see, in Fig. 14, a clear tendency for lung cancer rates, with or without correction for smoking prevalence, to decrease with increasing radon exposure, in sharp contrast to the increase expected from LNT, shown by the lines labeled "Theory". These data have been analyzed for over 500 possible confounding factors, including socioeconomic, geographic, environmental and ethnic associations (Cohen 2000), and the possible effects of an unrecognized confounding factor were investigated (Cohen 2006), but the conclusion remains firm that LNT fails very badly by grossly over estimating the cancer risk from low level radiation.

What has been interpreted as conflicting results were derived from a pooled study of seven case-control studies (Krewski et al. 2005); shown in Table 4. We see there that none of the data points give a very statistically significant excess lung cancer risk, but the pattern suggests an excess risk from radon exposures, although not necessarily increasing with exposure at least for the four lowest points, which comprise the region of significance in Fig. 14. A pooled study includes many complicated

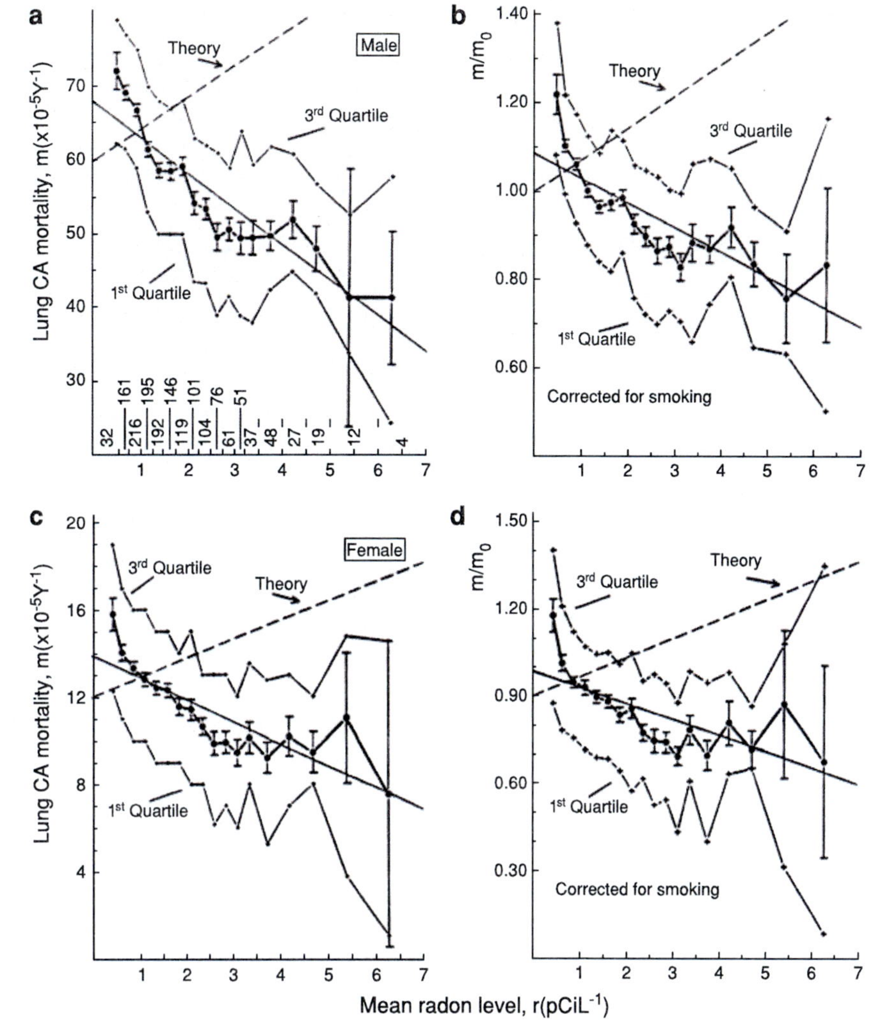


**Fig. 14** Age-adjusted lung cancer mortality rates, with and without correction for smoking prevalence, versus average radon level in homes for U.S. counties (Cohen 1995). See explanations in text. **a** and **c** are without smoking correction, for males and females respectively, and **b** and **d** are with smoking correction for males and females respectively

adjustments for differences among the different studies in the pool, and potential confounding factors with the adjustments for the few of them that are recognized might be a problem. If there is a conflict with Fig. 14, each of the several attempts to explain it as a problem with the latter have been shown to be completely implausible (Cohen 2006). Actually it is not clear that there is a conflict, because Fig. 14 is not a dose–response relationship for individuals exposed to radon, but rather is an experimental observation with extremely high statistical significance, to be compared with the prediction from LNT. That comparison indicates that the theory fails very badly, grossly over-estimating the risk from low level exposure. The results in Table 4 can hardly be interpreted as a test of LNT.

Results similar to those in Fig. 14 have been reported in more recent studies of radon versus lung cancer in the U.S. (Thompson et al. 2008) and Germany (Conrady et al. 2010).

## 6.3 Dependence of Latent Period on Dose

There is a substantial body of data, both on animals and on humans, indicating that the latent period between radiation exposure and cancer death increases with decreasing exposure; these have been reviewed by Cohen (1980) and by Raabe (1994). An example of results for dogs injected with alpha particle emitters (Dougherty and Mays 1969) is shown in Fig. 15. These

**Table 4** Odds ratios for lung cancer versus residential radon exposure from seven pooled case–control studies (Krewski et al. 2005)

| Radon level (Bq/m$^3$) | Odds ratio (95% C.I.) |
|---|---|
| <25 | 1.00 |
| 25–49 | 1.13 (0.95–1.35) |
| 50–74 | 1.09 (0.89–1.34) |
| 75–99 | 1.16 (0.91–1.48) |
| 100–149 | 1.248 (0.96–1.60) |
| 150–199 | 1.22 (0.87–1.71) |
| >199 | 1.37 (0.98–1.92) |

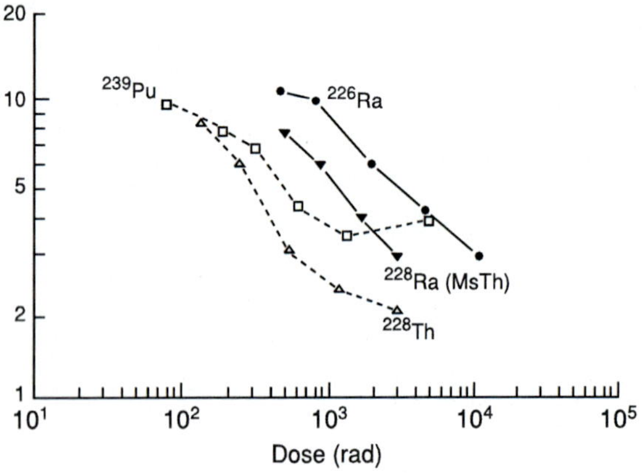


**Fig. 15** Survival time for beagle dogs who developed bone cancer from injections of various alpha emitting radioactive isotopes, versus dose to their bone at one year before death (Dougherty and Mays 1969)

observations lead to the obvious conclusion that for low enough exposures, the latent period exceeds the normal life span, so no actual cancers develop. Thus there is an effective threshold.

It has also been shown (Mitchel 2007) that the latent period before cancer death from a high dose exposure is delayed substantially by a preceding low dose exposure, even in situations where the probability of eventual cancer death is not affected.

This extended latency effect alone, even in the absence of all considerations discussed previously, would invalidate LNT as applied to low level radiation.

## 7 Other Side of Background

LNT predicts that biological effects of radiation below background levels should be less than those experienced at normal background. The few experiments to date (Smith et al. 2011) have shown that absence of background radiation has deleterious rather than beneficial effects.

## 8 Conclusion

The conclusion from the evidence reviewed in this paper is that the LNT fails very badly in the low dose region, grossly over-estimating the risk from low level radiation. This means that the cancer risk from the vast majority of normally encountered radiation exposures is much lower than given by usual estimates, and may well be zero or even negative.

**Acknowledgment** The author acknowledges a great debt to Myron Pollycove, Jerry Cuttler, and James Muckerheide for help in pointing out references involved in this paper.

## References

Anderson RE (1992) Effects of low dose radiation on the immune response. In: Calabrese EJ (ed) Biological effects of low level exposures to chemicals and radiation, Lewis, Chelsea, pp 95–112

Aurengo A et al (2005) Dose–effect relationship and estimation of the carcinogenic effects of low dose ionizing radiation. http://cnts.wpi.edu/rsh/docs/FrenchAcads-EN-FINAL.pdf

Azzam EI, de Toledo SM, Raaphorst GP, Mitchel REJ (1996) Low dose ionizing radiation decreases the frequency of neoplastic transformation to a level below spontaneous rate in C3H 10T1/2 cells. Radiat Res 146:369–373

Berrington A, Darby SC, Weiss HA, Doll R (2001) 100 years of observation on British radiologists; mortality from cancer and other causes, 1897–1997. Br J Radiol 74:507–519

Blankenbecker R (2010) Low dose pre-treatment for radiotherapy. Dose Response 8:534–553

Bonner WN (2004) Phenomena leading to cell survival values which deviate from linear-quadratic models. Mutation Res 568:33–39

Boothman DA et al (1996) Altered G1 checkpoint control determines adaptive survival responses to ionizing radiation. Mutation Res 358:143–153

Brooks AL (2011) Is a dose rate effectiveness factor needed following exposure to low total radiation doses delivered at low dose rates. Health Phys 100:262

Cai L, Liu SZ (1990) Induction of cytogenic adaptive response of somatic and germ cells in vivo and in vitro by low dose X-irradiation. Int J Radiat Biol 58:187–194

Cardis E et al (1995) Effects of low dose and low dose rates of external ionizing radiation: Cancer mortality among nuclear industry workers in three countries. Radiat Res 142:117–132

Cardis et al (2007) The 15 country collaborative study of cancer risk among radiation workers in the nuclear industry. Radiation Res 167:396–416

Chaffey JT, Rosenthal DS, Moloney WC, Hellman S (1976) Total body radiation as treatment for lymphosarcoma. Int J Radiat Oncol Biol Phys 1:399–405
Chen WL et al (2004) Is chronic radiation an effective prophylaxis against cancer?, J Am Physicians and Surgeons 9:6–10
Choi NC, Timothy AR, Kaufman SD, Carey RW, Aisenberg AC (1979) Low dose fractionated whole body irradiation in the treatment of advanced non-Hodgkin's lymphoma. Cancer 43:1636–1642
Cohen BL (1980) The cancer risk from low level radiation. Health Phys 39:659–678
Cohen BL (1995) Test of the Linear no-threshold theory of radiation carcinogenesis for inhaled radon decay products. Health Phys 68:157–174
Cohen BL (1998) The cancer risk from low level radiation. Radiat Res 149:525–526
Cohen BL (2000) Updates and extensions to tests of the Linear no-threshold theory. Technology 7:657–672
Cohen BL (2006) Test of the Linear no-threshold theory; rationale for procedures. Dode Response 3:369–390
Coleman MA et al (2005) Low dose irradiation alters the transcript profiles of human lymphoblastoid cells including genes associated with cytogenic radioadaptive response. Radiat Res 164:369–382
Conrady J, Lermbcke J, Thai DM (2010) Kritische Stellungnahme zu den epidemiologischen Grundlagen der emofohlenen Richtwerte der Radonkonzentration in Wohnungen-Ergebnisse einschlägiger Srudien in Sachsen RADIZ Schlema e.V.; Tagungsband der 5. Biophysikalischen Arbeitstagung in Bad Schlema, 10. - 20. Juni 2010: Biologische Wirkung niedriger Strahlendosen- Natürliche Strahlenexposition, Radonbalneotherapie und Strahlenschutz
Davis HG, Boice JD, Hrubec Z, Monson RR (1989) Cancer mortality in a radiation-exposed cohort of Massachusetts tuberculosis patients. Cancer Res 49:6130–6136
Dougherty TF, Mays CW (1969) In: Radiation Induced Cancer, International Atomic Energy Agency. Medical Physics Publishing Madison, p 361ff
Duport P (2001) A data base of cancer induction by low-dose radiation in mammals: overview and initial observations, Second Conference of the World Council of Nuclear Workers (WUNOC). Dublin, 2001
Evans RD (1974) Radium in man. Health Phys 27:497–510
Feinendegen LE (2005a) Evidence for beneficial low level radiation effects and radiation hormesis. Brit J Radiol 78:3–7
Feinendegen LE (2005b) Low doses of ionizing radiation: relationship between biological benefit and damage induction, a synopsis. World J Nuc Med 4:21–34
Feinendegen LE, Brooks AL, Morgan WF (2011) Biological consequences and health risks of low-level exposure to ionizing radiation: Commentary on the Workshop. Health Phys 100:247–259
Finkel MP, Biskis BO (1969) Pathological consequences of radiostrontium administered to fetal and infant dogs. Radiation biology of the fetal and juvenile mammal, AEC Symposium Series, vol. 17. In: Proceedings of the 9th Hanford Biology Symposium, pp 543–565
Finkel MP, Biskis BO (1962) Toxicity of Plutonium in mice. Health Phys 8:565–579
Finkel MP, Biskis BO (1968) Prog Exp Tumor Res 10:72ff
Finkel T, Holbrook NJ (2000) Oxidants, oxidative stress, and the biology of aging. Nature 408:239–247
Fornalski KW (2010) The healthy worker effect in nuclear industry workers. Dose Response 8:125–147
Fritz-Niggli H, Schaeppi-Buechi C (1991) Adaptive response to dominant lethality of mature and immature oocytes of D. Melanogaster to low doses of ionizing radiation: effects in repair-proficient and repair deficient strains. Int J Radiat Biol 59:175–184
Ghiassi-nejad M, Mortazavi SMJ, Beitollahi M, Cameron JR et al (2002) Very high background radiation areas of Ramsar, Iran: preliminary biological studies and possible implications. Health Phys 82:87–93
Gilbert ES, Petersen GR, Buchanan JA (1989) Mortality of workers at the Hanford site: 1945–1981. Health Phys 56: 11–25
Golder-Novoselsky E, Ding LH, Chen F, Chen DJ (2002) Radiation response in HSF cDNA microarray analysis, DOE Low dose radiation research program Workshop III. U.S. Dept. of Energy, Washington, DC
Gridley G et al (1999) Is there a healthy worker effect for cancer incidence among women in Sweden? Am J Ind Med 36:193–199
Hashimoto S, Shirato H, Hosokawa M et al (1999) The suppression of metastases and the change in host immune response after low-dose total body irradiation in tumor bearing rats. Radiat Res 151:717–724
Health Physics Society (HPS) (1996) Radiation Risk in Perspective: Position Statement of the Health Physics Society (adopted January 1996). Health Physics Society Directory and Handbook, 1998–1999, p 238. Also at http://www.hps.org
Heidenreich WF, Paretzke HG, Jacob B (1997) No evidence for increased tumor risk below 200 mSv in the atomic bomb survivor data. Radiat Envoron Biophys 36:205–207
Howe GR (1995) Lung cancer mortality between 1950 and 1987 after exposure to fractionated moderate dose rate ionizing radiation in the Canadian fluoroscopy cohort study and a comparison with lung cancer mortality in the atomic bomb survivors study. Radiat Res 142:295–304
Hwang SL et al (2008) Estimates of relative risks for cancer in a population after prolonged low dose rate radiation exposure. Radiat Res 170:143–148
Ina Y, Sakai K (2005) Activation of immunological network by chronic low dose rate irradiation in wild type mouse strains: analysis of immune cell populations and surface molecules. Int J Radiat Biol 81:721–729
Ina Y et al (2005) Suppression of thymic lymphoma induction by life-long low dose rate irradiation accompanied by immune activation of C57BL/6 mice. Radiat Res 163:153–158
Jaworowski J (2010) Observations on the Chernobyl disaster and LNT. Dose Response 8:148–171
Kaminski JM (2011) Non-radiation causes of carcinogenesis in the atomic bomb survivors. Health Phys 100:309
Kelsey KT, Memisoglu A, Frenkel A, Liber HL (1991) Human lymphocytes exposed to low doses of X-rays are less susceptible to radiation induced mutagenesis. Mutat Res 263:197–201
Kondo S (1993) Health effects of low level radiation. Medical Physics Publishing, Madison, pp 85–89

Koshurnikova NA et al (2002) Studies of the Mayak nuclear workers: health effects. Radiat Environ Biophys 41:29–31
Kostyuchenko VA, Krestina LY (1994) Long term irradiation effects in the population evacuated from the East-Urals radioactive trace area. Sci Total Environ 142:119–125
Krewski D et al (2005) Residential radon and risk of lung cancer: a combined analysis of 7 North American case–control studies. Epidemiology 16:137–145
Le XC, Xing JZ, Lee J, Leadon SA, Weinfeld M (1998) Inducible repair of thymine glycol detected by an ultrasensitive assay for DNA damage. Science: 280:1066–1069
Liu SJ (1992) Multilevel mechanisms of stimulatory effect of low dose radiation on immunity. In: Sugahara T, Sagan LA, Aoyama T (eds) Low Dose Irradiation and Biological Defense Mechanisms. Amsterdam, Elsevier Science, pp 225–232
Liu SZ (2003) Non-lineardose–response relationship in the immune system following exposure to ionizing radiation: mechanisms and implications, Nonlinearity in Biology, Toxicol Med 1:71–92
Liu SZ (2007) Cancer control related to stimulation of immunity by low-dose radiation. Dose–Response 5:39–47
Makinodan T, James SJ (1990) T cell potentiation by low dose ionizing radiation: possible mechanisms. Health Phys 59:29–34
Makinodan T (1992) Cellular and sub-cellular alteration in immune cells induced by chronic intermittent exposure in vivo to very low dose of ionizing radiation and its ameliorating effects on progression of autoimmune disease and mammary tumor growth. In: Sugahara T, Sagan LA, Aoyama T (eds) Low dose irradiation and biological defense mechanisms. Amsterdam, Elsevier Science, pp 233 237
Matanoski GM (1991) Health effect of low level radiation in shipyard workers, Final report. Report No. DOE DE-AC02–79 EV10095; U.S. Dept of Energy See Tables 3.6B and 3.6D
Matanoski GM (2008) Risk of radiation in U.S. shipyard workers. J. Radiation Res.49:83–91
Michel REJ (2010) The dose window for radiation protective adaptive response. Dose Response 8:192–208
Miller AB, Howe GR, Sherman GJ et al (1989) Mortality from breast cancer after irradiation during fluoroscopic examinations in patients being treated for tuberculosis. N Engl J Med 321:1285–1289
Miller RC, Randers-Pehrson G, Geard CR, Hall EJ, and Brenner DJ (1999) The oncogenic transforming potential of the passage of single alpha particles through mammalian cell nuclei. Proc Natl Acad Sci 96:19–22
Mitchel REJ, (2006) Low doses of radiation are protective in vitro and in vivo: Evolutionary origins. Dose-Response 4:75–90.
Mitchel REJ (2007) Low doses of radiation reduce risk in vivo. Dose Response 5:1–10
Mitchel REJ et al (2003) Low doses of radiation increase the latency of spontaneous lymphomas and spinal osteosarcomas in cancer prone, radiation sensitive Trp53 heterozygous mice. Radiat Res 159:320–327
Mohan AK et al (2003) Cancer and other causes of mortality among radiologic technicians in the United States. Int J Cancer 103:259–267
Monson RR (1986) Observations on the healthy worker effect. J Occup Med 28:425–433
Morgan WF (2011) Radiation induced genomic instability. Health phys 100(3):280–281
Pierce DA, Shimizu Y, Preston DL, Vaeth M, Mabuchi K (1996) Studies of the mortality of atomic bomb survivors, Report 12, Part 1, Cancer: 1950–1990. Radiat Res 146:1–27
Pollycove M, Feinendagen L (2001) Biologic responses to low doses of ionizing radiation: detriment vs hormesis; Part 1. J Nuclear Med 42:17N–27N
Preston DL et al (2004) Effect of recent changes in atomic bomb survivor dosimetry on cancer mortality risk estimates. Radiat Res 162:377–389
Raabe OG (1994) Three dimensional models of risk from internally deposited radionuclides. In: dosimetry internal adiation, Raabe OG (eds) Madison. Medical Physics, WI, pp 633–656
Redpath JL, Antoniono RJ (1998) Induction of a rapid response against spontaneous neoplastic transformation in vitro by low dose gamma radiation. Rad Res 149:517–520
Redpath JL, Lu Q, Lao X, Molloi S, Elmore E (2003) Low doses of diagnostic X-rays protect against neoplastic transformation in vitro. Int J Radiat Biol 79:235–240
Rodgers BE, Holmes KM (2008) Radio-Adaptive Response to Environmental Exposures at Chernobyl. Dose Response 6:209–221
Rogel A et al (2005) Mortality of workers exposed to ionizing radiation at the French National Electricity company. Am J Ind Med 47:72–82
NCRP (2001) Evaluation of the linear non-threshold dose–response model for ionizing radiation, NCRP Publication 136. Bethesda, MD
NCRP (National Council on Radiation Protection, Measurements) (1995) Principles and application of collective dose to radiation protection, NCRP Publication 121. Bethesda, MD
Sakamoto K, Myogin M, Hosoi Y et al (1997) Fundamental and clinical studied on cancer control with total and upper half body irradiation. J Jpn Soc Ther Radiol Oncol 9: 161–175
Scott BR (2010) Special issue introduction. Dose–Response 8:122–124
Shadley JD, Dai GQ (1992) Cytogenic and survival adaptive responses in G-1 phase human lymphocytes. Mutat Res 265:273–281
Smith GB, Grof Y, Navarette A, Guilmette RA (2011) Exploring biological effects of low level radiation from the other side of background. Health Phys 100:263–265
Tanooka H (2001) Threshold Dose–Response in radiation carcinogenesis: an approach from chronic beta-irradiation experiments and a review of non-tumor doses. Int J Radiat Biol 77:541–551
Thompson RE, Nelson DF, Popkin Z (2008) Case-control study of lung cancer risk from residential radon exposure in Worcester County. Massachusetts Health
Tokarskaya ZB, Okladlnikova ND, Belyaeva ZD, Drozhko EG (1997) Multifactorial analysis of lung cancer dose–response relationships for workers at the Mayak Nuclear Enterprise. Health Phys 73:899–905
Tubiana M, Aurengo A (2005) Dose effect relationship and estimation of the carcinogenic effects of low doses of ionizing radiation. Int J Low Radiat 2:1–19

Ullrich RL, Storer JB (1979) Influence of gamma radiation on the development of neoplastic diseases in mice: II solid tumors. Radiat Res 80:317–324

UNSCEAR (United Nations Scientific Committee on Effects of Atomic Radiation) (1994) Report to the General Assembly, *Annex B: Adaptive Response*. United Nations, New York

Voelz GL, Wilkinson CS, and Acquavelle JF (1983) An update of epidemiologic studies of plutonium workers. Health Phys 44 Suppl (1):493–503

Wang JX et al (2002) Cancer incidence and risk estimation among medical X-ray workers in China, 1950–1995. Health Phys 82:455–466

Yamaoka K (1991) Increased SOD activities and decreased lipid peroxide in rat organs induced by low X-irradiation. Free Radical Biol Med 11:3–7

Yin E et al (2005) Gene expression changes in mouse brain after exposure to low-dose ionizing radiation. Int J Radiat Biol 79:759–775

Yoshinaga S et al (2004) Cancer risks among radiologists and radiologic technologists: review of epidemiologic studies. Radiology 233:313–321

Yukawa O et al (2005) Induction of radical scavenging ability and suppression of lipid peroxidation in rat liver microsomes following whole body low dose X-irradiation. J Radiat Biol 81:681–688

Zaichkina SI et al (2003) Low doses of radiation decrease the level of spontaneous and gamma induced chromosomal mutagenesis in bone marrow cells of mice in vivo. Rariats Biol Radioecol 43:153–155

# Image Quality in CT: Challenges and Perspectives

Thomas L. Toth

## Contents




T. L. Toth (✉)
GE Healthcare, Brookfield, WI, USA
e-mail: Thomas.toth@plexar.com



**Abstract**

This chapter discusses an overview of the complexities of CT image quality. It focuses primarily on the image quality of conventional CT scanners in common clinical use and includes some references to emerging new technologies and reconstruction methods. A review of the fundamental physics of a CT image is provided along with an explanation of why low kV scanning can be a useful dose reduction strategy if approached cautiously. Measurable image characteristics for spatial resolution, image noise and low contrast detectability are discussed along with a summary of image artifacts. Particular emphasis is given to CT noise and low contrast detectability, since these are the image quality characteristics most influenced by dose usage. Noise and detectability are the essence of the clinical dose dilemma: what do I need to detect and how much dose is necessary to be able to confidently detect its presence or absence?


## 1 Introduction

CT Image quality is a complex topic with different meanings and emphasis that depends on the individual, their experience, area of expertise and issues of the moment. Image quality (IQ) is a non-specific term that is used to describe in qualitative way the goodness of an overall image or the goodness of some image characteristic. For CT images of human anatomy, the radiologist has an intuitive expectation of image quality based on training and experience.


D. Tack et al. (eds.), *Radiation Dose from Multidetector CT*, Medical Radiology. Diagnostic Imaging,
DOI: 10.1007/174_2011_482, © Springer-Verlag Berlin Heidelberg 2012

For an image scientist or physicist, image quality usually takes the form of measurable image characteristics. The reality of a CT image (ideal image) is based on the physics of how X-rays interact with matter and the mathematical reconstruction processes used to produce images from the X-ray projections. In this chapter we first provide a simplified understanding of what a CT image represents and why Hounsfield Units (HU) do not necessarily have constant values. We then discuss measureable image characteristics and artifacts and how they relate to clinical diagnostic challenges and dose management.

Imaging scientists generally classify characteristics of CT image quality in terms of: HU accuracy, spatial resolution, noise, low contrast detectability and artifacts. Spatial resolution relates to how well small object features are preserved in the image. Noise is generally considered to be undesired random variations that are imposed upon the ideal image. Noise has a definite texture or look that depends on various factors. Noise depends on the intensity of the post patient detected X-rays and is inversely associated with dose and the efficiency of the scanner and its image reconstruction process. These factors influence the appearance and intensity of the noise contained in the image. Image noise obscures small low contrast objects and is the most important characteristic associated with dose utilization. Artifacts are systematic distortions and misrepresentations of features within an ideal image that are generally not associated with how much dose is used.

In this chapter we will focus primarily on image quality for conventional CT systems that are in widespread medical practice. We will discuss the ideal CT image, spatial resolution, noise and artifacts; how they are measured and give some indication of how they affect diagnostic radiology and what can be done to minimize detrimental effects. As is the case with many multi-dimensional situations there are often difficult trade-offs that improve some aspects of image quality while degrading others. We will also briefly discuss some of the emerging technologies (dual energy scanning, nonlinear filtering and iterative reconstruction methods) that will have a profound effect on many of the IQ issues associated with current conventional CT.

## 2 The Ideal CT Image: The Simplified Physics of a Conventional CT Image

It is important to understand that the ideal CT image is not a constant even if unaffected by spatial resolution blurring, noise or artifacts. HU values that comprise the image will have a range of values that depend on various factors associated with fundamental X-ray physics principles (McCollough 1975). HU values that are used as indicators for various medical conditions can have a range of acceptable values that could overlap with unacceptable values. CT images reconstructed by conventional kVp energy integrating systems are most susceptible to HU variations. Emerging dual energy acquisition and reconstruction methods allow an image to be produced at a specific photon energy and hence, the HU variation can be substantially controlled.

### 2.1 The CT Image

A CT image (Fig. 1) represents a cross-sectional map of effective X-ray linear attenuation coefficients of the patient's anatomy. A linear attenuation coefficient (designated by the symbol $\mu$) is a measure of how photons interact with matter. $\mu$ represents the exponential probability that an X-ray photon will be absorbed or scattered from its path. The value of $\mu$ is dependent on the material, its density and the energy of the X-ray photons. The matrix of effective $\mu$ values that comprise a CT image are estimated from a set of X-ray measurements using a mathematical reconstruction process.

The CT attenuation map is generated in terms of Hounsfield Units (HU), named after Sir Godfrey Hounsfield, who built the first CT scanner in 1971 based on the theoretical underpinnings of CT scanning developed by Allan Cormack in 1963. HU values are the ratio of the effective $\mu$ of each image pixel relative to the $\mu$ of water $\mu_w$) times 1000−1000.

Hence air, with a $\mu$ of virtually zero, has a CT value of −1000 HU and water has a value of 0 HU. Most human soft tissues are in the range of −50 to 100 HU. Dense bone is generally above 900 HU and metal prosthesis and dental fillings may exceed 3000 HU.

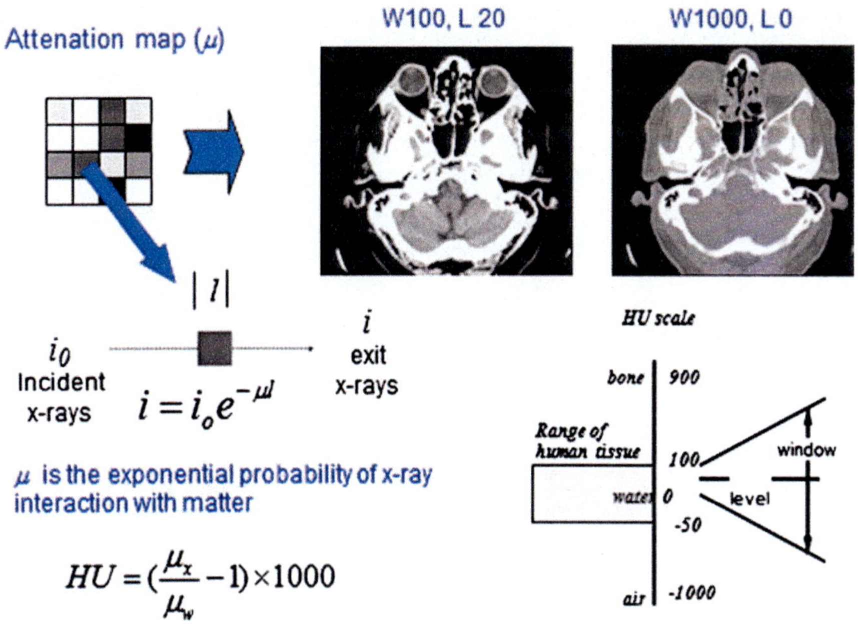


**Fig. 1** The physical meaning of a CT image

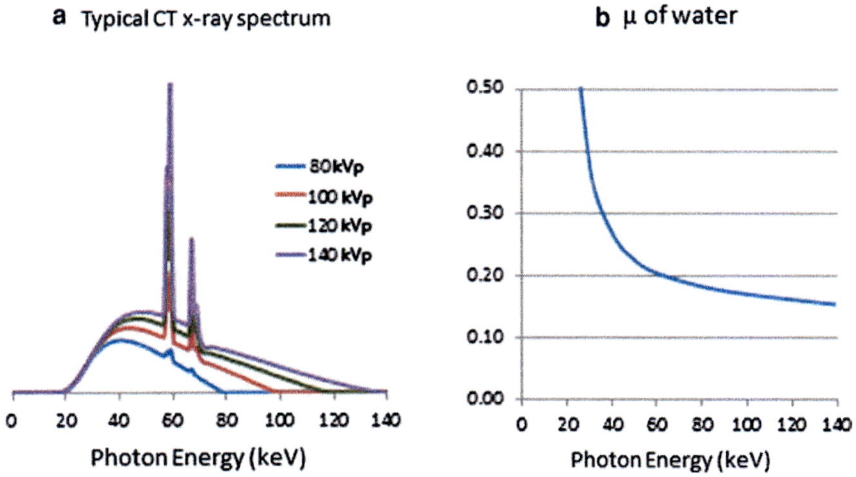


**Fig. 2** Typical CT X-ray spectrum and linear attenuation coefficient (μ) of water

## 2.2 HU Values: Why They are not Constants

HU values are not constants since the X-ray tube output consists of a range of photon energies and $\mu$ is not a constant but is a function of photon energy. A typical CT X-ray spectrum along with the μ for water is shown in Fig. 2. Since μ for water increases at lower energies, more lower energy photons are removed than higher energy photons as X-rays pass through increasing lengths of material. This effect is referred to as beam hardening. Since the effective energy of the beam is increasing with increasing lengths of material, the beam is harder to stop. As a result, the effective μ of water (Fig. 3a), as well as μ for other materials is not constant.

Since a CT image is a map of effective μ values relative to the μ of water, CT reconstruction algorithms apply a water beam hardening correction to force the effective μ of water to be a constant. Otherwise water phantom images would be cupped (See Fig. 10a in the artifacts section). The effective μ of other materials relative to water will depend on the μ of the material and the effective energy of the beam.

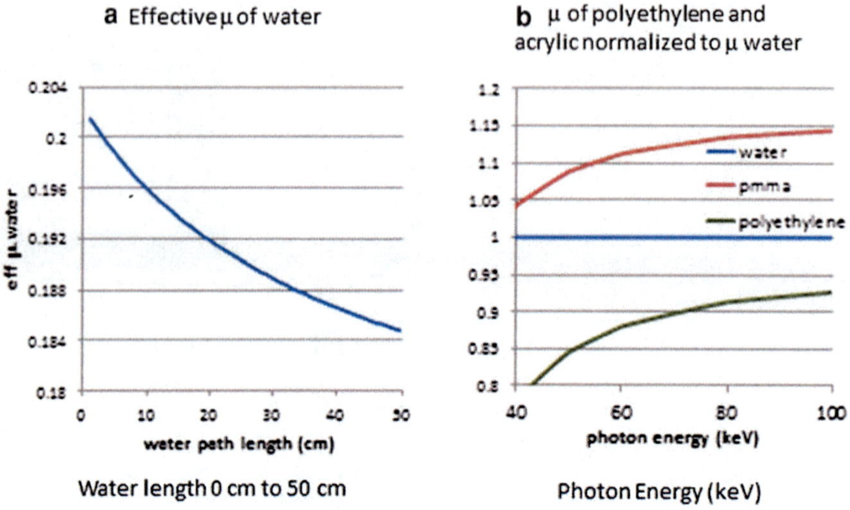


**Fig. 3** Effective μ of water, polyethylene and acrylic for a typical 120 kVp CT X-ray beam spectrum

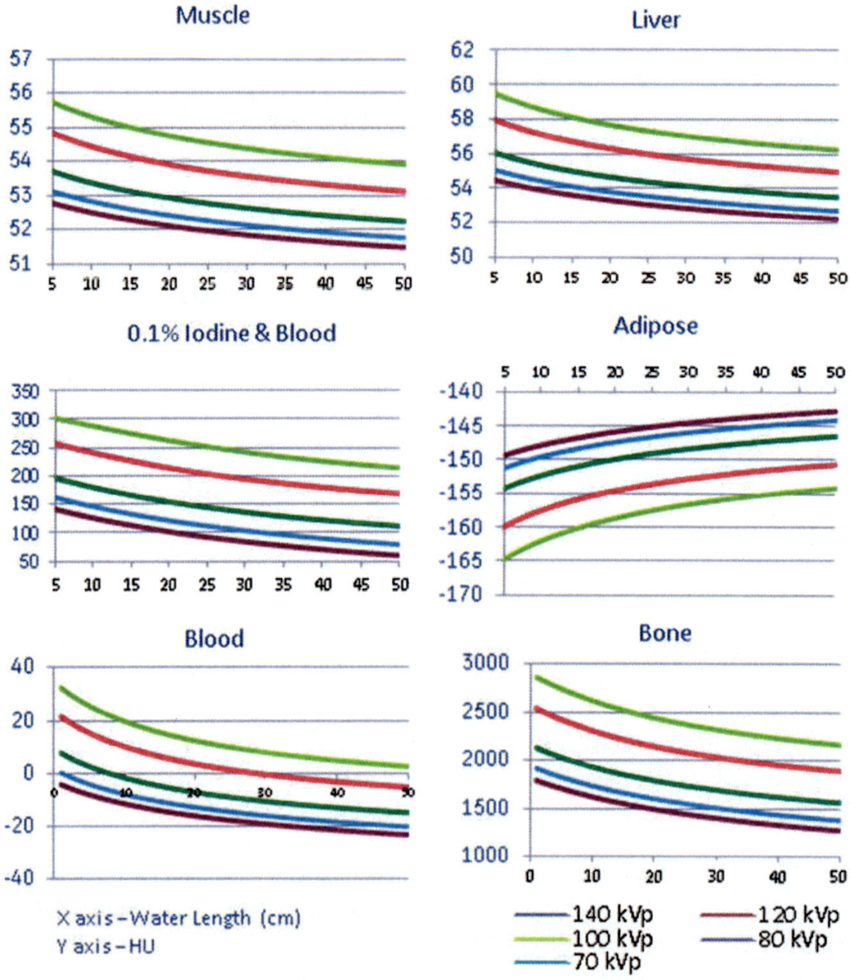


**Fig. 4** Computer-simulated HU values for various ICRU 44 tissue models and kVp settings for a typical CT X-ray beam spectrum. The values represent a 1 cm diameter sample of the tissue at the center of a water cylinder with a range of diameters from 5 to 50 cm. This figure is intended to demonstrate a model of the CT physics and should not be used as an explicit predictor of in vivo tissue

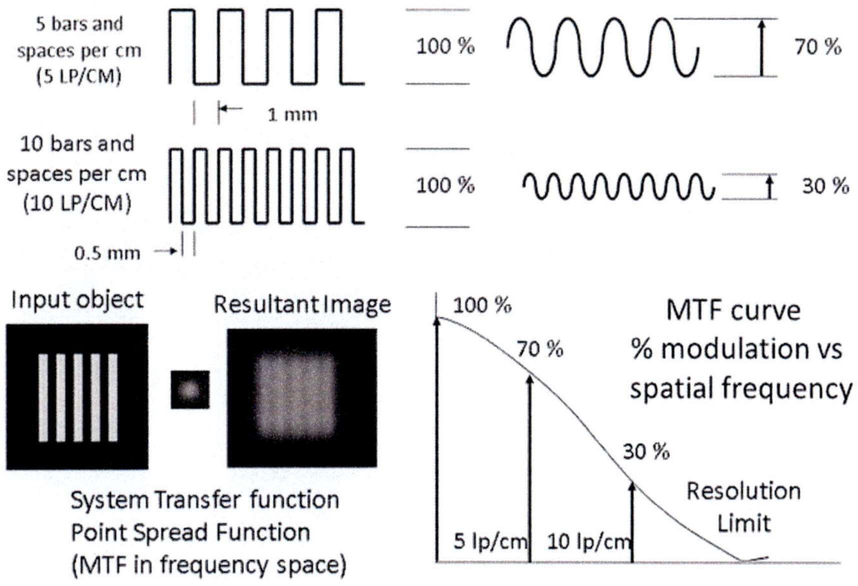


**Fig. 5** The spatial transfer function of the CT system blurs the spatial detail of the resulting image. The spatial resolution is a measure of the spatial transfer function and is typically given as a system MTF

As shown in Fig. 3b, the μ of Acrylic and polyethylene increases relative to water as the effective energy increases. The effective energy is dependent on the selected kVp, X-ray filtration (materials and tissue in the path of the beam) and the size of the patient being scanned. Generally the effective energy for a typical CT image ranges between 50 and 80 keV.

The implication for human tissue is summarized in Fig. 4 which shows simulated CT values for various tissue models based on ICRU report 44. The simulations assume a typical CT source filtration of 7 mm aluminum equivalent and a one cm diameter sample of the tissue at the center of a water cylinder with a range of diameters from 5 to 50 cm. For each chart, the Y axis is the HU value and the X axis is the length of water beam hardening for the effective energy. The different colors represent kVp selections from 70 to 140 kVp. Figure 4 is intended to demonstrate a model of the CT physics and should not be used as an explicit predictor of in vivo tissue.

In each case the difference in HU value (contrast relative to water) decreases with increased kVp settings and larger water cylinder diameters since these changes increase effective energy. These HU variations in the image are a normal result of the behavior of the X-ray physics processes and can be employed to reduce dose. The increased contrast with lower kVp on smaller patients can provide the same contrast-to-noise ratio (CNR) in the image at a lower dose, depending on the diagnostic problem. In general, the contrast-enhanced tissues and bone will provide the greatest contrast-to-noise ratio increase.

For example, note that for a 20 cm water cylinder, the model for unenhanced blood increases by 25 HU at 70 kVp relative to 120 kvp. However, contrast-enhanced blood modeled with a 0.01% Iodine solution increases by 140 HU for the same kvp change. If the mA is increased at the 70 kVp setting to achieve the same CNR for the contrast-enhanced blood as at 120 kVp, a dose savings will result.

Be aware, however, that the same CNR means that the image noise increases along with the contrast. In addition, the non-contrast enhanced tissue will have a reduced CNR so the full dose reduction may not be possible since the CNR does not increase in the same way for all tissue in the image. The nosier appearance of the image may be helped somewhat by increasing in viewing window width setting. Readjusting the window will help maintain the same gray scale relationship with the CNR, at least for those tissues for which the contrast has increased.

Although not shown, the effective energy also increases with effective target angle. The target angle is the angle between the ray path to a detector row and the surface of the X-ray tube target. The detector rows

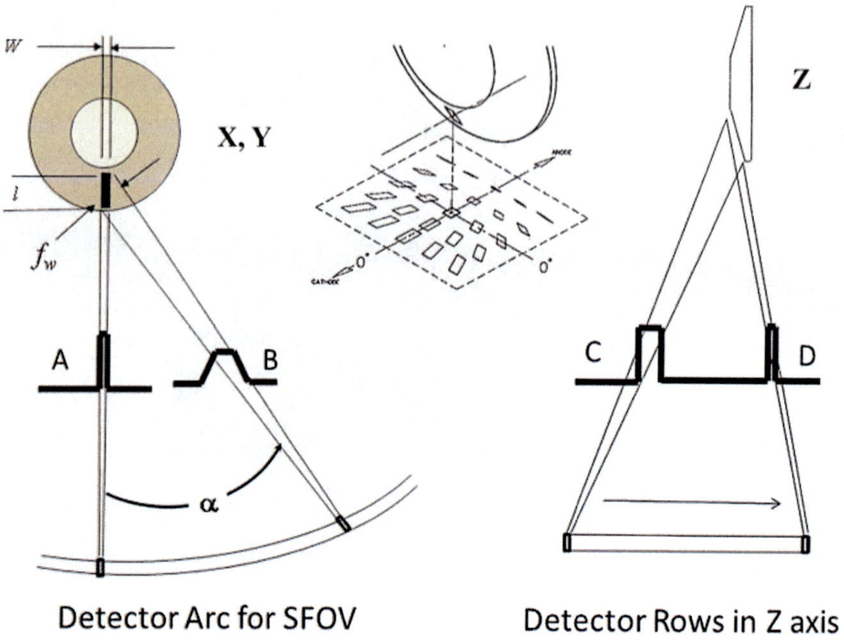


**Fig. 6** Effect of the X-ray tube focal distribution function on spatial resolution

toward the anode side (Fig. 6d), can have a somewhat higher effective energy. This can result in HU variations for contrast-enhanced tissue as a function Z-axis position along the patient.

## 3 In-plane Spatial Resolution

In-plane spatial resolution is a measure of the ability of the system to reproduce small features within the image slice plane. The input object is convolved or blurred by the point spread function (transfer function) of the CT system (Yester and Barns 1977). The spatial resolution of a CT system (sometimes called the high contrast resolution) is typically specified in terms of a modulation transfer function (MTF). An MTF response curve represents the modulation factor as a function of spatial frequency. For example, the 1 mm bars and spaces, shown in Fig. 5, have a spatial frequency of 5 line pairs per centimeter (lp/cm) since 5 cycles of bar and space pairs are contained in a one cm. If the system transfer function at a spatial frequency of 5lp/cm is a factor of 0.7 times the original amplitude, then the modulation at this spatial frequency would be 70%. This means that only 70% of amplitude of the input object at this spatial frequency is transferred to the image. The curve of the % modulation as a function of spatial frequency is the MTF curve (Fig. 5). The resolution limit is where the MTF approaches the first zero crossing.

Data sheets for CT systems will usually state the spatial response in terms of the spatial frequency at some percent modulation; for example 4lp/cm at 50% MTF. Such specifications are only a simple single statement of the overall resolution response of the system. Although these specifications have some utility in comparing systems, they are only a sample of the overall performance of the system. The point spread function is a two-dimensional function that cannot be fully represented by a one-dimensional MTF chart or by a simple specification such as the 50 or 10% modulation point. In addition, the spatial resolution is not generally symmetric but changes as a function of location within the scan field of view (SFOV).

The resolution in the image is a function of a number of factors relating to the design of the scanner and the selected protocol operating parameters. The focal distribution function (size and shape of the focal spot), the detection function (active width of the detector pixels), the sample spacing between rays in a projection, number of projections per gantry revolution and the reconstruction process including the selected algorithm.

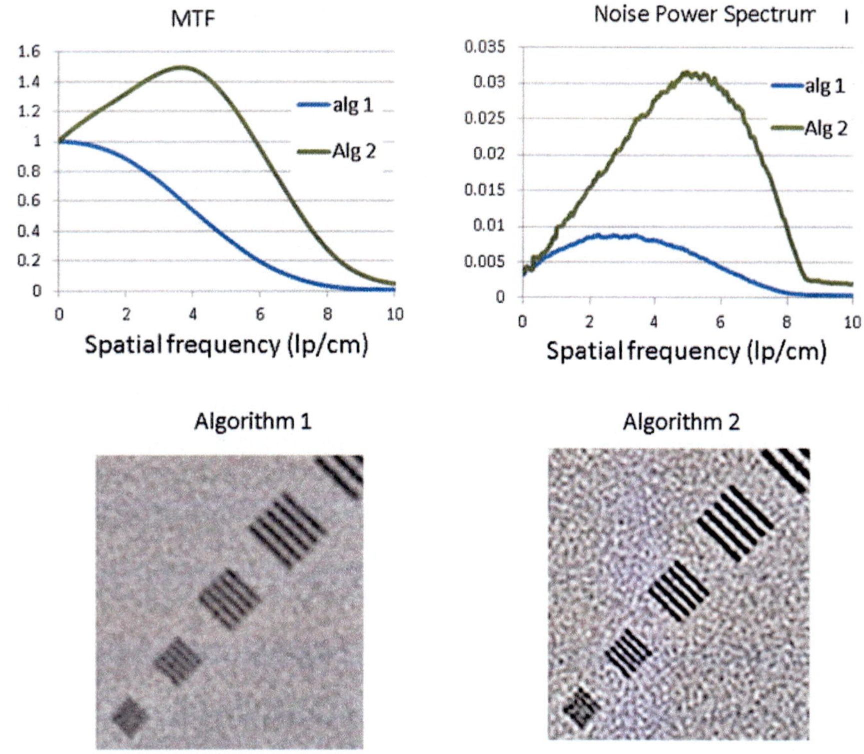


**Fig. 7** Example reconstruction algorithms and the effect on the image

The projected focal distribution function is primarily responsible for the variable (non-stationary) nature of the spatial resolution within an image. The X-ray target is sloped at an angle (typically from 7 to 14°) as in Fig. 6. This is done to spread the heat on the target to allow high tube currents to be applied while maintaining a small projected focal spot size. A small size is needed to maintain good resolution. The central ray in Fig. 6a has the narrowest width and thus the best inherent spatial resolution. The envelope between the focal distribution function and a detector is called the X-ray optical function. A small object (a point for example) within the X-ray optical function cannot be resolved any smaller than the width and sensitivity of the sampled beam at that location. As the fan angle distance increases from the SFOV center (isocenter), the projected width of the focal spot increases as shown in Fig. 6b. Thus the radial resolution in the image is reduced as the distance from isocenter increases. Spatial resolution is generally decreased throughout the image for the larger focal spot sizes that may be required when higher tube currents are employed.

The azimuthal resolution may also have a tendency to decrease with increasing distance from isocenter depending on the number of views sampled during one gantry revolution. Consider a ray though isocenter. The distance between successive angular view samples depends on the number of views (projections) per rotation and increases with the distance from isocenter. Since the acquisition system is effectively integrating (accumulating a measurement) over the duration between samples, there is an increase in azimuthal blurring with distance from isocenter since the azimuthal spatial distance between samples is increasing. Thus, the spatial resolution will generally be highest near isocenter and degrade with increasing distance. This effect can be reduced by choosing modes that increase the number of views per rotation since this reduces the sample spacing. In addition, resolution is generally best within the central SFOV region. This is another reason that centering the patient can be important.

The reconstruction algorithm, sometimes called the reconstruction filter or kernel, also has a significant effect on the resolution available in the image.

These algorithms can reduce or enhance the spatial resolution of edges but they cannot increase the resolution beyond the inherent X-ray optical response limit. Two example algorithms are shown in Fig. 7. The MTF for algorithm 1 is typical for routine scans while algorithm 2 is edge-enhanced and includes a slight resolution increase (zero crossing of the MTF occurs at a slightly higher spatial frequency). The smallest resolution pattern is not resolved with algorithm 1. Although the smallest pattern is resolved in algorithm 2, the larger patterns are darker due to increased modulation intensity while the surrounding area is lighter due to an overshooting effect from the edge enhancement. The noise pattern is also much more intense with algorithm 2 as seen in the noise power spectrum (discussed later). High resolution algorithms, especially edge-enhanced algorithms, amplify both the MTF and the noise. They can significantly change the appearance of an image but generally cannot change the inherent signal-to-noise ratio or increase the inherent spatial resolution limit. The inherent spatial resolution limit is the zero crossing of the lowest spatial frequency element of the image chain.

## 4 Z-Axis Resolution (Slice Sensitivity Profile)

Spatial resolution in the Z axis is also a critical aspect of CT image quality especially for reformatted 3D image representations. Although Z-axis spatial resolution could be described by an MTF curve in the same manner as for in-plane resolution, it is often simply referred to as the slice thickness. The slice thickness is the full width at half maximum intensity of the slice sensitivity profile (SSP). For multislice CT systems, the ray envelope in the Z axis between the focal spot and a detector cell is essentially responsible for the fundamental Z-axis resolution limit in much the same way as for in-plane ray samples. Z-axis resolution is also not a constant over all detector rows, but is altered by the projected length of the focal distribution function. The detector rows toward the cathode side of the tube (Fig. 6c) will see a larger focal spot than the rows toward the anode side (Fig. 6d) and thus the cathode side rows will have a wider inherent slice sensitivity profile and reduced Z-axis resolution.

Reconstruction processing also affects the slice sensitivity profile. The most notable example is helical scanning where combinations of detector row data are weighted and included in the reconstructed image to produce larger slices than the inherent detector row aperture limitation. The weighting of various detector row data defines the shape of the slice sensitivity profile and hence determines the Z-axis resolution. Not so obvious, are the effects of three-dimensional axial reconstruction algorithms for multislice systems. Three-dimensional back projection algorithms weight and combine data rows from the larger cone angles as a function of distance from isocenter. Three-dimensional reconstruction methods significantly reduce cone beam artifacts (discussed later) but can cause the outer detector rows to have larger slice sensitivity profiles than the rows near the center of the detector where the X-ray samples are more perpendicular to the detector face.

In addition to the Z-axis spatial resolution, the SSP can affect the contrast of objects within the image. The contrast of an object will be reduced if it is smaller than the extent of the SSP. This reduction in contrast occurs due to partial volume averaging of the contrast of the object with the contrast of the surrounding region within the slice. Thus the contrast of small ellipsoid objects within an image is often increased by using narrower slices. This contrast increase is slightly offset however by the increased noise with narrower slices. Narrower slices are noisier since fewer photons contribute to the generation of the image.

## 5 Detectability, Image Noise and Dose

The image science regarding object detectability in the presence of noise is a very complicated topic and even a simple review is well beyond the scope of this chapter. Although we risk oversimplifying the subject, we will try to provide an intuitive understanding of some of the basic principles. A good review of concepts related to medical imaging can be found in (ICRU54 1996). A comprehensive study of the subject can be found in the textbook by Harrison Barrett and Kyle Myers (Barrett 2004).

The ability to detect small low contrast features in CT images is one of the primary reasons that CT has

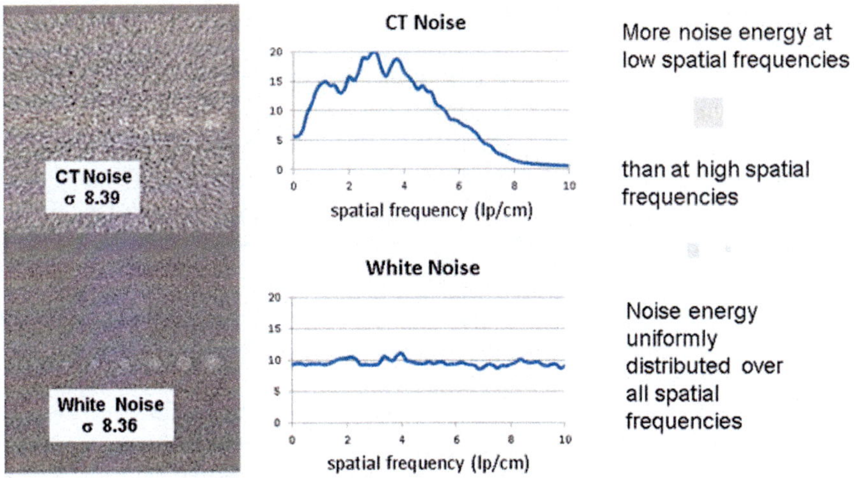


**Fig. 8** CT image noise compared to white noise with the same standard deviation

become such an integral part of medical practice (Hsieh 2003). It allows subtle low contrast tumors and lesions to be detected in soft tissue that may not otherwise be apparent using other diagnostic X-ray imaging methods. The low contrast detectability (LCD) performance of a CT system is a very important characteristic since it is a measure of the ability to identify low contrast features at a low X-ray dose. This is the essence of the clinical CT dose reduction problem: what do I need to detect and how much dose is it necessary to use to be able to confidently detect its presence or absence.

The inherent detectability of a low contrast object in an image is related to its shape, size, contrast and the noise and background environment within which it resides. Noise can obscure small subtle low contrast features. When such features are clinically important, noise must be low enough to permit correctly identifying them from the background. Noise in a CT image is the random variation imposed on the true HU values of each pixel and is related to dose as well as other factors associated with the design and conditions of operation of the scanner. As the dose is increased, the noise decreases approximately with the inverse square root of the X-ray intensity. The use of insufficient dose subjects the patient to the risk of an inaccurate diagnosis if the noise is too high; however, the use of too much dose subjects the patient to unnecessary radiation. Thus, noise and its effects on LCD is one of the most vital characteristics of a CT image.

## 5.1 The Nature of CT Noise

Image noise was carefully studied and characterized in conjunction with the development of television by Albert Rose while at RCA in the 1940s (Rose 1974). Many of Rose's early findings are directly applicable to X-ray images. Rose found that the diameter and contrast of an object must be 5 times greater than the noise in a uniform background for 100% detectability confidence. The noise that Rose studied is referred to as white noise since the noise energy is uniformly distributed as a function of spatial frequency. That is, if you think of noise as random blobs of various sizes, the intensity is similar for the largest to the smallest size blobs for white noise. The small blobs are the higher spatial frequencies while the larger blobs are the lower spatial frequencies. As discussed above, spatial frequencies in CT are generally presented on a line pair per centimeter scale (l p/cm). For example, a spatial frequency of 5 line pairs per centimeter means that five pairs of 1 mm light and 1 mm darker blobs will fit into a 1 cm length. White noise can be accurately characterized by a simple standard deviation measurement and used to predict detectability in accordance with the Rose criteria. Although it is common to state CT noise as a standard deviation value, this practice can be very misleading since CT image noise is not white noise as studied by Rose.

The CT image noise spectrum is colored by the filtered back projection image reconstruction process such that the noise intensity changes as a function of spatial frequency. The consequences of this are demonstrated in Fig. 8.

The two noise patterns in Fig. 8 both have a standard deviation of about 8.4 yet the small low contrast objects surrounded by white noise are much easier to see than in the CT noise. This occurs since the CT noise spectrum, in this example, is more intense at the lower spatial frequencies than it is for the white noise. As a result, the larger noise blobs (lower spatial frequencies) are similar in size and intensity to the small diameter low contrast regions. To recognize these objects, they must be different from the background environment. The small objects in this example are similar in appearance to the noise and therefore they are effectively camouflaged and hidden. In addition the higher intensity of the low frequency noise content makes the edges of the larger low contrast regions appear more ragged. Since the noise at the low spatial frequencies for the white noise is less intense than for the CT noise in Fig. 8, the same small low contrast objects are more visible in the white noise. Thus, standard deviation as a measure of image noise is not very useful metric to compare dose utilization of CT systems or to assume that it relates to LCD performance. Standard deviation is useful for comparing the relative changes in noise intensity only when the spatial frequency shape remains unchanged. It is deceptive to compare the standard deviations of image noise with different spatial frequency shapes.

The noise power spectrum (NPS) shown in the charts of Fig. 8 is a more complete description of the image noise. The NPS shows the intensity of noise as a function of spatial frequency. Unfortunately, the NPS is not a simple single value such a standard deviation. The complexity of the NPS, however, can be more completely described indirectly in terms of a low contrast detectability (LCD) specification. An LCD specification identifies an object, generally of a specific diameter and contrast, that is detectable in a noise field at some dose. Unfortunately, the methods and the confidence of detectability used for LCD claims are not standardized and are not usually fully disclosed. Since conditions of operation and measurement methods vary, it is virtually impossible to objectively compare LCD performance and dose efficiency.

## 5.2 Feature Detectability and Noise

In Fig. 8 we provided an explanation of why the smaller low contrast objects were more difficult to detect in CT noise than in white noise even though both have the same standard deviation. A meaningful metric related to detectability is the signal-to-noise ratio (SNR) (Judy 1981). The signal can be thought of as the information about the object that is transferred to the image. The signal is defined by those spatial frequencies that provide information about the object. The signal competes with the noise within the range of spatial frequencies that describe the object. Spatial frequencies beyond those describing the object are considered excess bandwidth and usually do not have a significant effect on object detectability unless they are saturating the gray scale range of the image.

The SNR is related to the power of the spatial frequency content of the object divided by the power of the spatial frequency content of the noise. There are a number of variations of SNR such as the ideal Bayesian observer (IBO SNR) or the non pre-whitening SNR (NPW SNR) (ICRU54 1996). The NPW SNR may also employ a filter that models the effect of the human eye (Rose 1948). The IBO SNR describes the inherent image content while the NPW SNR (especially with an eye filter) is a better model of the content that influences the performance of a human observer.

Another method to more completely indicate noise content is to filter a uniform CT noise image with a kernel that removes those spatial frequencies that are not associated with an assumed object to be detected (Chakraborty and Eckert 1995) (Chao 2000). The standard deviation of the filtered noise image (SDF) indicates the variability of the noise that competes with a defined object and is a better measure than the raw unfiltered pixel standard deviation. A statement about detectability for the defined object can also be made based on the SDF. For example, if one wants 95% confidence that a region of the image contains or does not contain the object, the object contrast would need to be about 3.3 times the SDF. (Recall that Rose found that the object contrast to be 5 times the SDF for 100% accurate detectability.)

Other methods to determine LCD are the use of an object template or NPW matched filter (Gagne 2006). Essentially these methods try to estimate the required contrast difference between the object to be detected and its background noise environment.

Task-based LCD methods such as receiver operating curve (ROC) analysis attempt to measure how well a human observer can correctly determine if an object is or is not present (Barrett 2004; Popescu 2007). Although the measurement of human task-based activities, if done correctly, provides a virtual ground truth statement regarding detectability for a stated set of conditions, these methods require a careful design of experiments considering all factors, a sufficient number of observations and appropriate statistical analysis tools. Hence, they are not economically practical for most purposes.

On the other hand, although the use of phantoms with fixed low contrast objects is perhaps the simplest way to try to measure LCD, these methods can only measure subjective opinions of what objects the viewer thinks may or may not be detectable. Such opinions have been found to be highly variable even when the same observer grades the same image in a random presentation (Levinson 1968; Keat 2003). Thus such phantoms have very limited utility in evaluating LCD of an image (ICRU54 1996).

The best practical solution for comparing LCD performance and dose efficiency likely lies between these two extremes and would utilize some form of analytically measured SNR or LCD calculation based on imaging a set of test objects under a variety of attenuation conditions similar to the range of typical patients.

## 5.3 Noise Relationship to Operating Parameters, Patient Size and Dose

Now that we have some understanding of CT noise and how it relates to detectability of small low contrast objects, we will discuss the factors the affect the amount of noise in the image. X-ray generation at the surface of the X-ray tube anode is a random Poisson process. Thus, the mean number of X-rays received by a detector channel during a measurement interval is not always the same even when the materials between the source and the detector are unchanged. The measured value, related to the number of photons weighted times their energy, will vary from the mean approximately as the inverse square root of the mean number of photons. This variation is referred to as the X-ray quantum noise.

The X-ray samples that make up the projections contain X-ray quantum noise and sometimes noise from electronic or other sources as well. Noise in the image is a function of tube current, scan time, helical pitch, slice thickness, kVp, image reconstruction processing, filtration and patient characteristics regarding size, shape and anatomy.

### 5.3.1 Tube Current

The noise in a CT image can be reduced by increasing the tube current. The number of photons in the image and dose to the patient is proportional to the tube current. If the tube current is increased by a factor of four, the number of X-ray photons at all energies increases by a factor of four. Thus, in this example, the image noise would be reduced by one half (the inverse square root of four). However, since we increased the tube current by four in our example, the dose would also be increased by a factor of four. On some scanners, increasing the tube current setting above some value causes the system to switch to a larger focal spot. This larger focal spot can reduce spatial resolution, especially away from isocenter.

### 5.3.2 Scan Time

The scan time is the time for the gantry to make one revolution. The number of photons in the image (as well as patient dose) is proportional to the scan time in the same manner as tube current. Thus it is common to use milliamp seconds (mAs) as a relative indication of the number of X-ray photons. Of course increasing the scan time to reduce image noise increases the risk of anatomic patient motion artifacts.

### 5.3.3 Helical Pitch

The number of X-ray photons (as well as patient dose) is inversely related to the helical pitch. The helical pitch is the ratio of the patient table travel per gantry revolution divided by the total Z-axis detection aperture at isocenter. Some CT vendors use the term effective mAs to describe the mAs divided by helical pitch as a relative indicator of the number of photons.

### 5.3.4 kVp

The selected kVp for the scan has a large influence on the number of X-ray photons as well as on other image characteristics. As shown in Fig. 2(A), the

140 kVp spectrum not only provides photons at increased energy, it also increases the photon intensity over all photon energies. The increased number of photons reduces the noise in the image but also increases the dose to the patient. Also, recall that the contrast (HU values) of human tissue relative to water is decreased at increased kVp settings as shown in Fig. 3. Thus, although the noise is reduced at higher kVp values, the contrast-to-noise ratio for features of interest may actually decrease for the dose used; especially for Iodine contrast-enhanced tissue or blood. Thus, it can be more dose efficient to use lower kVp settings provided that the patient is small enough for sufficient X-ray penetration (acceptable image noise) and any associated increase in artifacts are acceptable.

### 5.3.5 Slice Thickness

Another way to reduce the noise in the image is to increase the slice thickness. The wider slice includes more X-ray photons in the data for reconstructing the image and thus is similar to increasing the tube current regarding image noise. Although increasing the slice thickness reduces noise without a typical increase in patient dose, it reduces the z-axis resolution of the image and may lead to a reduction in contrast-to-noise ratio due to volume averaging of small features. The noise is generally reduced in accordance with the inverse square root of the slice thickness unless significantly affected by data weighting of the reconstruction process.

### 5.3.6 Reconstruction Algorithm

The reconstruction algorithm (sometimes called the reconstruction filter or kernel) changes the spatial frequency content of the image noise as well as the image features. This can have a substantial effect on the standard deviation. For example in Fig. 7, algorithm 1 has a standard deviation of 3.1 and algorithm 2 has a standard deviation of 12.5 even though both were reconstructed from the same data. However, in many cases the reconstruction algorithm does not significantly influence the detectability of a small low contrast object. The reason is somewhat complex. The reconstruction algorithm boosts or reduces the frequency content of both the object and noise in a similar manner, and thus does not substantially alter signal-to-noise ratio. However, the object can appear somewhat more distinct if excess bandwidth is limited. Excess bandwidth is the spatial frequencies of the noise that are substantially greater than that of the object. For example spatial frequencies beyond 5lp/cm do not contribute substantially to the information content of a 2 mm object, and hence using a reconstruction algorithm that limits these spatial frequencies may allow objects of this size to be somewhat more visible (Hanson 1977). Ultimately the choice of algorithm depends on the imaging task (Wagner 1979) and/or the preferences and experience of the human viewer.

### 5.3.7 NonLinear Image Reconstruction Methods

Nonlinear adaptive image filtering and iterative image reconstruction methods can reduce the impact of X-ray quantum noise on CT images and allow lower dose while preserving clinical diagnostic utility (Kalra 2003), (Singh 2011). These methods attempt to preserve or enhance data that is statistically unlikely to be noise and reduce the intensity of data that is statistically likely to be noise. In this way signal-to-noise ratios are improved for image features of clinical of interest. Model-based iterative reconstruction methods, that are now just being introduced, have the potential of very significantly reducing dose while preserving diagnostic capabilities. These methods offer significant opportunities to reduce the effects of X-ray quantum noise on the clinical quality of CT images and thereby provide comparable diagnostic quality at substantially lower doses than today. The challenge for these methods is to reduce reconstruction time and to maintain the integrity of the image information.

Nonlinear adaptive image filtering and iterative reconstruction methods also present significant challenges regarding objective measurements such as MTF, NPS and LCD. The MTF and NPS of these systems may be variable as a function of object contrast, shape and the surrounding noise environment. Thus a single MTF, NPS or LCD measurement may not be representative of an overall image quality statement. It may be necessary to specify SNR values based on measured signal response and noise as a function of object contrast, size and surrounding noise environment. Ultimately, the clinical utility of these methods will need to be carefully explored.

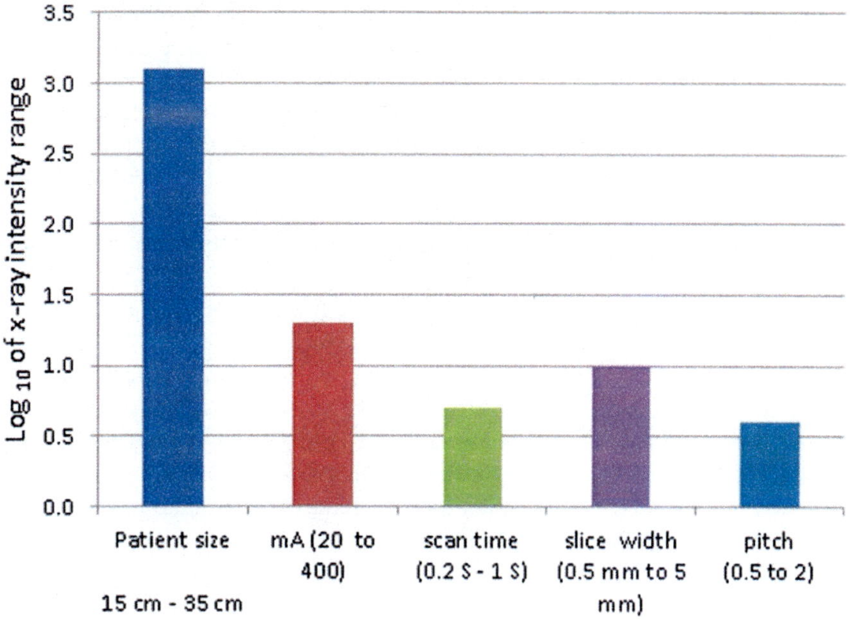


**Fig. 9** The log of the X-ray intensity range for patient size compared to typical CT scan control parameters

### 5.3.8 Patient Size

Figure 9 compares the X-ray intensity range as a log value for the range of typical patient sizes and various scanner parameter settings. The total X-ray intensity range for all factors is a factor of over five million. Patient size and anatomy, however, account for about one-half of the total X-ray intensity range and hence the patient has the greatest influence on image noise. The wide range of patient sizes require the user to make substantial adjustments in mA or other parameters for each patient in order to maintain appropriate image noise for the diagnostic task. In turn, the right dose is the lowest dose necessary to provide acceptable noise and object detectability for the diagnostic task.

CT manufacturers have simplified the patient size variation problem by introducing automatic tube current modulation (ATCM) systems. ATCM systems are also called AEC or automatic exposure control systems. These systems adapt to patient size and decrease mA for smaller patients and increase mA for larger patients. This can significantly reduce dose for smaller patients compared to using a fixed technique that is not adapted to size. However, users must be sure they fully understand the ATCM system on their make and model scanner since significant operating differences can exist.

Some ATCM systems will attempt to hold the image noise constant regardless of patient size while others will allow the noise to decrease somewhat with smaller patient sizes and increase with larger patients. Radiologists prefer somewhat lower noise on smaller patients, probably due to increased fatty tissue surrounding the organs of larger patients (Wilting et al. 2001). Hence, radiologists desire a somewhat increased SNR for small patients compared to larger patients. Technique charts and protocols developed for specific scanners and clinical tasks can provide guidance; however, the required SNR as a function of patient size for common diagnostic tasks is not rigorously known since an objective SNR metric has not yet been adapted to record clinical opinions (Rohler 2010). Thus it is difficult to reproduce results on different make and model scanners in clinical practice since results are expressed indirectly in terms of operating parameter settings for that particular scanner. Since ATCM systems for different scanners operate differently, users must take special care to learn how to properly operate the ATCM system for their scanner and follow the diagnostic task protocol charts developed for that scanner. Otherwise the potential dose savings offered by ATCM systems may not be fully achieved.

### 5.3.9 Patient Shape and Anatomy

In addition to the patient size, the shape and anatomy of the patient also has a significant effect on image noise. The noise in highly asymmetric attenuation regions, such as the patient's shoulders or pelvis, will be most strongly dominated by the X-ray views in the direction of the highest attenuation. The low intensity of detected X-rays and the associated high quantum noise and electronic noise exposure results in laterally elongated or streaky noise patterns. Since the low noise views in the AP direction do little to reduce overall image noise that is dominated by the excessively noisy lateral views, the mA can be reduced for the AP views to save dose without having a detrimental effect on image noise. This strategy is exploited by x–y ATCM modulation and can reduce dose up to 40% without a perceptible noise penalty (Kalender 1999).

Streaky noise patterns from highly attenuating directions (Fig. 10g), due to insufficient detected photons and subsequent effects of electronic noise interference are also often dealt with in the reconstruction process by adaptively filtering the excessively noisy data. This significantly reduces the streaking noise patterns in the image. Although there is a reduction in spatial resolution in a direction perpendicular to the long axis, this is generally a small price to pay for the dramatic improvement in images of highly attenuating asymmetric patient regions.

In addition to the patient shape, the patient's anatomy has a significant influence on the X-ray attenuation and noise. For example the patient's lungs are less dense than the abdomen or pelvis. So even if the external dimensions of the patient and technique settings are the same, the noise can be significantly lower in the chest since fewer X-rays are attenuated than in the abdomen or pelvis. Patient attenuation is a direct measure of how X-rays interact with matter. Protocol adjustments based on attenuation are therefore more accurate than using external patient characteristics such as patient age, weight, BMI or external dimensions (Menke 2005). ATCM systems provided by CT manufacturers uses patient attenuation information from the CT radiograph scan and thus can produce the most consistent results provided that the user understands how to appropriately set the controlling parameters for their particular scanner.

### 5.3.10 Electronic and Other Noise Sources

All data acquisition systems produce some small amount of electronic noise. Generally this noise is insignificant compared to the quantum noise variation and does not affect image noise. However, electronic noise can become a significant contributor to image noise when X-ray levels are low due to large or very asymmetric patient regions. Data-dependent filters, discussed earlier, can mitigate the effects of electronic noise. Proper patient centering and the use of appropriate dose for large patients also minimize electronic noise contribution.

Another noise source occurs when scattered X-rays from regions outside the intended X-ray sample paths impinge on the detector. Since scattered X-rays do not contribute to the image information, the signal variations they cause are a source of noise. Scattered X-rays can be a significant problem for wide beam scanners since large regions of the patient are producing scatter. It should be noted that scatter correction algorithms that help minimize artifacts do not reduce scatter noise. To reduce the effects of scatter induced noise, CT vendors employ detector collimation to block scattered X-rays from being detected.

### 5.3.11 Bowtie Filters and Patient Centering

Pre-patient X-ray beam shaping filters (bowtie filters), used on virtually all CT scanners, help reduce surface dose without a significant image noise impact if certain precautions are followed. X-ray path lengths are generally shorter for those rays away from the center and toward the edge of the patient. Therefore, X-ray intensity can be reduced to better balance the detected signals for improved dose efficiency. However, the patient must be appropriately centered within the SFOV to achieve the desired improvement. If the patient is off center, the most attenuating part of the patient combines with the increase bowtie attenuation to reduce the X-ray intensity. Noise increases of up to 15% can occur for adult abdominal patients that are 6 cm off center (Toth 2007). If patients are typically miscentered, then technique factors may likely be set somewhat higher to compensate for the increase in image noise.

Patient centering is also important with regard to ATCM systems. Z-axis ATCM requires information about the patient prior to the CT scan to forecast tube current utilization and dose. This information is

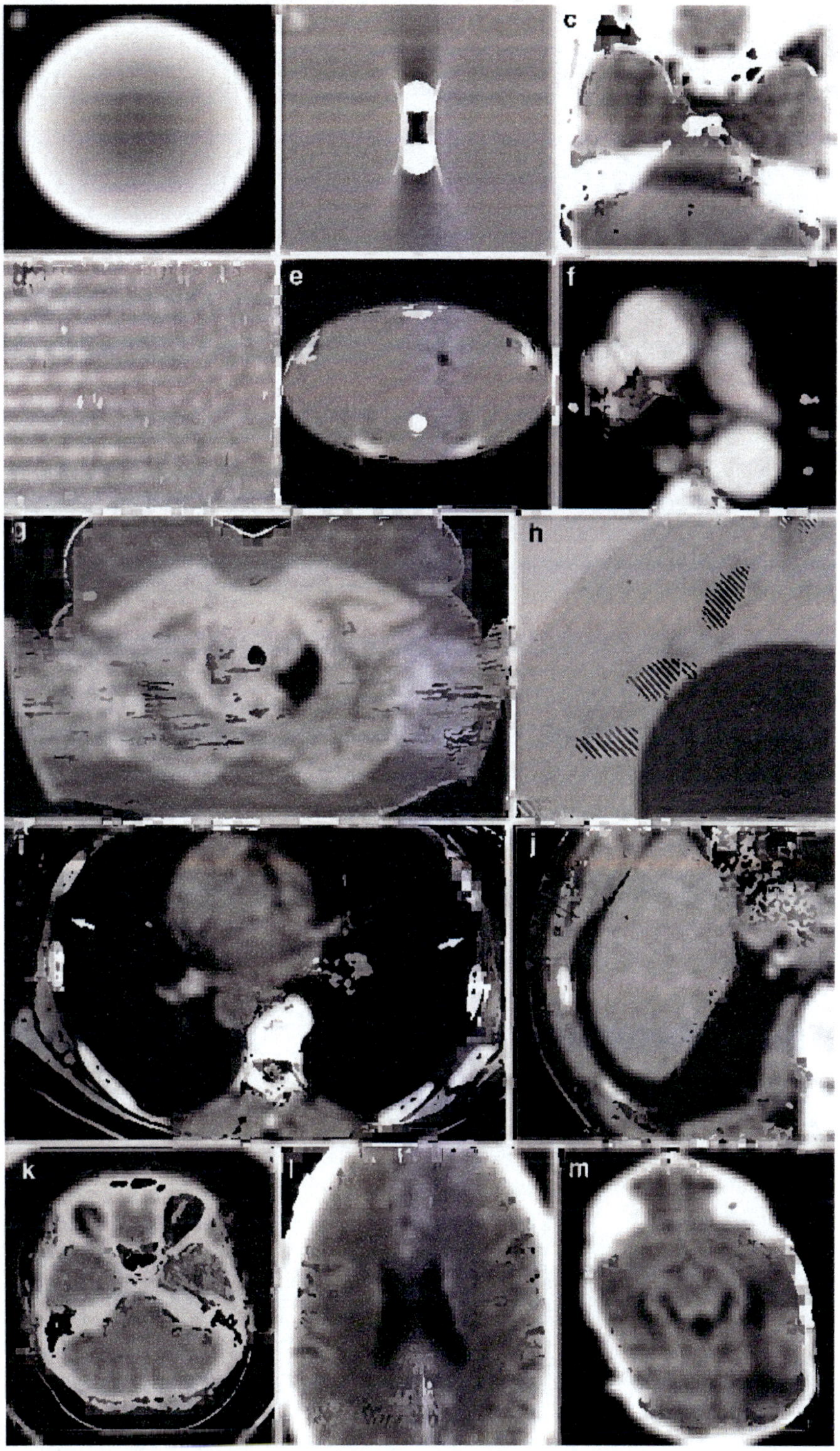


**Fig. 10** Summary of CT artifacts. **a** Water Beam hardening. **b** Bone beam hardening and/or scatter. **c** Partial volume, bone beam hardening and/or scatter. **d** Patient Motion. **e** 3D artifacts. **f** Helical and cone beam. **g** Low signal streaks. **h** Aliasing artifacts. **i** Off focal radiation. **j** Tube arcing (spit). **k** Vibration. **l** Electromagnetic interference (EMI). **m** Detection/calibration artifacts

typically obtained from the CT radiograph data. Since the fan beam magnification for the projections are dependent on the distance of the patient from the source, the patient will appear larger when closer to the source and smaller when further from the source. The most accurate mA predictions by the ATCM system occur when the patient is reasonably well centered so that source to patient distances and resultant magnification are consistent.

### 5.4 The Clinical Diagnostic Problem with Noise and Dose

In summary, the clinical diagnostic problem is to determine if an abnormal medical condition does or does not exist within otherwise normal human anatomy. The image noise and associated dose to accomplish a given clinical diagnostic task with acceptable confidence is difficult to measure. Almost all such studies to date employ qualitative opinions of image quality graded on an arbitrary scale of 1–5 for example. However, the determination is best measured with task based experiments that systematically vary or control all significant clinical factors, including dose, and objectively score the accuracy of the clinical outcome results. Such studies require a complicated design of statistical experiments that must be carefully targeted with a sufficient number of cases and observations in order to determine how one or more factors such as dose may or may not influence detectability.

The need to use artificial CT noise addition methods that accurately simulate dose reductions in clinical images or the use of cadavers further complicates these studies since subjecting live human patients to unnecessary multiple scans at various dose levels is clearly out of the question. In addition, assuming that acceptable diagnostic accuracy outcomes can be accurately determined with suitable statistical significants, the results are known only as a function of the conditions of operation, patient population and the make and model scanner that was used. Thus, in spite of the experimental cost and complexity of such research endeavors, the knowledge is limited since it generally cannot be used to duplicate results on other make and model scanners.

The use of $CTDI_{vol}$ or DLP as an indirect indicator of image quality also has significant limitations since it is only one of the significant factors effecting image quality. $CTDI_{vol}$ and DLP are only an indication of the dose delivered by the scanner to a fixed size reference phantom. A size specific dose estimate (SSDE) that provides adjustment factors for $CTDI_{vol}$ based on patient dimensions would be an improvement (AAPM 2011). However, $CTDI_{vol}$ or even SSDE does not indicate how much of the X-ray is detected or how efficiently the X-rays are processed to produce the image. These factors can be very different for various make and model scanners. Thus different scanners or operating conditions may require different dose values to achieve the same clinical image quality. $CTDI_{vol}$ should only be used as a very rough guide for establishing protocol notification and warning limits for a given clinical task and range of patient sizes.

## 6 Image Artifacts

Image artifacts are systematic distortions and misrepresentations of features within an ideal image that are generally not associated with how much dose is used. There are a wide variety of artifacts which are summarized in the collage of Fig. 10. We will discuss each of the artifacts, shown in Fig. 10 in the following paragraphs.

### 6.1 A: Water Beam Hardening

This image shows how a water phantom would look if the reconstruction process did not apply beam hardening corrections for water. Since the effective attenuation decreases with increasing lengths of material, a cupping artifact would be produced where the HU values at the center would be lower as the effective decreases due to beam hardening. A water beam hardening artifact, beyond the CT vendors specification, should never be seen in a properly functioning CT system.

### 6.2 B: Bone Beam Hardening and/or Scatter

Even though beam hardening is corrected for water, other materials with high atomic numbers, especially bone or a metal prostheses will not be properly corrected in the data. Such beam hardening results in inconsistencies in the data that produces shading artifacts between bones or adjacent to the skull in head images. The shading in the soft tissue region of the head image in Fig. 10c is another illustration of how bone beam hardening might appear. Although corrections for beam hardening are generally included for some CT reconstruction modes, especially for head scanning, (Joseph 1982) (Chen 2001) these corrections usually do not completely eliminate such artifacts. In theory, dual energy CT can virtually eliminate beam hardening artifacts; however, similar looking artifacts can still be present due to scatter contamination of the measurements or partial volume errors.

Scattered X-rays can produce similar looking shading artifacts in the image. Since highly attenuated samples are filled in by scattered X-rays it produces data inconsistencies similar to the beam hardening due to high atomic number materials. Scatter correction algorithms are often used to minimize these artifacts, especially for wide beam scanners that can produce more scattered X-rays than scanners with smaller Z-axis detector coverage.

## 6.3 C: Partial Volume, Bone Beam Hardening and/or Scatter

In addition to bone beam hardening or scatter, discussed above, broad shading artifacts can be caused by partial volume errors as well. Artifacts due to partial volume effects can be indistinguishable from beam hardening; however, such artifacts were much more common on older single slice CT scanners. Multislice scanners, with narrow slices are less prone to partial volume artifacts since larger width slices are summations from narrow individual detector row data after the log correction step.

## 6.4 D: 3D Artifacts

Sometimes artifacts will show up in reformatted images even if they are not obvious in the axial CT images. An example is this stripe artifact in a MIP image that is due to asymmetric noise in the axial images. Special algorithms are often employed to minimize such issues.

## 6.5 E: Helical and Cone Beam

Helical or spiral scanning with continuous table motion is very common for body and chest procedures. Helical scans can produce artifacts near dense features that change rapidly within the slice plane such as near the angled rods that simulate ribs in this image. These artifacts are intensified at high pitch rates. The pitch is the table travel per gantry revolution divided by the total length of the active detector rows. These artifacts generally do not exist in axial scan modes; however, a similar artifact can occur near such features due to the cone beam effects for images reconstructed from detector rows away from the center of the detector in wide beam scanners. CT vendors employ proprietary reconstruction methods to minimize cone beam and helical artifacts.

Helical artifacts can also be minimized in scanners that dynamically alternate the focal spot position in the Z axis (Flohr 2007). This approach requires that the Z-axis source collimation be opened sufficiently to accommodate both focal spot positions, increasing the potential for X-ray scatter as well as patient dose. It is not possible to track the rapid focal spot movements required by this technique with a dynamic collimator as it is in conventional helical scanning (Toth 2000).

## 6.6 F: Patient Motion

Patient motion artifacts are caused by organ movement (such as an aortic dissection artifact) or patient movement. Patient motion can cause shading, blurring, false features and/or streaking. Movement of patient anatomy while scan data is being collected causes inconsistencies that violate the mathematical integrity of the reconstruction process. Increased scan speeds and/or function anatomic gating can help minimize such artifacts with a cost of increased image noise.

## 6.7 G: Low Signal Streaks

Streaky noise artifacts occur for large asymmetric patient regions with low detected photon counts. The low photon counts and electronic noise can cause severe issues since signals are approaching zero into the log operation during image reconstruction. Electronic noise contamination occurs when the detected X-ray signal is low such as through the long axis of dense regions. Since electronic noise is generally relatively constant and is a small value compared to the detected signal plus the X-ray quantum variations, it will not have a significant effect except when the detected X-ray signal is weak due to a large patient and/or low technique factor settings.

Electronic noise is most evident as lateral streaks in scans through the shoulders or when the patient's arms are positioned at their sides. Scanner vendors generally apply mitigation algorithms (often in the form of low pass filters) that become active for projections contaminated by electronic noise and low signal levels. This reduces resolution but can substantially improve an otherwise unacceptable image.

## 6.8 H: Aliasing Artifacts

The fine line patterns are aliasing artifacts that are caused in this case by insufficient channel spatial samples within the projection. Aliasing is when higher frequencies are misrepresented as lower frequencies due to insufficient sample frequency. An example of aliasing is when wheel spokes appear to be improperly rotating (stopped, too slow, or rotating backward) in a video of a moving vehicle. In this case the frame rate of the video is not fast enough to capture the spoke before it crosses half the distance toward the next spoke so the spoke can appear to move backward in the next frame relative to the last position of the spoke ahead of it. In CT the spatial sampling, between detector cells can cause spatial frequency aliasing. This can manifest in the form of fine streaking patterns from sharp high contrast objects or edges.

CT vendors typically employ a clever quarter offset detector alignment strategy that reduces aliasing (La Rivière 2004). The focal spot can also be dynamically positioned to double the effective number of detector cell channels in a view (Flohr 2007). Significant aliasing in an image generally means that the system requires servicing.

## 6.9 I: Off Focal Radiation

Off focal radiation from the X-ray tube can cause the tissue near ribs to disappear and tissue at the bone brain interface for heads to become shaded. Off focus X-rays are produced as some of the electrons that are accelerated toward the anode are backscattered and then re-attracted indiscriminately by the positive potential of the anode. X-ray tubes with metal frames and electron collectors for backscatter can minimize most of this off focus radiation. Glass frame X-ray tubes generally have higher levels of off focus radiation that produce a very broad low intensity blurring. This blurring is generally not apparent except at edges with high attenuation transitions such as brain tissue near the skull or the tissue around the ribs near the lungs. Corrections for off focal radiation are sometimes employed to minimize these effects for tubes with significant off focal radiation. Even if minimized by reconstruction corrections, off focal radiation also slightly adds to the patient dose.

## 6.10 J: Tube Arcing (Spit)

During the normal course of operation X-ray tubes can exhibit micro arcs (tube spit) in response to particles or gas released from materials within the vacuum chamber. Normally these events are so brief they do not cause any observable effects in the image. In extreme circumstances, there can be multiple tube spits that can affect the image. Severe tube spits can appear as a spray of fine streaks generally pointing to the position of the tube at the time of the arc. Excessive spitting can be a sign that servicing is required.

## 6.11 K: Vibration

Normally the focal spot moves only slightly due to thermal effects, centripetal force and gravity. These minor motions generally have little effect on the image or are compensated by active feedback control such as focal spot positioning and/or beam tracking systems. However, in extreme cases such as X-ray tube bearing failure, erratic focal spot vibrations can be intense enough to cause the broad streak patterns such as those shown in the brain tissue of this image.

## 6.12 L: Electro-Magnetic Interference

Electro-magnetic interference (EMI) is when stray magnetic or electric fields are picked up by the data acquisition system. Depending on the EMI frequency and scan conditions of operation, various swirling and/or hash mark patterns as shown here can be added to the image. Such patterns are an indication that scanner servicing is needed.

### 6.13 M: Detection/Calibration Artifacts

The appearance of rings, bands or center artifacts can occur when one or more detector channels is not properly corrected during the image reconstruction process. The center channels of the detector are particularly sensitive to errors. Calibration and corrections for center channels must be within 0.05% to avoid center artifacts. Errors can result if routine calibrations are skipped, if a detector channel has excessive drift, or if small particles or imperfections exist in the pre-patient collimation and bowtie filter mechanisms. These types of artifacts can be an indication that the system requires calibration or servicing.

## 7 Summary

CT image quality is a complex topic with multiple competing characteristics. In general, changing the dose affects only the image noise intensity which in turn affects the ability to visualize low contrast features. Use of lower kVp, can improve the contrast-to-noise ratio of image features and thus can allow the use of lower dose depending on the diagnostic problem and patient size. In general spatial resolution and image artifacts are not affected by dose. However, there are some exceptions. For example, if increasing the dose output requires using a larger size focal spot, then spatial resolution will be reduced. The wide range of patient sizes requires a wide range of tube current adjustments to maintain appropriate signal-to-noise ratios. The range of patient sizes can be managed by understanding and properly using the AEC and dose reduction features provided by the CT vendor.

We would like to leave the reader with a final thought regarding CT image quality. The required image quality for a clinical diagnostic task depends on the question: what do I need to detect and how much dose is it necessary to use to be able to confidently detect its presence or absence? A precise answer and expert agreement may never be achieved, but our challenge is to keep pushing back the curtain of ignorance.

## References


AAPM (2011) Report 204, Size Specific Dose Estimates (SSDE) in Pediatric and Adult Body Examinations

Barrett HH, Myers KJ (2004) Foundations of image science. Wiley

Chakraborty D, Eckert M (1995) Quantitative versus subjective evaluation of mammography accreditation phantom images. Med Phys 22(2):133–143

Chao EH, Toth TL, Bromberg NB, Williams EC, Fox SH, Carleton DA (2000) A statistical method of defining low contrast detectability. Radiology 217:162

Chen CY, Chuang KS, Wu J, Lin HR, Li MJ (2001) Beam hardening correction for computed tomography images using a post reconstruction method and equivalent tissue concept. J Digit Imaging 14(2):54–61

Flohr TG, Stierstorfer K, Süss C, Schmidt B, Primak AN, McCollough CH (2007) Novel ultrahigh resolution data acquisition and image reconstruction for multi-detector row CT. Med Phys 34(5):1712–1723

Gagne R, Gallas B, Myers K (2006) Toward objective and quantitative evaluation of imaging systems using images of phantoms. Med Phys 33(1):83–95

Hanson KM (1977) Detectability in the presence of computed tomographic reconstruction noise, SPIE vol 127 Optical instrumentation in medicine VI

Hsieh J (2003) Computed Tomography principle design, artifacts, and recent advances. SPIE press, Bellingham

ICRU Report 54 (1996) Medical Imaging—The assessment of image quality, April 1996

Joseph PM, Spital RD (1982) The effects of scatter in X-ray computed tomography. Med Phys 9(4):464–472

Judy PF, Swensson RG (1981) Lesion detection and signal-to-noise ratio in CT images. Med Phys 8(1)

Kalender WA, Wolf H, Suess C, Gies M, Greess H, Bautz WA (1999) Dose reduction in CT by on-line tube current control: principles and validation on phantoms and cadavers. Eur Radiol 9:323–328

Kalra MK et al (2003) Can noise reduction filters improve low-radiation-dose chest ct images? pilot study. Radiology

Keat N (2003) Edyvean S. Low contrast detail detectability measurements on multi-slice CT scanners, RSNA

La Rivière PJ, Pan X (2004) Sampling and aliasing consequences of quarter-detector offset use in helical CT. IEEE Trans Med Imaging 23(6):738–749

Levison M, Restle F (1968) Invalid results from the method of constant stimuli. Percept Psychophys 4:121–122

McCollough EC (1975) Photon attenuation in computed tomography. Med Phys, vol 2 No. 6, No7./Dec

Menke J (2005) Comparison of different body size parameters for individual dose adaptation in body CT of adults. Radiology 236:565–571

Popescu LM (2007) Nonparametric ROC and LROC analysis. Med Phys 34(5):1556–1564

Rohler DP, Toth TL, McNitt-Gray M, Maniyedath A, Izen SH (2010) Extended image quality index (ExIQx) relating image quality and dose over the full CT operating range and for all patient sizes, RSNA, SSK15-01, Physics (CT dose optimization)

Rose A (1974) Vision: human and electronic. Plenum Press, New York

Rose A (1948) The sensitivity performance of the human eye on an absolute scale. J Opt Soc Am 38(2):196–208

Wagner RF, Brown DG, Pastel MS (1979) Application of information theory to the application of computed tomography. Med Phys 6(2):83–94

Singh S, Kalra MK, Gilman MD, Hsieh J, Pien HH, Digumarthy SR, Shepard JO (2011) Adaptive statistical iterative reconstruction technique for radiation dose reduction in chest ct: a pilot study. Radiology 259(2):565–573

Toth TL, Bromberg NB, Pan TS, Rabe J, Woloschek SJ, Li J, Seidenschnur GE (2000) A dose reduction X-ray beam positioning system for high-speed multislice CT scanners. Med Phys 27:2659

Toth TL, Ge Z, Daly M (2007) The influence patient size, and patient centering on CT dose and noise. Med Phys 34(7): 3093–3101

Wilting J, Zwartkruis A, van Leeuwen M, Timmer J, Kamphuis A, Feldberg M (2001) A rational approach to dose reduction in CT: individualized scan protocols. Eur Radiol 11: 2627–2632

Yester MV, Barnes GT (1977) Geometrical limitations of computed tomography (CT) scanner resolution. Proc SPIE Appl Opt Instr In Med VI 127:296–303

# Radiation Dose Metrics and the Effect of CT Scan Protocol Parameters

Sue Edyvean, Maria Lewis, and Alan Britten

## Contents



The address of the authors (Sue Edyvean and Maria Lewis) will be in existence until September 2011 and further correspondence can be done with their mail address.

S. Edyvean (✉) · M. Lewis · A. Britten
Department of Physics and Clinical Engineering, St. George's Hospital, ImPACT CT Scanner Evaluation Centre, London, SW170QT, UK
e-mail: sue.edyvean@gmail.com; sue@impactscan.org

**Abstract**

The CT scanner consists of many hardware and software features that affect patient dose. Many of these are controlled by the user, or are implicit within organ specific scan protocols. To understand many of these features and their implications on radiation dose to the patient, it is valuable to understand the CT dose indices that are commonly used and their limitations. This chapter begins by reviewing currently used, and accepted, dose descriptors for CT scanners, and outlines some of the limitations of these parameters whilst still advocating their valid use in the description of dose characteristics of CT scanners, and specifically in the comparison of CT scan protocols. The second part of the chapter discusses the effect of the scanner and scan protocol parameters on the dose to the patient. Specifically these are separated into some key hardware features, and then parameters which are usually selectable by the user within a scan protocol. A brief description and overview of these features are given, as well as aspects of their implications on image quality.

## 1 Introduction

The CT scanner consists of many hardware and software features that affect patient dose. Many of these are controlled by the user or are implicit within

D. Tack et al. (eds.), *Radiation Dose from Multidetector CT*, Medical Radiology. Diagnostic Imaging,
DOI: 10.1007/174_2012_542, © Springer-Verlag Berlin Heidelberg 2012 

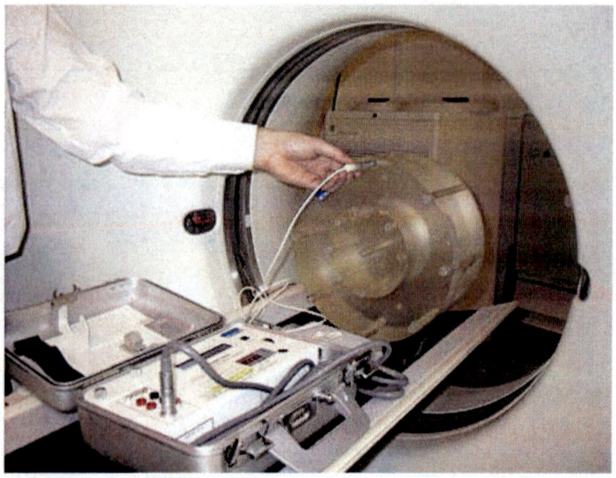

**Fig. 1** Standard-sized CTDI PMMA phantoms (14 cm axial length. diameters: 16 head, and 32 cm body), also showing 100 mm ion chamber and electrometer. This body phantom is made up of the head phantom, and an additional annulus to form the body phantom

organ-specific scan protocols. To understand many of these features and their implications on radiation dose to the patient it is valuable to understand the CT dose indices that are commonly used and to understand their use and their limitations.

The first part of this chapter reviews dose descriptors for CT scanners, and outlines some of the limitations in the currently used and accepted parameters.

The second part of this chapter discusses the effect of scanner and scan protocol parameters on the dose to the patient.

## 2 Radiation Dose Metrics in CT

Unlike a conventional diagnostic X-ray where the surface entrance radiation dose is the highest, and decreases through the patient, in CT the radiation dose is more uniformly distributed throughout a scanned object or patient since it is irradiated from all angles.

The radiation dose distribution from a CT scanner is a complex pattern determined in the scan plane by the nature of the X-ray fan beam, passing through a shaped filter, and irradiating all angles around a patient. Along the $z$-axis (patient axis) this distribution is determined by the spacing of the axial scans, or the spiral pitch in helical scanning. This presents particular challenges for identifying suitable dose parameters to describe the nature of the radiation dose to a patient.

The absorbed dose descriptor widely used in CT is the volume computed tomography dose index ($CTDI_{vol}$) (mGy) calculated from measurements in standard phantoms. The total amount of absorbed dose from a CT examination can be characterised by taking into account the $CTDI_{vol}$ and the physical length of the examination, and this product is described as the DLP (mGy.cm). Any scan parameter that affects the $CTDI_{vol}$ will affect DLP in the same way.

The $CTDI_{vol}$ and the DLP are standardised parameters, and are displayed on the scan console as required by the IEC standards on safety in CT (IEC 2009).

Radiation dose is measured in order to obtain some information about the effect on the patient, and in order to do this the effective dose, E, Sievert, (Sv) is defined, as a measure of the risk of cancer induction in the patient from the effects of the radiation. In CT the effective dose can be estimated by the product of the $CTDI_{vol}$ value and the exposure length to obtain the DLP from which the related radiation risk, as measured by E, can be calculated using tabulated factors that depend upon the radiation sensitivity of the organs covered in the scan.

### 2.1 Computed Tomography Dose Index ($CTDI_{vol}$)

The general form of the $CTDI_{vol}$ is a value of radiation dose that represents the absorbed dose (energy imparted per unit mass, generally quoted in milliGray (mGy)) to the central slice region of a scanned volume. It is calculated, and derived, from a measurement using a single slice exposure.

It can be measured in air, generally at the isocentre, and quoted as $CTDI_{free\ air}$, or measured in standard composition (polymethylmethacrylate (PMMA), acrylic, Perspex$^{TM}$ or Lucite$^{TM}$) and size phantoms, of 14 cm length and 16 and 32 cm diameter, representing head and body respectively (Fig. 1), and is quoted as the $CTDI_w$ or the $CTDI_{vol}$ (AAPM 2008, IEC 2009, IPEM 2003). It is usually measured with a 100 mm pencil ionisation chamber.

The $CTDI_{free\ air}$ is a useful parameter for characterising the radiation output of the scanner at the isocentre.

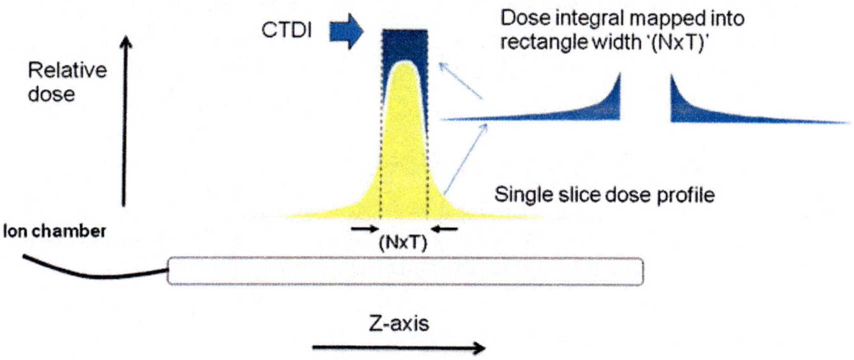


**Fig. 2** Graph of the single slice dose profile, showing the 100 mm CT pencil ion chamber used to measure the integral dose, and a demonstration of the calculation of the computed tomography dose index ($CTDI_{100}$)

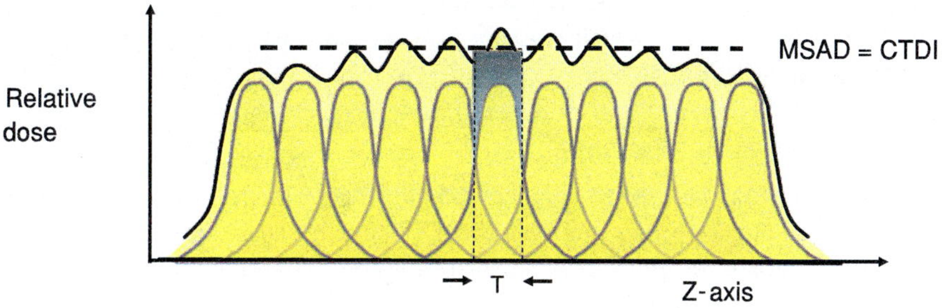


**Fig. 3** The relationship between the CTDI value and the multiple slice average dose (MSAD) where the integration length for the CTDI matches the scanned length for the MSAD

The $CTDI_{vol}$ is useful for characterising the radiation absorbed dose to a phantom from a typical scan protocol.

The general form of the CTDI, whether measured in phantoms or air, consists of three components; the dose integral (D), the integration limits ($\pm L/2$) (where $L$ is length of the detector active volume) and the nominal beam width ($N \times T$), where $N$ is the number of simultaneously acquired data (or image) slices and $T$ is the nominal data acquisition (or slice) width:

$$\mathrm{CTDI} = \frac{1}{N \times T} \int_{-L/2}^{+L/2} D(z)\mathrm{d}z \qquad (1)$$

It is generally known as the $CTDI_{100}$ when measured with the 100 mm pencil ion chamber, giving an integration distance of 100 mm.

$$\mathrm{CTDI}_{100} = \frac{1}{N \times T} \int_{-50}^{+50} D(z)\mathrm{d}z \qquad (2)$$

This is shown schematically in Fig. 2, whereby the 'tails' of the integral are folded into a rectangle whose width is the nominal beam width ($N \times T$).

When calculated from measurements made in the standard phantoms, the $CTDI_w$ is given as the weighted average of the dose at the central position and the peripheral positions. It is weighted by one-third of the central position to two-thirds of the peripheral position (Leitz et al. 1995). The aim is to represent the average dose across the whole of the phantom cross-section.

$$\mathrm{CTDI}_w = \frac{1}{3}\mathrm{CTDI}_c + \frac{2}{3}\mathrm{CTDI}_p \qquad (3)$$

Where
$CTDI_C$ = $CTDI_{100}$ measured in the central phantom position
$CTDI_P$ = $CTDI_{100}$ measured in the periphery phantom positions

The concept of the $CTDI_w$ is to represent the average dose in the central slice region of a scanned volume of length 100 mm, as though the phantom were scanned with a pitch of 1 or contiguous axial slices, and can be interpreted as the multiple scanned average dose (MSAD), Fig. 3.

To give an indicator dose for volumes that are scanned with non-contiguous slices, or with a pitch P not equal to one, a correction factor is applied to the $CTDI_w$ to give the $CTDI_{vol}$ (mGy).

$$\mathrm{CTDI}_{vol} = \frac{1}{P}\mathrm{CTDI}_w \qquad (4)$$

$CTDI_{vol}$ per mAs is sometimes given as the normalised $CTDI_{vol}$, ($_n CTDI_{vol}$). This can be a useful way of characterising a scanner but should not be used to compare protocol doses due to different applications of mAs.

### 2.2 The Dose Length Product (DLP)

While the $CTDI_{vol}$ is a measure of the absorbed dose at the central slice region of a 100 mm scanned volume, some consideration needs to be given for the extent of the patient receiving this dose. The DLP takes into account the length of patient scanned. It is a value representing the total amount of radiation dose imparted. It is the $CTDI_{vol}$ multiplied by the scanned length ($L$), in units of mGy.cm.

$$\mathrm{DLP} = \mathrm{CTDI}_{vol} \times L \tag{5}$$

The $CTDI_{vol}$ can be used to compare the absorbed dose for specific protocols, however the DLP considers all aspects of the protocol and so can be used to determine the radiation risk.

### 2.3 Effective Dose (E)

The effective dose (E) is a measure of the risk of cancer induction in the patient from the effects of the radiation. It takes into account the total amount of absorbed dose received and averages it to give a whole body effective dose. Special attention is given to organs that are particularly sensitive to radiation, and the absorbed dose to these sensitive organs is weighted as having a greater potential effect to the patient.

Effective dose may be estimated by measurements made in anthropomorphic phantoms, or by using numerical simulations using the Monte Carlo technique. Both require time and specialist expertise, and publications of reference results allow users to estimate E for their own protocols. Such publications are from the National Radiological Protection Board (NRPB) in the United Kingdom (Jones and Shrimpton 1991) or the Institute of Radiation Protection (GSF) in Germany (Zankel et al. 1991). Packages are available to carry out organ dose and effective dose estimates. Some are available for purchase, or a free Excel spreadsheet can be downloaded from www.impactscan.org which is used together with the NRPB organ dose coefficients (McCollough et al. 2000) (AAPM 2008).

A generic calculation methodology has been proposed by the European Working Group for Guidelines on Quality Criteria in Computed Tomography (Jessen et al. 2000), and using this methodology E can be estimated from the DLP which is usually reported on the console of most clinical CT systems. Effective dose values calculated from the NRPB Monte Carlo organ coefficients (Jones et al.) were compared to DLP values for the corresponding clinical exams to determine a set of conversion coefficients ($k$), where

$$E(mSv) \cong k \times \mathrm{DLP} \tag{6}$$

The most commonly used factors are given by the NRPB (Shrimpton et al. 2005) and also quoted by the AAPM (2008). These references give values for both adults and paediatrics. For adults the $k$-factors for the head and neck region are based on scanning in head mode, and utilising the 16 cm diameter CTDI phantom. These are: head and neck 0.0031, head 0.0021, and neck 0.0059. The $k$-factors for adult body scanning are based on the 32 cm CTDI phantom, and are: chest 0.014, abdomen and pelvis 0.015, and the trunk region 0.015.

It should be noted that there are different values published in other literature, in particular for the chest region. Also, the values given above are based on organ weighting factors given in ICRP 60. Newer organ weighting factors published in ICRP 103 result in different $k$-factors (Huda and Magil 2011).

Caution must however be taken not to consider that an effective dose is an accurate or appropriate measure of risk for an individual patient, since it is based upon assumptions relating to an average population. It is a broad measure of risk, and as such is useful for comparing the relative risks of different scan protocols or CT scanner systems.

## 3 Limitations of the $CTDI_{vol}$

The two descriptors, the $CTDI_{vol}$ and DLP, have limitations in their application, and must be used with a clear understanding of these limitations. The $CTDI_{vol}$ represents the average absorbed dose to a PMMA phantom, at the central slice region of a series of scans or helically scanned volume. It is not patient dose (McCollough et al. 2011). This would only be true if the patient consists of PMMA, is of the same diameter as the phantom at 16 or 32 cm, about 14 cm long, and the scanned volume is 100 mm in length,

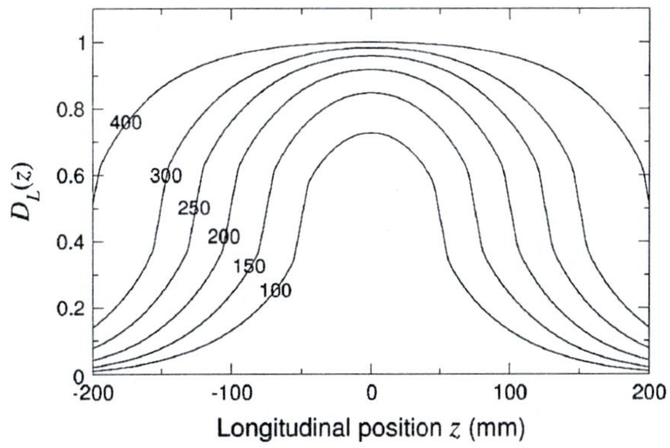


**Fig. 4** The dose profiles from multiple contiguous slices, with the scan length shown on each profile from 100 to 400 mm (reproduced with permission)

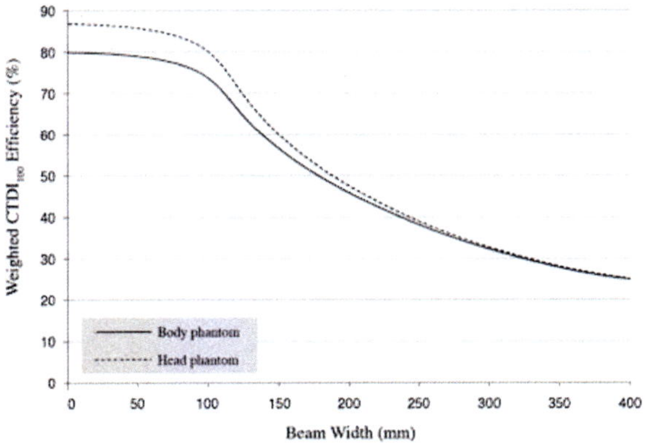


**Fig. 5** Showing the $CTDI_{100}$ efficiency as a function of beam width. The percentage weighted CTDI100 efficiency is the weighted $CTDI_{100}$ as a percentage of its equilibrium value weighted $CTDI_{\infty}$ (reproduced with permission)

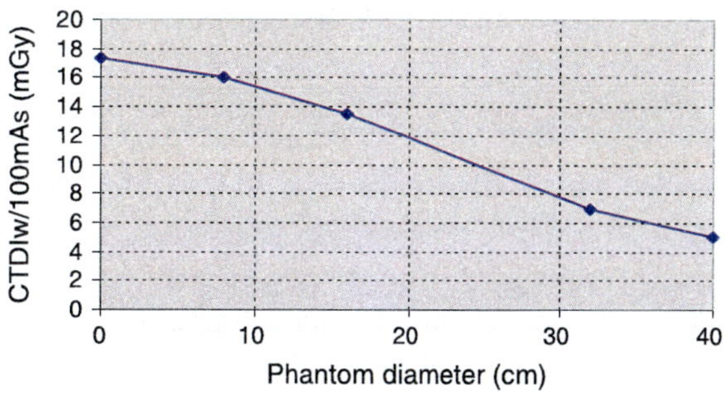


**Fig. 6** Relationship between phantom diameter and $CTDI_w$

all of which are clearly not true. Wide beams also present problems for the measurement and interpretation of $CTDI_{vol}$. However, despite the fact that the $CTDI_{vol}$ does not give direct patient dose, it is measured in a standardised manner which is easily repeatable in the clinical environment, and it produces values which can be related to patient dose and therefore used to optimise clinical protocols.

## 3.1 Limitations of CTDI: Scanned Length

The average dose to the central slice region of a series of slices increases with increased scan length, as shown in Fig. 4 (Nackonechny et al. 2005; AAPM 2010). This is because the scatter tails of the dose profiles extend to a considerable distance and therefore contribute to the dose of the central slice. The height of this cumulative dose profile rises to an equilibrium value at around 350 mm of irradiated length.

The average dose to the central slice region from a series of slices extending over 100 mm is equivalent to the $CTDI_{100}$ value, and it is seen (Fig. 4) that this value will underestimate the dose for scans of more than 100 mm length. As an example, for a scan of 200 mm length the dose is underestimated by about 30%. It should be noted that $CTDI_{100}$ also overestimates dose for scan lengths of less than 100 mm, though this is a less common occurrence than longer scans.

## 3.2 Limitations of CTDI: Beam Widths

The development of wide beam scanners causes a problem for the CTDI as a radiation dose metric, since the phantom and chamber lengths, 140 and 100 mm respectively, were designed to be long compared to the beam width and that is no longer the case with current scanners. The error introduced may be described as the "CTDI efficiency" (Boone 2007), shown in Fig. 5. The $CTDI_{100}$ efficiency relates to the errors arising from the short length of the phantom and chamber. For beams wider than 40 mm the efficiency of $CTDI_{100}$ starts to drop gradually as the beam width increases, until at 80 mm the efficiency decreases rapidly. In conclusion, the current $CTDI_{100}$ metric is not an accurate representation of dose for all beam widths. However, for beam widths less than 40 mm, the inaccuracies are at least consistent, and so doses for beam widths up to this length can be directly compared using $CTDI_{100}$.

## 3.3 Limitations of CTDI: Patient Size

$CTDI_{vol}$ represents the absorbed dose to specific-sized phantoms. The same scan protocol used on two patients, one small and one large, will have the same $CTDI_{vol}$ value, but will result in different absorbed doses. The actual dose to the large patient (absorbed energy per mass) will be lower. It will also be apparent that the image noise in the larger patient will be higher. However, if the larger patient were scanned with a higher mAs, to give a more equivalent image noise as that in the standard-sized patient, the $CTDI_{vol}$ would be higher, though this does not necessarily mean that the patient dose would be higher, since this can only be determined by further calculations based on the actual size of the patient.

This can perhaps be best shown in relation to the phantom sizes used to quote $CTDI_{vol}$ (Fig. 6). As an example, using a given body scan protocol, measurements show that the 16 cm diameter phantom will receive a dose of about 14 mGy as given by the $CTDI_{vol.}$ However the scanner will show a $CTDI_{vol}$ for the 32 cm phantom, for which the value is 7 mGy. Clearly then, the dose to the smaller phantom will be underestimated. This has general implications for assumptions about dose to patients of differing sizes, but also especially to paediatric patients. From this simple illustration we see that when comparing CT scan protocols using the $CTDI_{vol}$ it is essential that the protocol for a standard-sized patient is used. An additional cautionary observation is that some manufacturers quote CTDI values for paediatric body protocols using the 16 cm 'head' phantom.

### 3.3.1 Summary: Limitations of $CTDI_{vol}$

The $CTDI_{vol}$ is an index of absorbed dose from a calculation of a dose integral over 100 mm, so it does not represent the dose for scan lengths longer, or shorter, than 100 mm. It is therefore not representative of the actual dose from other scanned lengths. It is also measured in standard PMMA phantoms of given diameters and is not representative of the patient. However, as a tool to compare protocol doses it is eminently suitable.

Although the effective dose $E$ is the value used to describe patient risk, we may use $CTDI_{vol}$ as a protocol and scanner comparator, since $E$ is directly proportional to the $CTDI_{vol}$ value for the same scan length and body region scanned. Furthermore, the measurement of $CTDI_{vol}$ is defined and standardised, is presented on the scanner console by the scanner manufacturer, and uses equipment commonly found in Radiology and Medical Physics Departments, and so can easily be measured by users.

The DLP is also easily obtained once the $CTDI_{vol}$ for the protocol is known. The DLP can then be used to estimate effective dose and risk from standard tables for the organs exposed during the scan.

## 4 CT Scan Protocol Parameters Affecting Radiation Dose—Overview

This section deals with the parameters that can be selected when performing a CT scan, and how they impact the image quality and radiation dose to the patient.

The absorbed radiation dose is the energy per unit mass absorbed from the X-ray photons interacting with the patient. It is proportional to the incident number of photons per unit mass, and will vary with any scan parameter that affects that number. This is influenced by scanner hardware and software features. The operator has control over these features, both at the time of purchase through selection of the make and model of the scanner, and on a daily basis through the choice of scan parameters for each patient.

The scanner has a number of hardware components, inherent to the system, that affect patient dose; sometimes these are changed automatically by the scan protocol set up and sometimes they are selected by the user.

CT scan protocol parameters have a key influence in determining the radiation dose of an examination. These parameters can be divided into two broad categories, scan parameters and reconstruction parameters. Scan parameters have a direct effect on radiation dose. Reconstruction parameters have an indirect effect in that they do not directly affect the radiation dose, but may affect image quality, and therefore the user may then wish to change the exposure parameters to achieve a certain image quality.

When discussing patient dose, and factors that affect the dose, we also need to be aware of the effects on image quality, and this is the subject of the other chapters in this book. In its simplest form, radiation dose to the patient can be considered as the photons

**Table 1** MDCT Hardware parameters not usually directly selected, affecting patient dose

| Parameter | Effect on patient dose[a] | Effect on image quality[a] |
|---|---|---|
| X-ray tube filtration (flat and bow-tie) | Generally decreases with increasing tube filtration | Optimised bow-tie filter will give more uniform distribution of image noise. Increased filtration will reduce iodine contrast |
| Focal spot size (mm × mm) | Marginal increase in dose with larger focal spot may be seen | Limiting spatial resolution decreases with increasing focal spot size |

[a] Effect of each parameter, assuming other parameters are kept constant

being absorbed by the patient, and image quality by the photons being absorbed by the detectors.

Optimisation is the process of the selection of appropriate scan and reconstruction parameters to answer the diagnostic question at the lowest radiation dose. This will vary according to scanner model, diagnostic task and patient characteristics. Initial scan protocols are usually provided by the manufacturer's application specialist, but are often adapted to local requirements, either at the time of applications training, or at a later date.

Although radiation doses depend on scanner design characteristics, greater variations are usually encountered due to differences in user selection of scan and reconstruction parameters. This chapter therefore focuses on the effect of user selectable parameters on radiation dose.

The following sections will review, in the context of radiation dose to the patient, together with related image quality effects,

- Scanner hardware characteristics.
- Scan protocol parameters

Scan reconstruction and viewing parameters will be briefly addressed.

## 5 Scanner Hardware Characteristics

There are many physical features of the scanner that affect radiation dose and image quality. Some can only be chosen at the time of purchase, since they are characteristics of the manufacturer and model construction and operation. Such "fixed" characteristics are gantry size (scanner geometry), filtration, beam shaping filters and focal spot. Some of these parameters will change by default according to the type of scan, region-specific scan protocols, or other parameters that are set by the user. For this reason it is essential to ensure that the patient is scanned with the appropriate scan protocol, and to be aware of other features that may change (Table 1).

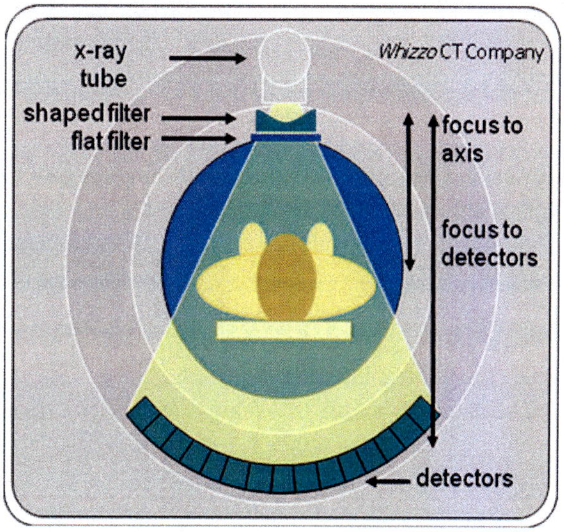


**Fig. 7** Schematic cross-sectional view of a third generation ct scanner

### 5.1 Gantry Size (Scanner Geometry)

The tube to isocentre, and the tube to detector distances are relevant to the patient dose and to the dose to the detectors respectively (Fig. 7). The inverse square law dictates that the further away from an X-ray source, the less the radiation is received. It is a common misconception that shorter geometry scanners give higher dose to patients. However the ratio of these two distances tends to be similar for most current scanners, approximately 0.67. Therefore the tube can be run at a lower tube current on smaller gantry scanners for the same image quality and a similar patient dose as on larger gantry scanners, though skin dose needs careful consideration particularly for procedures such as CT fluoroscopy.

For this reason for a given protocol the tube current, or a value of the normalised $CTDI_{vol}$ per mAs should not be used as comparison between scanners, as the values will reflect the geometry, and not the actual doses given for a particular scan.

## 5.2 X-Ray Tube Filtration (Flat and Bow-Tie Filters)

CT scanners generally utilise a greater amount of filtration than conventional X-ray units, in order to minimise the amount of beam hardening that occurs as the beam passes through the patient. The tube assembly for modern CT scanners usually has between 1 and 3 mm aluminium with an additional flat filter of 0.1 mm copper, giving a total filtration of between 5 and 6 mm Al equivalent. However, some scanners will have more filtration of about 0.2 mm copper giving rise to a total beam filtration of between about 8 and 9 mm Al equivalent, and sometimes up to about 12 mm Al equivalent (Nagel 2000).

As on conventional X-ray units, the filtration comprises inherent and added filtration. The added filtration generally constitutes a flat filter and a shaped filter, the latter sometimes referred to as 'bow-tie filter', 'beam shaping filter' or 'wedge' (Fig. 7).

The flat filters ensure that some of the softer X-rays are filtered out rather than being absorbed superficially by the patient and therefore redundant for provision of imaging information.

The shaped filters, made from polytetrafluoroethylene (PTFE), aluminium, or other materials and composites, ensure that more radiation is filtered from the edges of the field of view where the head or body shape tends to attenuate less of the beam. They are shaped in the transverse, X–Y plane, such that they become thicker with increasing distance from the isocentre along the *x*-axis. This ensures a more even photon flux to the detectors, and a more uniform photon spectrum in order to ensure optimum calibration, and results in a more uniform distribution of dose and image noise in the scan plane.

Modern scanners typically have two or three different filters available, and those used when scanning smaller patients or anatomical regions generally have bow-tie filters that are more shaped. These will be automatically implemented for the clinical scan under consideration. Therefore it is essential for good dose and image quality management that the protocol used matches the body part being imaged (e.g. adult, paediatric, head, large body, small body, cardiac etc.), or field of view selection.

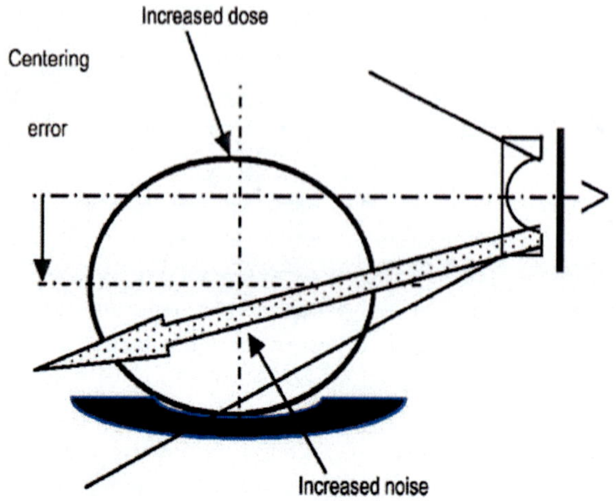


**Fig. 8** Patient that is mis-centred in the scan field of view can be expected to have degraded bow-tie filter performance with an undesired increase in both dose and noise (reproduced with permission)

Since the use of bow-tie filters reduces the dose to the peripheral regions of the patient, when a specific organ in the field of view is of particular interest, such as in cardiac scanning, then selection of a small SFOV is recommended as this can result in dose reduction due to the use of a more shaped filter. However it should be noted that changing the SFOV does not affect the extent of the angle of the fan beam. Any change in dose due to a change in SFOV will be the result of using a different bow-tie filter.

Since there are variations in total filtration, the CTDI for a given tube current (CTDI per mAs) should not be used as an indicator of patient dose between different scanners, or even different protocols wherein these use different filters. In all cases the tube current recommended will be according to the requirement of image quality in terms of photons at the detectors. Therefore, it is the actual $CTDI_{vol}$ for any protocol that should be considered and not the normalised $CTDI_{vol}$.

The use of bow-tie filters on CT scanners means that it is important to centre the patient accurately in the beam, otherwise the aim of the bow-tie filter is negated. Non-centring can result in an increase of both dose and noise in the image (Fig. 8). Phantom studies have demonstrated that a 41% increase in surface dose can occur with a 60 mm offset from the isocentre, and retrospective analysis of patients showed a maximum offset of 60 mm and a mean offset of 23 mm with a corresponding dose penalty of 33% (Toth et al. 2007).

#### 5.2.1 Summary: Beam Filtration

- Use the clinical scan protocol appropriate for the patient size and scanned region to ensure that the correct shaped filter is used.
- Ensure that the patient is centred in the scan field, this ensures that the patient is centred according to the shaped filter, and it is used to its maximum advantage in terms of image quality and reduced dose.
- CTDI should be the metric for comparison, and not CTDI per mAs, since filtration has a significant effect.

### 5.3 Focal Spot Size

On CT scanners there are usually two focal spot sizes available. These are not generally user selectable, but are determined by other scanning parameters. On some scanners the focal spot size will be determined by the total X-ray beam power (mA × kV), measured in watts. On these scanners, above a pre-determined power the focal spot will change from 'small' to 'large' to prevent overheating of the anode. On other scanners the focal spot selection may be defined by other parameters such as the slice thickness or mode (e.g. if there is a "high resolution" mode of acquisition then a fine focal spot may be selected).

The focal spot size generally does not have a very large effect on dose, though a larger focal spot may give a slightly higher dose since it gives a less defined dose profile. This effect may be magnified with narrow collimation settings, where the effect of the larger penumbra with the large focal spot can lead to significantly higher doses.

#### 5.3.1 Summary: Focal Spot

- Small focal spots ensure that the best spatial resolution is achieved when it is required. They are sometimes only available for thin slice data acquisition, or limited power settings.
- Larger focal spots give broader profiles which may be a factor for increased dose with narrow beam collimations.

## 6 Scan Protocol Parameters (Direct Effect on Dose)

The parameters described here are normally selectable by the operator of the scanner. A summary is given in Table 2.

### 6.1 Scan Mode

The first aspect to consider is the type of scan. There are two fundamental scan modes, sequential (axial) scanning and helical scanning, as well as specialised types of scanning for perfusion, fluoroscopy, cardiac and dual energy imaging.

CT acquisition is either performed by an axial scan whereby the couch is stationary and the tube and detectors rotate around the patient collecting the relevant data for image reconstruction. The patient support then moves along the $z$-axis to the next position and a subsequent set of data acquisition is undertaken. This mode is also known as 'step and shoot' or sequential scanning. Where the whole of the organ (e.g. the heart or brain) is covered by the wider beam scanners, this can be done in a single wide cone beam rotation. Helical scanning involves continuous couch translation with simultaneous data acquisition, and may allow whole body coverage within a breath hold.

Sequential scans have the advantage that only the required image volume is irradiated, and have the disadvantage that images can only be reconstructed in the scanned slice positions. Helical scanning on the other hand allows for reconstructions of overlapping slices at any $z$-axis position, with no additional irradiation. The disadvantage of helical scanning is the extra irradiation at either end of the helical run, which is required in order to provide data to be interpolated to reconstruct an image at each end of the image volume. With the larger beam widths that are increasingly available on modern scanners, this means that there is a significant extra irradiation beyond the imaged volume. An additional disadvantage is the

**Table 2** MDCT selectable scan parameters, affecting patient dose

| Parameter | Effect on patient dose[a] | Effect on image quality[a] |
|---|---|---|
| Scan mode (axial or helical) | Axial: no extra irradiation at each end of image volume<br>Helical: extra irradiation at end of imaged volume | Greater flexibility of reconstructed slice position<br>Greater flexibility of reconstructed slice position |
| Tube kilovoltage (kV) | Increases with increasing kV. Approx $\propto$ kV$^2$ | Noise decreases and iodine contrast decreases with increasing kV. Potential beam hardening and photon starvation artefacts at low kVs |
| Tube current (mA) | Increases linearly with increasing mA | Noise decreases with increasing mA. Noise $\propto 1/\sqrt{mA}$<br>Potential photon starvation artefacts if mAs is too low |
| Gantry rotation time (s) | Increases linearly with increasing gantry rotation time | Noise decreases with increasing rotation time. Noise $\propto 1/\sqrt{s}$ Potential photon starvation artefacts if mAs is too low |
| Pitch | Decreases with increasing pitch if mA remains constant | Noise generally increases with increasing pitch if mA is kept constant. Relationship dependant on reconstruction algorithm and effect on slice thickness profile. Potential increase in helical artefacts |
| *z*-axis X-ray beam collimation (mm) | Generally decreases with increasing *z*-axis collimation | Increasing *z*-axis collimation may lead to reduced *z*-axis resolution if detector acquisition width is affected |
| Scan length (cm) | Increasing scan length has no effect on absorbed dose (CTDI) but total energy absorbed (DLP) increases approximately linearly with scan length | No effect on image quality |

[a] Effect of each parameter, assuming other parameters are kept constant

appearance of the so-called 'helical artefact' although this has been greatly reduced with the newer 3-D reconstruction algorithms.

The specialised modes of scanning will not be addressed in detail here, as they are large topics in themselves and addressed elsewhere. In CT fluoroscopy and CT perfusion the same region of the patient is repeatedly imaged, and therefore irradiated. Most scanners operate with a lower mA in this mode, however as in traditional X-ray fluoroscopy, it is important to be aware of the total time of exposure and the mAs that is used on the specific region of the patient, since very high doses may be delivered in continuous exposure. Dual energy scanning often requires the use of two scans at different kVs, and therefore dose considerations are important. Cardiac scanning is a special application which in certain scan modes will operate at a high dose, though more recent techniques ensure that lower doses are achieved.

## 6.2 X-Ray Tube Potential (kV)

There are generally three or four discrete tube potential (kV) settings available on a CT scanner, typically between 80 and 140 kV. One manufacturer has recently made a 70 kV setting available. Varying the tube kilovoltage setting determines the number of X-rays generated and their mean energy, and so their penetrating power (Fig. 9).

Lower kilovoltage settings will therefore result in lower patient dose at the same mAs, but because fewer X-ray photons reach the detectors this will lead to higher image noise levels. However, lowering the kilovoltage will also increase the image contrast, particularly for materials with a high atomic number (Z), such as iodine.

Historically, a tube potential of 120 kV has been most commonly used in most routine adult scanning protocols. The relationship between dose and tube

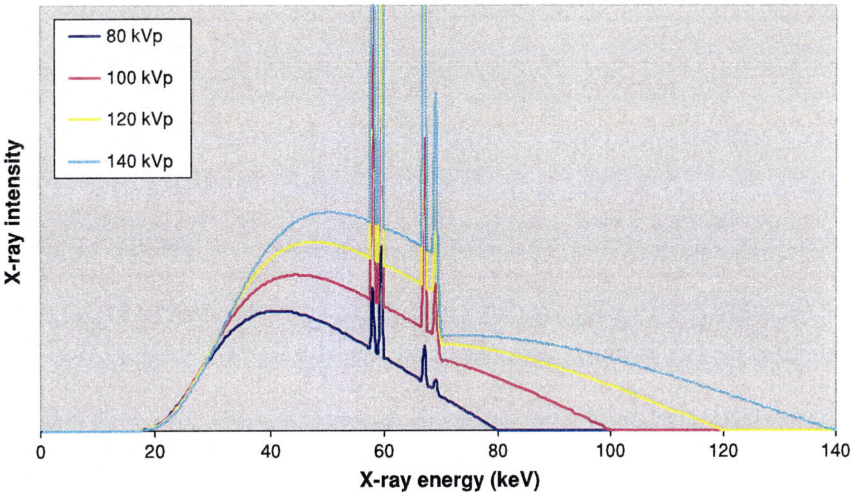


**Fig. 9** X-ray spectra at different X-ray tube potentials

potential is not linear, but dose is approximately related to the square of the kV. The exact relationship will depend on the X-ray tube type and added filtration, so will vary with scanner model and also with patient size (Siegel 2004). Table 3 shows an example of how the relative absorbed dose varies with tube kilovoltage for one particular scanner model in the standard CTDI phantoms.

As image noise is inversely related to the square root of patient dose, lowering the kV will be reflected in an increased image noise and if maintaining the noise level is a requirement of the clinical task, then the mAs must be increased. For babies or paediatric patients, the same noise level may be achieved at a reduced dose by lowering the tube potential from 120 to 100 or 80 kV and adjusting the mAs appropriately. However, for adolescent and adult patients, using this strategy will lead to higher doses. In an adult patient with an effective diameter of 40 cm, the dose for the same noise level will be almost three times higher at 80 than at 120 kV (Yu et al. 2011). For large patients it may even be advisable to increase the tube kilovoltage to 140 kV to reduce the image noise if low contrast resolution is the diagnostic requirement.

As stated earlier, lowering the kV increases the image contrast for high *z* materials, so in iodine contrast studies the same contrast to noise ratio (CNR) can generally be achieved at a reduced dose for most patient sizes (Yu et al. 2011), with the dose reduction particularly marked for small patients.

Lowering the tube potential, results in the following benefits in image quality and patient dose:

**Table 3** Variation of absorbed dose with tube kilovoltage setting

| Tube kilovoltage (kV) | Relative $CTDI_w^a$ |
|---|---|
| 80 | 0.4 |
| 100 | 0.7 |
| 120 | 1.0 |
| 140 | 1.4 |

[a] From $CTDI_w$ data for GE LightSpeed VCT in 16 and 32 cm diameter PMMA phantoms

- Increase in iodine attenuation due to increased photoelectric interactions in high atomic number (Z) materials, resulting in increased contrast between iodine and tissue.
- If all other parameters are kept constant, a decrease in patient dose due to reduced number of photons and lower mean energy of the photons.

These advantages need to be balanced by the following considerations:

- An increase in image noise due to reduced number of photons reaching the detectors.
- Potential for increase in artefacts due to reduced photon flux
- Increase in tube load where a higher tube current is required to compensate for the reduced photon flux.

Selecting the optimal kV for each diagnostic task is not straightforward, as it is dependant on both patient size and diagnostic task. One manufacturer has recently introduced software for automatic selection of kV to enable optimisation. The topic of kV selection is dealt with more fully in the chapter on 'Kilovoltage adjustment for dose optimization'.

### 6.2.1 Summary: X-Ray Tube Potential kV

- Lowering the kV increases iodine contrast and reduces dose at the same mAs, but increases noise and potentially artefacts.
- Lowering the kV is recommended in situations where the CNR can be preserved or increased at a reduced dose whilst maintaining other aspects of image quality i.e. noise and artefacts at acceptable levels. This is generally the case in studies involving iodine contrast, and on smaller patients.

## 6.3 X-Ray Tube Current (mA) and Gantry Rotation Time (s)

The patient absorbed dose, $D_P$ is proportional to both the X-ray tube current (mA) and the gantry rotation time (s), and so these are considered together, as the tube current—gantry rotation time product (mAs). Note that this is the mAs per rotation, and the total exposure time must also be taken into account for studies with multiple rotations at the same site such as in fluoroscopy, some perfusion protocols or cardiac protocols.

$$D_P \quad \propto \quad \text{mAs} \tag{7}$$

Doubling the mAs doubles the number of photons incident on the patient in one rotation, and therefore also the patient dose to that region.

The aspect of image quality affected by mAs variations is image noise, i.e. the standard deviation of CT numbers. Quantum noise, $\sigma$, generally plays the dominant role in determining image noise, and for a given set of scanning conditions, is related to the mAs, in the following manner:

$$\sigma \quad \propto \quad \frac{1}{\sqrt{\text{mAs}}} \tag{8}$$

From this relationship there will be the following effect of changes in mAs, and therefore dose, on image noise:

- Reducing the mAs to one-fourth of its value will double the image noise.
- Increasing the mAs, by a factor of 4 will halve the image noise.

For a particular diagnostic task the mAs must be carefully selected to achieve the appropriate level of image noise. In general, studies where a good low contrast resolution is required will need higher mAs values. Contrast resolution defines the ability to differentiate between structures of similar CT numbers, and therefore is highly dependant on the image noise.

If more attenuation is present in the path of the beam, fewer photons will reach the detectors and therefore a higher mAs is required to achieve the same image noise level. Traditionally, the appropriate mAs for patients of different sizes had to be selected manually, so as not to overdose small patients, or to avoid excessively noisy images on large patients.

Modern CT scanners, however, are equipped with automatic exposure control (AEC) systems which adjust the tube current according to patient attenuation to maintain the required level of image noise and aid in dose optimisation. There are three dimensions to this control (Fig. 10):

- Automatic adjustment for patient size
- Automatic adjustment for the cross-sectional shape at any 1 slice position
- Automatic adjustment for dimensional changes along the $z$-axis

Each manufacturer has slightly different ways of achieving the goal of a specified image quality using an appropriate radiation dose. This can be with respect to a given image noise on a phantom or standard-sized patient. It is important to remember that automatic exposure control systems can lead to increased dose, as well as lower dose, compared to a non-AEC protocol. It should be carefully noted that the parameters used under AEC control may lead to a higher $\text{CTDI}_{\text{vol}}$, but that the absorbed dose to the patient may not increase since the patient size exceeds that of the reference phantom in which CTDI is measured.

In helical scanning the mAs is sometimes quoted as the 'effective mAs', which takes into account the pitch value, and is calculated by dividing the true mAs by the pitch value, (Table 4). The effective mAs gives an indication of average dose to the region scanned. Care must be taken when calculating $\text{CTDI}_{\text{vol}}$ values to ensure that the true mAs is used, since $\text{CTDI}_{\text{vol}}$ already takes account of the pitch.

A fast gantry rotation speed minimises any artefacts due to patient movement, and also enables the examination to be carried out in the shortest time

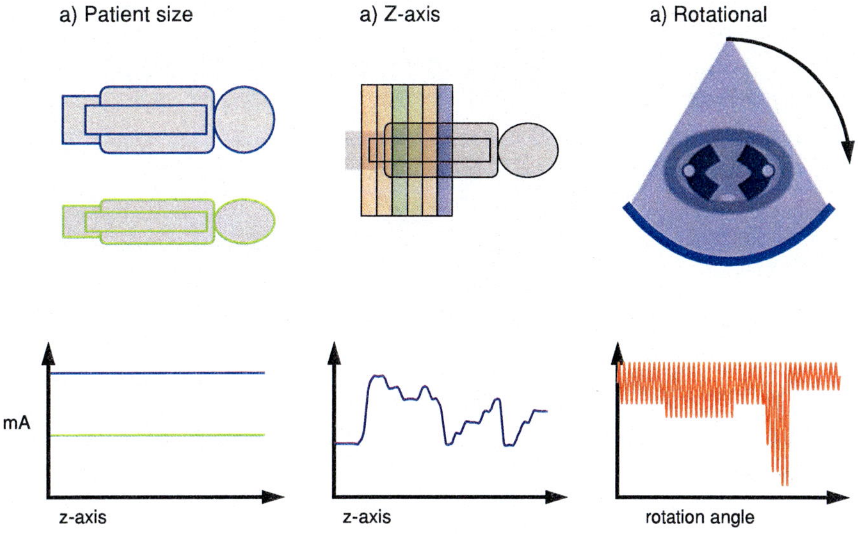


**Fig. 10** Schematic view of different AEC modulation approaches demonstrating the change in tube current with (**a**) different patient sizes, (**b**) patient dimension along the z-axis, (**c**) angular cross-section around the patient. The oscillation in (**c**) reflects the change with each rotation.

**Table 4** Example of Effective mAs values

| mA | Gantry rotation time | True mAs | Pitch | Effective mAs = true mAs/pitch |
|---|---|---|---|---|
| 200 | 0.5 | 100 | 1 | 100 |
| 200 | 0.5 | 100 | 0.5 | 200 |
| 200 | 0.5 | 100 | 2 | 50 |

possible which is advantageous for movement and breath hold considerations, and patient comfort. The gantry rotation time selected in a given protocol is generally therefore the shortest allowed within the constraints of generator power and X-ray tube load. For example, if a high mAs is required, this may lead to excessive X-ray tube load. In this circumstance it would be necessary to increase the rotation time in order to achieve the required mAs at a lower mA setting.

### 6.3.1 Summary

- The tube-current time product (mAs) directly affects the dose in a proportional relationship, and the image noise by an inverse square root relationship.
- 'Effective mAs' takes into account the pitch used in helical scanning, and is the effective mAs per length of patient.
- Automatic exposure control ensures that the mAs used is appropriate for the patient size and shape, at the required image quality. Dose values, as given by $CTDI_{vol}$ may go up but this may not result in a rise in absorbed dose to the patient.
- $CTDI_{vol}$ values between scanners must be quoted directly, and not per mAs since there are other factors determining the radiation dose (filtration, kV, scanner geometry size)

## 6.4 Pitch

The pitch is a parameter that is applicable in helical (spiral) scan mode. The standard definition of pitch in CT is given in Eq. (9).

$$\text{Pitch} = \frac{\text{Table translation per rotation (mm)}}{z-\text{axis } X-\text{ray beam width (mm)}} \quad (9)$$

This is illustrated in Fig. 11.

For a given collimation, the pitch is determined by the table speed. The advantage of using a higher pitch is that the scan is completed in a shorter time.

It is often stated that increasing the pitch can be used as a method of dose reduction, as, for a fixed tube current, radiation dose is inversely proportional to pitch, due to the shorter time of radiation exposure over the given volume. However, the effect of an increased pitch on image quality must also be considered, and there is always a loss of image quality of some form if the dose is reduced.

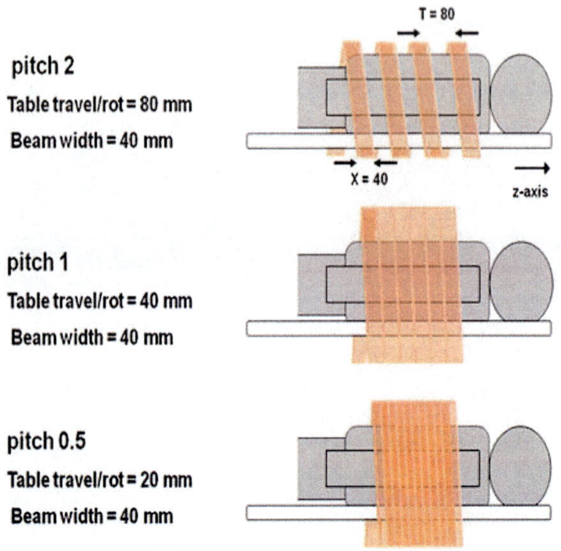


**Fig. 11** Illustration of different values of pitch

On single slice CT scanners the tube current remains unchanged when the pitch is increased, and therefore the dose does decrease proportionally with increasing pitch. However, the expense is a wider imaged slice, i.e. a reduced *z*-axis spatial resolution, resulting from an increased slice profile width, as the data required to reconstruct the slice are more separated in the *z*-axis. Image noise remains constant as the pitch changes, as the same amount of data is used to create the final image.

Multislice CT scanners, make use of different spiral interpolation algorithms than those used for single slice models and utilise the multiple data channels, so the slice profile width remains constant, or relatively constant, as the pitch changes. In this case therefore, the image noise will increase as pitch increases. However this is not true if the mAs is adjusted to compensate for the increased pitch, keeping the effective mAs constant. Some scanners will perform this adjustment automatically and therefore neither noise nor dose change with changes in pitch.

Another aspect of image quality that should be considered when selecting the pitch is that of helical artefacts. Generally, helical artefacts will increase with higher pitch values (Taguchi and Aradate 1998), although developments in reconstruction algorithms have led to these artefacts becoming less pronounced. In general, to cover a given volume in the same time, for optimal image quality it is preferable to use a higher pitch with a narrower slice width, than use a lower pitch with a wide slice width.

### 6.4.1 Summary: Pitch

- Increased pitch will speed up an examination, but may give greater interpolation artefacts
- Single slice scanners will have a lower average absorbed dose for a higher pitch. The image slice width however will be broader.
- Some multislice scanners automatically adjust the tube current to ensure that the effective mAs (and therefore the average absorbed dose, shown in the $CTDI_{vol}$) remains constant with changing pitch.

## 6.5 X-Ray Beam Collimation Along *Z*-Axis (mm)

The *z*-axis X-ray beam collimation can be varied to determine the volume of tissue irradiated in one gantry rotation. This is often called the 'beam width' even though it describes the length of patient being irradiated in one go. The maximum beam widths available vary from 10 mm on single slice scanners, through to around 40 mm on 64 detector bank scanners, and up to 160 mm on one 320 detector bank scanner.

### 6.5.1 Single Slice

For single slice scanners the detector dimension in the *z*-axis direction extends beyond the beam width, and the imaged slice width is determined by the beam collimation at the X-ray tube. In most cases, on single slice scanners the 'irradiated slice' is usually synonymous with the imaged slice thickness, the exception being where post-patient *z*-axis collimation is used to achieve very narrow slices.

On single slice scanners, generally the absorbed dose, as measured by CTDI, does not vary with *z*-collimation. The exception in some cases is with 1 and 2 mm nominal *z*-collimations. For these narrow slices the actual collimation can be wider than the nominal value resulting in a higher CTDI value. In these instances post-patient collimation is sometimes used to achieve the desired image slice thickness.

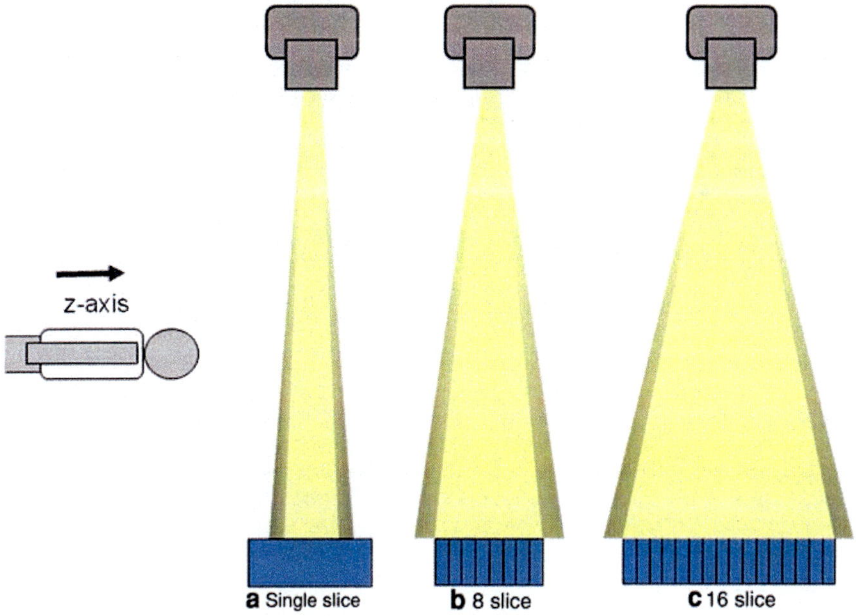


**Fig. 12** Demonstration of (**a**) the full use of the penumbra with single slice scanners, and the proportionally less wasted penumbra with wider beams in multislice scanners (**b**) 8 slice and (**c**) 16 slice scanner, both utilising the same-sized detector element in this example

### 6.5.2 Multislice

On multislice CT scanners, the imaged or reconstructed, slice thickness is selected independently of the collimated beam width. The imaged slice thickness is determined by the detector configuration, and the beam extends beyond the full extent of the detectors used for imaging (Fig. 12).

On some scanners, particularly those which are limited in their number of data slices, for example 16 slices and below, the detector array may be built to allow 16 slices of approximately 1 mm width slices utilising the full extent of the detector, and 16 submillimetre slices using the central portion of the detector array along its *z*-axis extent. Therefore the required data slice thickness will determine the extent of the detector utilised, and therefore the beam width. Table 5 shows data from 16 slice scanner models, demonstrating the smaller detector length used (and therefore smaller beam width) for narrow image slice thicknesses.

On multislice CT scanners, the collimated beam width is generally a few millimetres greater than the nominal collimation. For example when imaging 4 × 5 mm slices with a 20 mm nominal collimation, the actual *z*-collimation will be about 23 mm. The increased collimation is required to ensure uniform irradiation of all detector banks, and excluding the X-ray beam penumbra to outside this area. The dose from the penumbra region results in reduced dose efficiency (referred to as *z*-axis geometric efficiency) because it is not utilised for imaging. Because the extent of the penumbra is fixed, the amount of 'wasted' dose constitutes a greater percentage of the total dose for narrower collimations, leading to higher CTDI values at smaller *z*-collimations (Fig. 13). There are exceptions to these rules, particularly when a multislice scanner is operating in a single slice mode, or a dual slice mode, which are sometimes required for special scan protocols.

On multislice CT scanners it is usually preferable to use the widest collimation available because of the reduced time required to cover a given volume and the higher *z*-axis geometric efficiency. However, wide beam collimations result in more scattered radiation and on some scanners their use may limit the *z*-axis spatial resolution. There are two reasons for not selecting the widest beam width available on a given scanner.

First, as mentioned above, on some scanners of up to 16 slices, it may not be possible to achieve the narrowest data slice acquisition at the widest X-ray beam width, and so the *z*-axis spatial resolution will be limited. In these instances it is better to use the narrower beam, although the dose cost will be a little higher. This can also be the case even if a wider imaged slice is required, wherein the use of a thinner acquired data slice will lead to improved image quality due to a reduction in partial volume artefact.

**Table 5** Details of detection systems from 16 slice scanners showing the number of detectors and lengths of detector arrays

| | GE LightSpeed16 | GE LightSpeed Pro16 100 | Philips Brilliance CT 16 Power | Siemens Emotion 16 slice | Siemens Sensation 16 Straton | Toshiba Aquilion 16 CFX |
|---|---|---|---|---|---|---|
| Maximum number of simultaneously acquired data sets (no. of slices) | 16 | 16 | 16 | 16 | 16 | 16 |
| Number of elements along *z*-axis | 24 | 24 | 24 | 24 | 24 | 40 |
| Effective length of each element at isocentre (mm) | 16 × 0.625<br>8 × 1.25 | 16 × 0.625<br>8 × 1.25 | 16 × 0.75<br>8 × 1.5 | 16 × 0.6<br>8 × 1.2 | 16 × 0.75<br>8 × 1.5 | 16 × 0.5<br>24 × 1.0 |
| Total effective length of detector array at isocentre (mm) | 20 | 20 | 24 | 19.2 | 24 | 32 |
| Total effective length of detector array at isocentre (mm) for narrow slices | 10 | 10 | 12.0 | 9.6 | 12 | 8 |

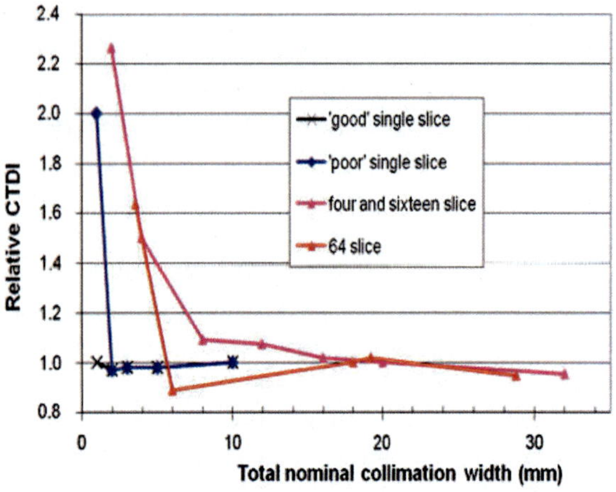


**Fig. 13** Relative CTDI for two single slice scanners (*'poor'*, requiring post patient collimation for the narrowest slice, *'good'* not requiring post patient collimation) and the data from the beam widths from a 4 and 16 slice scanner. This demonstrates the higher dose from multislice scanners, due to the non-use of the penumbra for imaging

The second situation where it may be advantageous to use a narrower beam is for scanning short lengths. This applies to both sequential and helical scan modes. In sequential (axial) scanning a wide beam may result in significant over-irradiation of the volume that requires imaging. In helical scanning some additional data, and therefore irradiation, is required at each end of the imaged volume in order to provide data for interpolation in the reconstruction process to create the end slices. With larger beam widths the extent of irradiation is greater and for short scan lengths the contribution to dose overrides the dose reduction gained from the increase in geometric efficiency.

Modern scanners have a feature known as 'adaptive' or 'dynamic' *z*-collimation, by which the unnecessary dose at the extremities of the scan volume is dynamically reduced at the beginning and end of the helical run.

### 6.5.3 Summary: X-Ray Beam Collimation

- On multislice scanners use the widest beam width compatible with the required scan length and thin data acquisition slices
- Consider sequential mode when wishing to avoid certain regions such as the eyes in head scanning

## 6.6 Scan Length (cm)

On a CT scanner the user defines the limits of the volume to be imaged. This is usually done from the scan projection radiograph (SPR), referred to as Scoutview, Scanogram or Topogram by the different CT scanner manufacturers.

The planned scan length is defined by the start and end positions selected by the user. On some scanners the start and end are defined as the centre of the *z*-axis collimation, so even in sequential (axial) scan mode the irradiated scan length is longer than the planned scan length. On other scanners the start position is defined by the trailing edge of the X-ray beam, and the end position by the leading edge. In this case, in sequential scan mode the planned scan length is equal to the irradiated scan length. The difference between these two alternative ways of defining the scan length becomes more significant for bigger *z*-collimations and for short scan lengths. In helical scan mode there is some additional irradiation in excess of the planned scan length due to the need for data interpolation, as explained in the section on *z*-collimation. Again this 'over-irradiation' is more significant at bigger *z*-collimations and for short scan lengths.

The scan length does not affect the absorbed dose ($CTDI_{vol}$), only the total energy absorbed as measured by the DLP or effective dose (*E*). The actual irradiated scan length is directly proportional to the DLP. However, for the planned scan length there will be some loss of proportionality due to the additional irradiation required at either end of the imaged volume in order to interpolate data to create the end images (described in the previous paragraph). As an approximation, for most adult body scanning, the DLP can be considered to be proportional to the scan length.

### 6.6.1 Summary: Scan Length

- Scan length does not affect the absorbed dose.
- Scan length does affect the total energy absorbed, the Dose Length Product and the effective dose, and therefore the risk calculated to the patient.

## 7 Reconstruction Parameters (Indirect Effect on Dose)

This chapter deals with the parameters that have a direct effect on exposure to the patient, while making it clear that the dose to the patient has a direct effect on the image quality.

The image quality from the reconstruction of acquired data must be optimised for the diagnostic task, and this is explained in other sections of this work. If the user's choices of reconstruction parameters (such as slice width, matrix size, filter, reconstruction method—such as iterative or filtered back projection, or other features), achieve a statistical noise per pixel that is lower than that required, then the radiation exposure may be reduced; or if the statistical noise per pixel is higher than required then the exposure must be increased. The parameters controlling exposure, described in this chapter, can then be varied to obtain the required statistical image noise, with a subsequent effect on patient dose.

## 8 Conclusion

There are well-established metrics of the radiation dose from CT scanners, with the $CTDI_{vol}$ value being clearly defined and with values widely available and easily measured. The $CTDI_{vol}$ is used with the examination scan length, to obtain the DLP, and this allows estimation of the effective dose and radiation risk.

Although the $CTDI_{vol}$ is not the same as patient dose, its value is directly related to absorbed dose for the same body region scanned and patient size, and so it provides a practical metric that can be used to compare between protocols during optimisation.

As with any metrics, the user needs to be aware of limitations, arising mainly from wide beam widths and longer scan lengths. These issues provide interesting theoretical challenges, but do not invalidate the use of $CTDI_{vol}$ as long as the indices are used for comparison rather than as absolute measures. It is expected that publications in 2012 from the IEC, AAPM and IAEA will further address these practical issues.

The user has the choice at the time of purchase to select the CT scanner technology with the desired features and functions that affect dose, but the main control the user has is in the selection of the scan protocol parameters for each patient. The selection of parameters affecting dose needs to be closely related to the optimisation of image quality, and the use of $CTDI_{vol}$ and image quality measures are key to overall scan protocol optimisation.

## References

American Association of Physicists in Medicine (2008) The measurement, reporting, and management of radiation dose in CT, AAPM Rep. 96, New York

American Association of Physicists in Medicine (2010) The measurement, reporting, and management of radiation dose in CT, AAPM Rep. 111, New York

Boone JM (2007) The trouble with CTDI 100. Med Phys 34 (4):1364–1371

Huda W, Magill D (2011). Medical Physics, Vol. 38 (3): 1261-5

International Electrotechnical Commission (2009) Medical electrical equipment—part 2-44 edition 3: particular requirements for basic safety and essential performance of X-ray equipment for computed tomography. IEC-60601-2-44—Edition 3, IEC Geneva

Institute of Physicists and Engineers in Medicine (2003) Measurement of the performance characteristics of diagnostic systems used in medicine, report No. 32 part III Computed Tomography CT scanners, 2nd edn, York

Jessen KA, Panzer W, Shrimpton PC (2000) EUR 16262: European guidelines on quality criteria for computed tomography. Office for Official Publications of the European Communities, Luxembourg

Jones DG, Shrimpton PC (1991) Survey of CT practice in the UK. part 3: normalised organ doses calculated using monte carlo techniques. National Radiological Protection Board, Oxon

Leitz W, Axelsson B, Szendro G (1995) Computed tomography dose assessment: a practical approach. Radiat Prot Dosim 57:377–380

McCollough CH, Schueler BA (2000) Calculation of effective dose. Med Phys 27(5):828–837

McCollough CH, Leng S, Yu L, Cody D, Boone J, McNitt-Gray MF (2011) CT dose index and patient dose : they are not the same thing. Radiology 259(2): 311–316

Nakonechny KD, Fallone BG, Rathee S (2005) Novel methods of measuring single scan dose profiles and cumulative dose in CT. Med Phys 32(1):98–109

Nagel HD (2000) Radiation exposure in computed tomography—fundamentals, influencing parameters, dose assessment, optimisation, scanner data, terminology, 2nd edn. COCIR (European Coordination Committee of the Radiological and Electromedical Industries), Hamburg

Shrimpton PC, Hillier MC, Lewis MA, Dunn M (2005) NRPB-W67: doses from computed tomograpy (CT) examinations in the UK—2003 review. HPA, Chilcot, Oxon

Siegel MJ, Schmidt B, Bradley D, Suess C, Hildebolt C (2004) Radiation dose and image quality in paediatric CT: effect of technical factors and phantom size and shape. Radiology 233:515–522

Toth T, Ge Z, Daly MP (2007) How patient centering affects CT dose and noise. Med Phys 34(7):3093–3101

Taguchi T, Aradate H (1998) Med Phys 25(4):550–561

Yu et al (2011) Optimal tube potential for radiation dose reduction in paediatric CT: principles, clinical implications and pitfalls. Radiographics 31(3):835–848

Zankl M, Panzer W, Drexler G (1991) The calculation of dose from external photon exposures using reference human phantoms and Monte Carlo methods. part VI: organ doses from computed tomographic examinations: GSF—forschungszentrum fur Umwelt und Gesundtheit. Institut fur Strahlenschutz, Neuherberg, Germany

# Scan Parameters and CT Radiation Dose

Sarabjeet Singh and Mannudeep K. Kalra

## Contents




S. Singh (✉) · Mannudeep K. Kalra
Department of Radiology, Harvard Medical School, Massachusetts General Hospital, Boston, MA 02114, USA
e-mail: mkalra@partners.org



**Abstract**

The most important parameter for reducing radiation dose is ensuring appropriate clinical indication for CT scanning. Once appropriateness of clinical indication for CT has been established, radiologists, physicists and radiologic technologists should work closely to adapt individual scanning parameters that affect radiation dose. Establishing dose-efficient CT protocols is by no means a task simpler than orchestrating a symphony where scan parameters have to be in sync in order to yield satisfactory results. This chapter briefly describes scan parameters that affect radiation dose in CT.


Radiation dose associated with CT examination is governed by several scan parameters. Set of these scan parameters for particular clinical indication or body region make a CT scanner protocol. Since image quality requirements for CT vary with desired clinical information and body region being scanned, optimal CT practice should have several different protocols systematically saved and documented for easy use when the need arises. Adjustments in scanner protocols to patient age or size in particular for pediatric CT should be absolute prerequisite for any good practice. This chapter succinctly defines scanner parameters and summarizes their practical effects on radiation dose or CT image quality. For more detailed technical descriptions, please refer to Online only chapter on scanning parameters affecting radiation dose.


D. Tack et al. (eds.), *Radiation Dose from Multidetector CT*, Medical Radiology. Diagnostic Imaging,
DOI: 10.1007/174_2012_543, © Springer-Verlag Berlin Heidelberg 2012

## 1 Radiation Dose Metrics

Surface or skin entrance dose used for conventional radiography cannot be used for representing radiation dose associated with CT (Kalra et al. 2004). Therefore, in CT, two dose descriptors are used to represent radiation dose—CT Dose Index volume (CTDIvol) and Dose Length Product (DLP). These descriptors represent the scanner output doses and do not represent actual patient exposure. CTDIvol represents the average scanner output radiation dose for specific scan protocol. It is measured as the average "absorbed" dose within the scan volume for standardized circular plastic phantoms (16 or 32 cm). The SI units for CTDIvol are milli-Gray (mGy). Since patients rarely come in standard 16 or 32 cm size, recently, the American Association of Physicists in Medicine Task Group has come up with size-specific dose estimates in order to normalize the scanner output CTDIvol to actual patient size or more specifically patient diameter (SSDE 2011).

DLP represents the overall or total absorbed energy deposited from a given scan protocol. It is measured by multiplying CTDIvol with the prescribed scan length in centimeters. The SI unit for DLP are mGy * cm.

Estimated Effective radiation dose (commonly known as effective dose) is the dose descriptor which reflects the biological effects or sensitivity to absorbed radiation dose. It is estimated as the product of DLP and coefficient factor for specific body regions and age. These coefficient factors take into account the weighted radiation sensitivity of various organs scanned in particular body regions as well as the age of the patient scanned. The units of effective dose are Sieverts, more commonly millisieverts (mSv).

It is important to understand that CTDIvol and DLP do not represent actual patient absorbed dose but serve an important function. Since the method used for their estimation is similar, these indices can be used to compare radiation doses between different CT protocols and CT equipments. These indices have been used as benchmark, alert or notification values to avoid excessive radiation doses. Generally, CTDIvol and/or DLP values are displayed on the user interface of the scanner prior to actual scanning of the patient, so that inadvertent under- or over-exposure to radiation dose can be avoided due to oversight.

## 2 Localizer Radiographs

Localizer radiograph (vendor terms: scout, topogram, surview or scanogram) is single projection digital images acquired with stationary X-ray tube position and moving scan table. Localizers are divided into various groups depending on the position of the X-ray tube, for example, for a supine patient position, X-ray tube positioned above the patient or 12'o clock position is the Antero-Posterior (AP) view, 3'o clock position is called the "lateral" view, whereas 6'o clock position of the X-ray tube is referred to as Postero-Anterior (PA) view.

Localizer information is crucial to adjust the patient centering in the gantry as well as to prescribe scan volume. Whereas AP view allows users to check the "$x$" axis centering (horizontal centering on the gantry table), the lateral view helps in "$y$" axis centering (height of the table) of the patient. As discussed in "Patient Centering in MDCT: Dose Effects" on patient centering in MDCT, appropriate patient centering in gantry isocenter is crucial for proper functioning of beam shaping filters and AEC technique. Another advantage of localizer radiograph is to prospectively select the scan and display Field Of View and optimal image center.

## 3 Tube Current

The most commonly used scan parameter to optimize radiation dose is the tube current (Kalra et al. 2004). It determines the number of electrons flowing through the cathode filament per unit time. Number of electrons striking the anode eventually determines the number of photons emanating from the focal spot of the X-ray tube per unit time. Tube current is measured in Amperes (A), which is the SI unit for electric current. X-ray tubes designed for CT usually work in the range of 0.001–1A; hence more commonly used unit for tube current is milli Amperes (mA). Patient dose is determined by not only by the amount of incident photons but also by taking time of exposure of these photons into consideration. When questioning radiation dose and image quality of CT examination, we need to be aware of two other definitions related to tube current, mAs and effective mAs. While

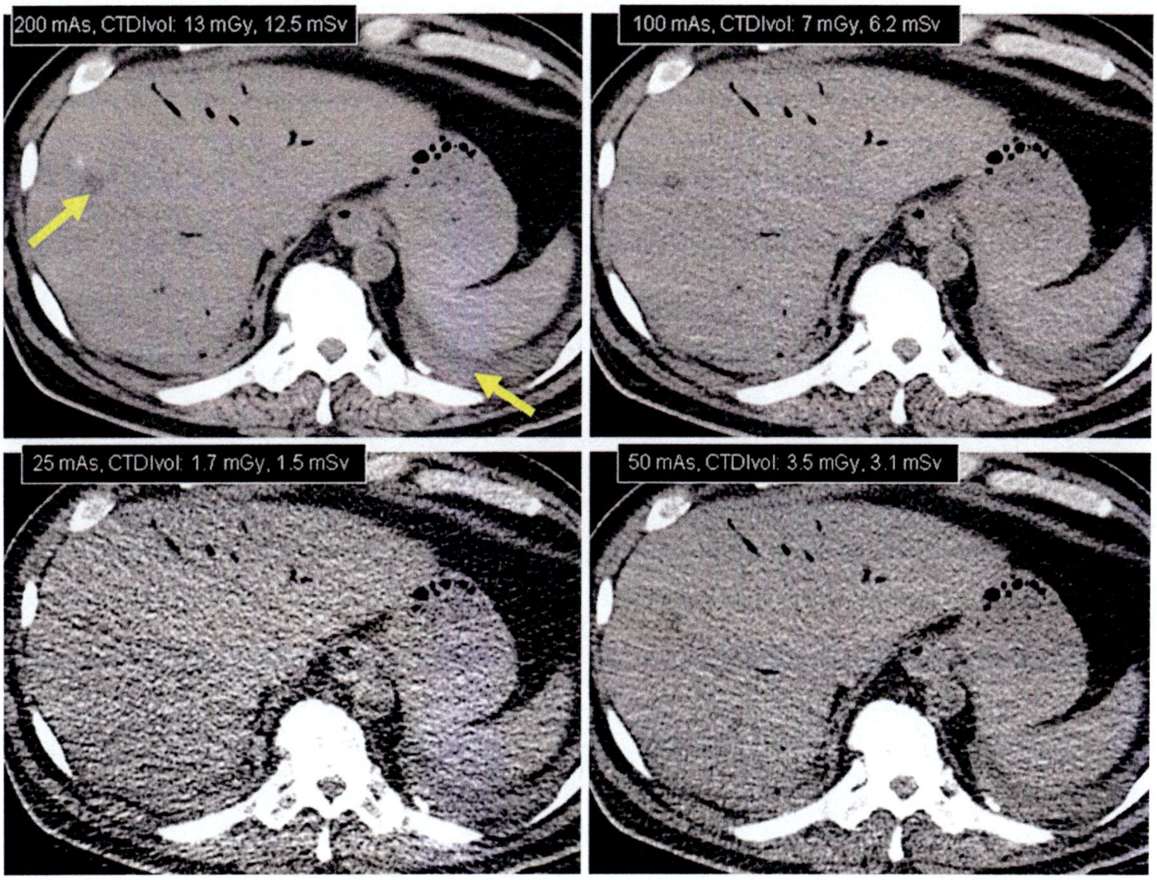


**Fig. 1** Transverse post mortem abdominal CT images acquired at various tube current levels (200, 150, 100 and 50 mAs) show a linear drop in radiation dose, as the tube current is lowered. Lower mAs images show higher image noise and impaired visibility of low attenuation hepatic lesion and the delineation of pleural effusion from consolidated lung (*arrow*)

"mA * s" is defined as the product of tube current and gantry rotation time (the time it takes for the X-ray tube to complete one full revolution), effective mAs takes pitch of the helical scanning mode into account and is defined as mAs divided by the selected pitch. Technical advances in MDCT gearing toward faster rotation of X-ray tube and higher pitch values for shorter scan time makes it all the more pertinent to use mAs and effective mAs for fair comparison across different scans and scanners.

Tube current has direct and linear relationship with associated radiation dose of the scan. It is the most easiest and convenient parameter to fine tune radiation dose. For example, radiation dose for a 100 mAs acquisition with CTDIvol of 10 mGy can be lowered by 50% or to 5 mGy by decreasing the tube current to 50 mAs (if all other parameters are kept constant). Also the other way around 30% increase or 13 mGy could be achieved by increasing the tube current to 130 mAs. This linear relationship is helpful while optimizing CT image quality.

As we lower tube current there is increase in image noise in reduced dose CT images (Fig. 1). Traditionally or before introduction of automatic exposure technique (AEC), tube current was optimized by manually prescribing a value for tube current, which was fixed or constant for the whole scan length. AEC on the other hand automatically optimizes the tube current based patient's size or attenuation, primarily from the information obtained from the localizer radiograph image. Details of the AEC technique are discussed in "Automatic Exposure Control in

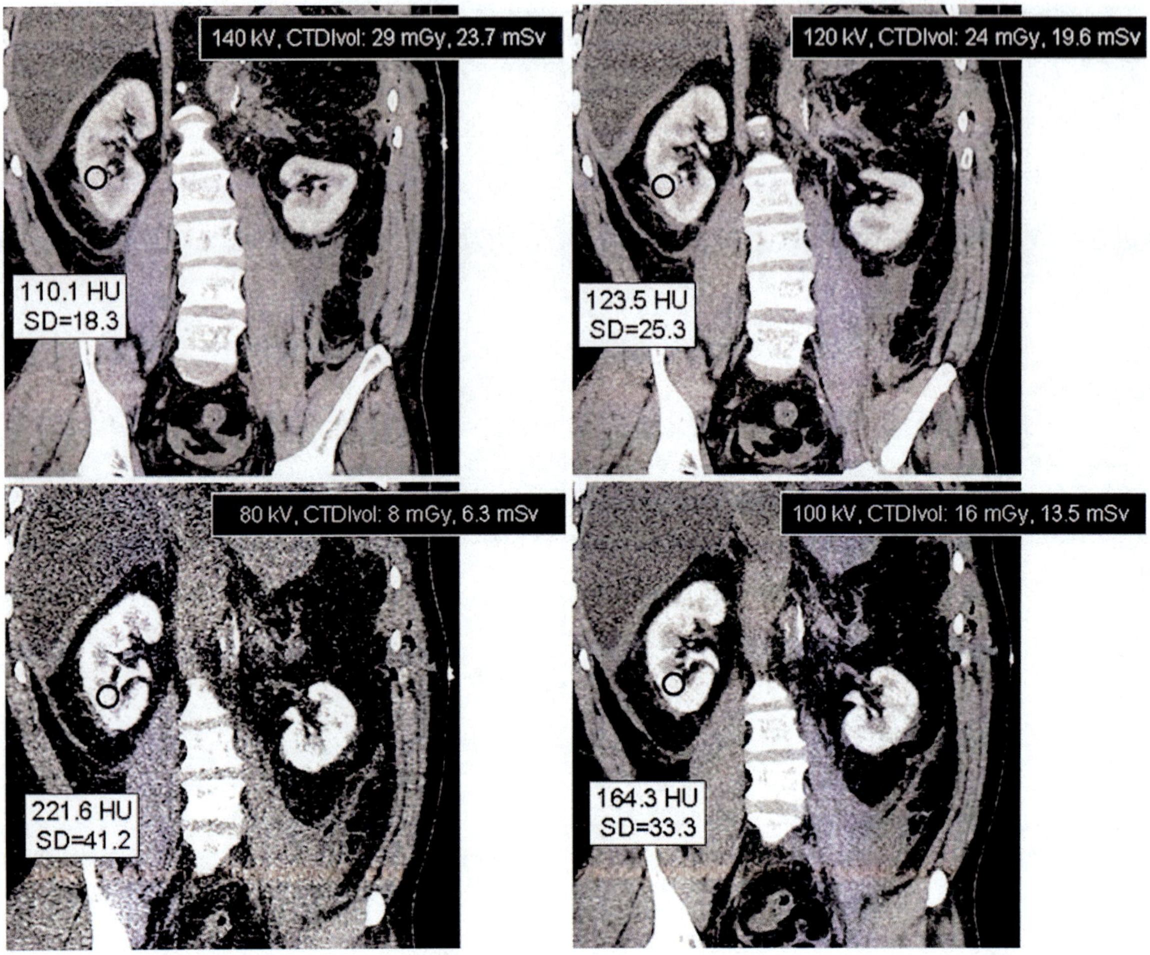


**Fig. 2** Coronal abdominal CT images acquired at different kV settings (140, 120, 100 and 80 kV) in post mortem settings shows increased image noise in hepatic parenchyma and psoas muscles. However, lower kV images also show increased attenuation values of contrast enhanced renal parenchyma which helps to improve the contrast to noise ratio

Multidetector-Row Computed Tomography" To reduce radiation dose for body CT, AEC should be employed in most patients. However, when there is lack of understanding of AEC or when very low dose CT is required, fixed mAs can be applied to achieve radiation dose reduction as well.

## 4 Tube Potential

Tube potential is defined as potential difference between cathode and anode of the X-ray tube, which drives electrons across X-ray tube. It is measured as kilo voltage (kV) and affects primarily the energy or the quality of electrons. Tube potential also affects the quantity of electrons, though not as much as the tube current. Traditionally 120 kV has been the most commonly applied tube potential, although with higher power X-ray tubes on modern MDCT scanners, there has been a shift toward lower kV, particularly with contrast enhanced CT where increase in noise can be offset by increase in image contrast. The advantage of using tube voltage reduction is that attenuation of iodine increases as tube voltage decreases, because the energies of the emitted X-rays move closer to the k-edge of iodine. However the disadvantage of tube reduction is the decrease in the amount of transmitted X-rays and increase in image noise (Fig. 2). Therefore, for contrast enhanced CT or in very small patients, reduction of kV may be a more prudent approach to dose reduction as compared to dose reduction in average or large patients undergoing a non-contrast CT. For example, beneficial feature of increased iodinated contrast enhancement with low kV technique is used for performing CT angiography at lower kV (Kalva et al. 2006; Wintersperger et al. 2005). For small children and smaller adults, lower kV could be used for smaller kids, as lower energy photons could pass through the smaller patients without much increase in image noise (Singh et al. 2009). Tube potential is discussed in greater details in "Pericardial Disease" on "Kilovoltage adjustment for dose optimization"

## 5 Gantry Rotation Time and Scan Time

Gantry rotation time is defined as time taken by the X-ray tube to complete one full circle or a 360° revolution. The demand for higher temporal resolution is driving the technical advances in MDCT for faster gantry rotation or shorter rotation time. Advantage of a faster gantry rotation is of course quicker capture of images/frames and hence fewer motion artifacts for moving anatomical parts (such as coronary arteries), dynamic evaluation of contrast enhancement in vessels and organs, and in some cases less need for sedation or anesthesia of patients who cannot or will not lie still during CT image acquisition. Another advantage of shorter gantry rotation time is reduction in exposure time and radiation dose. For example, CT examination performed with 200 mA, beam pitch 1:1 and gantry rotation time of 1 s, results in effective mAs of 200, whereas same scan performed with faster gantry rotation time of 0.3 s ends up with effective mAs of 60 if all other scanning parameters are held constant. Some of the present day MDCT scanners are able to achieve gantry rotation time lower than 300 ms. Faster gantry rotation is difficult to achieve as scanners are reaching the mechanical limits of rotation due to the centrifugal forces depending on the mass of gantry contents and the acceleration. To circumvent this limit and attain higher temporal resolution, one vendor has recently introduced dual X-ray tube or source MDCT scanner which combines data from two simultaneously operating X-ray tube-two detector panel assembly in order to reduce the total time required to generate CT images. This feature is exploited to reduce radiation dose and improve temporal resolution.

In general, on modern MDCT scanners, a faster gantry rotation time (0.5 s or less) should be preferred in most patients to avoid motion artifacts and decrease radiation dose. Although in some large patients or thicker or denser anatomical regions (head CT), a slower rotation times of up to 1 s are often used. Slower gantry rotation speed may also be a necessity on earlier generation MDCT scanners which cannot go beyond 440 mA at 120 kV, in particular for abdominal CT in larger patients. On the other hand, to maximize temporal resolution, fastest gantry rotation speeds are selected for cardiac CT procedures.

## 6 Detector Configuration and Table Speed

SSCT comprised of large number of detectors (750 or more) in X-ray fan beam direction, however in the z-direction they had single detector row which was generally 10 mm thick and some time as wide as 20 mm (Goldman 2008). Major limitation of SSCT was X-ray tube heating while acquiring thin slice images. Two different approaches were taken to overcome this constraint, either develop X-ray tube with higher heat efficiency or effectively use the available X-ray beam. Multiple rows or more than one detector in the z-direction were employed to effectively capture more than one slice at a time. Hence commonly used terms MSCT (Multi-Slice CT) or more descriptive term MDCT (Multi Detector row CT). Different vendors have taken different approaches in assembling these detector rows in the detector array (which is the term used for detectors available in the matrix of detectors). Detectors arrays are of two types—Fixed arrays where all detectors are of the same size and the Variable arrays which comprise of detectors rows with different thicknesses with thinner central detector rows and wider peripheral ones. For example, GE 64 or Philips 64 slice MDCT have fixed detector array of 64 rows of 0.625 mm fixed detector row thickness (64 * 0.625 mm). On the other hand, Siemens 16 slice CT has central 16 rows of 0.75 mm detectors and four on each side of 0.5 mm detector width. Selected detector configuration has direct effect in beam collimation or the width of the X-ray beam. For 64 slice GE or Philips scanner, one should use 64 * 0.625 mm detector configuration or 40 mm beam collimation for scanning, as wider X-ray beams have higher dose efficiency. However, when only small length or body region have to scanned, a thinner X-ray beam or narrower detector configuration such as 32 * 0.625 or 20 mm is more efficient. Also on variable detector arrays, thinner detector configuration (such as 16*0.75 mm) may be necessary although less dose efficient than wider configuration (such as 16*1.5 mm) if sections less than 1.5 mm are required. Vendors have recently introduced much wider detector arrays with 128, 256 or 320 detector rows.

Beam collimation, pitch and gantry rotation time has a direct effect on the table speed. For helical scanning, the table speed is directly proportional to the pitch and beam collimation. The beam collimation is determined based on selected detector geometry or configuration. Faster table speed implies faster scanning and less motion artifacts (Mahesh et al. 2001). In axial mode, table "increment" is defined as distance travelled by the table in one 360° rotation of the X-ray tube, which is measured in millimeters. Whereas in helical mode, table "feed" is defined as distance traveled by the table in one 360° rotation of the X-ray tube and measured in mm/rot. In general, highest number of data channels and fastest gantry rotation should be used to cover longer scan lengths.

## 7 Pitch

Beam pitch is defined as ratio of table travelled per gantry rotation to the total X-ray beam width. Both the table travel distance per gantry rotation time and the beam collimation are represented in millimeters. Hence, pitch is expressed as a ratio with no units (Mahesh et al. 2001).

Most scanners are now set to automatically adjust the tube current when pitch is changed so that there is less significant advantage of increasing or decreasing the pitch for primarily achieving dose reduction. For instance, a drop in the pitch is associated with automatic decrease in tube current and an increase in pitch is associated with increase in tube current. Thus, pitch should be adapted according to desired scanning speed or image quality. Many scanners also have evolved reconstruction approaches to result in similar image quality with change in pitch. In general for most routine body CT examinations, a pitch close to or higher than 1:1 should be used. For regions with rapidly changing anatomy such as skull base, a smaller pitch is preferred to minimize artifacts and improve image quality at the skull base.

Also, for single source MDCT, a much smaller and overlapping pitch is preferred for helical scanning to ensure that there is possibility of image reconstruction in different phases of cardiac cycle. This does increase radiation dose to the patients undergoing CT scanning and calls for ECG controlled tube current modulation to reduce radiation dose. Alternatively, for single source CT scanners, administration of beta blockers to slow the heart rate can help acquire prospectively triggered cardiac CT or make the ECG controlled tube current more efficient. These techniques are extensively discussed in chapter on cardiac CT procedures.

For dual source CT, however, much higher non-overlapping beam pitch (1.5–3.6:1) with substantial dose reduction are possible with very fast table travel speed for cardiac CT due to filling of "missing data" from the two complementary X-ray sources. Such high pitch values at high associated table travel speed also allow substantial reduction in motion artifacts and need for sedation in patients who can not or will not lie still for CT scanning.

## 8 Axial Versus Helical Mode

CT projection data can be acquired with two different modes; Axial or Helical. Axial or "step and shoot" mode comprises of two alternating phases of data generation ("shooting of X-rays") and patient positioning (stepping the patient or gantry table to scan location). During data generation phase, X-ray tube and detector assembly rotates around the stationary patient to acquire a complete set of projections at the prescribed scanning location. During patient positioning phase no data are generated and patient is positioned to next scan location (Hsieh 2003). Head CT is frequently performed with axial mode of scanning. Another application of axial scanning mode is in high resolution of lungs where thin images are acquired at 10–20 mm intervals to reduce radiation dose while sampling portions of lungs with high image quality. In cardiac CT, axial scanning is often used for calcium scoring and not infrequently for coronary CT angiography as well. Typically, axial scanning with prospectively triggered ECG tagged data acquisition is associated with up to 80% lower dose compared to retrospectively gated acquired helical CT data of coronary angiogram. Most commonly the axial or sequential coronary CT exams are limited to subjects with lower and regular heart rates as other cardiac phase images cannot be reconstructed if there are motion artifacts. However, some vendors overcome this limitation by allowing user to add "padding" to the prescribed or desired phase of cardiac in each cardiac cycle. Arrhythmia recognition software has also been introduced or some equipment to enable prospectively triggered ECG gated coronary CT angiography with axial scanning mode in order to reduce radiation dose.

Helical (or spiral) mode on the other hand comprises of continuous acquisition of CT data while the table is simultaneously moved at constant speed. Helical mode of scanning therefore allows volumetric data acquisition with reduced acquisition time. However, helical mode requires more advanced reconstruction algorithms to avoid image artifacts. Most body CT examinations on modern MDCT are performed with helical scanning mode.

## 9 Reconstruction Mode

Generally on most CT scanners, every data channel contributes to at least one CT image for image reconstruction with helical data acquisition. However, due to technical limitations of some scanners, multislice scanning and helical view weighting algorithms, few data channels at the beginning and end of helical scan are not used for CT image reconstruction.

For example, some scanners (such as 16, 32 and 64-row MDCT scanners from GE Healthcare) supplement the ability to select additional views or projection of data to reconstruct an image (Discovery™ CT750 HD). This in turn allows the users to optimize radiation dose, slice profile and helical artifact in two modes referred to as "Plus" and "Full" modes. The "Plus" mode requires slightly increased exposure time to acquire the additional views and is associated with wider slice profile (roughly 20% more than "Full mode") at 15–20% lower tube current for the same amount of noise. At the same mA, Plus mode provides reduced image noise and helical artifacts. "Full" mode has a better slice profile but requires 10–15% more tube current than "Plus" mode for similar image noise. Both "Full" and "Plus" modes can be used prospectively and retrospectively. CT raw data acquired in "Plus" mode can be retrospectively reconstructed in "Full" mode or vice versa.

## 10 Scan Length

Anatomical length covered in the z-direction constitutes the scan length for a particular CT examination. User defines the scan length based on the acquired localizer radiograph. Radiation dose from a CT examination is estimated from the DLP, measured in mGy * cm, which is the product of CTDIvol (measured in mGy) and scan length. Trimming the scan length to the region of interest directly lowers the radiation dose. For example, 50 cm scan length, when clipped to 25 cm results in 50% reduction in radiation dose. With rapid scanning capabilities of modern MDCT, tendency to extend beyond the desired target region of interest must be avoided. A shorter scan length does imply lower dose if all other scan parameters are held constant.

## 11 Scan Field of View

SFOV is defined as the in-place size (in X–Y or transverse direction) of the irradiated area, which is used to acquire a complete set of projections. It is measured in centimeters. Smaller SFOV provides better spatial resolution and less radiation dose to the patients, for example cardiac, extremities, spine CT examinations can be performed at smaller SFOV. Bow tie filters or beam shaping is chosen based on the selected SFOV. More aggressive beam shaping filters are used when smaller SFOV is selected. SFOV is differentiated from reconstruction FOV (RFOV) or display FOV (DFOV). RFOV is the size of the SFOV that is reconstructed to get the final images. DFOV is the actual display size of the CT images, and can be equal to or less than SFOV, but cannot exceed the SFOV. Too much "zooming" or excessive decrease in DFOV size compared to size of SFOV can impair visual perception of anatomy and lesions (Yamaguchi et al. 2011). Therefore it is important to select an appropriate a priori. Contrary to DFOV which can be altered post-acquisition of CT data, SFOV has to be prescribed a priori prior to CT data acquisition, since modern MDCT scanners are equipped with more than one type of beam shaping filters which are automatically selected by scanner based on selected SFOV, it is important to keep SFOV close to patient size or targeted area of interest (such as in cardiac CT or when imaging smaller body regions). In addition, in children use of 16 versus 32 cm phantom size for CTDIvol estimation may be confounded if larger SFOV is selected or prescribed for small size children.

## 12 Window Width and Window Level

Typically, display monitors use eight bit gray scales which represent 256 different shades of gray ($2^8$). Hounsfield units of air is −1,000, water as 0 and bone or contrast as, somewhere around 1,700. Therefore, compression of dynamic range of 2,700 HU values to a range of 256 shades of gray is needed, which can lead to unacceptable loss of details (Hsieh 2003). Modified gray scale helps avoid this limitation with use of window width and window level. The window width (WW) is the number of selected gray shades and window level (WL) is the mid point of the selected gray scale.

These window settings determine the spread of the CT attenuation values to the displayed pixels in the image. A broader window width is used for assessing anatomical structures with widely different HU values (for example, aerated lungs are generally seen at WW 1,500 and WL of about −600), whereas a narrower window width is used when assessing structures with smaller variations in HU values (for example, brain soft tissues with low HU differences are assessed at narrow WW 80 and WL of 40). These window settings should be adjusted according to the body region, anatomical region of interest and also individual radiologist preference to achieve the best image "display" contrast.

For low contrast lesions or structures (for example, liver and brain), narrow WW and lower WL accentuate lesion and detail visualization although image noise is also accentuated from a visual perception point of view thus relatively higher dose is generally needed at least for the primary scan acquisition whereas use of wider WW and WL in high contrast structures or lesions (such as lungs, bones and large to medium vessel CT angiography) decreases visual perception of image noise and therefore relatively lower dose can be employed.

## 13 Reconstruction Kernel

In computing domain, kernel is the main component of any operating system. In CT, "kernel" influences the smoothness and sharpness of images. They are also defined as software that processes the acquired CT raw data projections to generate images with particular image quality. All scanners allow users to select an appropriate kernel based on image quality or anatomical or pathological entities of interest. These kernels vary in strengths of sharpness or spatial frequency from lowest (with smoothest images) to sharpest (with high image noise). According to our experience, reconstruction kernels are perhaps the most under-utilized parameters to improve image quality particularly when it comes to low dose CT or CT of very large patient. When appropriately (particularly when not looking for small anatomical or pathology details) a softer or smoother kernel can be used to improve image noise in lower dose CT images.

Smoother or softer side of the kernels helps lower noise at the expense of poorer edge delineation. Sharper kernels provide better edge delineation and spatial resolution with trade off of higher image noise (Fig. 3). Theses features are further fine-tuned to optimize kernels for specific anatomy and function or even size.

## 14 Section Thickness and Section Interval

Section thickness is defined as the nominal width (in mm) of reconstructed image in the longitudinal axis. Section interval or increment (in mm) is defined as the distance between two consecutive reconstructed images. Thinner section contains higher image noise but less partial volume averaging. In general 50% decrease in section thickness doubles the image noise. Acquiring thin slices and reconstructing thick slices for viewing could reduce image noise and accept lower dose images (Fig. 4). With modern MDCT, general use of thinner sections for routine interpolation should be avoided as thinner sections do have

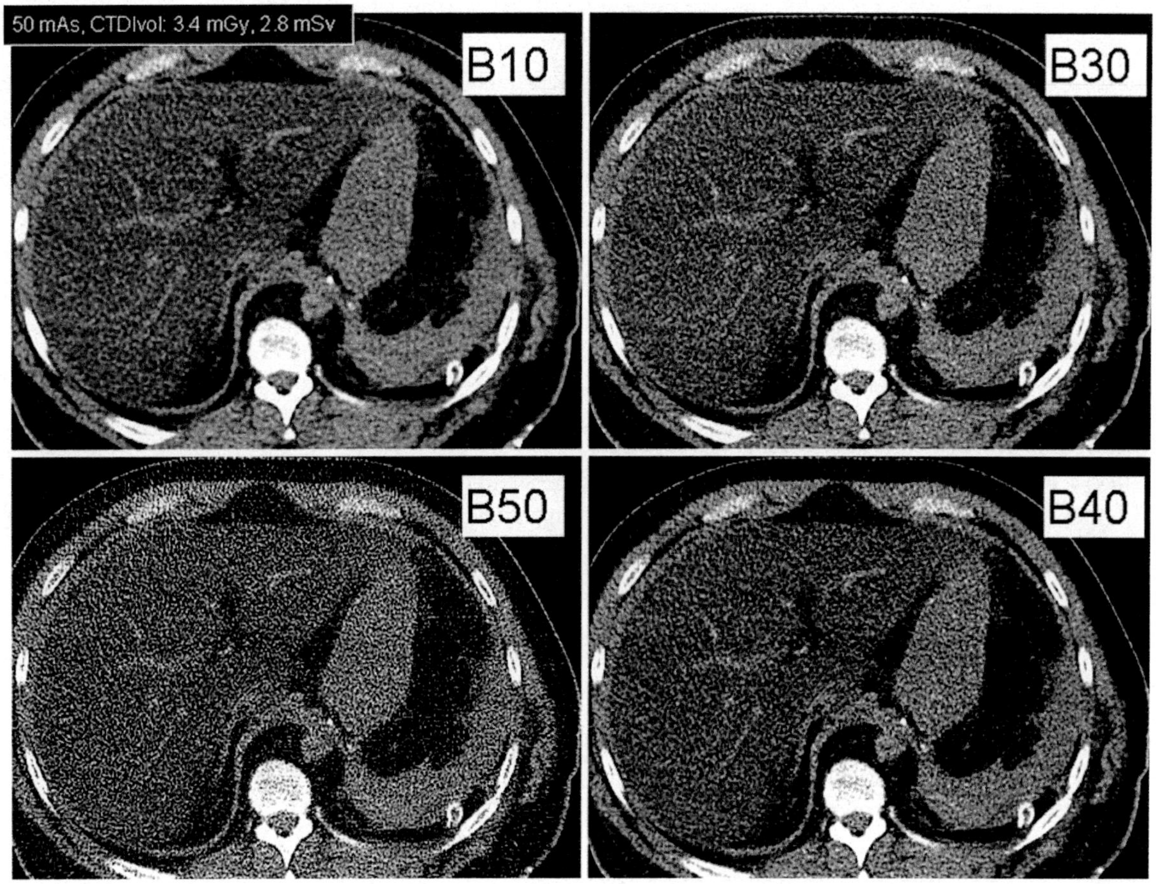


**Fig. 3** Transverse abdominal CT images reconstructed with various kernels (B10, B30, B40 and B50, Siemens Healthcare). B10 kernel (*smooth*) image shows reduced noise and smoother edges as compared to B50 kernel

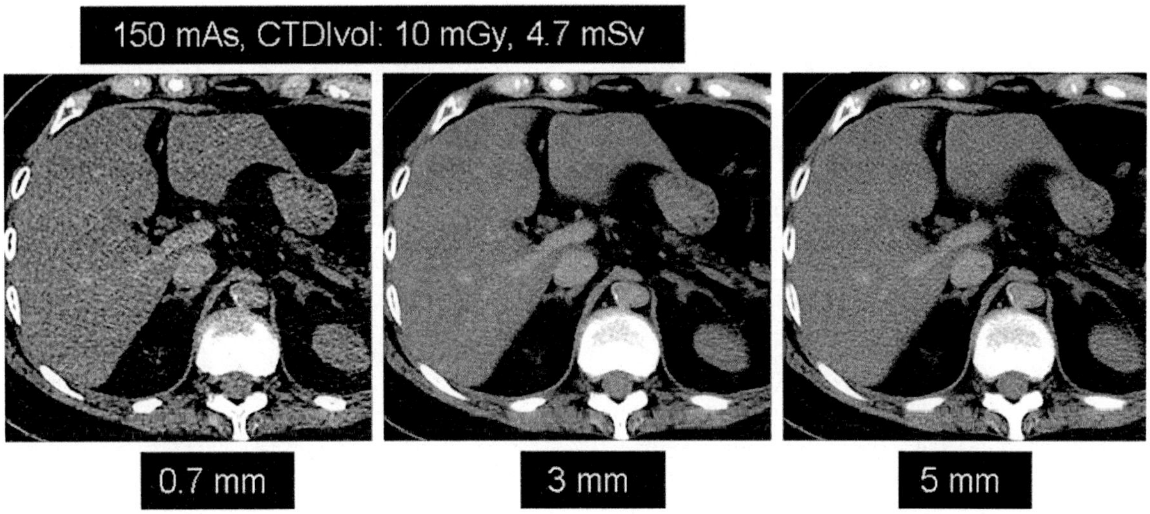


**Fig. 4** Transverse abdominal CT images reconstructed with at various section thicknesses (0.75, 3 and 5 mm). As slice thickness decreases, there is increase in image noise, so for primarily interpretation of routine studies, thicker sections must be used

higher image noise and may trigger need for higher dose CT data acquisition. On some scanners prospective prescribed section thickness has profound effect on automatic exposure control can lead to high doses, if careful attention is not paid. For example, on GE Healthcare's AEC technique (Auto mA), let us prescribe 20 noise index for 5 mm section thickness and get a CTDIvol of 10 mGy. If you change the section thickness to 1.25 mm, the system automatically increases the noise index to maintain 10 mGy, but if user over writes the noise index to original 20 for 1.25 mm section thickness, the CTDIvol will increase substantially as higher dose is necessary to obtain image noise in 1.25 mm sections that is equal to image noise in 5 mm sections. Other scanners are "section-neutral" and do not change radiation dose based on section thickness change.

## 15 Image Post Processing

Image post processing is defined as an additional phase of altering or improving the CT image quality, after CT images have been generated from the scanner. These mathematical algorithms are designed optimize image noise, image contrast, spatial resolution and finally artifacts. Prime focus of the process is to reduce or filter image noise while retaining contrast and spatial resolution; hence the common name image noise reduction filters. Image post processing filters are particularly very helpful in salvaging noisy or "bad" scan, for example, in an obese patient or in general very low dose CT examination and avoid any repeat acquisition in patients. CT manufacturers and 3rd party vendors or the non CT manufactures has take various approaches to lower image noise, technical details and types of these filters are discussed in depth in "Image Noise Reduction Filters".

## 16 Other Scanning Techniques

Recent studies have also demonstrated that image post processing 3D techniques, such as average intensity weighted reformats can result in substantial reduction in image noise and increase in acceptability of lower dose images (Lee et al. 2006). When appropriate, this routine image reformation must be employed to reduce radiation dose. Details of iterative reconstruction techniques are presented in "Conventional and Newer Reconstruction Techniques in CT" by Homer Pien and Colleagues. These techniques allow low dose CT data to be reconstructed with much lower noise and in some cases less artifacts. Substantial dose reduction is therefore feasible when using these techniques (Hara et al. 2009; Singh et al. 2010, 2011; Sagara et al. 2010; Prakash et al. 2010; Gervaise et al. 2011; Pontana et al. 2011; Honda et al. 2011).

## 17 Conclusion

In summary, CT scanning and radiation dose optimization involves working with several intricately-related scanning parameters. Understanding of general scan parameters and reconstruction approaches can help optimize and manage radiation dose in a more appropriate manner.

## References

Discovery™ CT750 wHD, Learning and reference guide. Operator manual, English 5308208-1EN revision: 2 (10-08). GE Healthcare, London

Gervaise A, Osemont B, Lecocq S, Noel A, Micard E, Felblinger J, Blum A (2011) CT image quality improvement using adaptive iterative dose reduction with wide-volume acquisition on 320-detector CT. Eur Radiol 22:295–301

Goldman LW (2008) Principles of CT: multislice CT. J Nucl Med Technol 36(2):57–68 quiz 75–76

Hara AK, Paden RG, Silva AC, Kujak JL, Lawder HJ, Pavlicek W (2009) Iterative reconstruction technique for reducing body radiation dose at CT: feasibility study. AJR Am J Roentgenol 193(3):764–771

Honda O, Yanagawa M, Inoue A, Kikuyama A, Yoshida S, Sumikawa H, Tobino K, Koyama M, Tomiyama N (2011) Image quality of multiplanar reconstruction of pulmonary CT scans using adaptive statistical iterative reconstruction. Br J Radiol 84:335–341

Hsieh J (2003) Computed tomography: principles, design, artifacts, and recent advances. SPIE Press, Bellingham

Kalra MK, Maher MM, Toth TL et al (2004) Strategies for CT radiation dose optimization. Radiology 230:619–628

Kalva SP, Sahani DV, Hahn PF, Saini S (2006) Using the K-edge to improve contrast conspicuity and to lower radiation dose with a 16-MDCT: a phantom and human study. J Comput Assist Tomogr 30(3):391–397

Lee KH, Kim YH, Hahn S, Lee KW, Kim TJ, Kang SB, Shin JH (2006) Computed tomography diagnosis of acute appendicitis: advantages of reviewing thin-section datasets using sliding slab average intensity projection technique. Invest Radiol 41(7):579–585

Mahesh M, Scatarige JC, Cooper J, Fishman EK (2001) Dose and pitch relationship for a particular multislice CT scanner. AJR Am J Roentgenol 177(6):1273–1275

Pontana F, Duhamel A, Pagniez J, Flohr T, Faivre JB, Hachulla AL, Remy J, Remy-Jardin M (2011) Chest computed tomography using iterative reconstruction vs filtered back projection (Part 2): image quality of low-dose CT examinations in 80 patients. Eur Radiol 21(3):636–643

Prakash P, Kalra MK, Digumarthy SR, Hsieh J, Pien H, Singh S, Gilman MD, Shepard JA (2010) Radiation dose reduction with chest computed tomography using adaptive statistical iterative reconstruction technique: initial experience. J Comput Assist Tomogr 34:40–45

Singh S, Kalra MK, Moore MA, Shailam R, Liu B, Toth TL, Grant E, Westra SJ (2009) Dose reduction and compliance with pediatric CT protocols adapted to patient size, clinical indication, and number of prior studies. Radiology 252(1): 200–208

Singh S, Kalra MK, Hsieh J, Licato PE, Do S, Pien HH (2010) Abdominal CT: comparison of adaptive statistical iterative and filtered back projection reconstruction techniques. Radiology 257:373–383

Singh S, Kalra MK, Gilman MD, Hsieh J, Pien HH, Digumarthy SR et al (2011) Adaptive statistical iterative reconstruction technique for radiation dose reduction in chest CT: a pilot study. Radiology 2011(259):565–573

Sagara Y, Hara AK, Pavlicek W, Silva AC, Paden RG, Wu Q (2010) Abdominal CT: comparison of low-dose CT with adaptive statistical iterative reconstruction and routine-dose CT with filtered back projection in 53 patients. AJR Am J Roentgenol 195:713–719

Size-Specific Dose Estimates (SSDE) In Pediatric and Adult Body CT Examinations. AAPM report 204, 2011. http://www.aapm.org/pubs/reports/RPT_204.pdf. Accessed 27 Dec 2011

Wintersperger B, Jakobs T, Herzog P, Schaller S, Nikolaou K, Suess C, Weber C, Reiser M, Becker C (2005) Aorto-iliac multidetector-row CT angiography with low kV settings: improved vessel enhancement and simultaneous reduction of radiation dose. Eur Radiol 15(2):334–341

Yamaguchi M, Fujita H, Bessho Y, Inoue T, Asai Y, Murase K (2011) Investigation of optimal display size for detecting ground-glass opacity on high resolution computed tomography using a new digital contrast-detail phantom. Eur J Radiol 80(3):845–850

# Optimization of Tube Potential for Radiation Dose Reduction in CT

Lifeng Yu, Joel G. Fletcher, and Cynthia H. McCollough

## Contents



**Abstract**

Tube potential is an important scanning parameter that should be optimized in clinical CT in order to improve image quality or reduce radiation dose. The main benefit of lower tube potentials is the improved enhancement of contrast materials relative to higher tube potentials. However, there is usually increased image noise at lower tube potentials, especially for larger patient sizes. This tradeoff between contrast enhancement and noise requires that patient size and diagnostic task be carefully considered when selecting the optimal tube potential for radiation dose reduction. In addition, CT x-ray tube and generator limitations, scanning speed, and artifacts must also be considered. This chapter describes the basic principles of optimal tube potential for radiation dose reduction in CT and provides a summary of recent development on automatic selection of optimal tube potential.

## 1 Introduction

Concerns with the potential risk of cancer induction resulting from the radiation dose in CT exams have arisen with the drastically increased use of CT (Brenner and Hall 2007; Einstein et al. 2007; Huda 2007). Although the existence of such risk remains controversial for the level of radiation doses typically received in diagnostic CT (Little et al. 2009; Tubiana et al. 2009), consensus is that patients should receive radiation dose as low as reasonably achievable (ALARA).

A commonly used method to reduce radiation dose is automatic exposure control (AEC), which automatically adapts the tube current in both angular

L. Yu (✉) · J. G. Fletcher · C. H. McCollough
Department of Radiology,
Mayo Clinic College of Medicine,
200 First Street SW, Rochester,
MN 55905, USA
e-mail: yu.lifeng@mayo.edu

D. Tack et al. (eds.), *Radiation Dose from Multidetector CT*, Medical Radiology. Diagnostic Imaging,
DOI: 10.1007/174_2011_490, 

and longitudinal directions according to patient attenuation to achieve predefined image quality (Gies et al. 1999; Kalender et al. 1999; Kalra et al. 2004a, b). Another important technique is to adjust tube potential. Many researchers have studied this technique (Huda et al. 2000; Boone et al. 2003; Siegel et al. 2004; Cody et al. 2004; Ertl-Wagner et al. 2004; Sigal-Cinqualbre et al. 2004; Funama et al. 2005; Frush and Herlong 2005; Wintersperger et al. 2005; Holmquist and Nyman 2006; Schueller-Weidekamm et al. 2006; Waaijer et al. 2007; Kalva et al. 2006; Frush 2008; Leschka et al. 2008; Kalender et al. 2009; Schindera et al. 2008). A common critical finding in these studies was that the appropriateness of using lower tube potential is highly dependent on patient size and diagnostic task. For smaller patients and some types of contrast-enhanced studies such as CT angiography (CTA), the dose reduction can be 50% or even higher. But for bigger patient sizes and other exam types, the image quality may become unacceptable if using the lower tube potential even without any radiation dose reduction. Selection of an optimal tube potential should take into account both the patient size and diagnostic task. In clinical practice this non-trivial task demands a quantitative approach that can automatically determine the optimal tube potential for an individual patient along with the amount of radiation dose reduction. Automatic selection of tube potential can be incorporated into the AEC in addition to the automatic tube current modulation in order to provide a convenient approach to optimizing the dose efficiency of scanning technique without much user interaction (McCollough 2005).

In this chapter, we first describe the basic principles of selecting the optimal tube potential for radiation dose reduction. Then we provide a summary on recent developments in automatic techniques to select the most dose-efficient tube potential. Special considerations when using lower tube potential are also discussed.

## 2 Principles of Optimal Tube Potential in CT

### 2.1 Contrast

Most CT exams involve the use of iodinated contrast media. The different energy dependence of the linear attenuation coefficients for iodine and water leads to different CT numbers for iodine at different tube potentials (Fig. 1). The increase of the CT number of iodine at lower tube potentials provides more iodine signal and hence improves the conspicuity of hypervascular or hypovascular pathologies (Schindera et al. 2008; Macari et al. 2010). Figure 2 shows a clinical example that demonstrates the benefit of the increased iodine signal at lower tube potential.

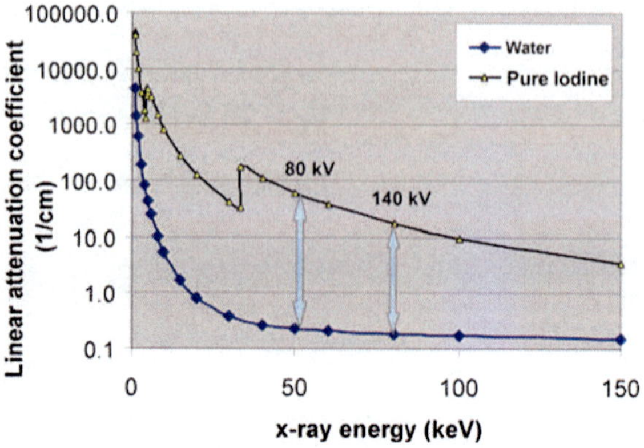


**Fig. 1** Linear attenuation coefficients of iodine and water as a function of X-ray energy. The *arrows* indicate the difference of linear attenuation coefficients between iodine and water at the mean energy of a typical 80 kV and 140 kV X-ray beam. Data are from National Institute of Standards and Technology (NIST) website: http://www.nist.gov/physlab/data/xraycoef/index.cfm

Figure 3 displays CT images of three water phantoms scanned using four different tube potentials available on a 128-slice scanner (Definition Flash, Siemens Healthcare). The lateral widths of the three phantoms were 25, 35, and 45 cm, representing typical attenuation levels for a small, average, and large sized adult, respectively. For each phantom size, the scanning technique (in quality reference mAs) was adjusted so that the radiation output, represented in terms of $CTDI_{vol}$, was matched for the four tube potentials (25 cm: 6.6 mGy; 35 cm, 15.3 mGy; 45 cm, 37.0 mGy). AEC was turned on. Several different contrast materials were placed inside the water to allow for measurement of material contrast. Figure 4 plots the contrast of iodine (the sample with an iodine concentration of 6.9 mg/cc, see arrows on 120 kV images) at the four tube potentials. On average, the iodine contrast of 80 kV was about 70 and 100% higher than that of 120 and 140 kV, and the iodine contrast of 100 kV was about 25 and 50% higher than that of 120 and 140 kV, respectively. The increase of iodine contrast at lower tube potential varies with the phantom size due to beam hardening.

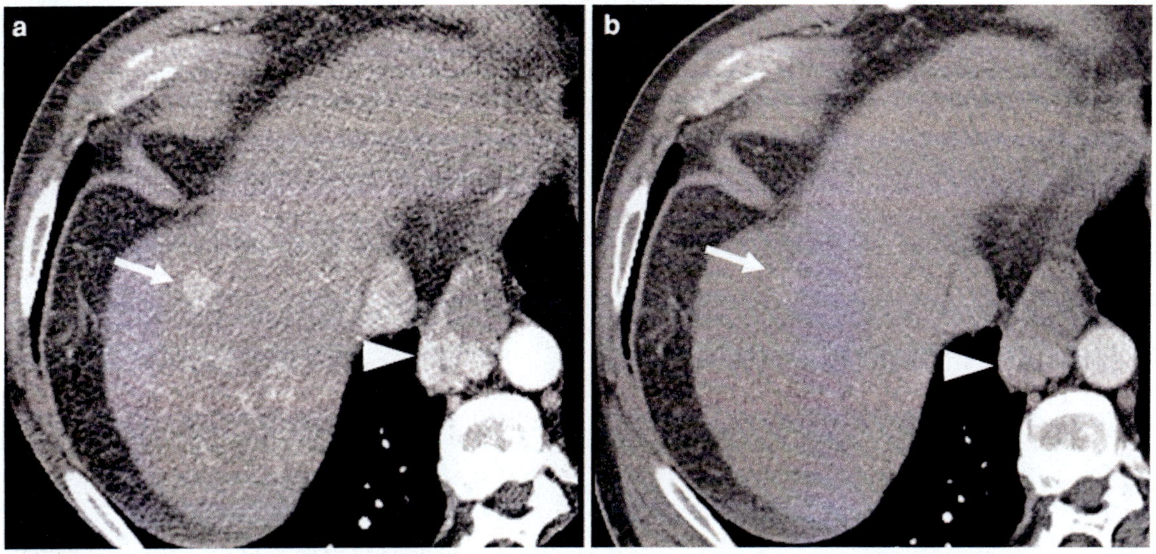


**Fig. 2** A 56 year-old female with contrast-enhanced dual-energy CT performed in the late arterial phase, demonstrating an hypervascular hepatocellular carcinoma at 80 kV (**a**) and 140 kV (**b**). The tumor (*arrows*) and esophageal varices (*arrowhead*) are much more conspicuous at 80 kV

## 2.2 Noise

Noise is another important factor that greatly influences image quality. Here we only discuss how noise level (expressed as the standard deviation of the CT numbers in a uniform region) is affected by tube potential and patient size. Noise spatial correlation and higher-order statistics also contribute significantly to the image quality, but they remain similar at different tube potentials provided that other factors such as reconstruction algorithms are the same. Figure 5 shows the noise level measured on the three phantom sizes at each of the four tube potentials (data from the same measurements as in Fig. 4). Note that the $CTDI_{vol}$ was matched for each of the four tube potentials when scanning the same phantom. For the 25 cm phantom size, the noise level was similar at 100, 120, and 140 kV and there was a slight increase at 80 kV. For the 35 and 45 cm phantom, noise increases substantially on the 80 kV images. In addition, significant photon-starvation artifacts appeared in the 80 kV images of the large phantom, due to the decreased penetrating capability of the lower energy photons and electronic noise (Guimaraes et al. 2010).

## 2.3 Contrast to Noise Ratio

Contrast to noise ratio (CNR) is typically used to represent the combined effect of contrast and image noise—both of which are important image quality metrics. CNR cannot be used to quantify the absolute image quality of an image as it does not take into account the effect of system spatial resolution, noise texture, and object size. However, if all other factors are the same, then CNR can serve as a relative measure to compare image quality. CNR is often expressed in terms of iodine contrast divided by noise in the background structures because iodine is the most widely used contrast material in CT. Figure 6 shows the iodine CNR at each of the four tube potentials for the three phantoms. The improvement of iodine CNR for the 25 cm phantom at lower tube potentials was very significant (almost doubled). The amount of increase in iodine CNR as tube potential was decreased was smaller for bigger phantoms. The iodine CNR at 80 kV for the 35 cm phantom still increased, but it dropped slightly for the 45 cm phantom. Based on Fig. 6, it appears that 80 or 100 kV images are still very close to 120 kV images in terms of iodine CNR. However, the actual image

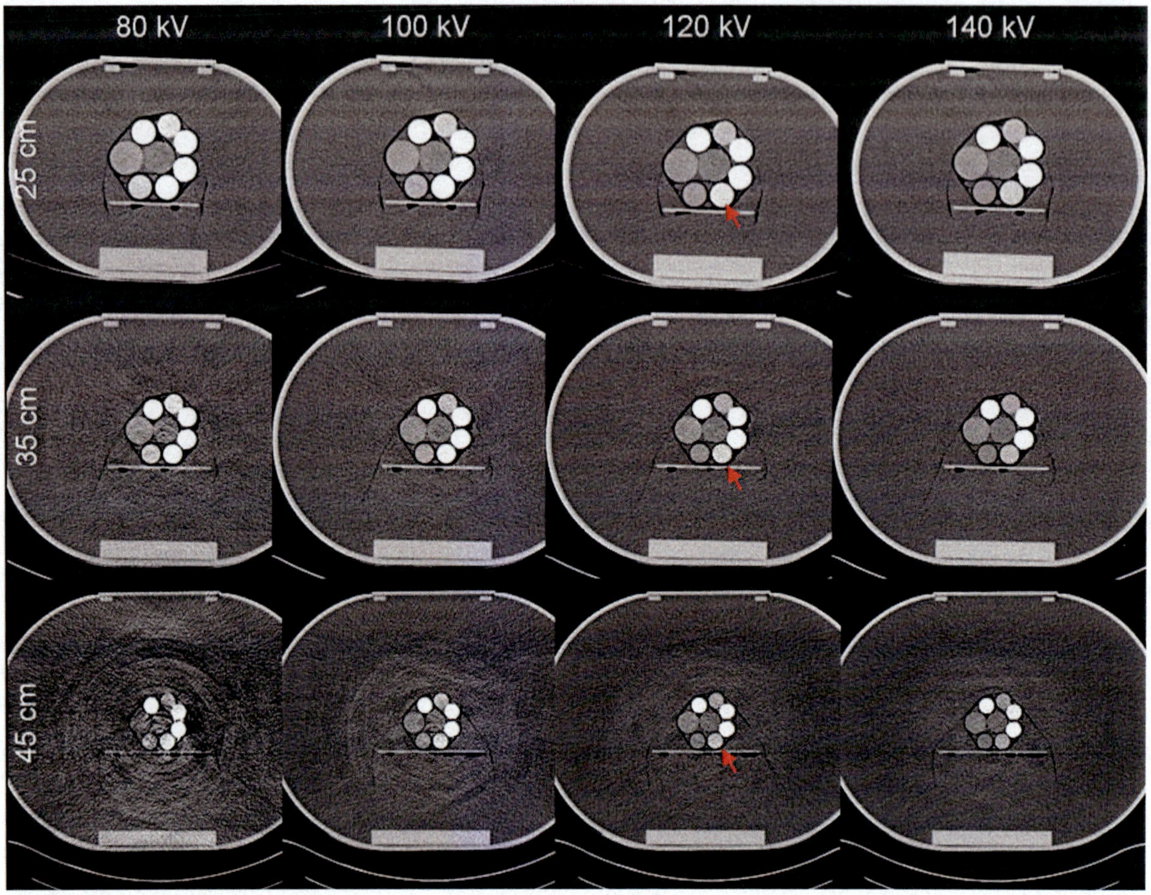


**Fig. 3** CT images of three water phantoms scanned with four tube potentials at the same $CTDI_{vol}$ for a given phantom size. The phantom lateral widths were 25, 35, 45 cm. For each phantom size, the prescribed $CTDI_{vol}$ was matched across the four tube potentials (25 cm: 6.6 mGy; 35 cm, 15.3 mGy; 45 cm, 37.0 mGy)

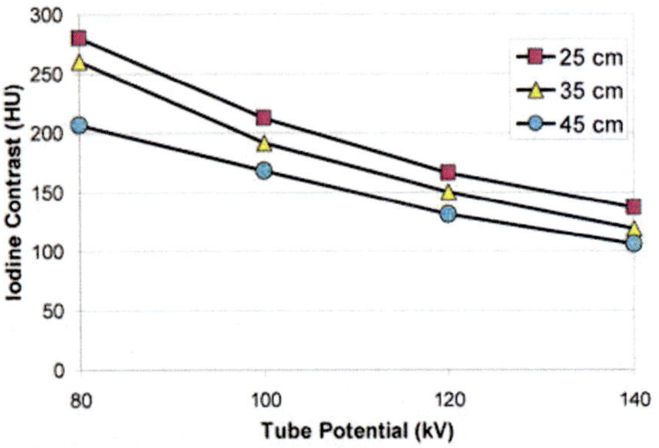


**Fig. 4** The change of iodine contrast with tube potential for different phantom sizes. For each phantom size, the $CTDI_{vol}$ was held constant as tube potential varied

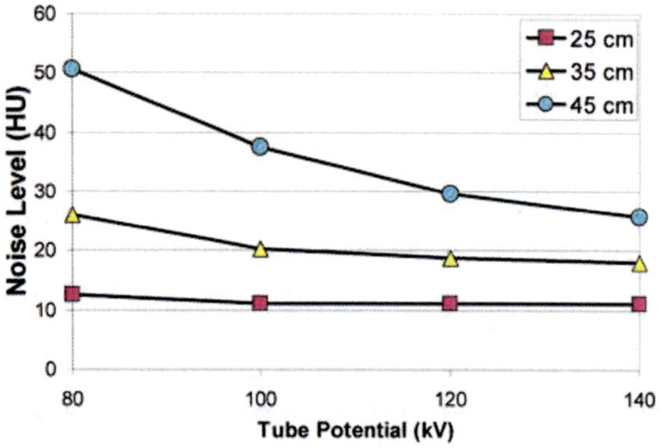


**Fig. 5** The change of noise level with tube potential for different phantom sizes. For each phantom size, the $CTDI_{vol}$ was held constant as tube potential varied

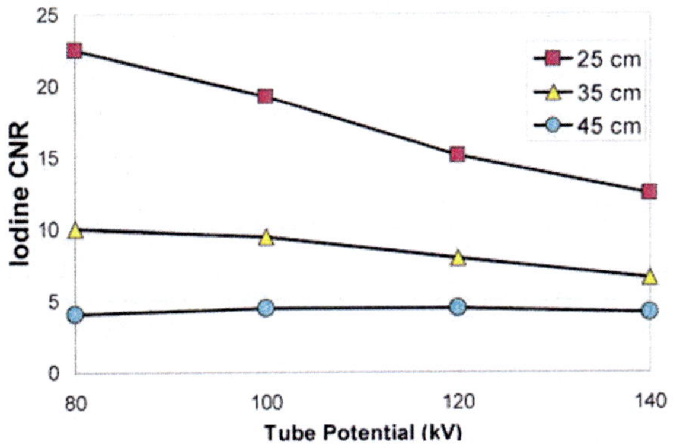


**Fig. 6** The change of iodine CNR with tube potential for different phantom sizes. For each phantom size, the $CTDI_{vol}$ was held constant as tube potential varied

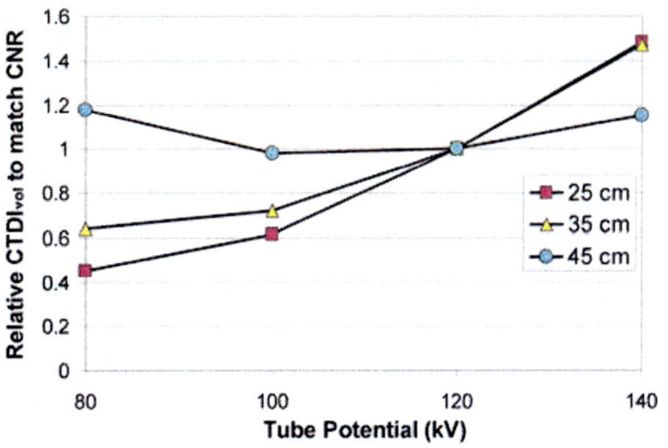


**Fig. 7** The relative radiation output required at each tube potential to obtain the same iodine CNR for the three phantoms

quality degradation at lower tube potentials for the large phantom actually cannot be fully characterized by the iodine CNR. As shown in Fig. 3 there were very severe photon starvation artifacts in the 80 kV image for the 45 cm phantom. Because of this reason, lower tube potentials should not be used for large patients.

## 2.4 Radiation Dose Reduction if Iodine CNR is to be Matched

To quantify how much radiation dose can be reduced, one should set up a target image quality using an appropriate image quality metric. By comparing the radiation dose needed at each tube potential to achieve the target image quality, one can determine the most dose-efficient tube potential. This section discusses the situation when iodine CNR is used as the image quality metric. Because of the increased iodine CNR at lower tube potentials, one could reduce the radiation dose and achieve similar or improved iodine CNR relative to the more commonly used 120 kV. Figure 7 displays the relative $CTDI_{vol}$ at each tube potential if the same iodine CNR is to be achieved. For the 25 cm phantom, the $CTDI_{vol}$ needed for identical CNR relative to that at 120 kV is 46% at 80 kV and 62% at 100 kV. The potential for dose reduction decreases with increasing phantom size. For the 35 cm phantom, 64% at 80 kV and 72% at 100 kV are needed. For the 45 cm, one needs 18% more dose at 80 kV than at 120 kV in order to match the iodine CNR. In this chapter we use $CTDI_{vol}$ to quantify the radiation level of the scanning technique and calculate the amount of radiation dose reduction. It should be noted that $CTDI_{vol}$ can only represent the weighted average dose measured in a standard CTDI phantom and it is not the radiation dose in patients. Knowing the patient attenuation, the radiation dose in each individual patient can be estimated using empirical methods or calculated using Monte Carlo-based methods (American Association of Physicists in Medicine Task Group 204, 2011; Li et al. 2011). For the purpose of estimating the relative radiation dose reduction among different tube potentials for the same patient, using $CTDI_{vol}$ is sufficient.

Based on the above phantom results, for small patient sizes, it appears that a significant amount of radiation dose can be saved using lower tube potential if matching iodine CNR is the goal. However, this is not necessarily correct for all clinical tasks. For example, consider the situation when the iodine CNR is matched for each tube potential. For the 25 cm phantom, the contrast at 80 kV is about 70% higher than at 120 kV. Therefore, if the iodine CNR were matched between the two tube potentials, the resulting noise at 80 kV would also be 70% higher than at 120 kV. For some diagnostic tasks, such as CTA for the evaluation of relatively large vessels, the increased iodine contrast may be sufficient to compensate for the increased noise level. However, for diagnostic tasks that involve the characterization of organs or structures without much iodine uptake, the benefit of brighter iodine at lower tube potential may not compensate sufficiently for the increase in noise. For these types of diagnostic tasks, the strategy of reducing radiation dose by matching the iodine CNR

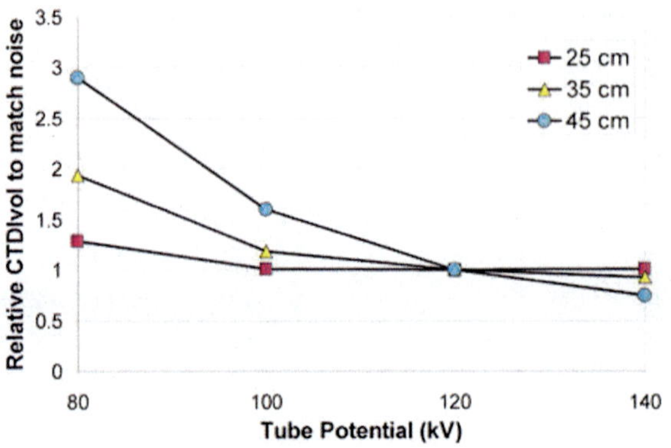


**Fig. 8** The relative radiation output required at each tube potential to obtain the same noise level for the three phantoms

is not appropriate (Yu et al. 2010). To select the most dose-efficient tube potential, noise must be considered independently from iodine CNR.

## 2.5 Radiation Dose Reduction if Noise is to be Matched

Based on measurements of noise at equivalent doses, the relative dose that is required at each tube potential in order to achieve the same noise level can be estimated. Figure 8 clearly demonstrates that if the image noise of a 120 kV image is to be matched, the potential for dose reduction at lower tube potentials is very limited or non-existent. Even for the 25 cm phantom that represents the attenuation of a very small adult, a 29% dose increase is required at 80 kV in order to match the noise. For the 35 cm phantom, representing the attenuation of a medium-sized adult, a 94% dose increase at 80 kV and a 18% dose increase at 100 kV is required achieve the same noise level. The increase in dose required for 45 cm phantom at lower tube potentials is even more dramatic.

## 2.6 Radiation Dose Reduction When Both Iodine CNR and Noise are Incorporated

One can see that the selection of the most dose-efficient tube potential and the estimate of the amount of dose reduction possible are highly dependent on the image quality metric that is used for matching at different tube potentials. The appropriate image quality metric is determined by the clinical task to be performed. When the task only involves the evaluation of highly iodine-enhanced vessels or structures, iodine CNR may be an appropriate image quality metric to use. If the diagnostic task involves evaluation of non-enhanced or poorly-enhanced soft tissue structures, then matching noise is more appropriate and the dose reduction is quite restricted using a lower tube potential. Many diagnostic tasks, such as routine contrast-enhanced abdomen/pelvis exams, are somewhere between these two scenarios. Lower tube potentials bring some benefit on the contrast enhancement of iodine, but the noise cannot be too high. A scheme that can utilize the benefit of the contrast enhancement at lower tube potentials but also can control the noise level is necessary to accommodate different diagnostic tasks. Therefore, an image quality index that can allow flexible adjustment between matching iodine CNR and matching noise is attractive to determine the most dose-efficient tube potential.

## 2.7 A General Strategy for Calculating the Most Dose-Efficient Tube Potential

To provide the flexibility between matching noise and matching iodine CNR, a novel image quality index, "noise-constrained iodine contrast to noise ratio (NC_iCNR)", was proposed to quantify the different levels of image quality required by different clinical applications for a reference dose level and tube potential (Yu et al. 2010). This quality index requires that iodine CNR and noise at the new settings of tube potential and dose level satisfy the following two conditions:

$$\mathrm{CNR} \geq \mathrm{CNR}_{\mathrm{ref}} \;\&\; \sigma \leq \alpha\sigma_{\mathrm{ref}},$$

where $\mathrm{CNR}_{\mathrm{ref}}$ and $\sigma_{\mathrm{ref}}$ denotes the iodine CNR and the noise level obtained in a reference scanning technique (e.g., a reference tube potential and mAs), respectively; $\alpha$ is a coefficient that specifies the level of noise constraint, which can be adjusted according to the diagnostic task. Maintaining a constant noise ($\alpha = 1$) or iodine CNR ($\alpha > 2$) are two special cases of this general image quality index. The relative $\mathrm{CTDI}_{\mathrm{vol}}$ at each tube potential to achieve the target image quality can then be determined as a function of

**Table 1** Optimal tube potential for different phantom sizes (lateral width) in abdomen CT exams when different noise constraints are applied. Recommended exam types for each noise constraint level are also listed. CTE = CT enterography; CTU = CT urography; CTA = CT angiography

| Noise Constraint | Recommended exam types | 25 cm | 30 cm | 35 cm | 40 cm | 45 cm | 50 cm | 55 cm |
|---|---|---|---|---|---|---|---|---|
| Very weak $\alpha$=1.00 | Routine non-contrast exams | 120 | 120 | 120 | 120 | 120 | 120 | 140 |
| Weak $\alpha$=1.15 | Liver, pancreas exams | 100 | 100 | 100 | 120 | 120 | 120 | 140 |
| Average $\alpha$=1.25 | Routine contrast-enhanced exams | 100 | 100 | 100 | 100 | 120 | 120 | 140 |
| Strong $\alpha$=1.50 | CTE, CTU, stone, or some CTA exams | 80 | 80 | 100 | 100 | 100 | 120 | 140 |
| Very strong $\alpha$=2.00 | CTA only involving large vessels | 80 | 80 | 80 | 100 | 100 | 120 | 140 |

patient attenuation $\Omega$, and the noise-constraint parameter $\alpha$, which is given by Yu et al. (2010)

$$RD(\Omega,kV)=\min\left\{\frac{C(\Omega,kV)}{C(\Omega,kV_{\text{ref}})},\alpha(\Omega,kV)\right\}^2\cdot\frac{k(\Omega,kV)}{k(\Omega,kV_{\text{ref}})}$$

where $k$ is a coefficient that relates the noise to radiation dose, which is a function of patient attenuation and tube potential. Here we use a general noise-constraint parameter that can vary as a function of both tube potential and patient attenuation.

This new image quality index applies a noise constraint when matching the iodine CNR. By adjusting the noise constraint parameter, the maximally increased noise level at lower tube potential, relative to the reference tube potential, can be adjusted based on the image quality requirements for different diagnostic tasks. One can see that, in this general image quality index, the noise constraint is compared to the relative contrast gain $\frac{C(\Omega,kV)}{C(\Omega,kV_{\text{ref}})}$ at each tube potential. This is equivalent to applying a constraint on the contrast gain at each tube potential relative to the reference tube potential.

Table 1 displays the optimal tube potential for seven different abdominal phantom sizes (in terms of lateral width) at five different noise constraint settings using the general strategy described above. The recommended noise constraint parameters for different exam types are also listed.

## 3 Clinical Implementation of Optimal Tube Potential

As described in the above basic principles, selecting the optimal tube potential that can use the least radiation dose to achieve the target image quality is a complicated task. There are two methods to implement the optimal tube potential: one is to implement a manual kV-mAs technique chart, the other is to implement a software tool on the scanner that can automatically select the optimal tube potential.

### 3.1 Manual kV-mAs Technique Chart

A convenient way to implement optimal tube potential is to use a patient weight or size-based kV-mAs chart, which specifies the tube potential and tube current (or mAs or effective mAs or reference mAs) for different patient weight or size ranges. The selection of the tube potential and the mAs level can be based on empirical evaluation or quantitative measurements on phantoms. According to the phantom results and the general strategy for automatic tube potential selection described above, Table 2 provides two example kV-mAs charts implemented on a 128-slice scanner (Definition Flash, Siemens Healthcare). One is for contrast enhanced routine abdomen/pelvis

**Table 2** Example kV-mAs technique chart for (a) contrast-enhanced routine abdomen/pelvis exams and (b) abdominal CTA exams, implemented on a 128-slice scanner (Definition Flash, Siemens Healthcare) according to the phantom measurements and the general strategy for automatic tube potential selection. Note that the relative $CTDI_{vol}$ is beyond the reduction of radiation dose allowed by CAREDose4D, the automatic exposure control (AEC) software on Siemens CT scanners. The further dose reduction beyond AEC for smaller patients was enabled by the use of lower tube potential (80 or 100 kV)

| Patient lateral width (cm)—mid liver | Optimal kV | Quality reference mAs | Helical pitch | Relative $CTDI_{vol}$ (versus use of 120 kV and CAREDose 4D) |
|---|---|---|---|---|
| (a) | | | | |
| <30 | 80 | 580 | 0.5 | 0.70 |
| 30–40 | 100 | 330 | 0.8 | 0.85 |
| 41–50 | 120 | 240 | 0.8 | 1.00 |
| >50 | 140 | 165 | 0.8 | 1.00 |
| (b) | | | | |
| <33 | 80 | 440 | 0.6 | 0.50 |
| 33–43 | 100 | 300 | 0.6 | 0.75 |
| 44–53 | 120 | 250 | 0.6 | 1.00 |
| >53 | 140 | 170 | 0.6 | 1.00 |

exams, the other for abdominal CTA exams. Note that for both protocols, the reduced $CTDI_{vol}$ at lower tube potential for smaller patients compared to the reference technique at 120 kV is in addition to the radiation dose reduction determined by CAREDose4D, the AEC software on Siemens CT scanners. The further dose reduction beyond AEC was enabled by the use of lower tube potentials (80 or 100 kV). The dose reduction increases with the decrease of the patient size. For large patients, no dose reduction is allowed compared to the reference 120 kV technique. As explained in the basic principles of optimal tube potential, CTA exams allow more dose reduction at lower tube potentials because the primary organ of interest is iodine-enhanced vessels. A relatively stringent noise constraint was applied in the kV-mAs chart for routine abdomen/pelvis exams, which resulted in a smaller dose reduction than CTA exams at lower tube potentials.

## 3.2 An Automatic kV Selection Tool Implemented on a Clinical Scanner

An obvious disadvantage of the manual kV-mAs technique chart is its approximate determination of the patient attenuation level. Patient lateral width or other measures (weight, perimeter, etc.) measured by technologists based on the scout or topogram are not always accurate representations of the true patient attenuation at each anatomic level in the scan range. In addition, using a manual chart like in Table 1, one has to prescribe a fixed amount of dose reduction for a certain patient size range (e.g., 30–40 cm), which should be gradually varied based on the patient attenuation level. The manual selection of the techniques may also be more susceptible to human error. Therefore, the selection of the optimal tube potential should be implemented on the CT scanner so that the software can automatically recommend the optimal tube potential and the reduced dose for each individual patient and each specific diagnostic task. The same strategy as describe above can be implemented in the automatic software.

One such software was recently developed by one of the major CT manufacturers (CAREkV, Siemens Healthcare). An example of using this software to select the optimal tube potential and to prescribe the dose-reduced technique is provided in Fig. 9. The reference technique was at 120 kV and 250 quality reference mAs. A strength setting was configured for the exam through a slider bar, as shown in the user interface, which corresponds to a contrast gain constraint setting, equivalent to the noise constraint described above. The software automatically determines the optimal tube potential and the dose-reduced technique.

In a recent study with 101 CTA (CT angiography) exams (162 scans) and 91 contrast-enhanced abdomen-pelvis CT exams (113 scans) performed using

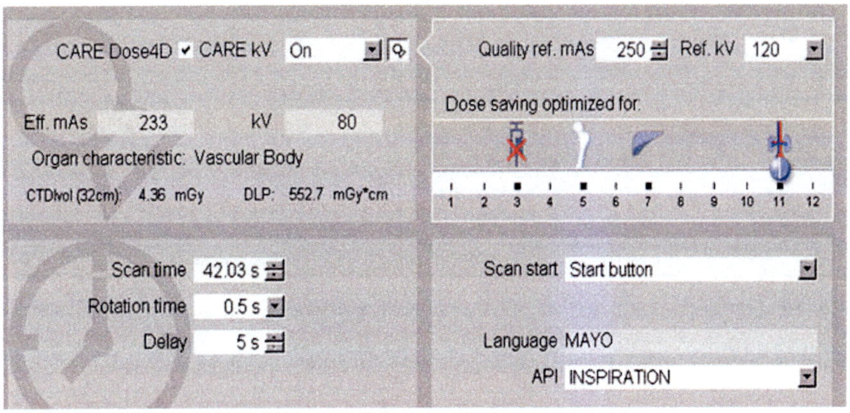


**Fig. 9** Example of using an automatic software to select the optimal tube potential and to prescribe the dose-reduced technique (CAREkV, Siemens Healthcare). The reference technique was at 120 kV and 250 quality reference mAs. The slider bar position, which corresponds to a strength setting, was at 11. 80 kV was identified as the optimal tube potential

the automatic tube potential selection tool (Yu et al. 2011a, b), 80 or 100 kV was automatically used for 73% of the CTA scans and 54% of the abdomen-pelvis scans. Overall radiation dose reductions of 29.6 ± 17.0% and 17 ± 15% compared with the reference 120 kV protocols were achieved for CTA scans and abdomen-pelvis scans, respectively. All exams were considered to have acceptable quality in terms of sharpness and diagnostic confidence. The automatic tube potential selection tool provided an efficient and quantitative way to guide the selection of the most dose-efficient tube potential in a busy practice of abdominal CT and CTA. Figure 10 provides image examples from an abdominal CTA case. In this case, the patient size was relatively small (lateral width 28 cm across the mid liver and 33 cm across the pelvis). The original reference technique was at 120 kV and 250 quality reference mAs, which would have resulted in a $CTDI_{vol}$ of 11.2 mGy. With the kV selection software, 80 kV was identified as the most dose efficient tube potential, and the $CTDI_{vol}$ was substantially reduced to 5.7 mGy, a 49% reduction from the reference technique.

## 4 Other Considerations When Adjusting Tube Potential

*First,* scan time and tube current limits are two important factors that need to be considered when adjusting tube potential (Yu et al. 2011c). CT systems have a limit to the maximum tube current, and consequently the maximum radiation output. A tradeoff typically exists between scanning speed and the maximum achievable radiation output. High scanning speed usually involves a fast rotation time and a high helical pitch, which limits the maximum radiation output, especially for lower tube potentials. For example, in body mode, the $CTDI_{vol}$ per 100 effective mAs (i.e. mAs/pitch) on a 64 slice scanner (Sensation 64, Siemens Healthcare) is 2.0 mGy for 80 kV, 4.5 mGy for 100 kV, and 7.6 mGy for 120 kV. For a typical 0.5 s rotation time, a 1.0 helical pitch, and a tube current limit of 500 mA, the maximum $CTDI_{vol}$ is only 5 mGy, which is much lower than what is typically required for a small to medium adult in a routine abdomen/pelvis exam (10–20 mGy). One may use a longer rotation time (e.g., 1.0 s) and/or a lower helical pitch (e.g., 0.5) to increase the maximum radiation output, which, however, will substantially increase the scan time. Therefore, when a fast scanning speed and a short scan time are desired, the lower tube potential may not be appropriate, even for small-sized patients. In addition to the image quality consideration, it is essential to take into account the scan time and tube current limit in order to select the most appropriate tube potential.

*Second,* artifacts are another important factor to consider. There are two types of artifacts that tend to appear in scans acquired with lower tube potentials. One is the photon starvation artifacts caused by insufficient penetrating photons. In Fig. 3, one can see that the image obtained with 80 kV for the 45 cm phantom contains much more severe photon starvation artifacts compared to the 120 kV image when the $CTDI_{vol}$ was matched at a standard level, suggesting that 80 kV should not be used at all for this patient size. The other type of artifact that could be of a potential concern for lower tube potentials is streaking and dark shadow or banding artifacts when dense

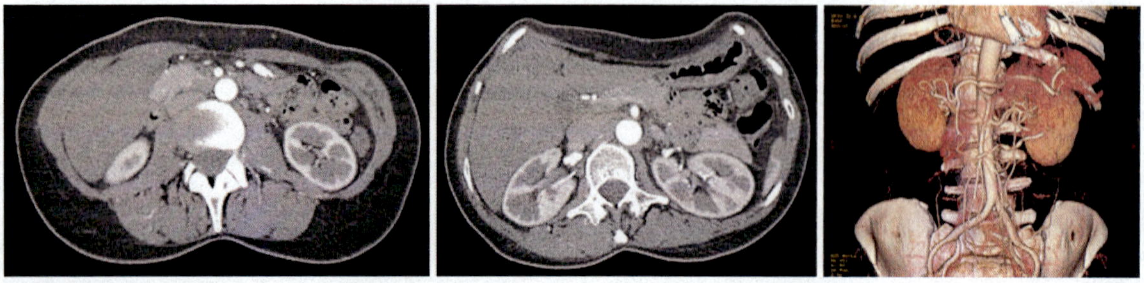

**Fig. 10** Images acquired with the automatic tube potential selection tool in an abdominal CTA exam. For this relatively small patient, 80 kV was identified as the optimal tube potential and the $CTDI_{vol}$ was dropped to 5.7 mGy, a 49% reduction from the reference technique

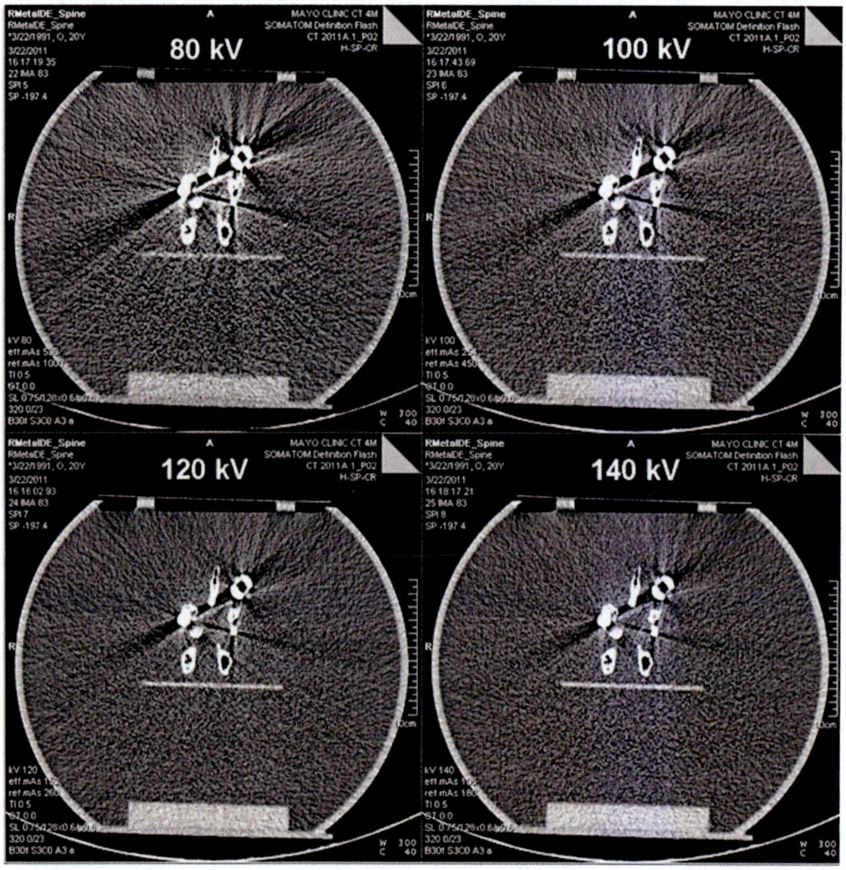


**Fig. 11** Image quality comparison at different tube potentials when a metal implant is present. The $CTDI_{vol}$ was held constant. The image acquired with the highest tube potential at 140 kV appears to contain the least streaking artifacts

materials (e.g., highly concentrated iodine contrast media or metal) are present. Due to the higher attenuation of dense materials at lower tube potential, beam hardening, scattering, and non-linear partial volume effects are more severe than at higher tube potentials. Therefore, if the scan range includes dense materials, a higher tube potential may be more appropriate. Figure 11 compares the image quality at different tube potentials when a metal implant is scanned inside a water tank (30 cm lateral width).

The same $CTDI_{vol}$ was used. The image acquired with the highest tube potential at 140 kV contains the least streaking artifacts.

*Finally*, optimal tube potential can also be used for improving image quality or reducing the volume of iodine contrast used in the CT exam. For some challenging exams, one would rather generate the best possible image quality instead of reducing radiation dose in order to make a confident diagnosis on subtle pathologies. In this situation, one can use the optimal tube potential to maximize the image quality, with no need to reduce the radiation dose. This strategy is particularly important for diagnostic tasks where the imaging performance is suboptimal or when the potential for medical benefit is high (e.g., detection of hepatocellular carcinoma or pancreatic adenocarcinoma). For some patients with difficult intravenous access or suboptimal renal function, one can also utilize the benefit of optimal tube potential to reduce the volume of iodine contrast injected to the patient (Hough et al. 2011).

## 5 Conclusions

This chapter describes the basic principles and clinical implementations of optimal tube potential selection for radiation dose reduction in CT. The appropriateness of tube potential selection and dose reduction is dependent on patient size and diagnostic task, and is also affected by the system tube current limits and scanning speed requirements. The use of lower tube potential should be carefully evaluated for each exam type in order to achieve an optimal tradeoff among contrast, noise, artifacts, and scanning speed.

**Acknowledgments** This work was partially supported by a research grant from Thrasher Research Fund. CHM and JGF have received research support from Siemens Healthcare. The authors would like to thank Ms. Kristina Nunez for her help with manuscript preparation.

## References

American Association of Physicists in Medicine. Size-Specific Dose Estimates (SSDE) (2011) In: Pediatric and Adult Body CT Examinations (Task Group 204).

Boone JM, Geraghty EM, Seibert JA, Wootton-Gorges SL (2003) Dose reduction in pediatric CT: a rational approach. Radiology 228:352–360

Brenner DJ, Hall EJ (2007) Computed tomography—an increasing source of radiation exposure. N Engl J Med 357:2277–2284

Cody DD, Moxley DM, Krugh KT, O'Daniel JC, Wagner LK, Eftekhari F (2004) Strategies for formulating appropriate MDCT techniques when imaging the chest, abdomen, and pelvis in pediatric patients. AJR Am J Roentgenol 182: 849–859

Einstein AJ, Henzlova MJ, Rajagopalan S (2007) Estimating risk of cancer associated with radiation exposure from 64-slice computed tomography coronary angiography. Jama 298:317–323

Ertl-Wagner BB, Hoffmann RT, Bruning R et al (2004) Multi-detector row CT angiography of the brain at various kilovoltage settings. Radiology 231:528–535

Frush DP (2008) Pediatric abdominal CT angiography. Pediatr Radiol 38(Suppl 2):S259–266

Frush DP, Herlong JR (2005) Pediatric thoracic CT angiography. Pediatr Radiol 35:11–25

Funama Y, Awai K, Nakayama Y et al (2005) Radiation dose reduction without degradation of low-contrast detectability at abdominal multisection CT with a low-tube voltage technique: phantom study. Radiology 237:905–910

Gies M, Kalender WA, Wolf H, Suess C (1999) Dose reduction in CT by anatomically adapted tube current modulation. I. Simulation studies. Med Phys 26:2235–2247

Guimaraes LS, Fletcher JG, Harmsen WS et al (2010) Appropriate patient selection at abdominal dual-energy CT using 80 kV: relationship between patient size, image noise, and image quality. Radiology 257:732–742

Holmquist F, Nyman U (2006) Eighty-peak kilovoltage 16-channel multidetector computed tomography and reduced contrast-medium doses tailored to body weight to diagnose pulmonary embolism in azotaemic patients. Eur Radiol 16: 1165–1176

Hough D, Yu L, Shiung M et al (2011) The lymphoma follow-up CT: age-appropriate individualization to decrease IV contrast dose or radiation dose. In: 97th Scientific assembly and meeting of the radiological society of North America, Chicago

Huda W (2007) Radiation doses and risks in chest computed tomography examinations. Proc Am Thorac Soc 4:316–320

Huda W, Scalzetti EM, Levin G (2000) Technique factors and image quality as functions of patient weight at abdominal CT. Radiology 217:430–435

Kalender WA, Wolf H, Suess C (1999) Dose reduction in CT by anatomically adapted tube current modulation. II. Phantom measurements. Med Phys 26:2248–2253

Kalender WA, Deak P, Kellermeier M, van Straten M, Vollmar SV (2009) Application- and patient size-dependent optimization of X-ray spectra for CT. Med Phys 36:993–1007

Kalra MK, Maher MM, Toth TL et al (2004a) Techniques and applications of automatic tube current modulation for CT. Radiology 233:649–657

Kalra MK, Maher MM, Toth TL et al (2004b) Strategies for CT radiation dose optimization. Radiology 230:619–628

Kalva SP, Sahani DV, Hahn PF, Saini S (2006) Using the K-edge to improve contrast conspicuity and to lower radiation dose with a 16-MDCT: a phantom and human study. J Comput Assist Tomogr 30:391–397

Leschka S, Stolzmann P, Schmid FT et al (2008) Low kilovoltage cardiac dual-source CT: attenuation, noise, and radiation dose. Eur Radiol 18:1809–1817

Li X, Samei E, Segars WP et al (2011) Patient-specific radiation dose and cancer risk estimation in CT: part I. development and validation of a Monte Carlo program. Med Phys 38:397–407

Little MP, Wakeford R, Tawn EJ, Bouffler SD, Berrington de Gonzalez A (2009) Risks associated with low doses and low dose rates of ionizing radiation: why linearity may be (almost) the best we can do. Radiology 251:6–12

Macari M, Spieler B, Kim D et al (2010) Dual-source dual-energy MDCT of pancreatic adenocarcinoma: initial observations with data generated at 80 kVp and at simulated weighted-average 120 kVp. Am J Roentgenol 194:27–32

McCollough CH (2005) Automatic exposure control in CT: are we done yet? Radiology 237:755–756

Schindera ST, Nelson RC, Mukundan S Jr et al (2008) Hypervascular liver tumors: low tube voltage, high tube current multi-detector row CT for enhanced detection—phantom study. Radiology 246:125–132

Schueller-Weidekamm C, Schaefer-Prokop CM, Weber M, Herold CJ, Prokop M (2006) CT angiography of pulmonary arteries to detect pulmonary embolism: improvement of vascular enhancement with low kilovoltage settings. Radiology 241:899–907

Siegel MJ, Schmidt B, Bradley D, Suess C, Hildebolt C (2004) Radiation dose and image quality in pediatric CT: effect of technical factors and phantom size and shape. Radiology 233:515–522

Sigal-Cinqualbre AB, Hennequin R, Abada HT, Chen X, Paul JF (2004) Low-kilovoltage multi-detector row chest CT in adults: feasibility and effect on image quality and iodine dose. Radiology 231:169–174

Tubiana M, Feinendegen LE, Yang CC, Kaminski JM (2009) The linear no-threshold relationship is inconsistent with radiation biologic and experimental data. Radiology 251:13–22

Waaijer A, Prokop M, Velthuis BK, Bakker CJ, de Kort GA, van Leeuwen MS (2007) Circle of Willis at CT angiography: dose reduction and image quality—reducing tube voltage and increasing tube current settings. Radiology 242:832–839

Wintersperger B, Jakobs T, Herzog P et al (2005) Aorto-iliac multidetector-row CT angiography with low kV settings: improved vessel enhancement and simultaneous reduction of radiation dose. Eur Radiol 15:334–341

Yu L, Li H, Fletcher JG, McCollough CH (2010) Automatic selection of tube potential for radiation dose reduction in CT: a general strategy. Med Phys 37:234–243

Yu L, Fletcher JG, Grant K et al (2011a) Automatic kV selection for radiation dose reduction in contrast-enhanced abdominal CT. In: 97th Scientific assembly and meeting of the radiological society of North America, Chicago

Yu L, Fletcher JG, Vrtiska T et al (2011b) Automatic kV selection for radiation dose reduction in ct angiography. In: 97th Scientific assembly and meeting of the radiological society of North America, Chicago

Yu L, Bruesewitz MR, Thomas KB, Fletcher JG, Kofler JM, McCollough CH (2011c) Optimal tube potential for radiation dose reduction in pediatric CT: principles, clinical implementations, and pitfalls. Radiographics 31:835–848

# Conventional and Newer Reconstruction Techniques in CT

Homer Pien, Synho Do, Sarabjeet Singh, and Mannudeep K. Kalra

## Contents



**Abstract**

Heightened concerns over increasing radiation dose from CT scanning have highlighted limitations of real-time image reconstruction methods using conventional filtered back-projection techniques. Significant advances in computational power have enabled commercial availability of several iterative approaches for CT image reconstruction and processing. These techniques enable radiation dose reduction, as well as opportunity to improve scanner resolution, while reducing some image artifacts. In this chapter, we review the technical basis of conventional and newer reconstruction techniques for CT.

## 1 Introduction

In a CT system the data acquired is the projection of the X-ray beam passing through the patient and impinging on the detector array. Each such projection measurement represents the total integrated attenuation of the X-ray along this path. As the gantry rotates, projections from different directions about the patient are acquired. Image reconstruction, then, is the process of creating an image from these integrated projections such that the value of each pixel in the image represents the X-ray attenuation at that pixel location.

Image reconstruction plays a major role in image quality. Image reconstruction dictates how sharp an image appears, how much noise there is, how apparent boundaries are between tissue types, how noticeable certain artifacts are, etc. In this context

H. Pien (✉) · S. Do · S. Singh · M. K. Kalra
Department of Radiology,
Massachusetts General Hospital,
Boston, MA, USA
e-mail: hpien@partners.org

D. Tack et al. (eds.), *Radiation Dose from Multidetector CT*, Medical Radiology. Diagnostic Imaging,
DOI: 10.1007/174_2011_520, 

**Fig. 1** Fourier transform pairs for both one- and two-dimensions. The signal is $f(x)$ (or $f(x,y)$ in 2-D). The Fourier Transform is $F(u)$ (or $F(u,v)$ in 2-D)

| | FOURIER TRANSFORM | INVERSE FOURIER TRANSFORM |
|---|---|---|
| 1-D | $F(u) = \int_{-\infty}^{\infty} f(x)e^{-j2\pi ux}\,dx$ | $f(x) = \int_{-\infty}^{\infty} F(u)e^{j2\pi ux}\,du$ |
| 2-D | $F(u,v) = \iint_{-\infty}^{\infty} f(x,y)e^{-j2\pi(ux+vy)}\,dxdy$ | $f(x,y) = \iint_{-\infty}^{\infty} F(u,v)e^{j2\pi(ux+vy)}\,dudv$ |

image reconstruction is comprised of two separate steps—an algorithm to estimate the attenuation coefficient at every pixel and a filter to control the level of noise and sharpness. In most clinical CT scanners, these two steps are implemented as a single "reconstruction kernel," where the user can select from a library of kernels representing different types of filtering to be applied. While this is true today, it is likely that newer CT scanners and reconstruction algorithms will—at least to a degree—decouple these functions to provide the user with control over both reconstruction algorithms and the filtering applied. Since the topic of reconstruction kernels is covered in Chapter 8, the focus of this chapter is on the tomographic reconstruction algorithms.

Two system parameters dictate the radiation dose received by the patient—voltage and flux. Voltage, measured in units of kilo-electron-volts (kV), is the amount of energy (or more precisely, the electrical potential difference between anode and cathode) contained in the X-ray emanating from the X-ray tube. Increasing the voltage increases tissue penetration and radiation dose, but decreases tissue contrast, image noise, and the presence of certain artifacts. Frequently, voltage is denoted by the peak instead of average voltage and is denoted by kVp. Flux, measured in units of milli-Amperes (mA), is the number of photons emanating from the X-ray tube. Increasing flux not only mproves the signal-to-noise ratio of the image and increases tissue contrast, but also increases radiation dose. From a low-dose CT imaging perspective, since voltage has a nonlinear effect on dose absorption, for the most part it is the flux that is currently used in clinical settings to lower the radiation dose. As a consequence, the primary factors that must be dealt with in low-dose imaging are elevated noise level and decreased tissue contrast.

Because of the importance of radiation dose, a deeper understanding of how reconstruction algorithms deal with dose-dependent image quality issues is critical. Image reconstruction algorithms can be broadly categorized into two groups: analytical algorithms and iterative reconstruction algorithms. At present the vast majority of image reconstruction algorithms are analytical—they tend to be fast, are well understood, but are susceptible to the noise issues that arise in low-dose imaging. Iterative reconstruction algorithms, on the other hand, appear to confer several advantages in low-dose imaging, but suffer from high computational demand. Recently, hybrid algorithms have come on the scene as a compromise between these two broad classes of algorithms. In this chapter, we provide an overview of the assumptions and techniques that underlie these algorithms at an intuitive level, and we hope to provide the reader with an understanding of the tradeoffs and compromises with these approaches.

## 2 Analytical Reconstructions

Analytical reconstruction algorithms are non-iterative techniques based on the Fourier transform (see Fig. 1). Intuitively, the Fourier transform computes the frequency content of 1D, 2D, or higher dimensional signals. Figure 2 shows a number of 1D signals and their corresponding frequency domain representation. In these frequency plots, the middle of the graph represents low frequency, with higher positive frequency towards the right, and higher negative frequency toward the left. The Fourier transform of 2D signals (i.e., images) follows analogously from its 1D counterpart (see (Gonzalez and Woods 2002) or other image processing texts for a more thorough discussion of frequency domain processing).

In prospective ECG-triggering mode, as a CT gantry revolves around the patient, the signal is recorded as a function of both the angle of the gantry as well as the detector position (Fig. 3) (see Swindell and Webb 1988). More precisely, the received

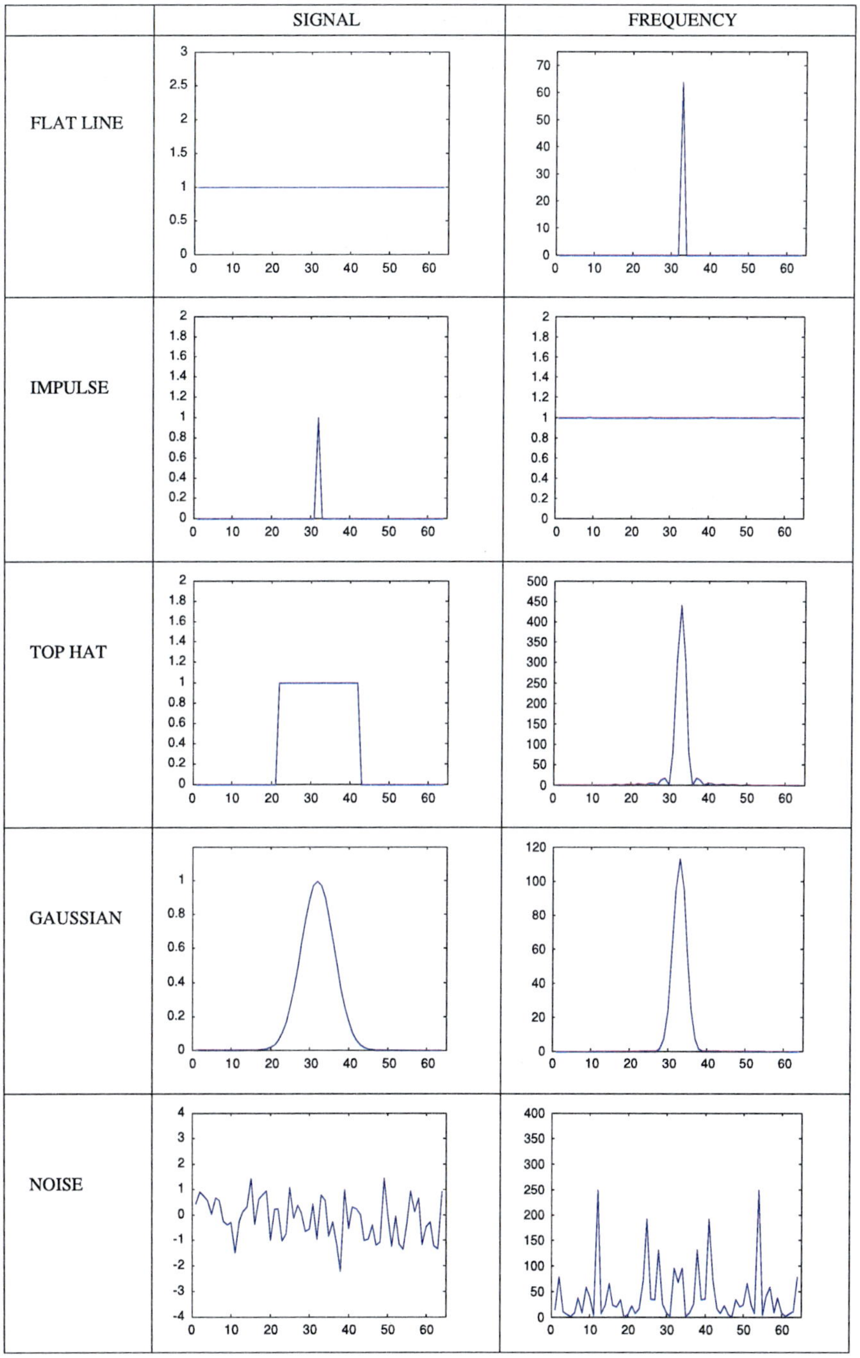


**Fig. 2** Examples of signals and their frequency domain representations. In a frequency domain representation the zero frequency is at the center, with higher frequencies (both positive and negative) away from the center. The zero frequency point is referred to as the DC (direct current) component, and it represents the total energy (area under the curve) of the signal. A flat line has no frequencies associated with it, and therefore it transforms to an impulse—there is only the DC component and no other frequencies. Conversely, an impulse signal has a single infinitely sharp discontinuity, and therefore it transforms to a frequency representation in which it is constant in all frequencies. In a top hat function, because of the sharp rise and fall of the signal, it creates side lobes in the frequency representation. A smoothly continuous curve such as the gaussian transforms to a smoothly continuous curve (in this case another gaussian). In particular, a broad gaussian (i.e., lots of low frequency gradual changes), transforms to a sharp gaussian in frequency domain (i.e., only lower frequency components); and similarly a narrow gaussian signal has more abrupt transitions, and thus transforms to a broader gaussian in frequency to encompass more high frequency components. Random noise has numerous frequencies associated with it—there is the appearance of both structure (oscillations) and sharp discontinuities. The frequency domain representation of this noise therefore has both lower frequencies (peaks near the middle) and higher frequencies

projection signal $p\ (\tau,\ \theta)$ represents the total attenuation integrated along the beam $R_{\tau,\theta}$. That is,

$$p(\tau,\theta) = \int_{R_{\tau,\theta}} f(x,y)d\tau.$$

This equation is most commonly written in a form that uses the Dirac delta function $\delta$ as defined by

$$\delta(x) = \begin{cases} +\infty \text{ if } x = 0 \\ 0 \quad\ \text{if } x \neq 0 \end{cases}.$$

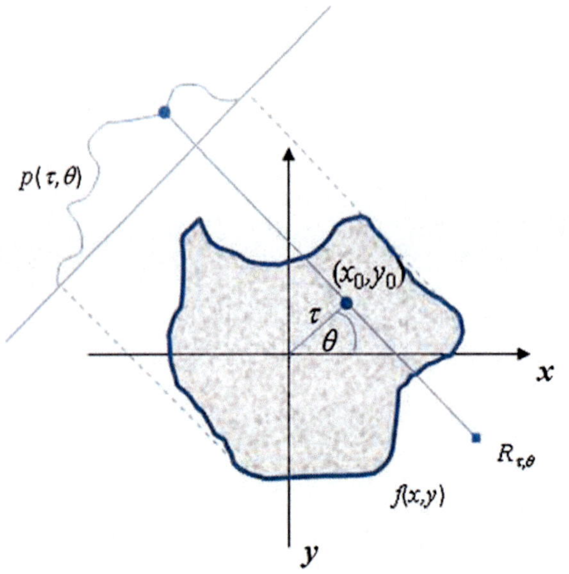


**Fig. 3** The CT projective geometry. A beam of X-ray $R$ shoots through the body $f(x, y)$ to produce the projection $p$. The ray $R$ is characterized by its projection angle $\theta$, and the particular detector element $\tau$. As the CT gantry rotates around the body, $\theta$ goes from 0 to 180° (or 360°, although when there's no motion the data acquired from 180 to 360° is the same as that from 0 to 180°). The set of projections $p$ that is acquired at different $\theta$s form the projection sinogram. The point of CT image reconstruction is to recover the attenuation coefficients of the body $f(x,y)$, given the projection sinogram $p(\tau,\theta)$

Recognizing that the ray $R_{\tau,\theta}$ passing through point $(x, y)$ must satisfy the equation $\tau = x\,\cos\theta + y\,\sin\theta$, or equivalently $x\,\cos\theta + y\,\sin\theta - \tau = 0$, the Dirac delta function can be used to restrict the integration along this ray, and the projective equation can be written as

$$p(\tau, 0) = \iint f(x, y) \cdot \delta(x\,\cos\theta + y\,\sin\theta - \tau)dxdy.$$

This equation is sometimes referred to as the *forward -projection* equation, and $p\,(\tau,\theta)$ is referred to as the projection sinogram. Figure 4 shows an example of the Shepp-Logan phantom, and the corresponding sinogram taken over 180 angles from 0° to 179°. Conversely, the *back-projection* equation, integrated along all possible angle $\theta$, can be written as

$$f_{bp}(x,\ y) = \int_0^{\pi} p(x\,\cos\theta + y\,\sin\theta, \theta)d\theta.$$

Intuitively, the back-projection operation simply propagates the measured (forward) projection signal back into the image space along the original projection path. This forward- and back-projection pair of equations is also known as the Radon transforms and the inverse Radon transform, respectively.

Given a sinogram, the inverse Radon transform—consisting of both a back-projection part and a filter part—is able to reconstruct the image $f(x, y)$. That is, applied directly, the back-projection transform reconstructs images that are blurred. Imagine an image on a very coarse grid, and the sinogram is acquired over thousands of angles spanning 180°. Now consider the pixel at the center of the image—projections from every angle will pass through that point. For all pixels one away from the center, fewer projections will end up passing through these pixels. Fewer projections still will pass through pixels further away from the center. As such, during back-projection, the centermost pixel will receive the greatest amount of back-projection, followed by those 1-pixel away, etc. The effect, in frequency domain, is a low-pass blur. To compensate for this blur, a high-pass filter is used. Since the blurring, in frequency domain (in 1D) follows $u$, the high-pass filter that is used is $1/u$. This is known as the ramp filter, or the Ram-Lak filter. Figure 5 shows an example of the effect of back-projection transform without filtering, and the inverse Radon transform with both back-projection and the Ram-Lak filter. It is for this reason that this technique for image reconstruction is called *filtered* back-projection, or FBP. Note that reconstruction kernels are simply variations of the Ram-Lak filter designed to have particular effects on the image, such as exaggeration of low frequency components to reduce noise, or exaggeration of frequencies corresponding to edges between anatomical structures.

Implicit in the discussion of FBP is the importance of the number of projections—the number of projections has a direct bearing on image quality. In Fig. 6 reconstructions using 1, 2, 5, 10, 30, 60, 100, and 180 angles are shown. Note that even with 100 angles there is undesired texturing in the output. For this reason, modern clinical CT scanners use more than 1,000 projections per 360° rotation.

In general terms, FBP requires three steps: compute the intersection of rays with pixels to accumulate partial-pixel contributions to the integration along each ray, filter the result, and back-project. Technically speaking, the Radon transform assumes that rays are parallel to each other. As such, in fan-beam geometries, the intersection of each ray with different pixels is interpolated so that parallel integrations can be

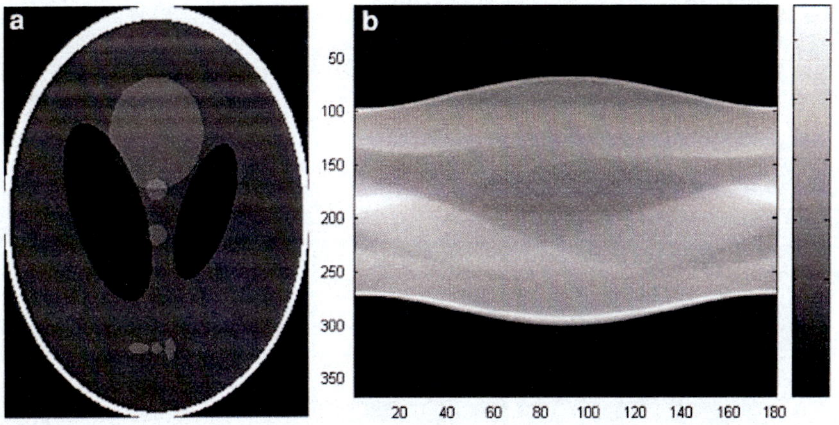


**Fig. 4** Projection sinogram. **a** The Shepp-Logan phantom. **b** The projection sinogram $p(\tau, \theta)$, shown with detector element ($\tau$) along the vertical axis, and the acquisition angle ($\theta$) along the horizontal axis

performed. While FBP works well in 2D (single-slice and step-and-shoot), computation of the partial pixels along each ray—referred to as the weighting matrix—is more complex for volumetric cone-beam CTs. The extension of FBP to circular cone-beam geometry is the FDK (also referred to as the Feldkamp) algorithm (Feldkamp et al. 1984). FDK conceptually follows the same three steps as FBP, although the computation of the weighting matrix becomes more complex.

Modern clinical CT scanners introduce other complications for reconstructions. When the number of rows in multi-row detector CT systems was low, the small cone-beam angles were negligible and FDK was sufficient. As cone-beam angles got larger, however, complex interpolation schemes had to be developed. Furthermore, the introduction of helical scanning meant that projections which are 180° apart no longer see the same anatomy. Numerous algorithms were devised to accommodate these new scanning geometries; algorithms such as PI and PI-SLANT take into account the 3D geometry during forward- and back-projections. An alternative approach, exemplified by the advanced single-slice re-binning (ASSR) algorithm, seeks to find the most appropriate 2D planes with the least amount of interpolation errors and artifacts (Kohler et al. 2002). To varying degrees, different versions of these algorithms have been implemented in various CT scanners including clinical scanners, micro-CT, materials inspection systems, and security screening CT scanners.

In the context of large-volume, cone-beam, helical CT scanners, the algorithms discussed thus far are all approximation algorithms—interpolations and approximations have to be made in order to satisfy the mathematical conditions which make the Radon transform valid. In the past decade, considerable attention has been given to *exact* reconstruction algorithms; these algorithms promise to deliver images that are free of various reconstruction artifacts (Katsevich 2002, 2004). However, due to implementation difficulties, these exact-solution algorithms have not made their way into routine use.

## 3 Iterative Reconstructions

Iterative reconstructions are also variously known as algebraic reconstructions or statistical reconstructions. Two concepts lie at the heart of these algorithms—reconstructing images by solving system of equations, and system modeling to capture scanner geometry.

Using the simplified diagram shown in Fig. 7, we assume that projections are obtained vertically (to obtain integrated values $p_a$ and $p_b$), diagonally (to obtain $p_c$), and horizontally (to obtain $p_d$ and $p_e$), then the set of attenuation coefficients which gave rise to these projection values can be solved by the system of equations shown on the right of Fig. 7. With larger detector arrays, the equations will involve many more variables. Conversely, with more projection angles, more equations are involved. Lastly, note that at angles other than the special angles shown, X-ray beams will propagate through small fractions of pixels, and any accurate implementation of iterative reconstruction needs to properly account for these fractional contributions to the integrated projections.

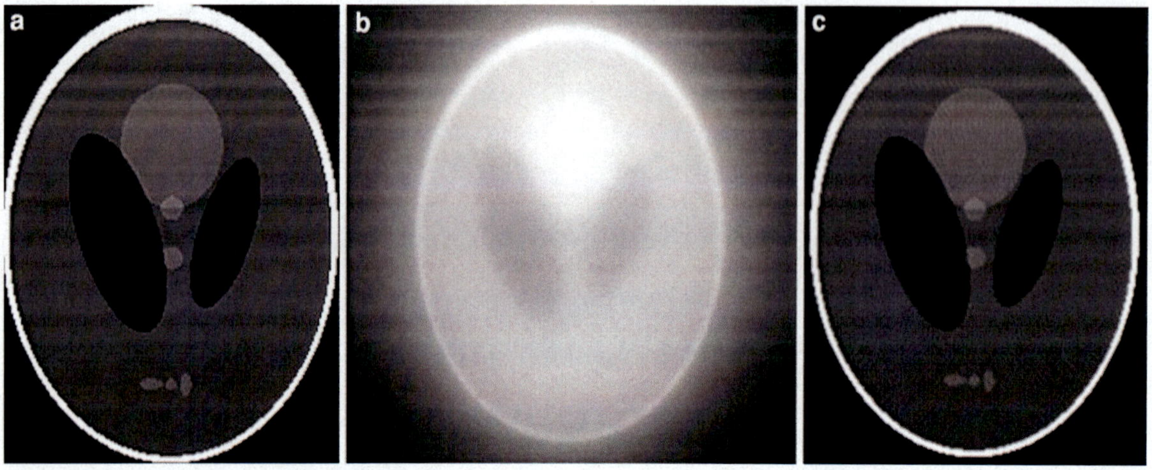


**Fig. 5** The effect of filtering on back-projection. **a** Shepp-Logan phantom image. **b** Back-projection when no filtering is used creates a blurred reconstructed image. **c** Back-projection with the Ram-Lak filter recreates the original phantom image. Note that this is true only when there is no noise. When noise is present, the Ram-Lak filter accentuates the high frequency noise and results in very noisy reconstructed images. Various reconstruction kernels are used to balance between image sharpness and noise, for different anatomic regions

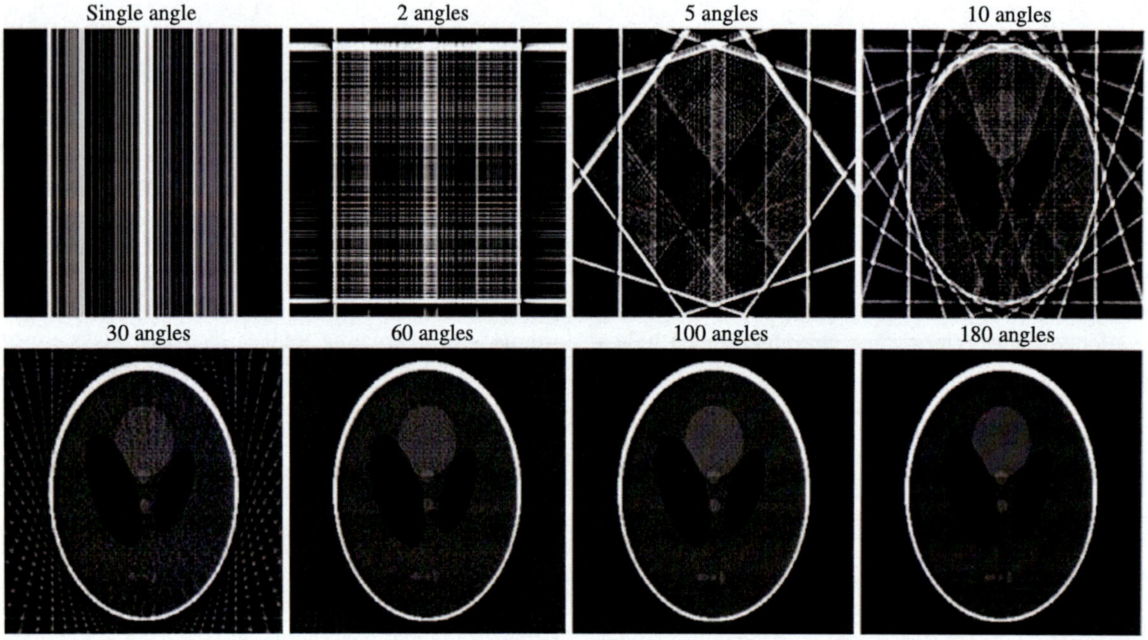


**Fig. 6** The effect of projection angles. The quality of FBP reconstructions depends in part on the number of projection angles used. Radon transform is used to illustrate this dependency. Specifically, an equal number of angles over a 0–180° range is used in these reconstructions (with the Ram-Lak filter). Even in the case of 100 angles, a small amount of texturing is apparent in the image

Modern CT scanners incorporate numerous geometrical properties, these include the distance from the source to the isocenter of the scanner, distance from isocenter to the detector array, the shape of the detector array, the size of each detector (which may not be uniform), the size of each detector row (which may not be uniform), the use of flying focal spot, the use of quarter-detector offset, and so on. Collectively, these geometrical properties make it very difficult to describe the projection process in simple mathematical terms,

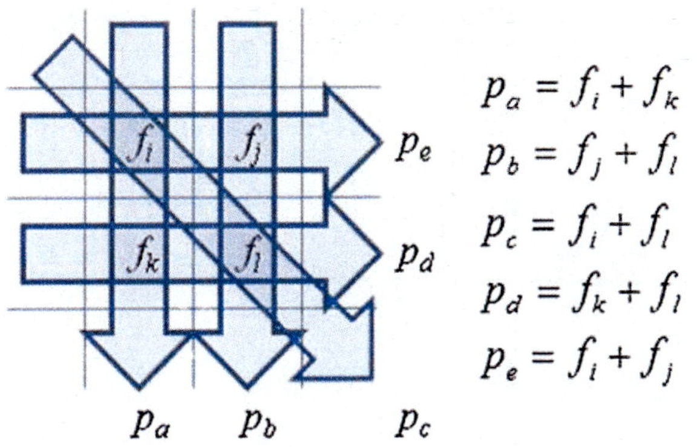


**Fig. 7** Iterative reconstruction algorithms can be viewed as solving a system of equations. In this simple example, the $f$'s denote the attenuation coefficients to be computed, $p$'s denote the values of the projections, and five projection values are used to determine the four attenuation coefficients (figure adapted from Buzug 2008)

and for this reason iterative reconstruction algorithms essentially simulate the path of an X-ray beam to calculate the fractional pixels contributing to a single projection. Thus, one factor which significantly impacts the accuracy of an iterative reconstruction algorithm is the fidelity with which these geometrical factors are modeled.

Intuitively, iterative reconstruction algorithms work as follows. The algorithm begins by hypothesizing the tissue attenuation values—these can be all zeros, random values, or initialized to filter-back-projection results. Subsequently, given a particular source location, the algorithm simulates a beam of X-ray emanating from the X-ray tube, propagating through the body, and impinging on the detector array. This simulated value is then compared to the actual value obtained by the CT scanner, and any discrepancy is used to update the solution to the system of equations of estimated tissue attenuation values, and the process repeats until the simulated projections are sufficiently close to actual projections.

Consider the simplified example in Fig. 7 in greater detail. Let $f_j$ denote the $j$th pixel in the data, where it is assumed that different rows of the data are strung together to form one long chain of pixels, and there are $N$ pixels in total. Let $p_i$ denote the $i$th ray in the projection (i.e., the detector element, or $\tau$ in Fig. 3), and assume there are $M$ such rays in the projection. Pixel $f_j$ is related to projection $p_i$ by the projection function $H$—this function dictates how each pixel is "fractionated" by the ray passing through it. More precisely

$$pi = \sum_{j=1}^{N} H_{i,j} f_j,\ i = 1, \ldots, M$$

Or in more concise notation, $\rho = Hf$. In an iterative reconstruction algorithm, the values of $f$ are estimated repeatedly, each time the values get closer to the desired solution, until finally it has converged sufficiently for the algorithm to stop. During each iteration, then, a correction factor needs to be added to the previous estimate of $f$. Let $f^k$ denote the estimate of $f$ on the $k$-th iteration, then the error in the $k$-th iteration is given by $\rho - Hf^k$. Intuitively, the correction for the next update is some function of the current error, or

$$f^{k+1} = f^k + g\left(p - Hf^k, \lambda\right).$$

That is, the correction is some function $g$ of the error, with a "relaxation" term $\lambda$ which controls how much correction to make on every iteration. In one of the first iterative reconstruction algorithms developed in the early 1970s—the Algebraic Reconstruction Techniques (ARTs)—this is precisely how the algorithm works (Gordon et al. 1970; Gordon and Herman 1971).

Two variants of ART have played a prominent historical role. In Simultaneous Iterative Reconstructive Technique (SIRT), instead of updating one pixel at a time, the corrections are held off until all updates for that pixel have been computed, and the average of all these updates becomes the new correction value. This leads to a less aggressive update strategy, which leads to better images but at the expense of slower convergence. In Simultaneous Algebraic Reconstruction Technique (SART), numerous strategies—including a different update function and the use of a filtering window—are used to improve the performance of the algorithm. A detailed description of ART, SIRT, and SART can be found in (Kak and Slaney 1988).

In another approach, the image acquisition process is modeled and used as part of the iterative reconstruction process. Specifically, the acquisition process can be represented by:

$$p = Hf + \eta;$$

that is, the projection data $p$ is related to the true data (i.e., the attenuation coefficients of the anatomy) $f$ through a CT projection process $H$ as well as detector noise $\eta$. Note that model-wise, this is the

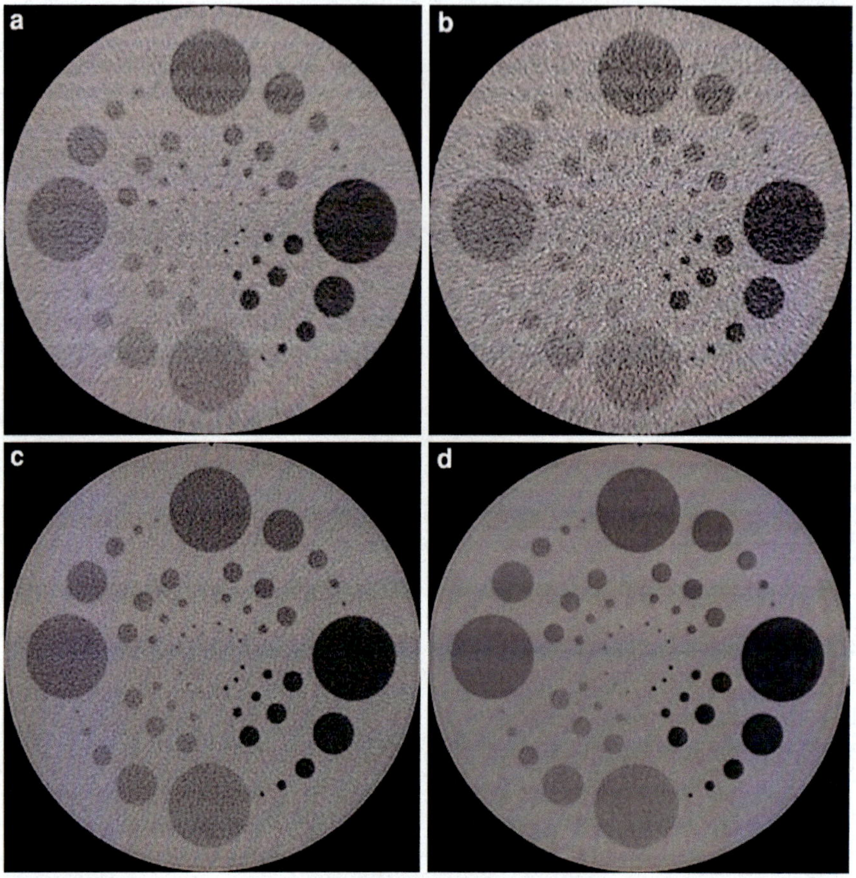


**Fig. 8** An illustration of the effect of various terms in a simple iterative reconstruction algorithm. **a** FBP image of a contrast phantom acquired at high dose (120 kVp, 319 mA, 330 ms rotation period). **b** FBP image acquired at low dose (120 kVp, 81 mA). **c** The least squares iterative reconstruction (i.e., no prior term) of the low-dose image. **d** A simple iterative reconstruction solution

same as the ART model but with the addition of a noise term. In the most simplistic version, the estimate of $f$, denoted by $\widehat{f}$, is achieved by

$$\widehat{f} = \min_{f} \{\| p - Hf \|^2 + R(Df)\}.$$

That is, $f$ is such that a simulated beam of X-ray following the CT forward model $H$ passing through $f$ must be close to the observed projection $p$. Furthermore, because of noise, $f$ should be smooth, and the most common way of inducing smoothness is to impose some constraint $R$ on the derivative of $f$ (we denote the derivative of $f$ by $Df$)—typically this is done by minimizing $\| Df \|$ or $\| Df \|^2$ or some other variation on derivatives, since smooth curves have smaller derivatives (integrated across the entire curve) than noisy curves. In this formulation, the first part of the expression is the data term, and the second is the prior term (also known as the regularization term). Intuitively, the data term constrains the estimation of $f$ to solutions that fit the observed data $p$, and the prior term indicates how the nonidealities of the scanner (noise in this example) are dealt with.

Some examples serve to illustrate the nature of each term. First, consider what happens if there is no data term, and the prior term is just the first derivative:

$$\widehat{f} = \min_{f} \{\| Df \|\}.$$

In this case, the smoothest $f$ is just a flat plane because the derivative of a constant is 0, so the final minimum solution is an image of a constant value. Now consider when there is only a data term:

$$\widehat{f} = \min_{f} \{\| p - Hf \|^2\}.$$

This is referred to as the least squares solution (i.e., the sum of the squares of the errors are minimized). This solution is shown in Fig. 8c. As can be seen, by virtue of having an accurate system model, the least-squares approach can generate high quality images, although due to the lack of regularization noise within

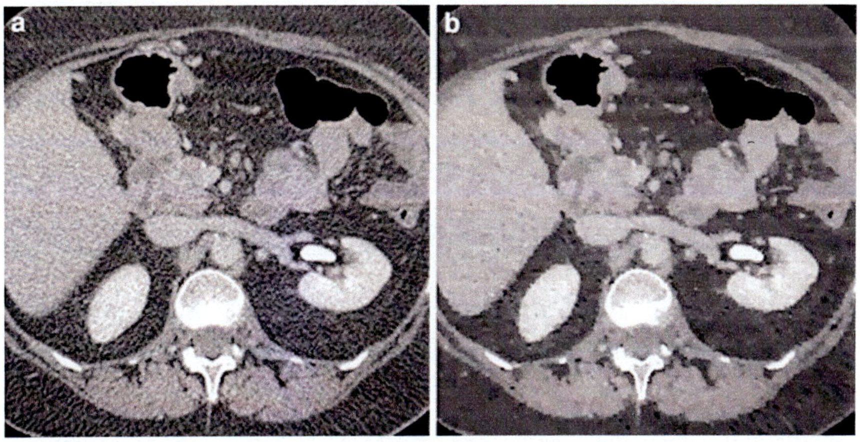


**Fig. 9** An example of overregularization. **a** A low-dose abdominal CT image created with FBP. **b** An iterative reconstruction solution in which the prior term is intentionally over-emphasized to create the patchy or blocky texture

uniform disks is visible. Now consider the case where both data and prior terms are invoked (Fig. 8d); in this case the prior term is used to reduce the noise in the image, resulting in a smooth image—in fact, this low-dose reconstructed image has higher signal-to-noise and contrast-to-noise ratios than the high-dose FBP image in Fig. 8a. Different variations on the data and prior terms give rise to different behaviors, including robustness to noise from low-dose imaging, and the mitigation of certain artifacts (cf. (Do et al. 2010, 2011)).

It is worthwhile noting that the use of the data and prior terms can have a dramatic impact on the appearance of an image. In the context of very low-dose imaging, noise becomes severe, and it is logical to think that this noise can be overcome by simply increasing the emphasis of the prior smoothing term. A prior term based on minimizing the derivatives of $f$ creates an $f$ that is "piece-wise smooth". That is, small noise bumps within a region are smoothed towards some mean value, but when there is an intensity change between regions, the next region will be smoothed toward a different mean value. The result of overemphasizing the prior term is that the image texture is altered, and the image takes on a "patchy" or "splotchy" appearance. This is shown in Fig. 9, and some approaches to dealing with this texture problem are discussed later in this chapter.

In yet another approach, the statistical characteristics of the X-ray flux are modeled; this set of approaches is generally referred to as *statistical* models. In essence, instead of treating the arrival of the X-rays as a deterministic process as we have described previously, these models characterize the statistical distribution of the X-ray photon arrival process, most often using the Poisson distribution. Arrival processes are often modeled by the Poisson distribution—the distribution (as a function of time) of runners completing a race, the arrival of customers at a bank teller's window, or the number of photons hitting a detector all tend to follow the Poisson distribution (Fig. 10). This approach first gained popularity in the reconstruction of emission tomography images due to the low-photon count of such systems, and is gaining acceptance for low-dose CT imaging (Shepp and Vardi 1982).

Consider the case in which, over $M$ projections, the probability that the random variate $P$ of X-rays equals the true (observed) projection $p$. This can be written as the conditional probability

$$\Pr(P = p|f) = \prod_{i=1}^{M} \frac{\overline{p}_i^{\,pi} e^{-\overline{p}i}}{p_i!},$$

where $\overline{p}_i$ denotes the expected value of the $i$th projection. By comparing against Fig. 10a, it is clear that the right hand side of this expression is a product of Poisson distributions—the number of X-rays hitting a detector for every one of the $M$ projections is modeled as a Poisson distribution. In other words, instead of asking, for the data term, what is the $f$ that gives rise to data which most closely resemble the observed projection values (as we did in the previous model), statistical models ask, given $f$, what is the most likely distribution of X-rays that result from it, and whether the expected value of this distribution matches the observed projection value. Implicit in this expression is the fact that $f$ and $p$ are related by the CT projection matrix $H$, just like in the previous approach.

a

$$Q(k;\lambda) = \frac{\lambda^k e^{-\lambda}}{k!}$$

b

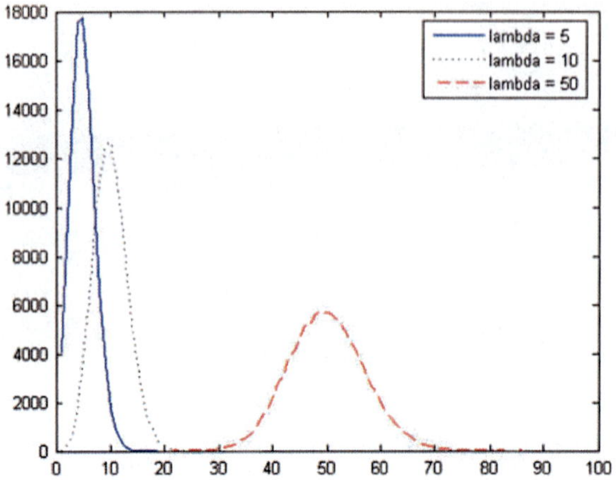


**Fig. 10** The Poisson distribution. **a** In a Poisson distribution, if the expected number of occurrences of an event in any given interval is $\lambda$, then the probability that there are exactly $k$ occurrences is given by $Q(k;\lambda)$. **b** The Poisson distribution for $\lambda = 5$, 10, and 50

## 4 Hybrid Reconstruction Algorithms

We briefly mention that although the separation of reconstruction algorithms into analytical and iterative reconstructions works in abstraction, in practice hybrid algorithms are sometimes used. These hybrid algorithms come in at least two flavors. In one case, an analytical reconstruction can be used to create an initial image, and post-processing algorithms iteratively reduce the noise in the resulting image until specific criteria are reached (such as a sufficiently high signal-to-noise ratio). In another case, an initial image can be formed using analytical reconstructions, while a more aggressive algorithm is used to reduce the noise. Since such aggressive algorithms may introduce unwanted textures (such as Fig. 9), the user is given the opportunity to "blend" these two images to produce one that has sufficiently reduced noise yet retains the desirable textures of conventional reconstructions.

## 5 Commercial Implementations

Due to concerns over radiation exposure for CT patients, all of the major clinical CT vendors have implemented algorithms on CT scanners which permit the use of low-dose scanning protocols. In particular, these algorithms are designed to be robust with respect to the higher noise levels that occur with lower voltage (kVp) and flux (mA). In order to deploy these low-dose processing techniques as quickly as possible, several CT vendors have adopted a two-phase approach. In their first-generation algorithms, vendors have deployed primarily post-processing-based algorithms for reducing the appearance of noise. At the time of this paper, several vendors are also in the process of commercially deploying iterative reconstruction algorithms that may permit further lowering of radiation dose as part of their second generation of low-dose CT algorithms. A sampling of these low-dose image reconstruction and processing packages—as commercialized by CT vendors–is shown in Table 1. Sample images are also shown in Figs. 11, 12, 13, 14 these are discussed next.

**Table 1** A sampling of current commercial low-dose image reconstruction algorithms by CT scanner vendors

| Vendor | First generation product name | Second generation product name |
|---|---|---|
| General electric | ASIR | Veo |
| Philips | $\text{iDose}^4$ | IMR |
| Siemens | IRIS | SAFIRE |
| Toshiba | QDS and Boost3D | AIDR 3D |

In Fig. 11 images processed using algorithms created by GE are shown. These low-dose axial abdominal images were acquired at 100 kVp, 50 mAs, 0.5 s gantry rotation speed, 0.9:1 beam pitch, and 5 mm section thickness. CTDIvol = 2.5 mGy, DLP = 105 mGy-cm, resulting in a dose exposure of 1.5 mSv. Shown are the original FBP, ASIR (Adaptive Statistical Iterative Reconstruction) algorithm, and Veo (a model-based iterative reconstruction) algorithm. While ASIR is a hybrid algorithm which provides the user with the ability to "blend" FBP and iteratively reconstructed images, Veo is a statistical reconstruction fully iterative algorithm (Thibault et al. 2007). Figure 11b was generated with a blending of 50%. Veo received FDA clearance in September 2011.

Results of low-dose processing using Philips' algorithms are shown in Fig. 12. Philips' first-generation product, $\text{iDose}^4$, operates in both sinogram and image space, and is designed to both reduce

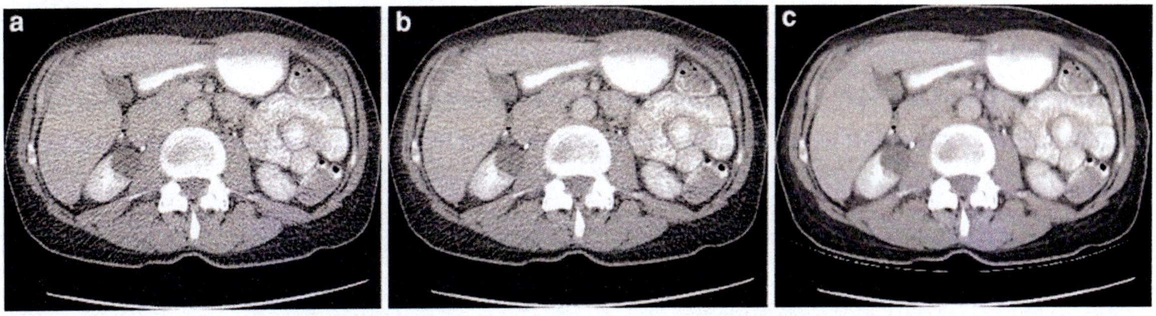


**Fig. 11** Low-dose reconstructions from GE. CT data acquired at 100 kVp, 50 mAs with 0.5 s gantry rotation speed, 0.9:1 beam pitch, and 5 mm slice thickness. CTDIvol = 2.5 mGy, DLP = 105 mGy-cm, resulting in a dose of 1.5 mSv. Shown are **a** FBP, **b** ASIR-50, and **c** Veo

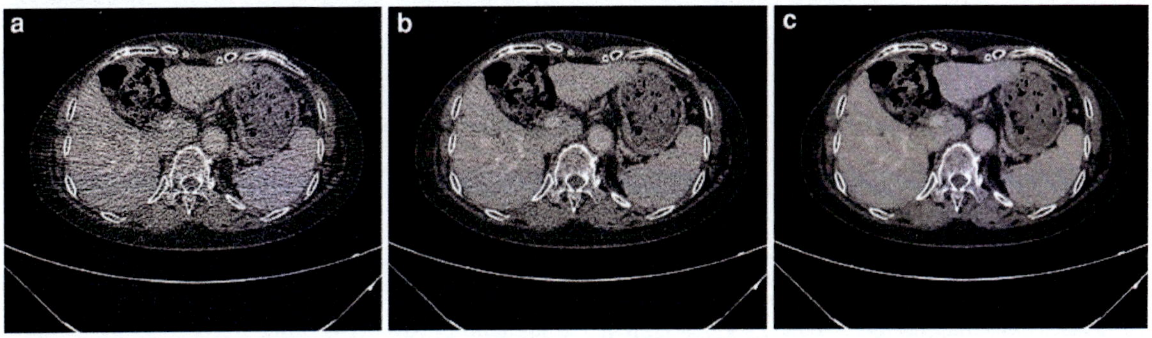


**Fig. 12** Low-dose reconstructions from Philips. Acquisition was performed at 120 kVp, 21 mAs, 0.75 s rotation time, 1 mm slice reconstruction thickness. CTDI = 1.275 mGy, DLP = 25.5 mGy-cm, resulting in a dose exposure of 0.38 mSv. Shown are (**a**) the analytical reconstruction image, (**b**) the iDose image, and (**c**) the IMR image. Images courtesy of Kevin Brown of Philips

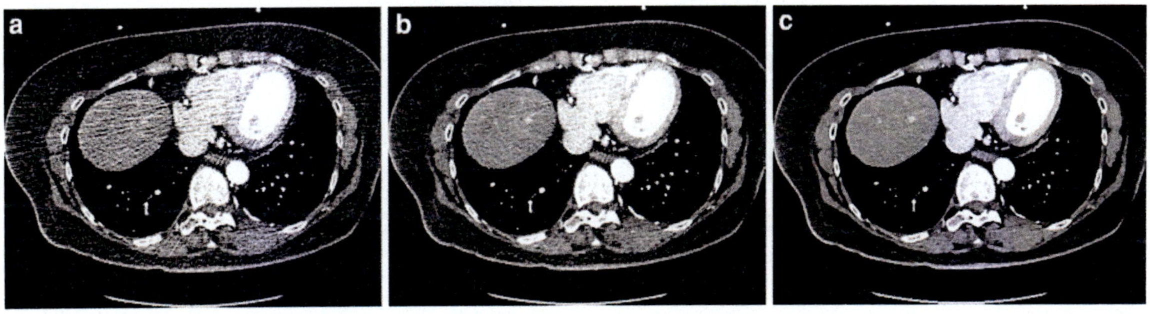


**Fig. 13** Low-dose reconstructions from Siemens. This contrast-enhanced chest dataset was acquired at 100 kVp, 107 mAs, 3.4:1 beam pitch, gantry rotation speed of 0.285 s, 0.6 mm section thickness. The CTDIvol = 3.5 mGy, DLP = 53 mGy-cm, which results in a dose exposure of 0.74 mSv. Shown are (**a**) FBP, (**b**) IRIS image, and (**c**) SAFIRE image, obtained with a setting of 4. Images courtesy of Thomas Flohr and Rainer Raupach of Siemens

artifacts and decrease noise, while preserving the noise power spectrum (Leipsic et al. 2011). IMR (Iterative Model Reconstruction) is a more recent advancement that uses knowledge-based models to perform global data optimization, and represents Philips' second-generation algorithm. The data shown in Fig. 12 was acquired at 120 kVp, 21 mAs, 0.75 s gantry rotation, and 1 mm reconstruction thickness.

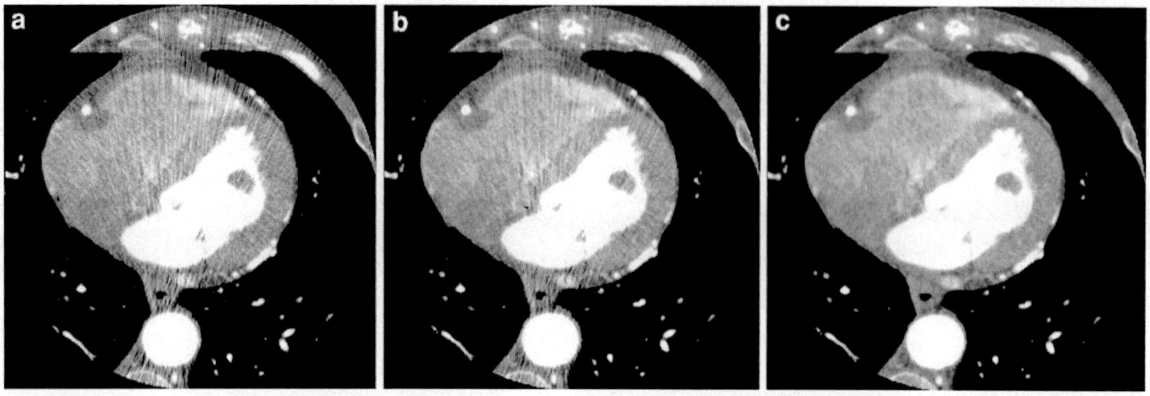


**Fig. 14** Low-dose reconstructions from Toshiba. The contrast-enhanced cardiac acquisition was performed with 80 kVp and 120 mA, 0.35 s rotation time, with prospective gating. The BMI of the subject was 20. The resulting DLP is 29.0 mGy-cm, with a CTDI of 2.1 mGy, resulting in a dose of 0.4 mSv. Shown are **a** analytical reconstruction image, **b** QDS/Boost image, and **c** AIDR 3D image. Images courtesy of Associate Professor Sujith Seneviratne of MonashHeart, and Erin Angel of Toshiba

The resulting CTDIvol = 1.275 mGy, DLP = 25.5 mGy-cm, which yields an exposure dose of 0.38 mSv. Shown are the FBP, iDose$^4$, and IMR results.

Results from Siemens' low-dose CT processing algorithms are shown in Fig. 13. This contrast-enhanced axial chest dataset was acquired at 100 kVp, 107 mAs, gantry rotation speed of 0.285 s at a pitch of 3.4:1; CTDIvol = 3.5 mGy, DLP = 53 mGy-cm, and the resulting exposure dose is 0.74 mSv. Siemens' first-generation product is named IRIS (Iterative Reconstruction in Image Space), where an initial sinogram domain reconstruction is computed, after which iterations in the image domain are used to decrease noise (Nelson et al. 2011). In Siemens' second- generation product, SAFIRE (Sinogram Affirmed Iterative Reconstruction), reprojections of the image data back into the sinogram domain are used in conjunction with image domain iterations to form the final image. SAFIRE received FDA clearance in November 2011. Figure 13 shows the FBP, IRIS, and SAFIRE reconstructions.

For Toshiba, its first-generation low-dose imaging product consists of two algorithms—QDS and Boost3D. QDS (Quantum Denoising Software) works in the image domain by selectively adapting the strength of smoothing or edge enhancement to the presence of edges. On the other hand, Boost3D operates in the sinogram domain to reduce the effect of structured (non-random) noise such as photon starvation and streaking. Toshiba's second-generation product is AIDR 3D (Adaptive Iterative Dose Reduction), which combines a statistical model-based reconstruction in the sinogram domain with an iterative image-based noise reduction algorithm (Gervaise et al. 2011). Figure 14 shows a low-dose contrast-enhanced cardiac CT example, in which the data was acquired at 80 kVp and 120 mA, 0.35 s rotation time, with prospective gating. The CTDI is 2.1 mGy, DLP = 29.0 mGy-cm, resulting in a dose of 0.4 mSv.

In addition to these (and other) vendor-specific implementations of low-dose image reconstruction algorithms, third-party vendors have also developed algorithms (cf. SafeCT, MedicVision, Isreal) which primarily work in the post-processing domain to reduce the appearance of noise. While vendor-specific implementations offer the advantages of seamless integration with their equipment for both workflow and service, for institutions with equipment from multiple vendors, the cost of procuring low-dose packages from each vendor can be high.

## 6 Discussions

Since the invention of CT, image reconstructions have undergone considerable evolution. Although the very first CT images were generated using iterative techniques, the computational advantages of analytical reconstructions made FBP, FDK, ASSR, and other analytical approaches the gold standard in commercial CT scanners for the next 30 years. More recently, with larger volume coverage and larger cone angles, along with increasing concerns over radiation exposure, and vast improvements over the speed of computation, iterative and hybrid reconstructions have been gaining clinical acceptability. These approaches, however, process the data in very different ways from conventional analytical reconstructions, and make very different assumptions about the nature of the scanner geometry and acquisition process. As such, it is important to have an intuitive understanding of how these algorithms work, what assumptions they make, the parameters which control them, and the ways in which they may introduce unwanted artifacts. And while the newest generation of iterative techniques appears to be very promising for improving image quality from low-dose CT, these algorithms continue to be significantly slower than analytical techniques, and likely will be for a few more years.

Although there are several published studies comparing the first-generation iterative approach to the standard or filtered back-projection techniques, there is a distinct lack of comparison between different iterative reconstruction techniques. From the point of view of their actual use in clinical practice, users must remember that these iterative reconstruction techniques do not reduce dose themselves *per se*, but rather allow users to acquire images at lower radiation dose levels and then these techniques process the acquired low-dose and higher noise images to improve image quality. As such, users have to determine the fractions of dose reductions for given patient sizes, body regions, and clinical indications with adjustment of scanning parameters. Typically, dose reduction with use of iterative approach is achieved with use of lower tube current and/or tube potential. Actual dose reduction in comparison with the standard or filtered back-projection reconstruction techniques has been extensively discussed in Part III of this textbook on practical dose reduction approaches. At the Massachusetts General Hospital, some of the first-generation iterative approaches (ASIR and IRIS) are used to obtain up to 30–75% dose reduction compared to the standard filtered back-projection techniques (Kalra et al. in press; Prakash et al. 2010a, b, c; Singh et al. 2010, 2011, in press).

Another practical aspect of applying iterative approach involves selection of settings for these iterative algorithms. For example, for applying ASIR, one must select 10–100% level of ASIR for image reconstruction. Selection of 10% ASIR implies that resulting image will have 10% ASIR blended with 90% filtered back-projection and will have higher noise compared to application of ASIR 90% which will have lower noise as 90% ASIR will be blended with just 10% filtered back-projection data. Other techniques such as IRIS, Veo, and AIDR 3D are on/off options with no user control for strength of noise reduction in the image datasets (although QDS/Boost and AIDR 3D provide some manual adjustability for research purposes). In short, each institution needs to understand and appreciate the implications of different reconstruction algorithms, and recognize the need to optimize protocols for specific low-dose imaging needs as they relate to patient, anatomy, and indications.

## References


Buzug TM (2008) Computed tomography: from photon statistics to modern cone-beam CT. Springer, Berlin

Do S, Karl WC, Kalra MK, Brady TJ, Pien H (2010) A variational approach for reconstructing low dose images in clinical helical CT. IEEE Int'l Symp Biomed Imaging

Do S, Karl WC, Liang Z, Kalra M, Brady TJ, Pien H (2011) A decomposition-based CT reconstruction algorithm for reducing blooming artifacts. Phys Med Biol 56:7109–7125

Feldkamp LA, David LC, Kress JW (1984) Practical cone-beam algorithm. J Opt Soc Am A1:612–619

Gervaise A, Osemont B, Lecocq S, Noel A, Micard E et al (2011) CT image quality improvement using adaptive iterative dose reduction with wide-volume acquisition. Eur Radiol [epub ahead of print]

Gonzalez RC, Woods RE (2002) Digital image processing 2nd edn. Prentice-Hall, Upper Saddle River

Gordon R, Bender R, Herman GT (1970) Algebraic reconstruction techniques (ART) for three dimensional electron microscopy and X-ray photography. J Theor Biol 29:471–481

Gordon R, Herman GT (1971) Reconstruction of pictures from their projections. Commun Assoc Comput Mach 14: 759–768

Kak AC, Slaney M (1988) Principles of computerized tomographic imaging. IEEE Press, New York

Kalra MK, Niels W, Woisetschläger M, Singh S, Lindblom M, Choy G et al Radiation dose reduction with Sinogram Affirmed Iterative Reconstruction Technique for abdominal CT. Radiology (to appear)

Katsevich A (2002) Theoretically exact FBP-type inversion algorithm for spiral CT. SIAM J Appl Math 62:2012–2026

Katsevich A (2004) An improved exact filtered backprojection algorithm for spiral computed tomography. Adv Appl Math 32:681–697

Kohler T, Proksa R, Bontus C, Grass M (2002) Artifact analysis of approximate helical cone-beam CT reconstruction algorithms. Med Phys 29:51–64

Leipsic J, Heilbron BG, Hague C (2011) Iterative reconstruction for coronary CT angiography: finding its way. Int J Cardiovasc Imag [epub ahead of print]

Nelson RC, Feuerlein S, Boll DT (2011) New iterative reconstruction techniques for cardiovascular computed tomography: how do they work, and what are their advantages and disadvantages? J Cardiovasc Comput Tomogr 5:286–292

Prakash P, Kalra MK, Kambadakone AK, Pien H, Hsieh J, Blake MA et al (2010a) Reducing abdominal CT radiation dose with adaptive statistical iterative reconstruction technique. Invest Radiol 45:202–210

Prakash P, Kalra MK, Ackman JB, Digumarthy SR, Hsieh J, Do S et al (2010b) Diffuse lung disease: CT of the chest with adaptive statistical iterative reconstruction technique. Radiology 256:261–269

Prakash P, Kalra MK, Digumarthy SR, Hsieh J, Pien H, Singh S et al (2010c) Radiation dose reduction with chest computed tomography using adaptive statistical iterative reconstruction technique: initial experience. J Comput Assist Tomogr 34:40–45

Shepp LA, Vardi Y (1982) Maximum likelihood reconstruction for emission tomography. IEEE Trans Med Imag MI-1:113–122

Singh S, Kalra MK, Gilman MD, Hsieh J, Pien HH, Digumarthy SR et al (2011) Adaptive statistical iterative reconstruction technique for radiation dose reduction in chest CT: a pilot study. Radiology 2011(259):565–573

Singh S, Kalra MK, Hsieh J, Licato PE, Do S, Pien HH (2010) Abdominal CT: comparison of adaptive statistical iterative and filtered back projection reconstruction techniques. Radiology 257:373–383

Singh S, Kalra MK, Bhangle AS, Saini A, Gervais DA, Westra SJ et al Pediatric CT protocols: Radiation dose reduction with hybrid iterative reconstruction. Radiology (in press)

Singh S, Kalra MK, Do S, Thibault JB, Pien H, Connor OJ et al Comparison of hybrid and pure iterative reconstruction techniques with conventional filtered back projection: dose reduction potential in the abdomen. J Comput Assist Tomogr (in press)

Swindell W, Webb S (1988) X-ray transmission computed tomography. In: Webb S (ed) The physics of medical imaging. IOP Publishing, Philadelphia

Thibault JB, Sauer KD, Bouman CA, Hsieh J (2007) A three-dimensional statistical approach to improved image quality for multislice helical CT. Med Phys 34:4526–4544

# Image Noise Reduction Filters

Sarabjeet Singh and Mannudeep K. Kalra

## Contents



S. Singh · M. K. Kalra (✉)
Department of Radiology, Harvard Medical School,
Massachusetts General Hospital, 55 Fruit street,
Boston, MA 02114, USA
e-mail: mkalra@partners.org

**Abstract**

With the expanding use of CT and growing concerns for radiation related risks, several efforts have been made in scientific community to lower radiation dose without compromising the image quality (Berrington de González et al. Arch Intern Med 169:2071–2077, 2009; Schauer and Linton Health Phys 97:1–5, 2009; UNSCEAR Health Phys 79(3):314, 2000). In this chapter, we discuss application of image post processing filters to low radiation dose CT, as one of the technical advances for lowering radiation dose.

Image quality is the major driving force for the success of any imaging modality. While technical or the physics side of the imaging community has always guided efforts to achieve "pretty" images/ better image quality, medical community on the other hand attempts to achieve "clinically acceptable" image quality. CT image quality has many aspects, which are influenced by various scanning and reconstruction parameters.

Image quality in CT is generally governed by four basic factors: image noise, image contrast, spatial resolution and artifacts. In the realm of subjective assessment of CT image, noise is defined as the graininess, speckled or salt and pepper look on the images. Region of interests (ROI) can be drawn over homogeneous areas of images to objectively measure image noise by calculating the standard deviation of the pixel values with in the ROI. As for CT images the pixel values primarily represents the distribution of X-ray attenuation values in the scanned tissue slice, represented as Hounsfield units (HU). Image noise is

D. Tack et al. (eds.), *Radiation Dose from Multidetector CT*, Medical Radiology. Diagnostic Imaging,
DOI: 10.1007/174_2011_460, © Springer-Verlag Berlin Heidelberg 2012

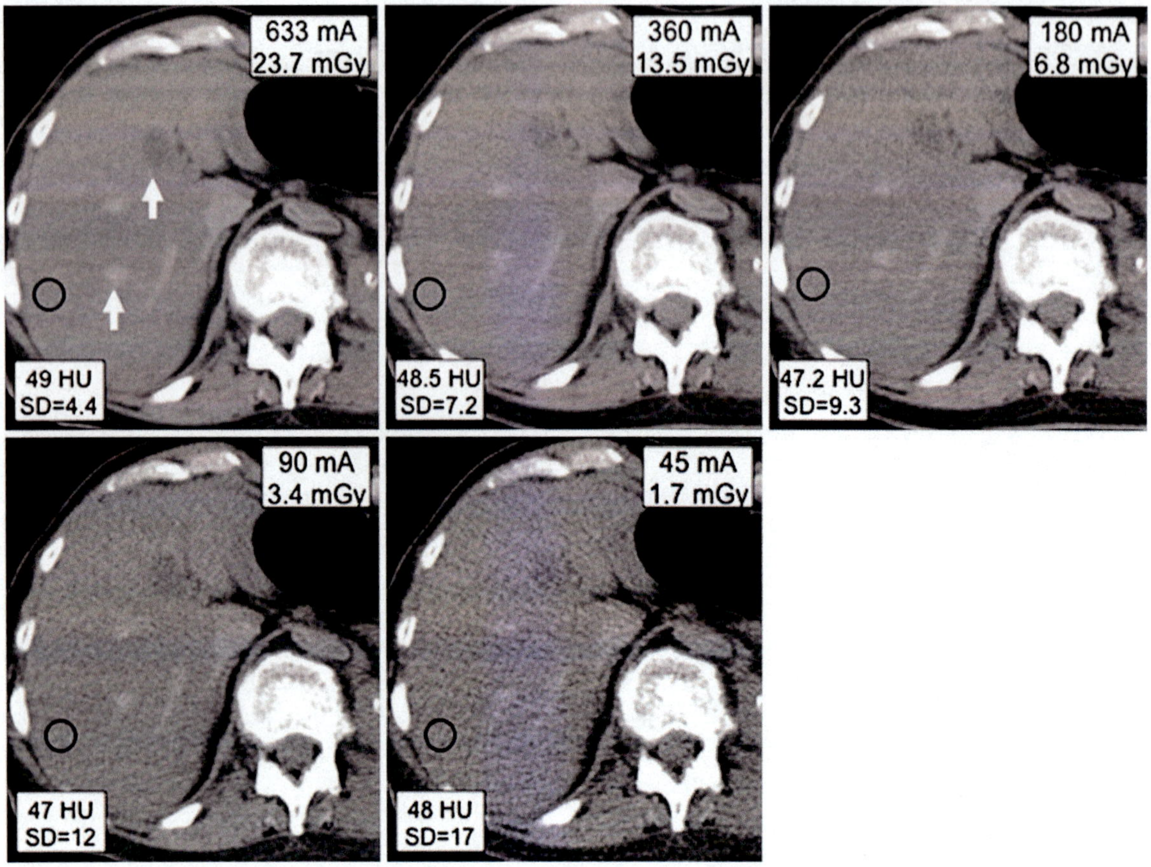


**Fig. 1** Postmortem abdominal CT (55 kg patient weight) at 120 kV and different tube current levels (315, 180, 90, 45, 22 mAs) resulting in CTDIvol of 24.0, 14.0, 7.0, 3.4, and 1.7 mGy, respectively. Image noise increases with decrease in the tube current and CTDIvol resulting in poor visualization of the margins of liver lesion and hepatic vessels

measured as the random variation in the HU values in the selected ROI.

CT image noise results from both quantum and electronic noises (AAPM 2011). Electronic noise is due to the random variation in signals before the image reconstruction and after the photons detection. Quantum noise on the other hand arises from the fluctuations in detection of the X-ray quanta. Low radiation dose CT examinations have lower number or energy of photons and hence have greater image noise. Scan parameters, including tube current (mA) and the selected tube potential (kVp) are important factors that influence the number and energy of X-ray photons and hence also the image noise. If all other scan parameters (for example, tube potential, rotation time, slice thickness) are kept constant and reducing the tube current by 50% results in increase the image noise by a factor of the square root of two (Kalender 2000) (Fig. 1).

Image contrast is defined as the ability to distinguish between differences in intensities or the HU values of the structure and its background. Image contrast is governed by differences in the HU values in the area of interest and the background. Reduction in tube potential lowers photon energy and results in greater X-ray attenuation and image contrast from iodine and some other structures due to higher photoelectric effect at lower kVp (Kalva et al. 2006). However, increase in image contrast at lower kVp is associated with increase in image noise as well (Fig. 2).

Spatial resolution is defined as the ability to resolve or distinguish small closely spaced structures in an image. Resolution of CT images is usually guided by the detector size or also called as aperture

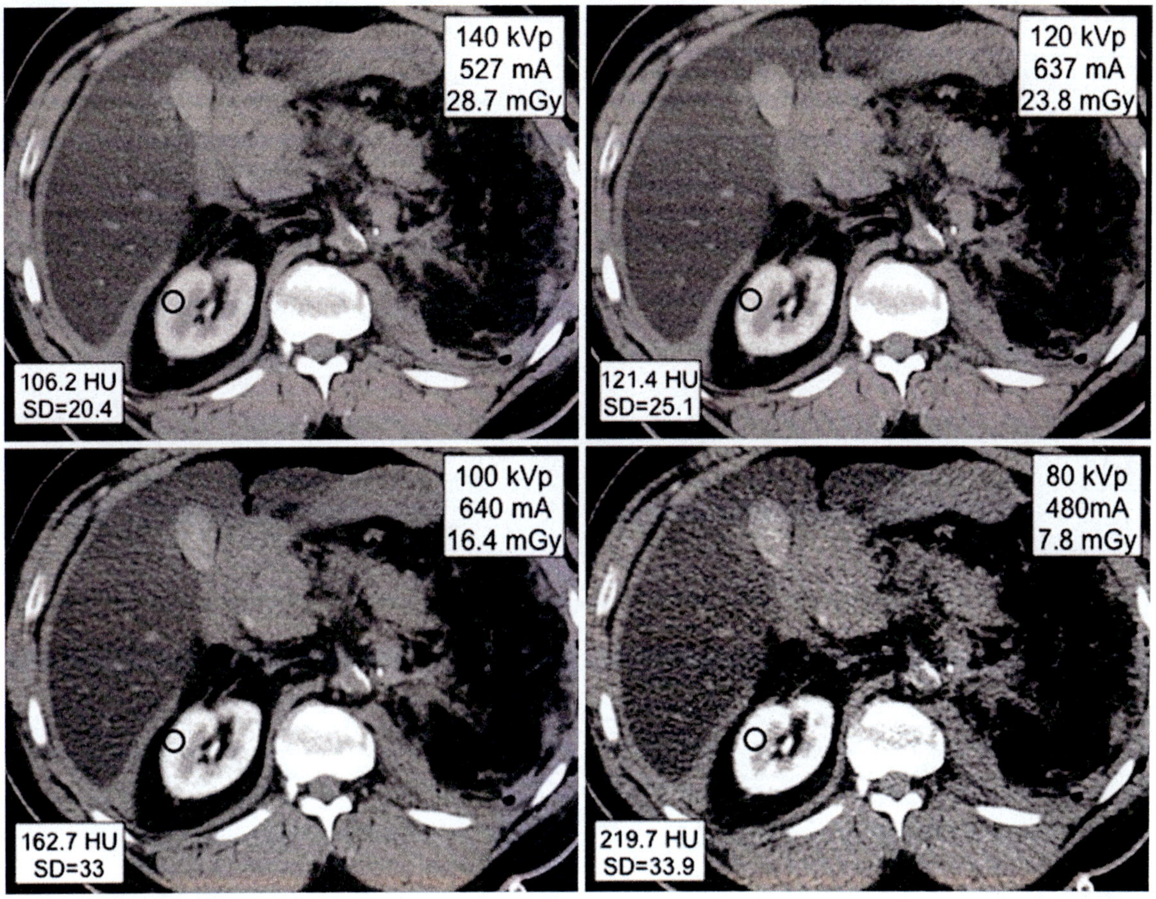


**Fig. 2** Postmortem abdominal CT (95 kg patient weight) images demonstrating severe diffuse hepatic steatosis at 140, 120, 100 and 80 kV. Image noise increased as the tube potential was decreased (20.4 at 140 kVp, 25.1 at 120 kVp, 33 at 100 kVp and 33.9 at 80 kVp). Also noted was the increase in the Hounsfield units as the tube potential was dropped from 140 to 80 kVp (106.2 HU at 140 kVp, 121.4 HU at 120 kVp, 162.7 HU at 100 kVp and 219.7 HU at 80 kVp). Postmortem nephrogram in bilateral kidneys is from pre-mortem contrast enhanced abdominal CT in this patient with renal failure

size and the spacing of the detector measurements. Other factors affecting the resolution include focal spot size, motion and displayed pixel size.

Artifacts are subjectively defined as any structure seen in the image, which is not a part of actual anatomy in that region. Quantitatively, image noise is "random" uncertainties in the HU values whereas artifacts are defined as any "systematic" uncertainties in CT numbers or the pixel values (AAPM 2011). They are primarily caused by discrepancies in acquired projection data, which could be due to motion, either voluntarily or involuntarily such as heart beat or lungs while breathing, mechanical scanner malfunction, projection data under sampling or photon starvation. Common CT artifacts are discussed in "Image Quality in CT: Challenges and Perspectives" on CT image quality by Thomas Toth.

CT image quality is finally guided by the combination of these four parameters. This delicate balance of radiation dose and image quality has to be carefully maintained without affecting the diagnostic information on the CT examinations. In the past several attempts have been made to lower image noise while maintaining other image quality attributes with the help of image post processing filters. (Berrington de González et al. 2009; Schauer and Linton 2009; UNSCEAR 2000)

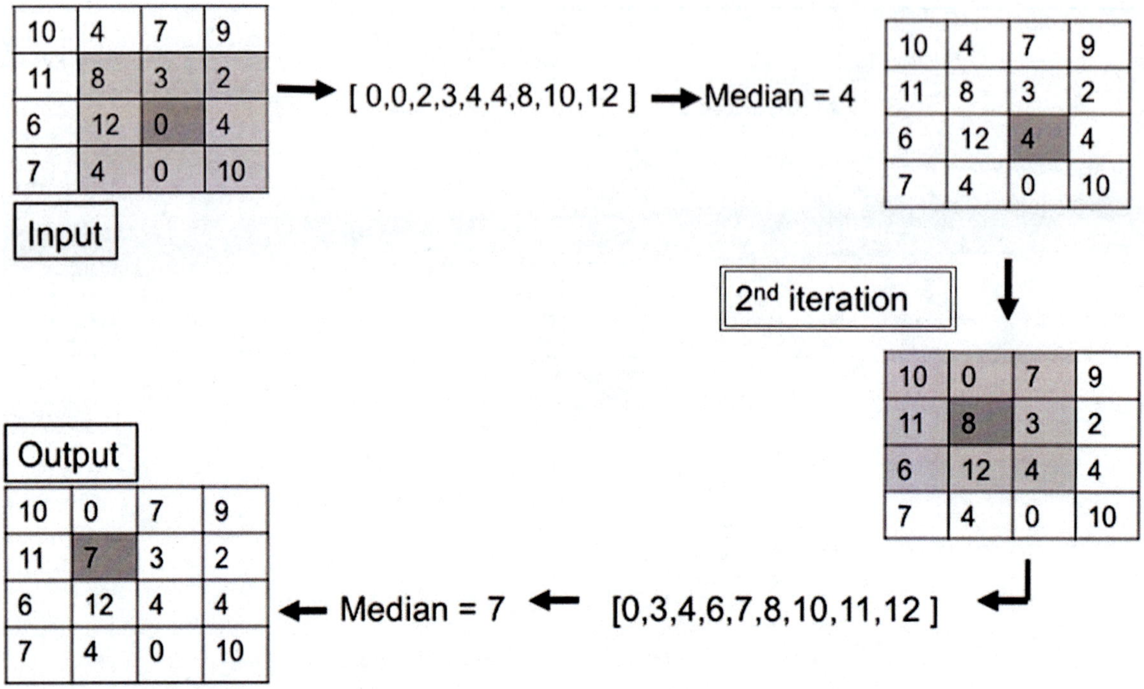


**Fig. 3** Simplified illustration of "median" nonlinear filter where the input images are processed to replace the pixel values by median values. Median nonlinear filter selects a central pixel and defined number of surrounding pixels (For example, 8 in this algorithm), calculates the median values for pixel values and finally replaces the central pixel with the median values. Median nonlinear filters perform selected number of iterations to obtain final output post processed images

## 1 Types of Image Processing Filters

Several image post processing filter based approaches have been implemented to improve image quality of CT images acquired with lower radiation doses. These include linear and nonlinear filters.

Image noise in CT due to quantum and electronic noise have wide range of frequency components and a linear low-pass filter can separate out the high frequency components from the noise. This image processing can reduce image noise. Anatomical or structural edges seen in the image domain consists of high frequency signal components in frequency domain and hence linear low-pass filters can separate these signals and result in blurring at tissue margins or interfaces while lowering image noise.

Whereas linear filters process the scan data as a whole without looking at individual data points such as tissue interfaces, nonlinear filters examine each data point or pixel and then decide whether that pixel is noise or a valid signal. If the pixel is noise, then it is replaced with estimate based on the surrounding pixel values. For example a "median non linear" filters first selects center pixel values and 8 surrounding pixels to calculate the median of those the 9 pixels and finally replace the center pixel with the estimated median value (Fig. 3). These functionalities of the nonlinear processing help in selective noise reduction in the regions of the image (where it needed the most) while retaining sharpness at the tissue interfaces. The nonlinear filters take into account the location and orientation of edges while processing for noise reduction.

Keselbrener et al. (1992) evaluated both average and median filter on high and low contrast phantom images. Their averaging filters adapted the smoothening strength based on the linking patterns of neighboring pixels (NLK filter). They also assessed shape and size of selected window and k parameter (number of neighboring pixels) for K-nearest neighbor median filter (KNNM filter). Authors found that results of NLK filters were more promising than the KNNM. Also NLK filters were able to reduce image noise to the same magnitude as the linear filter and

**Table 1** Tabulated summary of some approaches to noise reduction image and raw data filters

| Type/name | Authors | Vendor | Technique (domain) |
|---|---|---|---|
| ATM | Hsieh (1998) | GE healthcare | Adaptive Trimmed Mean filter (raw data domain) |
| MAF | Kachelriess et al. (2001)<br>Baum et al. (2003) | Siemens healthcare | Multidimensional adaptive filtering (raw data domain) |
| NRF | Kalra et al. (2003a)<br>Kalra et al. (2003b)<br>Kalra et al. (2004) | GE healthcare | Segmentation, reduce noise & preserve structures (image domain) |
| 3D ORA | Rizzo et al. (2005)<br>Seifarth et al. (2005) (3D-ORA plus)<br>Bai et al. (2009) | Siemens healthcare | 3 dimensional optimized reconstruction algorithm (image domain) |
| Adaptive NRF | Funama et al. (2006), Jan | | Noise reduction and edge preservation (image domain) |
| QDS | Okumura et al. (2006) | Toshiba | Quantum denoising system (image domain) |
| Boost 3D | Kazama et al. (2006) | Toshiba | Compensate for low quantum intensity (shoulders and pelvis) |
| NOVA | Schilham et al. (2006) | | Noise variance nonlinear filter (image domain) |
| ANR-3D | Wessling et al. (2007) | Siemens healthcare | 3D edge detection + 2D axial filter |
| NLAF | Martinsen et al. (2008)<br>Leander et al. (2010)<br>Martinsen et al. (2010)<br>Ledenius et al. (2010) | ContextVison, Inc. | 2D-nonlinear adaptive filter (image domain) |
| BF and NLM | Manduca et al. (2009)<br>Giraldo et al. (2009)<br>Guimarães et al. (2010) | | Bilateral filtering (BF) and non-local means (NLM): weighted smoothening and edge preservation (image domain) |

also preserve the resolution of high contrast images. In the low contrast images, NLK processing also lowered image noise as compared to linear filters.

## 1.1 Two-Dimensional Image Filters

There are different approaches reported in the medical literature on 2-D image processing. We review some of these approaches in this section (Table 1).

Noise reduction filters (NRF, GE Healthcare) (Kalra et al. 2003a, 2004) work in image domain and uses a gradient analysis method to separate the image into structured and nonstructured regions. Algorithm incorporates a threshold parameter to control this segmentation process. The nonstructured regions are isotropically filtered with a low-pass filter. The structured regions on the other hand are directionally filtered with a smoothing filter operating parallel to the edges and with an enhancing filter operating perpendicular to the edges. Finally a blending parameter regulates the recombination of the structured and nonstructured segments. Six different settings or combinations of segmentation and blending are made available to optimize the filters. These filters settings are stratified as; filter A, normal-low; filter B, normal-medium; filter C, normal-high; filter D, special-low; filter E, special-medium; and filter F, special-high. NRF helps to reduce image noise while preserving the qualitative appearance of the noise without perceptible loss of definition of anatomic structures.

Two-dimensional nonlinear adaptive filters (2D-NLAF, SharpView/ContextVision, Linkoping, Sweden) (Leander et al. 2010; Ledenius et al. 2010) are based on the concept that CT image contain anatomical structures of various sizes and image data can be resolved into different frequency bands containing similar size structures. Depending on the scanner type and the anatomy of the scanned region, CT image is divided into a defined number of bands. Each band usually contains similar size structures, which allows it to process anatomical structures by size. Low-pass band consists mainly of the amplitude of the 2D signal and low frequent variations, whereas the high-pass band contains predominantly small structures and noise. The remaining band cover structures of mid size and low frequent noise. These 2D-NLAF filters process each frequency band separately and merge the enhanced bands to produce final enhanced image. At the pixel level, these filters examine each pixel in relation to its neighboring pixels. Subsets of filters are used to assess the predefined local features by running these subsets of filters in different directions. The filters are designed so that the combined filter response is completely rotational invariant. A number of features are estimated during the estimation of these subsets of filter responses including variance, orientation, phase and energy. Feature estimation is performed on higher abstraction level, to produce more accurate and robust results. This information is used to decide whether the pixel is a part of same structure as its neighbors. Finally based on the calculated set of these features, the contextual information for every location in the image is formed. This contextual information is merged to produce a specific filtering method, which adapts to image signal at every pixel location and individually optimizes it. The distinct quality of 2D-NLAF is the likelihood of adapting desired behavior to the image content and hence allowing both noise reduction as well as edge enhancement. This feature can help in selective noise reduction in low contrast soft tissue regions as well as edge enhancement in high frequencies areas such as lungs and bones within a single image. Lastly, the 2D-NLAF parameters noise reduction and edge enhancement can be optimized for the anatomy of the scanned region. The enhancement is performed in different intensity value ranges, corresponding to tissue-type-specific Hounsfield Units (HU). Also these parameters can be adjusted based on user preference, as some radiologists prefer smooth images while others prefer sharp, crispy image.

Adaptive 2D noise reduction filter evaluated by Funama et al. (2008) varied the convolution kernel for every image pixel. Size of applied convolution kernel is selected on the basis of noise or the standard deviation of every pixel. Pixels with larger deviation were processed with larger kernel. The investigators suggested that with conventional filters amount of processing is determined by the distance from the center pixel which makes the edge or the boundaries of structures indistinct whereas their approach adapted the filter settings based on the standard deviation of pixel to obtain both smooth and sharpened data. Finally these data were combined appropriately to generate the final image.

## 1.2 Adaptive Noise Reduction Filter

Yanaga et al. (2009) evaluated adaptive noise reduction filter for low kilovoltage CT data. This algorithm first separates the image into several components to which independent filtering kernels are applied. Input image is split into Laplacian pyramid (Burt and Adelson 1983). This step allows the filter to produce various spatial frequency sub-bands and adapt to different sized anatomic structures in the image. For each spatial resolution level, algorithm then establishes three different classes; A, weakly textured regions or organs in the image; B, linear or elongated structures, for example blood vessels, ducts and tubes and C, organ boundaries. For example in CT urography, psoas muscles is designated as organs and ureter as elongated structures and margins of area with or without contrast irrigation as class C or organ boundaries. Different process settings are performed on these classes with isotropic smoothening with in the organs, directional smoothing and enhancement of elongated structures and fine outlining of the organ boundaries to avoid introduction of new artifacts.

## 1.3 Three-Dimensional Image Filters

The two-dimensional nonlinear smoothing performs filtration in the x–y or axial plane only, where position and orientation of edges is determined and an arbitrary one-dimensional filtration is performed along these edges. Since these 2D filters do not take into account information in the direction perpendicular to the x–y plane, smaller structures crossing the x–y plane can be loose details or become invisible because of partial-volume artifact.

The 3D filtration method, namely 3D optimized reconstruction algorithm (3D-ORA, Siemens Healthcare) (Rizzo et al. 2005; Bai et al. 2009) generalizes the two-dimensional nonlinear smoothing technique in all three directions (x, y, and z axes) to avoid loss of contrast and sharpness of small structures. 3D ORA filters reduce image noise while maintaining the spatial resolution, as measured by modulation transfer function (MTF). The 3D Advanced Noise Reduction (ANR-3D, Siemens Healthcare) (Wessling et al. 2007) filters analyze the initial input data to determine the orientation of edges in the images by estimating linear variance in different directions in 3D spaces. This approach assumes minimum variance to be tangential to the edge/contour. Three different filters are then employed based on the calculated variance. Intermediate datasets are generated by post processing with one 2D fixed axial filter working in frequency domain and two one-dimensional adaptive filters in different directions. Finally results from these filters are combined to obtain maximum nose reduction and least deterioration of information.

Quantum Denoising System (QDS) algorithm (Okumura et al. 2006) also works in image domain with three simultaneous mathematical processes. These processes include structure edge detection and analysis, smoothing of image, and enhancement of edge structure. The first process of edge detection and analysis includes a detailed interrogation of the input image for edge structures to determine the local edge strength so that edges can be maintained. This extracted edge information is used to estimate an optimal blending ratio for smoothened and sharpened image based on the edge sensitivity curve. The second part of QDS utilizes a low-pass smoothing filter to attenuate noise elements to reduce overall image noise. Third part of QDS applies a high-pass sharpening filter to enhance edges and fine structures in the input image. All of these three filtration processes function in the 3D space. Eventually, the images are locally blended based on determined local edge strength. The QDS lowers image noise by increasing the blending ratio of smoothening in low edge intensity areas and increasing the blending ratio of sharpening in area of high edge intensity. Hence, output image after QDS post processing results in lower pixel noise while enhancing the fine edge structures.

Noise variance nonlinear (NOVA) filter (Schilham et al. 2006) uses an estimate of the spatially dependent noise variance in an image. It comprises of moving average (MA) filter with window of $5 \times 5 \times 5$ voxels, which basically replaces the voxel value with the average of voxel values in the selected window around the voxel. In addition to the MA filter component, NOVA algorithm incorporates a weighting function of the intensity difference, between a voxel in averaging window and the intensity in the center of the window and the variance of the noise at the center of the window. This approach alters its noise reduction strength based on the estimated local standard deviation of noise.

Manduca et al. (2009) and Yu et al. (2010) evaluated the denoising algorithm based on bilateral filtering, which smoothens values using a weighted average in a local neighborhood, with weights determined according to both spatial proximity and intensity similarity between the center pixel and the neighboring pixels. This filtering is locally adaptive and can preserve important edge information in the sinogram, thus maintaining high spatial resolution. A CT noise model that takes into account the bowtie filter and patient-specific automatic exposure control effects is also incorporated into the denoising process.

## 1.4 Raw Data Domain Filters

Filters in the image space domain cannot make use of the measured attenuation values and the photon statistics from the raw data. These filters are considered as post processing techniques, since they operate on reconstructed DICOM images. The raw data filters work on sonogram or raw data domain.

Hsieh (1998) evaluated an adaptive trimmed mean filter that adapts to the detected photon starvation. This filter also applies smoothening to individual measured projections in the raw data. The selected level of smoothening is inversely proportional to the detected photon signal or the X-ray flux. For example, projections running through shoulders and pelvis have more attenuation and less detected signal at the detectors, hence requiring more smoothening. Whereas when detected signal is high, as in lungs filled with air, there is less or no need to apply filtering to these projections.

Contrary to one-dimensional adaptive filters assessed by Hsieh (1998), Kachelriess et al. (2001) evaluated raw data based multidimensional adaptive filter (MAF) which works in various planes, including detector plane, projection plane as well as along the long axis of the patient. The multidimensional adaptive filter preserves the boundaries of structures by adapting the kernel size, amount of smoothing and edge enhancement based on the calculated standard deviation of the CT number in the local region. To address the concern of additional time involved in processing in the raw data domain, these filters use local raw data i.e. within ±90° of the projections to adjust the filter settings. This approach allows the processing to take place in real time during data acquisition.

Yu et al. (2008) developed a locally adaptive algorithm for noise control in CT based in bilateral filtering. This technique processes projections in the raw data domain to account for local structural details in order to preserve the edges and maintain spatial resolution. The algorithm adapts its strength based on the detected number of photons from each projection. Noise reduction in raw data domain relies on the appropriate CT noise model, which eventually requires an estimate of the number of photons. Detected photons vary for each projection due to the use of automatic exposure control (AEC) and also vary across the X-ray beam due to the beam shaping/bow tie filter. These parameters are taken into consideration while processing the raw data to preserve the noise texture and improve the low contrast detectability.

The cross-section of most human bodies is often oval rather than completely circular, with lateral diameter greater than the anteroposterior diameter. As a result, there is a higher attenuation of the X-ray beam in the lateral projections compared to the anteroposterior projections. The lateral projections photons travel greater distance in the body than anteroposterior projections and greater photon starvations and eventually increased quantum noise. This effect is prominently seen in the area of thick bones, for example in shoulders, scapulae and pelvic region or in obese patients. Boost 3D filter (Toshiba Medical Systems) (Kazama et al. 2006) is also useful in projections with extremely high absorption of X-rays as in metallic implants and devices. These high density regions lower the detector output count and hence projections are affected by photon noise. Boost 3D software analyses the stochastic noise in each projection and optimizes the scan raw data in all 360° projections. For example, high stochastic noise in the projection due to either low radiation dose or high attenuation through thick bones is compensated by Boost 3D. This algorithm is programed to seek high X-ray absorption projections from the raw data and then process with raw data smoothening filter in the detector row direction ($z$-direction) and the axial plane ($x$–$y$ direction). The processed images have lower noise and less streak artifacts.

## 2 Clinical Application of Filters

### 2.1 Abdominal and Pelvis CT

Kalra et al. (2003a) have evaluated six different settings of noise reduction filters for dose reduction in abdominal CT examinations. They acquired images at 140 kVp, 240–300 mA in the portal venous phase (CTDIw: 17.8–22.2 mGy) and 4 additional low dose images acquired at 140 kVp, 120–150 mA (CTDIw: 8.4–10.5 mGy) in the equilibrium phase. Low dose post processed images (120–150 mA) have substantially lower image noise without any significant improvement in sharpness and contrast as opposed to unprocessed low dose images.

Another group of investigators (Funama et al. 2008) evaluated the role of adaptive noise reduction filters in low dose abdominal CT for various patient sizes who underwent biphasic hepatic CT (hepatic arterial phase at 140–180 mAs (CTDIw: 10.7–13.8 mGy), equilibrium phase at 60–100 mAs (CTDIw: 4.6–7.6 mGy). Equilibrium phase low dose images were post processed with specific filter settings adapted to three different weight groups (<50 kg, 50–70 kg, and >70 kg). Authors found no difference between low dose post processed and standard dose unprocessed images, in terms of graininess, tumor conspicuity, portal vein enhancement homogeneity and overall image quality. However, they did report statistically significant lower scores for the sharpness of liver contours.

Baum et al. (2003) have also demonstrated improved visualization of rectal wall and perirectal lymph nodes with better image quality when pelvic CT examination were post processed with multidimensional adaptive filters.

To generate multiple radiation dose levels in the same patient, investigators have added image noise using noise projection software on CT images with liver lesion to generate simulated low dose images (Wessling et al. 2007; Funama et al. 2006; Kröpil et al. 2010; Giraldo et al. 2009). Wessling et al. (2007) post processed simulated low dose images with ANR 3D and demonstrated noise was significantly lowered with superior image quality and no difference in liver detection was noted. Kröpil et al. (2010) evaluated simulated images of multi modal anthropomorphic phantom at various tube currents (100–500 mAs) and tube potential (80–140 kVp) for mesenteric low contrast lesion, hepatic blood vessels, liver and renal cysts. They found that 2D NLAF could help improve image quality of CT images acquired with to 50% radiation dose reduction. They divided the study group in high dose (CTDI >20 mGy), middle dose (CTDI 10–20 mGy or estimated effective dose 5–8 mSv) and low dose with CTDI values of less than 10 mGy (estimated effective dose 1–5 mSv). Results of this study showed improvement of subjective image quality, particularly the detection of low contrast mesenteric lesions and hepatic veins improved with post processing of middle dose group (CTDI 10–20 mGy or estimated effective dose of 5–8 mSv).

Another group of investigators simulated low radiation dose abdominal CT images by inserting Poisson noise in the raw data domain, before image reconstruction. They finally processed the low dose images with Bilateral Filtering (BF) and Non-local means (NLM) to enhance the image quality. BF and NLM both lowered image noise while preserving the sharpness in the high contrast regions of the images. However, there was slight amount of smoothening in low contrast areas of the abdominal CT images (Giraldo et al. 2009). Manduca et al. (2009) evaluated the noise-resolution properties of bilateral filtering incorporating similar CT noise model in phantom studies. They also tested this algorithm on one patient with CT colonography protocol at 120 kVp and 100 "quality reference mAs", resultant CTDIvol of 7 mGy. They selected the edge between air and stool on the bowel wall to assess the noise and resolution profile. When compared to the convolution kernels, bilateral filtering lowered image noise with much less affect on spatial resolution.

Several prior studies have been performed to assess the effect of noise reduction filters on lesion detection and conspicuity. Although noise reduction filters have effectively shown the potential of lowered image noise, this post processing can lead to smoothening of organs and noticeable loss of anatomic structural margins or edge definition. In particular, liver is the focus of image post processing due to the low contrast lesions. Kalra et al. (2004) have evaluated 2D nonlinear filters for lesion evaluation and found decreased lesion conspicuity on aggressive noise reduction settings. Authors concluded that their filters may be more useful in high contrast settings like evaluation of renal stones, CT urography and CT colonography (Fig. 4).

In fact application of nonlinear Gaussian filter algorithm to CT colonography images of porcine colon (acquired at 100 and 10 mAs, estimated CTDIvol = 0.5–5 mGy) with simulated lesion ranging from 1–8 mm resulted in 50–70% image noise reduction for 10 mAs images. Although all simulated lesions were seen on post processed images with reconstructed slice thickness of 1.25 mm, definition of lesion size and shape was more "accurate" with 100 mAs scans (Branschofsky et al. 2006).

Another study has reported the use of liver phantom with simulated hepatic lesions (Funama et al. 2006). In this study, Funama et al. generated an inhomogeneous phantom of upper abdomen simulating diffuse and chronic liver disease. This "virtual liver phantom" comprised of liver, stomach with air, kidneys, vertebral bodies, ribs and peritoneal fat and contained simulated nodules of various sizes and attenuation. Authors found that detectability of 80 mAs (CTDIw = 4.6 mGy) post processed images was equivalent to 160 mAs (CTDIw = 12.2) unprocessed image. Rizzo et al. (2005) evaluated 3D ORA in an IRB approved study to acquire additional images in 40 patients undergoing abdominal CT examinations at 140 kVp and combined tube current modulation (CARE Dose4D) with quality reference mAs of 120 ($n = 6$, CTDIvol: 11.9 mGy) and 160 mAs ($n = 34$, CTDIvol: 15.9 mGy). Post processing with 3D ORA lowered image noise with significant reduction in image contrast at higher strengths of filtration which was also associated with lower lesion conspicuity in 9/40 cases. They reported missing six focal liver lesions at such higher levels of noise

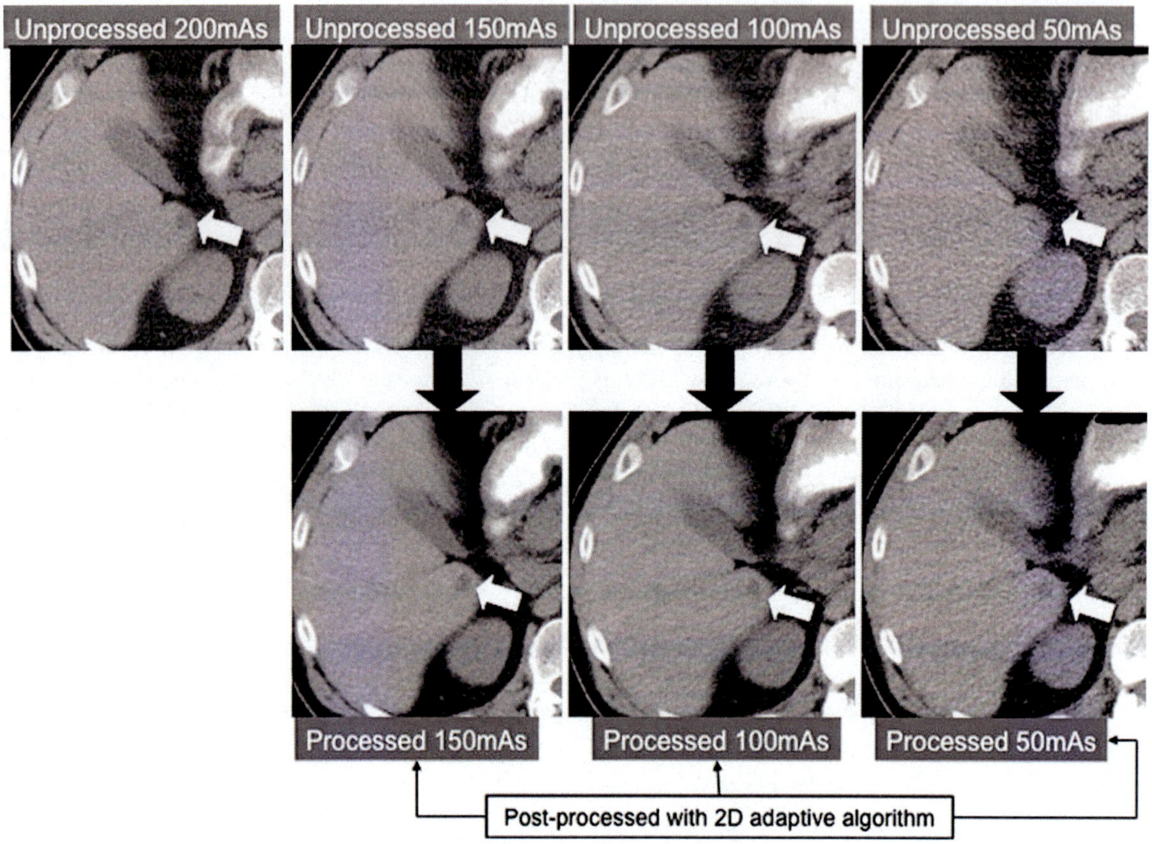


**Fig. 4** Abdominal CT images acquired at 200, 150, 100 and 50 mAs in the same patient with a limited scan length of 10 cm shows a low attenuation liver lesion. Post processed images with 2D nonlinear adaptive filters in lowered image noise and improved visibility of the liver lesion

reduction as well as appearance of pseudolesions/ artifacts.

Wessling et al. (2007) evaluated 40 known benign and malignant liver lesions, including benign hepatic cysts, liver metastasis, hemangiomas, hepatocellular carcinomas, choloangiocarcinomas and hepatic abscesses. Authors added quantum noise to raw data to simulate low dose abdominal CT images. These images were then post processed with ANR-3D and evaluated for lesion detection, image noise and delineation of hepatic veins, portal veins, contrast between vessels and liver parenchyma. Compared to standard dose of 180 mAs (CTDIw: 11.4 mGy), detection rate was the same for unfiltered images at 105 mAs (CTDIw: 6.6 mGy) and filtered images at 80 mAs (CTDIw: 5.1 mGy). Post processing with ANR 3D allowed detection of low contrast lesions (mean diameter of 5–28 mm) at 80 mAs and high contrast lesions (mean diameter of 4–13 mm) at all mAs settings.

Lowering of tube potential, results in increased signal from iodine which eventually improves signal to noise ratio. For example reduction in tube potential from 120 to 80 kVp, results in increase in signal by a factor of 1.7. Yanaga et al. (2009) acquired CT urography images at 80 and 120 kVp and processed the lower kVp (80 kVp; estimated effective dose of 2.9 mSv) images with adaptive noise reduction filters for comparison with 120 kVp (estimated effective dose of 7.0 mSv). CT urography images were assessed for homogeneity of urinary tract, which is important for detecting any filling defect due to urinary tract stones or tumors. Post processed 80 kVp images were found to be comparable to 120 kVp in terms of diagnostic confidence.

Guimarães et al. (2010) acquired CT Enterography images on dual energy scanner with automatic exposure control settings turned on. Original raw data was processed with commercial reconstruction kernel of B40 (routinely used for abdominal CT on Siemens CT equipment) and sharper B45f kernel. Raw data were also processed with projection space-based bilateral filtering as well as with 3D ORA filters following image reconstruction. Images generated with projection space denoising had lower noise and were superior to 3D ORA filters. However, slight blurring resulted in minor false increase in bowel wall thickening (1.8–9.4%) on post processed images which was not statistically or clinically significant.

## 2.2 Head CT

In head CT images, higher image noise can affect visibility of low contrast details such as gray white matter differentiation and conspicuity of the cortical ribbon (Fig. 2). Other subtle details affected by low radiation dose include sharpness of the subarachnoid space, delineation of the ventricular margins, septum pellucidum and ability to visualize anatomical details in the posterior fossa.

Baum et al. (2004) evaluated the potential of the multidimensional adaptive filtering technique by investigating its effects on image noise and quality in head and neck CT examinations. Authors selected various settings of the filters called as the modification fraction, which was defined as the measure of maximum projection of data points that were modified during the filter processing. They concluded that multidimensional adaptive filters do not lead to any loss of detailed information or resolution with modification fractions up to 15%. Authors also found some loss of sharpness and delineation of anatomical details with 20% modification fraction, hence emphasizing the need for appropriate filter setting. Neuro 3D filters have shown about 50% radiation dose reduction with minimum deterioration of spatial resolution in both phantom and clinical studies (Nakashima et al. 2010).

Kakeda et al. (2010) evaluated 3D denoising (QDS/quantum denoising filter) on anthropomorphic vascular phantom designed to imitate cerebral aneurysms. They implanted aneurysms (3 mm, 6 mm) and blebs (2 mm in diameter) in the phantom. Various combinations of tube potential and tube currents were chosen (100 kVp: 150, 200, 250 mAs; 120 kVp: 100, 150, 200 mAs; 135 kVp: 100 mAs). CTA images acquired at 120 kVp and 200 mAs (CTDIw = 48 mGy) were considered as standard radiation dose. Three different strengths of QDS, namely Q04, Q06, Q08, were selected to process the images, where Q06 and Q08 were stronger filter settings in terms of noise reduction and sharpening. QDS post processed CTA images with settings Q08 (highest strength) acquired at 100 kVp, 250 mAs (CTDIw = 39.8) and 120 kVp, 100 mAs (CTDIw = 36.0) showed better image quality scores and CNR. Authors also estimated the Wiener noise power spectra (NPS) and found that Q08 filter lowers the image noise the most, especially in the low spatial frequencies. Modulation transfer function (MTF) showed no change with post processing. Results of NPS and MTF suggest that spatial resolution of structured objects was retained and noise reduction was achieved successfully in the non-structured regions of the images. Another group of investigators investigated QDS for enhancement of non-contrast head CT images for ischemic stroke. They evaluated both low contrast phantom and clinical images of 10 patients with chronic ischemic stroke for contrast to noise ratio. QDS improved CNR by up to 24% and similar enhancement of signal to noise ratio of head CT images.

Further clinical investigations are needed in head CT for effect of filters on detection of tiny low contrast lesions, such as subtle cortical infarcts. Although noise reduction filters lower noise, they also cause smoothening of images, which may interfere with detection of lacunar infarcts or small subarachnoid hemorrhages or petechiae.

## 2.3 Chest CT

Chest CT images are viewed at wider window width and length due to high inherent background contrast due to inflated lungs. Diagnostic interpretation due to image noise is less affected in the lungs as compared to abdominal and head CT. However, other soft tissues in the chest such as small mediastinal structures like lymph nodes or small vessels may be adversely affected by higher image noise in very low radiation dose images.

Kalra et al. (2003b) acquired two sets of additional four images in the equilibrium phase at 140 kVp and mA of 220, 240, 240, 280 (estimated CTDIvol = 9.5, 10.3 and 12.1 respectively) followed by low dose images of 110, 120, 120, 140 mA (estimated CTDIvol = 4.7, 5.2 and 6.0 respectively). They processed low dose images (110–140 mA) with 2D noise reduction filters at six different settings. Authors reported lower image noise at the expense of significant loss of sharpness of small vasculature in the peripheral lungs, especially with the filter settings that resulted in highest reduction in image noise.

Martinsen et al. (2010) compared effect of 2D nonlinear adaptive filters (2D-NLAF, ContextVison, Inc. CT) on low dose (30 mAs, CTDIvol = 1.8 mGy) chest CT images compared to higher dose images (200 mAs, CTDIvol = 8 mGy) in 8 patients with known or suspected thoracic malignancies. Post processed CT images were given higher image quality scores as compared with unprocessed low dose images without loss of structural details reported on some of the prior studies.

Emphysema presents as low attenuation air pockets on chest CT. Depending on the size and distribution of these air pockets, visual grading is possible (at threshold of less than −960 to −910 HU). With these threshold HU values, emphysema is quantified as percent of lung volumes below the threshold, also called as the pixel index (PI). However very low radiation dose images in the lung windows can have artifactual tiny low attenuation holes and confound assessment of very low dose chest CT images. Schilham et al. (2006) applied Noise Variance filter (NOVA) on 15 mAs images of 25 patients who were also scanned at 150 mAs. Compared to unprocessed 15 mAs images, the PI scores of processed low dose images were significantly close to PI scores at 150 mAs images. No blurring of edges, especially for long structures like vessels, and walls of small bronchi was noted following application of NOVA filters.

Kubo et al. (2006) have evaluated multidimensional adaptive filters for both streak artifact reduction and visibility of peripheral blood vessels. Authors acquired low dose chest CT images at 25 mAs in 12 patients and increased tube current to 50 mAs in 2 patients with suspected parenchymal disease. The low dose images following application of multidimensional filters had significantly lower streak artifacts in upper and lower thoracic regions without any deterioration in visibility of peripheral blood vessels.

Kubo et al. (2008) have also applied another 3D adaptive raw data filter (Boost 3D, Toshiba) on low dose chest CT raw data (50 mAs, CTDIvol = 8.2 mGy) of 58 patients who were also scanned at 150 mAs (CTDIvol = 24.5 mGy). Authors also reported lower image quality for lingula and left lower lobe as compared to right middle and lower lobes, attributing to motion artifacts by cardiovascular pulsation. Paul et al. (2010) have evaluated application of QDS and BOOST 3D (Toshiba) to chest CT images in the regions of thoracic inlet and mediastinal structures. Chest CT images were acquired at 120 kVp and 100–200 mA as standard dose (CTDIvol = 4.2–8.5 mGy) and low dose at 50 mA (CTDIvol = 2 mGy) and ultra low dose at 20 mA (0.82 mGy). They reported 5% dose reduction with BOOST 3D, 30% dose reduction for QDS and up to 35% dose reduction when QDS and BOOST 3D were combined for image processing.

## 2.4 Cardiac CT

Adequate contrast to noise ratio (CNR) is required to detect tiny low contrast details, such as non-calcified atherosclerotic plaques in the coronary arteries. Previous studies have also application of noise reduction filters for noise and radiation dose reduction in cardiac and vascular CT protocols (Khullar et al. 2005; Szucs-Farkas et al. 2011; Seifarth et al. 2005; De Geer et al. 2011).

In cardiac CT angiography, coronary stents leads to blooming artifacts which leads to limited evaluation of in-stent stenosis or luminal patency. Seifarth et al. (2005) evaluated the ability to visualize the stent lumen patency with use of appropriate convolution kernel and role of 3D ORA plus filters (Siemens Healthcare). CT images were acquired at effective 550 mAs, 120 kVp, pitch 0.28 (estimated CTDIvol = 44.7 mGy) and reconstructed with medium smooth body kernel (B30f) and edge enhancing kernel (B46f).

Although, B46f reduced the blooming artifacts around structures with high attenuation values, for example, stents or calcified plaques, there was a significant increase in image noise. Application of 3D ORA plus filter to B46 images reduced image noise and improved the visibility of stent lumen and any low contrast structures within the stent lumen.

De Geer et al. (2011) evaluated 2D nonlinear adaptive filters to improve image quality of cardiac CT angiography. They acquired two radiation dose levels in dual source scanner with maximum dose

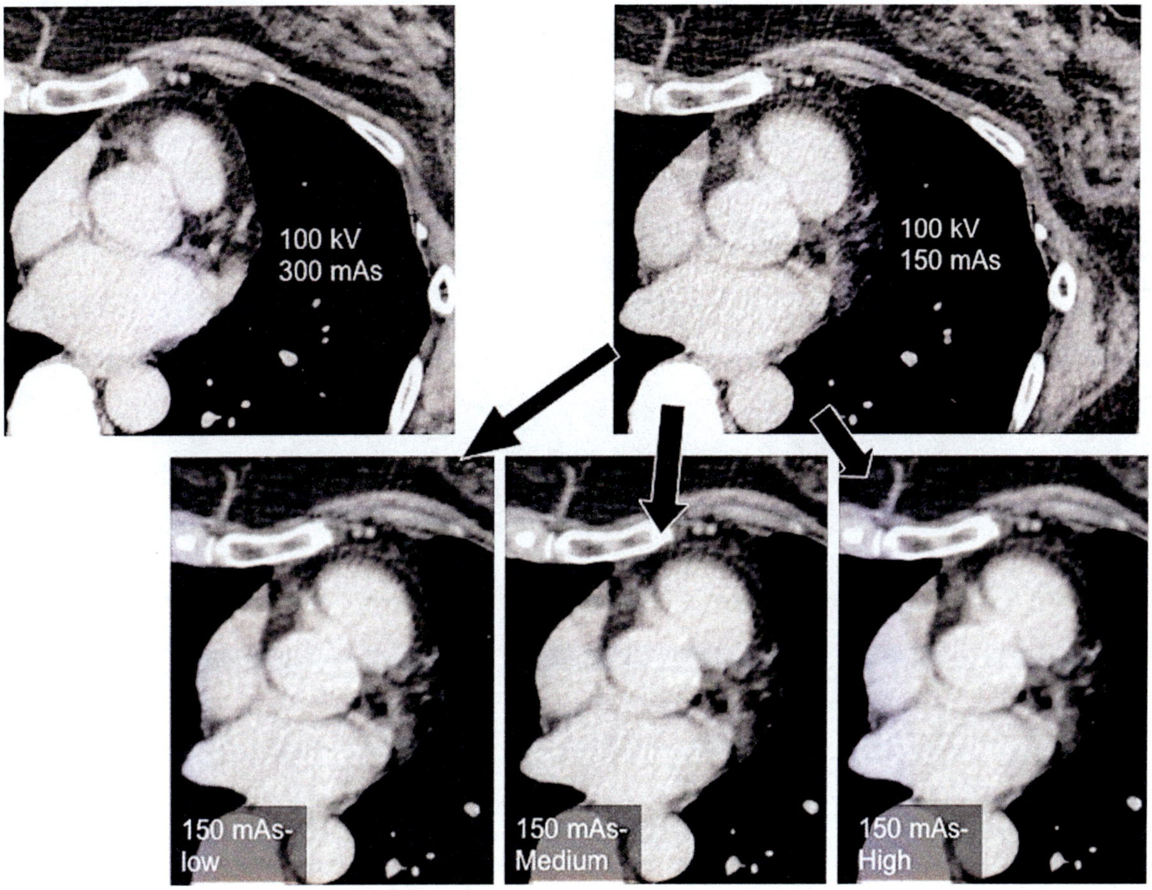


**Fig. 5** With use of ECG modulated tube current, coronary CT angiography was performed with lowered radiation dose at 85% R–R interval with scan parameters of 120 kV and 164 mAs as compared to 120 kV and 279 mAs at 65% R–R interval. These low dose images when post processed with 2D nonlinear adaptive filters resulted in lowered image noise without any significant change in the image contrast

during diastole and 80% reduced dose during systole. Lower dose images were post processed with 2D NLAF and assessed using visual grading of image quality, as well as objective noise and HU measurements in ascending and descending aorta. Compared to the baseline unprocessed images, low dose post processed or filtered images had better image quality with lower image noise (Fig. 5).

## 2.5 Obesity and CT Image Quality

Abdominal CT examinations of obese patients pose various clinical challenges due to increased image noise and artifacts. Schindera et al. (2011) evaluated CT images of intermediate (30 cm) and large (40 cm) liver phantom to assess the effect of large patient size on detection of hypovascular liver lesions. Phantom was customized to imitate liver during portal venous phase and comprised of lesions of various sizes (5, 10, 15 mm). Authors reported 42% noise reduction and 47–69% improvement in CNR with application of 3D ORA filters. The 5 mm lesions were missed in unfiltered low dose images of the large phantom. Although post processing with 3D ORA improved detection of 5 mm lesions, however this improvement did not reach statistical significance ($p = 0.054$).

For thoracic inlet imaging with CT in very large patients, Baum et al. (2004) have suggested role of higher filter settings of multidimensional adaptive filters by up to 20% modification fraction to lower image noise.

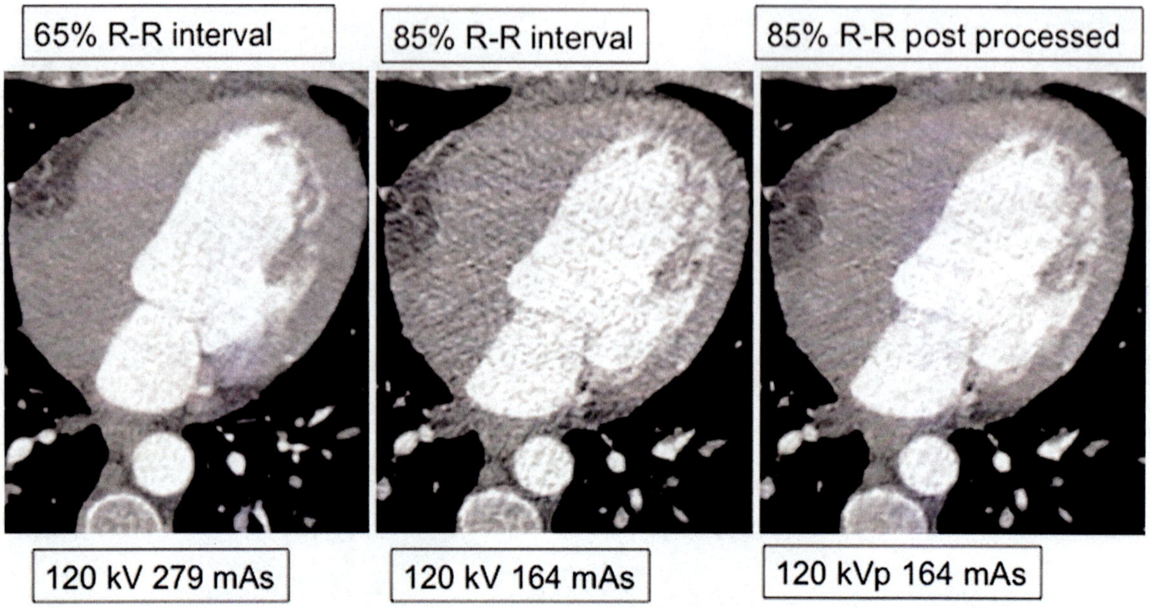


**Fig. 6** Chest CT examination was performed at 100 kVp and 300 mAs and additional images were acquired at low dose (100 kVp and 150 mAs) with limited scan length. Post processing of low dose images with image filters incorporated in a PACS at three different settings (low, medium and high) resulted in lowered image noise, with least amount of noise in high filter setting

### 2.6 Pediatric CT

Nishimaru et al. (2010) assessed the 3D post processing algorithm, using specific combination of 1D median filters for simulated low dose pediatric CT examination. They reconstructed same raw data with different display field of views (DFOV) and compared NLK (neighborhood linking) (Keselbrener et al. 1992) and QDS. They found that NLK and QDS do not lower image noise for small diameter DFOV less than 15 cm, and hence will be ineffective for small premature babies or infants.

Ledenius et al. (2010) evaluated pediatric head CT images after adding artificial noise to simulate low dose images and stratifying brain in two levels (upper representing lateral ventricles and and basal ganglia; lower level for posterior fossa and fourth ventricle). Simulated low dose images (CTDIvol = 23 mGy in upper level and 28 mGy in lower level) were processed with 2D-NLAF separately. Authors reported that 2D-NLAF can allow 13–15% dose reduction for head CT imaging when compared to standard dose head CT (CTDIvol = 27 mGy in upper level and 32 mGy in lower part) (Fig. 6).

## 3 Workflow

Most CT vendors have some noise reduction filters available during image reconstruction or for image post processing on the CT console. Convolution/reconstruction kernel available on the scanner console could be used to optimize image quality as per the selected protocol. Smoother kernels (for example, "B10" or "B20" from Siemens or "Soft" from GE) can be used to lower image noise in abdominal CT examination, whereas sharper kernels can be implemented for greater sharpness in lungs or bones. Some vendors combine their reconstruction kernels with noise reduction post processing filters to reduce noise in images. Filters may also be offered as image post processing features (noise reduction filters (GE Healthcare), advanced smoothening algorithms (Siemens)). These filters can be applied for different strengths of noise reduction (such as low, medium and high).

Some image or PACS workstations are also armed with noise reduction or edge enhancement filters which only work on DICOM image domain and not on projection space or raw data domain (Fig. 7).

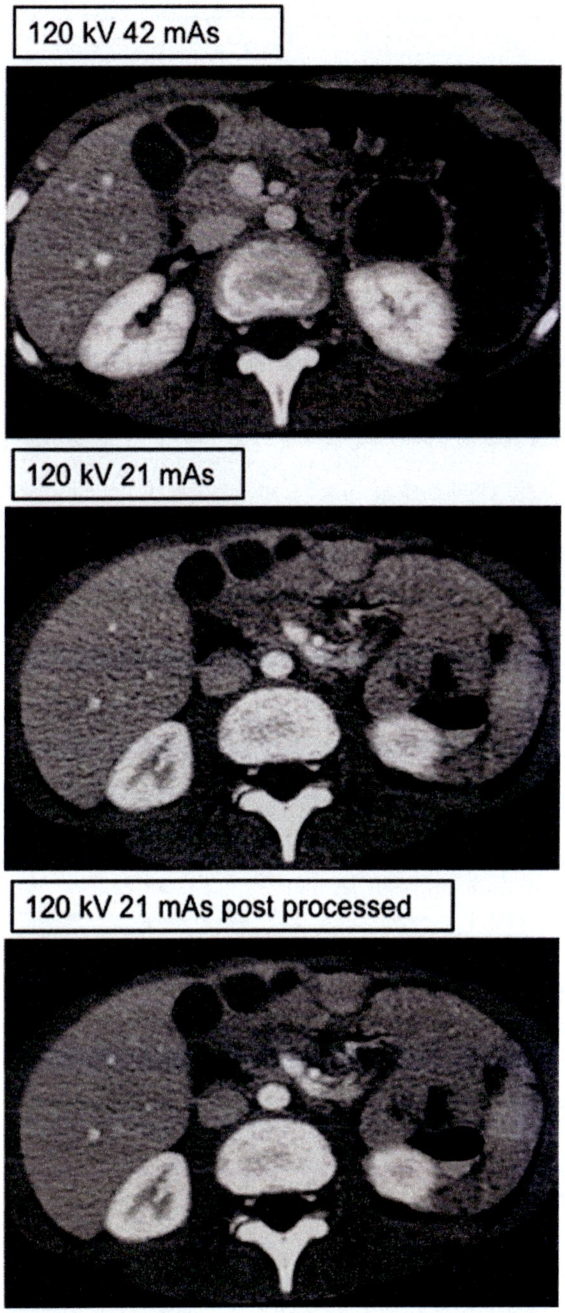


**Fig. 7** 6-year-old boy with known history of partial small bowel obstruction underwent follow up abdominal CT at lower tube current of 21 mAs, as compared to prior 42 mAs. These low dose images when post processed with 2D NLAF resulted in lower image noise and acceptable diagnostic image quality

Finally some "3rd party" vendors provide there own algorithms which are generally scanner and vendor independent and "sit" between the CT console and the PACS. They process DICOM images during their transit from CT console to the PACS. This workflow setting does involve at least some processing time but can be automated according to the scanning protocols based on preference of the interpreting radiologists.

## 4 Limitations

Although image noise reduction filters have shown effective noise reduction, many prior studies suggest that there is a delicate balance between strength of noise reduction and smoothening or blurring of edges. In addition, some strong filter settings can give an entirely different look or appearance to the images, which may not be something that radiologists are comfortable to interpret with confidence (Kalra et al. 2003a).

While most image space noise reduction filters function in real time, some raw data based filters may add to the processing time for images. For example, application of 3D algorithm proposed by Nishimaru et al. can take 150 s to process 200 images with slice thickness of 1.25 mm and DFOV of 10 cm on 2.4 GHz Intel Core Duo processor (Schindera et al. 2011 Jun). Adaptive NRF evaluated by Funama is image domain filter, but specific for parameters for the Hitachi scanners with estimated processing time of 0.2 s for each image with pixel size of 512 × 512 on Pentium III processor: 1,100 MHz (Funama et al. 2008).

Another limitation of these filters is that only while few image enhancement algorithms are available with the scanners or PACS, other elective filters on the scanner or the third party algorithms come with licensure and maintenance costs. Some of these third party filters do require additional time from the radiologists to select optimal settings of the algorithms, as well as from the hospital or departmental IT team to set up and maintain running DICOM entity in between PACS and CT scanner.

Finally with recent availability of partial and fully iterative reconstruction techniques may have changed the dynamics for application of noise reduction filters. While in the older serving CT scanners without iterative capabilities, noise reduction filters may retain their position, newer scanners with iterative reconstruction techniques will likely limit application of at least some of the noise reduction filters or processing.

At the time of writing of this manuscript, we are aware of any direct comparison between the two techniques of image quality improvement for low radiation dose CT.

## 5 Conclusion

In conclusion, use of noise reduction filters has been well documented for reducing radiation dose associated with CT scanning. When used correctly, noise reduction filters can help in substantial dose reduction with noise suppression without inadvertent loss of anatomical details or lesion conspicuity.

## References

AAPM (2011) AAPM Report # 39 specification and acceptance testing of computed tomography scanners. Accessed from http://www.aapm.org/pubs/reports/RPT_39.pdf on August 17, 2011

Bai M, Chen J, Raupach R, Suess C, Tao Y, Peng M (2009) Effect of nonlinear three-dimensional optimized reconstruction algorithm filter on image quality and radiation dose: validation on phantoms. Med Phys 36(1):95–97

Baum U, Noemayr A, Reissig A, Lell M, Cavallaro A, Kachelriess M, Riedel T, Kalender WA, Bautz W (2003) Improvement of the image quality of MSCT of the pelvis with a raw data-based, multidimensional filter. Rofo 175(11): 1572–1576

Baum U, Anders K, Steinbichler G, Lell M, Greess H, Riedel T, Kachelriess M, Kalender WA, Bautz WA (2004) Improvement of image quality of multislice spiral CT scans of the head and neck region using a raw data-based multidimensional adaptive filtering (MAF) technique. Eur Radiol 14(10):1873–1881

Berrington de González A, Mahesh M, Kim KP, Bhargavan M, Lewis R, Mettler F, Land C (2009) Projected cancer risks from computed tomographic scans performed in the United States in 2007. Arch Intern Med 169:2071–2077

Branschofsky M, Vogt C, Aurich V, Beck A, Mödder U, Cohnen M (2006) Feasibility of ultra-low-dose multi-detector-row CT-colonography: detection of artificial endoluminal lesions in an in vitro-model with optimization of image quality using a noise reduction filter algorithm. Eur J Med Res 11(1):13–19

Burt P, Adelson E (1983) The Laplacian pyramid as compact image code. IEEE Trans Commun 31:532–540

De Geer J, Sandborg M, Smedby O, Persson A (2011) The efficacy of 2D, non-linear noise reduction filtering in cardiac imaging: a pilot study. Acta Radiol 52(7):716–722

Funama Y, Awai K, Miyazaki O, Nakayama Y, Goto T, Omi Y, Shimonobo T, Liu D, Yamashita Y, Hori S (2006) Improvement of low-contrast detectability in low-dose hepatic multidetector computed tomography using a novel adaptive filter: evaluation with a computer-simulated liver including tumors. Invest Radiol 41(1):1–7

Funama Y, Awai K, Miyazaki O, Goto T, Nakayama Y, Shimamura M, Hiraishi K, Hori S, Yamashita Y (2008) Radiation dose reduction in hepatic multidetector computed tomography with a novel adaptive noise reduction filter. Radiat Med 26(3):171–177

Giraldo JC, Kelm ZS, Guimaraes LS, Yu L, Fletcher JG, Erickson BJ, McCollough CH (2009) Comparative study of two image space noise reduction methods for computed tomography: bilateral filter and nonlocal means. Conf Proc IEEE Eng Med Biol Soc 2009:3529–3532

Guimarães LS, Fletcher JG, Yu L, Huprich JE, Fidler JL, Manduca A, Ramirez-Giraldo JC, Holmes DR Jr, McCollough CH (2010) Feasibility of dose reduction using novel denoising techniques for low kV (80 kV) CT enterography: optimization and validation. Acad Radiol 17(10):1203–1210

Hsieh J (1998) Adaptive streak artifact reduction in computed tomography resulting from excessive X-ray photon noise. Med Phys 25(11):2139–2147

Kachelriess M, Watzke O, Kalender WA (2001) Generalized multi-dimensional adaptive filtering for conventional and spiral single-slice, multi-slice, and cone-beam CT. Med Phys 28(4):475–490

Kakeda S, Korogi Y, Ogawa M, Otsubo K, Morishita Y (2010) Reduction of the radiation dose for multidetector row CT angiography of cerebral aneurysms using an edge-preserving adaptive filter: a vascular phantom study. AJNR Am J Neuroradiol 31(5):827–829

Kalender WA (2000) Computed tomography. MCD, München, p 137

Kalra MK, Maher MM, Sahani DV, Blake MA, Hahn PF, Avinash GB, Toth TL, Halpern E, Saini S (2003a) Low-dose CT of the abdomen: evaluation of image improvement with use of noise reduction filters pilot study. Radiology 228(1):251–256

Kalra MK, Wittram C, Maher MM, Sharma A, Avinash GB, Karau K, Toth TL, Halpern E, Saini S, Shepard JA (2003b) Can noise reduction filters improve low-radiation-dose chest CT images? Pilot study. Radiology 228(1): 257–264

Kalra MK, Maher MM, Blake MA, Lucey BC, Karau K, Toth TL, Avinash G, Halpern EF, Saini S (2004) Detection and characterization of lesions on low-radiation-dose abdominal CT images postprocessed with noise reduction filters. Radiology 232(3):791–797

Kalva SP, Sahani DV, Hahn PF, Saini S (2006) Using the K-edge to improve contrast conspicuity and to lower radiation dose with a 16-MDCT: a phantom and human study. J Comput Assist Tomogr 30(3):391–397

Kazama M, Tsukagoshi S, Okumura M (2006) Image quality improvement and exposure dose reduction with the combined use of X-ray modulation and Boost3D. Proc SPIE Int Soc Opt Eng 6142:847–855, 61422G. doi:10.1117/12.653092

Keselbrener L, Shimoni Y, Akselrod S (1992) Nonlinear filters applied on computerized axial tomography: theory and phantom images. Med Phys 19(4):1057–1064

Khullar D, Subramanyan K, Johnson P (2005) Evaluation of a noise-reduction contrast-enhancement algorithm for CT cardiac angiography. Proc SPIE 5749:310–318

Kröpil P, Lanzman RS, Walther C, Röhlen S, Godehardt E, Mödder U, Cohnen M (2010) Dose reduction and image quality in MDCT of the upper abdomen: potential of an adaptive post-processing filter. Rofo 182(3):248–253

Kubo T, Nishino M, Kino A, Yoshimura N, Lin PJ, Takahashi M, Raptopoulos V, Hatabu H (2006) 3-dimensional adaptive raw-data filter: evaluation in low dose chest multidetector-row computed tomography. J Comput Assist Tomogr 30(6): 933–938

Kubo T, Ohno Y, Gautam S, Lin PJ, Kauczor HU, Hatabu H (2008) iLEAD study group: use of 3D adaptive raw-data filter in CT of the lung: effect on radiation dose reduction. Am J Roentgenol 191(4):1071

Leander P, Söderberg M, Fält T, Gunnarsson M, Albertsson I (2010) Post-processing image filtration enabling dose reduction in standard abdominal CT. Radiat Prot Dosimetry 139(1–3):180–185

Ledenius K, Stålhammar F, Wiklund LM, Fredriksson C, Forsberg A, Thilander-Klang A (2010) Evaluation of image-enhanced paediatric computed tomography brain examinations. Radiat Prot Dosimetry 139(1–3):287–292

Manduca A, Yu L, Trzasko JD, Khaylova N, Kofler JM, McCollough CM, Fletcher JG (2009) Projection space denoising with bilateral filtering and CT noise modeling for dose reduction in CT. Med Phys 36(11):4911–4919

Martinsen AC, Saether HK, Olsen DR, Skaane P, Olerud HM (2008) Reduction in dose from CT examinations of liver lesions with a new postprocessing filter: a ROC phantom-study. Acta Radiol 49(3):303–309

Martinsen AC, Saether HK, Olsen DR, Wolff PA, Skaane P (2010) Improved image quality of low-dose thoracic CT examinations with a new postprocessing software. J Appl Clin Med Phys 11(3):3242

Nakashima J, Takahashi T, Takahashi Y, Imai Y, Ishihara Y, Kato K, Nakazawa Y (2010) Radiation dose reduction using a non-linear image filter in MDCT. Nihon Hoshasen Gijutsu Gakkai Zasshi 66(5):515–524

Nishimaru E, Ichikawa K, Okita I, Tomoshige Y, Kurokawa T, Nakamura Y, Suzuki M (2010) Development of a noise reduction filter algorithm for pediatric body images in multidetector CT. J Digit Imaging 23(6):806–818

Okumura M, Ota T, Tsukagoshi S, Katada K (2006) New method of evaluating edge-preserving adaptive filters for computed tomography (CT): digital phantom method. Nihon Hoshasen Gijutsu Gakkai Zasshi 62(7):971–978

Paul NS, Blobel J, Prezelj E, Burey P, Ursani A, Menezes RJ, Kashani H, Siewerdsen JH (2010) The reduction of image noise and streak artifact in the thoracic inlet during low dose and ultra-low dose thoracic CT. Phys Med Biol 55: 1363–1380

Rizzo SM, Kalra MK, Schmidt B, Raupach R, Maher MM, Blake MA, Saini S (2005) CT images of abdomen and pelvis: effect of nonlinear three-dimensional optimized reconstruction algorithm on image quality and lesion characteristics. Radiology 237(1):309–315

Schauer DA, Linton OW (2009) NCRP report no. 160, ionizing radiation exposure of the population of the United States, medical exposure–are we doing less with more, and is there a role for health physicists? Health Phys 97:1–5

Schilham AM, van Ginneken B, Gietema H, Prokop M (2006) Local noise weighted filtering for emphysema scoring of low-dose CT images. IEEE Trans Med Imaging 25:451–463

Schindera ST, Torrente JC, Ruder TD, Hoppe H, Marin D, Nelson RC, Szucs-Farkas Z (2011) Decreased detection of hypovascular liver tumors with MDCT in obese patients: a phantom study. Am J Roentgenol 196(6):W772–W776

Seifarth H, Raupach R, Schaller S, Fallenberg EM, Flohr T, Heindel W, Fischbach R, Maintz D (2005) Assessment of coronary artery stents using 16-slice MDCT angiography: evaluation of a dedicated reconstruction kernel and a noise reduction filter. Eur Radiol 15(4):721–726

Szucs-Farkas Z, Bensler S, Torrente JC, Cullmann JL, Vock P, Schindera ST (2011) Nonlinear three-dimensional noise filter with low-dose CT angiography: effect on the detection of small high-contrast objects in a phantom model. Radiology 258(1):261–269

UNSCEAR ( 2000) The United Nations scientific committee on the effects of atomic radiation. Health Phys 79(3):314

Wessling J, Esseling R, Raupach R, Fockenberg S, Osada N, Gerss J, Heindel W, Fischbach R (2007) The effect of dose reduction and feasibility of edge-preserving noise reduction on the detection of liver lesions using MSCT. Eur Radiol 17(7):1885–1891

Yanaga Y, Awai K, Funama Y, Nakaura T, Hirai T, Roux S, Yamashita Y (2009) Low-dose MDCT urography: feasibility study of low-tube-voltage technique and adaptive noise reduction filter. Am J Roentgenol 193(3):W220–W229

Yu L, Manduca A, Trzasko J, Khaylova N, Kofler JM, McCollough CH, Fletcher JG (2008) Sinogram smoothing with bilateral filtering for low-dose CT. Progress in Biomed Optics Imaging Proc SPIE 6913, article 691329

Yu L, Manduca A, Jacobsen M, Trzasko JD, Fletcher JG, DeLone DR, McCollough CH (2010) Adaptive modulation of bilateral filtering based on a practical noise model for streaking and noise reduction in multi-slice CT. Proc SPIE 7622:76222O

# Hardware Developments for Radiation Dose Reduction

Rich Mather

## Contents



**Abstract**

The evolution of CT has created systems that scan faster, use thinner sections, and cover more patient anatomy in a single rotation. These developments have not only opened the spectrum of CT applications but have also driven the need for new methods of radiation dose reduction. By analyzing the imaging chain from X-ray tubes and collimators to detectors and data acquisition systems, we examine the various hardware-based dose reduction strategies in the modern CT system. As part of a concerted effort between clinicians, physicists, and manufacturers, hardware innovation and system design play a significant role in optimizing the radiation dose in CT.

## 1 Introduction

As the use of X-rays is central to the design of a CT scanner, there will necessarily be some degree of radiation exposure to the patient. The magnitude of that exposure is dependent on factors that are inherent to the scanner design, the operator's choice of protocol parameters, as well as on factors that are independent of the scanner itself. Some of the scanner-independent factors include: patient size and density, the presence of exogenous contrast material, and, most importantly, the nature and requirements of the clinical task. The necessary image quality depends heavily on the diagnostic question being asked, and the magnitude of the radiation dose is directly proportional to the required level of image quality. While low noise and good low-contrast resolution are

R. Mather (✉)
Toshiba Medical Research Institute,
706 N Deerpath Dr, Vernon Hills, IL 60061, USA
e-mail: rmather@tmriusa.com

D. Tack et al. (eds.), *Radiation Dose from Multidetector CT*, Medical Radiology. Diagnostic Imaging,
DOI: 10.1007/174_2011_477, © Springer-Verlag Berlin Heidelberg 2012

important when assessing pancreatitis or imaging non-calcified plaque in the coronary arteries, significantly more noise can be tolerated for a virtual colonoscopy exam or for kidney stone detection. Once the required image quality of an examination is determined, it is critical to minimize the dose necessary to achieve the necessary image quality and accomplish the diagnostic task. A significant amount of attention has been paid recently to the topic of dose reduction in CT imaging. However, a better focus is on the optimization of the use of radiation in CT. Many of the advances in CT scanner hardware have been developed for precisely this purpose: minimize the radiation risk to the patient by optimizing the use of X-rays in CT.

## 2 CT Evolution

CT imaging has been constantly evolving since its inception. The technology has moved from single-detector-row imaging to multi-detector-row and from relatively slow rotation speeds to fast rotation speeds. The rise of multi-detector-row scanners allowed for significantly thinner slice sensitivity profiles and opened up the door to volumetric imaging with CT, enabling anatomy to be imaged as three-dimensional volumes rather than just two-dimensional cross sections. While a single-row helical system with a 5 mm slice thickness and a one second rotation time can only cover approximately 150 mm in a 30 s acquisition, a four-row helical system with a 0.5 s rotation time can cover more than a meter with a 3 mm slice thickness. This was a significant advance in CT imaging and enabled new volumetric clinical applications that were previously impossible or impractical. However, with 4-row CT the operator was forced to tradeoff between the amount of volumetric coverage and the slice thickness that was achievable. Furthermore, 4-row CT scanning using the thinnest slices had a dose penalty (Bushberg et al. 2002). In order to ensure a uniform flux of X-rays across each of the detector rows, the width of the X-ray beam had to be larger than width of the detectors. The part of the beam that does not fall on the active portion of the detectors is called the penumbra. Typically, the penumbra depends on the acquired slice thickness, with more penumbra necessary for thin slices, and not on the total collimation. Since the penumbra is relatively fixed, it comprises a much larger percentage of the total collimation with thin slices compared to thick ones.

With the introduction of the 16-detector-row scanners, some of these limitations were greatly mitigated. For example, the thin slice dose penalty was minimized, allowing for most scans to be acquired using 1 mm slices or less. Also, with the increased coverage per rotation, the entire body was able to be imaged in 30 s or less with those same thin slices. The introduction of CT angiography was one of the major benefits of thin slice imaging as near-isotropic spatial resolution (Mahesh 2002) and reduced partial volume artifacts allowed the visualization of small vessels, even in the presence of metal prostheses (Fig. 1). Finally, with faster rotation times, the potential to image the coronary arteries using a third-generation CT scanner was clinically possible (Achenbach et al. 2003). Overall, the 16-detector-row systems were more dose-efficient and versatile CT scanners compared to their 4-row predecessors.

CT technology has continued to evolve rapidly over the last five years. All vendors continued past 16-detector rows to wider coverage in the z-direction with thin image sections between 0.5 and 0.625 mm. All of these >16 row systems are capable of fast rotation times from 0.33 to 0.4 s which allows routine cardiac imaging on most clinical patients. This breed of scanner is typically referred to as a "64", reflecting either the number of detector rows or the number of "slices" produced with flying focal spot technology.

## 3 Vendor State-of-the-Art

While the primary technology for the 64-row systems is fairly similar for all vendors, technology beyond 64 rows marked an exploration of different technological direction from the manufacturers. The state-of-the-art scanners from each company have unique properties that reflect the different directions of the current expansion of CT innovation.

General Electric (GE) introduced a new detector technology called Gemstone on their Discovery HD750. This detector technology allowed increased sampling rates over earlier detectors. This enabled dual energy scanning with fast (approximately 0.5 ms) kV switching (Lin et al. 2011). "The Discovery HD750, a 64 detector row system, was the first modern CT

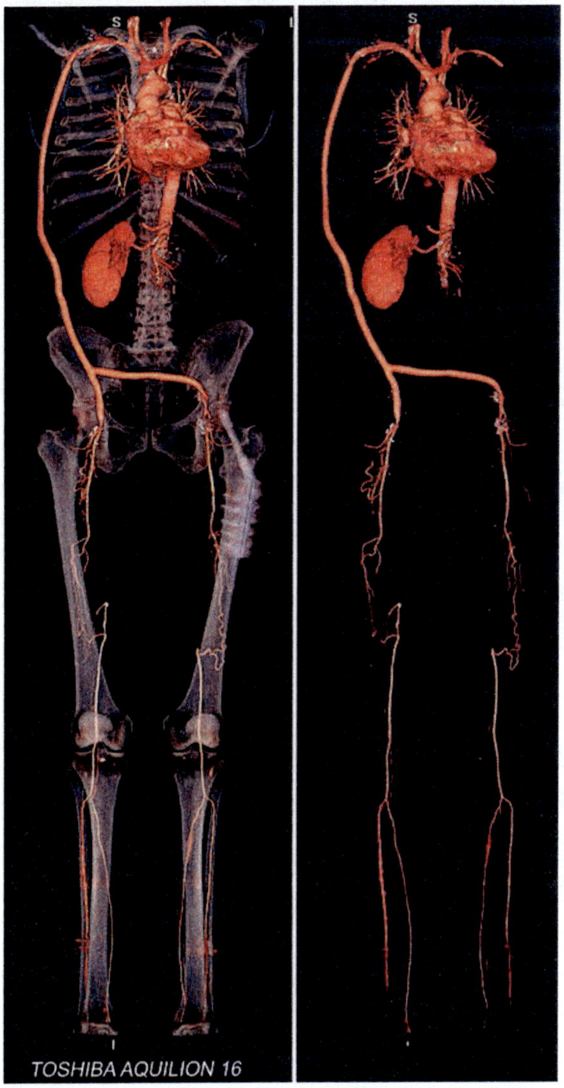


**Fig. 1** 16-row angiography with metal prosthesis. (Images courtesy of Toshiba America Medical Systems)

scanner to introduce iterative reconstruction technology to the market. Their latest Food and Drug Administration cleared version is called Veo or MBIR (model based iterative reconstruction)".

Philips' current top-of-the-line system is the Brilliance iCT. This scanner has 128 detector rows covering 8 cm of anatomy in the z-direction at isocenter. It uses flying focal spot technology to acquire 256 slices of data and has a rotation time of 0.27 s (Bardo et al. 2009) which is the fastest in the industry. Philips' iterative reconstruction, called iDose[4], is available on the iCT.

Siemens' flagship system is called the Definition Flash. The Flash is a dual source scanner with two X-ray tubes and 2 detector arrays offset by 90°. By using both sources, this system is able to improve its temporal resolution to 75 ms (Flohr et al. 2009), the lowest in the industry, without using multisegment reconstruction. Each detector array has 64 rows which can read out 128 slices using flying focal spot technology. Furthermore, the system is capable of scanning with high helical pitch up to 3.4 for fast anatomic coverage. Siemens' iterative reconstruction algorithm, IRIS (iterative reconstruction in image space) is available on the Definition Flash.

Toshiba's premium system is the Aquilion ONE. The Aquilion ONE has 320 detector rows covering 16 cm of anatomy in the z-direction at isocenter (Rybicki et al. 2008), the widest coverage in the industry, in one rotation of the gantry. This system can image entire organs, such as the head or the heart, with no table motion. Furthermore, real-time dynamic volumetric imaging is available through multiple acquisitions taken in one 16 cm stationary location. Toshiba's iterative reconstruction algorithm, AIDR (Adaptive Iterative Dose Reduction), is available on the Aquilion ONE.

## 4 Hardware Dose Reduction

Every step forward in the evolution of computed tomography technology, from the first commercial single-detector-row machine to today's sophisticated, state-of-the-art scanners, has brought with it changes in hardware design that have altered the definition of what is considered the optimal radiation dose. Many technological improvements, such as mA modulation (Mastora et al. 2001), have made CT technology fundamentally more dose-efficient. On the other hand, some advanced clinical applications and levels of image quality made possible by advancing CT technology have brought forth new tradeoffs and challenges in radiation dose management. In order to maintain image quality and minimize radiation dose with these thinner and faster CTs, new hardware solutions also had to be developed. These hardware innovations and their effect on dose optimization in CT are best explained in the context of where each innovation affects the imaging chain. The imaging chain begins with the generation of photons in the

X-ray tube, then proceeds through the filtration and collimation of the X-ray beam, and concludes with the absorption of X-rays by the detector and subsequent generation of a corresponding electronic signal that is passed along by data acquisition system (DAS).

At the beginning of the imaging chain, the X-ray tube generates the photons that are the basis of the projectional imaging techniques employed by computed tomography. As in all electronics, a CT X-ray tube contains both a negatively charged side, the cathode, and a positively charged anode side, typically made of Tungsten. In a conventional X-ray tube the X-ray generation process begins when a high current, on the order of 50–600 milli-amperes (mA), is put through the cathode filament. The electric current results in high temperatures that free electrons from the cathode. The electrons are then accelerated by a high voltage field toward the anode. The strength of the electric potential across the tube is typically 120 kilo-volts (kV) but can range from 70 to 140 kVp. When these accelerated electrons strike the tungsten anode they are forced to suddenly slow down, creating X-rays through a process called bremsstrahlung ("breaking radiation"). The choice of mA and kVp has a large impact on photon flux at the detector as well as patient dose, as will be discussed later. However, let us start our discussion of X-ray tube hardware by examining the impact of the anode itself on dose optimization.

As discussed earlier, a modern CT scanner is capable of rotating at speeds >3 revolutions per second. In order to dissipate heat and extend the time period in which X-rays can be generated before the tube needs to cool, the anode itself also rotates. These forces can result in vibrations of the anode which in turn leads to instabilities and variations in the position of the anode and the photons coming off it. In order to get a stable, uniform photon flux at each of the detector elements, the presence of anode vibration leads to the need for a wider collimation and increased penumbra. Penumbra is the portion of the X-ray beam that exceeds the dimension of the detector but which is necessary to accommodate the inherent divergence of the X-ray beam and any other sources of non-uniform photon flux, such as anode vibration. Penumbra, sometimes called "overbeaming" contributes to patient dose but, because penumbra exceeds the dimensions of the detector, it does not directly contribute to image formation (Seeram 2001). In order to minimize penumbra and reduce patient dose while maintaining image quality, an early advancement in X-ray tube technology was the addition of bearing supports on both ends of the anode axis. These bearings supports ensure uniform photon flux, thus minimizing extra patient dose from unnecessary penumbra.

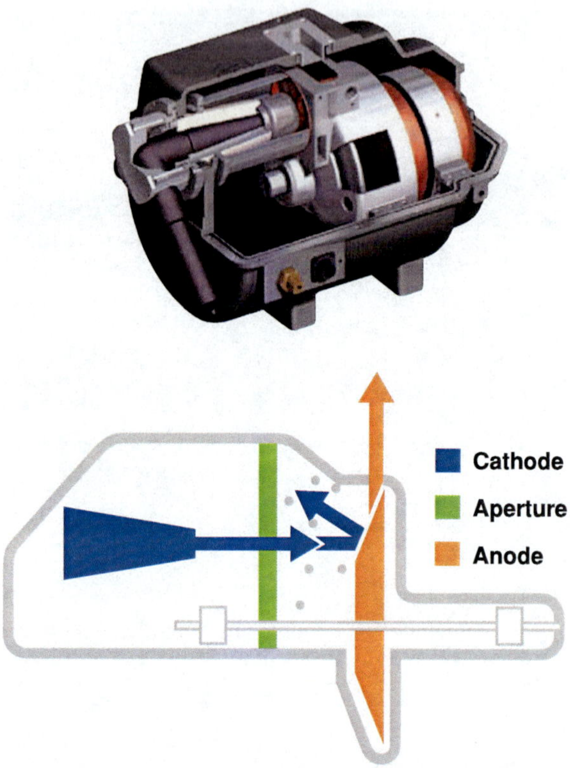


**Fig. 2** X-ray tube design showing anode, cathode, and double-support bearings. Recoil electrons are captured by a positively charged aperture or grid to prevent them from striking the anode away from the focal spot, increasing patient dose and X-ray tube heating. (Images courtesy of Toshiba America Medical Systems)

Another source of extraneous patient dose and impaired image quality that can occur in the X-ray tube is the presence of off-focal electrons. Off-focal electrons are electrons that have been knocked into trajectories that produce X-rays outside of the anode focal spot. These wayward electrons produces X-rays that result in blurring, artifact, and unnecessary patient dose. Therefore, another advance in X-ray tube technology comprised the introduction of a positively charged grid that captures off-focal electrons (Fig. 2). By fitting this positively charged grid

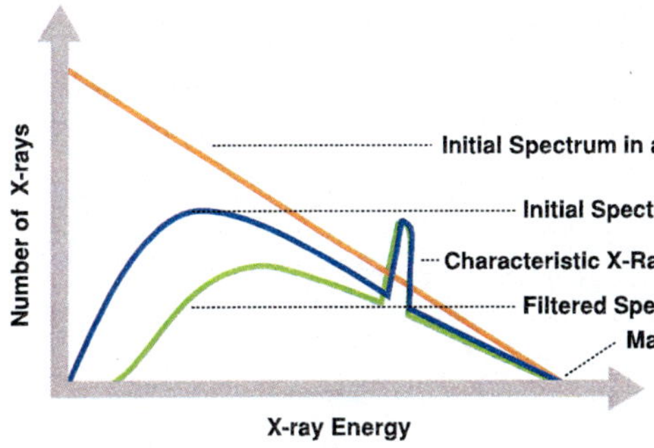


**Fig. 3** Typical bremsstrahlung spectrum with and without filtration. The initial spectrum (*orange*), in a vacuum, steadily decreases up to the kV setting in air, the lowest energy X-rays are filtered out, but a large number of low energy X-rays remain (*blue*). Many of the lowest energy X-rays will not penetrate a patient and only contribute to dose. All CT scanners employ a certain amount of additional filtration to "harden" the beam and remove the low energy X-rays (*green*)

near the electrically grounded anode, any secondary, off-focal electrons are captured and removed from the system, thus reducing radiation dose and improving image quality (Seeram 2001).

The introduction of anode support bearings and positively charged grid represent two technological advances that improved dose optimization by both reducing radiation dose and improving image quality. The relationship between the mA and kVp in the X-ray tube and dose optimization is more complex. Let us start by examining kVp. It is important to note the X-rays generated by the bremsstrahlung process are not of a single energy. Instead, a spectrum of photon energies are produced based on the particular interactions of the electrons with the exact anode material used in the tube. Therefore, the X-rays that leave the anode have a spectrum (Fig. 3) of energies that range from near zero up to a maximum energy equal to the kV (the "p" in kVp stands for "peak", a reference to the peak energy outputted). In general, very low energy X-ray photons do not penetrate through the body often and contribute almost exclusively to patient dose. On the other hand, the highest energy photons in some cases can pass too readily through the patient and fail to generate signal contrast. Image formation relies upon photons that fall into a "medium" energy range where they can potentially be absorbed by patient or by the detector depending on the material in the beam, resulting in contrast between the tissues and organs being imaged. Because this ideal "medium" energy range will depend on the imaging task and the age and size of the patient, an essential component to CT hardware is the availability of a variety of X-ray tube kilovoltages. Currently, kVp settings ranging from 70 to 140kVp are available. To prevent useless low energy X-rays from contributing to patient dose without contributing to image quality, all CT scanners also add a certain filtration technology outside the X-ray tube to block the low energy X-rays from leaving the X-ray tube (Szulc and Judy 1979). There is, however, a tradeoff involved applying filtration: in the process of removing low energy X-rays, some desirable, medium and high energy X-rays will be removed as well, decreasing the overall output of the tube in the desired energy range. This means that higher mA values are needed to realize a given flux at the detector. Furthermore, the higher overall beam energy may compromise the system's ability to generate contrast differentiation. While all manufacturers employ some amount of fixed filtration to harden their beam to the desired amount, at least one company has implemented selectable filtration technology that can further increase the hardness of the beam when clinically appropriate, such as when scanning an obese patient. By carefully targeting the X-ray energy range to the task at hand, via kVp selection and/or filtration, dose optimization can be improved.

Modern CT technology also improves dose efficiency by accommodating the shape of the patient. The best image quality is achieved when the photon flux at the detector is uniform (non-uniformities can lead to shading and other artifacts that can hinder clinical diagnosis). Because most clinical subjects scanned are roughly round or ovoid in shape, the path that the X-rays take through the edges of the subject will be significantly shorter than the path taken by the X-rays through the center. Therefore, in order to achieve uniform X-ray flux at the detector, the beam must be shaped to reduce the number of photons leaving the edges the X-ray tube assembly relative to the number of photons at center (Fig. 4). This beam shaping is accomplished by shaping the physical filter in the X-ray tube such that the filter is thicker at the edges than in the center; a so-called bowtie filter. A properly shaped bowtie filter improves dose optimization by improving image and reducing unnecessary radiation dose at the peripheries. As patients and

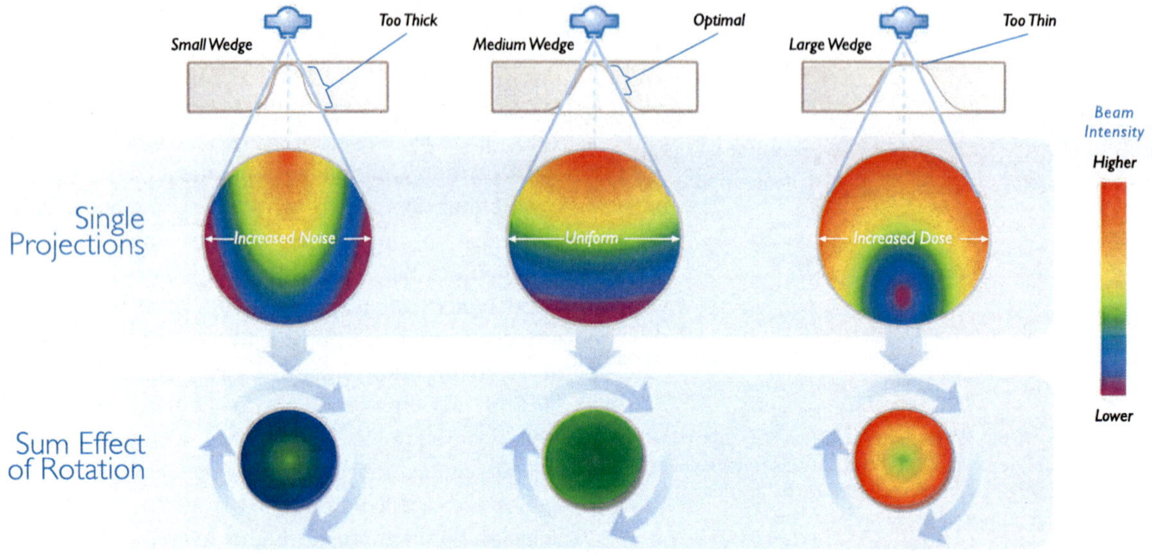


**Fig. 4** Bowtie filter. Matching the bowtie to the object that is being scanned (*middle*) creates a uniform dose distribution. If the bowtie is too small (*left*), the images will have increased noise toward the periphery. If the bowtie is too large (*right*), it is dose inefficient as the periphery is exposed to extra radiation that does not improve image quality. (Graphic courtesy of Philips Healthcare)

body regions come in a variety of sizes, all scanners allow a selection of bowtie filter hardware so that the bowtie can be matched to the patient.

After the X-ray beam is shaped in the X–Y direction by the bowtie filter, it is appropriately sized in the z-direction by the collimators. The collimators are designed to allow the width of the X-ray beam to be no greater than the size of the detection and any necessary penumbra. In the past, the collimators were fixed and stationary. The advent of helical CT presented a new challenge to collimation technology. Helical CT relies upon interpolated data from adjacent z-axis locations to generate an image at a particular z position: therefore, extra rotations are needed at each end of the desired scan range to obtain enough data. These extra rotations are called "over-ranging" or helical overscan (Tzedakis et al. 2005). While over-ranging is necessary, only about half of the projection data gathered during the extra rotations are needed to complete the reconstruction of the image at each end of the scan range. Therefore, a significant portion of the extra rotations contribute unnecessary patient dose. The relative contribution of the overscan region to the total patient radiation dose is a function of the length of the acquired volume, the helical pitch, and the detector configuration (van der Molen and Geleijns 2007). The percentage of dose that is contributed by the overscan region increases with shorter volumes. For narrow X-ray beams, the increase in radiation dose from over-ranging was accepted, given the improvements in image quality and increased amount of diagnostic information made possible by helical CT. But as CT technology has evolved from narrow beam to wide beam helical scanning this tradeoff in radiation dose became larger and less acceptable, creating an opportunity for collimator technology to advance in order to better optimize the use of radiation dose. In order to ameliorate the effect of over-ranging on radiation dose, all manufacturers have developed active collimation. Active collimators are not fixed with respect to the X-ray tube assembly, but rather move to block the unnecessary portion of the beam during over-ranging by opening or closing independently of each other. Since only the projections that contribute to image formation at the edge of the helical volume are necessary, the collimation can block off the X-rays in the regions outside the helical volume. As the table moves the helical volume into the complete Z-direction view of the tube and detectors, the collimators open to their full size consistent with the current detector configuration. Finally, as the table moves the helical volume out of the Z-direction view of the tube and detectors, the collimators begin to close again, cutting off much of the over-ranging at the end of the scan. These dynamic collimators minimize the dose contributed by over-ranging (Deak et al. 2009), however high helical pitch and fast rotation times can limit the overall effectiveness.

As the X-rays pass through the subject, one of three things can happen. They are either completely absorbed by the subject, be transmitted through the subject with no interaction, or be scattered and change direction. The completely absorbed and completely transmitted X-rays are the responsible for the contrast and signal in the CT image. Since scattered photons change direction on their way through the subject, they appear to have come from a different direction and only contribute to noise and shading within the image. In order to minimize the effects of scatter, all MDCT systems place thin septa between their detector channels (Bushberg et al. 2002). The X-ray tube and detector rotate together around the subject. Consequently, each detector's view of the focal spot is limited to a narrow angle and it can be expected that any primary, non-scattered photon will arrive at that detector from that narrow angle. The septa act like blinders for the detector channel to prevent scattered photon from reaching the detector. Most CT systems place these septa only in the X–Y direction. However, one wide detector system employs a two-dimensional anti-scatter grid to minimize the effects of scatter in the Z-direction. The tradeoff with all septa and grids is that while they reduce the overall scatter in the system, they also create "dead spots" in the detector leading to a reduced geometric efficiency.

No single hardware aspect of a scanner has more influence on dose than the efficiency of the detection system. The detector's ability to catch the X-ray, convert it to light, transmit that light, and convert it to an electrical signal with minimal loss defines the overall detection efficiency of the detector. Detectors that can efficiently capture and convert the X-ray signal help to lower patient dose for a given level of image quality. While many CT scanners used Xenon filled detectors in the past, all modern scanners use some form of solid scintillator. Most MDCT scanners use a form of Gadolinium Oxysulfide (GOS) ceramic (Fig. 5). The base form of GOS has relatively low light output. However, by "doping", or adding to, the ceramic with some rare-earth elements such as Praesodynium and/or Cerenium, the light output can be increased. Each manufacturer uses a proprietary formula and sintering process to create their ceramic (Okumura et al. 2002). One manufacturer uses a garnet crystal as their scintillator allowing the detector to be read with a high frequency for fast kV switching dual energy imaging. The detector material, whether ceramic or crystal, is one of the most proprietary hardware components in a CT scanner and significantly contributes to the dose efficiency to the system as a whole.

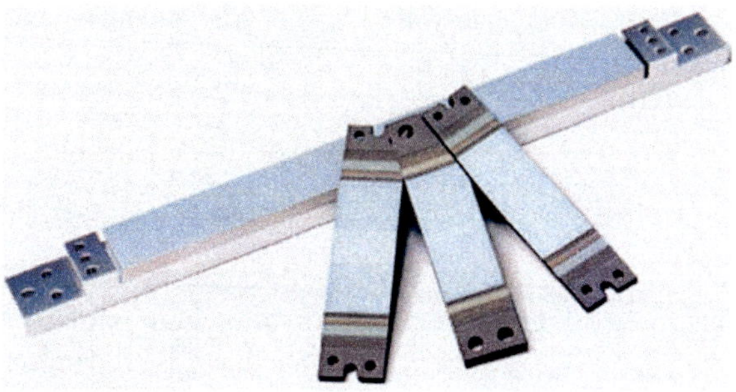

**Fig. 5** Multi-detector CT detector modules. Each module consists of rows of detector elements of various sizes. Each module covers 24 channels in the X–Y direction as well as a number of rows in the Z-direction. By combining multiple modules in the X–Y direction, the entire detector array can be constructed

Once the X-rays are captured and turned into light by the detectors that signal must be digitized, collated, and passed to the reconstruction system. This process is governed by the data acquisition system (DAS) which has to be capable of reading the detector signals rapidly, typically between 1000 and 4000 times per second. In the digitization and transfer of the X-ray signal, electronic noise can be introduced to the measured data. Through the use of high-end digital electronic pioneered by the audio industry, the amount of corruption of the signal with electronic noise can be minimized.

At this point in the imaging chain, the influences of scanner hardware are complete and the reconstruction process takes over. Innovations such as adaptive filtering in the raw-data and image domain as well as iterative reconstruction algorithms further optimize image quality by minimizing image noise. Ultimately dose reduction is a combination between optimization in the scanner hardware and in the scanner and reconstruction software.

## 5 Conclusion

While there are many important scanner innovations that help to optimize image quality and minimize patient dose, it is important to note that dose reduction is a process that extends beyond the CT scanner itself. There are multiple stakeholders in this process, and each contributes to the task of minimizing dose. The radiologist, technologist, and medical physicist at the clinical site must optimize the scanner protocols for the local patient population and clinical practice. The manufacturer's applications specialists and development engineers collaborate to develop best practices for their systems and continuously innovate to optimize image quality and dose. Finally, the academic and industry researchers collaborate to develop new technologies and clinical approaches to dose optimization. All of these stakeholders has a role to play in ensuring that an appropriate examination is conducted on an appropriate patient with an appropriate radiation dose. By combining scanner hardware and software with expert users and optimized clinical practices, CT dose will continue to be optimized.

## References

Achenbach S, Ropers D, Pohle K et al (2003) Clinical results of minimally invasive coronary angiography using computed tomography. Cardiol Clin 21:549–559

Bushberg JT, Seibert JA, Leidholdt EM, Boone III JM (2002) Ch 13 Computed Tomography. In: The essential physics of medical imaging, 2nd edn. Lipincott Williams and Wilkins, pp 367–369

Bardo DM, Asamato J, Mackay CS, Minette M (2009) Low-dose coronary artery computed tomography angiogram of an infant with tetralogy of fallot using a 256-slice multidetector computed tomography scanner. Pediatr Cardiol 30:824–826

Deak PD, Langner O, Lell M, Kalender WA (2009) Effects of adaptive section collimation on patient radiation dose in multisection spiral CT. Radiology 252:140–147

Flohr TG, Leng S, Yu L et al (2009) Dual-source spiral CT with pitch up to 3.2 and 75 ms temporal resolution: image reconstruction and assessment of image quality. Med Phys 36:5641–5653

Lin XZ, Miao F, Li JY et al (2011) High-definition CT Gemstone spectral imaging of the brain: initial results of selecting optimal monochromatic image for beam-hardening artifacts and image noise reduction. J Comput Assist Tomogr 35:294–297

Mastora I, Remy-Jardin M, Suess C et al (2001) Dose reduction in spiral CT angiography of thoracic outlet syndrome by anatomically adapted tube current modulation. Eur Radiol 11:590–596

Mahesh M (2002) Search for isotropic resolution in CT from conventional through multiple-row detector. Radiographics 22:949–962

Okumura M, Tamatani M, Igarishi K (2002) Development of X-ray Detector for Multi-slice CT with 0.5 mm. Slice thickness and 0.5 second revolution. Proc SPIE 4682:14

Rybicki FJ, Otero HJ, Steigner ML et al (2008) Initial evaluation of coronary images from 320-detector row computed tomography. Int J Cardiovasc Imaging 24:535–546

Seeram E (2001) Computed tomography: physical principles, clinical applications, and quality control. 2nd edn. Saunders, Philadelphia

Szulc M, Judy PF (1979) Effect of X-ray filtration on dose and image performance of CT scanners. Med Phys 6: 479–486

Tzedakis A, Damilakis J, Perisinakis K et al (2005) The effect of z overscanning on patient effective dose from multidetector helical computed tomography examinations. Med Phys 32:1621–1629

van der Molen AJ, Geleijns J (2007) Overranging in multisection CT: quantification and relative contribution to dose–comparison of four 16-section CT scanners. Radiology 242:208–216

# Application of Shielding in CT Radiation Dose Reduction

Shima Aran, Sarabjeet Singh, and Mannudeep K. Kalra

## Contents



**Abstract**

In-plane shields have been shown to reduce CT radiation dose to some of the most radiosensitive organs. However, potential for artifacts and changes in attenuation numbers make their universal use controversial for radiation protection purposes. In this chapter, we discuss advantages and disadvantages of use of in-plane shielding for reducing radiation dose associated with CT scanning.

Introduction of CT scanning in the early 1970s marked a revolution in non-invasive imaging of the human body. Since then, CT has been applied extensively in urgent and life threatening situations, routine rule out indications as well as for guiding diagnostic and therapeutic procedures. There is little doubt that CT provides important information for detection, diagnosis and staging of several clinical maladies. As a result, there has been a phenomenal increase in use of CT scanning with over 62 million CT examinations performed in the United States alone each year (Brenner and Hall 2007). On one hand this number documents widespread availability of a useful technology for medical benefits, on the other hand these numbers also magnify the associated radiation doses with CT scanning especially when the scanned subject is young or a child or when the expected benefits do not sufficiently outweigh potential long-term risks of associated radiation dose (Mukundan et al. 2007).

Appropriateness or justification of clinical indications for CT scanning should therefore be the primary strategy for CT radiation dose reduction. Thereafter special care should be taken when imaging children or young adults with CT in order to maintain a radiation

S. Aran · S. Singh · M. K. Kalra (✉)
Department of Radiology, Harvard Medical School, Massachusetts General Hospital, Boston, MA, USA
e-mail: mkalra@partners.org

D. Tack et al. (eds.), *Radiation Dose from Multidetector CT*, Medical Radiology. Diagnostic Imaging,
DOI: 10.1007/174_2011_450, © Springer-Verlag Berlin Heidelberg 2012

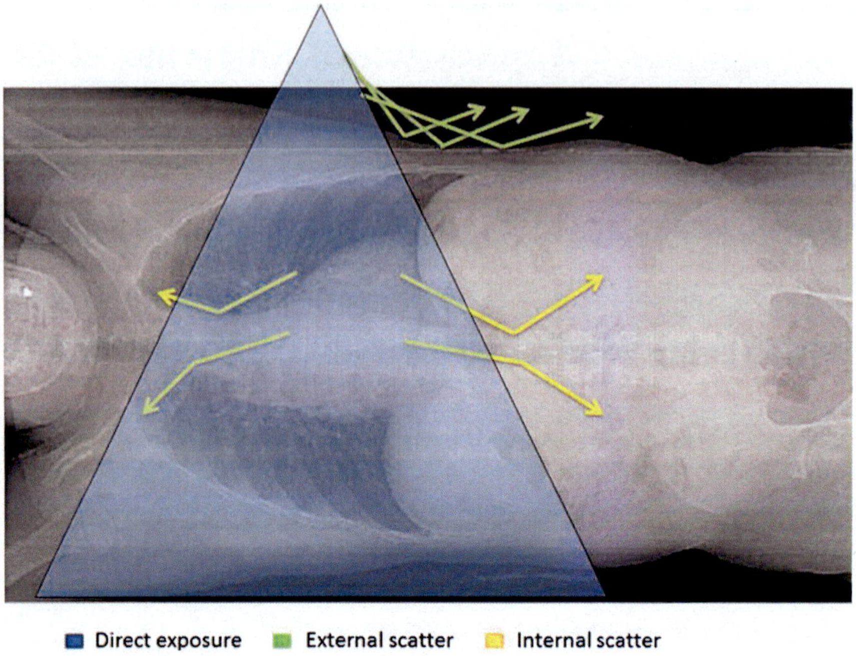


**Fig. 1** Direct and scattered (internal and external) sources of radiation exposure to the organs

dose that is just sufficient to obtain required diagnostic information. Tailoring of radiation dose individual examination or protocol type should always retain at least the basic required diagnostic information from the CT procedure.

Several adjustments to scanning procedures and parameters have been shown to reduce radiation dose associated with CT scanning while retaining the diagnostic information but none precedes use of barrier or shields in radiation-based medical imaging. In conventional radiography, lead shields have been in use for several years to protect both patients and radiographers from scattered radiation dose. Tight X-ray beam collimation in CT scanning is also associated with some scattered radiation exposure, which may originate from interaction of the X-ray photons with air or body surface (external scattered radiation) or from deflection of X-ray photon when it is traversing within the body (internal scattered radiation) (Fig. 1). In this chapter, we discuss the application of radioprotective shields for protecting patients undergoing CT scanning.

## 1 Radiation Sensitivity

As stated above, infants and young children are at several fold higher risk of radiation-induced carcinogenesis as compared to adults (Fricke et al. 2003). Within the human body, certain organs or tissues are more radio-sensitive as compared to the others. The most radiosensitive organs such as the eye, lung, breast, thyroid gland and testes have highest cell multiplication or metabolic rate, or represent undifferentiated or well-nourished cell types (Rubin 1968). These tissues are more sensitive to radiation exposure with significantly smaller threshold values compared to other organs. The risk is greater in children and young adults compared to older individuals.

For example, the pediatric thyroid gland is one of the most radiosensitive organs with an excess relative risk per Gray (Gy) of 7.7 and an excess absolute risk of 4.4 per 10,000 person-years per Gy when radiation exposure occurs before age of 15 years (Schonfeld et al. 2011). The adult exposure is associated with a small increased risk of thyroid cancer. Prior studies have correlated increase of breast cancer to radiation doses of less than 0.1 Gy (Yi et al. 2010). Paradoxically, lungs are the most radiosensitive organs in the thorax with a greater weighting factor (than breasts) in the most recent recommendations from the International Commission on Radiological Protection (ICRP 2007; Dauer et al. 2007). For eye lens, the threshold for cataract induction in adults is 0.5–2 Gy (Mukundan et al. 2007). Children are more susceptible to cataract induction at less than half of this dose of radiation. While these radiation dose levels far

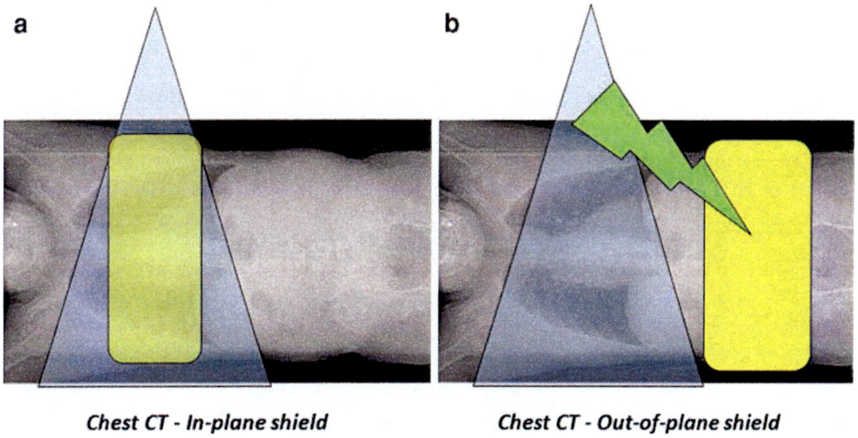


**Fig. 2** In-plane (**a**) and conventional out-of-plane (**b**) shields: For chest CT, a breast shield will serve as in-plane shield, where as a lead shield over the abdomen will protect from external scattered radiation

exceed radiation dose associated with most CT procedures, it is important to remember that increased risk of cancer with radiation is a stochastic risk and that radiation from multiple CT exams can accumulate to reach or exceed some of these "threshold" levels. Application of a shielding device for reducing radiation exposure to some of the radiosensitive organs is feasible and convenient due to their superficial anatomic location (thyroid, breasts and testes).

The developing fetus is very sensitive to radiation due to the proliferating nature of the cells and the process of differentiation. The risk of different radiation side effects vary with gestational age. Generally, CT radiation doses would not meet the thresholds required to induce congenital defects or mental retardation. Thus, the most significant effect of antenatal radiation exposure is increased risk of childhood cancer, especially leukemia (Chatterson 2011). Compared to other fetal effects of radiation, the risk for carcinogenesis does not appear to change with the gestational age (ICRP 2003; National Radiological Protection Board RCoR 1998). Protection of the fetus with appropriate scanning practices is thus important.

## 2 Classification of the Shields

Traditionally, shields have been used in conventional radiography and CT scanning for protection from external scattered radiation. These shields may be classified as the in-plane and the conventional shields. The purpose of the in-plane shielding is to reduce the radiation exposure to the underlying tissue within the scan field by partially blocking the X-ray beam, while allowing enough beam to generate a diagnostic CT image. With conventional or out-of-plane shielding, particular areas outside the scan field are completely protected from external scattered radiation (Fig. 2).

The conventional shields may be external (generally made of lead such as lead apron) or internal (barium sulfate) shields. The conventional or out-of-plane shielding is mostly performed for the thyroid (Beaconsfield et al. 1998) and breast (Beaconsfield et al. 1998; Brnic et al. 2003) during head CT scanning and for the testes (Romanowski et al. 1994; Price 1999; Hohl et al. 2005) for abdominal CT and fetus (Chatterson et al. 2011; Iball et al. 2008; Kennedy et al. 2007) for chest CT examinations, where a relevant dose reduction to the organ can be achieved (Fricke et al. 2003; Hohl et al. 2006).

Due to tight collimation of X-ray beams in modern CT scanners, most scattered radiation dose with CT is from internal scattering of X-rays when they are traversing through the body. While keeping surface covering lead shields may protect against minor external scattered radiation dose to fetus from chest CT of the pregnant mother, external shielding will do little to protect against internal scattering. Thus, some investigators have cleverly employed oral barium sulfate as an internal shield to protect the fetus (Yousefzadeh et al. 2006) from internal scattered radiation from a chest CT examination of the pregnant mother. By using this technique, scattered radiation dose was decreased by 13 and 21% with 2% barium sulfate and 87 and 96% with 40% barium sulfate, as calculated in the near (representing the uterine dome at near term) and far (representing the uterine position

**Table 1** Tabulated summary of major studies on radiation protection with use of shields during CT scanning

| Author (year) | Organs assessed | Patient/ phantom | Shield material | Organ dose reduction | Conclusion |
|---|---|---|---|---|---|
| Chatterson et al. (2011) | Fetus (1st–3rd trimester uterus) | Phantom | Lead and bismuth-antimony | 53–73% (Lead) | Reducing voltage and limiting z-axis is more effective than shields |
| | | | | 45–72% (Bismuth) | No significant difference between lead and bismuth-antimony |
| Lee et al. (2011) | Thyroid | Adult phantom | Bismuth | 3–27% | Thyroid shield significantly reduced superficial radiation dose to the neck |
| | | | | | No remarkablenoise increase with increase in CT attenuation |
| Chang et al.(2010) | Eye lens, thyroid, breasts | Phantom | Bismuth | 1–55% | No significant difference between bismuth and lead |
| | | | | | No influence on image quality if distance between shield and organ >1 cm |
| Raissaki et al. (2010) | Eye lens and thyroid | Patient and phantom | Bismuth | 29–32% | Shield artifacts are superficial and diagnostically insignificant in Head CT |
| | | | | | Shields should be placed 1 cm above the eyes |
| | | | | | Shield wrinkling should be avoided |
| Catuzzo et al. (2010) | Thyroid, eye lens and breasts | Patient and phantom | Bismuth | 30–60% | Effectively reduces dose to pediatric patients |
| | | | | | No significant influence on image quality |
| Lee et al. (2010) | Thyroid, eye lens and breasts | Adult phantom | Bismuth | 20% (eyes) and 12% (thyroid) and 22% (breast) | Combined use of ATCM and in-plane shielding reduced the CT dose more than the use of one technique |
| Kalra et al. (2009) | Breasts | Phantom | Bismuth | 37–41% | Shields reduce radiation dose regardless of off-centering |
| | | | | | ATCM did not increase radiation dose when using a shield |
| Takada et al. (2009) | Breasts | | Bismuth, zinc, copper, iron | 6% bismuth | Other materials are more effective than bismuth in dose reduction |
| | | | | 12–13% for Cu, Fe | |
| | | | | 13% zinc | |
| Leswick et al. (2008) | Thyroid and breasts | Phantom | Bismuth | 42% (shield) | Z-axis ATCM is more effective than shields at reducing thyroid radiation ATCM and shield combination slightly further reduces the dose |
| | | | | 83–85% (Shield + ATCM) | |
| Coursey et al. (2008) | Breasts | Pediatric phantom | Bismuth | 26% (Shield), 52% (shield + ATCM) | Bismuth breast shield + z-axis ATCM further reduces radiation dose Greatest reduction when shield is placed after the localizer radiograph |
| Ngaile et al. (2008) | Eye lens and thyroid | Patient and Phantom | Lead | 44% eye | Not significantly compromising image quality |
| | | | | 51% thyroid | |

(continued)

**Table 1** (continued)

| Author (year) | Organs assessed | Patient/ phantom | Shield material | Organ dose reduction | Conclusion |
|---|---|---|---|---|---|
| Iball et al. (2008) | Fetus | Phantom | Lead | Reduced radiation, decreases to 1/4 by 0.35 mm lead | Specifically designed lead shield could reduce fetal dose more efficiently, while reducing patient discomfort as well |
| Doshi et al. (2008) | Fetus (1st–3rd trimester uterus) | Phantom | Lead | 35% | Substantial dose reduction with use of lead shield<br>Important to restrict scan volume<br>Localizer radiograph should be stopped before direct irradiation of fetus |
| Keil et al. (2008) | Eye lens | Phantom | Bismuth versus Bi, Sb, Gd, W alloy | 38% Bismuth<br>48% new alloy | The new protector material shows a significantly higher dose reduction in contrast to bismuth shield |
| Parker et al. (2008) | Breasts | Adult phantom | Tungsten | 56–61% | An externally applied shield can reduce exposure<br>Image quality not evaluated |
| Vollmar and Kalender (2008) | Breasts | Phantom | Bismuth | 50% | Bismuth shield significantly reduced radiation exposure |
| Mukundan et al. (2007) | Eye lens | Pediatric phantom | Bismuth | 42% | Artifacts from shield occur outside diagnostic area of interest |
| Kennedy et al. (2007) | Fetus | Phantom | Lead | 55% | Artifacts not evaluated for shield<br>Reducing the kVp or mAs with shields increases the noise |
| Dauer et al. (2007) | Testes | Adult phantom | Lead (1 mm wrap-around) | 58% (scatter exposure) and 97% (direct exposure) | Lead shields are not recommended for in-plane shielding due to severe artifacts and the difficulties in positioning the shields |
| Yilmaz et al. (2007a, b) | Breasts | Adult patient and phantom | Bismuth | 40% (patient) and 17% (phantom) | No qualitative changes in image quality |
| Yilmaz et al. (2007a, b) | Breasts | Patient | Bismuth coated latex | 37% | Routine use of breast shields in female patients undergoing calcium scoring with MDCT is recommended |
| Geleijns et al. (2006) | Eye lens, brain, thyroid, breasts, and lungs | Phantom | Bismuth | 27% lens, 1% brain, 26% thyroid, 30% breast, 15% lungs | The application of in-plane selective shielding is discouraged.<br>More effective dose reduction with mA reduction |
| Heaney and Norvill (2006) | Thyroid, eye lens and breast | Phantom | Bismuth | 48% eye, 47–55% thyroid, 23% breast | Angling the gantry to avoid orbits is more effective in reducing dose to eyes<br>Thyroid shields for all neck CT work<br>Breast shields for all pediatric patients and all females are recommended |

(continued)

**Table 1** (continued)

| Author (year) | Organs assessed | Patient/ phantom | Shield material | Organ dose reduction | Conclusion |
|---|---|---|---|---|---|
| Yousefzadeh et al. (2006) | Fetus | Adult phantom | Barium sulfate internal shield ± Lead | 13–21 (2% barium sulfate) and 87–96% (40% barium sulfate) and 99% (Lead) | 30–40% barium sulfate shield attenuates scattered photons as effectively as a 1-mm lead shield |
| Neeman et al. (2006) | Thyroid, eye lens, breasts, ovaries, and testes | Adult and pediatric phantoms | Tungsten-antimony (light weight polymer sheet) | 87–92% (to patient) and 85–93% (to operator) | The use of double-layer lead-free gloves resulted in a maximum radiation dose reduction of 97% |
| Parker et al. (2006) | Breasts | Adult phantom | Bismuth and tungsten-antimony | 37–56% (bismuth) and 43–73% (tungsten-antimony) | Shield significantly reduces the exposure<br>Image quality not evaluated |
| Hohl et al. (2006) | Thyroid and breasts | Phantom | Bismuth | 47% thyroid and 32% breast | No qualitative changes in image quality |
| Perisinakis et al. (2005) | Orbits | Pediatric patient and phantom | Bismuth | 38% orbits, 33% whole head, 34% entire eye, 20% partial eye | Shield significantly reduces dose when there is direct exposure to eyes<br>Despite low mA, shields had no effects on diagnostic confidence |
| Hohl et al. (2005) | Testes | Patient | Lead | 87% scatter exposure | Not significantly compromising image quality |
| Colombo et al. (2004) | Breasts and eye lens | Patient and phantom | Bismuth | 34% (breast) and 50% (eye lens) | Does not excessively affect image quality |
| Fujibuchi et al. (2004) | Head and chest (to skin surface and uterus) | Phantom | Protective seat | 50% to chest, uterus (small difference) | Effective radiation differs between institutions.<br>Institutions should determine best protocol optimization for each individual |
| McLaughlin and Moorey (2004) | Eye and thyroid | Patient | Bismuth | 18% eye, 57% thyroid | Thyroid shield is recommended<br>Eye shields do not produce as marked a reduction in radiation dose |
| Fricke et al. (2003) | Breasts | Pediatric patient and neonatal phantom | Bismuth | 29% | No qualitative or quantitative changes in image quality |
| Brnić et al. (2003) | Breasts | Patients | 0.35 mm lead apron | 57% (6–82%) scattered radiation | The higher the patient BMI, the higher the percentage of internal scatter in total breast dose |
| Hein et al. (2002) | Eye lens | Patient and phantom | Bismuth | 40% | No significant artifacts |
| Hopper (2002) | Thyroid, eye lens and breast | Patient and phantom | 1T, 2T, 3T Bismuth coated latex | 48.5–65.4% (orbit) and 67.3–74.2% (thyroid) and 52.4% (breast) | No significant artifacts |

(continued)

**Table 1** (continued)

| Author (year) | Organs assessed | Patient/ phantom | Shield material | Organ dose reduction | Conclusion |
|---|---|---|---|---|---|
| Hopper et al. (2001) | Eyes | Patient and phantom | 1T, 2T, 3T Bismuth coated latex | 48.5–65.4% (1T–3T shields) 40% patient, 49% phantom | No significant artifacts |
| Price et al. (1999) | Testes | Phantom | Lead (1 mm rubber wrap-around) | 77–93% (scattered radiation) and 93%(direct radiation) | Considerable image degradation from streak artifact from in-plane lead shield |
| Beaconsfield et al. (1998) | Thyroid and breasts | Patient | Lead | 45% (thyroid) and 76% (breast) | Image quality not evaluated |
| Hopper et al. (1997) | Thyroid, eye lens, breasts and testis | Patient and phantom | Bismuth | 57% breast, 60% thyroid, 40% eye, 51% testes | No significant artifact |
| Hidajat et al. (1996) | Uterus, ovaries, testes and thyroid | Phantom | Lead | Testes (95%) thyroid (23%) | For abdominal CT, testis capsule reduces testes dose |
| | | | | | Lead apron does not reduce exposure to uterus and ovaries |
| | | | | | For head CT, thyroid collar reduces the scattered exposure to the thyroid |
| Romanowski et al. (1994) | Testes | Phantom | Lead | 85.70% (testes) | Shield significantly reduces the scattered exposure |

during early gestation) fields. Authors reported that a 30–40% barium sulfate in the stomach attenuates scattered photons as effectively as a 1-mm lead shield. Thus, administering a small amount of oral 30–40% barium sulfate to a pregnant woman prior to chest CT can substantially reduce radiation dose to the conceptus regardless of the gestational age. The range of dose reduction using conventional shielding is variable according to the previous studies, ranging from 6 to 99% for lead shields (Brnic et al. 2003; Hohl et al. 2005; Kennedy et al. 2007; Yousefzadeh et al. 2006; Doshi et al. 2008).

The in-plane shields are mostly made of bismuth, tungsten-antimony or lead. The bismuth and lead shields have shown similar performance as shielding materials (Chang et al. 2010). Other metallic shields with lower atomic numbers such as zinc, copper and iron have been also assessed for dose reduction. Common examples of in-plane shields include eye shield for head CT to protect the eye lenses (Hopper et al. 1997, 2001; Hein et al. 2002; Hopper 2002; McLaughlin and Mooney 2004; Perisinakis et al. 2005), breast shield for chest CT (Fricke et al. 2003; Hopper et al. 1997; Hopper 2002), thyroid shield for neck, cervical spine (Hopper et al. 1997) and chest CT (Hopper 2002; McLaughlin and Mooney 2004) and testes shield for abdominopelvic CT (Dauer et al. 2007; Price et al. 1999; Kalra et al. 2009). The amount of dose reduction with use of in-plane shields depends on several factors such as scanning parameters and techniques, as well as the material used for shielding. Dose reduction ranges with in-plane shields have been reported to be 1–74.2% for bismuth, 43–92.3% for tungsten-antimony, 44–97% for lead and 12–13.3% for other shielding materials (Table 1).

## 3 Shield Thickness and Layers

Hopper et al. have evaluated shields with different ply thickness of bismuth (1-, 2-, 3- and 4-ply in thickness; 1 ply thickness of bismuth is equivalent to 0.85 g of bismuth per square centimeter) (Hopper et al. 1997). In general, greater the ply thickness, greater is the dose reduction with up to 56% dose reduction with 4-ply bismuth shield. However, greater ply thickness will also have greater beam attenuation and effect on image quality although further studies did not report any significant artifacts associated with eye shields regardless of ply thickness (Hopper et al. 2001).

**Table 2** Tabulated summary of studies documenting adverse effect of in-plane bismuth shields on CT image quality

| Author (year) | Shielded organs | Phantoms assessed | Image quality |
|---|---|---|---|
| Chatterson et al. (2011) | Fetus (1st–3rd trimester uterus) | Female phantom | Substantial artifacts in images below the diaphragm |
| Lee et al. (2010) | Eyes, thyroid and breasts | Adult male and female phantoms | Degraded image quality when shield is in contact with the phantom. Increased image noise and CT numbers at the phantom surface |
| Kalra et al. (2009) | Breast | Chest phantom | Increased image noise, attenuation values and streak artifacts |
| Leswick et al. (2008) | Thyroid and breasts | Phantom | Increased image noise when shields combined with longitudinal automatic exposure control |
| Coursey et al. (2008) | Breasts | Pediatric phantom ("5 year old") | Increased image noise |
| Vollmar and Kalender (2008) | Breasts | Phantom | 40% increase in image noise<br>Artifacts impaired image quality |
| Geleijns et al. (2006) | Eye lens, brain, thyroid, breasts, and lungs | Phantom | Dominant increase in noise with breast and thyroid shield |
| Heaney and Norvill (2006) | Eye lens, thyroid and breasts | Phantom | Local artifact with eye shield |

Greater ply thickness can be useful for patients undergoing multiple CT examinations and children (Hopper 2002).

Fricke et al. have reported use of a 2-ply bismuth shield in order to maintain the image quality (Fricke et al. 2003). They achieved 29% radiation dose reduction with their 2-ply (1.7 g of bismuth per square centimeter) shield which was in line with the 28% reduction seen with 2-ply shields used by Hopper et al. To avoid image artifacts, Fricke et al. recommended the use of the 2-ply rather than the 4-ply bismuth shields (Fricke et al. 2003).

As stated above, out-of-plane lead shields are often used to protect conceptus from external scattered radiation dose when pregnant mother is undergoing a non-abdominal CT examination (such as chest, head or neck CT). Although greater ply thickness of lead shields will decrease the external scattered radiation dose, amounts greater than 0.7 mm thickness is not recommended due to concerns over increased patient discomfort with little benefits in terms of significantly higher dose reduction. Unlike conventional radiographs, for CT, the lead shields must be positioned around the patients and should cover up to the caudal edge of the scan volume (Kennedy et al. 2007).

## 4 Effect of Shields on CT Image Quality

Several studies have reported effect of in-plane shields on image quality with CT. There is little doubt that in-plane shielding reduces radiation doses to some radiosensitive organs but they also alter CT numbers (HU values), compromise the image quality as well as result in streak and beam hardening artifacts (Mukundan et al. 2007; Dauer et al. 2007; Chatterson et al. 2011; Price et al. 1999; Kalra et al. 2009; Lee et al. 2010; Geleijns et al. 2010; Leswick et al. 2008; Coursey et al. 2008; Vollmar and Kalender 2008; Geleijns et al. 2006; Heaney and Norvill 2006) (Table 2). Unfortunately, many prior investigations of these shields have not evaluated image quality effects but merely restricted themselves to documentation of dose reduction potential (Beaconsfield et al. 1998; Brnic et al. 2003; Romanowski et al. 1994; Iball et al. 2008; Yousefzadeh et al. 2006; Doshi et al. 2008; McLaughlin and Mooney 2004; Kojima et al. 2011; Takada et al. 2009; Keil et al. 2008; Parker et al. 2008; Yilmaz et al. 2007a; Parker et al. 2006; Neeman et al. 2006; Hidajat

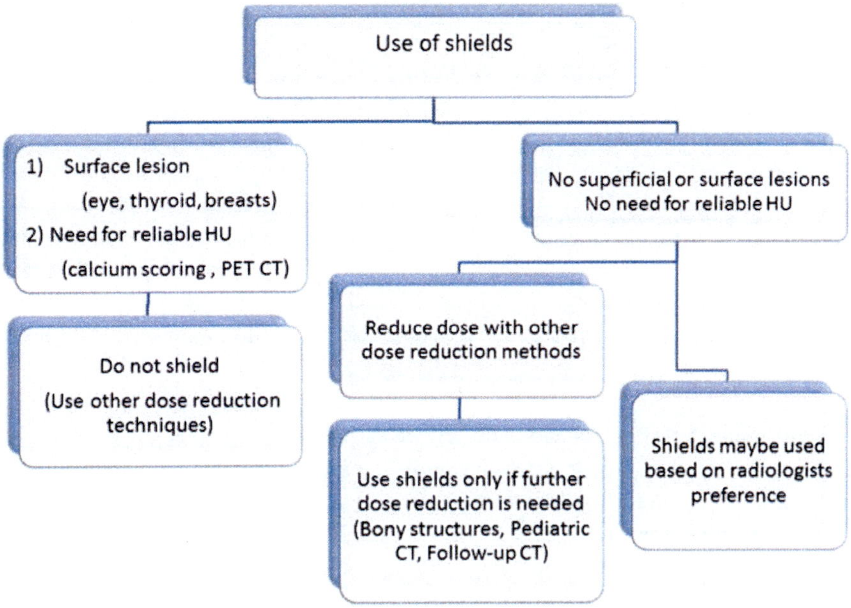


**Fig. 3** Decision tree that may be used for determining role of in-plane shielding based on region of interest and radiologists' comfort and acceptability of effects of in-plane shielding to reduce radiation dose

et al. 1996). On the other end of the spectrum which claims no deterioration in the image quality with use of in-plane shielding (Fricke et al. 2003; Hopper et al. 1997, 2001; Hohl et al. 2005, 2006; Kennedy et al. 2007; Chang et al. 2010; Hein et al. 2002; Hopper 2002; Perisinakis et al. 2005; Dobbs et al. 2011; Lee et al. 2011; Raissaki et al. 2010; Catuzzo et al. 2010; Kim et al. 2010; Ngaile et al. 2008; Yilmaz et al. 2007b; Colombo et al. 2004; Fujibuchi et al. 2004). It is generally stated that the in-plane shields should not be placed on the body surface to avoid inadvertent increase in CT numbers at the surface and streak artifacts from the shields. At least 1 cm gap between the shield and the body surface should be maintained to avoid negative effect on image quality (Chang et al. 2010; Raissaki et al. 2010).

## 5 Distance Between the Shield and Skin

The increase in image noise and streak artifacts with use of in-plane shields can be limited by applying a spacer or gap between the shield and patient surface or skin. Direct contact should be avoided in all situations because the maximum increase in CT number and image noise is noted when there is direct contact between shield and patient surface. This also implies that in-plane shields should not be used when CT is being performed for evaluation of the areas in the vicinity of the surface over which the shields are to be placed. Such conditions may include abnormalities of breast, subcutaneous tissues, thyroid gland and testes. In such cases, other methods of radiation dose reduction should be employed or the distance between the shield and the surface must be increased (Hohl et al. 2006; Chang et al. 2010; Kalra et al. 2009).

## 6 Cost-Benefit Analysis for Shields

The cost of the shields is another factor that can truly impact the feasibility of using this radioprotective device. Bismuth shields are costly especially, the eye, breast and thyroid shields that are labeled as single-use by the manufacturer in order to reduce the rate of infection. According to one website, costs for one adult bismuth breast, thyroid and eye shield in United States dollars are $100, $12.50 and $6.25, respectively (http://www.barrieronline.com/radiation/ct-shields.php). This cost makes it prohibitive to most healthcare practices to use these shields as disposable items (Heaney and Norvill 2006; Dobbs et al. 2011). In fact, most users, we have spoken with, employ these shields as reusable items on multiple patients. They take precautions to avoid contact of the shield with patient surface with use of a spacer.

Some patients find use of eye shield uncomfortable or unacceptable, which may increase the possibility of patient movement during the CT scanning. In its extreme scale, the discomfort and anxiety with the eye shields, especially in pediatric patients, may necessitate need for general anesthesia.

## 7 Alternative Methods to the Use of Shields

Several scanner techniques can help reduce radiation dose associated with CT scanning. For example, automatic tube current modulation (ATCM) or automatic exposure control (AEC) (Kalra et al. 2009, 2004; Lee et al. 2010; Leswick et al. 2008; Coursey et al. 2008), organ-sensitive dose protection (X-CARE) (Vollmar and Kalender 2008), adaptive dose shields and reduction of tube current time product (mAs) and peak-voltage (kVp) (Kennedy et al. 2007) as well as changing the gantry angle (Heaney and Norvill 2006; Keil et al. 2008).

The ATCM has been increasingly applied as a tool to decrease radiation dose and is considered by some investigators to be superior to in-plane shielding in adults (Geleijns et al. 2010). However, the achieved dose reduction by this technique may be lower in children and neonates (Coursey et al. 2008). This technique has been shown to reduce radiation dose to breast by approximately 50% without any significant effect on image quality or altering the accuracy of CT numbers (Geleijns et al. 2010).

Combined use of ATCM and shielding device can result in additional radiation dose reduction. When using in-plane shields with ATCM, it is important to place the shield after acquisition of the planning or localizer radiographs which will maximize dose benefits from both shielding and automatic exposure control technique. However, use of in-plane shield with ATCM can also result in additional increase in image noise in comparison to use of constant tube current (Leswick et al. 2008; Coursey et al. 2008). Thus, simultaneous use of shield with ATCM may be limited to clinical situations where a low CT dose is unlikely to compromise desired diagnostic information. Additionally, the in-plane shield should be placed at least 1 cm apart from the patient when applying AEC technique (Kalra et al. 2009; Lee et al. 2010).

The organ-sensitive dose protection or X-CARE (Siemens Healthcare) is a partial angle scan technology which selectively reduces the radiation exposure of the radiosensitive organs. In this technique the tube current is reduced or switched off during the rotation phase in which the anatomical region of interest is most directly exposed to radiation. In this way, it is possible to reduce the radiation exposure of individual anatomical regions by up to 40% while maintaining image quality and homogeneous distribution of noise (Vollmar and Kalender 2008; Kim et al. 2010). Unfortunately use of this technique for reducing breast dose with chest CT results in slight increase in lung dose, which is also a radiosensitive organ. However, this technique can still be safely used for CT imaging of other organs such as thyroid. In this case, there will be slight increase in radiation to the spinal cord and neural branches; however, the nervous system is considered the least radiosensitive tissue (Rubin 1968).

To decrease radiation dose from scan over-ranging which results from X-ray beam falling beyond the detector rows at the start and end of the scanning location, some vendors have introduced adaptive dose shields. These adaptive shields block the X-rays that fall either beyond the start location or after the end location of the prescribed scan range (Kojima et al. 2011). The dose reduction with the use of these shielding mechanisms depends on gantry rotation speed, scan length and pitch factor with higher dose reduction at slower gantry rotation and smaller pitch factor. This technique results in greater dose saving for short scan ranges (such as coronary CT angiography) as compared to long scan ranges (such as CT angiography of the entire chest).

## 8 Conclusion

In conclusion, in-plane shields can reduce CT radiation dose to some of the most radiosensitive organs of the body. However, artifacts and increase in image noise can be concerning to some radiologists, who can also achieve similar dose reduction with other methods that have less impact on the image quality. In our practice, we do not use the in-plane shields during CT scanning. In order to assess the feasibility of shielding in radiation protection, both beneficial and harmful effects of shielding as well as availability of other dose reduction methods should be assessed to determine if shields should be used for additional radiation dose reduction (Fig. 3).

## References


Beaconsfield T, Nicholson R, Thornton A, Al-Kutoubi A (1998) Would thyroid and breast shielding be beneficial in CT of the head? Eur Radiol 8(4):664–667

Brenner DJ, Hall EJ (2007) Computed tomography—an increasing source of radiation exposure. N Engl J Med 357(22):2277–2284

Brnic Z et al (2003) Efficacy of breast shielding during CT of the head. Eur Radiol 13(11):2436–2440

Catuzzo P et al (2010) Dose reduction in multislice CT by means of bismuth shields: results of in vivo measurements and computed evaluation. Radiol Med 115(1):152–169

Chang KH et al (2010) Dose reduction in CT using bismuth shielding: measurements and Monte Carlo simulations. Radiat Prot Dosimetry 138(4):382–388

Chatterson LC, Leswick DA, Fladeland DA, Hunt MM, Webster ST (2011) Lead versus bismuth-antimony shield for fetal dose reduction at different gestational ages at CT pulmonary angiography. Radiology 260(2):560–579 (Epub ahead of print)

Cohnen M et al (2003) Effective doses in standard protocols for multi-slice CT scanning. Eur Radiol 13(5):1148–1153

Colombo P et al (2004) Evaluation of the efficacy of a bismuth shield during CT examinations. Radiol Med 108(5–6): 560–568

Coursey C et al (2008) Pediatric chest MDCT using tube current modulation: effect on radiation dose with breast shielding. AJR Am J Roentgenol 190(1):W54–W61

Dauer LT et al (2007) Radiation dose reduction at a price: the effectiveness of a male gonadal shield during helical CT scans. BMC Med Imaging 7:5

Dobbs M, Ahmed R, Patrick LE (2011) Bismuth breast and thyroid shield implementation for pediatric CT. Radiol Manage 33(1):18–22 quiz 23–4

Doshi SK, Negus IS, Oduko JM (2008) Fetal radiation dose from CT pulmonary angiography in late pregnancy: a phantom study. Br J Radiol 81(968):653–658

Fricke BL DL, Frush DP, Yoshizumi T, Varchena V, Poe SA, Lucaya J (2003) In-plane bismuth breast shields for pediatric CT: effects on radiation dose and image quality using experimental and clinical data. Am J Roentgenol 180(2):407–411

Fujibuchi T et al (2004) Shielding effect of protective seats during CT examination. Nippon Hoshasen Gijutsu Gakkai Zasshi 60(12):1730–1738

Geleijns J et al (2006) Quantitative assessment of selective in-plane shielding of tissues in computed tomography through evaluation of absorbed dose and image quality. Eur Radiol 16(10):2334–2340

Geleijns J, Wang J, McCollough C (2010) The use of breast shielding for dose reduction in pediatric CT: arguments against the proposition. Pediatr Radiol 40(11):1744–1747

Heaney DE, Norvill CA (2006) A comparison of reduction in CT dose through the use of gantry angulations or bismuth shields. Australas Phys Eng Sci Med 29(2):172–178

Hein E et al (2002) Low-dose CT of the paranasal sinuses with eye lens protection: effect on image quality and radiation dose. Eur Radiol 12(7):1693–1696

Hidajat N et al (1996) The efficacy of lead shielding in patient dosage reduction in computed tomography. Rofo 165(5):462–465

Hohl C et al (2005) Radiation dose reduction to the male gonads during MDCT: the effectiveness of a lead shield. AJR Am J Roentgenol 184(1):128–130

Hohl C et al (2006) Radiation dose reduction to breast and thyroid during MDCT: effectiveness of an in-plane bismuth shield. Acta Radiol 47(6):562–567

Hopper KD (2002) Orbital, thyroid, and breast superficial radiation shielding for patients undergoing diagnostic CT. Semin Ultrasound CT MR 23(5):423–427

Hopper KD, King SH, Lobell ME, TenHave TR, Weaver JS (1997) The breast: in-plane X-ray protection during diagnostic thoracic CT—shielding with bismuth radioprotective garments. Radiology 205(3):853–858

Hopper KD et al (2001) Radioprotection to the eye during CT scanning. AJNR Am J Neuroradiol 22(6):1194–1198

Hurwitz LM, Yoshizumi T,, Reiman RE, Goodman PC, Paulson EK, Frush DP, Toncheva G, Nguyen G, Barnes L (2006) Radiation dose to the fetus from body MDCT during early gestation. AJR Am J Roentgenol 186(3):871–876

Hurwitz LM et al (2006b) Radiation dose to the female breast from 16-MDCT body protocols. AJR Am J Roentgenol 186(6):1718–1722

Iball GR, Kennedy EV, Brettle DS (2008) Modelling the effect of lead and other materials for shielding of the fetus in CT pulmonary angiography. Br J Radiol 81(966):499–503

ICRP (2003) ICRP publication 90: biological effects after prenatal irradiation. ICRP, Oxford, UK

Kalra MK et al (2004) Strategies for CT radiation dose optimization. Radiology 230(3):619–628

Kalra MK et al (2009) In-plane shielding for CT: effect of off-centering, automatic exposure control and shield-to-surface distance. Korean J Radiol 10(2):156–163

Keil B et al (2008) Protection of eye lens in computed tomography—dose evaluation on an anthropomorphic phantom using thermo-luminescent dosimeters and Monte-Carlo simulations. Rofo 180(12):1047–1053

Kennedy EV, Iball GR, Brettle DS (2007) Investigation into the effects of lead shielding for fetal dose reduction in CT pulmonary angiography. Br J Radiol 80(956):631–638

Kim S, Frush DP, Yoshizumi TT (2010) Bismuth shielding in CT: support for use in children. Pediatr Radiol 40(11): 1739–1743

Kojima H, Tsujimura A, Yabe H (2011) Usefulness of the adaptive dose shield for the infant CT. Nippon Hoshasen Gijutsu Gakkai Zasshi 67(1):57–61

Lee K et al (2010) Dose reduction and image quality assessment in MDCT using AEC (D-DOM & Z-DOM)

and in-plane bismuth shielding. Radiat Prot Dosimetry 141(2):162–167

Lee YH, Park ET, Cho PK, Seo HS, Je BK, Suh SI, Yang KS (2011) Comparative analysis of radiation dose and image quality between thyroid shielding and unshielding during CT examination of the neck. AJR Am J Roentgenol 196(3):611–615

Leswick DA et al (2008) Thyroid shields versus z-axis automatic tube current modulation for dose reduction at neck CT. Radiology 249(2):572–580

Mayo JR, Aldrich J, Muller NL (2003) Radiation exposure at chest CT: a statement of the Fleischner Society. Radiology 228(1):15–21

McLaughlin DJ, Mooney RB (2004) Dose reduction to radiosensitive tissues in CT. Do commercially available shields meet the users' needs? Clin Radiol 59(5):446–450

Mukundan S Jr et al (2007) MOSFET dosimetry for radiation dose assessment of bismuth shielding of the eye in children. Am J Roentgenol 188(6):1648–1650

National Radiological Protection Board RCoR (1998) Diagnostic medical exposures: advice on exposure to ionising radiation during pregnancy. NRPB, Didcot, UK

Neeman Z et al (2006) CT fluoroscopy shielding: decreases in scattered radiation for the patient and operator. J Vasc Interv Radiol 17(12):1999–2004

Ngaile JE et al (2008) Use of lead shields for radiation protection of superficial organs in patients undergoing head CT examinations. Radiat Prot Dosimetry 130(4):490–498

Parker MS, Chung JK, Fatouros PP, Hoots JA, Kelleher NM, Benedict SH (2006) Reduction of radiation dose to the female breast: Preliminary data with a custom-designed tungsten-antimony composite breast shield. Journal of Applied Research 6(3):230–239

Parker MS et al (2008) Absorbed radiation dose of the female breast during diagnostic multidetector chest CT and dose reduction with a tungsten-antimony composite breast shield: preliminary results. Clin Radiol 63(3):278–288

Perisinakis K et al (2005) Reduction of eye lens radiation dose by orbital bismuth shielding in pediatric patients undergoing CT of the head: a Monte Carlo study. Med Phys 32(4):1024–1030

Preston DL et al (2007) Solid cancer incidence in atomic bomb survivors: 1958–1998. Radiat Res 168(1):1–64

Price R, Halson P, Sampson M (1999) Dose reduction during CT scanning in an anthropomorphic phantom by the use of a male gonad shield. Br J Radiol 72(857):489–494

Raissaki M et al (2010) Eye-lens bismuth shielding in paediatric head CT: artefact evaluation and reduction. Pediatr Radiol 40(11):1748–1754

Romanowski CA, Underwood AC, Sprigg A (1994) Reduction of radiation doses in leg lengthening procedures by means of audit and computed tomography scanogram techniques. Br J Radiol 67(803):1103–1107

Rubin P, Casarett GW (1968) Clinical radiation pathology as applied to curative radiotherapy. Cancer 22(4):767–778

Schonfeld SJ, Lee C, Berrington de Gonzalez A (2011) Medical exposure to radiation and thyroid cancer. Clin Oncol (R Coll Radiol) 23(4):244–250

Takada K, Kaneko J, Aoki K (2009) Breast dose reduction in female CT screening for lung cancer using various metallic shields. Nippon Hoshasen Gijutsu Gakkai Zasshi 65(12):1628–1637

The 2007 recommendations of the International Commission on Radiological Protection. ICRP publication 103. Ann ICRP 37(2–4):1–332

Tsujino K et al (2003) Predictive value of dose-volume histogram parameters for predicting radiation pneumonitis after concurrent chemoradiation for lung cancer. Int J Radiat Oncol Biol Phys 55(1):110–115

Vollmar SV, Kalender WA (2008) Reduction of dose to the female breast in thoracic CT: a comparison of standard-protocol, bismuth-shielded, partial and tube-current-modulated CT examinations. Eur Radiol 18(8):1674–1682

Winer-Muram HT et al (2002) Pulmonary embolism in pregnant patients: fetal radiation dose with helical CT. Radiology 224(2):487–492

Yi A et al (2010) Optimal multidetector row CT parameters for evaluations of the breast: a phantom and specimen study. Acad Radiol 17(6):744–751

Yilmaz MH et al (2007a) Coronary calcium scoring with MDCT: the radiation dose to the breast and the effectiveness of bismuth breast shield. Eur J Radiol 61(1):139–143

Yilmaz MH et al (2007b) Female breast radiation exposure during thorax multidetector computed tomography and the effectiveness of bismuth breast shield to reduce breast radiation dose. J Comput Assist Tomogr 31(1): 138–142

Yousefzadeh DK, Ward MB, Reft C (2006) Internal barium shielding to minimize fetal irradiation in spiral chest CT: a phantom simulation experiment. Radiology 239(3):751–758

# Radiation Dose: Records and Audits

Tessa S. Cook, William W. Boonn, and Woojin Kim

## Contents




**Abstract**

As the utilization of computed tomography has grown in the past decade, so has the interest in being able to monitor doses of ionizing radiation received by patients. Until recently, the biggest obstacle to dose monitoring was the image-based dose sheet on which dose-related parameters are stored. While development of a new radiation dose structured report will promote dose monitoring and reporting in the future, a vast repository of legacy data with image-based dose sheets still exists worldwide. In this chapter, we discuss the challenges faced in CT dose monitoring as well as some solutions that have been developed to overcome the limitations of the image-based dose sheet. We also address the steps involved in designing and implementing an institutional dose monitoring program, and participation in regional and national dose registries. Finally, we discuss the recent advances in organ dose estimation using Monte Carlo simulations.


## 1 Introduction

Computed tomography (CT) utilization has increased dramatically in the last 10–15 years (Maitino et al. 2003; Levin et al. 2008). The proportion of *background* radiation in the United States attributed to medical imaging has increased from approximately 15% in 1987 to nearly 50% in 2009 (Sinclair et al. 1987; Kase et al. 2009). Furthermore, exposure to radiation as a result of medical imaging has occupied the spotlight in recent years, receiving attention from


T. S. Cook (✉) · W. W. Boonn · W. Kim
Hospital of the University of Pennsylvania, Philadelphia, PA, USA
e-mail: tessa.cook@uphs.upenn.edu



D. Tack et al. (eds.), *Radiation Dose from Multidetector CT*, Medical Radiology. Diagnostic Imaging,
DOI: 10.1007/174_2011_455,

professional organizations such as the American College of Radiology (ACR) and the American Association of Physicists in Medicine (AAPM), and more notably, from the US House of Representatives Subcommittee on Health (Congressional Subcommittee on Health 1910), as well as the lay press (Bogdanich 2010; Landro and Wall Street Journal 2010). Beginning in July 2012, radiologists in California will be required by statewide legislation to include CT dose parameters in their study interpretations (SB 1237).

A number of scientific articles have debated the potential for deleterious effects as a result of this increased utilization of imaging with ionizing radiation (Brenner and Hall 2007; Brody et al. 2007; Goske et al. 2008; Martin and Semelka 2006). However, the answers to these questions are not easily obtained. What is clear, though, is that increasing awareness of health care professionals—radiologists and non-radiologists alike—regarding imaging-related radiation dose is integral to improving patient care. The ACR's white paper on radiation dose states that "… there should be special attention paid to…education for all stakeholders in the principles of radiation safety, the appropriate utilization of imaging… the standardization of radiation dose data to be archived during imaging for its ultimate use in benchmarking, good practice, and finally, the identification and perhaps alternative imaging of patients who may have already reached threshold levels of estimated exposure…." (Amis et al. 2007). Studies have demonstrated that there is wide variability in estimated effective radiation dose among CT scans, even when performed at the same institution using the same protocols (de Gonzalez et al. 2009; Smith-Bindman et al. 2009). These observations only serve to further emphasize the need for reliable, accurate CT dose monitoring and reporting.

Multiple initiatives are underway to standardize the documentation and reporting of radiation dose information. The Digital Imaging and Communications in Medicine Structured Reporting (DICOM SR) standard contains dose objects dedicated to storing CT radiation dose information (DICOM 2007; DICOM Standards Committee 2008). Using these DICOM SR objects, the Integrating of the Healthcare Enterprise (IHE) initiative has developed a Radiation Exposure Monitoring (REM) profile to assist vendors in the implementation of standardized dose reporting by scanner software (Accessed March 15 2010). The ACR Dose Index Registry (DIR), part of the National Radiology Data Registry (NRDR), is actively collecting dose data from facilities across the nation, in an effort to standardize dose reporting and establish dose reference levels for all CT examinations (Amis et al. 2007; National Radiology Data Registry 2011). The initiative to reduce unnecessary radiation exposure from medical imaging was recently launched by the US Food and Drug Administration (FDA). A specific goal of the FDA's initiative is to "[e]stablish requirements for manufacturers of CT and fluoroscopic devices to record radiation dose information for use in patient's medical records or a radiation dose registry" (White Paper 1999). The NIH is also making efforts to track and report radiation dose for all patients imaged at the Institutes (Neumann and Bluemke 2010). As discussed later in the chapter on International Atomic Energy Agency perspectives and initiatives on CT radiation dose, the IAEA has initiated the Smart Card or Smart Rad Track project to track and monitor cumulative radiation doses.

However, these endeavors do not address the challenge posed by vast repositories of retrospective CT data that store dose parameters as an image-based dose sheet instead of structured data within the DICOM header. Furthermore, CT scanners currently in use may not have firmware amenable to incorporating radiation dose into image headers. To that end, a number of open-source and commercial software solutions for dose monitoring have been developed in the past 2 years. Many of these solutions also facilitate communication of data to registries such as the one sponsored by the ACR.

In this chapter, we discuss some of the relevant CT dose parameters, historic obstacles to effective CT dose monitoring, and some of the new solutions that have been implemented both for facility-based dose monitoring and reporting as well as for large-scale dose registries. We also discuss the future of dose monitoring with respect to organ dose estimation.

## 2 CT Dose Parameters and Their Effect on Patient Dose

An institutional review board (IRB)-approved survey revealed that 76% of radiologists and radiology trainees reviewed the image-based dose information sheet or page less than 10% of the time they performed or interpreted a CT examination. Despite these statistics, radiologists receive more physics training than their non-radiologist physician counterparts, and are best equipped to analyze and interpret the parameters that are typically reported. While there is considerable variation across CT scanner vendors with respect to the format of the dose sheet, there is a common subset of relevant parameters that is always reported. In this section, we briefly review these parameters and their impact on patient dose.

## 2.1 kVp: Tube Voltage

The kVp—or kilovolt peak—represents the maximum voltage potential across the X-ray tube. Dose varies as the square of the kVp, which means that small changes in kVp can have a significant effect on dose. The kVp represents the energy of the photons in the X-ray beam; higher energy photons will penetrate the patient and reach the detector array, while lower energy photons will get absorbed within the patient. However, the use of a lower kVp is advantageous for iodine-enhanced imaging, because the average energy of the X-ray spectrum comes closer to the k-edge of iodine (approximately 33 kiloelectron-volts) and results in increased attenuation. This has been demonstrated to be effective in body CT angiography procedures including coronary CTA (Luaces et al. 2009; Hausleiter et al. 2009) and CT perfusion studies. In larger patients, it is not practical to use a lower kVp because more of the lower energy photons will be absorbed by the tissues. However, in thinner patients and children, lower kVp imaging is more feasible and will result in substantial dose savings. Most vendors report the kVp on the image-based dose sheet.

## 2.2 mAs: Tube Current–Time Product

The mAs, or tube current (mA)-time (s) product, is a representation of the total number of photons used over the course of a CT examination. A higher total study mAs indicates that more photons were used to produce the image. Dose varies linearly with the mA, so using a higher mA will lead to a higher patient dose. Conversely, using a lower mA will result in increased image noise, because fewer photons were used to penetrate the patient and create the image. Some limitations can be placed on the mA by using tube current modulation, which chooses the tube current dynamically based on a reference prescribed before the scan begins. Very few dose sheets actually provide any information pertaining to the parameters used for different tube current modulation techniques. Details of automatic tube current modulation techniques are discussed in a separate chapter in this textbook.

## 2.3 $CTDI_{vol}$: Volumetric CT Dose Index

Multiple CT dose indices exist, however, the volumetric CT dose index is often the one reported on a CT dose sheet. The first relevant CT dose index is the $CTDI_{100}$, which is measured using a 100 mm pencil chamber placed at the center of a cylindrical acrylic phantom. When the 100 mm pencil chamber is used to make measurements both in the center and at the periphery of the phantom, a weighted CTDI or $CTDI_w$ is obtained. Dividing the weighted $CTDI_w$ by the pitch results in the $CTDI_{vol}$. It is important to remember that the $CTDI_{vol}$ and other CT dose indices are not measures of patient dose, but rather represent the energy output by the scanner measured in different ways. In fact, the $CTDI_{vol}$ is measured in milligray (mGy); 1 Gray is equal to 1 Joule/kilogram.

## 2.4 DLP: Dose-Length Product

The dose-length product (DLP) can be used to derive an estimate of the whole-body effective dose received by a patient during a CT scan. It is calculated by multiplying the $CTDI_{vol}$ by the scan length in centimeters, resulting in units of mGy-cm. The estimated whole-body effective dose, reported in millisieverts (mSv), can be calculated by multiplying the DLP by an anatomy-specific conversion factor, also known as a k factor. The k factors are derived from tissue weighting factors maintained by the International Commission on Radiological Protection (ICRP); the latter were most recently updated in 2007 (ICRP 2007).

## 2.5 Other Factors

Patient age, gender and size can also affect dose (Huda and Vance 2007; Kalra 2004). Younger patients are at higher risk of experiencing the adverse effects of radiation exposure because of more rapid turnover of cellular DNA and the higher potential for radiation-induced mutations. Breast tissue in women is similarly more susceptible. While larger patients may appear to receive a higher dose on the basis of DLP alone, for a given CT protocol, a thinner patient will receive a higher organ dose than a larger patient because of a smaller amount of attenuating subcutaneous tissue. CT examination protocols should not only be customized to answer the clinical question, but also adjusted for patient size, in order to optimize both diagnostic image quality and dose savings, and maximize the benefit-risk ratio of exposing patients to ionizing radiation.

# 3 Dose Reporting: Past and Present

## 3.1 Image-Based Dose Sheet

Historically, CT dose parameters have been recorded as pixels on an image-based dose sheet associated with each CT examination. The format and location of these dose sheets vary with CT scanner vendors, but at minimum a dose sheet typically reports the $CTDI_{vol}$ and DLP for each cross-sectional series within a CT examination. More detailed dose sheets may report the series name, kVp, total mAs, individual series mA settings and even the type of phantom used (e.g., 16-cm head phantom or 32-cm body phantom).

The image-based dose sheet has posed the greatest challenge to dose monitoring efforts thus far, as it mandates that the process begins with extraction of the values from the dose sheet. Successful automation of this process using optical character recognition has spurred the development of a number of open-source and commercial dose monitoring tools, some of which will be discussed here. Figure 1 shows a sample dose sheet for a pulmonary embolism chest CT examination from the Siemens Definition Flash scanner.

18-Sep-2011 15:23

Ward: ER
Physician: CHEST
Operator: JD

Total mAs 2545 Total DLP 340 mGycm

| | Scan | KV | mAs / ref. | CTDIvol* mGy | DLP mGycm | TI s | cSL mm |
|---|---|---|---|---|---|---|---|
| Patient Position F-SP | | | | | | | |
| Topogram | 1 | 120 | 34 mA | 0.14 L | 6 | 4.4 | 0.6 |
| PreMonitoring | 2 | 120 | 40 | 2.40 L | 2 | 0.5 | 10.0 |
| Contrast | | | | | | | |
| Monitoring | 3 | 120 | 40 | 7.21 L | 7 | 0.5 | 10.0 |
| PE | 6 | 100 | 193 / 150 | 7.98 L | 325 | 0.5 | 0.6 |

| Medium | Type | Iodine Conc. mg/ml | Volume ml | Flow ml/s | CM Ratio |
|---|---|---|---|---|---|
| Contrast | | 0 | 0 | 0.0 | 100% |
| Saline | | | 0 | 0.0 | |

*: L = 32cm, S = 16cm

**Fig. 1** Sample image-based dose sheet from a pulmonary embolism chest CT examination performed on the Siemens definition flash scanner. Note the dose parameters reported: total mAs, total DLP, series kV, series mA and reference mA (for tube current modulation), series CTDIvol and series DLP, among others. The phantom type is also indicated

## 3.2 Radiation Dose Structured Report

Recent work by the DICOM Standards Committee produced the DICOM Dose SR, or radiation dose structured report (RDSR), as it has come to be known (DICOM 2007, 2008). This structured report is an effort to standardize the reporting of dose parameters across vendors and also to facilitate large-scale dose monitoring by incorporating the report into the DICOM header. All four major CT vendors now support the RDSR in their newest scanners. While firmware updates for RDSR backwards-compatibility are now available for a number of recent older scanners, not all older models will be updated.

The RDSR includes data from the DICOM study header as well as accumulated dose data and data about individual irradiation events. The data elements from the DICOM header include the following: accession number, study date and time, institution name and address, station name (i.e., unique CT scanner identifier at a facility), scanner manufacturer and model, study and series description and patient demographics (gender, age, weight, etc.). The values for these data elements always exist within the DICOM header for a given study, regardless of whether or not the RDSR is generated. Accumulated dose data included within the RDSR represents a summary of a particular CT examination. These data include the total study DLP, total effective dose and phantom type.

An individual irradiation event within the RDSR is defined as a single series of a CT scan, regardless of whether that series represents a scout image or acquisition of cross-sectional data. Some of the data elements associated with an irradiation event include those CT acquisition parameters that are typically found on the image-based dose sheet: scan length, kVp, mA, $CTDI_{vol}$ and DLP. However, additional parameters are also reported, including pitch, $CTDI_w$, collimation width, number of X-ray sources, rotation time, X-ray modulation type and effective dose. In total, the RDSR provides a wealth of information beyond the image-based dose sheet, and has the added advantage of standardization across vendors.

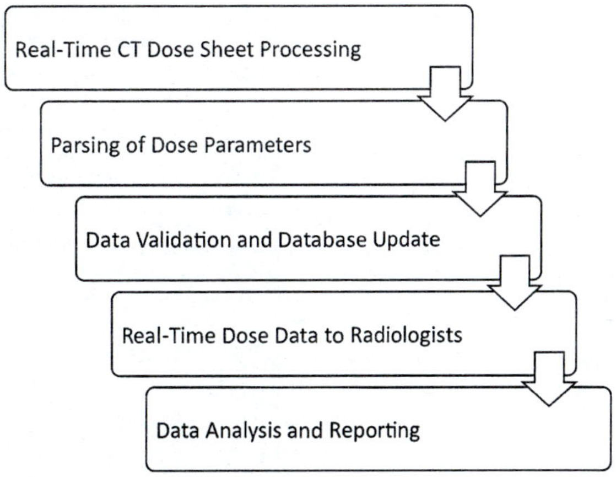


**Fig. 2** The RADIANCE processing pipeline. No manual user input is required, although the pipeline can also be triggered manually if desired

## 4 Facility-Level CT Dose Monitoring

Faced with the challenge of a vast repository of image-based dose sheets worldwide and the immediate need for CT dose monitoring, the radiology community has responded by developing a number of open-source and commercial dose monitoring tools. Among these is RADIANCE–Radiation Dose Intelligent Analytics for CT Examinations (Cook et al. 2010). Introduced in 2010, RADIANCE is a freely available, open-source software package (http://www.radiancedose.com) designed to extract dose-related parameters from image-based dose sheets as well as import them from the RDSR. The software is intended to be used by individual imaging facilities or a conglomerate health system with multiple hospitals or imaging centers for internal dose monitoring. Data collected at a facility is not transmitted to a central RADIANCE dose repository, but rather retained within the facility.

### 4.1 RADIANCE: Features

RADIANCE is configured as a processing pipeline which runs without requiring external user input. The pipeline is shown in Fig. 2. The input to the pipeline is usually the image-based dose sheet. The dose sheet often comprises one of the series of a CT examination, which simplifies retrieval from the picture archiving and communications system (PACS). It is typically a single page, although for some studies and with some manufacturers, it can extend to multiple pages. Some CT scanner manufacturers use a unique combination of series number and series description to identify the dose sheet, while others provide only a unique series description and vary the series number.

Pipeline operations begin with optical character recognition (OCR) of the dose sheet. This converts the pixel-based information into ASCII text (GOCR 2010), which is subsequently parsed to extract the relevant CT dose parameters. Additional information about the type of examination performed, the imaging facility, the scanner equipment and the patient is extracted from the DICOM study header. These data, together with the CT dose parameters, are stored in a searchable relational database.

Because each vendor's image-based dose sheet is unique, the source vendor for each dose sheet is identified before further processing occurs, in order to correctly parse the expected dose parameters. Once the parameters from a dose sheet are parsed, validated and stored in the RADIANCE database, the estimated whole-body effective dose is calculated by multiplying the total study DLP by the appropriate anatomy-specific *k* factor. At present, RADIANCE uses the *k* factors derived from International Commission on Radiologic Protection (ICRP) Publication 60 (ICRP 1990).

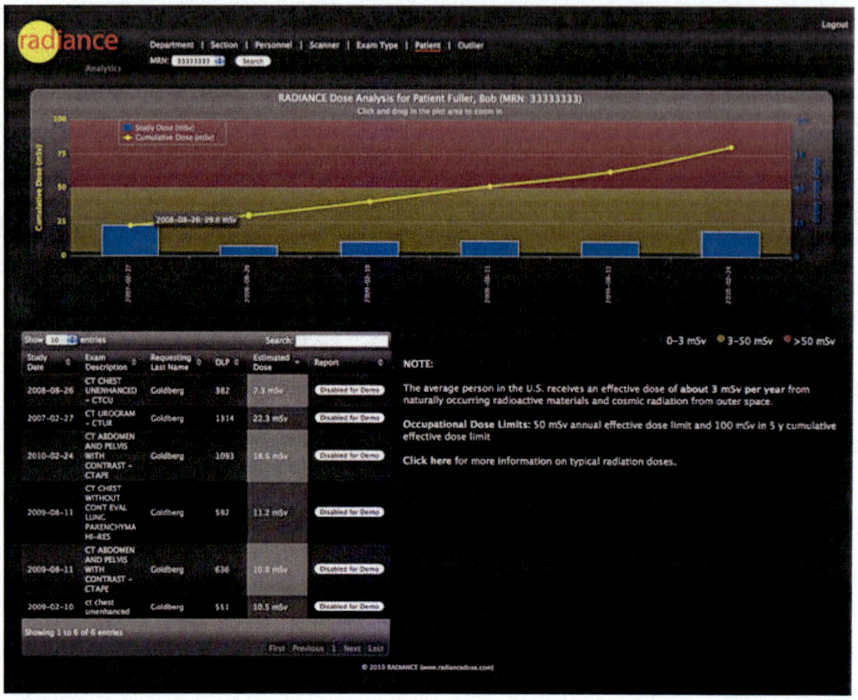


**Fig. 3** A real-time dose profile available to radiologists at the workstation during study interpretation. All CT examinations undergone by this patient within our health system are included, with estimated doses sourced either from image-based dose sheets, when available, or from published dose estimates for older examinations or those without available dose sheets. All displayed names have been anonymized

In addition to archival within the database, the information extracted from an image-based dose sheet can also be used to construct the RDSR representation of a CT examination. This is achieved using the PixelMed Java DICOM Toolkit (Clunie 2010). RADIANCE populates the structured report template with the data from its database, and generates an RDSR that can be automatically transmitted to the ACR's Dose Index Registry. This enables imaging facilities to automate transfer of their dose data to the Registry, obviating the need for manual data entry or manual transmission of dose reports. In addition to exporting RDSRs, RADIANCE can also import scanner-generated RDSRs into the database, to enable facilities to centralize their dose monitoring even if some of their scanners do produce the newer radiation dose structured reports.

In its current implementation at our institution, RADIANCE runs in real-time, searching for newly completed CT examinations that have not been included in the database. Once the image-based dose sheet for a study has been sent to the PACS, RADIANCE retrieves and processes the dose sheet via direct query of the PACS. Departmental radiologists can access a patient's estimated dose profile (Fig. 3) while interpreting a recent examination or determining a protocol for a subsequent examination (Cook et al. 2011).

RADIANCE has been shown to be compliant with the IHE REM Profile. This is discussed further in Sect. 5.1.

## 4.2 RADIANCE: Dashboard Analytics

To facilitate review of an imaging facility's dose data, we have designed a customizable dashboard built on the RADIANCE database schema and included in the open-source release. The dashboard provides a set of standard overview screens that summarize dose estimates by departmental section, scanner, personnel, patient and exam type. In addition, it allows users to identify those exams that exceed a prescribed threshold for estimated whole-body dose (in millisieverts). In addition to the predefined overview screens, the dashboard is customizable and enables users to add additional screens that organize the data differently for their individual facilities' requirements.

The patient dashboard indicates the dose estimates for each individual CT examination at a particular facility, as well as a cumulative lifetime dose estimate for that patient at that facility. This is the same patient dose profile that radiologists can view at the workstation during image interpretation or study protocoling (Fig. 3). Acknowledging the limitations of

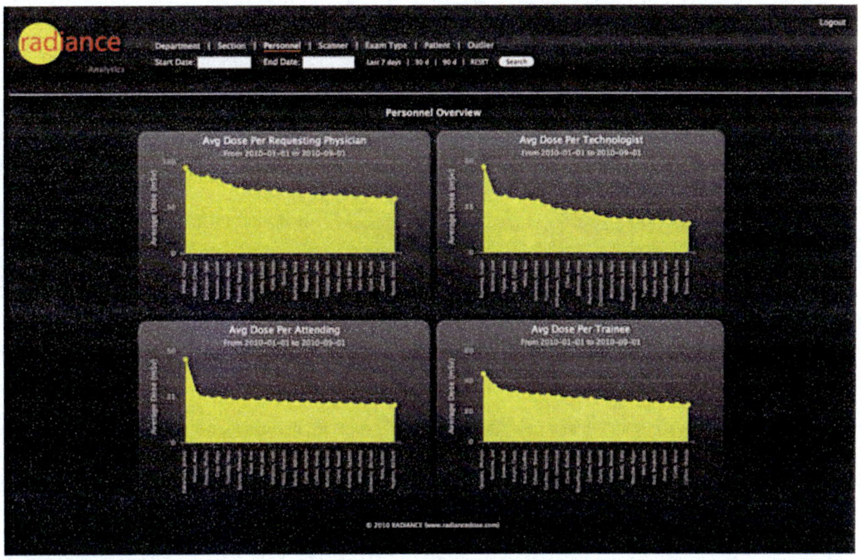


**Fig. 4** The personnel dashboard enables analysis of average dose estimates by provider–referring physician, performing technologist, reporting radiologist and consulting radiology trainee. All displayed names have been anonymized

summing individual dose estimates for CT scans of different body parts, this representation gives both the radiologist and the referring physician a sense of not only how many exams this patient has undergone, but also what types of studies were performed and by whom they were ordered.

A screenshot from the personnel overview is shown in Fig. 4. The personnel overview allows users to examine dose estimates by referring provider, performing technologist and reporting radiologist, to look for trends in ordering and reporting as well as compliance with protocol implementations. A screenshot from the scanner overview is shown in Fig. 5. This view is useful for identifying potential protocol differences between scanners for the same study type, or possibly a lack of adherence to prescribed protocols for a particular study.

## 4.3 RADIANCE: Monthly Scorecards

Scorecards—monthly dose summary reports—are generated for every radiologist, technologist, section chief and radiology administrator within the department. Each report is customized to the role of the individual to whom it is sent. For example, individual radiologist and technologist scorecards summarize average dose estimates for all interpreted or performed study types for the month, compared to that individual's doses for the previous month and the department's doses for the current month. The top 10 highest dose estimates overall as well as for patients under 50 are listed. The final interpretation and images for each of these studies are linked. Free-text comments can be added to explain the higher doses for these studies.

Individual radiologists and technologists are only shown dose estimates for exams with which they are involved, i.e., have personally interpreted or performed (Fig. 6). Section chiefs receive an overview to that described in the previous paragraph for all exams performed and interpreted within their section, as well as access to the data for all of their section radiologists and technologists. Finally, departmental administrators can access all these screens as well as individual dose estimates by study type. They receive a one-year review of the average and maximum dose estimates for a study type of their choice (Fig. 7). They can also review average doses by the radiologist and technologist in the department for a particular study type.

## 4.4 Other Open-Source Dose Monitoring Tools

In addition to RADIANCE, other open-source dose monitoring tools also exist. Each software package achieves the same goal—extraction of dose parameters from the image-based dose sheet, RDSR, or both—with unique and complementary features.

DoseUtility is an interactive, Java-based program that can interface directly with a PACS to retrieve and

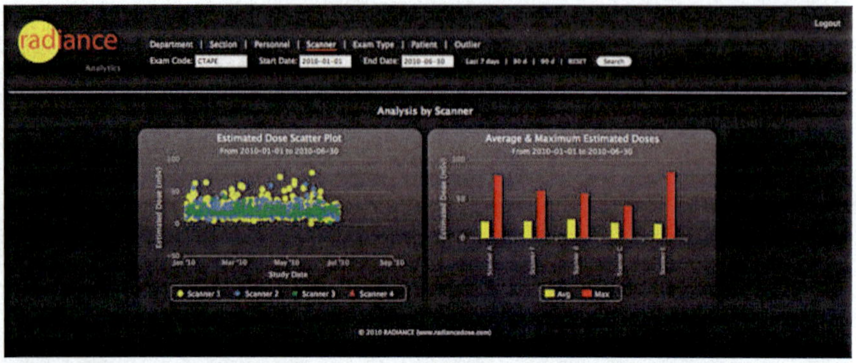


**Fig. 5** The scanner dashboard enables comparison of dose estimates for a particular type of CT examination when obtained on different scanner models. Such an analysis is useful for identifying protocol differences that may lead to higher doses on different scanners and can be optimized for dose savings across the board

interpret either image-based dose sheets or RDSRs (Clunie, accessed September 15, 2011). While DoseUtility does not archive the extracted dose parameters in a database, it is another useful tool for transferring data to the ACR's Dose Index Registry, particularly for facilities with scanners that still generate image-based dose sheets.

DoseRetriever is another interactive system, which can be run without any sophisticated hardware or software from a USB flash drive (Cheng 2011). It can also retrieve dose sheets directly from PACS and process the data before archival in a database. One unique feature of this software is the font library it uses to perform the OCR analysis of image-based dose sheets. This approach greatly minimizes the errors in the OCR extraction process and thus also decreases the amount of post-processing and validation necessary to ensure that the data are accurate.

Built on the PixelMed library, GROK–Generalized Radiation Observation Toolkit—is another Java-based dose monitoring package which attempts to solve the problem of how CT exams from different body parts are combined into a single dose sheet (Warden 2011). In addition, GROK includes early adjustment of dose estimates for patient body habitus.

Together, these open-source tools have facilitated dose monitoring and reporting for radiologists worldwide, and enabled participation in dose registries even for facilities without the newest CT scanner hardware or firmware.

## 4.5 Commercial Dose Monitoring Applications

In addition to open-source tools, there are an increasing number of commercial dose monitoring software applications. Many are similar to RADIANCE, in that they use some form of OCR extraction to remove the dose parameters from the image-based dose sheets, but also support RDSR parsing. Others only import the RDSR and provide reporting tools based on the imported data. More sophisticated applications include the organ dose estimation for comparison with the conventional DLP-based methods of dose monitoring.

A number of DLP-based products are currently available. Among them is Valkyrie, developed at Columbia University, which is a web-based application that uses OCR extraction and generates dose estimates adjusted according to patient weight (Barnes 2011). PEMNET, which stands for Patient Exposure Management NETwork and is produced by Clinical Microsystems, Inc. (http://www.pemnet.info), performs multi-modality radiation dose monitoring, and can track doses for radiography, CT and even fluoroscopy. DoseMonitor, a product produced by PACSHealth (http://www.dosemonitor.com), has built-in alerting features that monitor a patient's cumulative estimated effective dose and trigger alerts when specified thresholds are exceeded by subsequent studies. DoseMetrix, a product of Primordial, Inc. (http://www.primordialdesign.com/home.html), is a customized

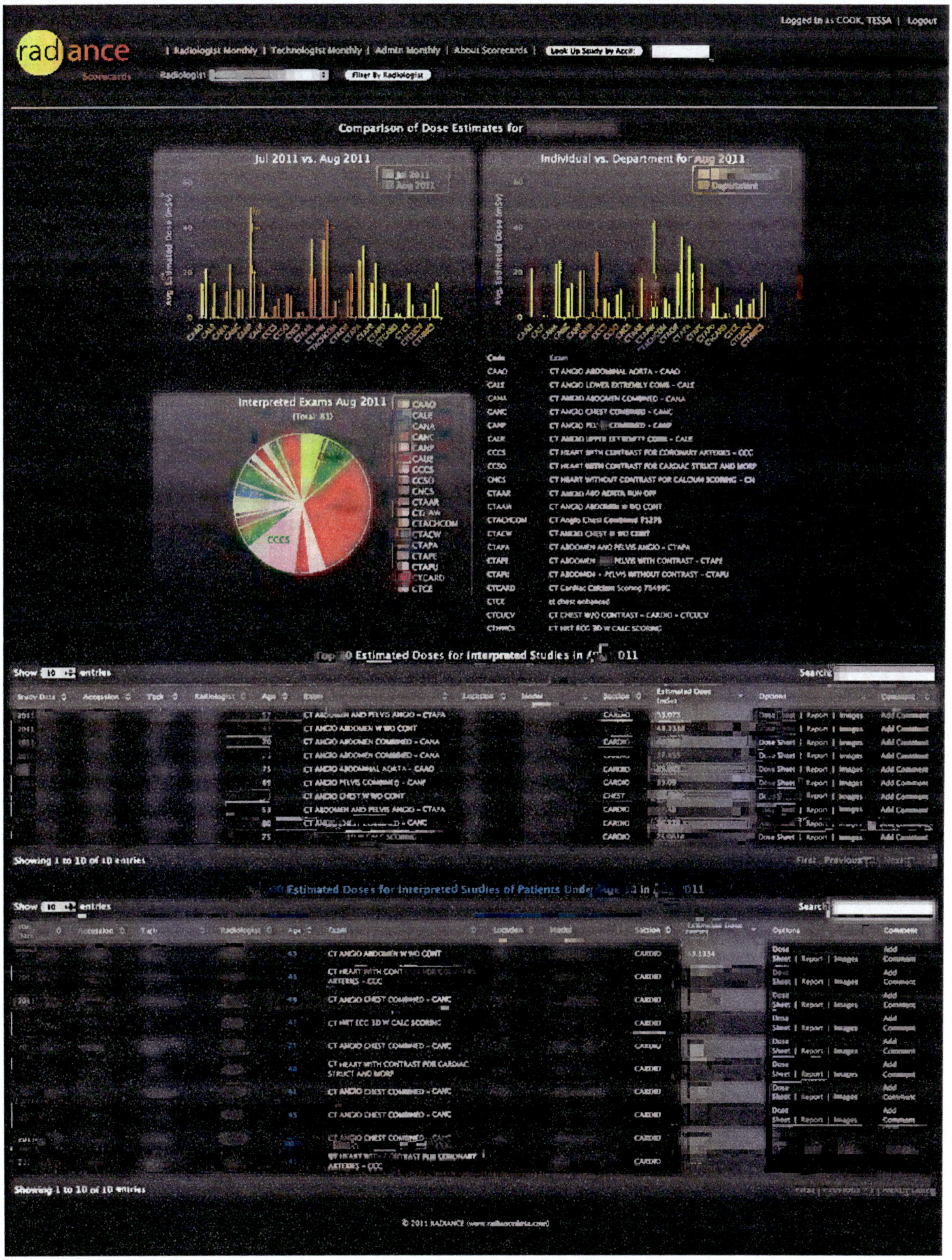


**Fig. 6** Monthly radiologist scorecard. The report summarizes dose estimates for studies interpreted during the recently completed month, and compares them to studies interpreted by that same radiologist during the preceding month, as well as by peer radiologists during the current month. For HIPAA compliance, some information has been blurred

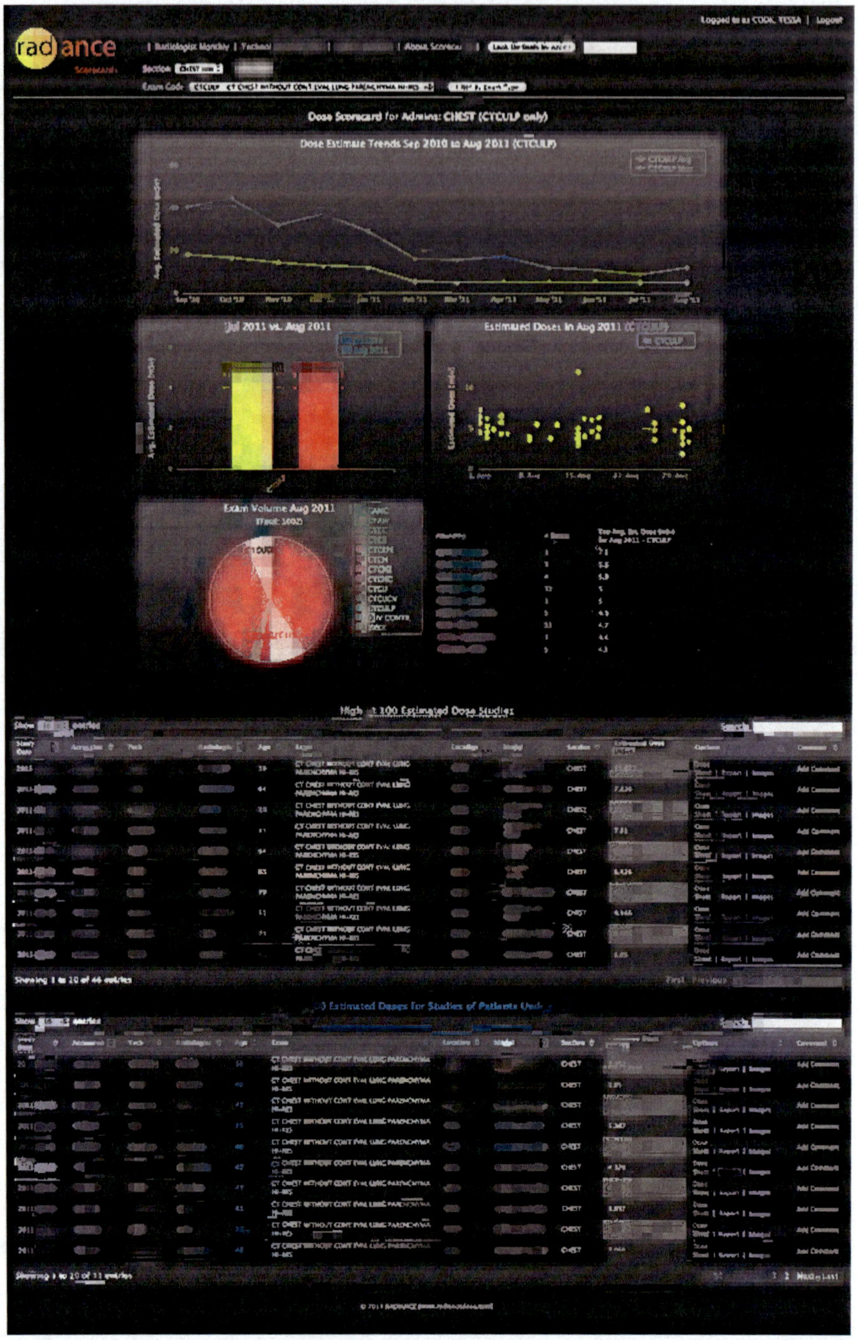


**Fig. 7** Monthly radiology administrator scorecard. One unique feature of the administrator-level scorecard is the 12-month retrospective review of average and maximum dose estimates for a particular study type. For HIPAA compliance, some information has been blurred

solution for dose monitoring. Imalogix (http://www.imalogix.com/) is a commercial solution which collects dose data at an off-site location and generates a variety of reports with respect to dose monitoring, scanner utilization and protocol compliance. Its latter two features are applicable to modalities in addition to CT.

An application called eXposure, developed by Radimetrics, Inc. (http://www.radimetrics.com), uses Monte Carlo simulations to reproduce the CT scan using the exposure parameters recorded in the DICOM study headers. eXposure calculates organ dose estimates using hermaphrodite mathematical phantoms (Cristy 1980), and also provides a number of convenient tools for protocol management as well as outlier detection and investigation.

# 5 Large-Scale CT Dose Monitoring Efforts

## 5.1 The IHE REM Profile

The IHE REM Profile is an implementation guide for both vendors and consumers that provides a set of standards for radiation dose monitoring. RADIANCE is compliant with the IHE REM Profile as both a dose information consumer and a dose reporter. As a dose information consumer, RADIANCE can be configured to query the PACS for CT dose sheets using standard DICOM query/retrieve operations. It is also able to read RDSRs produced by newer scanner models and import those data into the database. Since the database contains protected health information, it is password-protected and intended to reside behind an imaging center's firewall, rather than on a public network.

As a dose information reporter, the analytics dashboard built on the database schema allows users to scrutinize their dose data more carefully, and analyze dose estimates by departmental section, individual scanner, involved personnel or individual patient. Outlier identification is also possible, i.e., detecting studies whose dose estimates exceed a prescribed threshold. With the exception of the patient dashboard, which requires input of the patient's medical record number, all data presented by the dashboard are completely de-identified in keeping with the REM Profile. One of the actions of a dose information reporter in the REM Profile is to transmit dose information to a registry. Hence, RADIANCE is able to generate de-identified RDSR representations of legacy CT dose sheets, to enable users to participate in dose registries. Using secure FTP, RDSR representations of legacy CT dose sheets can be transmitted to the ACR's Dose Index Registry to demonstrate communication between a dose information reporter and a dose registry. Alternatively, they can be routed through the ACR's TRIAD (Transfer of Images and Data) Server, installed locally at each facility, and sent to NRDR-DIR.

## 5.2 Multi-Center Dose Registries

One of the ultimate goals of dose monitoring is to determine the appropriate range of dose estimates for a particular CT examination. Both the American College of Radiology (ACR) and the Society of Pediatric Radiology (SPR) are working towards this goal. The ImageWisely™ and ImageGently™ campaigns, respectively, are actively increasing awareness of the issues surrounding CT-related radiation among radiologists, referring physicians and patients and their families (Brink and Amis 2010; Goske et al. 2008). Furthermore, both groups are spearheading large-scale dose registries in order to collect dose estimates from a variety of patient populations for different CT examinations.

The ACR's Dose Index Registry (2011), was formally launched in May 2011 and is already receiving dose data from over 200 facilities nationwide. Biannual reports are generated for all participating facilities, summarizing the average DLP for individual study types as compared to other similar facilities (i.e., one teaching hospital to another or one outpatient community practice to another). The registry is able to accept data directly from scanners that produce RDSRs, or via intermediate software packages such as RADIANCE or DoseUtility that can generate RDSR representations of image-based dose sheets.

In conjunction with the ACR, the SPR is launching QuiRCC (Quality Improvement Registry for CT Scans in Children 2011), a registry specifically designed to collect data for CT in pediatric patients. Children are significantly more susceptible to adverse outcomes from excessive exposure to ionizing radiation than adults. Just as adult protocols are inappropriate for pediatric patients, so too are appropriate dose levels determined by studying CT dose estimates in adult patients. QuiRCC is carefully following not only dose estimates, but also CT acquisition parameters and patient size parameters at six pediatric hospitals in the United States.

Together, the efforts of the ACR and the SPR will go a long way towards defining reference dose levels for both adult and pediatric CT examinations.

## 6 Organ Dose Estimation: What the Future Holds

It is clear that educating both radiologist and non-radiologist physicians on this issue is paramount, as is the need for more accurate, reliable and routine tracking and monitoring of CT-related radiation dose. As discussed previously, the simplest method for dose estimation is to multiply the DLP by the appropriate anatomy-specific k factor. However, these k factors were derived using Monte Carlo simulations with a mathematical hermaphrodite phantom (Cristy 1980), specific scanner geometry conditions and the assumption that the patient was only imaged once (i.e., a single-phase examination). However, despite these constraints, k factors are universally used for CT dose estimation as they provide a real-time effective dose estimate and do not necessitate high-performance computing hardware.

While deriving effective dose from DLP provides a straightforward, practical estimate of patients' radiation exposure, it does not reflect patient size (McCollough et al. 2011). Menke demonstrated that a water-equivalent diameter, derived from a CT scout image by modeling the patient as a cylinder with the density of water, could be used to normalize dose estimates (Menke 2006). Using Monte Carlo simulations of CT scans and subsequent calculation of organ doses, researchers have demonstrated that DLP can underestimate dose for smaller patients, including children, and overestimate dose for larger adults (Brenner et al. 2006; Hurwitz et al. 2007).

It is critical to understand that CTDI and the associated dose indices do not represent actual patient dose (McCollough et al. 2011). This motivated the AAPM to develop correction factors for $CTDI_{vol}$ based on effective patient diameter (Size-Specific Dose Estimates 2011). Additional work has been done to normalize for inherent differences in scanner geometries and enable comparisons of dose estimates between scanners, however, these corrections still do not account for patient factors—size, gender, body habitus (Turner et al. 2010; Huda and Mettler 2011). Recent work using Monte Carlo simulations to calculate organ doses from anthropomorphic phantoms of different sizes has more clearly illustrated how much DLP can vary with patient size (Li et al. 2008, 2011). Research has shown that patient position, and in particular, arm position with respect to the torso, can affect dose estimation (Brink et al. 2008; Tack and Gevenois 2008).

However, computational needs render it impractical to model every patient individually. Depending on the type of phantom used, a single Monte Carlo simulation can take a few hours. This limitation motivates the need for standardized phantoms which can be used to quickly compute organ dose estimates. Alternatively, if these phantoms could be customized in some way to reflect a patient's body habitus, this would conceivably increase the accuracy of organ dose estimation. Ongoing work is centering on large-scale segmentation efforts in order to establish libraries of organ segmentations which can be used to build more realistic phantoms.

## 7 Conclusion

The exponential rise in CT utilization in recent years, coupled with notable instances of patients' overexposure to CT-related radiation, have spawned numerous parallel efforts to improve CT dose monitoring and reporting. The convenience of DLP-based dose estimation and the need for dose monitoring tools have led to the development of a number of freeware and commercial solutions for dose monitoring. In addition, large-scale as well as regional dose registries have been established in order to develop dose reference levels for different CT examinations. Ultimately, these efforts improve the care of our radiology patients and promote more responsible imaging. Until we fully understand the risks associated with repeated exposure to ionizing radiation, we must continue to maximize the benefit-to-risk ratio of imaging-related radiation exposure and strive to answer the clinical question with the most appropriate imaging modality.

## References

Amis JES, Butler PF, Applegate KE, Birnbaum SB, Brateman LF, Hevezi JM, Mettler FA, Morin RL, Pentecost MJ, Smith GG, Strauss KJ, Zeman RK (2007) American College of Radiology white paper on radiation dose in medicine. JACR 4:272–284

Barnes E (2011) Valkyrie software rides to rescue of CT radiation dose dilemma. http://www.auntminnie.com/index.aspx?sec=sup&sub=cto&pag=dis&ItemID=90460. Accessed October 31

Bogdanich W, Ruiz RR (2010) FDA to increase oversight of medical radiation. New York Times

Brenner DJ, Hall EJ (2007) Computed tomography: an increasing source of radiation exposure. NEJM 357(22): 2277–2284

Brenner DJ, McCollough C, Orton CG (2006) Is it time to retire the CTDI for CT quality assurance and dose optimization? Med Phys 33:1189–1191

Brink JA, Amis ES (2010) Image wisely: a campaign to increase awareness about adult radiation protection. Radiology 257(3):601–602

Brink M, de Lange F, Oostveen LJ, Dekker HM, Kool DR, Deunk J, Edwards MJR, van Kuijk C, Kamman RL, Blickman JG (2008) Arm raising at exposure-controlled multidetector trauma ct of thoracoabdominal region: higher image quality, lower radiation dose. Radiology 249(2): 661–670

Brody A, Frush D, Huda W, Brent R (2007) Radiation risk to children from computed tomogoraphy. Pediatrics 120(3):677

Cheng P (2011) CT Dose Retriever. http://www-hsc.usc.edu/phillimc/doseretriever/index.html. Accessed September 15

Clunie DA (2011) PixelMed Java DICOM Toolkit. http://www.dclunie.com/pixelmed/software/(2010) Accessed March 1

Clunie DA (2011) How to Use DoseUtility. http://www.dclunie.com/pixelmed/software/webstart/DoseUtilityUsage.html. Accessed September 15, 2011

Congressional Subcommittee on Health: Medical radiation: an overview of the issues. http://energycommerce.house.gov/index.php?option=com_content&view=article&id=1910: medical-radiation-an-overview-of-the-issues&catid=132: subcommittee-on-health&Itemid=72 (February 26, 2010). Accessed March 1, 2010

Cook TS, Zimmerman S, Maidment ADA, Kim W, Boonn WW (2010) Automated extraction of radiation dose information for CT examinations. J Am Coll Rad 7(11):871–877

Cook TS, Kim W, Boonn WW (2011) Integrated, On-Demand Retrieval of Cumulative CT Dose Estimates at the Workstation During Image Interpretation. In: SIIM

Cristy M (1980) Mathematical phantoms representing children of various ages for use in estimates of internal dose. Tech. Rep. NUREG/CR-1159, United States Nuclear Regulatory Commission

de Gonzalez AB, Mahesh M, Kim K, Bhargavan M, Lewis R, Mettler F, Land C (2009) Projected cancer risks from computed tomographic scans performed in the united states in (2007). Arch Intern Med 169(22):2071–2077

DICOM (2007) Standards Committee: DICOM Standard Supplement 127: CT radiation dose reporting

DICOM (2008) Standards Committee: DICOM Standard Part 16: content mapping resource

Dose Index Registry (2011) https://nrdr.acr.org/Portal/DIR/Main/page.aspx. Accessed September 15

GOCR. http:/gocr.sourceforge.net. Accessed March 1, 2010

Goske M, Applegate K, Boylan J, Butler P, Callahan M, Coley B, Farley S, Frush D, Hernanz-Schulman M, Jaramillo D et al (2008a) The Image Gentlycampaign: increasing CT radiation dose awareness through a national education and awareness program. Pediatr Radiol 38(3):265–269

Goske M, Applegate K, Boylan J, Butler P, Callahan M, Coley B, Farley S, Frush D, Hernanz-Schulman M, Jaramillo D et al (2008b) The Image Gentlycampaign: increasing CT radiation dose awareness through a national education and awareness program. Pediatr Radiol 38(3):265–269

Hausleiter J, Meyer T, Hermann F et al (2009) Estimated radiation dose associated with cardiac CT angiography. JAMA 301:500–507

Huda W, Mettler FA (2011) Volume CT dose index and dose-length product displayed: what good are they? Radiology 258:236–242

Huda W, Vance A (2007) Patient radiation doses from adult and pediatric CT. Am J Roentgenol 188(2):540–546

Hurwitz LM, Yoshizumi TT, Goodman PC, Frush DP, Nguyen G, Toncheva G, Lowry C (2007) Effective dose determination using an anthropomorphic phantom and metal oxide semiconductor field effect transistor technology for clinical adult body multidetector array computed tomography protocols. J Comput Assist Tomogr 31(4):544–549

ICRP (1990) Recommendations of the International Commission on Radiologic Protection. ICRP Publication 60. Ann. ICRP 21(1–3)

ICRP (2007) The 2007 Recommendations of the International Commission on Radiologic Protection. ICRP Publication 103. Ann. ICRP 37(2-4)

Kalra MK, Maher MM, Toth TL, Hamberg LM, Blake MA, Shepard J, Saini S (2004) Strategies for CT radiation dose optimization 230(3):619–628

Kase KR et al. (2009) Ionizing radiation exposure of the population of the United States. Tech. Rep. 160, National Council of Radiation Protection

Landro L (2010) Radiation risks prompt push to curb CT scans. Wall Street Journal

Levin DC, Rao VM, Parker L, Frangos AJ, Sunshine JH (2008) Recent trends in utilization rates of abdominal imaging: the relative roles of radiologists and nonradiologist physicians. JACR 5:744–747

Li X, Segars WP, Samei E, Sturgeon GM, Colsher JG, Frush DP (2008) Patient-specific dose estimation for pediatric chest CT. Med Phys 35:5821–5828

Li X, Samei E, Segars WP, Sturgeon GM, Colsher JG, Toncheva G, Yoshizumi TT, Frush DP (2011) Patient-specific radiation dose and cancer risk estimation in CT: part II. application to patients. Med Phys 38:408–419

Luaces M, Akers S, Litt H (2009) Low kVp imaging for dose reduction in dual-source cardiac CT. Int J Cardiovasc Imaging 25:165–175

Maitino AJ, Levin DC, Parker L, Rao VM, Sunshine JH (2003) Nationwide trends in rates of utilization of noninvasive diagnostic imaging among the medicare population between 1993 and 1999. Radiology 227:113–117

Martin D, Semelka R (2006) Health effects of ionising radiation from diagnostic CT. Lancet 367(9524):1712–1714

McCollough CH, Leng S, Yu L, Cody DD, Boone JM, McNitt-Gray MF (2011) CT dose index and patient dose: they are not the same thing. Radiology 259(2):311–316

Menke J (2006) Comparison of different body size parameters for individual dose adaptation in body CT of adults. Radiology 236:565–571

National Radiology Data Registry (2011) http://nrdr.acr.org. Accessed September 15

Neumann RD, Bluemke DA (2010) Tracking radiation exposure from diagnostic imaging devices at the NIH. JACR 7(2):87–89

Quality Improvement Registry for CT Scans in Children (2011) https://nrdr.acr.org/Portal/QuIRCC/Main/page.aspx. Accessed September 15

Radiation Exposure Monitoring (2010) http://wiki.ihe.net/index.php?title=Radiation_Exposure_Management. Accessed March 15

SB (2011) 1237–Radiation control: health facilities and clinics: records. http://info.sen.ca.gov/pub/09-10/bill/sen/sb_1201-1250/sb_1237_bill_20100929_chaptered.html. Accessed September 15

Sinclair WK, Adelstein SJ, Carter MW, Harley JH, Moeller DW (1987) Ionizing radiation exposure of the population of the United States. Tech. Rep. 93, National Council of Radiation Protection

Size-Specific Dose Estimates (SSDE) (2011) Pediatric and Adult Body CT Examinations. Tech. Rep. TG-204, American Association of Physicists in Medicine

Smith-Bindman R, Lipson J, Marcus R, Kim KP, Mahesh M, Gould R, de Gonzalez AB, Miglioretti DL (2009) Radiation dose associated with common computed tomography examinations and the associated lifetime attributable risk of cancer. Arch Intern Med 169(22):2078–2086

Tack D, Gevenois PA (2008) Efforts for lowering radiation dose delivered with CT: raising arms, or is there more? Radiology 249(2):413–415

Turner AC, Zankl M, DeMarco JJ, Cagnon CH, Zhang D, Angel E, Cody DD, Stevens DM, McCollough CH, McNitt-Gray MF (2010) The feasibility of a scanner-independent technique to estimate organ dose from MDCT scans: using CTDIvol to account for differences between scanners. Med Phys 37(4):1816–1825

Warden GI (2011) GROK–Generalized Radiation Observation Kit. http://dose-grok.sourceforge.net/. Accessed September 15

White Paper: Initiative to Reduce Unnecessary Radiation Exposure from Medical Imaging (2010) http://www.fda.gov/Radiation-EmittingProducts/RadiationSafety/RadiationDoseReduction/ucm199994.htm#_Toc253092884. Accessed March 15

# Collective Radiation Dose from MDCT: Critical Review of Surveys Studies

Georg Stamm

## Contents




**Abstract**

Large-scale surveys were used to establish reference dose levels (RDL) for typical CT examinations. The different findings in different countries will be compared and discussed with respect to the statistical values used. While the third quartile values of surveys are well-established to define dose levels that 75% of the users can easily maintain, it has been suggested by several authors to use the first quartile value for optimization processes defining those dose levels which can be achieved using modern technique, appropriate settings for the scan parameters and good practice. Interpretation of collected data and comparison of results of several surveys will be done with a special focus on pediatric issues. While RDLs for adult have been published frequently and have also been already updated using new data from either more recent surveys or by interpreting data from smaller samples it appears that RDL for CT examination of children have been rarely addressed in the past. Only more recent publications in 2008–2010 have recognized this issue and RDL for pediatric CT exams have now been published for a larger number of countries. For a quick estimate of patient dose and risk conversion factors from dose length product (DLP) to effective dose (f in mSv/(mGy*cm)) can be used. The various published values for children of different ages will be compared with respect to limitations and in correlation with the findings for adult patients. The effectiveness of surveys regarding dose reduction and optimization has been reviewed. The main conclusion is that although RDLs for conventional X-ray



G. Stamm (✉)
Medizinische Hochschule Hannover, Institut für Diagnostische und Interventionelle Radiologie, Carl-Neuberg-Str. 1, Hannover, 30625, Germany
e-mail: stamm.georg@mh-hannover.de


D. Tack et al. (eds.), *Radiation Dose from Multidetector CT*, Medical Radiology. Diagnostic Imaging,
DOI: 10.1007/174_2011_433, 

examinations have been remarkably decreased (in mean between 30 and 35%) the RDLs for CT exams have remained nearly constant in several countries or even slightly increased. Some new approaches for automatic extraction of dose values from DICOM metadata show great potential for continuous monitoring and optimization processes once all technical restrictions are solved or simplified.

## 1 Introduction

In the past years a lot of surveys have been carried out trying to estimate not only the collective dose of CT examinations but also the effective dose for specific scan regions. Only few surveys were carried out with a large sample size [UK 1999, 2001 and 2003 (National Radiological Protection Board 1999; Hart and Wall 2001; Shrimpton et al. 2005), Germany 1992–1995, 1999, 2002 (Bernhardt et al. 1995; Galanski et al. 2001; Brix et al. 2003), Switzerland 1998 (Aroua et al. 2000, 2004) and (Treier et al. 2010) Austria 2000 (Nowotny et al. 2005) while a larger number of surveys with smaller sample sizes can be found in the literature. The later ones were often focussed either on a limited number of scanners or on small number of scanner sites. (e.g. Greece, Italy, Wales, USA). These small surveys will always contain a bias in the data because they are not representative for all scanners and sites (Hiles et al. 2001; Shrimpton et al. 1998; Goddard and Al-Farsi 1999; Papadimitriou et al. 2003; Tsapaki et al. 2001; Scheck et al. 1998; Olerud 1997, 2001, 2003; Friberg 2003; Einarsson and Magnusson 2001; van Unnik 1997; Hatziioannou et al. 2003; Tsapaki et al. 2001; Origgi et al. 2006; Szendrö et al. 1995; Tung et al. 2011; Livingstone and Dinakaran 2009; Kharita and Khazzam 2010; Muhogora et al. 2010). A comprehensive review of adult patient radiation doses from CT examinations published in the literature can be found in Pantos et al. (2011) together with a comparison with reference dose levels.

Large-scale surveys are necessary to take into account the considerable variations in patient size and differences in scan parameters and settings even within the various sites.

The NEXT (nationwide evaluation of X-ray trends) surveys in the US (see for example Conway et al. 1992 ) are carried out nearly every year and are mostly focussed on a defined body region. Although this seems to be a very promising approach for obtaining reliable data the spectrum of typical examinations is very limited; a broad overview will be available only after several years when the first surveys are already out of date.

Surveys with small sample size showing only a snapshot of the current situation using scanners of only one or two vendors can be found more frequently in the literature of medical journals, the larger surveys are all carried out on behalf of national authorities such as NRPB (National Radiological Protection Board) in UK, BfS (Bundesamt für Strahlenschutz) in Germany or BMSG (Bundesministerium für soziale Sicherheit und Gesundheit) in Austria with a typical time frame of 5–15 years between updates.

The aim of this chapter will be to compare the results of the different surveys to stress on local or national specialities. It should be a critical review on current trends and help to read and interpret the results of those surveys more carefully.

The focus will be on European surveys and show a comparison of methods, results, outcomes and conclusions. Whenever possible also a comparison of different national surveys will be made. Publications from the US and Australia will be included as examples and do not necessarily meet the requirements of completeness. Also the mentioned small-sized surveys may not show up as a complete list.

The large-sized surveys always were used as base material to establish guidelines for scan techniques and parameter settings. But what is more important for future work is to introduce guidelines for optimization. The German survey form 1999 for example was used not only to produce reliable data on patient dose from CT examinations to set up national reference dose levels for CT. It also showed the direction and hints on how to optimize scan protocols that will be discussed later on.

Another main aim for future tasks should be to define acceptable image quality in relation to patient dose. The manufacturers have already shown that there is a possibility for an automatic exposure control (AEC) in CT. But the procedures to achieve this aim are rather different. The definition of an acceptable image quality should be more uniform and applicable to all different scanner models. This is especially important because the relation of $kV_p$, image quality and dose is a very complex task. Defining image

**Table 1** Number of CT examination per year and 1,000 people (values from UNSCEAR (2000) report if not mentioned otherwise)

| | |
|---|---|
| UNSCEAR health Level 1 | 57 |
| UNSCEAR health Level 2 | 1.5 |
| Germany | 64 |
| Germany (1990–92) | 55 |
| Germany (1999) | 90 |
| UK | 21 |
| USA | 91 |
| Sweden | 39 |
| Sweden (1991) | 24 |
| Australia (1994) | 60 |
| Austria (2000) | 76 |
| Switzerland (1998) | 46 |

quality only in terms of image noise (standard deviation of HU values) does not meet all requirements. A more sophisticated approach in terms of contrast-noise-ratios (CNR) defined for the various body regions is needed, in particular for low contrast examinations such as liver and abdomen.

## 2 Reference Dose Levels (RDL)

Looking at the frequencies of CT-examinations and their contribution to the annual collective dose (Tables 1, 2, 3 and Fig. 1) it is necessary to introduce so-called reference dose levels to clearly define thresholds that can be exceeded in individual cases but should not be exceeded in general.

A lot of surveys have been carried out in the past either to establish national reference dose levels according the EU quality criteria for CT [EUR16262 (European Commission 1999)] or to check if CT procedures in the different Member States comply with the EU RDL. RDLs can and should be included in guidelines for scanning techniques. While using projection radiography the consistency between the actual dose values and the RDLs can only be checked after the examination computed tomography offers solely the possibility to check compliance prior to starting the examination. Although RDLs do not represent individual exposure to the patient they represent an estimate of the mean collective dose to the patient for the corresponding body regions (Fig. 2).

Three major dose quantities can be used to serve as RDLs: first we have the two local dose values such asweighted CTDI ($CTDI_w$) and volume CTDI ($CTDI_{vol}$). The later one can be regarded as a measure for the mean dose within an examination region and is dependent on mAs product, kV settings, distance focus-to-axis-of-rotation. The dose length product (DLP) as the third quantity is an integral dose value and depends on the correct choice of scan length. A comparison of the estimated RDLs of different several surveys can be found in Tables 4 and 5.

## 3 Statistical Values and Their Meanings

The surveys provide a lot of data on examination or scan parameters. $CTDI_w$, $CTDI_{vol}$ and DLP can be interpreted and compared in different ways. Mean values of common or often used procedures may serve for a ranking of each scanner site in comparison with the results of the survey. Median values can be used to evaluate the distribution (for example the skewness or asymmetry) of the data. The results of the German 1999 (Galanski 2001) survey showed that there is no big difference between mean and median values. Of common interest are especially the 3rd quartile values that can serve as a threshold that should not be exceeded in general. These values also provide a well-established base for defining RDLs. 3rd quartile values mean that 75% of the participating institutes and scanner sites redeem these values while only 25% have to change their protocols or procedures.

Some examples of mean dose values for the different surveys as well as 3rd quartile values are presented in Tables 6 and 7.

Interpreting the data from the German 1999 survey in more detail we have found that the 1st quartile values are a good measure for an optimization process especially for new scanners. This has often been neglected in the past. Surveys should not only delineate the present state but also show possible improvements and ameliorations.

Boxplots are an expressive and convincing representation of data from surveys. Within only one figure they show not only the sometimes large variation between minimum and maximum values but also the important statistical parameters such as mean and

**Table 2** Frequencies of different CT procedures in percent (%), total number of exams per year and scanner and number of installed CT bases (see also Fig. 1)

| | Germany (1999) (Galanski et al. 2001) | UK (1997/98) (Radiological Protection Board National 1999) | Austria (Nowotny et al. 2005) | Italy (2006) (Hatziioannou 2003) | Switzerland (1998) (Aroua et al. 2000) | Netherlands (1998) (Meeuwsen et al. 2003) | Sweden (1991) (Szendrö et al. 1995) | Australia (1994) (Thomson and Tingey 1997) |
|---|---|---|---|---|---|---|---|---|
| Brain | 37 | 44.5 | 34.9 | 39 | 24 | 39 | 53 | 30.4 |
| Chest | 15 | 13.8 | 15.3 | 17 | 14.6 | 19 | – | 8.1 |
| Abdomen | 25 | 21.4 | 26.1 | 20 | 20.4 | 28 | 25[a] | 14.6 |
| Lumbar spine | – | 4.5 | – | 10 | 11.5 | 10 | 9.6 | 12.4 |
| Pelvis | – | 10 | – | 10 | – | 3 | – | 5.9 |
| No.of exams per scanner and year | 3,600 | – | 4,560 | – | – | – | – | – |
| Installed bases | 2,000 | – | 227 | 1,328 | – | – | 90 | – |

[a] Sweden examination of the trunk

median values and the two quartile values (see Fig. 3). The large variation between minimum and maximum values (sometimes the outlier in both direction is separated by a factor of up to 30 as can be seen in Table 8 showing the range and ratios of dose values found in different surveys) should not frighten because the majority of data are distributed within a factor of 2 or 3 of the mean value (an example can be seen in Fig. 4 which shows an histogram plot of the effective dose deduced for the examination of the abdomen/pelvis examination in the German 1999 survey).

## 4 Interpretation of Data and Pitfalls

Most surveys are only local studies and not spread nationwide. Sometimes they are restricted to only a few radiological centers. Therefore the collected data may include an unbalanced bias, which can lead to misinterpretation. For example using only data from selected institutes with good radiological practice will not represent the mean of all institutes. Including only few scanners will cause a bias based on the specialties of those scanners i.e. focus-axis-distance, filtration and limited pitch values. Other scanners that do not meet those technical parameters will show up as "dose slingshots". Looking at the values of the normalized $CTDI_w$ ($_nCTDI_w$) of the example in Table 9, scanner A seems to deliver a sixfold higher dose to the patient than scanner B. After estimating the corresponding effective dose we can conclude that they are nearly the same which can be explained taking into account the mAs settings for both scanners: scanner A needs only 1/6 of the mAs settings compared with scanner B. This is also a convincing example for "mAs is not dose".

The survey in 1999 was the first study in Germany where data for all scanners from all manufacturers was collected. The quota for returned questionnaires was more than 50% so that a reasonable analysis concerning the age of the scanners, the distribution among university hospitals and private practice was possible as well as taking into account the features of the rather new scanners.

The German survey of MDCT scanners in 2002 (Brix 2003) resulted in a snapshot of the present situation. It showed that the change from SDCT to MDCT was not smooth but resulted in an increase in dose. The main reason was an inadequate use of the new technique and a lack of intensive training of the users. For the future an additional survey has to be

**Table 3** Comparison of percentage of total collective dose delivered by CT examination (see also Fig. 1)

| | Germany (1990–92) (Bernhardt et al. 1995) | Germany (1999) (Galanski 2001) | UK (1997/98) (National Radiological Protection Board 1999) | Austria (2000) (Nowotny et al. 2005) | UNSCEAR (2000) HL1 (Bundesamt für Strahlenschutz 2003) | UNSCEAR (2000) HL2 (Bundesamt für Strahlenschutz 2003) | Switzerland (1998) (Aroua et al. 2000) | Netherlands (1998) (Meeuwsen et al. 2002) | Ireland (2009) (Health Service Executive 2011) | Iceland (1998) (Einarsson and Magnusson 2001) |
|---|---|---|---|---|---|---|---|---|---|---|
| Collective dose (%) | 35 | 40 | 39.7 | 40.4 | 41 | 5 | 27.8 | 42 | 67 | 54 |
| No.of exams (%) | 4 | 6 | 3.3 | 4.2 | 6 | 1 | 3.4 | 5.8 | – | 13.6 |
| No.of exams/ year | – | $7.2 * 10^6$ | $1.39 * 10^6$ | 620,000 | – | – | 328,000 | 494,000 | 211,728 | 25,762 |

carried out on a broader base and include those scanners with more than eight detector rows (N >8).

Reference dose levels are indicated in terms of weighted CTDI ($CTDI_w$), which is a local dose value (dose per slice) and in terms of the dose length product (DLP), which is an integral dose value (dose to the patient). The 2003 UK survey (Shrimpton et al. 2005) and the EU 2004 survey on MDCT (Shrimpton 2002) and CT Quality Criteria (2004) suggested specifying RDLs in terms of volume CTDI ($CTDI_{vol}$) in order to take into account new scanner technologies and the introduction and use of so-called "effective mAs" settings. The main aim of this concept introduced by the vendors in the early stages of MDCT starting with the four-slice scanners is to keep image quality constant and independent from the chosen pitch or table feed.

This has caused some irritation among the users because they were accustomed to notice a dose reduction when using pitch values >1. This was a common well-known rule when dealing with SDCT scanner but does not apply anymore for most of the MDCT scanners. Thus the introduction of a direct dose indicator was almost mandatory to solve this problem. More recent scanner models display the $CTDI_{vol}$ directly at the operator window according the IEC Standard 60601-2-44 (International Electrotechnical Commission (IEC) 2001). This would allow a direct comparison to RDLs prior to starting the examination if the RDLs were defined in terms of $CTDI_{vol}$. Unfortunately RDLs are defined in terms of $CTDI_w$, which means that the user has to multiply the displayed value with the corresponding pitch. This simple task will become complicated if this pitch value is not displayed in figures but as in descriptive terms such as "high quality" or "high speed". This behavior has been abandoned by the vendors as well as calling the displayed $CTDI_{vol}$ weighted CTDI. But those scanners are still in operation and the user must know about these possible pitfalls.

A revision of the EU RDLs seems to be necessary because they were established before the introduction of MDCT. The update should include the new dose value $CTDI_{vol}$ so that a direct comparison with the displayed value at the operator console is possible. First values for RDLs in terms of $CTDI_{vol}$ reported in the EU 2004 survey can be found in Tables 10 and 11.

A result of the survey in Switzerland (1998) (Aroua et al. 2000) was the suggestion of an update every 5 years in a so-called "mini survey" covering

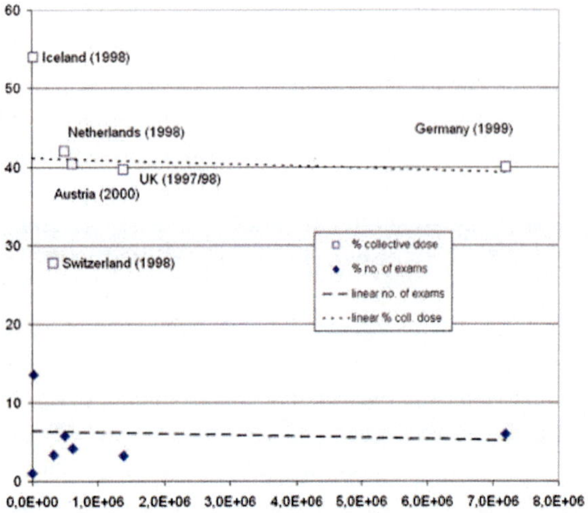


**Fig. 1** Contribution to total number of radiographic procedures and contribution to collective effective dose as a function of the total number of CT examination per year. Independent of total number of CT examinations the relative contribution to total number of radiographic procedures is about 6% while the relative contribution to collective effective dose is about 40% (see Table 2 for detail)

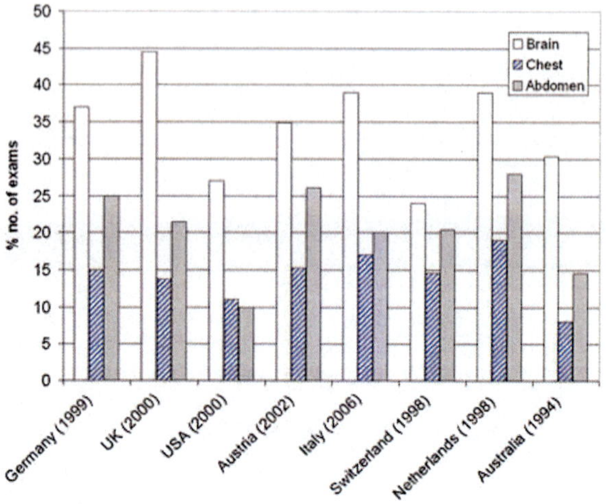


**Fig. 2** Relative distribution of the CT procedures brain, chest and abdomen in different countries

only about 10% of the volume of a complete survey. This should be sufficient for reliable data on examination frequencies and trends in dosimetric values. When looking at the rapid evolution of scanner technique this seems to be mandatory but on the other hand one has to bear in mind that a mini survey may produce only a snapshot of a rapid changing technique and usage that cannot be applied in general. The Swiss survey proposed a complete re-evaluation with the same sample size every 20 years, which is a rather long time period. But if the mini surveys produce reliable data and are focused on rapid evolving techniques it can be possible.

With regard to CT examinations, the characteristic features of the CT scanners and the optimization of examination protocols are important (number of passages, scanned volume, thickness and spacing of slices, etc.). They enable a significant reduction of the doses given (see the proposals of the recent German study).

## 5 Comparison of Different Surveys

The annual frequency of examinations, the contribution to collective dose as well as the corresponding relative numbers of examinations are presented in Tables 1, 2 and 3 and compared with the findings of the UNSCEAR report (2000). The different surveys carried out in past are listed in the Tables 4, 5 and 7 which compare the findings concerning RDLs in terms of $CTDI_w$ and DLP (Table 4 and 5). In Table 6 the mean of the different dose values including effective dose is compared while Table 7 shows the 3rd quartile that is commonly used as reference level.

The EUR16262 document introduced normalized dose values with respect to dose length product (conversion factor f = mSv/(mGy*cm)) to enable a quick and robust estimate of effective dose values. As can be seen from the figures in Table 12 these conversion factors only differ by about 10–20% among the different surveys. Different scan lengths for the listed procedures may cause these differences. As can be seen looking for example at the data from Shrimpton (whole trunk 0,015; chest 0,014; abdomen and pelvis 0,015) normalized values can be used for three anatomical regions head, neck and body, The conversion factors should be based on the phantom values of DLP and not on DLP free in air. With DLP displaying at the operator console of this value can be used for a quick evaluation of the effective dose and hence radiation exposure of the patient. Although the listed values suggest that these conversion factors may serve as a robust estimate one has always to bear in mind that those conversation factor were deduced from mean values. This means that they were averaged for all scanners and all different scan parameter

**Table 4** Comparison of reference dose levels (RDL) in terms of $CTDI_w$ (mGy) in different European countries compared with the EU directive EUR16262

| | Germany (1999)[a] (Galanski 2001) | Germany (2010)[b] (German National Radiation Protection Board 2010) | UK (2003) SSCT (Shrimpton et al. 2005) | UK (2003) MSCT (Shrimpton et al. 2005) | Austria[c] (2000) (Nowotny et al. 2005) | Syria (2009) (Kharita and Khazzam 2010) | EUR 16262 (European Commission 1999) |
|---|---|---|---|---|---|---|---|
| Routine head (brain) | 45 | 65 | 70 | 110 | 68, 9 | 60.7 | 60 |
| Face and sinuses | 25 | 20 | – | – | – | – | 35 |
| Routine chest | 13 | 12 | 13 | 18 | 18.9 | 22 | 30 |
| Chest HR | – | – | 22 | 50 | 28 | 30.5 | 35 |
| Routine abdomen | 15 | 20 | 20 | 20 | 19.8 | 24.1 | 35 |
| Liver and spleen | 15 | 20 | – | – | 20.6 | 24.1 | 35 |
| Lumbar spine | 30 | 42 | – | – | 40.7 | – | – |
| Routine pelvis | 18 | 20 | 17 | 20 | 23.5 | 27.5 | 35 |

[a] 1st quartile of the 1999 survey for comparison
[b] $CTDI_{vol}$ only as orientation not as RDL
[c] 3rd quartile of the 2000 survey

**Table 5** Comparison of reference dose levels (RDL) in terms of DLP (mGy * cm) in different European countries compared with the EU directive EUR16262

| | Germany (1999)[a] | Germany (2010)[b] | UK (2003) SSCT | UK (2003) MSCT | Austria[c] (2000) | Syria (2009) | EUR 16262 |
|---|---|---|---|---|---|---|---|
| Routine head (brain) | 520 | 950 | 760 | 930 | 1275 | 793 | 1050 |
| Face and sinuses | 190 | 250 | – | – | – | – | |
| Routine chest | 250 | 400 | 430 | 580 | 484 | 520 | 650 |
| Chest HR | – | – | 80 | 170 | 76 | 133 | 280 |
| Routine abdomen | 490 | 900 | 510 | 560 | 1109 | 721 | 780 |
| Liver and spleen | 210 | 450 | 460 | 470 | 763 | – | 900 |
| Lumbar spine | 170 | 250 | – | – | 495 | – | 800 |
| Routine pelvis | 300 | 450 | – | – | 589 | 542 | 570 |

[a] 1st quartile of the 1999 survey for comparison
[b] DLP per series
[c] 3rd quartile of the 2000 survey

settings (such as $kV_p$, mAs, scan length, slice and section thickness, pitch). So these values should and can be used whenever a quick estimate of effective dose is necessary. But one has to keep in mind that this is only a rough estimate and does not take into account gonads. For the neck region two values have to be considered, depending on whether body or head mode is used during the scan. And they should never

**Table 6** Mean dose values.

| | Germany (1999) (Galanski et al. 2001) | | | Germany (2002) (Brix et al. 2003) | | | Greece (2002) (Shrimpton et al. 1998) | | | Italy (2002) (Papadimitriou et al. 2003) | | | Italy (2006) (Origgi et al. 2006) | | UK (2003) (Shrimpton et al. 2005) | | |
|---|---|---|---|---|---|---|---|---|---|---|---|---|---|---|---|---|---|
| Region | $CTDI_w$ | DLP | E | $CTDI_w$ | DLP | E | $CTDI_w$ | DLP | E | $CTDI_w$ | DLP | E | $CTDI_w$ | E | $CTDI_w$ | DLP | E |
| Brain | 57 | 676 | 1.8 | 58.4 | 1016 | 2.8 | 68 | 919 | 2.1 | 59 | 707 | 1.6 | 59.6 | 1.7 | 57 | 690 | 1.5 |
| Upper adomen | 21 | – | – | – | – | – | 23 | 493 | 7.4 | 23 | 632 | 8.3 | 24.3 | 7.8 | 16 | 350 | 5.3 |
| Abdomen and pelvis | 21 | 770 | 13 | 15.6 | 790 | 14.4 | – | – | – | – | – | – | – | – | 16 | 470 | 7.1 |
| Pelvis | 23 | 480 | 8 | 17.1 | 398 | 7.2 | 27 | 540 | 10.3 | 24 | 434 | 8.2 | 24.9 | 8.9 | – | – | – |
| Chest | 18 | 420 | 6.5 | 14.8 | 350 | 5.7 | 21 | 430 | 7.3 | 21 | 480 | 6.2 | 19.7 | 8.0 | 14 | 400 | 5.8 |
| Lumb.spine | 39 | 230[a] | 2.8 | 30.3 | 445[b] | 8.1 | 39 | 470[b] | – | 36 | 303[c] | 4.7 | 34.1 | 4.5 | – | – | – |
| Sample size (sites) | 850 | | | 113 | | | 14 | | | 32 | | | 56 | | 118 | | |
| % of inst.bases | 45 | | | 50 | | | – | | | – | | | – | | 25 | | |

| | Austria (2000) | | | Switzerland (1998) (Aroua et al. 2000) | Oman (1999) (Hiles et al. 2001) | Iceland (1998) (van Unnik 1997) | Australia (1994) (Thomson and Tingey 1997) | Wales (1999) (Hiles et al. 2001) | |
|---|---|---|---|---|---|---|---|---|---|
| Region | $CTDI_w$ | DLP | E | E | E | E | E | $CTDI_w$ | DLP |
| Brain | 57.7 | 1,036 | 2.25 | 2.4 | 2.4 | 1.3 | 2.4 | 46 | 731 |
| Upper adomen | 17.5 | 877 | 14.7 | 10.3 | 9.5 | 13.2 | – | 22 | 745 |
| Abdomen + pelvis | – | – | – | – | – | – | 16.7 | – | – |
| Pelvis | 20.2 | 487 | 8.0 | 7.3 | – | 6.1 | 11.2 | 23 | 646 |
| Chest | 16.2 | 400 | 6.7 | 9.0 | 3.4 | 8.5 | 10.4 | 17 | 663 |
| Lumb.spine | 35.5 | 407 | 6.2 | 9.4 | – | | 12.4 | – | – |
| Sample size (sites) | 130 | | | – | 6 | 4 | 182 | 18 | |
| % of inst.bases | 57 | | | – | – | 80 | 55 | – | |

| | Nordic Pilot survey (2001) (Olerud et al. 2001) | | | Norway (1993) (Olerud 1997) | Sweden (1991) (Szendrö et al. 1995) |
|---|---|---|---|---|---|
| Region | $CTDI_w$ | DLP | E | E | E |
| Brain | 60 | 740 | 1.7 | 2.0 | 2.1 |
| Upper adomen | – | – | – | 12.8 | |
| Abdomen + pelvis | – | – | – | – | 10[d] |

(continued)

**Table 6** (continued)

| | Nordic Pilot survey(2001) (Olerud et al. 2001) | | | Norway(1993) (Olerud 1997) | Sweden(1991) (Szendrö et al. 1995) |
|---|---|---|---|---|---|
| Pelvis | – | – | – | 9.8 | – |
| Chest | 10.8 | 420 | 7.1 | 11.5 | – |
| Lumb.spine | 40 | 420 | 7.9 | 4.6 | 6 |
| Sample size (sites) | 25 | | | 49 | 90 |
| % of inst.bases | – | | | 50 | 100 |

Comparison of different surveys ($CTDI_w$ (mGy), dose length product DLP (mGy * cm) and effective dose E (mSv) for whole examination; DLP and E are mean values for male and female)

[a] Only one segment (= 6 cm scan length)

[b] Multiple segments

[c] Mean scan length 3.6 cm

[d] Sweden examination of the trunk

be used to compare different scanners because even if scan parameters are nearly identical other dose-influencing factors may differ. This includes focus-to-axis distance, beam filtration and beam shaper.

The main limitation of surveys is the quality of the reported data. It is necessary to check the returned questionnaires whether the scan parameters seem to be reasonable or not. In case of any doubts a validity check has to be made for the reported values of the scan parameters. The survey in Germany showed that the more complex the task of the survey is the more difficulties arise with the data quality. While the 1999 survey on single slice scanners was rather easy to set up and carry out the MSCT survey in 2002 was much more complex. Therefore it was necessary to distribute a manual on how to collect the necessary data. The survey on pediatric examinations started in 2006 was once again more complex for the user and also for the conductors of the survey. A lot of queries were necessary to improve the reported data. In the future these tasks will become more and more complex because scanning techniques and scanner techniques are rapidly changing and the differences in the user interfaces of different scanners are getting wider and wider. This means that for large-scale surveys one has to supply "translation tables" for each scanner family in order to help the user to spot the relevant and necessary data.

Some limitations and main findings of the different surveys are summarized in the following short quotations.

The survey in Iceland (IRPI) (Einarsson and Magnusson 2001) listed only of five CT bases and found an increase in number of CT exams from 1993 to 1998 by about 93%. The main conclusion was that "*…efforts to reduce dose should include optimization of both how CT examinations are performed and the criteria for requesting them*". This statement although deduced from a very small survey holds for every survey and will be discussed in a special section at the end of this chapter.

The Nordic survey (presented at the IAEA meeting in Malaga, Spain) (Olerud et al. 2001) included only five sites from each of the five countries (Denmark, Finland, Iceland, Norway and Sweden) and found that "*This Nordic pilot project shows that the EC quality criteria can be used as a collaborative inspection tool. However, the radiologists work within their own reference frames. That introduces a bias, and the*

**Table 7** 3rd quartile dose values.

| Region | Germany (1999) | | | Germany MSCT (2002) | | | Italy (2006) | | | UK (2003)[c] | | Syria (2009) | | Austria (2000) | | |
|---|---|---|---|---|---|---|---|---|---|---|---|---|---|---|---|---|
| | $CTDI_w$ | DLP | E | $CTDI_w$ | DLP | E | $CTDI_w$ | DLP | E | $CTDI_w$ | DLP | $CTDI_w$ | DLP | $CTDI_w$ | DLP | E |
| Brain | 66 | 783 | 2.2 | 76 | 1,149 | 3.3 | 68.7 | 915 | 2.1 | 66 | 784 | 60.7 | 793 | 57.7 | 1,036 | 2.25 |
| Upper adomen | – | – | – | – | – | – | 25.6 | 602 | 9.1 | 20 | 477 | 24.1 | 721 | 17.5 | 877 | 14.7 |
| Abdomen and pelvis | 24 | 941 | 15.7 | 18 | 1.029 | 18.9 | – | – | – | 19 | 534 | – | – | – | – | – |
| Pelvis | 28 | 603 | 10.3 | 20 | 455 | 8.3 | 28.9 | 501 | 9.5 | – | – | 27.5 | 542 | 20.2 | 487 | 8.0 |
| Chest | 22 | 540 | 8.2 | 20 | 442 | 7.2 | 25 | 627 | 10.7 | 15 | 488 | 22 | 520 | 16.2 | 400 | 6.7 |
| Lumb.spine | 47 | 319[a] | 3.1 | 39 | 575[b] | 10.3 | 41.7 | 367 | 6.2 | – | – | | | 35.5 | 407 | 6.2 |
| Sample size (sites) | 850 | | | 113 | | | 29 | | | 118 | | 30 | | 130 | | |
| % of inst.bases | 45 | | | 50 | | | | | | 25 | | 11.8 | | 57 | | |

Comparison of different surveys (CTDIw, dose length product DLP and effective dose E for whole examination; DLP and E are mean values for male and female)
[a] Only one segment (= 6 cm scan length)
[b] Multiple segments
[c] Values are for all scanners (SSCT and MSCT)

*survey design is not suitable for ranking*". These findings show that small surveys are often not suitable to represent the mean values for a whole country.

The main difficulty when comparing different surveys is that the setup of the surveys is often rather different. In some countries examination of the abdomen means whole abdomen in other it just means upper abdomen. Additionally also the definition of series is often quite different. In Germany for example examinations of the abdomen are mostly carried out as biphasic examinations while for the NRPB surveys only one series was taken into account.

Another difficulty is that dose values are calculated on base of axial examinations while other surveys use already spiral examinations. In the German 1999 survey (National Radiological Protection Board 1999) we tried to compare our data with data from 1999 NRPB survey (Galanski 2001). The differences found could be explained with different use of scan ranges and spiral technique.

## 6 Surveys Comparing MDCT and SDCT

When the first four slice scanners were established in the beginning of 2000 the reported dose values increased by a factor of 4 compared with those of single slice scanners. This behavior and the dramatic increase in dose to the patient were mainly a result of an inadequate experience of the users with these new technical possibilities. New concepts introduced by the vendors such as effective mAs and its influence on dose values were not sufficiently communicated to the users. In combination with the possibility of acquiring more and thinner slices this lead to the reported increase in dose. Now the users are more experienced and know how to deal with thin slices, the post-processing technique of image processing has improved and hence modern MSCT scanners should deliver a dose to the patient that is comparable to modern single slice scanners.

One main reason presented at the 2003 symposium on Radiation Protection of the North West RP Societies in Utrecht was: "*It has to be emphasized that the comparison of the dose data collected from the three time periods, reflecting the different CT scanner generations, is rough since the medical indications were not identical. The huge variation in doses for the*

**Table 8** Range and ratios of dose values found in serveral surveys.which indicates that there are possibilities of remarquable dose reductions

| | Germany (1999) (Galanski et al. 2001) | | | | UK[a] (1998) (National Radiological Protection Board 1999) | | EU 2004 $Q_C$ (CT Quality Criteria 2004) | | Norway (1993) (Olerud 1997) | Australia (1994) (Thomson and Tingey 1997) |
|---|---|---|---|---|---|---|---|---|---|---|
| | $CTDI_w$ (mGy) min (max) | DLP (mGy*cm) min (max) | E (mSv) min (max) | $E^b$ | $CTDI_w$ (mGy) Min (Max) | DLP (mGy * cm) min (max) | DLP (mGy * cm) | $E^b$ | $E^b$ | $E^b$ |
| Head | 14 (199) | 173 (2384) | 0.4 (14.5) | 36 | 21 (130) | 231 (2.087) | 204 (2.805) | 11.7 | 8 | 29 |
| Chest | 5.5 (66) | 100 (1766) | 1.35 (26.4) | 21 | 4 (46.4) | 72 (1.304) | 61 (1.322) | 14.4 | 19.5 | 64 |
| Abdomen and pelvis | 7.4 (66) | 105 (2767) | 2 (51.1) | 26 | 6.8 (46.4) | 115 (1.874) | 140 (1.475) | 10.6 | 13.3 | 25 |
| Pelvis | 6.9 (56.2) | 90 (1349) | 1.6 (23) | 14 | 6.8 (55.2) | 68 (1324) | – | – | 17.2 | 18 |
| Lumb.Spine | 9.4 (94.1) | 29 (821) | 0.35 (10.4) | 30 | – | – | – | – | – | – |

[a] Values were used for the European EU16262EN quality criteria

[b] Min/max ratio

[c] Head/cranium: acute stroke, chest: pulmonary embolism, abdomen/pelvis: rule out abscess [32]

**Table 9** Comparison of normalized $CTDI_w$, resulting effective dose and corresponding mAs settings for a male patient undergoing a CT examination of the abdomen

| Scanner | ${}_nCTDI_w$ (mGy/mAs) | E (mSv) | mAs |
|---|---|---|---|
| A | 0.25 | 7.3 | 74 |
| B | 0.043 | 7.9 | 267 |

*same medical indications indicates a potential for optimization of CT protocols in Norwegian hospitals. The best parameters to report for dose comparison would be $CTDI_{vol}$ and the total DLP* (Olerud)". This statement shows one of the main difficulties when comparing dose values from SDCT and MDCT. With the introduction of MDCT the indications for examination change and sometimes the adaptation of scan protocols does not change accordingly. If indications change with new scanner technology then exposure of the patient is really hard to compare. For example if combined protocols are possible with MDCT-like chest and abdomen or abdomen and pelvis or even chest and abdomen and pelvis it is hard to compare with SDCT examinations of only one of the mentioned regions. What is possible is to check whether the local dose values in the specified regions are nearly the same. Therefore the introduction of the $CTDI_{vol}$ as an average dose within a CT slice was important. This dose value reflects to some extent the scanner technology (detector efficiency) and the selected scan parameters ($kV_p$, mAs, pitch, etc.). The total dose for an examination as represented by the DLP reflects the scan length and number of series taken. Thus only examinations for nearly the same combination of scan regions can be compared. Nevertheless DLP is good and quick estimate of dose to the patient.

Also the German 2002 survey on MDCT (Brix et al. 2003) showed that the introduction of new scanner technologies first led to an increase in patient dose. After users had realized the pitfalls of the new

**Table 10** Median results of the 2004 survey on MSCT (CT Quality Criteria 2004) compared with the initial EUR16262 values (European Commission 1999)

| | $CTDI_{vol}$ [mGy] | DLP [mGy * cm] | E [mSv] | QC Criterion $CTDI_{vol}$ | EUR16262 $CTDI_w$ | EUR16262 DLP |
|---|---|---|---|---|---|---|
| Cranium[a] | 53 | 746 | 1.7 | 60 | 60 | 1050 |
| Chest, HR | 3 | 117 | 2.5 | 10 | 15 | 280 |
| Chest, pulm. embol. | 11 | 302 | 5.9 | 10 | 30 | 650 |
| Abdomen, rule out abscess | 11 | 551 | 9.3 | 15 | 35 | 780 |
| Abdomen, liver metastases | 13 | 643 | 9.5 | 25 | 35 | 900 |

[a] Cranium: acute stroke

technique the potential of the new technique dose values could be reduced to the same level as estimated in the 1999 survey of SDCT. This was mainly caused by new displaying modalities. Trading off the potential of MDCT means using thin slices whenever possible and/or rapid scanning of the selected region. Unfortunately thin slices always cause an increased noise in the resulting images because less photons reach the detectors and hence signal-to-noise ratios decrease. With the introduction of MDCT this lead to a pronounced increase in patient dose (factor of 2–4 compared with reported dose values for SDCT). Contemporary with the MDCT technique also the viewing technique or post processing of the image data improved rapidly. This allowed new so-called display modalities for diagnosis. The availability of thin slab technique allows the combination of several adjacent slices either by simply averaging or by a more sophisticated processing such as MIP (maximum intensity projection). This processing reduces image noise while keeping spatial resolution nearly constant. This was the main improvement for overcoming the dose trap of thin slices. Thus both scanning technique and review technique have changed and are used and trained to acquire thin slices with a dose to patient that is nearly identical. The ideal procedure is to scan the anatomical region with thin slices and to look at the resulting thin slice data set as a so-called secondary raw data set, which will be used for display.

Within the framework of the EU 2004 survey on MDCT(Shrimpton 2002) and (CT Quality Criteria 2004) only 53 questionnaires were evaluated. For examinations of the cranium the reported CTDI values and the 3rd quartile of the evaluated DLP were of the same order of magnitude compared with the RDL from EUR16242 ($CTDI_w = 60$ mGy, DLP = 1050 mGy * cm, see Tables 10 and 11).

For chest HR examinations the findings showed that "*the observed ratio of 5, 6 for 75-percentile and the 25-percentile of the effective dose indicates substantial interdepartmental variations in technique and suggests the potential for optimization* (Shrimpton 2002)".

As a conclusion the survey suggested that an evidence for an optimization could be deduced if "*a high ratio (> 3) between 75-percentile and 25-percentile indicates substantial variations in scan parameters and technique among the departments and suggests the need for protocol optimization* (Shrimpton 2002)".

In the German 2002 MDCT survey the reported increase in the local dose value $CTDI_{vol}$ was 17–60% compared with the single- and dual-slice systems.

The scan length increased with regard to examinations of the spine system up to 160% mainly caused by scanning the whole lumbar or cervical spine region instead of only a few segments. "*In general, however, the danger of an uncontrolled increase of patient exposure due to CT procedures has to be limited by a clear medical justification in each individual case, independent of whether a standard examination is carried out or a new MDCT application such as coronary angiography, coronary calcium scoring or virtual colonoscopy* (Brix et al. 2003)".

## 7 Pediatric Issues

Only few efforts have been made to estimate dose values to pediatric patients and to establish separate RDLs. This is a very important task because dose when using the same settings as for adults in children

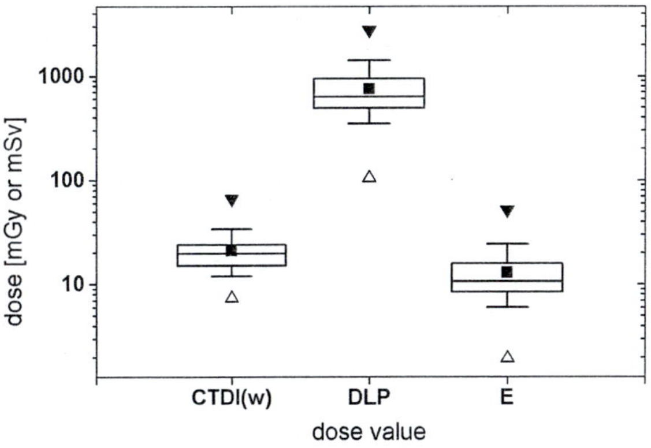


**Fig. 3** Boxplot of estimated dose values for examination "abdomen and pelvis". Reported values show a range of 30. Figure taken from the results of the German 1999 survey (Galanski et al. 2001)

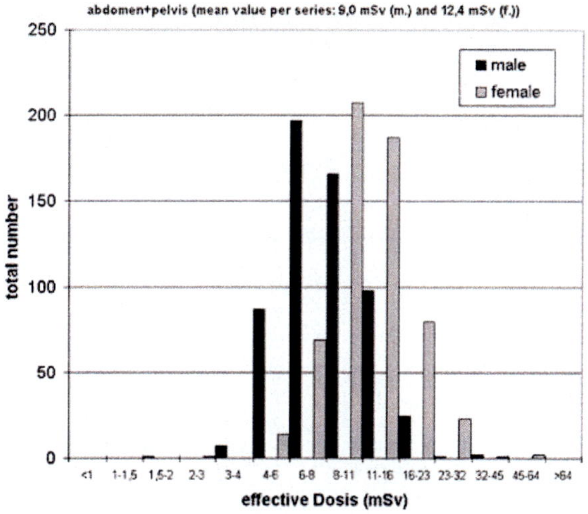


**Fig. 4** Distribution of effective dose for examination "abdomen and pelvis". Mean values were 9,0 mSv for male and 12,4 mSv for female. Figure taken from the results of the German 1999 survey (Galanski et al. 2001)

it results in a twofold to fourfold higher dose and hence a higher risk for radiation-induced cancer (Brenner et al. 2001). The diameters of small patients especially children are much smaller than those of standard sized adults. Also the dose-related risk is 2–3 times higher than that of an adult. A promising task would be to reduce dose (mAs settings of a specific scanner) by a factor corresponding to either size dependent or weight dependent. Some examples are given in Chapple et al. (2002), Vock (2005), Khurrsheed et al. (2002), Cody et al. (2004) , Pages et al. (2003), Boone et al. (2003), Paterson et al. (2001), Linton and Mettle(2003), Sandstede 2003; Verdun et al. (2004), Hollingsworth et al. (2003), Shrimpton and Wall (2000), Brenner et al. (2001), Donnelly et al. (2001), Suess and Chen (2002), Huda (2002).

While a lot of surveys have been carried out to establish reference dose values for adult only little effort has been made on searching for RDLs for children. The first survey covering especially values for children was the UK 2003 review published as NRPB-W67 (Shrimpton et al. 2005) (results for RDL values are presented in Table 15) and a national conference on dose reduction CT with emphasis on pediatric patients (Linton and Mettler 2003).

The assessment of effective dose for pediatric CT is particularly complicated. The EU 2004 survey introduced the concept of geometric scaling factors, conversions factors and pediatric enhancement factors to calculate effective dose from DLP values. The 3rd quartile values for the estimated $CTDI_{vol}$, DLP and effective dose in head and chest examinations can be found in Table 13 together with the corresponding values for adults. "*Effective doses are of the same order of magnitude when compared to values for the adult CT head acquisition (acute stroke). It seems feasible to restrict effective dose to about 1 mSv. Chest: The observed variations in CTDI and effective dose are substantial and they suggest a realistic potential for dose reduction* (Shrimpton 2002; CT Quality Criteria 2004)".

The survey also showed that there is a good agreement between effective dose and dose length product "*The linear relationship is expressed as conversion coefficients for the calculation of effective dose from dose length product* (Shrimpton 2002; CT Quality Criteria 2004)".

In Table 13 those normalized dose values are presented and compared with the values for adult (see also Table 12). To apply those values for dose estimation is rather simple and robust but does not include variations depending on scanner characteristics. The error when estimating dose values can be very large when the scanners have for example a different focus-axis-distance or different filtration. Thus calculated values should serve only as a rough estimate.

The values of Shrimpton (Shrimpton and Wall 2000) and Quality Criteria (2004) seem to be higher than estimated by Chapple et al. (2002) [with the

**Table 11** 2004 Quality Criteria MSCT versus SSCT (www.msct.info) (CT Quality Criteria 2004)

| | SSCT/CTDI$_w$ (mGy) | MSCT/CTDI$_{vol}$ (mGy) | Remarks |
|---|---|---|---|
| Cranium (acute stroke) | 60 | 60 | Pitch 1 or contigous scan |
| Chest HR | 35 | 10 | |
| Chest (pulm. embol. and pulm. metastases) | 30 | 10 | Pitch >1 |
| Abdomen/pelvis (rule out abscess) | 35 | 15 | |
| -(liver metastases) | 35 | 25 | |
| -(urolithiasis) | 35 | 10 | |

**Table 12** Normalized values of effective dose per dose length product (f = E/DLP in mSv/mGy * cm) for various body regions

| | Shrimpton (2004) (Shrimpton et al. 2005) | Italy (2006) (Origgi et al. 2006) | EUR16262 (European Commission 1999) | Germany (1999) (Galanski et al. 2001) | Germany (2002) (rix et al. B2003) | EU 2004[a] (CT Quality Criteria 2004) |
|---|---|---|---|---|---|---|
| Head and neck | 0.0031 | – | – | 0.0039 | 0.0038 | – |
| Head | 0.0021 | 0.0024 | 0.0023 | 0.0028 | 0.0028 | 0.0023 |
| Neck | 0.0059 | 0.0052 | 0.0054 | 0.0098 | 0.0061 | – |
| Chest | 0.014 | 0.0163 | 0.017 | 0.0154 | 0.0016 | 0.019 |
| Abdomen and pelvis | 0.015 | 0.0149 | 0.015 | 0.0174 | 0.0186 | 0,017 |
| Lumb. Spine | – | 0.0166 | – | 0.0125 | 0.0185 | – |
| Pelvis | – | 0.0175 | 0.019 | 0.0171 | 0.0185 | 0.017 |
| Trunk | 0.015 | – | – | – | 0.0177 | – |

Values from both German surveys based on mean values for E and DLP
[a] Cranium: acute stroke, chest: pulmonary embolism, abdomen/pelvis: rule out abscess

**Table 13** 75-percentiles of dose values for children and adult (from 2004 Quality criteria www.msct.info) (CT Quality Criteria 2004)

| Children | CTDI$_{vol}$ (mGy) | DLP (mGy*cm) | E (mSv) | Remarks |
|---|---|---|---|---|
| Head 1–12 month | 31 | 333 | 2.6 | |
| Head 4–6 years | 47 | 374 | 1.8 | |
| Chest 1–12 month | 5.8 | 78 | 5.9 | |
| Chest 4–6 years | 6.2 | 76 | 3.4 | |
| Adult | | | | |
| Head | 72 | 945 | 2.1 | Acute stroke |
| Chest | 14 | 549 | 8.4 | Pulm. embol. |

exception of values for the head for neonates]. Thus values of Shrimpton can be regarded as conservative values to estimate radiation dose using conversion factors. Values of Chapple were derived from measurements using pediatric anthropomorphic phantoms (thermo-luminescent dosimeters TLDs loaded inside and on the surface of the five phantoms). There may be a large uncertainty related with the fact that there are only two scanners included in this estimation. A graphical representation of those normalized effective dose values (conversion factors E/DLP in mSv/(mGy * cm) can be found in Fig. 5 (Fig. 5a

**Table 14** Normalized values of effective dose per dose length product (f = E/DLP in mSv/mGy * cm) for various body regions and patient ages (see also Fig. 5 a + b)

| | a | b | c | a | b | c | a | b | c | a | b | c | b | a | EUR 16262 | Germany (1999) |
|---|---|---|---|---|---|---|---|---|---|---|---|---|---|---|---|---|
| Age in years | 0 | | | 1 | | | 5 | | | 10 | | | 15 | Adult | Adult | Adult |
| Head and neck | 0.013 | – | – | 0.0085 | – | – | 0.0057 | – | – | 0.0042 | – | – | – | 0.0031 | – | 0.0039 |
| Head | 0.011 | 0.027 | 0.013 | 0.0067 | 0.008 | 0.008 | 0.004 | 0.004 | 0.005 | 0.0032 | 0.003 | 0.004 | – | 0.0021 | 0.0023 | 0.0028 |
| Neck | 0.017 | – | 0.023 | 0.012 | – | 0.015 | 0.011 | – | 0.010 | 0.0079 | – | 0.007 | – | 0.0059 | 0.0054 | 0.0098 |
| Chest | 0.039 | 0.034 | 0.057 | 0.026 | 0.022 | 0.038 | 0.018 | 0.014 | 0.026 | 0.013 | 0.011 | 0.019 | 0.01 | 0.014 | 0.017 | 0.0154 |
| Abdomen and pelvis | 0.049 | 0.043 | 0.050 | 0.030 | 0.019 | 0.031 | 0.020 | 0.013 | 0.021 | 0.015 | 0.011 | 0.015 | 0.01 | 0.015 | 0.015 | 0.0174 |
| Pelvis | – | 0.037 | – | – | 0.027 | – | – | 0.018 | – | – | 0.017 | – | 0.01 | – | 0.019 | 0.0171 |
| Trunk | 0.044 | – | 0.049 | 0.028 | – | 0.031 | 0.019 | – | 0.021 | 0.014 | – | 0.015 | – | 0.015 | – | – |

Data from UK 2003 (Shrimpton 2002), Shrimpton 2004 (Shrimpton et al. 2005) and EU MDCT Quality Criteria (CT Quality Criteria 2004)
Data from Chapple et al. (2002)
Data from Alesso and Phillips (2010)

shows the values for head examination, Fig. 5b for examination of the abdomen) together with the values for adult according the EUR16262 document and the results from the German 1999 survey.

In Germany the national authorities (BfS) initiated a survey at the end of 2005 to get reliable data on scan protocols for children helping to establish RDLs for children. This work started with a survey on age distribution and frequencies of pediatric CT examinations. After identifying those institutes with at least 100 pediatric CT examinations per year these institutes were included in a second survey to gather the data for the scan protocols of five most carried out type of examinations. The first results show that the distribution of pediatric CT examinations is by about 1–2% of all CT examinations. This may be true only for Germany so each country has to check the annual rate of pediatric CT examinations. It also turned out that the main indications for pediatric CT are examinations of the head/brain, chest, abdomen, NHH and spine. These findings compare with a recent study in Japan (Ono et al. 2011) where also head scans were identified as the most frequent CT examination. In contrast to the German findings, however, the frequency of CT-scanned body regions was highest for children in the age between 0 and 4 years.

A Nordic pediatric CT Survey was on going from 2005 to 2006; the survey focused on the scan regions such as brain, chest, abdomen and whole body which should be the main examinations carried out in pediatric CT as was already shown in the preliminary results of the German pediatric survey.

Those surveys are absolutely necessary because we have only few reliable data on dose of the patient for pediatric CT examinations. There are a lot of suggestions on minimizing radiation dose to children but those papers are not suitable to establish RDLs for children. Some strategies should be mentioned as follows:

Donnelly et al. 2001 suggested an adaptation of the tube current for pediatric patients according to the weight. Other authors (Boone et al. 2003; Verdun et al. 2004) recommended a matching according to patient circumference or diameter. Hollingsworth et al. (2003) focus on the $kV_p$ settings that should and can be lowered to 100 $kV_p$ or even 80 $kV_p$ for small children, "*Kilo-voltage of 120 may not be the optimal level for examining infants*".

**Table 15** pediatric reference dose levels from UK 2003 (Shrimpton) and Germany 2005/2006 (Galanski et al. 2006) survey

| Year | $CTDI_w$ (mGy) | $CTDI_{vol}$ (mGy) | | DLP (mGy*cm) | | E (mSv) [a] |
|---|---|---|---|---|---|---|
| | | UK | Germany[b] | UK | Germany[b] | |
| Head 0–1 | 35 | 35 | 27–33 | 270 | 300 | 2.5 |
| Head 5 | 50 | 50 | 40 | 470 | 500 | 1.5 |
| Head 10 | 65 | 65 | 50 | 620 | 650 | 1.6 |
| Chest 0–1 | 23 | 12 | 3–4 | 200 | 60 | 6.3 |
| Chest 5 | 20 | 13 | 7 | 230 | 130 | 3.6 |
| Chest 10 | 26 | 20 | 10 | 370 | 230 | 3.9 |
| Abdomen 0–1 | | | 5–7 | | 170 | |
| Abdomen 5 | | | 12 | | 330 | |
| Abdomen 10 | | | 16 | | 500 | |

[a] Mean values
[b] Published 2010 (German National Radiation Protection Board)

Suess and Chen (2002) suggest an adaptation of dose by changing the mAs-settings in relation to settings for adult. For examinations of the head they propose a variation with age (<6 month = 25%, >6 years = 100%), while for body protocols the variation should be done according to patient weight (<15 kg = 15%, >54 kg = 100%). Also defining a patient equivalent diameter can be used to set dose reduction factors (relative mAs-settings) with respect to a 28 cm patient diameter. According to Boone et al. (2003) this dose reduction factor may vary from 0.05 = 5% for a diameter of 12 cm (circumference = 38 cm) to 3.5 = 350% for a diameter of 35 cm.

The 16 cm CTDI phantom is not suitable to estimate/measure CTDI for new borns and children. As the displayed $CTDI_{vol}$ and DLP values at the operator console are based on phantom values for a 16 cm, a 32 cm phantom will be too high and cannot serve as a dose constraint with regard to RDLs.

When looking at survey data from UK 2003 (Shrimpton et al. 2005) and the MDCT quality criteria 2004 (Shrimpton; CT Quality Criteria 2004) there seems to at least a factor of 2 between the reference dose levels for adult and children. Thus more sophisticated surveys are necessary to define those RDLs and the corresponding image quality. Should the noise level for adults and children be the same when defining RDLs or do we have to deal with a lot of examinations where the detection of low contrast lesions is not of primary interest and importance?

The estimated values from the German 2005/2006 pediatric survey have been published as RDLs in 2010 and are listed for comparison in Table 15. A recent publication (Muhogora 2010) reported dose values for pediatric CT exams in 19 developing countries. The presented values for chest ($CTDI_w$ = 8.7–10.4 mGy, DLP = 153–194 mGy *cm) and abdomen ($CTDI_w$ = 8.5–13.8 mGy, DLP = 180–413 mGy *cm) are in good agreement with the dose values for 5 and 10 years old children in Table 15.

## 8 Optimization Processes

The main question remaining is how to change scanning protocols to meet the requirements of RDLs? As a result of the German 1999 survey the steps for an optimization process have been defined and reported (Nagel 2010).

This more practical guideline can serve as a first step to adjust scan parameters.

CT is a radiological procedure that has enough possibility for dose reduction although some efforts have already been made. The 3rd quartile values deduced from the different surveys can only serve as a first attempt of dose optimization. Users of older single slice scanners should redeem these values while users of modern single slice and multi slice scanners should follow the 1st quartile values for an optimization process. This approach has also been

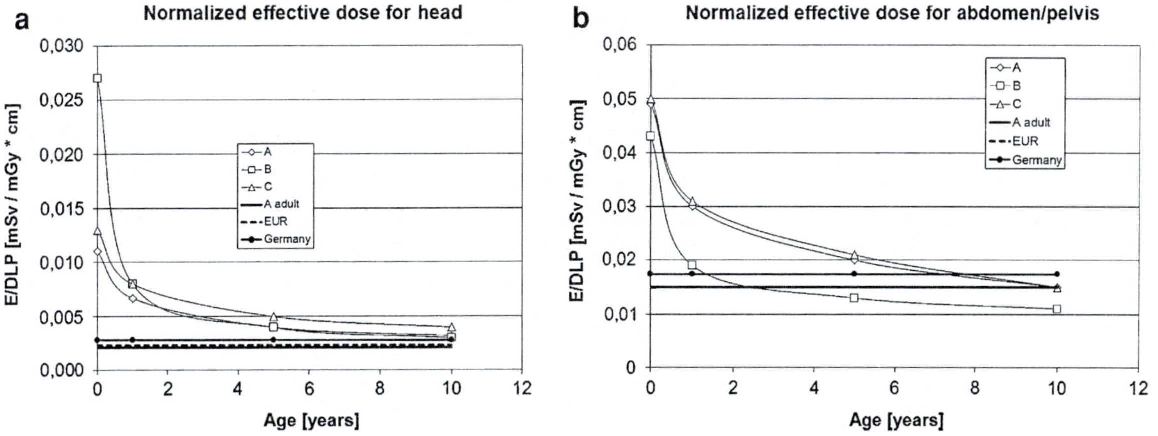


**Fig. 5** Normalized effective dose as a function of patient age for head (**a**) and abdomen/pelvis (**b**) region according to Table 14 with curve (A) representing data from UK 2003 (Shrimpton 2002), Shrimpton 2004 (Shrimpton et al. 2005) and EU MDCT Quality Criteria (2004), (B) data from Chapple et al.(2002) and (C) data from Alesso and Phillips (2010). Also included for reference are the values from the EUR16262 document and the German 1999 survey

mentioned in a recent survey and audit process in Switzerland (Treier et al. 2010) which shows that further reduction of patient doses is possible and is not bound to the 3rd quartile values.

The so-called achievable doses' mentioned in the 1999 NRBP vol. 10 document (National Radiological Protection Board 1999) are typically a factor of 2 or 3 lower than the RDLs. Dose optimization with respect to $CTDI_w$ will be mainly based on a reduction of the mAs settings. With respect to dose length product DLP the optimization has to be made on pitch factor and scan length or even on number of series. These scan parameters and their modifications are well known to radiologist and radiographers. Hence restricting scan length to the region of interest is the easiest way to avoid unnecessary radiation exposure of the patients.

Starting point for additional dose optimization should be the examination of the abdomen and pelvis. The first reason is that this examination is related with a high integral exposition, on the other hand there are high requirements for the image quality especially low contrast resolution.

Examinations with almost the same requirements for image quality and/or absorption should be done with the same values for $CTDI_w/CTDI_{vol}$. This holds for example for liver and kidney or for the abdominal aorta or head and neck.

The lower absorption in the chest region allows an obvious dose reduction compared to the values for the abdomen especially when using a wide window for image display ("lung/chest window"). To assure an adequate representation of the medastinum and tips of the lung, the adaptation should not be lower than half of the values for the abdomen. This also holds for the examinations of the thoracic aorta and the pulmonary vessels. For distinct high contrast examinations of the chest a reduction to 1/10 of the $CTDI_w$ value for the abdomen is possible. But this should be created as a special scanning protocol. Examinations of the pelvis are also related to a higher inherent contrast and allow a dose reduction to 2/3 of the $CTDI_w$ value of the abdomen. This also holds for an examination of the whole trunk.

## 9 Effectiveness of Surveys Regarding Dose Reduction and Optimization

Comparing the updates of national RDLs in Germany (Bundesamt für Strahlenschutz 2003; German National Radiation Protection Board 2010) and Switzerland (Aroua 2004; Treier 2010) it is interesting to note that there seems to be no great changes and dose reductions concerning CT examinations. While the RDL values for conventional X-ray examinations have been lowered by in mean 30–35%, the corresponding values for CT are more or less the same or have even increased (e.g. in Germany the DLP for abdomen with two series was 1,500 mGy*cm in 2003 and is 1,800 mGy*cm in 2010). Potential effects of surveys and RDLs can only be achieved if either optimization processes become mandatory, e.g. defining the 1st quartile as "good practice" and leaving the RDL (3rd quartile) as limit for "malpractice" or by coupling the participation in surveys or audit processes to reimbursements of health insurances.

The complexity of dose CT data collection for large patient samples has been addressed in a recent paper by Jahnen et al. (2011). A more or less automatized data collection is necessary and has been already proofed for smaller sample sizes. In Germany a similar discussion has been started by the control boards (so called "Ärztliche Stellen") for checking image quality, compliance with national RDLs and justification of X-ray examinations including CT. The check is up to now done manually on a regular time scale for every 2 years. If RDLs are exceeded frequently by the users and cannot be explained for example with an abnormal distribution of patient constitution the control board will not only remind the user of his malpractice and monitor whether the proposed improvements have been established but is also obliged to inform legal authorities. To simplify this time consuming process a project for automatic data extraction from the DICOM header metadata of the corresponding images has been started. Once finished this project will help to estimate and monitor dose levels continuously. It may also serve as an optimization tool if the online extraction can display the extracted and calculated dose values for a defined examination with respect to mean or quartile values from all collected data of the same type of examination.

But we have to have in mind that we are dealing with a rapidly evolving technique. Some examinations are now possible that we were not even thinking of some years ago. Thus optimization and adjustment of RDL will always be a task that will be in delay to current developments.

The swizz survey suggested three major steps for making RDLs a powerful tool for dose reduction and optimization:

"*These include* (1) *periodical on-site re*-audits, (2) *the establishment of a consulting service free of charge that provides expert advice to radiologists on CT protocol optimization and* (3) *the introduction of clinical audits to identify and eliminate unjustified CT examinations*" (Treier 2010).

## 10 Conclusion

Surveys are necessary to define RDLs. They should be carried out on a large-scale base because small-scale surveys just result in a snapshot of the current situation in the participating institutes. Also a bias related with the limited number of scanners and manufactures included in a small-scale survey can adulterate the findings. A comparison of different surveys should be made very carefully taking into account different scanning techniques (number of series, slice thickness, pitch) as well as different definitions of the region to be examined (upper and lower limit of scan region, different protocols for example in the head region axial vs. helical).

An update of important surveys to define RDLs in terms of new dose quantities such as $CTDI_{vol}$ seems to be necessary and has been reported in several surveys carried out in the last few years and more recently in some short notes (Early results from new dose survey unveiled at UKRC meeting 2011) and presentations (Meeson et al. 2011). Own experiences suggest that the setup the conduction and the evaluation of large-scale surveys will become more difficult in future because gathering all relevant scan parameters will become a more and more complex and time consuming task. This holds in particular for those scanners using AEC or any other option of modulating the tube current. The technical development is rapidly improving. This will unburden the users from carefully choosing the scan parameters adapted to each patient more or less individually but we are being surrendered to the technical developments. Verification of the dose estimates either displayed at the operators console or calculated retrospective will become more and more difficult.

Special surveys have to be carried out for defining RDLs for children. This task is even more complex to accomplish. Those surveys have to take into account several age groups (at least four namely <1 year, <5 years <10 years and <15 years) which means that the number of institutes executing a sufficient number of annual examination will be rather small (for example the in 2005/2006 finished survey in Germany (Galanski et al. 2006) listed only about 75 institutes carrying out at least 100 procedures each year).

Carrying out large-scale surveys on a frequent rate (e.g. once a year or even continuously) will lead to a huge amount of collected data where consistency and reliability has to be proved at least using adequate control samples. Therefor it seems to be more reasonable to check compliance with RDLs in other ways:

1. Using software tools to extract DICOM header metadata and online check compliance with reported mean and quartile values
2. Onsite audits to collect reliable data directly at the installed bases. This will eliminate the collection of wrong data and directly identify unjustified examinations.

Justification of X-ray and especially CT exams has to be addressed to education of radiologists and radiographers as well as to referring physicians in order to avoid unnecessary examinations and to improve efforts for optimization and compliance with the RDLs.

## References

### Large-Scale Surveys


Aroua A, Vader J-P, Valley J-F (2000) Survey on exposure by radiodiagnostics in Switzerland in 1998. www.hospvd.ch/public/instituts/ira

Bernhardt J, Veit R, Bauer B (1995) Erhebung zur Strahlenexposition der Patienten bei der Röntgendiagnostik. Z Med Phys 5:33–39

Brix G, Nagel HD, Stamm G, Veit R, Lechel U, Griebel J, Galanski M (2003) Radiation exposure in multi-slice versus single slice CT: results of a nationwide survey. Eur Radiol 13:1979–1991

Conway BJ, McCrohan JL, Antonson RG, Rueter FG, Slayton RJ, Suleiman OH (1992) Average radiation dose in standard CT examinations of the head: results of the 1990 next survey. Radiology 184:135–140

Galanski M, Nagel HD, Stamm G (2001) CT-Expositionspraxis in der Bundesrepublik Deutschland. Ergebnisse einer bundesweiten Umfrage im Jahre 1999. Fortschr Röntgenstr 173:R1–R66

Hart D, Wall BF (2001) Radiation exposure of the UK population from medical and dental X-ray exmaninations, NRBP-W4. http://www.hpa.org.uk/radiation/publications/w_series_reports/2002/nrpb_w4.htm

Meeuwsen E, Brugmans M (2002) Gegevens over medische stralingstoepassingen: van ziekenhuisquêtes tot zorgverzekeraars. RIVM Rapport nr. 610059 009, Bilthoven. http://www.rivm.nl/bibliotheek/rapporten/610059009.html

Meeuwsen E, Brugmans M (2003) Radiation exposure or the Dutch population from medical examinations. In: Proceedings of radiation protection symposium of the North West RP societies, Utrecht, pp 273–278

National Radiological Protection Board (1999) Guidelines on patient dose to promote the optimisation of protection for diagnostic medical exposures, documents of the NRPB, vol 10, no. 1

Nowotny R (2005) Entwicklung und Vergleich von Methoden zur Ermittlung und Überprüfung von Dosisreferenzwerten in der Röntgendiagnostik gemäß Patientenschutzrichtlinie EU 97/43 im Auftrag des Bundesministerium für Soziale Sicherheit und Generationen. http://www.bmgf.gv.at/cms/site/detail.htm?thema=CH0343&doc=CMS1065194276970

Shrimpton PC, Hillier MC, Lewis MA, Dunn M (2005) Doses from computed tomography (CT) examinations in the UK—2003 Review, NRPB-W67. http://www.hpa.org.uk/radiation/publications/w_series_reports/2005/nrpb_w67.htm

Shrimpton PC (2002) Assessment of patient dose in CT, NRPB-PE/1/2004. Chilton, NRBP. Also published as Appendix C or the 2004 CT Quality Criteria (MSCT, 2004). http://www.msct.info/CT_Quality_Criteria.htm

Thomson JEM, Tingey DRC (1997) radiation doses from computed tomography in Australia, ARL/TR 123


### Small-Scale Surveys


Einarsson G, Magnusson S (2001) Patient dose and examination frequency for diagnostic radiology in Iceland 1993–1998. In: Radiological protection of patients in diagnostic radiology, nuclear medicine and radiotherapy, proceedings of an IAEA-CN-85 international conference held in Malaga, Spain

Friberg EG (2003) Dual and multi slice CT—what about the doses, proceedings radiation protection, symposium of the North West RP societies, Utrecht, pp 193–196

Goddard CC, Al-Farsi A (1999) Radiation doses from CT in the Sultanate of Oman. BJR 72:1073–1077

Hatziioannou K, Papanastassiou E, Delichas M, Bousbouras P (2003) A contribution to the establishment of diagnostic reference levels in CT. BJR 76:541–545

Olerud HM (1997) Analysis of factors influencing patient doses from CT in Norway. Rad Prot Dosim 71:123

Olerud HM CT-dose surveys. In: Proceedings of radiation protection symposium of the North West RP Societies, Utrecht, pp 178–192

Olerud HM, Torp CG, Einarsson G et al (2001) Use of the EC quality criteria as a common method of inspecting CT laboratories—a pilot project by the Nordic radiation protection authorities. In: Radiological protection of patients in diagnostic radiology, nuclear medicine and radiotherapy, proceedings of an IAEA-CN-85 international conference held in Malaga, Spain

Origgi D, Vigorito S, Villa G, Bellomi M (2006) Survey of computed tomography techniques and absorbed dose in Italian hospitals: a comparison between two methods to estimate the dose-length product and the effective dose to verify fulfilment of the diagnostic reference levels. Eur Radiol 16:227–237

Papadimitriou D, Perris A, Manetou A et al (2003) A survey of 14 computed tomography scanners in Greece and 32 scanners in Italy: examination frequencies, dose reference values, effective doses and doses to organs. Rad Prot Dosim 104:47–53

Scheck R, Coppenrath EM, Bäuml A, Hahn K (1998)) Radiation dose and image quality in spiral computed tomography: results of a multicentre study at eight radiological institutions. Rad Prot Dosim 80:283–286

Hiles PA, Brennen SE, Scott SA, Davies JH (2001) A survey of patient dose and image quality for computed tomography in Wales. J Radiol Prot 21:345–354

Shrimpton PC, Jessen KA, Geleijns J, Panzer W, Tosi G (1998) Reference dose in computed tomography. Rad Prot Dosim 80:55–59

Szendrö G, Axelsson B, Leitz W (1995) Computed tomography practice in Sweden: quality control, techniques and patient dose. Rad Prot Dosim 57:469–473

Tsapaki V, Kottou S, Papadimitriou D (2001) Application of the European Commission reference dose levels in CT examinations in Crete, Greece. BJR 74:836–840

van Unnik JG, Broerse JJ, Geleijns J et al (1997) Survey of CT techniques and absorbed dose in various Dutch hospitals. BJR 70:367–371

## Guidelines, Reference Dose Levels

Bundesamt für Strahlenschutz (2004) Bekanntmachung der diagnostischen Referenzwerte für radiologische und nuklearmedizinische Untersuchungen vom 10. Juli 2003, Bundesanzeiger Nummer 143 vom 5.8.2003, pp 17503–7504

CT quality criteria (2004) (A 6th framework research project of the European Commission). http://www.msct.info/CT_Quality_Criteria.htm

European Commission (1999) European guidelines on quality criteria for computed tomography, Report EUR 16262 EN, Luxembourg, office for official publications of the European communities, pp 69–78. http://www.drs.dk/guidelines/ct/quality/

International Electrotechnical Commission (IEC) (2001) Medical electrical equipment–Part 2: particular requirements for the safety of X-ray equipment for computed tomography, IEC-Standard 60601-2-44 Ed. 2.0, Geneva

Nagel HD (2010) Leitfaden zur Bewertung und Optimierung der Strahlenexposition bei CT-Untersuchungen http://www.sascrad.de/attachments/File/Leitfaden_CT_(Ed_3).pdf

## Publications on Paediatric CT

Boone JM, Geraghty EM, Seibert JA, Wootton-Gorges SL (2003) Dose reduction in pediatric ct: a rational approach. Radiology 228:352–360

Brenner DJ, Elliston CD, Hall EJ, Berdon WE (2001) Estimated risks of radiation-induced fatal cancer from pediatric CT. AJR 176:289–296

Chapple C-L, Willis S, Frame J (2002) Effective dose in paediatric computed tomography. Phys Med Biol 47: 107–115

Cody DD, Moxley DM, Krugh KT, O'Daniel CJ, Wagner LK, Eftekhari F (2004) Strategies for formulating appropriate MDCT techniques when imaging the chest, abdomen, and pelvis in pediatric patients. AJR 182:849–859

Donnelly LF, Emery KH, Brody AS (2001) Minimizing radiation dose for pediatric body applications of single-detector helical CT: strategies at a large children's hospital. AJR 176:303–306

Hollingsworth C, Frush DP, Cross M, Lucaya J (2003) Helical CT of the body: a survey of techniques used for pediatric patients. AJR 180:401–406

Huda W (2002) Dose and image quality in CT. Pediatr Radiol 32:709–713

Khursheed A, Hillier MC, Shrimpton PC, WALL BF (2002) Influence of patient age on normalized effective doses calculated for CT examinations. BJR 75:819–830

Linton AW, Mettler FA Jr (2003) National conference on dose reduction in CT, with an emphasis on pediatric patients. AJR 181:321–329

Pages J, Buls N, Osteaux M (2003) CT doses in children: a multicentre study. BJR 76:803–811

Paterson A, Frush DP, Donnelly LF (2001) Helical CT of the body: are settings adjusted for pediatric patients? AJR 176:297–301

Sandstede J (2003) Pediatric CT. http://www.multislice-ct.com/www/

Shrimpton PC, Wall BF (2000) Reference doses for paediatric CT. Rad Prot Dosim 90:249–252

Suess Ch, Chen X (2002) Dose optimization in pediatric CT: current technology and future innovations. Pediatr Radiol 32:729–734

Verdun FR, Lepori D, Monnin P, Valley J-F, Schnyder P, Gudinchet F (2004) Management of patient dose and image noise in routine pediatric CT abdominal examinations. Eur Radiol 14:835–841

Vock P (2005) CT dose reduction in children. Eur Radiol 15:2330–2340

## New Reference for Second Edition

Alesso AM, Phillips GS (2010) A pediatric CT dose and risk estimator. Pediatr Radiol 40:1816–1821

Aroua A, Besançon A, Buchillier-Decka I et al (2004) Adult reference levels in diagnostic and interventional radiology for temporary use in Switzerland. Rad Prot Dosim 111:289–295

Early results from new dose survey unveiled at UKRC meeting (2011) http://www.auntminnieeurope.com/index.aspx?sec=sup&sub=cto&pag=dis&ItemID=605176

Galanski M, Nagel H.D, Stamm G (2006) Paediatric CT exposure practice in the federal republic of Germany, results of a nation-wide survey in 2005/2006. http://www.mh-hannover.de/7965.html

German National Radiation Protection Board (Bundesamt für Strahlenschutz) (2010). Diagnostic reference dose levels. http://www.bfs.de/de/ion/medizin/referenzwerte02.pdf

Health Service Executive (2011), Population dose from CT scanning 2009. http://www.hse.ie/eng/about/Who/medexpradiatonunit/PopulationDose.html

Jahnen A, Kohler S, Hermen J, Tack D, Back C (2011) Automatic computed tomography patient dose calculation using DICOM Header Metadata; Rad Prot Dosim, doi: 10.1093/rpd/ncr338

Kharita MH, Khazzam S (2010) Survey of patient dose in computed tomography in Syria 2009. Rad Prot Dosim 141: 149–161

Livingstone RS, Dinakaran PM (2009) Regional survey of CT dose indices in India. Rad Prot Dosim 136:222–227

Meeson S, Shrimpton PC, MacLachlan SA, Golding SJ (2011) Update on radiation exposure from CT: Early progress in the third UK CT dose survey. http://www.biophysicssite.com/Documents/Poster_4_web_secure.pdf

Muhogora WE, Ahmed NA et al (2010) Paediatric CT examinations in 19 developing countries: frequency and radiation dose. Rad Prot Dosim 140:49–58

Ono K, Ban N, Ojima M, Yoshinaga S et al (2011) Nationwide survey on pediatric CT among children of public health and school nurses to examine a possibility for a follow-up study on radiation effects. Rad Prot Dosim 146:260–262

Pantos I, Thalassinou S, Argentos S, Kelekis NL, Panayiotakis G, Efstathopoulos EP (2011) Adult patient radiation doses from non-cardiac CT examinations: a review of published results. BJR 84:293–303

Treier R, Aroua A, Verdun F et al (2010) Patient doses in CT examinations in Switzerland: implementation of national diagnostic reference levels. Rad Prot Dosim 142: 244–254

Tung CJ, Yang CH, Yeh CY, Chen TR (2011) Population dose from medical diagnostic exposure in Taiwan. Rad Prot Dosim 146:248–251

UNSCEAR Report (2000) Annex D, Medical radiation exposure, New York

# ALARA Concept for MDCT Optimization: What is Reasonable, What is Achievable?

Denis Tack

## Contents



D. Tack (✉)
Department of Radiology, RHMS Clinique Louis Caty, Rue Louis Caty 136, 7331, Baudour, Belgium
e-mail: denis.tack@skynet.be

**Abstract**

Almost all MDCT scanners are installed with default parameters providing a perfect image quality called "standard", and deliver the corresponding "standard dose". Optimization is a process by which a substantial proportion of the standard dose is eliminated without loss in diagnostic performance and/or confidence. The final "optimized dose" reached by this process is not clearly defined in the literature because it varies among manufacturers, scanner generation, and CT users. The ALARA principle implies setting the optimized dose at the lowest reasonable level. In this chapter, we describe possible methods for optimization and propose achievable and reasonable limits for CT scanning of the head, the chest, the abdomen, and the spine.

## 1 Introduction

In Western countries, CT is the largest source of medical radiation (Hricak et al. 2011) and may even be the largest source of all radiations. Each CT examination delivers 1–24 mSv, a dose that belongs to the range of low-level radiations. Deterministic effects (such as hair loss) can occur but only for very specific examinations and conditions (Smith-Bindman 2010). The deleterious effect of diagnostic CT is the risk of cancer. This carcinogenic effect of radiation risk of low-level radiation as that delivered by CT is a matter of debate and has been extensively described in "Clincical Expansion of CT and Radiation Dose" by Chadwick and Leernout. They advocate the use of

D. Tack et al. (eds.), *Radiation Dose from Multidetector CT*, Medical Radiology. Diagnostic Imaging,
DOI: 10.1007/174_2011_458, 

the linear-no-threshold (LNT) model of carcinogenesis. On the other hand Cohen lists in "Risks from Ionising Radiation" all the arguments against the LNT model and in favor of a threshold or even of a protective effect of low-level radiations that is named hormesis. Based on the precautionary principle, the LNT model is currently used for calculating the risks of cancer induction by CT. Because of the high number of CT examinations performed each year, the cancer risk for the population is a matter of concern (Brenner and Hall 2007). Thus, it is the responsibility of each CT user to minimize the dose delivered by each examination (Golding 2010). Reasons for excess of radiation dose delivered by CT are numerous, including inappropriate prescription—a problematic discussed in "Guidelines for Appropriate Use of CT Imaging" by Hinshaw—extended cephalo-caudal coverage (z-coverage), high number of acquisitions, and use of high default settings. Default settings as installed and proposed by manufacturers provide perfect image quality but have not been validated in patients. These settings result almost only from phantom studies where the noise is as low as possible, and the spatial reslution as high as possible. According to the ALARA principle, optimized CT parameters represent a compromise between image quality, diagnostic confidence, and radiation dose. As the dose should be as low as possible, a CT image without any artifact or noise cannot be considered as optimized. An optimization process should not be considered as finalized as long as image quality appears very good or perfect. As optimized CT parameters depend on the scanner characteristics, the body region scanned, and the clinical condition, absolute values applicable to any scanner and CT technique do not exist. In this chapter, we review and illustrate the methods, pitfalls, and tricks for optimization and provide up-to-date examples of optimized parameters for the head, sinus, cervical spine, chest, abdomen, and lumbar spine.

## 2 Definition of Terms for CT Qualifying the Dose

Terms qualifying radiation dose are not strictly defined. As an example, the dose of a so-called "low-dose" protocol in one CT center or one scanner could correspond to the one of a standard dose CT in another center or scanner. In the chest, the term low-dose is used for qualifying the dose delivered in the NSLT research trial (National Lung Screening Trial Research Team 2010) whereas this dose is higher than that routinely delivered in other radiology departments. Another confusion of this order can be seen with the introduction of iterative reconstructions, a denoising image reconstruction method replacing the filtered back projection kernels (FBP). The introduction of iterative reconstructions enables to reduce the CT dose by 30–70% (Singh et al. 2010, 2011) and this dose tends to be called "low". However, the reduced dose level achieved with iterative reconstructions in some investigations has been achieved from quite high standard dose settings that were not previously optimized. As a general rule outlined by Leng and Mc Cullough (Leng et al. 2010), iterative reconstruction should be applied on optimized doses hereafter defined as the lowest dose providing acceptable image quality. Because a strict definition of these terms does not yet exist, we introduce the following propositions.

### 2.1 Standard Dose

The term "standard dose'' refers to the dose usually recommended by CT manufacturers, very similar to the reference diagnostic levels (RDLs) defined by surveys (Stamm, "Collective Radiation Dose from MDCT: Critical Review of Surveys Studies" in the present edition) and often used in routine practice but that could be substantially reduced—to an optimized dose level—without deleterious effect on image quality. Table 1 lists typical CTDIvol values and RDLs for brain, chest, abdomen scanning.

### 2.2 Optimized Dose

The term "optimized dose" refers to a dose that provides adequate but not perfect image quality but not with excessive radiation, and is the practical application of ALARA (As Low As Reasonably Achievable) principle. At optimized dose, noise in images is higher than at standard dose but does not affect subjective evaluation of image quality. Table 2 lists achievable optimized dose settings for head, sinus, chest, abdomen, and lumbar spine. Optimized dose levels are often close to the 25th percentile observed in surveys (P25). These values can thus

**Table 1** Reference diagnostic levels (RDLs) for head, chest, and abdominal MDCT, representing upper limits of acceptable practice but not optimized or ALARA practice

| Body region | Year | Origin | CTDIvol (mGy) | DLP (mGy cm) |
|---|---|---|---|---|
| Head | 1999 | EUR 16262 | 60 | 1,050 |
| | 2010 | Germany | 65 | 950 |
| | 2010 | Switzerland | 65 | 1,000 |
| | 2002 | Sweden | 75 | 1,200 |
| Chest | 1999 | EUR 16262 | 23 | 650 |
| | 2008 | Switzerland | 15 | 450 |
| | 2010 | France | 15 | 475 |
| | 2005 | UK | 14 | 580 |
| Abdomen | 1999 | EUR 16262 | 25.0 | 1,100 |
| | 2002 | Germany | 14.6 | 635 |
| | 2003 | UK | 15.3 | 534 |
| | 2008 | France | 17.0 | 800 |
| | 2010 | Belgium | 17.1 | 830 |

*Note* Data are taken from EMAN European Medical ALARA Network 2011 report
Values are given for an average adult patient weighting 70–75 kg
RDLs correspond to the 75th percentile of observed dose values in survey
*CTDIvol* in mGy, is the computed tomography dose index volume (CTDIw/pitch)
*DLP* in mGy.cm is the dose-length product

reflect the actual objectives (upper limit) for optimization. The optimized—ALARA—dose level in a particular CT department and a specific CT scanner is not a priori known, and has to be found out by the user who is responsible for this process (Golding 2010).

## 2.3 Low Dose

The term "low dose" should be restricted to a dose not higher than that delivered by a set of plain films investigating the considered clinical condition. At low dose, image quality is lower but diagnostic accuracy is still preserved. At low dose, noise in images is clearly visible but does not impair the recognition of anatomy as well as positive and negative CT signs. Low dose should be the preferred method for scanning young patients and patients with potentially recurring disease and or pain. It has been extensively investigated in the sinonasal cavities (Mulkens et al. "Dose Optimization and Reduction in CT of the Head (Brain)" in the present edition), in the chest (Gevenois and Tack, "Dose Reduction and Optimization in Computed Tomography of the Chest" in the present edition) and in the abdomen (Keyzer and Tack in "Dose Optimization and Reduction in MDCT of the Abdomen" of present edition). DLP delivered by low-dose protocols for these examinations are listed in Table 2.

# 3 Methods for Dose Optimization

Optimization of CT dose should consider all available CT parameters that influence the dose including automatic exposure control (AEC) system, the tube current time product, reconstruction algorithm or kernel, tube potential, collimation, reconstructed slice thickness, pitch factor, and acquisition direction.

## 3.1 AEC System: Principles and Pitfalls

AEC systems aim to adapt the tube current to the absorption measured from one or from two scout views. The technical solution differs between manufacturers and should be understood by the users for appropriate optimization. AEC systems are described in "Automatic Exposure Control in Multidetector-Row Computed Tomography" by Kalra et al., and possible adverse effects of centering the patient in conjunction with bow-tie filters and AEC are described

**Table 2** Optimized and low-dose MDCT dose descriptors for head, sinus, chest, and abdomen in an average-sized adult patient scanned ALARA

| Body region | Year/quality[a] | Origin/reference | CTDIvol (mGy) | DLP (mGy.cm) |
|---|---|---|---|---|
| Head | 2006/OD | Tsapaki et al. (2006) | 40 | 520 |
| | 2011/OD | Mulkens et al. "Image Noise Reduction Filters" | 930 | 400 |
| Sinus | 2010/OD | Switzerland P25 | 10 | 150 |
| | 2010/OD | Belgium P25 | 5 | 70 |
| Chest | 2010/OD | Switzerland P25 | 5 | 250 |
| | 2010/OD | Belgium P25 | 5 | 240 |
| | 2010/OD | NLST | 3–5 | 120–180 |
| | 2011/OD | Singh et al. | 3,5 | 120 |
| | 2007/LD | Bankier et al. (2007) | 2 | 70 |
| | 2011/LD | Fig. 15 | 0.5 | 20 |
| | 2010/LD/Seq | O'Connor et al. (2010) | NA | 8–12 |
| Abdomen | 2010/OD | Switzerland P25 | 10 | 350 |
| | 2010/OD | Luxemburg P25 | 7.9 | 352 |
| | 2010/OD | Allen et al. (2010) | 8,7 | 400 |
| | 2010/OD | Kambadakone et al. (2010) | 5.9–8.9 | 250–400 |
| | 2009/OD | Seo H et al. | 6.0 | 240 |
| | 2004/LD | Keyzer et al. (2004) | 3.0 | 100–150 |
| | 2009/LD | Keyzer et al. (2009) | 2.0–3.0 | 80–150 |
| | 2009/LD | Platon et al. | 2.1 | 84 ± 10 |
| Lumbar Spine | 2010/OD | Luxemburg P25 | 20 | 400 |
| | 2010/OD | Switzerland P25 | 15 | 300 |
| | 2010/OD | Belgium P25 | NA | 475 |
| | 2007/OD | Bohy et al. (2007) | 26 | 400 |

*Note* For body MDCT, dose descriptors are suited for an average-sized adult patient in helical mode
[a] Quality refers to optimized dose (OD) as the result of ALARA and low-dose (LD) representing degraded image quality but with preserved diagnosis
*P25* 25th percentile of dose values as observed in nationwide surveys
*NA* non available
*NLST* national lung screening trial research team
*Seq* acquisition in sequential mode
CTDIvol are given in 16 cm phantom for Head and Sinus and in 32 cm phantom for body-MDCT

in "Patient Centering in MDCT: Dose Effects" by Kalra et al. As a general rule, AEC systems are the most appropriate to warrant constant image quality throughout the acquisition. They are the only ones able to adapt the dose in the three directions (X, Y, and/or Z directions) and to adapt the tube current to the measured patient's absorption that is directly linked to his habitus. Thus, AEC systems should always be activated, whatever the scanner protocol and the CT machine. Basically, two concepts of AEC exist: those that warrant constant image noise (GE and Toshiba scanners) and express the index of image quality as a noise index (NI), and those that warrant a constant image quality but not constant noise and express the index of image quality in terms of "quality reference effective mAs" (Philips and Siemens). Differences in AEC concepts may have important consequences on patient's dose, in particular in obese patients as shown in Fig. 1. This figure shows that for a constant noise index in all patients and the same CTDIvol in a standard patient, the dose delivered in obese patients may be higher with AEC systems warranting a constant noise than with those warranting a constant "quality". The difference in

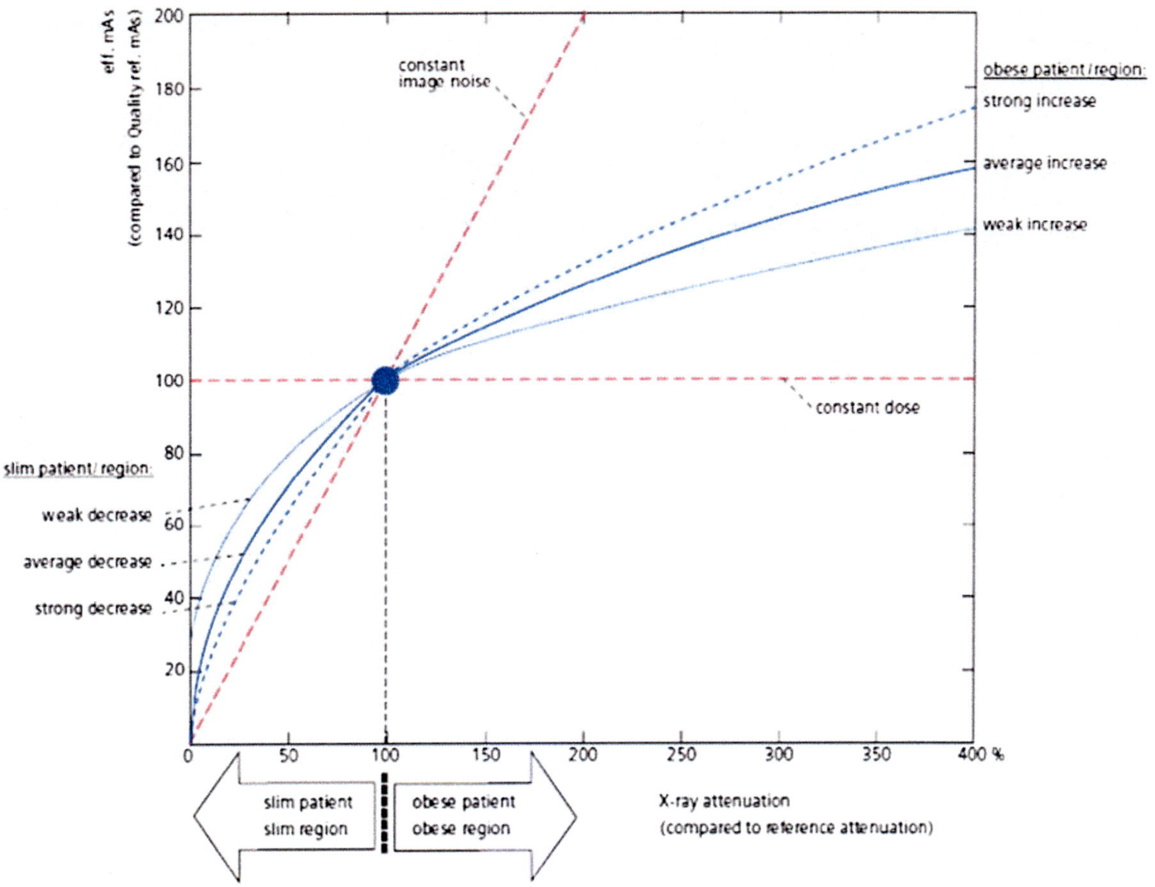


**Fig. 1** Chart representing the relationship of dose and obesity depending on the automatic exposure control (AEC) system used. The strongest increase in dose is seen with AEC warranting a constant noise (GE and Toshiba scanners), whereas the dose increase may be moderate or reduces in AEC tolerating more noise in obese (Siemens and Philips scanners). For chest and abdominal CT, specific protocols for obese using higher noise index are recommended with AEC warranting constant noise. On the other hand, for CT scanning of the lumbar spine, specific protocols with higher image quality (lower noise) in obese are recommended when using Siemens AEC system (Care-Dose 4D)

dose delivered as a function of body weight or body mass index (BMI) has been investigated by Meason et al. (2010). They showed that the relationship between CTDIvol and the cross-sectional area is logarithmic rather than linear when using AEC warranting a constant noise. It is to note that in obese patients with abundant fat, higher noise fat can be tolerated without giving the impression of impaired image quality as compared to standard patients. In order to avoid an excessively increased dose in obese patients when scanning the trunk, specific protocols with higher noise index should be used on GE and Toshiba scanners.

For lumbar and cervical spine scanning however, the amount of fat in the region of interest of the spine does not differ significantly between standard and obese patients. Only thin layers of fat tissue are present in the spinal canal. Thus, AEC systems that do not warrant constant noise (Siemens) but tolerate higher noise in obese do not provide sufficient image quality in the spine of obese patients when using the same quality reference effective mAs setting. With these scanners, obese-specific protocols should exist for the lumbar spine and include higher quality reference effective mAs or a higher tube potential or a combination of both. Figure 1 shows that Siemens AEC system (Care dose 4D) can be set up with three different curves of dose increase as a function of absorption on the topogram. The one used in almost all CT units and that gives satisfactory image quality for scanning abdomen and chest is called "average"

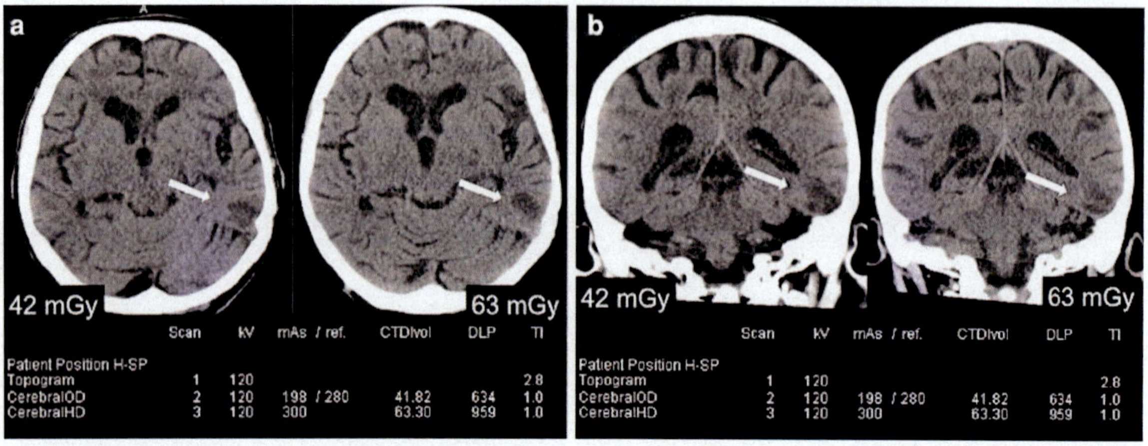


**Fig. 2** Brain CT performed in two consecutive acquisitions obtained at 120 kV (64 × 0.6 mm) in a 70-year-old man with acute stroke. *Arrows* show a hypoattenuated area in the left parieto-temporal region. **a** shows side-by-side comparison of representative axial slices with 3 mm thickness. The *left one* is acquired at CTDIvol of 42 mGy with tube current modulation switched on. The reference image quality index is at 280 mAs. The mean delivered effective tube current time product is at 198 mAs. The second acquisition displayed at the *right side* is obtained without tube current modulation with an effective tube current time product at 300 mA and the corresponding CTDIvol value is at 63 mGy. **a** displays the corresponding side-by-side comparison in coronal orientation at the level of the hypoattenuated region. Dose report is displayed at the *bottom* of the figure. Images obtained at 63 mGy (displayed on the *right* are reconstructed with Kernel H30, whereas those obtained at 42 mGy are reconstructed with a slightly smoother algorithm H20. Note: Tube current modulation is only active in the Z-axis for brain CT with Philips and Siemens scanners

(Fig. 1). At a constant tube potential of 120 kV, this curve does not provide adequate image quality in obese patients for spine examinations. Two or three others exist, the smooth and the strong ones, almost never used. From 2011, it is possible to choose one specific curve for each body region to be scanned. We have thus tested the strong curve for lumbar spine at 120 kV, in addition to the iterative reconstruction technique. Examinations in obese performed earlier at 140 kV and with CTDIvol at 80 are now obtained at 120 kV and CTDIvol at approximately 50 mGY.

## 3.2 Practical Application of Optimization Using AEC

### 3.2.1 Step by Step Reductions

The easiest way to optimize CT dose is to lower the tube current time product step by step by modifying the AEC index of image quality, i.e. by increasing the noise index with GE and Toshiba scanners or by decreasing the Quality Reference mAs with Siemens and Philips scanners. This was recently achieved in a university department for CT of the brain. The initial settings were 120 kV, 400 mAs effective (quality reference mAs), corresponding to a CTDIvol of 63 mGy. The quality reference mAs were then reduced stepwise by means of 10 mAs once a week. Radiologists were asked to give their feedback on all possible problems related to image quality. After 14 weeks, the quality index was at 260 mAs, corresponding to a CTDIvol of 42 mGy, and image quality was still considered as acceptable. The next week, further 10 mAs reduction was no more accepted as image quality deterioration began to stimulate the debate on acceptable or unacceptable noise in images. It is to note that during such a process, the reconstruction algorithm (Kernel) should also be adapted with preference to a smoother one—see hereafter.

### 3.2.2 Side-by-Side Comparisons of Standard and Optimized Scans

Knowing the approximate dose level of an optimized acquisition, a rapid and immediate way to optimize standard CT is to compare the standard and the optimized acquisitions for the same patient. Numerous solutions exist for this process:

- Scanning the patient twice with identical settings unless the CTDIvol, set at standard level for one acquisition and at optimized level

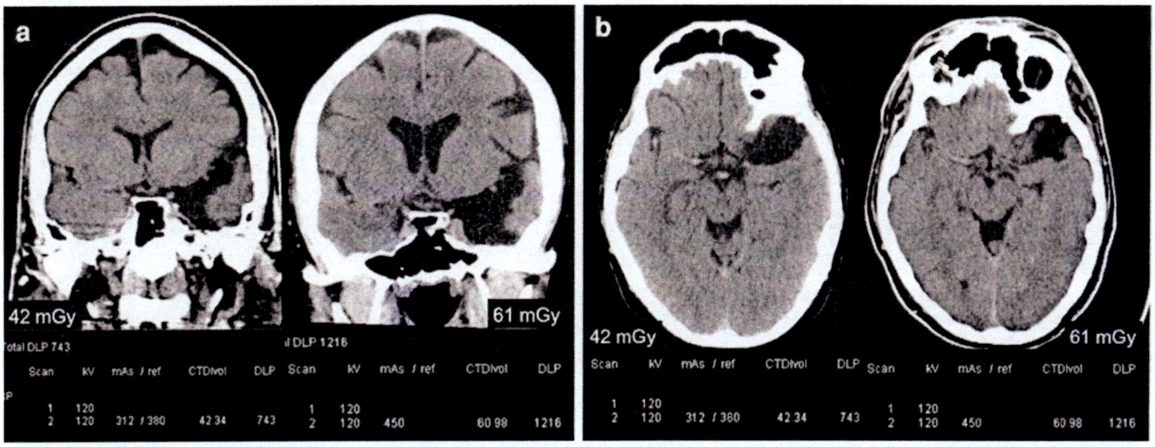


**Fig. 3** Two consecutive brain CT examinations with 3 months' interval (the first one is displayed on the right) in a 42-year-old man who had a motor vehicle accident. Acquisitions were obtained at 120 kV and with a collimation of 16 × 0,6 mm. The right one was obtained with fixed tube current at 450 effective mAs and resulted in a CTDIvol of 61 mGy. The *left one* (a control scan 3 months after the injury) was obtained with tube current modulation, reference quality image setting at 380 mAs, and mean effective tube current time product of 312 mAs resulting in a CTDIvol reduced at 42 mGy. **a**, **b** show *axial* and *coronal* representative images. An arachnoid cyst is seen in the left temporal region. Images obtained at 61 mGy (displayed on the *right* are reconstructed with Kernel H30, whereas those obtained at 42 mGy are reconstructed with a slightly smoother algorithm H20. Note: Tube current modulation is only active in the Z-axis for brain CT with Philips and Siemens scanners

(typically standard minus 40%, range −30 to −50%) for the other acquisition. An example for a CT of the head is shown in Fig. 2.

- Using a scan from the archives as reference standard and scanning the patient once with optimized parameters.—An example for a CT of the head is shown in Fig. 3.
- If a multiphase examination of the liver is clinically indicated, using standard parameters for portal phase, and optimized ones for unenhanced and/or arterial phase.

### 3.2.3 Tube Current–Time Product

The radiation dose is proportional to the tube current time product. Thus, optimization by means of reduction of mAs seems the easiest way to go. However, as tube current time product is best adapted to the patients' absorption by enabling the AEC system, direct modifications of the tube current time product for dose optimization is not recommended for CT dose optimization. This however needs two comments for possible exceptions:

- With GE and Toshiba scanners, it is mandatory to set appropriate upper and lower values of tube current time products (mAs) as limits for the AEC system. The lowest limit intends to warrant a minimal image quality in very small patients. The highest value intends to avoid radiation dose excess in obese patients. The AEC system modulates the tube current within these two limits. If the mAs gap between these limits is too small, the tube current will either be at the upper limit in large patients or at the lower limit in small patients. In both situations, AEC is practically disabled and tube current modulation in X–Y–Z axes will not occur even with an AEC function switched "ON". Before each acquisition, the AEC system enables to check the mAs table displaying the mAs per slice along the Z axis. A table with constant mAs values indicates inadequate mAs limits. In our experience of clinical audit in CT dose optimization (Tack et al. 2011), CT protocols as installed by the manufacturer often suffer from a narrowed mAs window. If the mAs table shows constant mAs values for a given mean CTDIvol, the mA window should be widened, and the NI adjusted to maintain the CTDIvol at a similar value.
- With Siemens and Philips scanners, the image quality index is expressed in "quality reference effective mAs" or in effective mAs. This is a source of huge confusion among users who are not aware of the design of the AEC system.

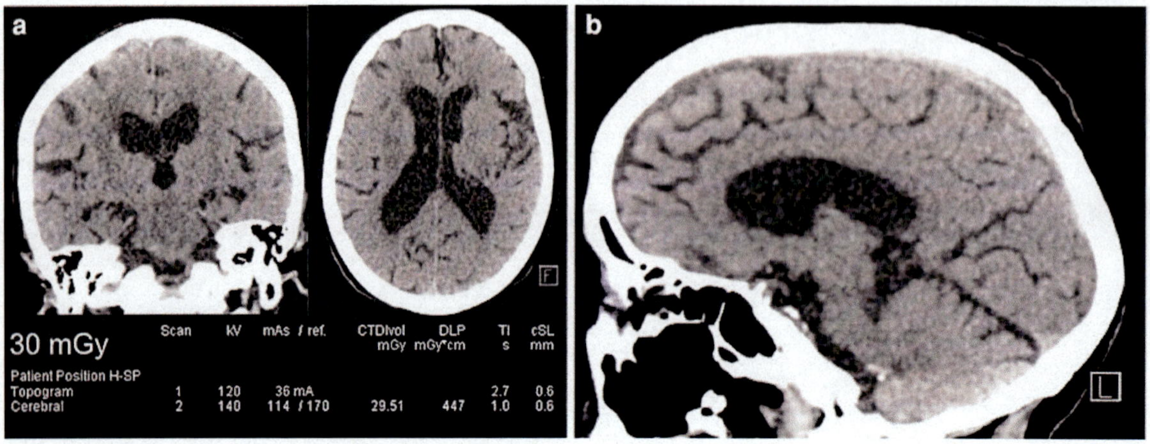


**Fig. 4** Optimized Brain CT acquisition obtained with 40 × 0.6 collimation, 140 kV, activated tube current modulation (in Z-axis), image quality reference mAs at 170. The resulting delivered tube current time product is at 114 effective mAs and the CTDIvol is at 30 mGy. **a** shows axial and coronal slices with dose report and (**b**) shows a sagittal reformat

### 3.2.4 Reconstruction Algorithm or Kernel

The historical kernels provided by manufacturers are based on filter back projection technique (FBP). Recently, iterative reconstruction algorithms have been introduced in CT (they were used since the eighties for scintigram reconstructions. Iterative reconstruction is now proposed by all manufacturers as options for improving CT reconstructions. The variety of FBP kernels available to CT users differs between manufacturers and cannot be easily compared. Typically, each manufacturer provides three or more FBP algorithms called soft, standard, and high-resolution (or bone). The noise represented by the standard deviation of Hounsfield units (HU) within a region of interest (ROI) and the spatial resolution increase from soft to Hi-Res. Siemens scanners offer a larger variety of algorithms, typically eight or nine, numbered B10 to B90 for the body and H10 to H 90 for the head. As a general rule, the noise linked to high-resolution algorithms is very similar to the noise resulting from reductions in tube current time product. Most importantly, default algorithms for soft tissues are often the "standard" ones, generating more noise than the soft algorithms but without significant increase in spatial resolution for slices of 3 mm thickness or less.

The optimization process must thus consider the appropriate reconstruction algorithm. Typically, in an average patient weighting 75 kg, a mediastinum scanned at 9 mGy and reconstructed with standard algorithm (Siemens B30 or B40) could be scanned at 5 mGy and reconstructed with a soft algorithm (Siemens B10 or B20) and produce very similar images. A comparison between two acquisitions with optimized dose and reconstruction algorithm is shown in Figs. 2, 3 and 4 for the brain.

### 3.2.5 The Tube Potential

The influence of the tube potential on the radiation dose is very important as the dose varies as a function of the 2.5–2.8 power of the tube potential. Optimization through tube potential reductions may thus provide substantial dose savings. However, as the relationship between tube potential and image quality is complex and not linear, and as the available tube potential settings are restricted to few predefined values (typically 80, 100, 120, and 140 kV), optimization rarely includes modifications in tube potential. The only currently widely admitted recommendation of tube potential reduction from 120 to 100 or 80 kV is CT angiography (Sigal-Cinqualbre et al. 2004, Schueller-Weidekamm et al. 2006, Szucs-Farkas et al. 2009a). Table 1 lists a series of CT protocols and their corresponding tube potentials. Default tube potential is often set at 120 kV. At lower tube potentials of 100 or 80 kV, the absorption of iodine is much higher than that obtained at 120 kV. A tube potential at 100 kV can be used for CT angiography in patients with body weight up to 100 kg (Schindera et al. 2009, Szucs-Farkas et al. 2009b), and for routine CT of the head in children up to 10 years of age, and for routine enhanced abdominal CT in patients with abdominal diameter up to 35 cm and body weights lower than 80 kg (Guimarães et al. 2010). A tube potential as high as 140 kV has been routinely used for scanning chest or abdomen in adults and in children because image quality gave satisfaction and "lower" tube currents could be used, with the direct economical advantage of saving tube's life (Tack and Gevenois 2009, Jaffe 2009). If Tube potential as high as 140 kV is preferred, the tube current should be dramatically decreased as shown hereafter for chest and abdomen MDCT. For iodine enhanced examinations, 140 kV does not represent optimized or best possible practice as lower tube potential takes the advantage of high iodine absorption.

### 3.2.6 The Collimation and Reconstructed Slice Thickness

The "scan thin–read thick" principle consists in using thin collimations at acquisition, reconstruct thin CT slices (ideally slightly thickened and use multiplanar reformations in order to eliminate the noise on such near-isotropic data sets (EMAN 2011). The principle is that noise in thin section volumetric data sets can be reduced or eliminated electronically by multiplanar reformations (MPR), maximum intensity projection (MIP), and volume rendering techniques (VRT). This principle has widespread applications in CT protocols since it retains spatial resolution within the imaging plane while reducing noise by increasing the thickness of the reconstructed image. The "scan thin–read thick" principle avoids to increase the radiation dose because of thin sections.

The thickness of the original thin sections has to be adapted to the required spatial resolution in z-direction. In general, higher resolution (i.e. a minimum section collimation) is used for skeletal structures or the chest, while a slightly lower resolution (2x minimum collimation) is acceptable for the abdomen. This is important because dose efficiency of many scanners (<64-slice) is higher for the slightly wider collimation (EMAN 2011).

The thinnest possible collimation at acquisition often preferred with MDCT scanners is 0.6 or 0.625 mm (0.5 mm with Toshiba scanners). This is appropriate for most CT protocols and in particular for those from which thin sections are needed as in the chest for bone examinations. A valuable alternative for abdominal CT is to use a 1.20 (Siemens) or 1.25 mm (GE) collimation by electronical sampling to pairs of adjacent detector rows. With unchanged remaining parameters, the 1.2 and the 1.25 collimations save 12% of the CTDIvol as compared respectively to the 0.6 and 0.625 mm collimations.

Once the collimation is chosen, the slice thickness of the first reconstructed series has a marginal influence on the dose-length product because of overranging effect of helical scanning (less than 1%).

### 3.2.7 The Pitch Factor

A modification of the table feed by rotation and of the pitch factor has no direct influence on the dose on Siemens and Philips scanners because while the table feed is doubled, the CT automatically doubles the tube current and keeps the effective mAs and CTDIvol constant.

With GE and Toshiba scanners, a modification of the table feed by rotation or of the pitch factor has a direct and proportional effect on the dose. Doubling the pitch factor reduces the dose (CTDIvol) values by the same factor of 2. Increasing the table feed by rotation is not the easiest way to optimize the dose. As a general rule, the pitch factor should be appropriate to the clinical conditions in order to avoid apnea of more than 15–20 s and to follow the iodine enhancements along the investigated vessels (aorta, carotid arteries, run off). The pitch factor proposed by the vendor is usually set at an appropriate level with 64 or more detector-row scanners.

### 3.2.8 The Acquisition Direction

The acquisition direction has almost no effect on the radiation dose. However, because of the design of AEC systems with online tube current modulation (Care-Dose 4D—Siemens) and of their 180° latency for adapting the bub current to the measured absorption, scanning the cervical spine in cephalo-caudal direction will result in a lower dose but higher artifacts as compared to the cuado-cranial direction that should be preferred.

## 3.3 Recommendations in Optimization Process

- Do not use the reference Diagnostic Levels (RDLs) from surveys as reference for dose optimization. These values listed in Table 1 are typically

**Table 3** CT parameters and dose descriptors in optimized and low-dose MDCT of the abdomen as a function of body weight

| | *Optimized MDCT of the Abdomen in Adult Patients* | | | |
|---|---|---|---|---|
| Patient's Weight (Kg) | Tube potential (KV) | Example | CTDIvol (mGy) | DLP (mGy.cm) |
| >120 | 140 | Fig. 16 | 12.0–15.0 | 600–1000 |
| 100–120 | 120–140 | NA | 8.0–12.0 | 400–600 |
| 80–100 | 120–140 | Figs. 17, 26 | 4.0–8.0 | 300–400 |
| 60–80 | 100–120 | Figs. 18, 28 | 3.0–4.0 | 200–300 |
| | *Low-dose MDCT of the abdomen in adult patients* | | | |
| Patient's weight (Kg) | Tube potential (KV) | Example | CTDIvol (mGy) | DLP (mGy.cm) |
| >120 | 140 | Fig. 19 | 6.0–10.0 | 300–500 |
| 100–120 | 120–140 | Fig. 20 | 3.5–6.0 | 120–300 |
| 80–100 | 120–140 | Fig. 21 | 2.0–4.0 | 150–200 |
| 60–80 | 100–120 | Fig. 22 | 1.5–3.0 | 100–150 |
| | *Low-dose MDCT of the abdomen in small adults and in children* | | | |
| Patient's weight (Kg) | Tube potential (KV) | Example | CTDIvol (mGy) | DLP (mGy.cm) |
| 40–60 | 100 | Figs. 23, 24 | 1.5- 3.0 | 50–100 |
| <40 | 80 | Fig. 25 | 1.0–2.0 | 25–50 |

*Note* AEC current modulation should always be activated
The choice of the tube potential is dependent on the use of iodine contrast and on the body weight
Low-Dose protocols suppose accepted higher noise levels as compared to routine optimized MDCT acquisitions
In adults, DLP values are given for an optimized acquisition length of 30 cm, set from the top of the kidneys to the superior aspect of the symphysis pubis
In children, acquisition length is 25 cm in those weighting <40 kg and 30 cm in all others
These protocols can be applied on most MDCT scanners
Using newly developed scanners (GE HD750, Siemens Definition, and Philips ICT) and using iterative reconstruction algorithms, noise can be reduced, enabling further significant dose reductions by 30–50%

standard dose settings and should rather be considered as the upper limits of acceptable practice, in other words, the limit of radiation malpractice.

- As objective for optimization refer to Table 2 and in particular to the 25th percentile of surveys. With a modern scanner, the first percentile observed in surveys is the adequate objective. As stated by Georg Stamm in "Software for Calculating Dose and Risk", the first percentile of surveys could be considered as the achievable objective with the newest scanners and software.
- For imaging young patients with benign disorders, such as acute appendicitis with low-dose MDCT, refer to low-dose values in Table 3.
- Read the dose reports generated by the CT scanner for each examination you interpret to become familiar with the CTDIvol and DLP values,
- Take the appropriate time necessary for optimization
- Keep the AEC switched on unless for sequential mode with large x-ray beam of 16 cm (Acquilion One–Toshiba).
- Select a standard-sized patient for starting optimization (1 m70 and 70–75 kg),
- Select an appropriate kV setting depending on the patient's diameter (see above).
- Check mAs that limit AEC: on GE and Toshiba scanners, make sure that the mA window is widely opened enabling tube current to be significantly reduced in small individuals and increased in obese. For this purpose, reduce the lowest possible mAs limit to 20, and increase the upper limits of the scanner generator. Before acquisition, check the mAs table in order to make sure that the AEC system is acting in varying the mAs from slice to slice. Adapt the index of image quality stepwise while decreasing the CTDIvol displayed on the CT screen. This index of image quality corresponds to the noise index with GE and Toshiba scanners, to

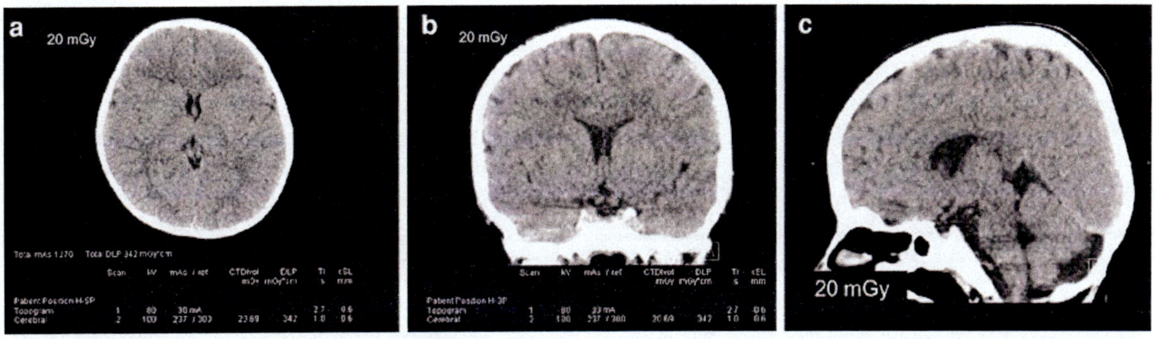


**Fig. 5** Optimized Brain CT acquisition in a 8-year-old boy with 100 kV, activated AEC and image quality set at 300 mAs. The resultant tube current time product is at 237 effective mAs and the CTDIvol at 20 mGy. **a, b** show representative *axial* and *coronal* views with dose report, and (**c**) shows sagittal reformat. Slice thickness is at 3 mm

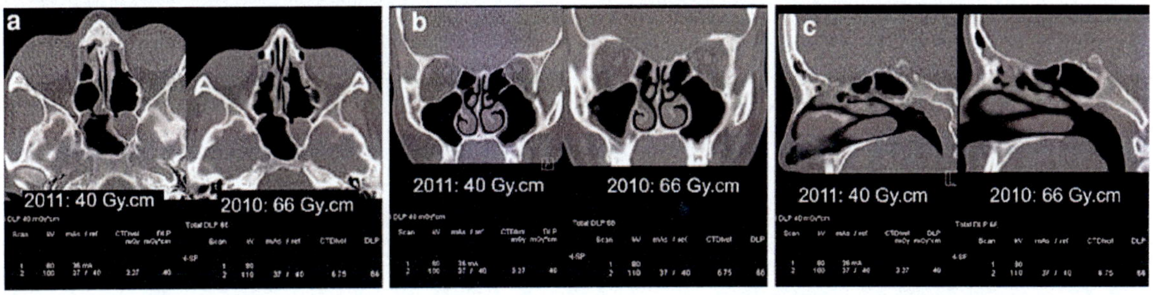


**Fig. 6** Side-by-side comparison of axial (**a**), coronal (**b**), and sagittal (**c**) reformats on the sinonasal cavities in a 34-year-old woman. The *left-sided* images were obtained in 2011 with a scanner of the latest MDCT generation (Siemens Definition AS series) and delivered a CTDIvol of 3.27 mGy and a DLP of 40 mGy.cm. The *right-sided images* were obtained 3 months earlier in 2010 on a 16-slice scanner (Siemens Emotion 16) through an acquisition delivering a CTDIvol of 6.75 mGy and a DLP of 66 mGy.cm

**Fig. 7** Axial 3 mm slices at the level of lung bases obtained in two male patients weighting 85 kg, similar chest wall thickness and 33 cm in lateral chest diameter. Figure 3a was reconstructed from a non-optimized CT acquired with a CTDIvol at 28.3 mGy. Figure 3b was reconstructed from an optimized CT acquired with a CTDIvol a 7.7 mGy. Image noise was 11UH in Fig. 3a and 15 UH in Fig. 3b

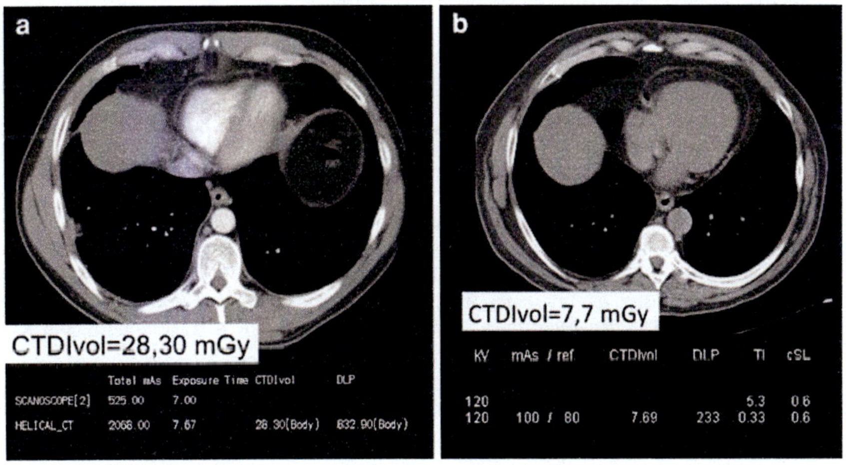

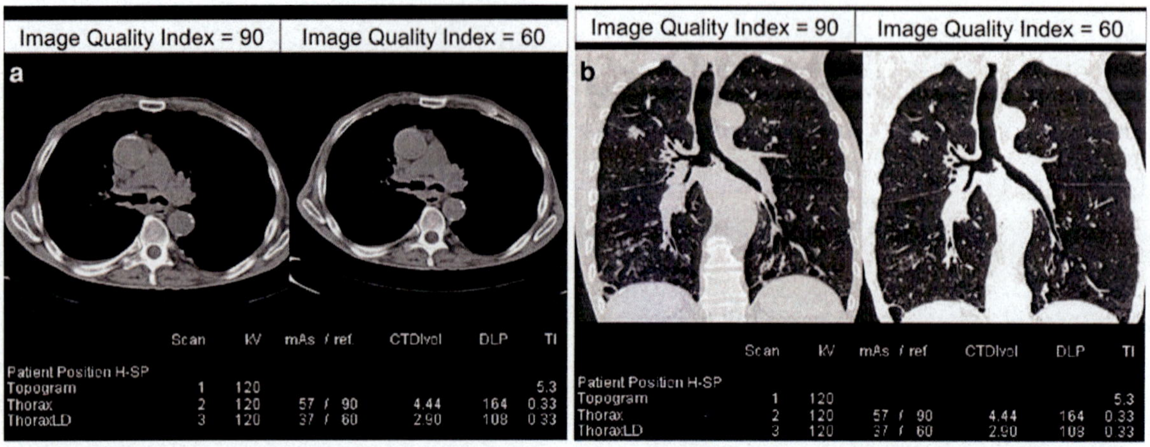


**Fig. 8** Side-by-side comparisons of unenhanced CT scans obtained in a 70-year-old underweight male patient with stage IV colon cancer and a BMI at 21 kg/m$^2$. The only modified parameter is the image quality index of the tube current modulation system. The first acquisition is performed with an index at 90 mAs (standard dose), whereas the second is obtained with the index set at 60 mAs (optimized dose), and a dose reduced by one-third. **a** shows axial views in mediastinal window with comparable and acceptable image quality and (**b**) shows coronal slices in pulmonary window. Both normal and abnormal findings are equally seen on standard and optimized dose images. Note that the dose in this underweight patient is half the value of that delivered in the obese patient shown in Fig. 9

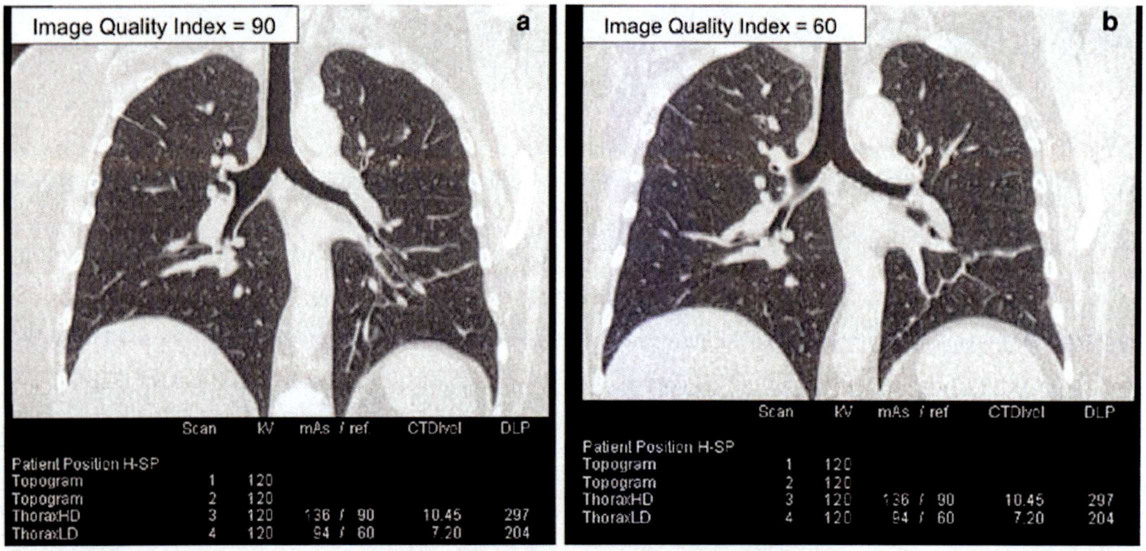


**Fig. 9** Side-by-side comparisons of unenhanced CT scans obtained in a 60-year-old obese woman with stage IV breast cancer and a BMI at 32 kg/m$^2$. As in Fig. 8, the only modified parameter is the image quality index of the tube current modulation system. The first acquisition is performed with an index at 90 mAs (**a**, standard dose) whereas the second is obtained with the index set at 60 mAs (**b**, optimized dose), the dose being reduced by one-third. Image quality is comparable and acceptable at optimized dose. Note that the mean tube current time product has been automatically increased by 50% by AEC system for both acquisitions as compared to the default settings

the "quality *reference eff. mAs*" with Siemens scanners, and to the eff. mAs with Philips scanners.

- Choose a slice thickness value slightly higher than the detector's nominal thickness, typically 1.5 mm for abdominal MDCT when acquired with 0.5, 0.6, or 0.625 mm. ("Scan thin, view thick"—see above),
- Use smoother reconstruction algorithms if possible unless for high-resolution data sets. Typically, with

a Siemens scanner, use B10 or B20 preferably to B30 or B40.

- Compare with previous acquisitions in the same patient.
- Discuss with your colleagues. If satisfied, process to a further optimization in the next standard-sized patient. If not satisfied, check parameters such as collimation and reconstruction thickness, and increase the dose by 10%. If this dose level is much higher than those displayed in Table 3 and Figs. 2, 3, 4, 5, 6, 7, 8, 9, 10, 11, 12, 13, 14, 15, 16, 17, 18, 19, 20, 21, 22, 23, 24, 25, 26, 27, 28, 29 and 30, contact your manufacturer for further support.
- In children, lower the KV settings to 100 if patient's weight ranges from 40 to 80 kg and down to 80 kV if weight is lower than 40 kg. Tube current time products may remain almost unchanged or slightly increased when lowering tube potential.

# 4 Examples of Optimized Parameters for CT Scanning

The purpose of this section is to illustrate standard and optimized CT images for the most frequent CT examinations.

## 4.1 CT of the Head

As shown in "Image Quality in CT: Challenges and Perspectives" by Georg Stamm in the present edition, reference diagnostic levels (RDL) expressed in CTDIvol for brain CT are usually around 60 mGy. Surveys show that the 25th percentile for brain CT is approximately at 50 mGy.cm. A CTDI at 40 mGy has been found to be the reasonable limit for optimized MDCT of the first and second generation (Tsapaki et al. 2006). The lowest CTDIvol observed in surveys for head CT in adults are approximately at 30 mGy. Examples of brain CT at 60, 40, and 30 mGy are given in Figs. 2, 3 and 4. An example of an optimized acquisition in an 8-year-old boy is shown in Fig. 5. As a general rule, AEC should be activated for brain CT. It may save at least 15% of the dose event if active in the Z direction only as for GE, Siemens, and Philips scanners. In adult patients, the tube potential may be set at 120 or 140 kV as in Fig. 4. In pediatric patients (below 12 years of age), 100 kV should be preferred as shown in the "Dose Optimization and Reduction in CT of Children" by P. Vock et al. Figures 2, 3, 4 and 5 refer to helical acquisitions. We show an acquisition with CTDIvol at 20 mGy in an 8-year-old boy in Fig. 5. In some departments, the sequential mode is preferred to the helical one. It offers the possibility to tilt the gantry while scanning, whereas tilting may not be possible with helical scans as with Philips, Toshiba, and Siemens scanners. Tilting the gantry has two advantages. First, it may reduce the scan height that is often higher than 15 cm without gantry tilt and can be reduced to 12 cm when tilting. Second, tilting enables to reduce the direct exposure to eye lens.

## 4.2 CT of Sinonasal Cavities

The natural contrast between structures within sinonasal cavities enables to use very low-dose settings as detailed by Tom Mulkens et al. in "Image Noise Reduction Filters" of the present edition. CTDIvol values (with head CTDI phantom—16 cm in diameter) may range between 4 and 8 mGy. Newest scanner generation and in particular the sequential mode of the 320 detector-row scanner enables further reductions while maintaining image quality at an acceptable level. A side-by-side comparison of a CT of the sinonasal cavities in the same patient with 3 months' interval is shown in Fig. 6 and illustrates the difference between the 16 slice scanner generation and the latest 128-slice scanner.

## 4.3 CT of the Chest

The chest is the body region with the highest risk and because it contains the most radio-sentitive organs such as the breast (Hricak et al. 2011; Deak et al. 2010; Huda et al. 2011). The high natural contrast between structures (air in the lungs and fat in the mediastinum) enables to reduce the dose by a factor of 4–10 while maintaining image quality at an acceptable level. Typically, a CTDIvol of 3.5 mGy in a standard patient weighting 70 kg is achievable without iterative reconstruction (Singh et al. 2011). Standard settings as installed by manufacturers are almost never optimized as shown in Fig. 7 that compared images of similar quality obtained with

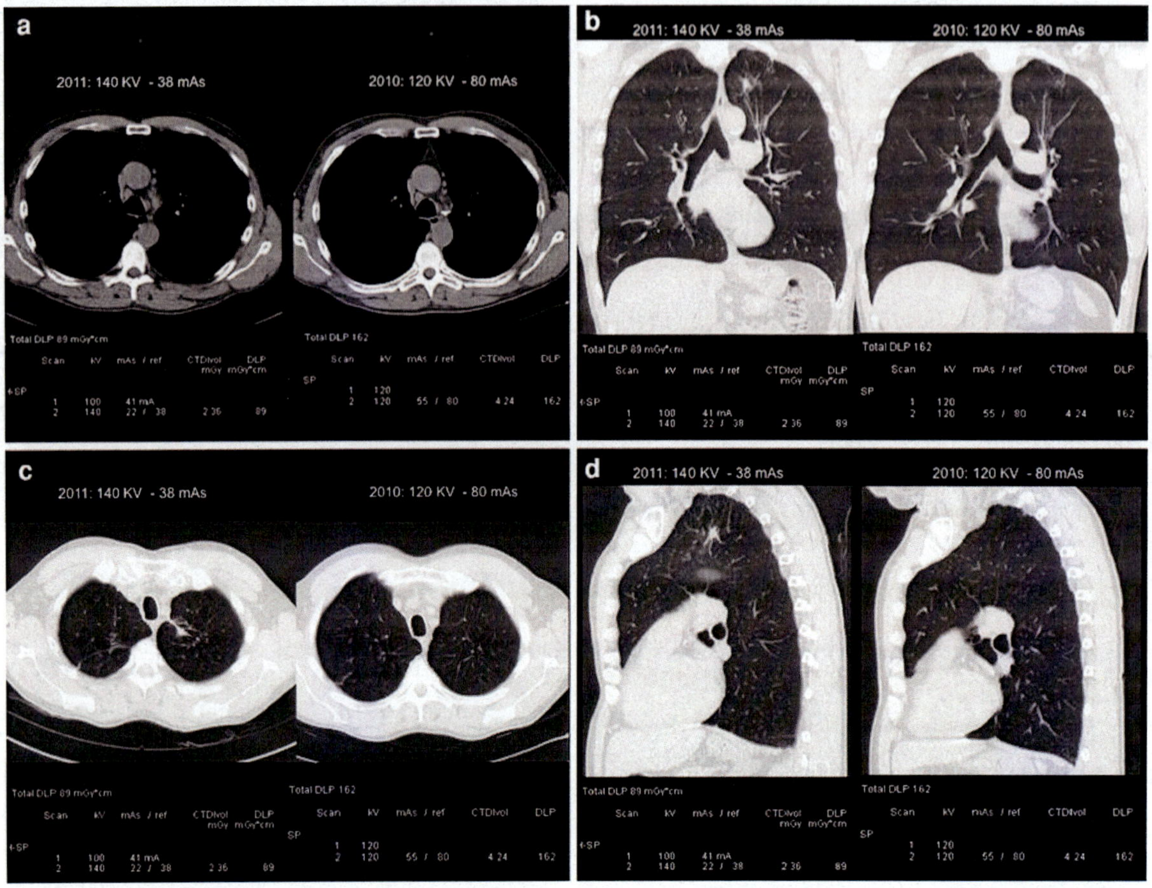


**Fig. 10** Consecutive chest CT examinations in the same patient with stable body weight of 65 kg obtained in 2010 and in 2011. A pulmonary lesion has appeared in 2011 in the left upper lobe. The 2010 acquisition was obtained with 120 kV and 80 mAs, whereas the second CT was obtained at 140 kV and 38 mAs default setting. The CTDIvol was reduced from 4.24 to 2.36 mGy (−45%). Image quality is very similar between both acquisitions as shown in mediastinal window in (**a**), and in pulmonary window in coronal (**b**), in axial (**c**), and in sagittal views (**d**)

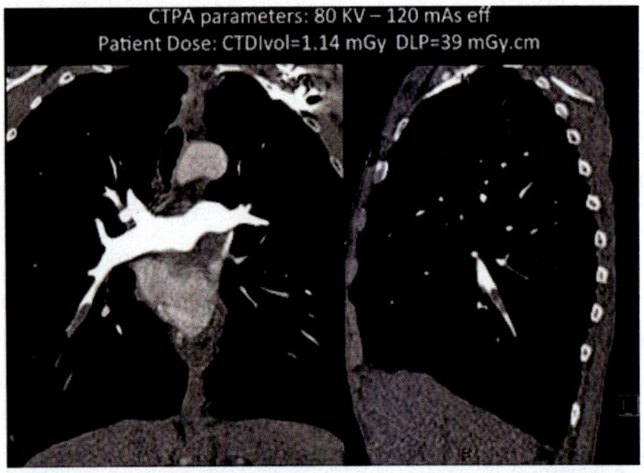


**Fig. 11** CTPA examination in a patient weighting 55 kg obtained at 80 kV. The CTDIvol of this acquisition is at 1.14 mGy and the DLP of the entire examination is 39 mGy.cm. Npte that the vessel enhancement is perfect

CTDIvol at 28 mGy non optimized) and at 7.7 mGy (optimized) in an 85 kg patient.

### 4.3.1 Tube Current Time Product and Noise Index Selection

Optimization of chest CT can be performed while comparing CT acquisition with different dose settings. Because AEC may have different effects in underweight and in obese patients, optimized settings have to be tested in patients with very different body weights and body mass index (BMI) as shown in Figs. 8 in an underweight patient, and in Fig. 9 in an obese patient. The dose in the obese patient shown in Fig. 9 is twice as high as that delivered to the patient displayed in Fig. 8. This AEC-dependent dose increase is reasonable and is not based on a constant noise.

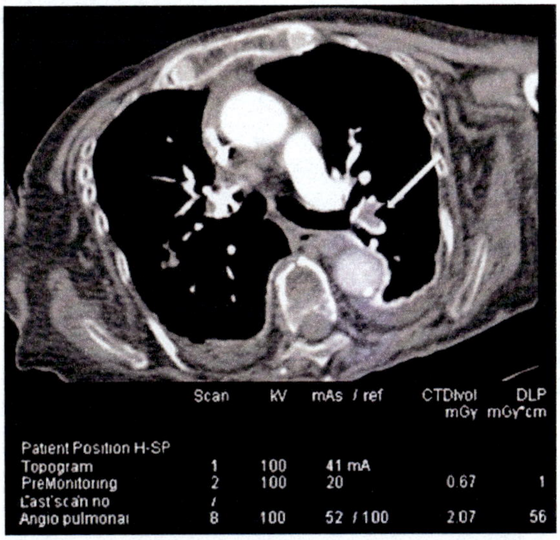


**Fig. 12** CTPA examination in a patient weighting 60 kg obtained at 100 kV. The CTDIvol of this examination is at 2.07 mGy and the DLP is 56 mGy.cm. A pulmonary embolus is seen in the left upper lobe (*arrow*)

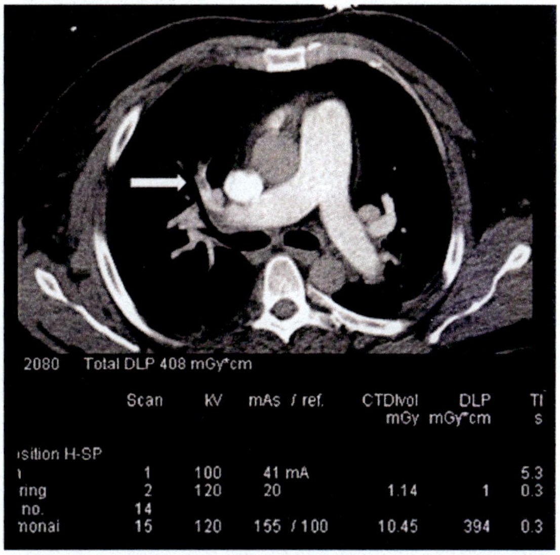


**Fig. 13** CTPA examination in a patient weighting 115 kg obtained at 120 kV. The CTDIvol of this acquisition is at 10.5 mGy and the DLP at 394 mGy.cm. The vessel enhancement is not excellent, probably because of tube potential at 120 kV. A pulmonary embolism is seen in right upper lobe (*arrow*). Note that this obese patient was exposed to a DLP that does not exceed the reference levels

### 4.3.2 Tube Potential Selection

- Unenhanced chest CT. High tube potential selection at 140 kV, in association with lowered tube currents can be recommended for unenhanced chest CT, whereas low tube potentials at 100 or at 80 kV are recommended (Sigal-Cinqualbre et al. 2004, Schueller-Weidekamm et al. 2006) for CT angiography. A comparison of consecutive acquisitions with 6 months' interval in the same patient is shown in Fig. 10. The first CT examination was acquired in 2010 at 120 kV and a quality reference mAs of 80. The second CT examination was acquired in 2011 at 140 kV and a quality reference mAs of 38 mAs. Patient's weight was stable at 65 kg between the two examinations. According to CT Expo software, a simultaneous change in KV from 120 to 140 and in mAs from 80 to 38 should result in a CTDIvol reduction from 5.4 to 3.8 mGy (−30%). In the patient shown in Fig. 10, the dose reduction was 45%. In a local survey on chest CT dose, the average DLP per examination using 140 kV and 38 mAs was 120 mGy.cm in 50 consecutive patients including obese, and a dose reduction by 45% was observed as compared to the 120 kV and 80 mAs settings used the year before. It is to note that high tube potential strategy for unenhanced chest CT is not dependent on the manufacturer and has been successfully tested during optimization processes on GE, Philips, and Siemens scanners at 140 kV and with Toshiba scanners at 135 kV, on patients with various BMI ranging from obese to underweight.
- CT pulmonary angiography (CTPA) requires the use of low tube potential at 100 or at 80 kV. The 120 kV setting is only recommended for CT angiography in obese patients. An example of a CTPA examination obtained at 80 kV in a patient weighting 60 kg is shown in Fig. 11. An acquisition with 100 kV obtained in a 62-year-old woman with spondylarthritis and acute pulmonary embolism is shown in Fig. 12. As previously demonstrated in the literature (Schueller-Weidekamm 2006) the vessel enhancement is significantly higher while using low KV settings. Unfortunately, their use is not often possible as patients who undergo CTPA are frequently obese because obesity is one of the risk factors for this disease (Tang et al. 2011). An example of CTPA at 120 kV obtained in an obese patient weighting 115 kg is shown in Fig. 13.
- Low-Dose unenhanced Chest CT. As shown in "Hardware Developments for Radiation Dose Reduction " of the present edition, CT scanning

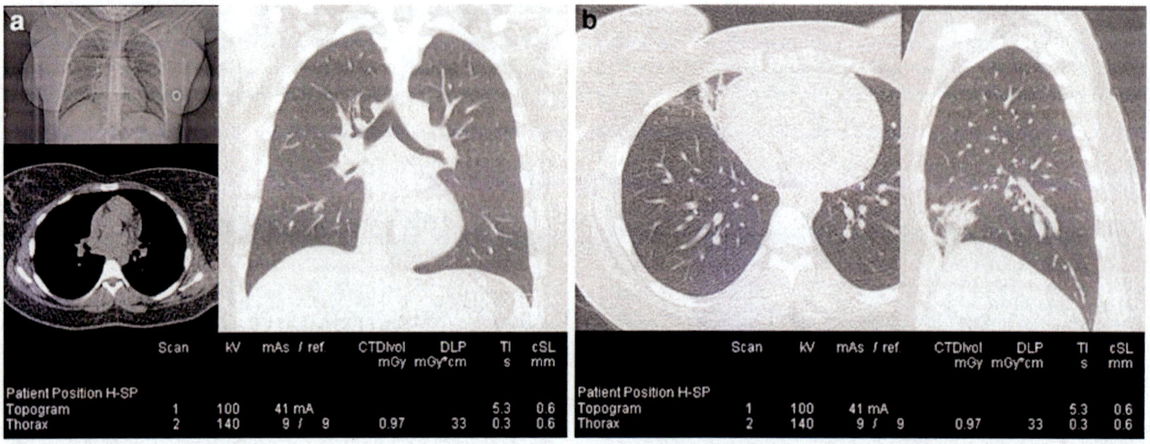


**Fig. 14** Low-Dose chest CT examination acquisition obtained in a 23-year-old teacher with suspected tuberculosis. Tube potential is at 140 kV, mean effective tube current time product is 9 mAs, and the CTDIvol is 0.97 mGy. DLP is at 33 mGy.cm. Three millimeter slices are reconstructed with iterative algorithm (IRIS—Siemens Healthcare Forchheim—Germany; Kernel are I26 for the mediastinum and I50 for the lungs). **a** shows scout view, mediastinal axil slice and coronal pulmonary reformat. **b** shows sagittal and axial pulmonary windows and an infiltrate in the right middle lobe

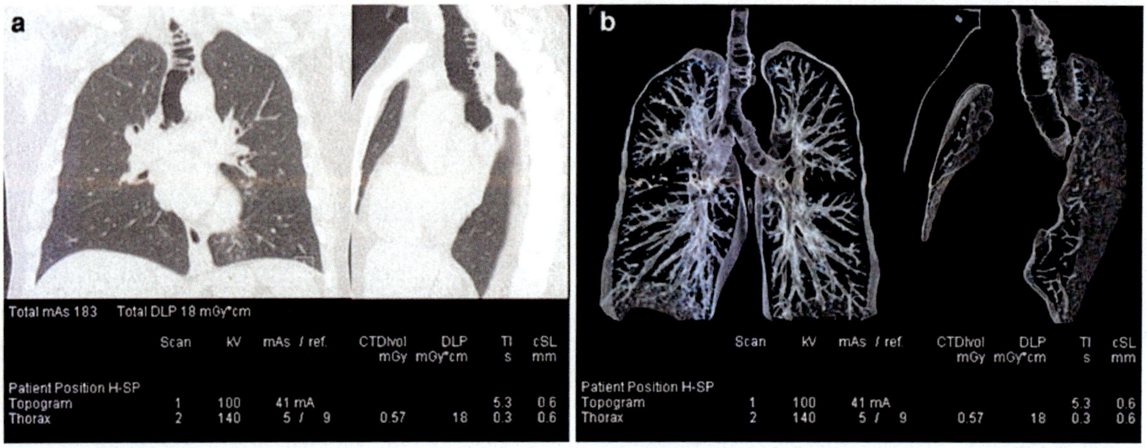


**Fig. 15** Low-Dose chest CT examination obtained in a patient weighting 65 kg with the same parameters as in Fig. 14 but with a mean effective tube current time product of 5 mAs. The CTDIvol is of 0.57 mGy and the DLP of 18 mGy.cm. A tracheobronchial diverticulosis can be seen in (**a**) in coronal and sagittal 3 mm slices and in (**b**) in virtual bronchography VRT reformats

of the lung parenchyma and of the mediastinum can be performed with so-called low-dose settings. Although the presented dose levels in Figs. 8, 9, 10, 11, 12 and 13 are not high, we do not name their radiation dose level as low because the image quality is still good. We prefer naming the dose level of 3–4 mGy for CTDIvol as optimized and call "low-dose" the settings associated with a low image quality characterized by noise. This image quality is reduced but it is still accurate for diagnosis. A low-dose acquisition can be obtained with a tube current time product divided by 3–6 as compared to the optimized one. This noise has to be reduced by any available solution, and in particular by iIterative reconstruction algorithms. An example is shown in Fig. 14 in an obese patient

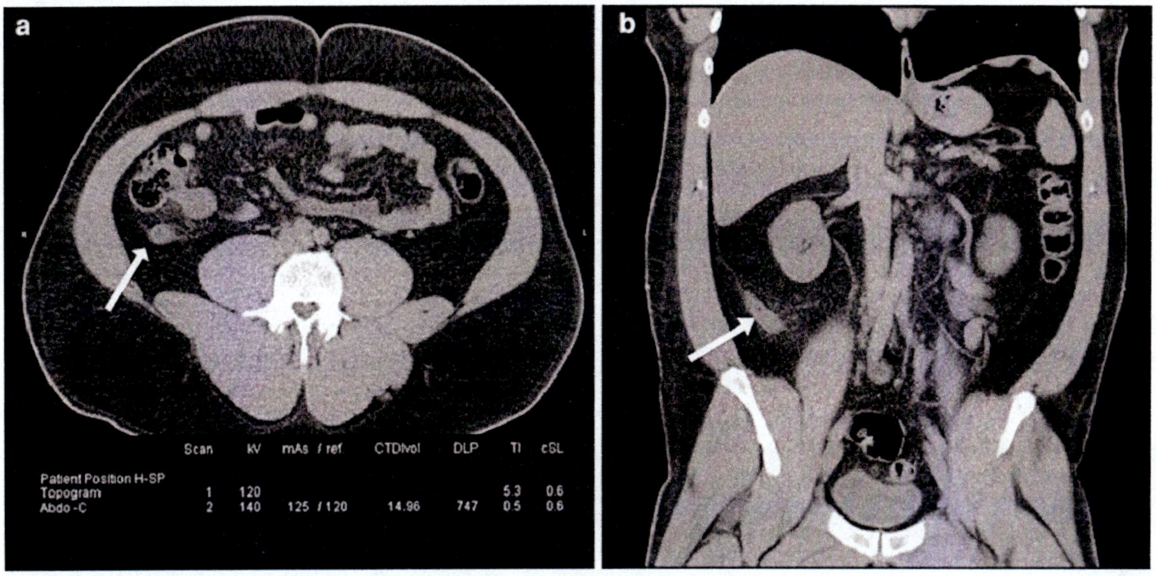


**Fig. 16** Optimized dose MDCT in an obese patient weighting 135 kg, with acute appendicitis. Tube potential at 140 kV is used. Dose-length product is as high as 747 mGy.cm. Transverse abdominal diameters are of 37 (P-A) and 43 (*lateral*) cm. Arrows in (**a**) (*axial plane*) and 16B (*coronal plane*) show enlarged appendix and fat stranding

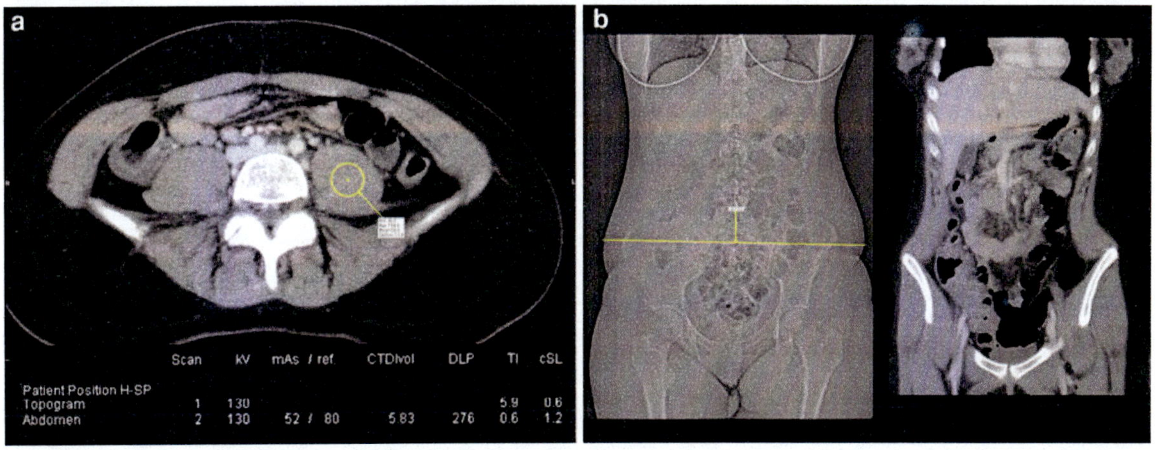


**Fig. 17** Optimized dose MDCT in a 28-year-old woman weighting 78 kg and with right lower quadrant pain. **a** shows standard deviation of UH measurements within a ROI placed in psoas muscle, representing image noise and corresponding to 16 UH. **b** shows the frontal scout view with measurement of patient's lateral diameter that is of 35 cm. In this figure, the coronal MRP shows a right colon thickening indicating colitis. Dose descriptors are the following: CTDIvol = 5.83 mGy and DLP = 276 mGy.cm

and resulted in a DLP of 33 mGy.cm. In a standard patient undergoing low-dose chest CT, the DLP is around 20 mGy.cm. Low-dose chest CT delivers a dose that is in the range of a two-views chest radiograph (Fig. 15).

### 4.4 CT of the Abdomen and Pelvis

The collective dose from abdominal CT examinations is the highest of all CT examinations because both the number of CTs performed on the abdomen and the

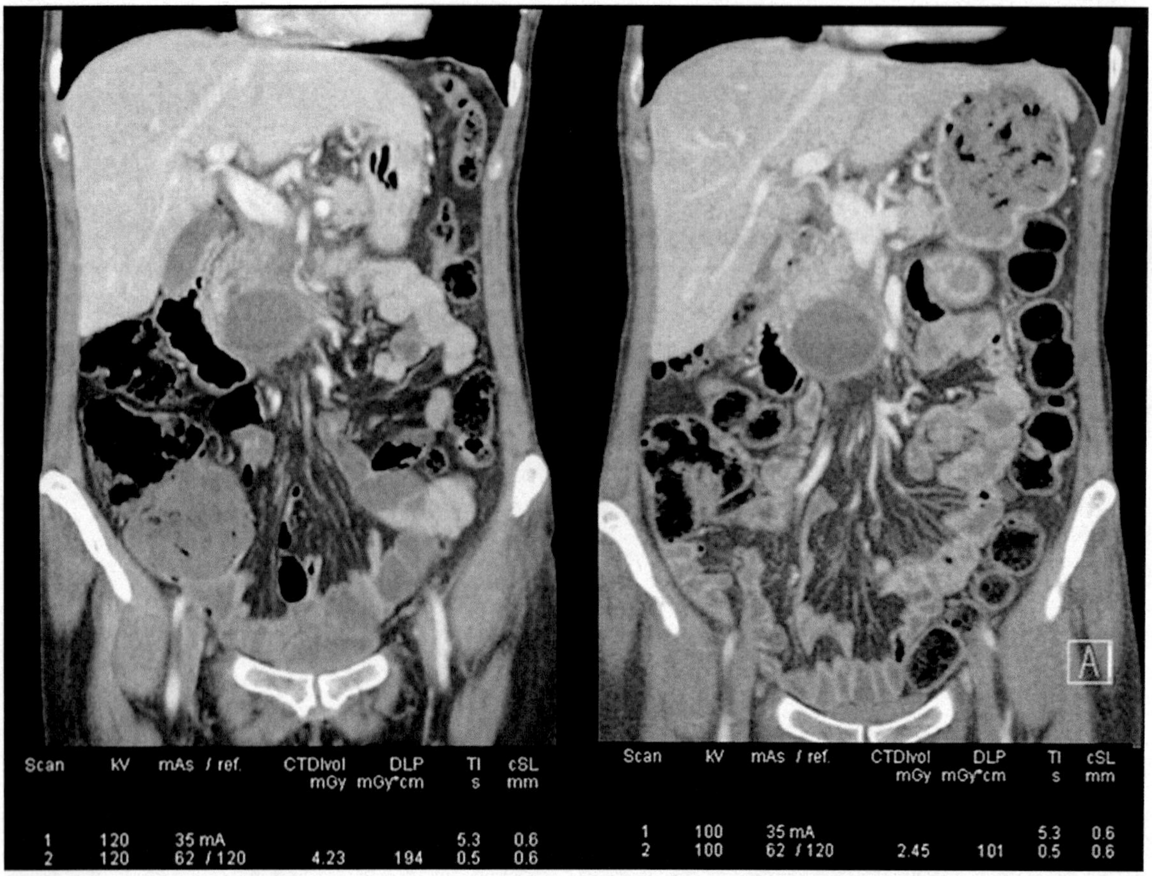


**Fig. 18** Tube potential optimization: advantage of using 100 kV in a patient weighting <80 kg. Two consecutive optimized dose abdominal MDCT examinations in portal venous phase are obtained in a 36-year-old patient with stable weight of 67 kg, for follow-up of acute pancreatitis with pseudocyst of the pancreatic head. Left coronal image is acquired at 120 kV and follow-up CT displayed right coronal image is acquired at 100 kV. CTDIvol has been reduced from 4.23 to 2.46 and the DLP has been reduced from 194 to 101 mGy.cm, whereas image quality is preserved. Note that index of image quality that is set at 120 has not been modified between the two examinations

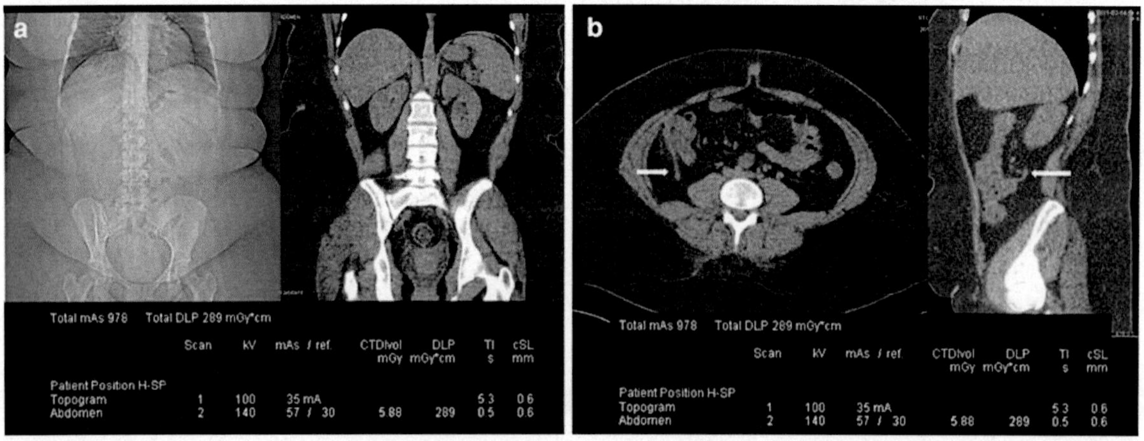


**Fig. 19** Low-Dose unenhanced MDCT of the abdomen in an extremely obese 22-year-old woman with right iliac fossa pain. Tube potential is at 140 kV and reference image quality index is set at 30 mAs. The mean delivered effective tube current time product is increased to 57 mAs. The CDTIvol is at 5,88, whereas the DLP is at 289 mGy.cm. **a** shows image quality (noise in fat is at 16 UH) and extreme obesity shape. **b** *Arrows* show normal appendix

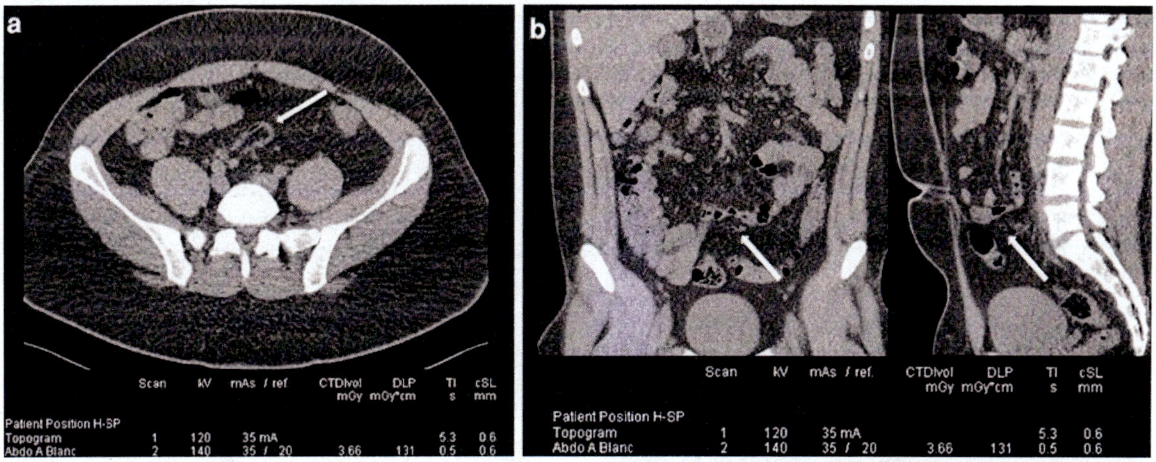


**Fig. 20** Low-Dose unenhanced MDCT of the abdomen in an obese 21-year-old man weighting 105 kg with suspected acute appendicitis. Tube potential is at 140 kV and reference image quality index is set at 20 mAs. The mean delivered effective tube current time product is increased to 35 mAs by the AEC system. The CDTIvol is at 3.66 mGy, whereas the DLP is at 131 mGy.cm. Normal aerated appendix and absence of fat stranding can be seen in axial (**a**), coronal and sagittal reconstructions (**b**). Note that the acquisition height has been limited to the kidneys and contributes to obtain a very low DLP as compared to that expected in patients weighting 105 kg

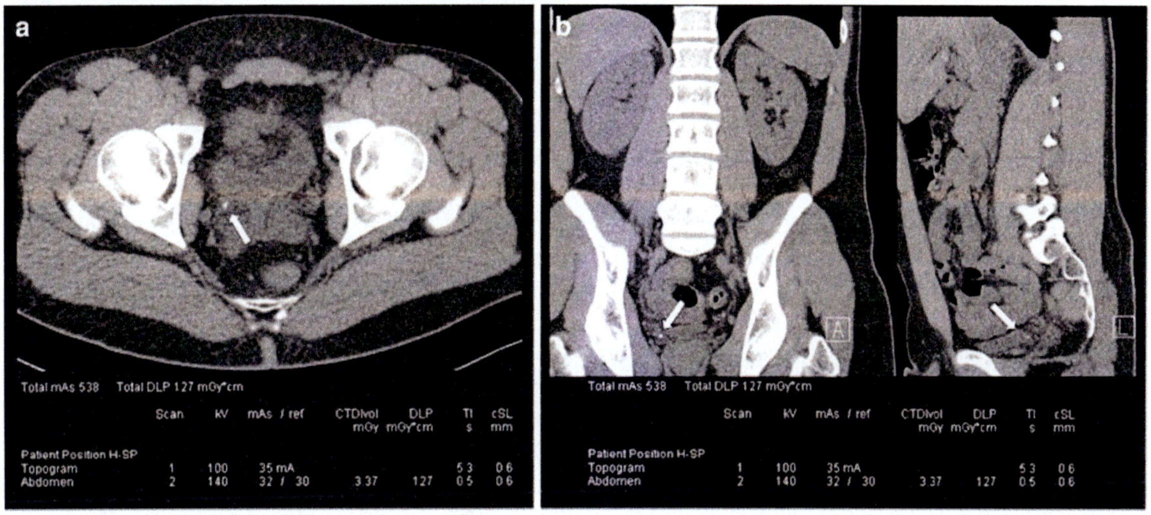


**Fig. 21** Low-Dose unenhanced MDCT of the abdomen in a 21-year-old man weighting 90 kg and 1m78 tall, with suspected acute left renal colic. Tube potential is at 140 kV and reference image quality index is set at 30 mAs. The mean delivered effective tube current time product is increased to 32 mAs by the AEC system. The CDTIvol is at 3.37 mGy, whereas the DLP is at 127 mGy.cm. A 2 mm large calcification is seen in the distal left ureter. This stone was later endoscopically retrieved

radiosensitivity of abdominal organs are high. Among all abdominal CTs performed, pain is the most frequent clinical context and can happen in old but also in young patients. Approximately half of the CT performed on the abdomen is obtained in patients aged less than 50 years (Hricak et al. 2011). For all these reasons, it is of utmost importance to optimize and further minimize the CT dose on the abdomen. Particular attention has to be paid to patient's diameter of weight, and in particular to obese patients. As explained above, obese patients should be scanned with specific protocols tolerating higher noise levels as standard patients in order to avoid dose excess from AEC systems warranting constant noise.

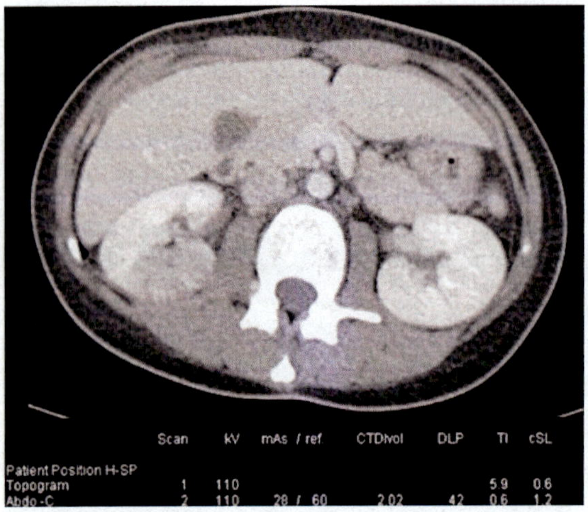


**Fig. 22** Low-Dose iodine enhanced MDCT of the upper abdomen performed in order to confirm acute left pyelonephritis in a 22-year-old woman. Tube potential is at 110 kV and reference image quality index is set at 60 mAs. This preset is reduced to 28 mAs effective by the AEC system. The resulting CTDIvol is at 2 mGy. Because the pelvis was not included in the scan range, DLP is at 42 mGy.cm only

Benchmarkings obtained from surveys can help in finding reference values for upper limits of inacceptable practice—shown in Table 1, and levels of optimized dose for abdominal CT shown in Table 2. The CT Parameters and dose descriptors in optimized and low-dose CT of the abdomen as a function of body weight are listed in Table 3 and illustrated in Figs. 16, 17, 18, 19, 20, 21, 22, 23, 24 and 25.

For unenhanced CT, the tube potential may be as high as 140 kV, but with low tube current time product (typically 60 efffective mAs in an 80 kg patient).

For enhanced CT, the tube potential should be at 120 kV if the body weight is higher than 80 kg in men and 70 kg in women, and at 100 kV in men weighting less than 80 kg and women weighting less than 70 kg.

Optimizing abdominal CT is often perceived as dangerous for the accuracy of the technique. Comparisons of different dose levels are thus necessary to be reassured and convinced of the potential for dose reduction. Examples of comparisons are shown in Figs. 26, 27 and 28.

With optimized parameters as displayed in this section on abdominal CT, the mean DLP per acquisition on 50 consecutive patients undergoing abdomino-pelvic CT is lower than 300 mGy cm, a dose lower than one half of the RDL.

### 4.5 CT of the Lumbar Spine

Optimizing the lumbar spine CT acquisitions is particularly difficult for various reasons. First, obesity is one of the main risk factors for low back pain. Second, the increased fat component in abdominal CT slices of obese patients enabling to tolerate higher noise is not present in the spinal canal. Thus, one cannot tolerate similar noise in lumbar spine imaging in obese as compared to abdominal imaging. Third, there is a trend to increase the acquisition height with MDCT in order to produce similar heights as for MRI. In some EU countries in which this trend is significant, the DLP for lumbar spine have at least doubled with MDCT as compared to single detector CT. Nevertheless, an investigation on tube current reductions on lumbar spine CT using noise simulating technique (Bohy et al. 2007) suggests that a mAs reduction by 35–50% is feasible. Interestingly, this study also confirms that the dose reduction has lower impact on image interpretation as compared to interobserver variability. This means that observers have to train and work together, not only for reproducible diagnoses but also for image quality acceptability. Figures 29 and 30 show examples of side-by-side comparisons of standard and optimized dose MDCT of the lumbar spine. Finally, the potential role of iterative reconstructions enabling to reduce the noise in lower dose MDCT of the spine is illustrated in Fig. 31.

## 5 Acquisition Height and Multiphasic Examinations

It is usually accepted that both the number of phases and the acquisition heights are too high in routine practice.

### 5.1 Number of Phases and Acquisition Height in Head CT

A very interesting study published in 1998 investigated the need for enhanced head CT after negative

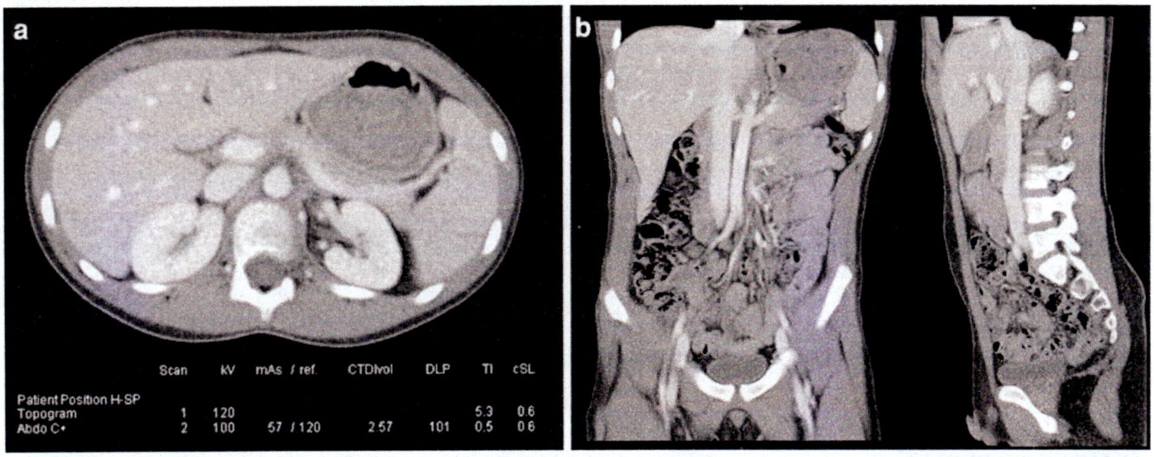


**Fig. 23** Iodine enhanced abdominal MDCT in a 12-year-old boy weighting 45 kg complaining of right iliac fossa pain. No sign of appendicitis was found by CT. Tube potential is at 100 kV and reference image quality index is set at 120 mAs. This preset is reduced to 57 mAs effective by the AEC system. The resulting CTDIvol is at 2,57 mGy and the DLP is at 101 mGy.cm. **a** shows a representative 3 mm *axial view* and **b** shows *coronal* and *sagittal* 3 mm views

unenhanced acquisition (Demaerel et al. 1998). The aim of this study was to define guidelines for intravenous contrast administration in cranial CT, as there were no recent guidelines based on a large series of patients. In 1,900 consecutive patients (1,480 adults and 420 children) pre- and post-contrast scan was analyzed in order to assess the contribution of contrast enhancement to the diagnosis. The findings were grouped according to whether abnormalities were seen on the pre- and/or post-contrast scan, or whether no abnormalities were seen at all. Sensitivity, specificity, positive predictive value, negative predictive value, and accuracy of a pre-contrast scan were used to determine validity. Results showed that intravenous contrast enhancement only contributes to the diagnosis if a suspicious abnormality is seen on the unenhanced scan or in the appropriate clinical setting (rule out metastases and pre-operative of carotid artery surgery—33.6% of the indications in this series). In the remaining patients (65.6%) there is no diagnostic contribution, except for a small number of abnormalities (0.8%). These are often anatomical variants and have no therapeutic impact. The authors conclude that the number of contrast-enhanced cranial CT examinations can significantly be reduced by using four general guidelines for contrast administration resulting in considerable cost savings without affecting the quality of service to the patient. These guidelines can be applied in any radiology department. In 2011, 13 years after this investigation was published, CT dose surveys show that the practice of systematic dual Head CT acquisitions is still observed in some departments.

Regarding acquisition height, the influence of both patient positioning and gantry tilting is important on the DLP of brain CT. Acquisition height is significantly increased if the gantry cannot be tilted and the patient does not flex the head in orbito-meatal orientation. In adition, sequential scanning with gantry tilting enables to reduce the dose to the eye lens significantly (Abdeen et al. 1998, 2010). Bismuth shields can also reduce the dose to the eye lens and is recommeneded at least in children (Raissaki et al. 2010).

## 5.2 Number of Phases and Acquisition Height in Chest CT

Chest CT is usually acquired in one single acquisition. Rarely, additional acquisitions are requested such as expiratory CT (Bankier et al. 2001). This is not part of routine practice. For CTPA, one single acquisition is sufficient. The appropriate acquisition height is however questionable. CTPA was first developed with single detector scanners (Remy-Jardin et al. 1992, 1996) and proved to have a negative predictive value as high as 98%. With single detector technique, the acquisition height was 15 cm, from the aortic arch to the diaphragm. CTPA examinations acquired with MDCT nowadays cover the entire chest

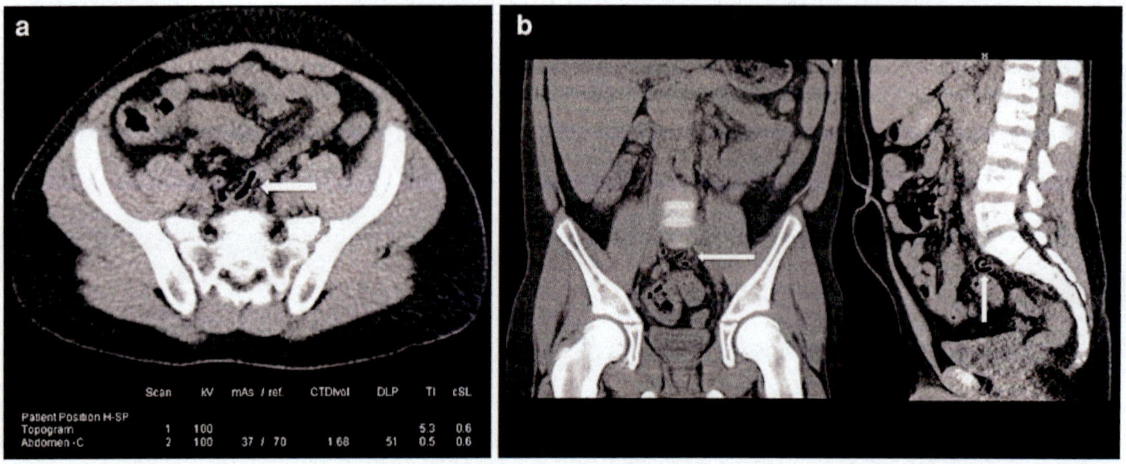


**Fig. 24** Low-Dose unenhanced MDCT of the abdomen in a 11-year-old boy weighting 40 kg and with right iliac fossa pain and inconclusive US. Tube potential is at 100 kV and reference image quality index is set at 70 mAs. This preset is reduced to 37 mAs effective by the AEC system. The resulting CTDIvol is at 1.68 mGy and the DLP is at 51 mGy.cm. This dose descriptor corresponds to the effective dose E of an abdominal plain film examination with 1 to 2 views. The appendix (*arrows*) is normal in axial (**a**) and in coronal and sagittal orientations (**b**)

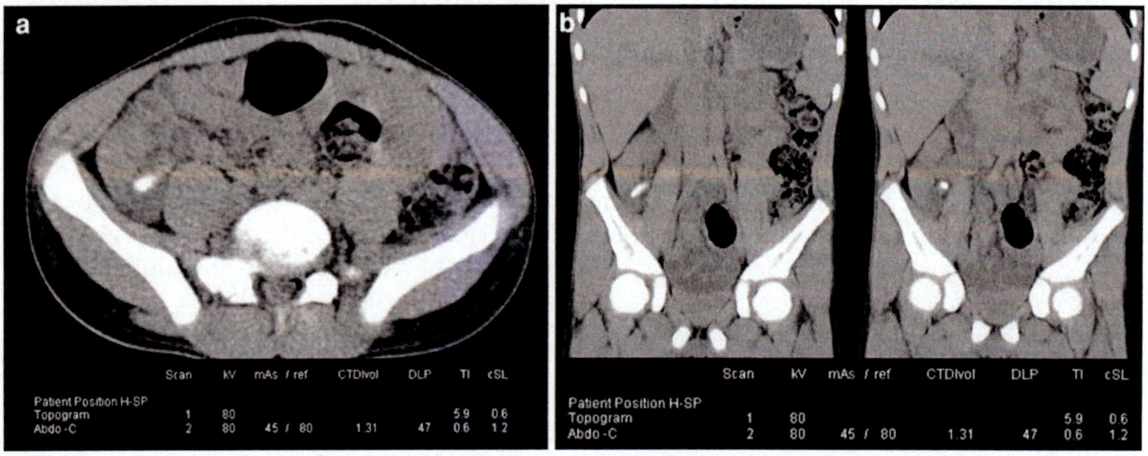


**Fig. 25** Unenhanced MDCT obtained at 80 kV in a 9-year-old boy weighting 34 kg after inconclusive ultrasound examination. Acute appendicitis is demonstrated by MDCT while CTDIvol is at 1.38 mGy only and DLP is lower than 50 mGy.cm. In case of inconclusive unenhanced CT, enhanced acquisition can be obtained with similar presets

with an acquisition height of 30–35 cm. However, MDCT has not yet been shown to provide a higher predictive value to CTPA as compared to the historical one. On the other hand, the influence of doubling the acquisition height on the benefit of MDCT in terms of alternative diagnoses has not yet been investigated. It is thus questionable whether one should acquire the entire chest or the middle portion of the chest for excluding pulmonary embolism.

## 5.3 Number of Phases and Acquisition Height in Abdominal CT

Both the number of phases and the acquisition height should be justified when scanning the abdominal cavity, and in particular in patients referred to CT for abdominal pain that corresponds to the most frequent reason for requesting a CT of the abdomen and affects both older and young or very young patients including

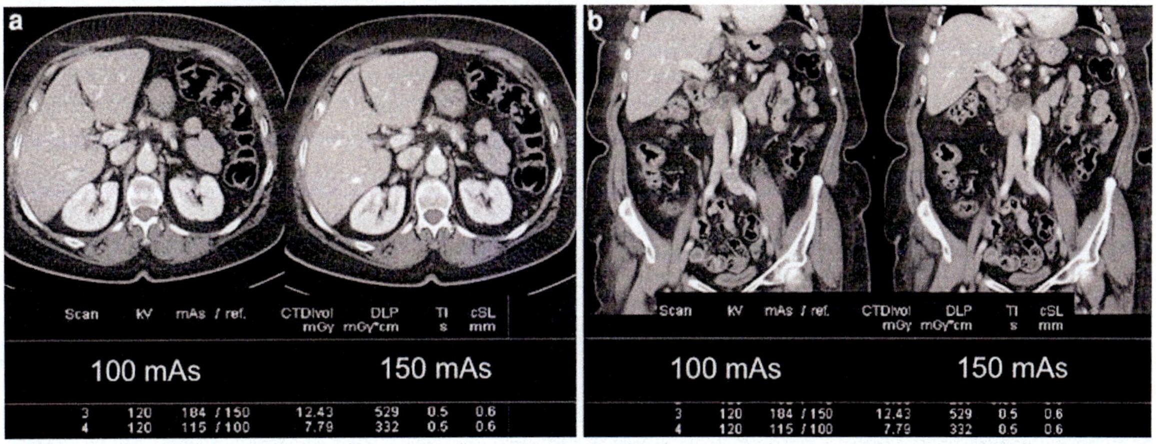


**Fig. 26** Comparison of two consecutive CT enhanced acquisitions of the abdomen with a dose reduction of 33% in an 88-year-old woman weighting 87 kg. The first is performed with 120 kV and 150 mAs effective, and the second with the same tube potential but 100 mAs. Slice thickness is 3 mm. Image noise is slightly higher in the 100 mAs *axial* (**a**) and *coronal* (**b**) orientations, but the 100 mAs images are of acceptable quality for the local radiologists

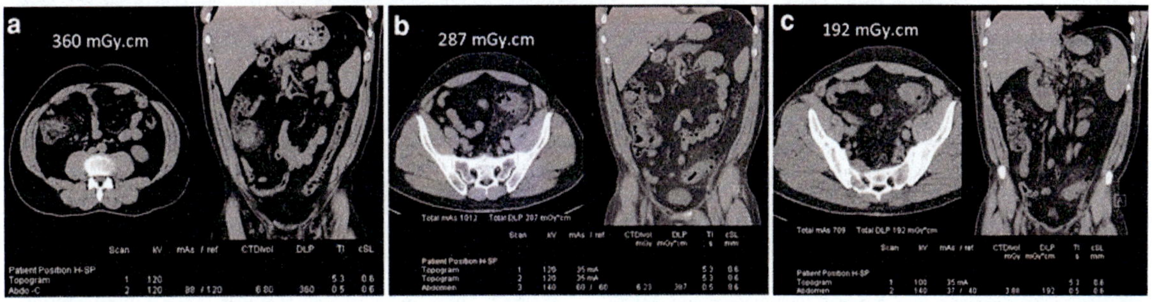


**Fig. 27** Comparison of three consecutive unenhanced examinations in the same 42-year-old man weighting 90 kg. **a** (Octobre 2010—*right* iliac fossa pain) shows 3 mm CT images acquired with a Sensation 64 scanner (Siemens healthcare—Forchheim, Germany) using 120 kV and 120 mAs (quality reference). CTDIvol is at 6.8 mGy and the DLP is 360 mGy.cm. CT shows *right* sided colitis. **b** (January 2011—*left* iliac fossa pain and suspected diverticulitis) 3 mm CT images acquired with a Definition AS 128 scanner using 140 kV and 60 mAs (quality reference). CTDIvol is at 6.23 and the DLP is 287 mGy.cm. **c** (February 2011—control of the acute uncomplicated *left* colon diverticulitis) from February 2011 shows 3 mm CT images at 140 kV and 40 mAs (quality reference). CTDIvol is 3.88, and DLP is 192 mGy.cm. This figure illustrates three important parameters of dose optimization; 1/for unenhanced CT, 140 kV with low tube current is an efficient way to optimize and preserve excellent image quality. 2/the acquisition height in patients with lower abdominal pain could be limited, and the cranial part of the liver may not be included in the scan range. 3/a control CT for acute divertivulitis can be obtained with lower tube currents as compared to the initial one

children (Hricak et al. 2011). A question that should be addressed prospectively is whether CT performed for lower abdominal pain should include the lung bases and the entire liver or only the kidneys. An acquisition height reduction by 20–25% could be achieved if the liver is not entirely included in the scan range. Similarly, there is no benefit in scanning patients referred for non-traumatic abdominal pain with multiphasic examinations. On should perform preferably one single acquisition, with or without iodine contrast injection.

## 5.4 Acquisition Height in CT of the Lumbar Spine

Default acquisition of the entire lumbar spine at MDCT with sagittal reformat is more and more frequently seen nowadays with acquisition heights of 20–22 cm. Unfortunately, ACR (2008) does not define criteria for acquisition height. In surveys, the mean acquisition height of lumbar spine CT examinations ranges from 14 to 22 cm. As a general rule, the height of acquisition

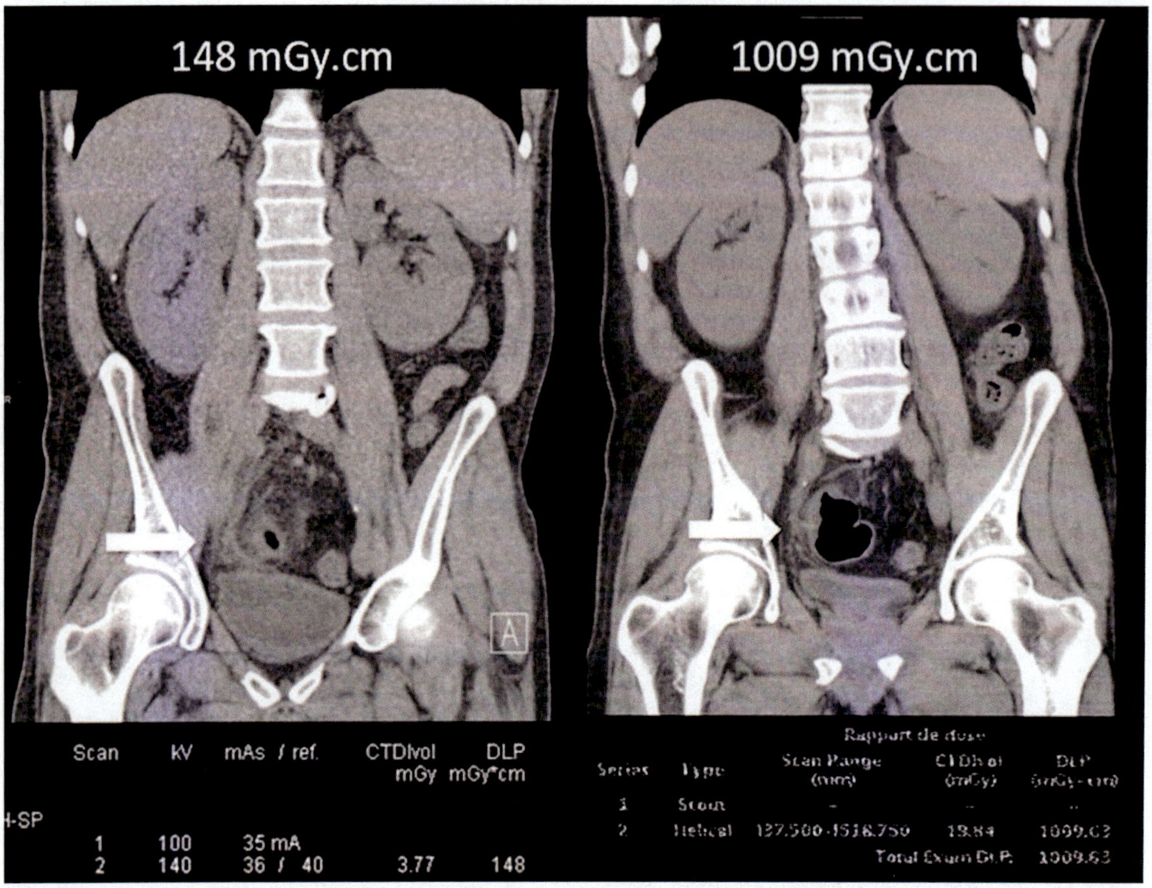


**Fig. 28** Comparison of two consecutive unenhanced MDCT in a 48-year-old man weighting 75 kg who had a sigmoid perforation on a foreign body that proved to be a swallowed toothpick. The toothpick is visible on the right-sided coronal reformat but had not been seen by the local radiologist who acquired the CT at 120 kV and a noise index of 10 UH for 1.25 mm slices. The resultant CTDIvol is at 19.84 mGy and the DLP is of 1.009 mGy.cm. The second scan displayed on the left acquired after endoscopical removal of the toothpick was acquired at 140 kV and 40 mAs (quality index) and automatically reduced to 36 mA by the AEC system, inducing a CTDIvol of 3.77 mGy and a DLP of 148 mGy.cm. This dose is seven times lower than the initial one. The 1.009 mGy.cm is above the RDL and typically corresponds to default parameters as installed by vendors on their CT machines

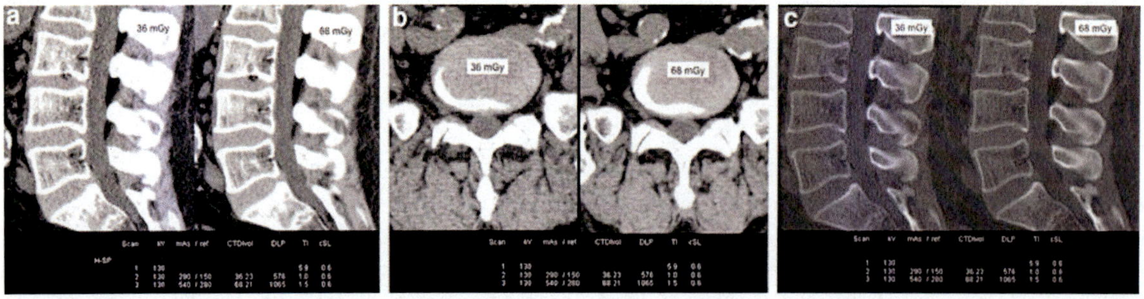


**Fig. 29** Side-by-side comparison of two consecutive unenhanced MDCT of the lumbar spine obtained in a 67-year-old patient weighting 92 kg, with stage IV colon carcinoma and complaining of low back pain. Two acquisitions are obtained, one at standard dose at 68 mGy CTDIvol, displayed on the right, and the second at optimized dose at 36 mGy CTDIvol, displayed on the left. **a** shows sagittal reformats in soft tissue algorithm and window, **b** shows *axial slices* and 29C sagittal reformats with bone algorithm and window

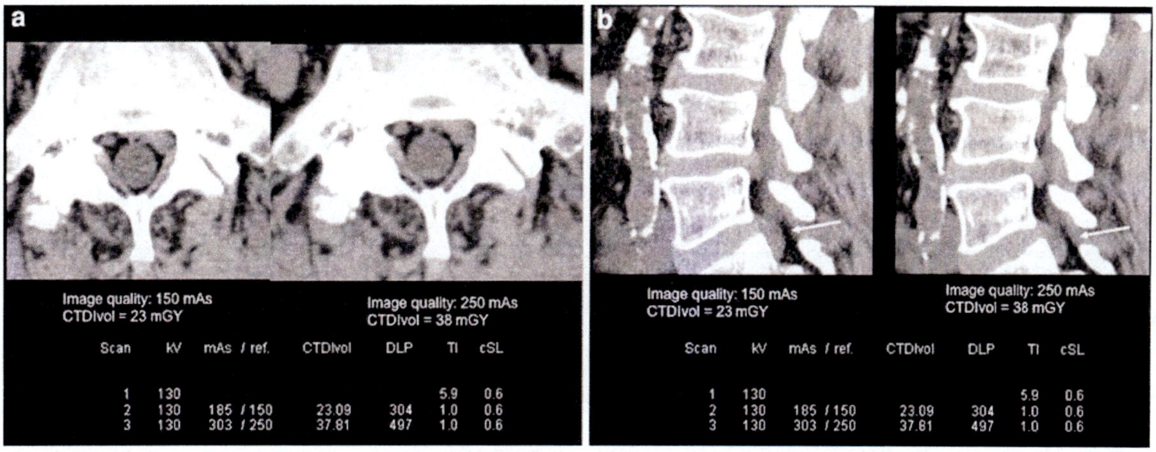


**Fig. 30** Side-by-side comparison of two consecutive unenhanced MDCT of the lumbar spine obtained in a 72-year-old man weighting 71 kg, with stage III non-small cell lung carcinoma who complained of low back pain. Two acquisitions are obtained, one at standard dose at 38 mGy CTDIvol, displayed on the right, and the second at optimized dose at 23 mGy CTDIvol, displayed on the left. **a** shows axial slices at the level of L5-S1 disk and shows a discal herniation. **b** shows the same herniation (*arrow*) in left para-sagittal orientation. sagittal reformats in soft tissue algorithm and window, (**b**) shows *axial slices* and 29C sagittal reformats with bone algorithm and window

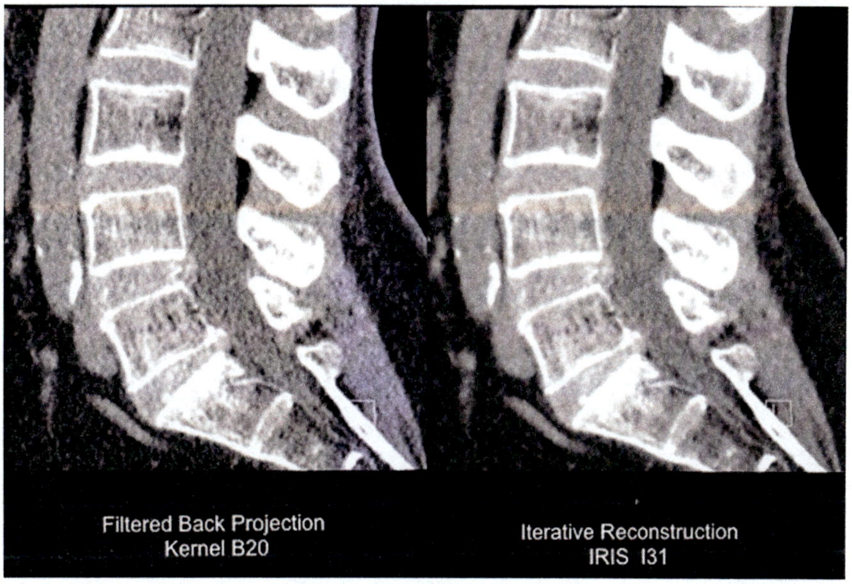


**Fig. 31** Side-by-side comparison of sagittal reformats of the lumbar spine showing the potential benefit of iterative reconstruction technique for imaging low back pain with CT. The *right one* is obtained with iterative reconstructions (IRIS I31 Kernel, Siemens healthcare, Forchheim, Germany) and the *left one* with usual filtered back projection technique (B20 Kernel). Noise in FBP reformat is significantly reduced in Iterative reformat

should be defined depending on the patient's symptoms as was done 20 years ago while using single detector CT in sequential mode.

## 6 Summary and Conclusion

Optimization is a part of everyday practice and has to be conducted by CT users responsible for the dose they deliver. Vendors are welcome to help in this process but the final decision on the ALARA image quality and dose relies on the radiologists. The historical references for radiation dose in CT (RDLs) are very high. Current CT technology enables to reduce standard dose by 50% of th RDLs, cvcn without iterative reconstruction. According to recent data from the literature (see "Image Noise Reduction Filters" by Kalra and Singh entitled "Image filters and radiation dose") iterative techniques may provide additional dose reductions. Automatic exposure control systems are helpful tools for maintaining the image quality at the ALARA level and should not be switched off. Low-dose protocols deliver nowadays a dose very close to that of radiographic examinations. These protocols should be default in young patients. A special attention has to be paid to justifying acquisition's height and to the number of acquisitions required.

## References


American College of Radiology (ACR) (2008) ACR Appropriateness Criteria®. Clinical Condition: Low Back Pain. Access at http://search.acr.org/

Abdeen N, Chakraborty S, Nguyen T, dos Santos MP, Donaldson M, Heddon G, Schwarz BA (2010) Comparison of image quality and lens dose in helical and sequentially acquired head CT. Clin Radiol 65:868–873

Allen BC, Baker ME, Einstein DM, Remer EM, Herts BR, Achkar JP, Davros WJ, Novak E, Obuchowski NA (2010) Effect of altering automatic exposure control settings and quality reference mAs on radiation dose, image quality, and diagnostic efficacy in MDCT enterography of active inflammatory Crohn's disease. AJR 195:89–100

Bankier AA, Schaefer-Prokop C, De Maertelaer V, Tack D, Jaksch P, Klepetko W, Gevenois PA (2007) Air trapping: comparison of standard-dose and simulated low-dose thin-section CT techniques. Radiology 242:898–906

Bankier AA, Van Muylem A, Knoop C, Estenne M, Gevenois PA (2001) Bronchiolitis obliterans syndrome in heart-lung transplant recipients: diagnosis with expiratory CT. Radiology 218:533–539

Brenner DJ, Hall EJ (2007) Computed tomography–an increasing source of radiation exposure. N Engl J Med 357: 2277–2284

Bohy P, de Maertelaer V, Roquigny A, Keyzer C, Tack D, Gevenois PA (2007) Multidetector CT in patients suspected of having lumbar disk herniation: comparison of standard-dose and simulated low-dose techniques. Radiology 244: 524–531

Deak PD, Smal Y, Kalender WA (2010) Multisection CT protocols: sex- and age-specific conversion factors used to determine effective dose from dose-length product. Radiology 257:158–166

Demaerel P, Buelens C, Wilms G, Baert AL (1998) Cranial CT revisited: do we really need contrast enhancement? Eur Radiol 8:1447–1451

EMAN European Medical ALARA Network (2011) WG1 :optimization of Patient CT Exposures—synthesis Document 31-03-2011—Page 53–71. Access on line at http://www.eman-network.eu/spip.php?article164

Golding SJ (2010) Radiation exposure in CT: what is the professionally responsible approach? Radiology 255: 683–685

Guimarães LS, Fletcher JG, Harmsen WS, Yu L, Siddiki H, Melton Z, Huprich JE, Hough D, Hartman R, McCollough CH (2010) Appropriate patient selection at abdominal dual-energy CT using 80 kV: relationship between patient size, image noise, and image quality. Radiology 257: 732–742

Hricak H, Brenner DJ, Adelstein SJ, Frush DP, Hall EJ, Howell RW, McCollough CH, Mettler FA, Pearce MS, Suleiman OH, Thrall JH, Wagner LK (2011) Managing radiation use in medical imaging: a multifaceted challenge. Radiology 258:889–905

Huda W, Magill D, He W (2011) CT effective dose per dose length product using ICRP 103 weighting factors. Med Phys 38:1261–1265

Jaffe TA (2009) Reply. AJR 192:W141–W141

Kambadakone AR, Prakash P, Hahn PF, Sahani DV (2010) Low-dose CT examinations in Crohn's disease: impact on image quality, diagnostic performance, and radiation dose. AJR 195:78–88

Keyzer C, Tack D, De Maertelaer V, Bohy P, Gevenois PA, Van Gansbeke D (2004) Acute appendicitis: comparison of low-dose and standard-dose unenhanced multi-detector row CT. Radiology 232:164–172

Keyzer C, Cullus P, Tack D, De MV, Bohy P, Gevenois PA (2009) MDCT for suspected acute appendicitis in adults: impact of oral and IV contrast media at standard-dose and simulated low-dose techniques. AJR 193:1272–1281

Leng S, Yu L, McCollough CH (2010) Radiation dose reduction at CT enterography: how low can we go while preserving diagnostic accuracy? AJR 195:76–77

Meeson S, Alvey CM, Golding SJ (2010) The in vivo relationship between cross-sectional area and CT dose index in abdominal multidetector CT with automatic exposure control. J Radiol Prot 30:139–147

National Lung Screening Trial Research Team (2010) The national lung screening trial: overview and study design. Radiology 258:243–253

Raissaki M, Perisinakis K, Damilakis J, Gourtsoyiannis N (2010) Eye-lens bismuth shielding in paediatric head CT: artefact evaluation and reduction. Pediatr Radiol 40: 1748–1754

Remy-Jardin M, Remy J, Wattinne L, Giraud F (1992) Central pulmonary thromboembolism: diagnosis with spiral volumetric CT with the single-breath-hold technique–comparison with pulmonary angiography. Radiology 185:381–387

Remy–Jardin M, Remy J, Deschildre F, Artaud D, Beregi JP, Hossein-Foucher C, Marchandise X, Duhamel A (1996) Diagnosis of pulmonary embolism with spiral CT: comparison with pulmonary angiography and scintigraphy. Radiology 200:699–706

Smith-Bindman R (2010) Is computed tomography safe? N Engl J Med 363:1–4

O'Connor OJ, Vandeleur M, McGarrigle AM, Moore N, McWilliams SR, McSweeney SE, O'Neill M, Ni Chroinin M, Maher MM (2010) Development of low-dose protocols for thin-section CT assessment of cystic fibrosis in pediatric patients. Radiology 257:820–829

Schindera ST, Graca P, Patak MA, Abderhalden S, von Allmen G, Vock P, Szucs-Farkas Z (2009) Thoracoabdominal-aortoiliac multidetector-row CT angiography at 80 and 100 kVp: assessment of image quality and radiation dose. Invest Radiol 44:650–655

Schueller-Weidekamm C, Schaefer-Prokop CM, Weber M, Herold CJ, Prokop M (2006) CT angiography of pulmonary arteries to detect pulmonary embolism: improvement of vascular enhancement with low kilovoltage settings. Radiology 241:899–907

Sigal-Cinqualbre AB, Hennequin R, Abada HT et al (2004) Low-kilovoltage multi-detector row chest CT in adults: feasibility and effect on image quality and iodine dose. Radiology 231:169–174

Singh S, Kalra MK, Hsieh J, Licato PE, Do S, Pien HH, Blake MA (2010) Abdominal CT: comparison of adaptive statistical iterative and filtered back projection reconstruction techniques. Radiology 257:373–383

Singh S, Kalra MK, Gilman MD, Hsieh J, Pien HH, Digumarthy SR, Shepard JA (2011) Adaptive statistical iterative reconstruction technique for radiation dose reduction in chest CT: a pilot study. Radiology 259: 565–573

Szucs-Farkas Z, Strautz T, Patak MA, Kurmann L, Vock P, Schindera ST (2009a) Is body weight the most appropriate criterion to select patients eligible for low-dose pulmonary CT angiography? Analysis of objective and subjective image quality at 80 kVp in 100 patients. Eur Radiol 19:1914–1922

Szucs-Farkas Z, Schaller C, Bensler S, Patak MA, Vock P, Schindera ST (2009b) Detection of pulmonary emboli with CT angiography at reduced radiation exposure and contrast material volume: comparison of 80 kVp and 120 kVp protocols in a matched cohort. Invest Radiol 44:793–799

Tang Y, Sampson B, Pack S, Shah K, Yon Um S, Wang D, Wang T, Prinz M (2011) Ethnic differences in out-of-hospital fatal pulmonary embolism. Circulation 123: 2219–2225

Tack D, Gevenois PA (2009) Body MDCT at 140 kV. AJR 192:W139–W140

Tack D, Jahnen A, Kohler S, Harpes N, Back C (2011) Clinical audit on optimization of radiation dose from mdct: effect on diagnostic reference levels for brain, sinus, cervical spine, chest, abdomen-pelvis, and lumbar spine examinations and on nationwide collective effective dose. ECR 2011, C-0066. Accessd on 13 June 2011, http://posterng.netkey.at/esr/online_viewing/index.php?module=view_postercoverpage&task=viewcoverpage&start=0&ls=authorlist&pi=105261&perid=216620&num=1&count=3&cid=ANY

Tsapaki V, Aldrich JE, Sharma R, Staniszewska MA, Krisanachinda A, Rehani M, Hufton A, Triantopoulou C, Maniatis PN, Papailiou J, Prokop M (2006) Dose reduction in CT while maintaining diagnostic confidence: diagnostic reference levels at routine head, chest, and abdominal CT–IAEA-coordinated research project. Radiology 240:828–834

# Automatic Exposure Control in Multidetector-row CT

Mannudeep K. Kalra

## Contents




**Abstract**

Automatic exposure control (AEC) is one of the most important aspects of radiation dose and image quality optimization for CT scanning. It is important to use this technique appropriately in order to obtain CT examinations with required image quality and/or radiation dose levels as improper use can lead to much lower or much higher radiation doses to patients undergoing CT examinations. There is similarity in basic principle behind different AEC techniques across different CT vendors but there are considerable differences between how the techniques are applied on platforms of different CT vendors. This chapter discusses various techniques of AEC available for use on clinical CT equipments.


*Confusion now hath made his masterpiece!*
William Shakespeare

*Confusion is a word we have invented for an order which is not yet understood.*
Henry Miller

William Shakespeare may have accidentally explained the premise for development of automatic exposure control (AEC) techniques, although Henry Miller may have summarized the issues related to the heterogeneous nomenclature of these techniques!

This chapter attempts to explore the rationale behind development of AEC for multidetector-row CT scanners and to describe mechanisms, clinical evidence and pitfalls of AEC techniques for radiation dose reduction or optimization.


M. K. Kalra (✉)
Department of Radiology,
Harvard Medical School,
Massachusetts General Hospital,
Boston, MA 02114, USA
e-mail: mkalra@partners.org



D. Tack et al. (eds.), *Radiation Dose from Multidetector CT*, Medical Radiology. Diagnostic Imaging,
DOI: 10.1007/174_2011_480, © Springer-Verlag Berlin Heidelberg 2012

## 1 Definition

AEC techniques have been defined as automatic adjustment of tube current in the x–y plane (angular AEC) or along the z-axis (z-axis AEC) or both (combined AEC) according to the size and attenuation characteristics of the body region being scanned in order to achieve constant CT image quality with lower radiation dose (Kalra et al. 2004a, b). The temporal automatic tube current modulation or the electrocardiography (ECG) controlled (pulsed) dose modulation is also a type of AEC technique used for cardiac and coronary CT angiography.

In simple terms, AEC techniques used for CT scanning behave like photo-timing used in conventional radiography (Kalra et al. 2005a, b). The photo-timing technique terminates exposure once adequate exposure has been achieved. In this way, photo-timing attempts to limit dose while making sure that adequate quality has been achieved, regardless of patient size and body region being assessed. Thus, it allows longer exposure time for X-ray projection of a larger, thicker and denser body part or patient, and shorter exposure time for thinner, smaller and less dense portion. On the other hand, CT scanning requires continuous exposure to X-rays, so instead of terminating exposure, the AEC techniques change tube current (mA) for different X-ray projections to maintain constant image quality (generally noise). Thus, AEC will decrease tube current for projections through smaller, less dense body regions (such as anterior–posterior projection at the level of the shoulders or chest) and will increase it for projections through larger, denser regions (such as lateral projection at the shoulder or abdomen). Ultimate objective of both the techniques, AEC and phototiming, is to ensure that no more and no less exposure is given to patients in order to acquire images with constant quality (Kalra et al. 2004b).

## 2 Rationale

Until recently, most CT studies were performed with fixed tube current technique (Kalra et al. 2004a). These fixed tube current values may be selected by technologists based on their arbitrary judgment or as per department protocols set by technologists, radiologists and/or medical physicists based on patient age and size, or study indication (Kalra et al. 2002, 2003a). However, the fixed tube current technique for multidetector CT scanning may be associated with following limitations:

- Lower dose efficiency: tube potential determines the photon energy and tube current influences the photon fluence or the number of photons. The proportion of X-rays used for image creation to the amount of incident X-rays determines dose efficiency of the scanner. In contradiction to the fixed tube current, the AEC techniques can improve dose efficiency while maintaining constant image quality by modulating tube current to apply required amount of photons during a single X-ray rotation (for different X-ray beam projections) and from one rotation to the next (for different z-axis or section locations) (Althen 2005; Terada 2005).
- Standardization issues: fixed tube current values have to be adjusted for different generations of multidetector-row CT scanners. Given the fact that on any given modern multidetector-row scanner, there are several ways to perform scanning, manual selection of fixed tube current may be difficult. In such circumstances, AEC techniques can automatically modulate mA to the selected combination of scanning parameters for obtaining CT images with required quality. In this context, the AEC techniques are being increasingly used for dose optimization with multidetector CT (Miyazaki et al. 2005).
- ECG control dose modulation or ECG pulsing: In contradiction of fixed tube current, ECG pulsing can reduce tube current during ventricular systole and increase tube current during relevant diastolic phase.

## 3 Nomenclature and Types of AEC Techniques

There is some confusion over the most appropriate nomenclature for AEC technique (Kalra et al. 2004b). Both AEC and automatic tube current modulation have been used to describe the same technique. Although automatic tube current modulation may actually represent the technique more accurately, AEC may be the more commonly accepted term for the technique.

Similarly, several terminologies have also been used to describe different subtypes of AEC techniques (Kalra et al. 2004b). In order to avoid confusion, most

**Table 1** Different types of AEC techniques available on current multidetector CT scanners

| Technique | GE | Hitachi | Philips | Siemens | Toshiba |
|---|---|---|---|---|---|
| Angular AEC | Smart mA | Adaptive mA | D-DOM | CARE Dose | SURE Exposure |
| Z-axis AEC | Auto mA | Not available | Z-DOM | Not available | Not available |
| Combined AEC | Auto mA 3D | IntelliEC | Work in progress | CARE Dose 4D | SURE exposure 3D |

(Z-DOM is a combination of Automatic Current Setting (ACS) and DOM technqiues)

commonly used or described terminologies have been specified and used in this chapter. Based on the scanning plane or direction in which AEC techniques are used for dose or tube current modulation, AEC techniques may be classified into x–y plane or angular, z-axis, and combined AEC techniques (Kalra et al. 2004b). The angular AEC techniques adapt tube current during each gantry rotation around the patient (Greess et al. 1999, 2001, 2002, 2004; Kopka et al. 1995). Thus, more than one tube current (mA) may be used during each gantry rotation. The angular AEC may estimate tube current during the first 180° gantry rotation and use this information for adapting tube current for the subsequent 180° gantry rotation. This has been labeled as real time or online angular AEC (CARE Dose, Siemens Medical Solutions, Forchheim, Germany; DOM, Philips Medical Systems, Netherlands) (Kalra et al. 2004b). The other type of angular AEC technique (Smart mA, GE Healthcare Technologies, Waukesha, Wisconsin, USA) uses a single localizer radiograph (the lateral projection) to obtain information for tube current modulation during the entire 360° rotation of X-ray tube around the patient.

In z-axis AEC, the tube current is adapted to maintain a constant specified image quality over the scan length. Some vendors have distinct standalone z-axis AEC techniques (Auto mA, GE Healthcare Technologies; Z-DOM, Philips Medical Solutions) while others such as Siemens Healthcare and Toshiba Medical Systems do not have z-axis AEC as separate entities but are available only as combined AEC techniques. The z-axis AEC changes tube current from one table position to the other based on information derived from a single localizer radiograph (Kalra et al. 2005b).

Lastly, the combined AEC techniques (Auto mA 3D, GE Healthcare Technologies; CARE Dose 4D, Siemens Medical Solutions) includes tube current modulation in both z-axis (z-axis AEC) and x–y plane (angular AEC) (Kalra et al. 2005a).

The different types of available AEC techniques on current multidetector CT scanners are summarized in Table 1 (Kalra et al. 2005b).

## 4 AEC Mechanisms

Before moving on to the mechanism of AEC, it may be helpful to understand some basic physics nomenclature of CT. Three axes of CT scanner in relation to the patients are explained in Fig. 1. Within each section position, there are several hundred projection angles from which X-ray beams begin their journey from X-ray source to the detectors through the patient body. These projection angles lie in the x–y plane of the scanner. With table feed, there is change in the z-axis section position of the patient.

Image noise, mottle or graininess, an important determinant of image quality, depends on applied tube current and X-ray beam attenuation (Kalra et al. 2004a). The latter depends on patient size, shape and attenuation characteristics (profile) of the body region being scanned. An increase in the tube current results in lower noise and a decrease in the tube current causes greater image noise. In general, an increase in attenuation profile results in greater image noise and vice versa. Thus, in order to maintain constant image noise in presence of changing attenuation profile, a region or projection with lower attenuation can be scanned with lower tube current compared with a high attenuation region or projection, which needs greater tube current. Although fixed tube current can be selected based on patient weight or size, use of fixed tube current does not allow adjustment of tube currents with in a given study (Fig. 2; Kalra et al. 2002, 2003a).

*Angular AEC.* The localizer radiograph-based angular AEC was the first AEC technique developed for radiation dose optimization in early 1990s for single-detector-row helical CT scanners (Kopka et al. 1995;

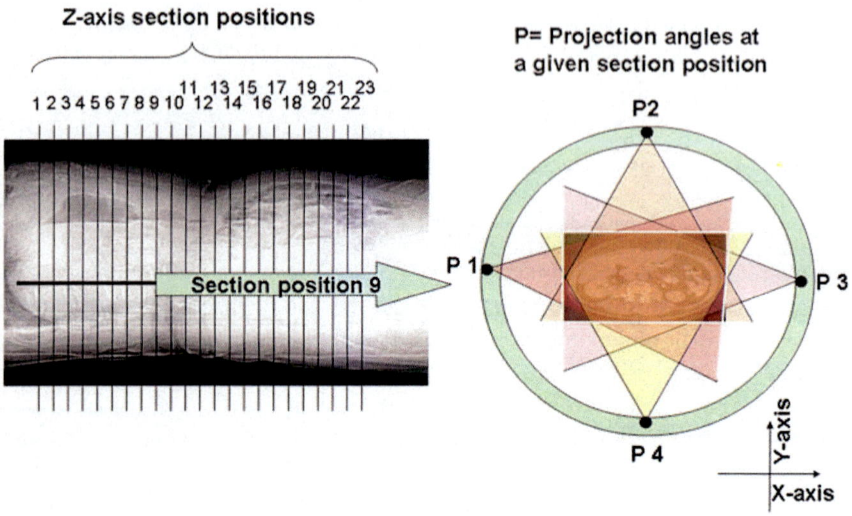


**Fig. 1** The three axes of CT. The z-axis section position implies slice location or slice position. The x–y axes plane lies within each z-axis section position and represents plane of X-ray beam projections during each gantry rotation

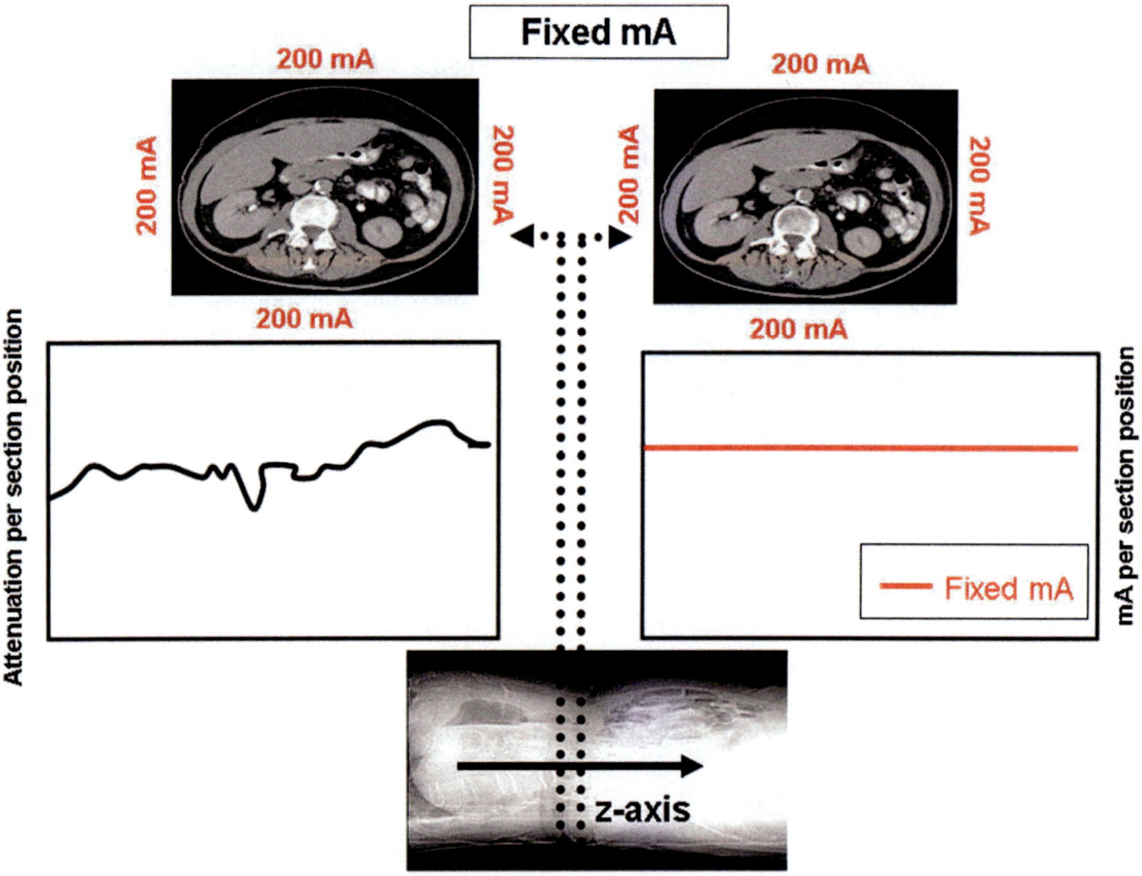


**Fig. 2** With fixed tube current, the scanner employs a single, specified mA value for all projections and section position for a given scan series acquisition. Although several CT centers adapt mA value with fixed tube current technique based on patient size and study indication, this technique cannot take into account the variability of attenuation in a section at different beam projections and at different z-axis section positions

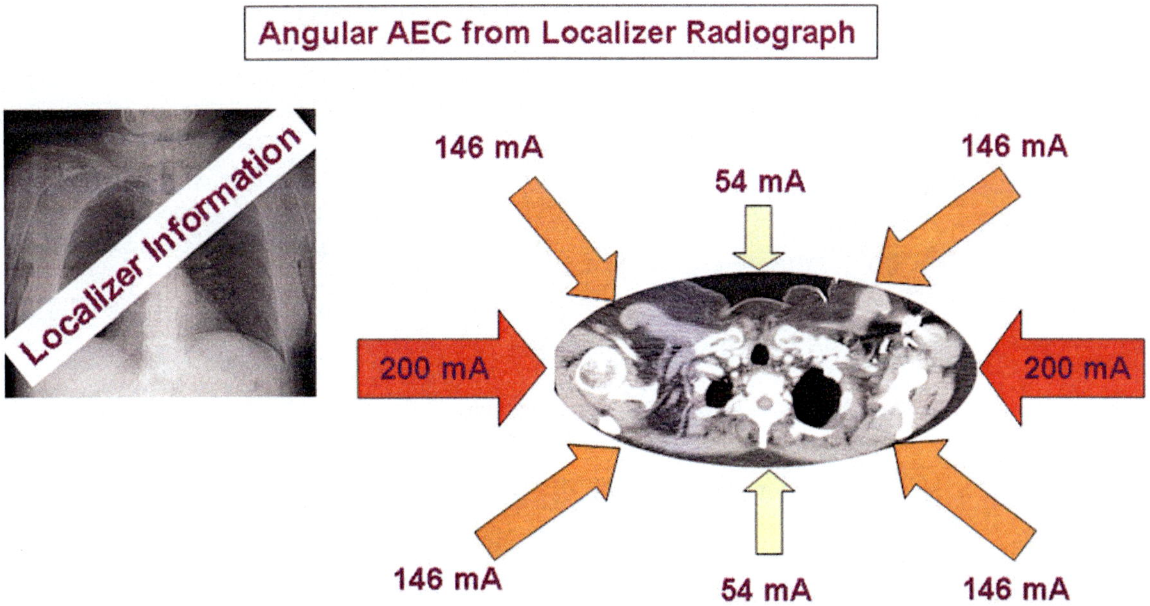


**Fig. 3** With localizer radiograph based angular AEC technique, information about attenuation profile at different beam projections with in each section position is collected from localizer radiograph. This information is used to modulate mA values at different beam projection angles during each X-ray tube revolution (the entire 360°). In an elliptical or asymmetric body cross-section, the technique will decrease mA values for beam projections in thinner portions or lower attenuation (such as in anterior–posterior or posterior–anterior projections) and increase mA values for beam projections passing through regions with greater attenuation or thicker portion (such as lateral projections)

Lehmann et al. 1997; Giacomuzzi et al. 1996). With angular AEC technique, the tube current is modulated to decrease X-rays in projection angles (or in the x–y plane), which will have less beam attenuation and contribute less to the noise in the overall image (Kalra et al. 2004b). This is especially helpful in reducing radiation dose to the non-circular or asymmetric body regions, such as the shoulders, where "non-lateral" projections (such as anterior–posterior projections) have less X-ray beam attenuation compared with the lateral projection (which is typically the projection with greatest attenuation and noise contribution). Therefore, angular AEC will reduce mA and dose in the "non-lateral" projections without affecting overall image noise.

The Smart mA technique is a localizer radiograph-based angular AEC technique, which determines the mA values from estimation of patient size, cross-sectional shape and regional attenuation information obtained from a single localizer radiograph (Fig. 3; Kopka et al. 1995; Lehmann et al. 1997; Giacomuzzi et al. 1996). For this technique, the technologists specify a mA value and the software automatically adjusts tube current for different X-ray beam projection angles for the entire 360° tube rotation. The specified mA value provides information about the desired image noise for lateral projections and this information is then used to reduce mA for other "non-lateral" projections.

On the other hand, the CARE Dose technique is an on-line, angular AEC technique that adapts mA in real time or "on-the-fly" from projection data, which tails 180° behind the initial projection angles of X-rays and uses attenuation profile data from initial half rotation (180°) to modulate mA values in real time for the following half rotation (180°) (Fig. 4; Kalra et al. 2004b; Greess et al. 1999, 2001, 2002, 2004). For this technique, the technologist selects an effective mAs value (product of tube current and gantry rotation time divided by the pitch) and the scanner automatically adapts the tube current during each tube rotation while using specified effective mAs as a reference for desired image noise in the lateral projections of first 180° rotation.

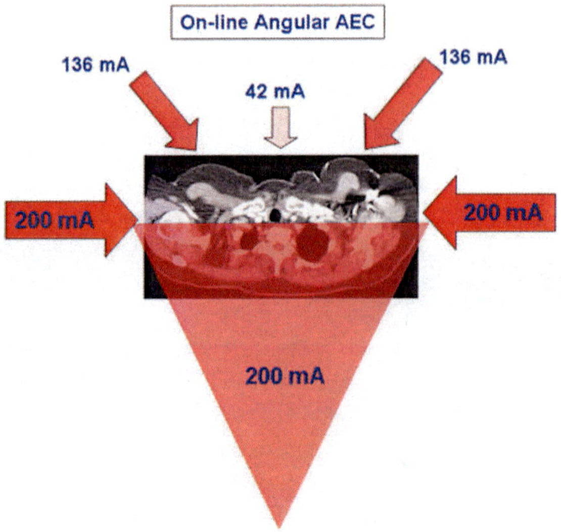


**Fig. 4** With on-line, real-time angular AEC technique, information about attenuation profile at different beam projections with in each section position is collected during first half rotation of X-ray tube around the patient. This technique assumes that beam for subsequent half rotation is a mirror image of the first half rotation and modulates mA values for the second half according to attenuation data collected from the first half rotation. As a result the on-line angular AEC modulates mA with 180° lag. In an elliptical or asymmetric body cross-section, the technique will use same prescribed mA (in present example 200 mA) in the first half rotation, and adapt the mA values for beam projections in the second half rotation based on beam attenuations

Regardless of its type, if used alone, all angular AEC techniques require specification of mA values and thus introduce an element of arbitrary or inappropriate selection of initial mA value. For example, selection of higher mA value for angular AEC will results in higher dose compared with use of a lower mA (Kalra et al. 2004b).

*Z-axis AEC.* The z-axis AEC techniques modulate mA for different z-axis section positions along the scanning direction based on the attenuation profile of the region being scanned (Fig. 5; Kalra et al. 2004d, e; Campbell et al. 2005; Chapman et al. 2005; Namasivayam et al. 2006). Contrary to the angular AEC, the z-axis AEC techniques adjust mA values to maintain image quality (noise index for Auto mA and reference image for Z-DOM) specified by the user at all z-axis section positions and do not change tube current for different projections angles. Using a single localizer radiograph, generally the lateral radiograph, the software estimates mA values required to obtain images with a specified noise level (Kalra et al. 2005b).

For the Auto mA technique, the technologist selects a noise index (which approximates the image noise desired for the study) and an acceptable tube current range (minimum and maximum mA values, with in which the technique will modulate the tube current) for the CT exam. Radiation dose with this technique depends on the specified noise index and patient size. A 5% decrease in noise index implies about 10% increase in dose, whereas a 5% increment in noise index causes approximately 10% dose reduction (Kalra et al. 2005b). The minimum and maximum mA values also influence radiation dose associated with Auto mA by limiting the extent of decrease or increase in mA at any given noise index.

Although z-axis AEC represents a step forward from angular AEC techniques, as it requires technologists or radiologists to specify desired image quality rather than a tube current value, appropriate image quality requirements have not been completely defined. Furthermore, image quality requirements may differ for different studies and for different patients (small versus large). Thus, selection of high image quality can result in better image quality and higher dose exam that may not necessarily provide higher diagnostic yield. Conversely, lower image quality selection with z-axis AEC can cause inadvertently higher image noise and may compromise diagnostic acceptability of CT exam.

*Combined AEC.* These techniques modulate tube current for each z-axis section position (z-axis AEC component) and for different projection angles in each X-ray tube rotation (angular AEC component) (Fig. 6; Kalra et al. 2005a; Rizzo et al. 2006). The angular AEC component of the technique may be based on attenuation profile information obtained from the localizer radiograph or from online estimation of attenuation at different projection angles.

The Auto mA 3D technique uses a single localizer radiograph to derive information for modulating mA at each slice position (Auto mA) and for different projection angles (Smart mA). As required for Auto mA technique, for this technique also, the user prescribes a noise index value with or without minimum and maximum mA limits (Kalra et al. 2004b).

CARE Dose 4D combines the on-line angular AEC (CARE Dose) with the z-axis AEC technique (ZEC) (Rizzo et al. 2006). This technique estimates size,

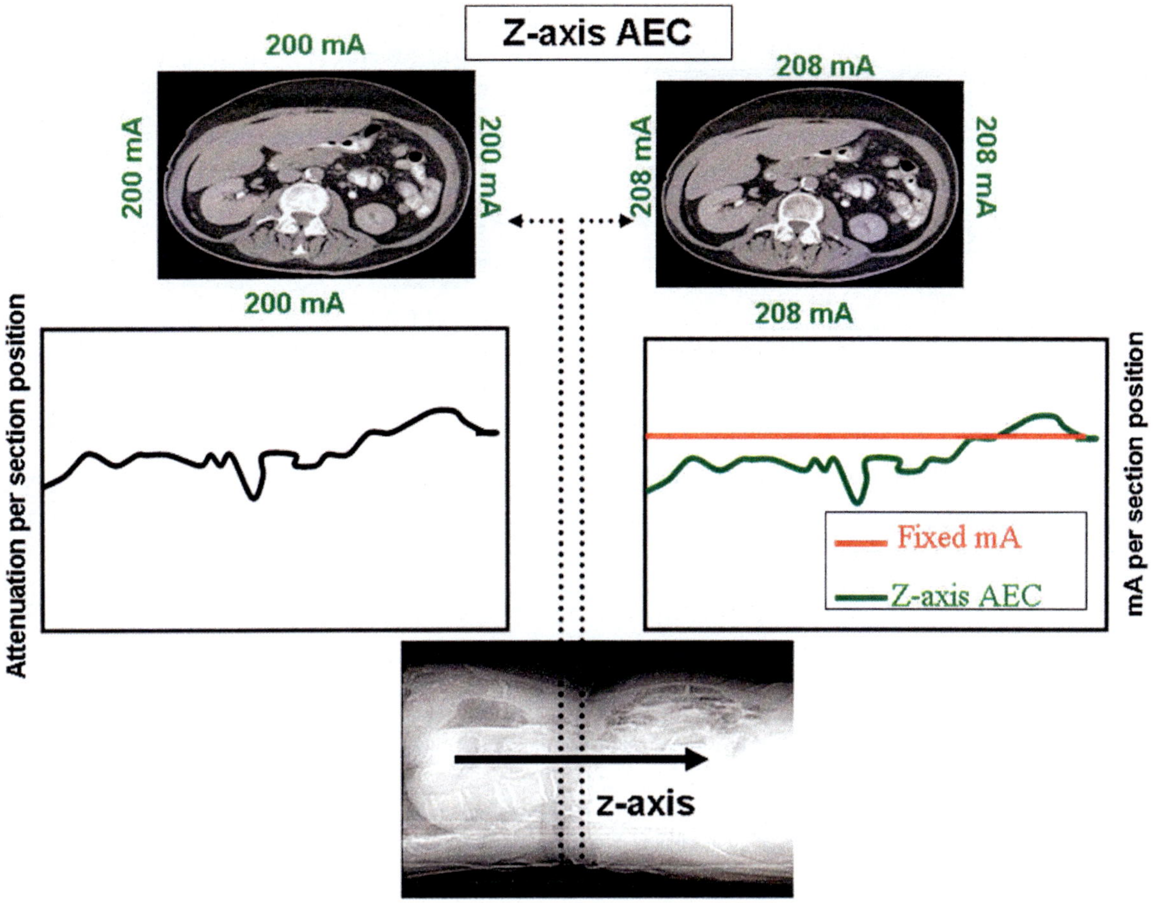


**Fig. 5** With z-axis AEC technique, attenuation for each z-axis section position is estimated from a single localizer radiograph. These data are used to estimate mA value for each z-axis section position in order to generate images with specified image quality at all sections positions (as selected by the user in terms of quality reference mAs or noise index). The mA values change from one section position to other but not for different projection angles as in angular AEC techniques

shape and attenuation profile over the scan length (z-axis) in the direction of projection as well in the perpendicular direction (in the x–y plane) using a mathematical algorithm. Axial mA values are determined from the estimation of these attenuation profiles and adapted to the patient size and attenuation profile. The mA adaptation is based on the user-specified quality reference mAs for z-axis AEC. Subsequently, these mA levels are used for on-line angular AEC according to the attenuation profile at different projection angles. The quality reference mAs value indicates the average effective mAs for a "reference patient." The reference patient is defined as a "typical adult" weighing 70–80 kg (for adult CT studies) or as a "typical child" weighing 20 kg (for pediatric CT studies) (Rizzo et al. 2006).

The diagnostic requirements of studies and radiologists' preferences determine the quality reference mAs value. Although the quality reference mAs value is not changed for patients of different size, for adjusting image quality or dose, the users can change the quality reference mAs or strength of AEC. The technique classifies the patient as "slim" or "obese" from a single localizer radiograph and adapts mA according to the user-specified modulation strength for "slim" or "obese." With CARE Dose 4D, effective mAs is decreased for "slim" patients and increased for "obese" patients and the extent of mA

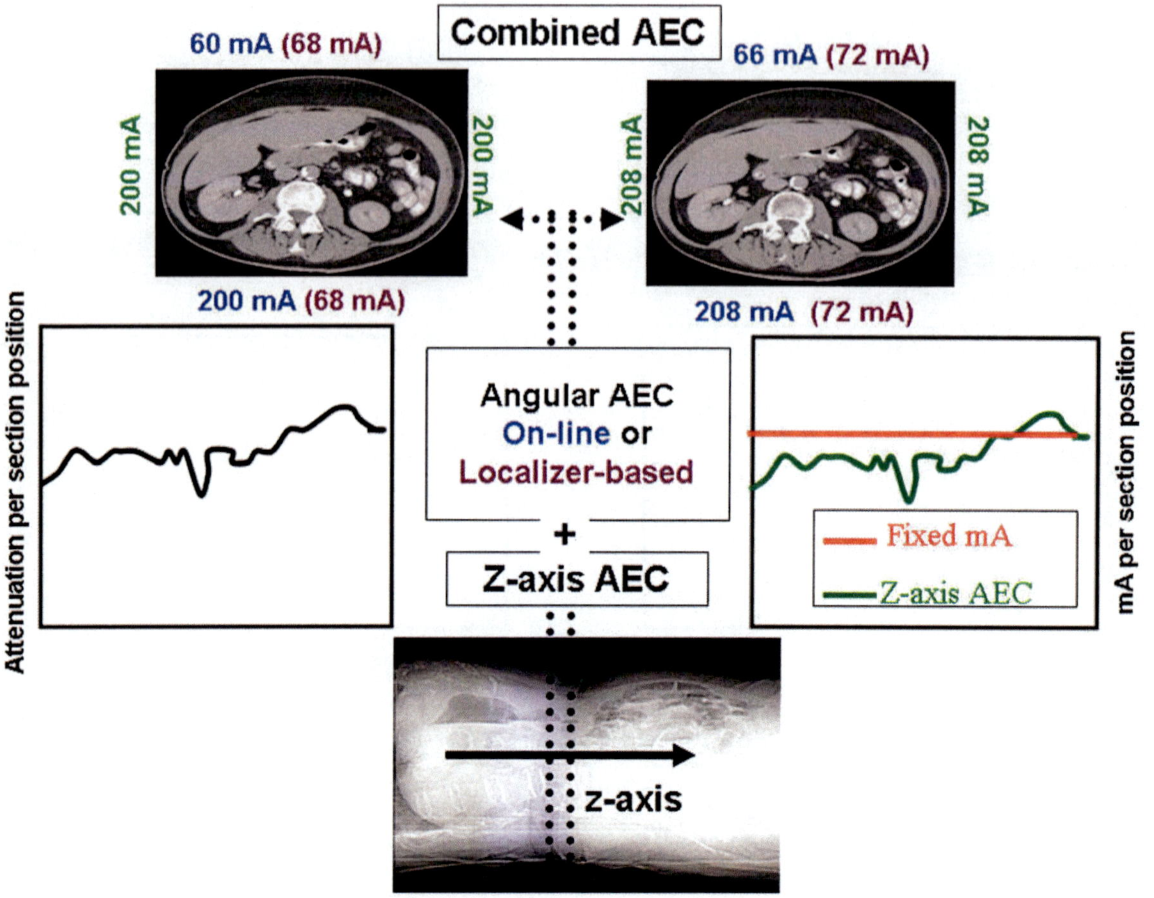


**Fig. 6** The combined AEC techniques initially use z-axis AEC to estimate mA values for each section position from a localizer radiograph. Subsequently, the mA values for angular AEC is also estimated based on mA values estimated from z-axis AEC and localizer radiograph (Auto mA 3D), or from z-axis AEC and on-line estimation of attenuation (CARE Dose 4D)

modulation can be controlled with use of appropriate modulation strengths (weak, average or strong).

The SURE Exposure 3D technique (Toshiba) uses standard deviation (standard, low dose or high quality) as image quality reference parameters for adapting tube current in angular and longitudinal directions.

*ECG dose modulation.* For coronary CT angiography studies, most image data are reconstructed in ventricular diastole so that influence of cardiac motion in the ventricular systole can be reduced. The ECG pulsing decreases the tube current substantially during ventricular systole, and increases it to the specified level during the diastolic phase, which is used for image reconstruction. This helps in reducing the overall dose to the patients. Thereby, the diastolic phase reconstructed image data will have no compromise in image quality whereas the systolic phase data will have more noise. With ECG pulsing, slower and regular heart rates allow greater and more precise dose modulation and reduction during ventricular systole, whereas faster and/or irregular heart rates will be associated with greater radiation dose to the patient.

In recent years, ECG tube current modulation techniques have evolved remarkably. In particular, improved gantry rotation speeds and development of dual source CT has helped increase feasibility of applying ECG triggered scanning or ECG tube current modulation technique in greater proportion of patients undergoing cardiac CT. While some scanners allow users to set the minimum mA for certain cardiac phases where full image quality is not necessary, typically to a value close to 20% of the maximum mA, other scanners allow user to specify minimum mA up to 4% of the maximum mA. Most scanners either automatically

**Table 2** Summary of mechanism of use of different ACE techniques

| AEC techniques | Mechanism of use |
|---|---|
| Angular AEC<br>Smart mA<br>DOM<br>CARE Dose | Specify<br>mA<br>mAs/slice<br>Effective mAs |
| Z-axis AEC (Auto mA) | Specify noise index as well as minimum and maximum mA thresholds for tube current modulation |
| Z-axis AEC (ZEC) | Specify quality reference mAs (rarely used without angular AEC also) |
| Z-axis AEC (Real EC) | Choose from four levels of image noise based on diagnostic requirement |
| Combined AEC (Auto mA 3D) | Specify noise index, minimum and maximum mA thresholds for current modulation |
| Combined AEC (CARE Dose 4D) | Specify quality reference mAs (modulation strength—weak, average, or strong, for small and large patients can be preset) |

recommend or allow user to specify a window of RR interval for application of maximum mA. In general smaller maximum mA window can be applied to patients with slower heart rate for higher radiation dose reduction compared to use of no ECG mA modulation. On the other hand, a wider window is necessary for patients with higher rates and therefore in these patients administration of negative chronotropic agents such as beta blockers can help not just increase number of evaluable coronary segments but also drive the radiation dose lower. With faster scanner, most specifically, dual source multidetector-row CT, the ramp up and ramp down times for change in mA have also decreased, which has further helped drive radiation dose lower (Table 2).

## 5 Clinical Evidence for AEC Techniques

In the past 10 years, several clinical studies have shown benefit of AEC techniques for managing radiation dose for single-detector-row helical CT as well as multidetector-row CT scanners (Greess et al. 1999, 2004; Kopka et al. 1995; Lehmann et al. 1997; Giacomuzzi et al. 1996; Kalra et al. 2004d, e; Campbell et al. 2005; Chapman et al. 2005; Namasivayam et al. 2006; Rizzo et al. 2006; Mastora et al. 2004; Mulkens et al. 2005; Tack et al. 2003). Compared to the fixed tube current technique, these techniques have been shown to reduce radiation dose for most patients without compromising diagnostic acceptability of CT studies and increase radiation dose in some large patients in order to maintain image quality at specified levels (Greess et al. 1999, 2001, 2002, 2004; Kalra et al. 2004d, e; Campbell et al. 2005; Chapman et al. 2005; Namasivayam et al. 2006; Rizzo et al. 2006; Mastora et al. 2004; Mulkens et al. 2005; Tack et al. 2003). Results of some clinical studies with AEC techniques have been summarized in Table 3.

Several studies have shown benefits of ECG pulsing for cardiac CT studies (Poll et al. 2002). Phantom studies have shown that substantial dose reduction can be achieved with use of ECG pulsing depending on the heart rate. Patients study also indicate high level of average radiation dose reduction for both males and females with ECG controlled tube current modulation compared to non-modulated coronary multidetector CT angiography (Jakobs et al. 2002).

Recently, Singh et al. have reported substantial dose reduction with use of combined modulation type of AEC technique (Auto mA 3D) based on tightly controlled minimum and maximum mA range for dose modulation (Singh et al. 2009). The authors emphasize need for clinical indication and number of prior CT examination-based optimization of AEC techniques for radiation dose reduction. Although AEC does adapt tube current to patient size, some AEC techniques do need adjustment or fine tuning for extreme patients sizes as well (Singh et al. 2009). A size proportionate reduction of tube current for the very small children may result in substantially noisy

**Table 3** Summary of reports on automatic exposure control techniques

| Study | Technique | Region | Dose reduction (%) |
|---|---|---|---|
| Greess et al. (1999) | CARE Dose | Shoulders | 38 |
| Greess et al. (2001) | CARE Dose | Chest (pulmonary nodules) | 21 |
| Greess et al. (2002) | CARE Dose | Neck<br>Chest<br>Abdomen | 20<br>23<br>23 |
| Tack et al. (2003) | CARE Dose | Chest<br>Abdomen | 17<br>20 |
| Mastora et al. (2004) | CARE Dose | Thoracic outlet | 35 |
| Kalra et al. (2004a, b, c, d, e) | Auto mA | Abdomen | 10–41 |
| Kalra et al. (2005a, b) | Auto mA | Chest | 18–26 |
| Kalra et al. (2005a, b) | Auto mA | Abdomen (renal stones) | 43–66 |
| Mulkens et al. (2005) | CARE Dose 4D | Chest<br>Abdomen-pelvis<br>Lumbar spine<br>Cervical spine | 20<br>32<br>37<br>68 |
| Namasivayam et al. (2006) | AutomA | Neck | 36 JJJJ |
| Rizzo et al. (2006) | CARE Dose 4D | Abdomen | 41–43 |

(Greess et al. 1999, 2001, 2002, 2004; Kalra et al. 2004d, e; Campbell et al. 2005, Chapman et al. 2005; Namasivayam et al. 2006; Rizzo et al. 2006; Mastora et al. 2004; Mulkens et al. 2005; Tack et al. 2003)

images as very small children have poor tissue contrast due to paucity of fat outlining the organs and also due to small field of view which tends to magnify the image noise. On the other hand, proportionate increase in large children may not take into account the high tissue contrast offered by abundant fat outlining the organs and tissues.

In an impressive study on comparison of z-axis AEC techniques from four different CT vendors, Soderberg and Gunnarsson have recently reported similar automatic exposure control (AEC) features between GE and Toshiba and also between Philips and Siemens CT systems (Söderberg and Gunnarsson 2010). These authors also reported substantial dose reduction with application of AEC in the range of 35–60% with an increase in image noise with substantial reduction in tube current in regions such as lungs (where noise is not a major factor affecting lesion detection any way).

## 6 Trouble-Shooting for AEC Techniques

- For all localizer radiograph-based AEC techniques (Smart mA, Auto mA, Auto mA 3D, Real EC, ZEC, CARE Dose 4D), localizer radiograph must include the entire region being scanned with AEC. Beyond the localizer radiograph, these techniques will not adapt tube current appropriately.
- As some AEC techniques rely on localizer radiographs, it is important to avoid patient movements after acquisition of first localizer radiograph (generally a single lateral localizer is used for most AEC techniques).
- AEC techniques will adapt tube current taking into account all other relevant scanning parameters such as section profile, beam pitch, detector configuration, gantry rotation time, and tube potential.
- Appropriate centering of patient in gantry isocenter, particularly in reference to table height, is extremely important in multidetector CT scanners, as surface dose to the patient and image noise can increase with off-centering (Personal communication with Thomas L. Toth, GE Healthcare Technologies).
- If arms are positioned by the side of patient undergoing body CT, AEC techniques can increase dose by as much as 30–35% (as they will compensate for increase in attenuation from arms) (Kalra et al. 2003b). In a recent patient study, additional dose to traumatized patients if one or two arms were lying along the torso was 18 and

45%, respectively (Brink et al. 2008). Thus, where possible, localizer radiographs must be acquired with appropriate positioning of the arms.

- Some AEC techniques ignore metallic implants from estimation of attenuation profile and tube current (such as CARE Dose 4D) (Dalal et al. 2005), where as others can increase tube current in the region of metallic prosthesis as they cannot exclude contribution of high attenuation from metallic prosthesis (Rizzo et al. 2005). In latter circumstances, set a lower desired image quality or use the fixed tube current technique.
- Pediatric and adult settings for desired image quality usually differ and must be set as such (Kalra et al. 2004c, d). For a large patient, an increase in tube current with AEC techniques may be insufficient to obtain desired or specified image quality (Kalra et al. 2004c, d). In such instances, user must be attentive to other scanning parameters such as table feed, gantry rotation time, and kVp.
- For low dose examinations, such as CT colonography and kidney stone CT, select lower "desired image quality" requirement for AEC techniques compared with routine indications.
- Some AEC techniques may not be applicable or appropriate in all body regions, such as in head or extremities, therefore, user must enquire about applicability and accuracy of AEC techniques from their vendors.
- With ECG pulsing, image data during systolic phase will be noisy and may impair the cardiac cine or functional assessment as well as visualization of incidental extra-cardiac thoracic findings. In some cases, reconstructing these image datasets at thicker sections and/or smoother reconstruction kernel settings may help.

## 7 Pitfalls

Despite commendable advances and efforts of the vendors to optimize radiation dose associated with CT scanning, there are some issues associated with use of AEC techniques in routine clinical practice. Most importantly, there are substantial differences between nomenclature and dose modulation with AEC techniques from different vendors. This implies that scanning method used with one AEC technique cannot be used on similar AEC technique on a scanner from a different vendor. Furthermore, presently most vendors recommend use of an "empirical" desired image quality for scanning. It is important to understand that AEC techniques will work only as efficient as the specified or desired image quality. If higher image quality is specified (for example, higher quality reference mAs for CARE Dose 4D or lower noise index for Auto mA), than system will use higher dose. Likewise, different desired image quality thresholds must be specified for different clinical indications for example, lower quality reference mAs must be used for kidney stone protocol compared with the routine abdominal CT protocols. Selection of inadvertently low image quality can lead to excessive dose reduction with AEC techniques and compromise diagnostic acceptability of the study. To facilitate appropriate use of AEC techniques, there is need to define threshold levels of "desired image quality" for different clinical indications and patient ages.

Although AEC techniques can automatically increase tube current and dose to large patients, it is important to realize that in large patients, increase in applied peak kilovoltage, gantry rotation time, or scan field of view, or decrease in beam pitch may also be necessary to obtain desired diagnostic information.

As with any new technique, there is a learning curve that radiologists and technologists must overcome in order to use these AEC techniques appropriately.

Not all body CT indications need to be scanned with use of AEC techniques. For indications where noise is not a major factor in detection, a very low fixed mA can perhaps easily achieve low radiation dose objective. For example, in case of lung nodule follow up or lung cancer screening protocol CT, very low fixed mAs of 10–40 are generally sufficient and simple to apply.

The CT dose index volume (CTDI vol) displayed on the user interface of the scanner is the average CTDI vol over the scan length. This is crucial to understand as CTDI vol changes over the scan length and can be higher or lower at different section positions in the scan range. Thus, estimation of local or organ-based effective doses with use of these average CTDI vol may not be accurate. A recent study by Papadakis et al. (2011) utilizes adult and pediatric phantoms has reported effect of AEC on estimated organ and effective doses. These authors caution users against extrapolating mAs reduction with AEC to reduction of absorbed dose to the organs. Furthermore, mAs reduction with AEC only provides a rough estimate for effective dose reduction and can be different by more than 15% in most cases.

Brisse et al. (2009) have reported assessment of organ and effective doses in pediatric anthropomorphic phantoms with and without use of AEC. According to their study, AEC does result in substantial dose reduction for thyroid, lungs, esophagus, and breasts in the ranging from 6 to 39%, but also leads to higher organ doses for salivary glands, urinary bladder and ovaries as high attenuation from the skull base and pelvic bones increases the mAs with the longitudinal AEC. The authors recommend caution when applying AEC in children for dose reduction in the latter body regions.

Estimation for applied mAs for z-axis or combined modulation types of AEC techniques comes from estimation of patient attenuation from the localizer radiograph which is acquired prior to administration of intravenous contrast. Not surprisingly, some studies have reported that there is slight increased noise (<3 HU) with application of AEC to contrast enhanced CT compared to non-contrast CT (Paul et al. 2011). Increase in image noise with AEC is much smaller for wider detector geometry CT (128-slice CT) as compared to smaller geometry CT (16- and 64-slice CT).

Wang et al. (2011) have also reported higher CTDI vol (mean increase of 11%) with positive enteric contrast material for abdominal and pelvic CT as compared to oral water as contrast agent. However, Lim et al. (2011) have reported no change in radiation dose with use of AEC in patients with stool and fluid tagging for low dose CT colonography.

## 8 Recent Updates to Automatic Exposure Control

### 8.1 Nomenclature of AEC

Under leadership of Dianna Cody, PhD and Cynthia McCollough Ph.D., the Working Group on Standardization of CT Nomenclature set up by the American Association of Physicists in Medicine (AAPM) has recently a consensus report on standardized terms for CT scanners (Cody and McCollough 2011). In this document, AEC has been described as preferred name for this technique. In this landmark document, angular tube current modulation, longitudinal tube current modulation, and angular and longitudinal tube current modulation techniques have been named as standard terms for angular AEC, z-axis AEC and combined AEC techniques, respectively.

### 8.2 Auto mA and Auto mA 3D

In order to reduce radiation dose, this technique now allows users to select percentage dose reduction compared to archived parameters for Auto mA. Thus after selecting noise index and minimum and maximum mA range, the users can specify a desired percentage dose reduction, which leads to automatic application of new higher noise index in order to obtain proportionate dose reduction. This feature is especially helpful in follow up imaging or with application of adaptive statistical iterative reconstruction (ASIR) technique for image reconstruction where dose reduction has to be applied with changes in scanning parameters (Prakash et al. 2010a, b).

### 8.3 CARE Dose 4D

Recently, the vendor for this technique has altered this technique on their newer multidetector CT scanners. First, the technique no longer refers to different size reference phantom for pediatric patients. Instead, the technique now uses single adult reference patient for tube current modulation in angular and longitudinal directions for both children and adult patients. This implies that users can now use the adult reference mAs (image quality metric for CARE Dose 4D) for both children and adults. Second, the technique now has five settings of modulation strengths (very weak, weak, average, strong, very strong) instead of three settings (weak, average, strong) in the older version. Finally, the vendor has also introduced an automatic kV selection (Care kV) feature on some of their scanners. Application of automatic kV selection technique recommends an appropriate kV based on selected image quality parameters and then automatically changes the required reference mAs (CARE Dose 4D) in order to achieve either dose reduction or image quality improvements with change in kV.

## 9 Summary

- Most modern multidetector-row CT scanners have AEC techniques.
- AEC techniques can aid in optimizing radiation dose for different patient sizes and clinical indications.
- Constant image quality at lower radiation dose can be achieved with AEC techniques in most patients.
- For different clinical indications, users must modify the scanning parameters for AEC in order to attain desired dose reduction or image quality.

## References


Althen JN (2005) Automatic tube-current modulation in CT—a comparison between different solutions. Radiat Prot Dosim 114:308–312

Brink M, de Lange F, Oostveen LJ, Dekker HM, Kool DR, Deunk J, Edwards MJ, van Kuijk C, Kamman RL, Blickman JG (2008) Arm raising at exposure-controlled multidetector trauma CT of thoracoabdominal region: higher image quality, lower radiation dose. Radiology 249:661–670

Brisse HJ, Robilliard M, Savignoni A, Pierrat N, Gaboriaud G, De Rycke Y et al (2009) Assessment of organ absorbed doses and estimation of effective doses from pediatric anthropomorphic phantom measurements for multi-detector row CT with and without automatic exposure control. Health Phys 97:303–314

Campbell J, Kalra MK, Rizzo SMR, Maher MM, Shepard J (2005) Scanning beyond anatomic limits of thorax in chest CT: findings, radiation dose and automatic tube current modulation. Am J Roentgenol 185:1525–1530

Chapman VM, Kalra MK, Grottkau BE, Albright M, Jaramillo D (2005) 16-Slice multidetector CT of the post-traumatic pediatric elbow: optimum parameters and associated radiation dose. Am J Roentgenol 185:516–521

Cody D, McCollough CM (2011) American association of physicists in medicine (AAPM) working group on standardization of CT nomenclature and protocols. AAPM CT Lexicon version 1.1 8/31/2011. http://www.aapm.org/pubs/CTProtocols/documents/CTTerminologyLexicon_2011-08-31.pdf. Accessed 3 Nov 2011

Dalal T, Kalra MK, Rizzo SM, Schmidt B, Suess C, Flohr T et al (2005) Metallic prosthesis: technique to avoid increase in CT radiation dose with automatic tube current modulation in a phantom and patients. Radiology 236:671–675

Giacomuzzi SM, Erckert B, Schopf T, Freund MC, Springer P, Dessl A et al (1996) The smart-scan procedure of spiral computed tomography: a new method for dose reduction. Rofo Fortschr Geb Rontgenstr Neuen Bildgeb Verfahr 165:10–16

Greess H, Wolf H, Baum U, Kalender WA, Bautz W (1999) Dosage reduction in computed tomography by anatomy-oriented attenuation-based tube-current modulation: the first clinical results. Rofo 170:246–250

Greess H, Baum U, Wolf H, Lell M, Nomayr A, Schmidt B et al (2001) Dose reduction in spiral-CT: detection of pulmonary coin lesions with and without anatomically adjusted modulation of tube current. Rofo 173:466–470

Greess H, Nomayr A, Wolf H, Baum U, Lell M, Bowing B et al (2002) Dose reduction in CT examination of children by an attenuation-based on-line modulation of tube current (CARE Dose). Eur Radiol 12:1571–1576

Greess H, Lutze J, Nomayr A, Wolf H, Hothorn T, Kalender WA et al (2004) Dose reduction in subsecond multislice spiral CT examination of children by online tube current modulation. Eur Radiol 14:995–999

Jakobs TF, Becker CR, Ohnesorge B, Flohr T, Suess C, Schoepf UJ et al (2002) Multislice helical CT of the heart with retrospective ECG gating: reduction of radiation exposure by ECG-controlled tube current modulation. Eur Radiol 12:1081–1086

Kalra MK, Prasad S, Saini S, Blake MA, Varghese J, Halpern EF et al (2002) Clinical comparison of standard-dose and 50% reduced-dose abdominal CT: effect on image quality. Am J Roentgenol 179:1101–1106

Kalra MK, Maher MM, Prasad SR, Hayat MS, Blake MA, Varghese J et al (2003a) Correlation of patient weight and cross-sectional dimensions with subjective image quality at standard dose abdominal CT. Korean J Radiol 4:234–238

Kalra MK, Maher MM, Saini S (2003b) What is the optimum position of arms for acquiring scout images for whole-body CT with automatic tube current modulation? Am J Roentgenol 181:596–597

Kalra MK, Maher MM, Toth TL, Hamberg LM, Blake MA, Shepard JA et al (2004a) Strategies for CT radiation dose optimization. Radiology 230:619–628

Kalra MK, Maher MM, Toth TL, Schmidt B, Westerman BL, Morgan HT et al (2004b) Techniques and applications of automatic tube current modulation for CT. Radiology 233:649–657

Kalra MK, Maher MM, Kamath RS, Horiuchi T, Toth TL, Halpern EF et al (2004c) Sixteen-detector row CT of abdomen and pelvis: study for optimization of Z-axis modulation technique performed in 153 patients. Radiology 233:241–249

Kalra MK, Maher MM, Toth TL, Kamath RS, Halpern EF, Saini S (2004d) Comparison of Z-axis automatic tube current modulation technique with fixed tube current CT scanning of abdomen and pelvis. Radiology 232:347–353

Kalra MK, Maher MM, Toth TL, Kamath RS, Halpern EF, Saini S (2004e) Radiation from "extra" images acquired with abdominal and/or pelvic CT: effect of automatic tube current modulation. Radiology 232:409–414

Kalra MK, Rizzo SM, Novelline RA (2005a) Reducing radiation dose in emergency computed tomography with automatic exposure control techniques. Emerg Radiol 11:267–274

Kalra MK, Naz N, Rizzo SM, Blake MA (2005b) Computed tomography radiation dose optimization: scanning protocols and clinical applications of automatic exposure control. Curr Probl Diagn Radiol 34:171–181

Kopka L, Funke M, Breiter N, Hermann KP, Vosshenrich R, Grabbe E (1995) An anatomically adapted variation of the tube current in CT: studies on radiation dosage reduction and image quality. Rofo Fortschr Geb Rontgenstr Neuen Bildgeb Verfahr 163:383–387

Lehmann KJ, Wild J, Georgi M (1997) Clinical use of software-controlled X-ray tube modulation with "Smart-Scan" in spiral CT. Aktuelle Radiol 7:156–158

Lim HK, Lee KH, Kim SY, Kim KJ, Kim B, Lee H et al (2011) Does the amount of tagged stool and fluid significantly affect the radiation exposure in low-dose CT colonography performed with an automatic exposure control? Eur Radiol 21:345–352

Mastora I, Remy-Jardin M, Delannoy V, Duhamel A, Scherf C, Suess C et al (2004) Multi-detector row spiral CT angiography of the thoracic outlet: dose reduction with anatomically adapted online tube current modulation and preset dose savings. Radiology 230:116–124

Miyazaki O, Kitamura M, Masaki H, Nosaka S, Miyasaka M, Kashima K (2005) Current practice of pediatric MDCT in Japan: survey results of demographics and age-based dose reduction. Nippon Igaku Hoshasen Gakkai Zasshi 65: 216–223

Mulkens TH, Bellinck P, Baeyaert M, Ghysen D, Van Dijck X, Mussen E et al (2005) Use of an automatic exposure control mechanism for dose optimization in multi-detector row CT examinations: clinical evaluation. Radiology 237:213–223

Namasivayam S, Kalra MK, Pottala K, Waldrop S, Hudgins PA (2006) Optimization of z-axis automatic exposure control for multidetector row CT evaluation of neck and comparison with fixed tube current technique for image quality and radiation dose. Am J Neuroradiol 27:2221–2225

Papadakis AE, Perisinakis K, Oikonomou I, Damilakis J (2011) Automatic exposure control in pediatric and adult computed tomography examinations: can we estimate organ and effective dose from mean MAS reduction? Invest Radiol 46:654–662

Paul J, Schell B, Kerl JM, Maentele W, Vogl TJ, Bauer RW (2011) Effect of contrast material on image noise and radiation dose in adult chest computed tomography using automatic exposure control: a comparative study between 16-, 64- and 128-slice CT. Eur J Radiol 79:e128–e132

Poll LW, Cohnen M, Brachten S, Ewen K, Modder U (2002) Dose reduction in multi-slice CT of the heart by use of ECG-controlled tube current modulation ("ECG pulsing"): phantom measurements. Rofo 174:1500–1505

Prakash P, Kalra MK, Kambadakone AK, Pien H, Hsieh J, Blake MA et al (2010a) Reducing abdominal CT radiation dose with adaptive statistical iterative reconstruction technique. Invest Radiol 45:202–210

Prakash P, Kalra MK, Digumarthy SR, Hsieh J, Pien H, Singh S et al (2010b) Radiation dose reduction with chest computed tomography using adaptive statistical iterative reconstruction technique: initial experience. J Comput Assist Tomogr 34:40–45

Rizzo SM, Kalra MK, Maher MM, Blake MA, Toth TL, Saini S (2005) Do metallic endoprostheses increase radiation dose associated with automatic tube-current modulation in abdominal-pelvic MDCT? A phantom and patient study. Am J Roentgenol 184:491–496

Rizzo S, Kalra MK, Schmidt B, Suess C, Flohr TG, Blake MA et al (2006) Comparison of angular and combined automatic tube current modulation techniques with constant tube current CT scanning of the abdomen and pelvis. Am J Roentgenol 186:673–679

Singh S, Kalra MK, Moore MA, Shailam R, Liu B, Toth TL et al (2009) Dose reduction and compliance with pediatric CT protocols adapted to patient size, clinical indication, and number of prior studies. Radiology 252:200–208

Söderberg M, Gunnarsson M (2010) Automatic exposure control in computed tomography—an evaluation of systems from different manufacturers. Acta Radiol 51:625–634

Tack D, De Maertelaer V, Gevenois PA (2003) Dose reduction in multidetector CT using attenuation-based online tube current modulation. Am J Roentgenol 181:331–334

Terada M (2005) Optimization of image quality by CT scanner automatic exposure control systems. Nippon Hoshasen Gijutsu Gakkai Zasshi 61:1384–1386

Wang ZJ, Chen KS, Gould R, Coakley FV, Fu Y, Yeh BM (2011) Positive enteric contrast material for abdominal and pelvic CT with automatic exposure control: what is the effect on patient radiation exposure? Eur J Radiol 79:e58–62

# Patient Centering in MDCT: Dose Effects

Mannudeep K. Kalra and Thomas L. Toth

## Contents




**Abstract**

Appropriate patient centering is of pivotal importance in CT scanning. Without good centering there can be increase in patient radiation dose and loss of image quality, effects that are especially pronounced with use of automatic exposure control techniques. This chapter discusses implications of off-centering of patients during CT scanning.


*I have expressed some ideas that point to the center; I have saluted the dawn in my way, from my point of view. He who knows the way should do the same, in his way, and from his point of view.*

Friedrich Von Schlegel

Although contribution of CT scanning to radiation dose was recognized prior to introduction of multidetector row CT scanners, ever expanding applications of multidetector row CT scanning in patient care and of late, use of CT for screening, have heightened concerns and awareness of radiation induced cancer from CT radiation dose and prompted development of strategies and techniques for dose reduction (Kalra et al. 2004a; Frush 2003). Technological innovations for dose reduction and optimization include prepatient beam collimation and beam shaping filters as well as automatic exposure control techniques (Kalra et al. 2004b). To obtain appropriate benefits of these techniques in terms of dose reduction without compromising on the image quality, it is important to appropriately center the patients in the scanner gantry isocenter (Kalra et al. 2004b).


M. K. Kalra (✉)
Department of Radiology,
Emory University School of Medicine,
1364 Clifton Road NE, Atlanta GA 30322, USA
e-mail: mkalra@emory.edu

T. L. Toth
General Electric Healthcare Technologies,
3000 North Grandview, Boulevard,
Waukesha WI 53188, USA



D. Tack et al. (eds.), *Radiation Dose from Multidetector CT*, Medical Radiology. Diagnostic Imaging,
DOI: 10.1007/174_2011_447,

In this chapter, we will discuss the effects and reasons of off-centering patients in the gantry isocenter, factors contributing to patient off-centering, rationale for precise patient centering, and strategies that can be adopted to obtain adequate patient centering prior to their CT examinations.

## 1 Patient Positioning and Centering

For the sake of simplicity, we have arbitrarily classified the process of patient placement on the gantry table into positioning and centering. Positioning alludes to proper placement of patient on the gantry table in the z-axis or along the length of patient for scanning a particular portion or region of the body. Improper positioning of the patient may necessitate acquisition of localizer radiograph beyond the region of interest and perhaps acquisition of repeat localizer radiograph (Namasivayam et al. 2006). A recent study from analysis of localizer radiographs for abdominal CT examinations performed in a single institution have reported that localizer radiographs extended 13 cm (average) beyond defined region of interest (Namasivayam et al. 2006). With regard to, patient positioning it is important to pay special attention to the position of patient's arms, particularly when automatic exposure control techniques are being used for scanning. Automatic exposure control techniques employ tube current based on beam attenuation data obtained from the localizer radiographs and/or "on the fly" during initial tube rotation around the patient. Therefore, for body CT, if arms are positioned by the side of patient, estimation of tube current with automatic exposure control techniques will be erroneous and can lead to substantial increment in radiation dose (Kalra et al. 2003).

On the other hand, centering alludes to appropriate placement of patient with respect to the scanner gantry, so that patient's center corresponds to the scanner gantry isocenter in the x–y plane or the transverse cross-section of patient. A recent study from evaluation of scanning practice in a single tertiary health care center has reported that 95% of patients undergoing chest and abdominal CT examinations were off-centered relative to the superior-inferior direction in the gantry (Namasivayam et al. 2006).

## 2 Effects of Off-Centering

Image noise, mottle or graininess, a principle determinant of image quality, affects the low contrast resolution of CT. A higher image noise may compromise low contrast resolution and impair diagnostic confidence. Conversely, a lower image noise may improve low contrast resolution at the cost of higher radiation dose.

As X-ray tube revolves around the patient, X-ray beams traverse through the body region being scanned from several projections. Each image pixel generated from CT scanning is contributed from attenuation of several X-ray projections. Image noise in an image pixel is derived from noise from all X-ray projections responsible for generation of that pixel. In general, less X-ray beam attenuation implies less image noise and vice versa. The beam attenuation is also directly related to the length of path that the beam traverses through portions in the body region being scanned. Therefore, shorter beam path at the peripheral portions will be associated with less image noise, compared to longer beam path at the central portions. In order to shape the primary X-ray beam to patient body habitus and thereby reduce associated radiation dose, scanners from most vendors have beam shaping or bowtie filters. Bow-tie filters take advantage of the geometry of patient cross-section by reducing X-rays in projections with short beam paths and improving radiation dose efficiency of the scanner (Fig. 1) (Toth et al. 2005). In other words, these filters shape the X-ray beam to the body, restricting X-rays for the peripheral, less attenuating portions, and allowing most X-rays for the central portions with greater attenuation and contribution to image noise. Some vendors employ permanently positioned filters, while others use filters with different shapes that can be selected based on the specified field of view (Mayo et al. 2003).

Bow-tie filters presume that the center of the body region being scanned coincides or approximates with the gantry isocenter. However, with off-centering relative to gantry isocenter, the bow-tie filters miss their target. As a result portions of body region being scanned other than the peripheral portion receive less X-rays and contribute to higher image noise (compromise image quality). Conversely, peripheral portions receive more X-rays resulting in higher

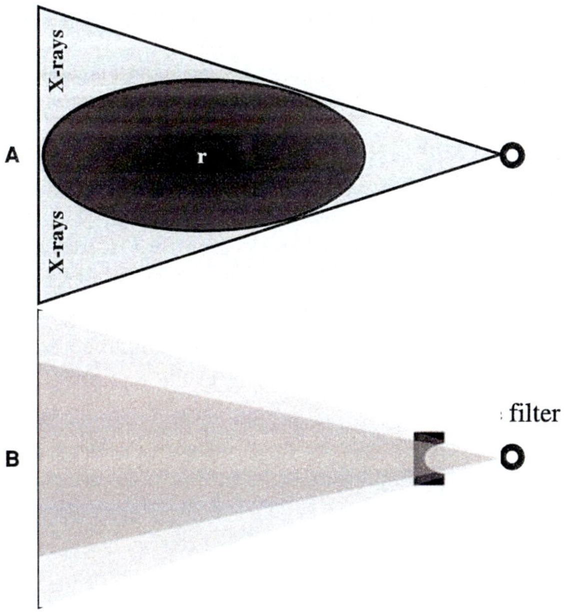


**Fig. 1** Without bow-tie filter (**a**), the homogeneous X-ray beam will lead to image with lower noise in the periphery and at the surface portions in the region being scanned (*r*). With bow-tie filter (**b**), the X-rays are reduced in the periphery (p) so that the peripheral and surface dose in the region being scanned increases and noise in these regions becomes similar to that in the central portions

peripheral and central radiation dose. These noise and dose effects assume importance in view of availability and use of automatic exposure control techniques on most modern multidetector row CT scanners. With use of fixed tube current for scanning, there was a tendency to use higher tube current for small patients and relatively lower tube current for larger patients. With precise dose adaptation using automatic exposure control techniques, substantial dose reduction was reported for small patients and dose increment was documented for larger patients (Kalra et al. 2004c; Mulkens et al. 2005). Use of lower dose for smaller patients with automatic exposure control techniques implies that off-centering of these patients can lead to disproportionate increase in image noise as well as the surface and peripheral radiation dose. Unfortunately, compared to large patients, there is "more room" to off-center a small patient in the scanner gantry.

Prior phantom studies to explore cause for suboptimal image quality in smaller patients undergoing abdominal-pelvic CT with automatic exposure control technique have shown that off-centering in the superior-inferior direction (y-axis of the gantry or table height related) with respect to the gantry isocenter increases image noise (Kalra et al. 2004d). Up to 30% increase in image noise was noted when the phantom was scanned at a position, which was 6 cm below the gantry isocenter. Therefore, in this chapter, all references to centering and off-centering are in related to patient placement in the superior-inferior direction of the gantry isocenter.

Subsequent studies have documented that up to 50% increase in surface and peripheral radiation dose can occur with 6 cm off-centering of a phantom (Li et al. 2006). Using Monte Carlo simulations in CT, Aviles Lucas et al. have also shown that variations of up to 30% can be noted in the air kerma to regions with in the American Association of Physicists in Medicine body phantom when its position is changed vertically in the gantry (Aviles Lucas et al. 2004). In a recent phantom study, Li et al., have recently reported that the peripheral and top surface (which will correspond to the anterior aspect of a supine patient) CT dose index (CTDI) increases by 12–18% with a 30 mm off-center distance and by 41–49% at a 60 mm off-center distance (Li et al. 2007).

Patients' studies show about 2–30% increase in surface and peripheral radiation dose from chest and abdominal CT examinations performed with off-centering of patients relative to gantry isocenter (Li et al. 2006). This increase in the surface radiation dose with off-centering can result in increased radiation dose to radiosensitive body parts such as the breasts, thyroid, eyes, and gonads.

## 3 Reasons for Off-Centering

Although no formal study has evaluated reasons for off-centering patients in the gantry isocenter, these may not be difficult to understand. Possible causes for off-centering patients undergoing CT scanning may include

- Awareness: Technologists and radiologists may not be aware of the importance of centering the patients appropriately in the gantry isocenter.
- Attention to details of centering: Inadequate attention to centering may be related to training of the technologists and radiologists, suboptimal use of laser assisted centering or increasing workload for multidetector row CT scanners with expanding

applications. This practice may be accentuated by acquisition of two orthogonal localizer radiographs for planning and ability to shift the display field of view (DFOV).

- Adjustment of DFOV: Modern scanners allow the technologists to shift the DFOV in all three planes (longitudinally or in z-axis along scan length and transversely or in xy axis for the section plane) on the localizer radiographs. Although this ability helps in displaying selected regions that are situated away from the gantry isocenter (for example, coronary CT angiography), it may also be responsible for lack of attention to centering as DFOV can be shifted to accommodate off-centering without increasing the size of the DFOV.
- Patient related factor: Patients seldom have a perfectly cylindrical shape. Thus, multi-region (such as neck, chest and abdomen) scanning in the same imaging session may make decisions related to patient centering difficult. Likewise, patients without circular cross-section are also difficult to center, in addition, to patients who cannot lie flat, cannot elevate their arms sufficiently above their heads (such patients are more likely to be centered below the gantry isocenter), have spinal curvature abnormalities, or need to elevate their head or chest relative to caudal portions of their body. Likewise, patients on life support systems or referred for emergent clinical indications may also be difficult to center optimally.
- Lack of automatic patient centering techniques: Such techniques may guide the users to center the patients correctly and inform them about off-centering and possible dose and noise penalty associated with scanning the patients who are not adequately centered in the gantry.

## 4 Strategies for Insuring Appropriate Patient Centering

In view of the importance of optimal patient centering in the gantry isocenter prior to their CT scanning, it is important to devise strategies to minimize patient off-centering. These may include:

- Education: Education of the technologists, radiologists, and medical physicists about importance of patient centering and implications of off-centering will facilitate attention to details of patient centering.
- Guidelines: Some guidelines can be given to the technologists for patient centering in the gantry isocenter. These may include importance of adjusting patient centering in the gantry rather adjustment of DFOV. Users must be instructed to pay particular attention to centering of children and small adults, especially when automatic exposure control techniques are being used for CT scanning or a low dose CT is being performed. For patients who can not rest their arms above their heads, body CT can be performed in "feet first" alignment so as to avoid inferior off-centering in these patients.
- Automatic patient centering software: This technique has not been commercially released at the time of writing this chapter. Initial assessment of this software (GE Healthcare Technologies, Waukesha, Wis.) has shown that this technique can help the users to center the patients with respect to the gantry (Li et al 2006). For body CT, this software estimates the patient center from the mean projection area data obtained from the entire lateral localizer radiograph. It recommends a correction factor (in mm) for patient table position which can be used to adjust table height in order to achieve appropriate patient centering. In addition, the technique also describes the surface and peripheral dose that can be saved with appropriate centering based on the recommended correction factor.
- It is interesting to note that at least one vendor now provides users an ability to correct patient off-centering from the scanner user interface without need for going back to the scanner gantry on some of their advanced CT systems (Siemens Definition Flash).

## 5 Recent Developments and Literature on Patient Centering

There is further evidence that patient centering is important for appropriate functioning of the automatic exposure control techniques in modern CT scanners. Gudjónsdóttir et al. have recently documented that there is up to 4.9% change in applied tube current with off-centering with horizontal or x-axis off-centering (Gudjonsdottir et al. 2009). With vertical or y-axis off-centering, a much greater change in tube current was noted for three CT scanners from different CT vendors (GE, Philips, and Siemens). This change in tube current with off-centering was associated with substantial change in image noise compared to scanning with object centered in the gantry isocenter. Matsubara et al. have reported a similar change in tube current with CT scanners from another major vendor (Toshiba) as well, with about 78–124% change in tube current with use of automatic exposure control technique for scanning of off-centered object (Matsubara et al. 2009).

Toth and colleagues analyzed adult body localizer radiographs and found that almost half of the patients are off-centered with a mean off-centering of 2.3 cm below the gantry isocenter resulting in up to 140% surface dose penalty with a mean dose penalty of 33% based on tube presumption of tube current increment to compensate for increased image noise from patient off-centering (Toth et al. 2007). In contradiction, Li et al., found that almost 95% of their patients were off-centered with a mean off-centering distance of about 3.3 cm (Li et al. 2008). Interestingly, almost 97% patients were centered below the gantry isocenter. One of the largest studies on off-centering from another tertiary healthcare center involving 397 patients recently reported that 81% patients were off-centered in just the vertical direction (Kim et al.). The authors also noted that the off-centered of patients undergoing CT leads to substantial unreliability in both CT numbers (HU) and image noise.

In addition, patient centering in the gantry isocenter is especially important for dual source CT scanners (Siemens) which have less than 35 cm field of view for scanning with dual X-ray source. This smaller field of view restriction also applies to high resolution or definition scanning with greater projections per rotation on single source CT scanner equipped with adaptive statistical iterative reconstruction (ASiR, GE Healthcare) technique.

In summary, perhaps the quotation from Friedrich Von Schlegel, a German philosopher, at the beginning of this chapter aptly emphasizes the importance of recognizing necessity of centering the patients for CT scanning too, in light of findings that support increased surface and peripheral dose to patients who are off-centered relative to the gantry isocenter as well as increased image noise. In future, automatic centering techniques may help the technologists and/or radiologists to achieve precise patient centering for CT scanning.

## References


Aviles Lucas P, Dance DR, Castellano IA, Vano E (2004) Monte Carlo simulations in CT for the study of the surface air kerma and energy imparted to phantoms of varying size and position. Phys Med Biol 49:1439–1454

Frush DP (2003) Responsible use of CT. Radiology 229:289–291

Gudjonsdottir J, Svensson JR, Campling S, Brennan PC, Jonsdottir B (2009) Efficient use of automatic exposure control systems in computed tomography requires correct patient positioning. Acta Radiol 50:1035–1041

Kalra MK, Maher MM, Saini S (2003) What is the optimum position of arms for acquiring scout images for whole-body CT with automatic tube current modulation? Am J Roentgenol 181:596–597

Kalra MK, Maher MM, Toth TL, Hamberg LM, Blake MA, Shepard JA et al (2004a) Strategies for CT radiation dose optimization. Radiology 230:619–628

Kalra MK, Maher MM, Toth TL, Schmidt B, Westerman BL, Morgan HT et al (2004b) Techniques and applications of automatic tube current modulation for CT. Radiology 233:649–657

Kalra MK, Maher MM, Toth TL, Kamath RS, Halpern EF, Saini S (2004c) Comparison of Z-axis automatic tube current modulation technique with fixed tube current CT scanning of abdomen and pelvis. Radiology 232:347–353

Kalra MK, Maher MM, Kamath RS, Horiuchi T, Toth TL, Halpern EF et al (2004d) Sixteen-detector row CT of abdomen and pelvis: study for optimization of Z-axis modulation technique performed in 153 patients. Radiology 233:241–249

Kim M, Singh S, Halpern E, Kalra MK. Relation between patient centering, mean CT numbers and noise in abdominal CT: Influence of anthropomorphic parameters. World J Radiology (in press)

Li J, Toth TL, Udayasankar U, Seamans J, Small WC, Kalra MK (2006) Automatic patient centering for MDCT: Effect on radiation dose. scientific paper at ARRS, Vancouver, Canada (in press)

Li J, Toth TL, Udayasankar U, Seamans J, Small WC, Kalra MK (2007) Automatic patient centering for MDCT: Effect on radiation dose. Am J Roentgenol 188:547–552

Li J, Udayasankar UK, Toth TL, Small WC, Kalra MK (2008) Application of automatic vertical positioning software to reduce radiation exposure in multidetector row computed tomography of the chest. Invest Radiol 43:447–452

Mayo JR, Aldrich J, Muller NL (2003) Fleischner Society Radiation exposure at chest CT: a statement of the Fleischner Society. Radiology 228:15–21

Mulkens TH, Bellinck P, Baeyaert M, Ghysen D, Van Dijck X, Mussen E et al (2005) Use of an automatic exposure control mechanism for dose optimization in multi-detector row CT examinations: clinical evaluation. Radiology 237:213–223

Matsubara K, Koshida K, Ichikawa K et al (2009) Misoperation of CT automatic tube current modulation systems with inappropriate patient centering: phantom studies. Am J Roentgenol 192:862–865

Namasivayam S, Kalra MK, Mittal P, Small WC (2006) Can radiation exposure associated with Abdominal and/or Pelvic CT be minimized with better practice? Initial results. scientific paper at ARRS, Vancouver, Canada (in press)

Toth TL, Cesmelia E, Ikhlef A, Horiuchi T (2006) Image quality and dose optimization using novel X-ray source filters tailored to patient size. In: Proceedings of SPIE 2005;5745:283-91. http://spiedl.aip.org/dbt/dbt.jsp?KEY=SISDG&Volume=5745&Issue=1&bproc=year&scode=2005. Accessed 16 Mar 2006)

Toth T, Ge Z, Daly MP (2007) The influence of patient centering on CT dose and image noise. Med Phys 34:3093–3101

# Part III

# Practical Approaches to Dose Reduction

# Dose Optimization and Reduction in CT of the Brain and Head and Neck Region

Tom Mulkens, Rodrigo Salgado, and Patrick Bellinck

## Contents



T. Mulkens (✉) · P. Bellinck
Department of Radiology, Heilig Hart Ziekenhuis,
Mechelsestraat 24, 2500 Lier, Belgium
e-mail: tom.mulkens@scarlet.be;
tom.mulkens@hhzhlier.be

R. Salgado
Department of Radiology,
Universitair Ziekenhuis Antwerpen,
Wilrijkstraat 10, 2650 Edegem, Belgium

**Abstract**

In this chapter an overview is given of different modalities for dose optimization and reduction in cranial CT and CT of the Head and Neck region. For adult cranial CT, the role of the justification process and the implementation of the use of imaging guidelines are discussed. Possibilities for dose reduction by use of diagnostic reference levels (RDLs) and the introduction of recent dose reduction techniques, like tube current modulation and iterative reconstruction, are overviewed. A separate part is dedicated to dose reduction in cranial CT of children. In the Head and Neck region, the main topics are use of low dose CT of the sinuses in adults and children and the recent introduction of cone beam CT as a low-dose alternative for conventional CT.

## 1 Introduction

Since its introduction in the 1970s, CT has played an increasingly important role in the imaging diagnosis of a variety of disorders. This is especially true in the field of neuroradiology, where CT made direct visualisation of neurological anatomy for the first time possible, thereby revolutionizing diagnostic imaging.

However, it is well known that CT-induced radiation dose is considered high compared with other (X-ray based) imaging techniques. For a CT examination of the same region, various authors have reported different dose values. This difference is due to variations in applied scan protocols, and in the different choice of units of measurements in which they expressed the dose. This hindered comparison

D. Tack et al. (eds.), *Radiation Dose from Multidetector CT*, Medical Radiology. Diagnostic Imaging,
DOI: 10.1007/174_2011_451, 

between studies and makes the correlation of CT with other radiological procedures difficult.

In routine practice, about 25–30% of all CT studies are studies of the head or brain, with a mean effective dose of 2 mSv (Van Unnik et al. 1997; Pantos et al. 2011). Effective dose of cranial CT is lower than that of the trunk, although individual organ dose for the head are considerably higher than for other parts of the body. This is owing to the uneven distribution of radiosensitive organs in the human body and the lower weighting factors for the head organs (Pantos et al. 2011).

Although magnetic resonance imaging (MRI) was expected to reduce the overall frequency of CT (especially in neuro imaging), this has not yet been the case completely (Rehani and Berry 2000; Hall and Brenner 2008). Indeed, the advent of helical and multidetector helical CT (MDCT) with rapid acquisition times and new diagnostic fields (e.g. CT angiography, perfusion CT, ...) has led to a further increase in CT examinations: over the last 25 years CT has risen 12-fold in the UK and more than 20-fold in the USA. Its contribution to the radiation dose is now responsible for 50% of the collective dose from medical X-rays in the UK (Hart and Wall 2004) and medical radiation exposure represents now, for the first time, the majority of the effective dose to which individuals in the USA are exposed (Hall and Brenner et al. 2008). This evolution has spurred a growing interest in CT dose optimisation and reduction in recent years.

MRI has superseded CT for examining the head, neck and spine, many parts of the musculoskeletal system and it offers an alternative for CT in the abdomen and pelvis. Nevertheless, the higher cost and the lower availability of MRI remains a problem.

CT remains the method of choice for evaluation of post-traumatic injuries of the head, spine, thorax, abdomen and pelvis, for detection and characterization of parenchymal lung disease and for staging of almost all solid malignancy, including lymphomas.

In the evaluation of cerebrovascular pathology, recent developments with diffusion and perfusion techniques have given MRI a higher sensitivity and specificity, although CT still plays a major role in evaluation of these disorders, due to its high sensitivity in detection of intracranial hemorrhage, faster image acquisition, wider availability, lower cost, ease of use—especially in critical patients—and fewer contraindications (Rehani and Berry 2000).

In CT, the effect of changing dose (e.g. by changing tube current or mAs settings) on the image quality is sometimes difficult to assess, as CT is a digital technique in which image acquisition and display are not related, i.e. the 'uncoupling effect'. Thus, unlike conventional plain-film radiography, excessive exposure will not result in overexposure of images and degradation of image quality. As a result, significant variations have been observed between individual scanners in the typical patient doses for common CT examinations and in large surveys from different countries (Van Unnik et al. 1997; Clark et al. 2000; Stamm 2007). Multiple studies concentrating on dose reduction, showed that low-dose CT is possible in high contrast imaging, e.g. imaging of the lungs, without loss of diagnostic information (Zwirewich et al. 1991). It remains however unclear whether dose reduction is also possible in areas with low contrast differences, like the intracranial brain structures.

This is nevertheless an important issue, since some patients, who are examined or treated for complex or chronic brain disease (e.g. malformation, tumors, trauma and cerebrovascular disease) often undergo multiple CT studies over time.

This also applies, for instance, for children with hydrocephalus with malfunctioning ventricular shunts or with follow-up of craniocerebral trauma. Although initial CT studies are oriented toward identification of subtle changes of intracranial structures, the main purpose of those control studies is to identify complications and gross morphologic changes. As this often involves structures with high contrast or large structures (e.g. follow-up of hemorrhage or ventricular size), a reduction of 'standard' scan parameters to lower dose settings seems possible in these CT studies (Cohnen et al. 2000).

## 1.1 Modalities for Dose Reduction in Head CT

### 1.1.1 Justification and Use of International Imaging Guidelines:

The system for radiation protection proposed by the International Commission on Radiological Protection (ICRP) is based upon three principles (ICRP report 60 1991): (a) justification; (b) optimization; and (c) individual dose and risk limits. The last principle does not apply to medical exposures.

Justification of a practice is defined as: 'No practice involving radiation exposure should be adopted unless it produces sufficient net benefit to the exposed individuals or society to overcome the possible detriment it causes'. Simplified, justification means that the benefits exceed the risks.

A useful (radiological) investigation is one in which the result—positive or negative—will alter clinical management and/or add confidence to the clinician's diagnosis.

Implementation of this justification process in clinical practice is mainly based on the implementation of referral guidelines for medical imaging, and this has been addressed by several organizations, both supranational, like the World Health Organization and European Community (European Commission 2008), as national, like the UK Royal College of Radiologists, Referral Guidelines (Royal College of Radiologists UK 2011) and the American College of Radiology, Appropriateness Criteria for Imaging (American College of Radiology 2011). These guidelines are regularly updated.

Clinical guidelines are systematically developed statements, which assist the clinician in decision making about appropriate healthcare for specific clinical conditions. The aim is to improve the diagnosis and treatment of a particular condition, to reduce variations in clinical practice and thereby improve the patient care in clinical practice and to encourage further research. Evidence-based guidelines are based on good research evidence of clinical effectiveness (Royal College of Radiologists UK 2011).

The problem with the implementation of the justification process by correct use of referral guidelines is that it is a very big challenge for the healthcare system, because it has large implications for the daily routine work of both prescribers and radiologists and both their training and the complete process is difficult to control.

Several studies have reported the inappropriate use of radiological examinations, according to the guidelines, especially CT examinations, whereby MRI should be a better option. Clarke et al. reported about the possibility to use MRI to replace CT examinations in a survey of 1,025 patients (Clarke et al. 2001) and concluded that more than 70% of the CT examinations could have been replaced by MRI and even more than 90% in examinations of the brain and (lumbar) spine, whereby such a policy can significantly reduce the CT collective radiation dose.

A survey of CT examinations in young patients under 35 years (Oikarinen et al. 2009) showed that, according to the European guidelines, 30% of the examinations were unjustified, whereby 77% in the CT lumbar spine, 36% in brain CT and 37% in abdomen CT, because mainly MRI, and sometimes ultrasound, were a better alternative.

MRI is today considered as the imaging 'gold standard' for evaluation of brain disease and brain CT is reserved for trauma evaluation, exclusion of non-traumatic intracranial hemorrhage and in critically ill patients (Oikarinen et al. 2009).

Nevertheless, brain CT still makes a large part of our daily clinical CT practice. There are several reasons. Strict implementation of the imaging guidelines is not so easy and straightforward : there is a problem with lower availability and higher cost of MRI. A long waiting time for MRI is not always accepted by referring clinicians and patients. Referring physicians do not know the 'radiological' guidelines and they sometimes do not like that radiologists change their request, unless an alternative imaging is performed immediately, so that the patient is helped immediately. CT scans are requested in the practice of defensive medicine (Hall and Brenner 2008).

In geriatric patients, the radiation risk is negligible, the clinician wants to exclude gross pathology and elderly patients are more frequently uncooperative, so that brain CT remains a good alternative for MRI.

### 1.1.2 Dose Reduction Possibilities in Head CT

Scan parameters of 'standard' examination protocols in cranial CT are usually implemented by manufacturers, and are oriented toward attaining the best image quality in order to meet the highest diagnostic criteria. For decades, neuroradiologists have welcomed the advances in depicting neuroanatomy by new imaging techniques and accepted physics theories and vendor advice that high signal-to-noise ratio concerns justify using recommended CT dose rates (Fox 2004). Indeed, image conspicuity for brain structures such as gray and white matter is in the category of 'low contrast'. Nevertheless, many neuroradiologists do not always pay attention to the doses used in their own CT suites. Their technologists usually receive training application from the CT vendors, which do not like to demonstrate routine work at minimal dose, because images with more noise will be presumed to show a vendor's product to be inferior (Fox 2004).

Only a few studies have focused on the possibility of lowering the dose for CT of the head.

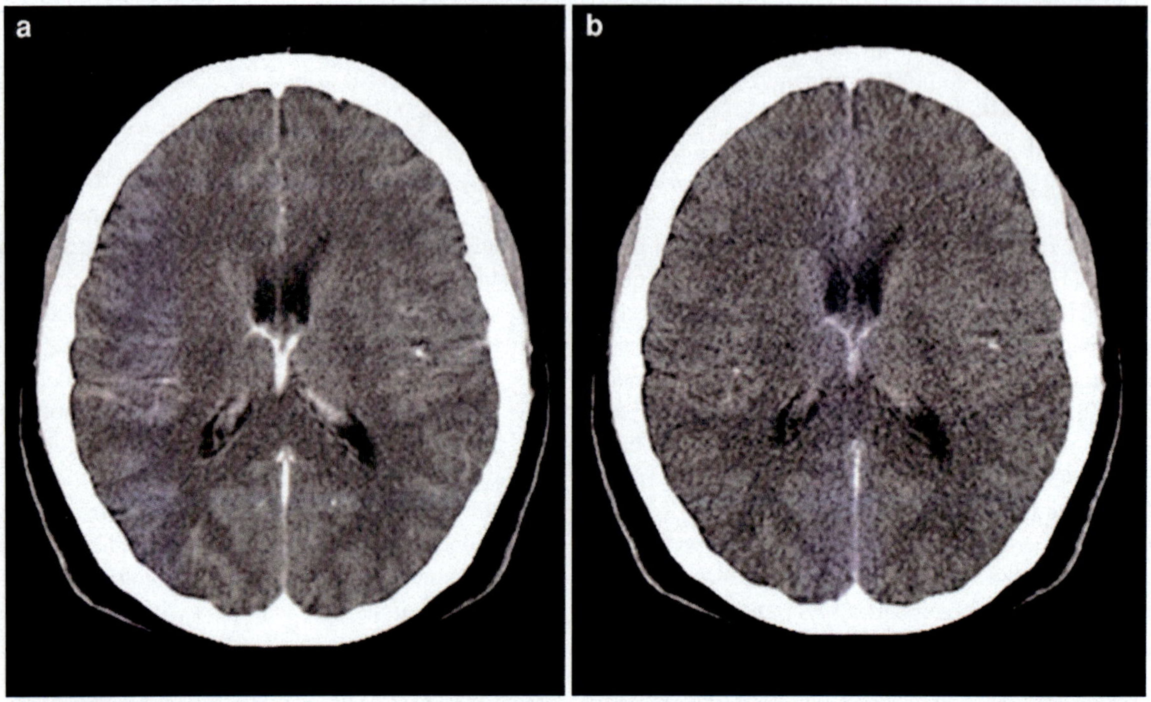


**Fig. 1** CT images of a 43-year-old woman with persistent headache since 3 weeks show normal brain structures at the level of lateral ventricles. Standard brain CT after I.V. iodine contrast with a 6-MDCT at 130 kV, 280 mAs, 1 s rotation, CTDI = 61.2 mGy, comparable to the 'EU reference level'. Calculated effective dose of 'standard' CT exam is 2.13 mSv; DLP = 820 mGy.cm: 5 mm axial image with 'standard' dose at 280 mAs (**a**) and additional 5 mm axial image at low-dose at 140 mAs (**b**) with 50% dose reduction the image is somewhat noisier but there is a clear delineation of the anatomical structures

In a study (Cohnen et al. 2000) to assess image quality changes on CT scans of the head using a formalin-fixed cadaver, the radiation dose was reduced by lowering both tube current and kilovoltage, and this on two different CT machines, both in conventional sequential mode and (single-slice) helical scanning. Five experienced readers independently evaluated subjective image quality, whereby no observable differences in image quality between scans obtained with doses from 100% ('standard mode') to 60% of standard settings were noted. In this study a linear inverse relation between image noise and dose was found. There was only a general assessment of subjective image quality in a cadaver head and no correlation with a clinical situation. Scans produced with a dose of more than 50% reduction in comparison with 'standard' settings were judged uninterpretable.

In a study (Mullins et al. 2004) in 20 elderly (>65 years) patients with a 4-MDCT helical CT exam of the head for routine indications, with 140 kV, 170 mAs, 1 s. scan time and pitch factor of 0.75 (CT Dose Index (CTDI) of 65 mGy), the scan was repeated for a limited volume by covering four 5 mm thick images at 90 mAs (CTDI of 34 mGy, other scan parameters identical) at four levels: posterior fossa, middle cranial fossa, corona radiata and centrum semiovale, with a dose reduction of 47% (Fig. 1). Gray matter (GM)–white matter (WM) conspicuity was not significantly different between the two dose groups. Main GM contrast-to-noise ratio (CNR) was 22% higher in the 170 mAs-group, which was statistically significant, but all 90 mAs images (although somewhat noisier) were considered of acceptable diagnostic image quality and sufficient resolution, as rated by three experienced neuroradiologists. They indicate that it is not unusual that in a hospital with an active neurologic intensive care and a stroke unit, some critically ill patients may receive multiple (sometimes daily) CT exams of the head for a period of some days or even weeks. The indications for these scans are frequently gross imaging findings, but which may change and affect management decisions:

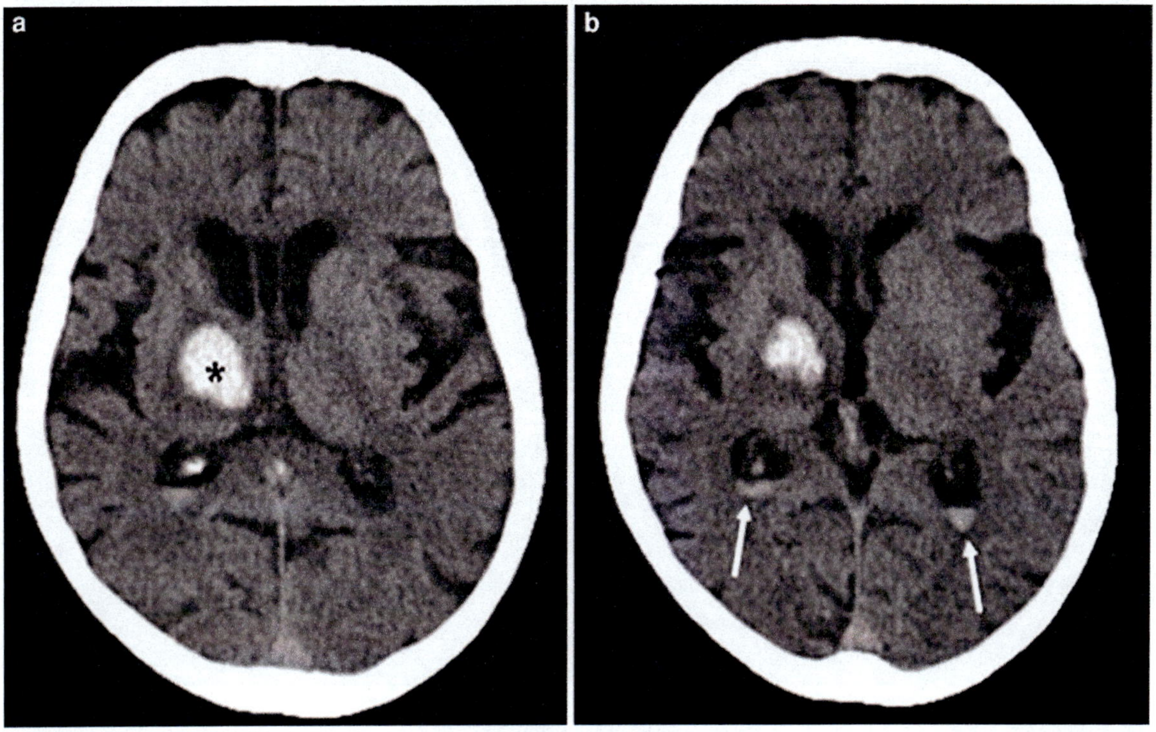


**Fig. 2** Control brain CT study with 50% dose reduction (CTDI of 30.6 mGy) in comparison with 'standard' settings by halving tube current in a 69-year-old woman with *right-sided* thalamus hemorrhage, one day after admission at the intensive stoke unit because of progressive somnolentia (same scan protocol as in Fig. 1**b**). Axial 5 mm images show clear visualization of hemorrhage (*asterisk*) (**a**) and presence of intraventricular extension with small blood–liquor levels (*arrows*) in both occipital horns (**b**). Calculated effective dose of low-dose CT exam is 1.12 mSv; DLP = 432 mGy.cm

traumatic or non-traumatic hemorrhage (Fig. 2), aneurysm rupture, stroke and hydrocephalus (Fig. 3).

For younger patients (and children) the difference of a scan with CTDI of 65 or 34 mGy seems significant, especially when this is repeated several times in a short period. Recommendation of a low-dose technique for initial workup seems inappropriate (at present), since there is no scientific backup from other low-dose studies showing its potential to detect subtle pathology (e.g. lacunar infarctions) accurately. However, objective measurements showed no statistical significant difference between standard and low-dose (about 50% less) images for GM-WM conspicuity, which is a far more subtle distinction in terms of Hounsfield units than the conspicuity of most lesions (Mullins et al. 2004).

Another study (Britten et al. 2004) reached similar results: they added spatially correlated statistical noise to standard images of CT of the head to simulate exposure reduction up to 50% in 23 elderly patients (>69 years). In this way, at 120 kV, starting from an initial scan at 420 mAs, they simulated images at 300, 260 and 210 mAs. They used the presence of periventricular low density lesions as an example of the effect of simulated dose reduction on diagnostic accuracy, which was not lowered significantly even with 210 mAs images (50% dose reduction), and used visualization of the internal capsule as measurement of image quality, which was obviously lowered with low-dose images.

In a third patient study Gündogdu et al. 2005 analyzed the effect of various tube current settings to optimize the image quality and dose for adult cranial CT in 60 patients. They examined three reference levels (posterior fossa, basal ganglia and centrum semiovale) and evaluated subjective image and noise quality scores and quantitative noise measurements. At 50% decreased dose protocol, starting from a CTDI of 58.2 mGy for the posterior fossa and 48 mGy supratentorially, there was no poor quality score at any level; at nearly 60% decreased dose protocol, poor quality scores were much higher, especially in the posterior fossa.

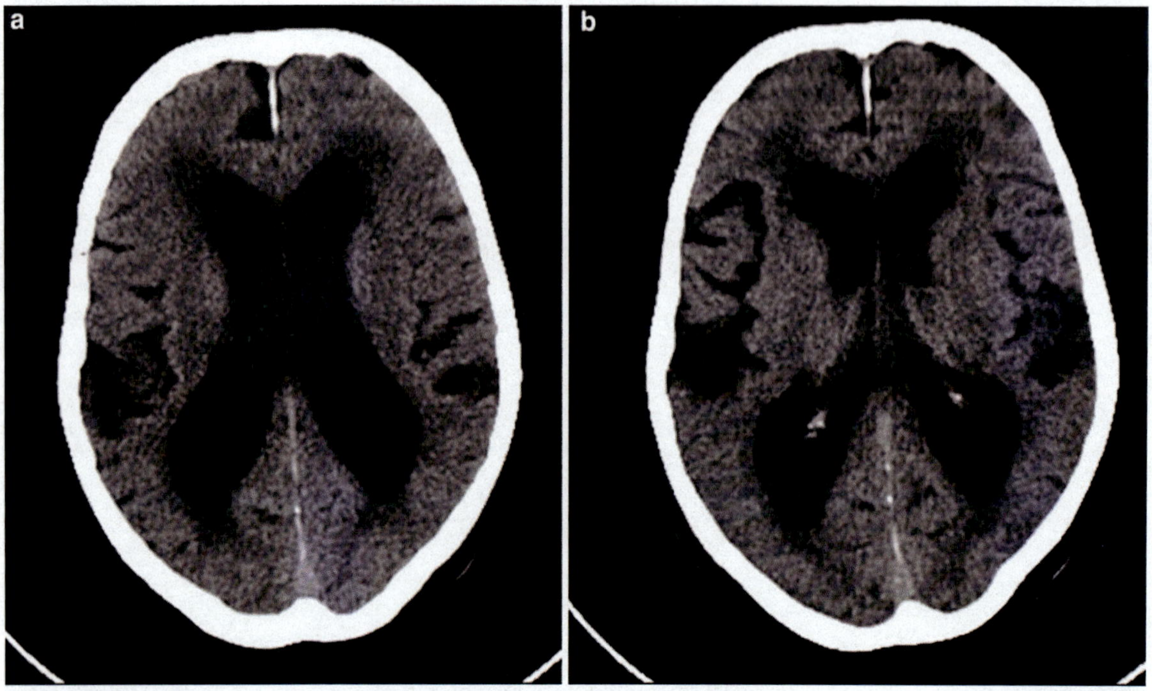


**Fig. 3** Follow-up brain CT study at low-dose (CTDI of 30.6 mGy) in a 79-year-old woman with (normal pressure) hydrocephalus. Low-dose axial CT images are of sufficient quality to compare the dilatation of both lateral ventricles (**a** and **b**) with previous CT studies. Calculated effective dose of low-dose CT exam is 1.05 mSv; DLP = 405 mGy.cm

The importance of these three studies (Mullins et al. 2004; Britten et al. 2004; Gündogdu et al. 2005) is that they indicate that there is a clinical feasibility for lowering the dose for 'standard' cranial CT examinations and that a dose reduction up to 50% seems to give no significant image quality loss. Their limitation is that they evaluated only morphological normal anatomic brain areas and the question remains of how much the resolution of low-contrast lesions will be affected by low-dose protocols.

In CT of the brain, the lens of the eye is of particular concern as cataract formation is a well-documented result of radiation damage. The use of a different scan plane (different beam angulation by gantry angulation) to avoid the orbits have been shown to reduce the eye lens dose by 87% (Yeoman et al. 1992), without affecting the severity of posterior fossa artifacts (beam hardening by the petrous bones). An international questionnaire survey in this study in more than 180 hospitals in the UK, USA, Australia and Europe, showed that only 32% of the hospitals routinely avoided the eye lens during cranial CT.

### 1.1.3 Use of Diagnostic Reference Levels in Head CT

For optimization and dose reduction in CT, one needs first to know the mean level of radiation of a 'routine' CT examination in a certain anatomic region.

In 1998, the European Commission (EC) proposed reference dose quantities or levels for CT (EC Working Document EUR 16262 1998), based on weighted CT Dose Index (CTDI w, mGy) and Dose-Length Product (DLP, mGy.cm). These EC 'dose reference levels' (DRL) for CT represent the third quartile values (75th percentile–P 75) of mean CT dose recorded for adequate samples of patients and have proved to be useful as reference diagnostic level (RDL) in initial surveys. For CT of the head, these reference values are 60 mGy for the CTDI w and 1050 mGy.cm for the DLP. This corresponds to a 'reference' effective dose for CT of the head of 2.2 mSv (Clark et al. 2000). The EC working document gives data that allow the values of DLP to be converted into effective dose by using conversion factors for broad regions of the body. For cranial CT this conversion value is 0.0021 mSv/mGy.cm. These reference doses are, in effect, investigation levels related to average practice, since they are derived from mean doses and are not applicable to individual patients. It is accepted that the use of these levels should not interfere with good clinical practice, but that they can be useful for comparing samples of patients from different centers. The goal or rationale behind these reference levels is the following: by setting the reference level on the third quartile values (P 75), the 25% hospitals or departments contributing to the highest dose above this p 75, should review their procedures and reduce their patient doses accordingly. This philosophy is now accepted in Europe.

A number of surveys have been carried out in Europe during the past ten years, both regional and national, mostly to establish whether regional and/or national dose levels comply with EU quality criteria, i.e. the reference 'EU DRL'. An overview of these surveys is given in another chapter of this book.

In Europe, the mean national dose values for head CT, in the period 1999–2006, varied from 57 to 68 mGy for CTDI (w) and from 676 to 1036 mGy.cm for DLP, generally only slightly less than the nowadays considered high reference EU levels and they observed a large dose variation, with a factor of 2 to 6 between the dose level of p 75 and the one of p 25 (Stamm 2007).

Initial surveys were done in the USA and United Kingdom (McCrohan et al. 1987; Shrimpton et al. 1991), which showed that minimum and maximum doses for brain CT examinations could vary by a factor up to 11-fold.

Inherent differences in scanner design have been shown to contribute to this dose variation between models by up to a factor of three at most. Hence, much of the wider variation observed was caused by the difference in local scanning technique and parameters employed (Shrimpton et al. 1991). They conducted a survey in which the CTDI was measured in scanners of a large number of English hospitals and effective doses of various standard examinations were calculated using organ-dose conversion factors. A Dutch survey showed similar findings (Van Unnik et al. 1997) and confirmed that the greatest single variable that determines the patient dose is the way the scan is performed. They found mean effective doses in a CT brain examination ranging from 0.8 to 5 mSv, with a mean of 2 mSv, whereby the large dose distribution can also be explained in part by the fact that a repeat scan with administration of iodine contrast doubles the dose. Although the reason for administration of contrast generally depends on the clinical situation, a large variation was shown, whereby in some hospitals nearly all patients were scanned without contrast and in others nearly all patients were scanned with contrast. Despite the clinical introduction of MRI for more than ten years, this Dutch survey showed that CT of the brain still represented about 35% of all CT examinations in 1997.

This is comparable with a local survey in our department which showed in 1997 that cranial CT compromised 37% of all CT examinations. Nevertheless, there is a declining amount of cranial CT exams in our department, which compromised 41 and 39% of all CT examinations in 1991 and 1995, respectively. This further lowered to 31 and 30% in 2002 and 2003, after introduction of an MR unit and further declined to around 25% in 2011, which is still a large part of our daily CT work. This declining trend in the use of CT of the head (in favor of MRI) is also reflected in the number of more than 50% brain CT exams of all CT examinations in the first US survey of 1987 (McCrohan et al. 1987).

Recent national surveys in Germany (update July, 2010) and Norway show still relatively high mean levels of DLP for head CT of 950 and 900 mGy.cm, respectively (Veit et al. 2010; Silkoset et al. 2010), which, more than 10 years after the introduction of the 'EU-DRL' of 1050 mGy.cm, is only a small dose reduction.

More local surveys (Hidajat et al. 2001; Hiles et al. 2001) and a multinational survey in a smaller patient population (Tsapaki et al. 2006) showed that lower values can be obtained for brain CT: CTDI: mean value of 46, 47.8 and 39 mGy (47 mGy for p 75) and mean DLP of 731, 544 and 587 mGy.cm, respectively. They conclude that dose reduction is possible while maintaining diagnostic confidence and that there is a need for revision of the EU-DRL, because they do not reflect anymore the technical improvements of modern CT, since the EU data were introduced before the introduction of helical and multidetector CT (Tsapaki et al. 2006). A meta-analysis of published studies of the radiation dose of the most common types of CT examinations from 1991 to the end of 2009 (Pantos et al. 2011) showed that mean effective dose for CT examinations of the head, chest and abdomen prior to 1995 were significantly higher than for the later studies, whereas over the period between 1996 and 2009 the mean effective dose of these examinations was virtually unchanged.

The problem with the strategy for reducing the collective dose by introducing DRL, proposed by the

**Table 1** Comparison of dose reference levels (DRL) in terms of dose-length-product (DLP, mGy.cm) for adult cranial CT, compared with the levels of the EU directive EUR16262

| CT head | EU | France | Belgium | Belgium | | Lier, Belgium [a] | |
|---|---|---|---|---|---|---|---|
| DRL | 1998 | 2004 | 2007 | 2007 | 2006 | 2009 | 2011 |
| DLP | P 75 | P 75 | P 75 | P 25 | mean | mean | mean |
| mGy.cm | 1050 | 1050 | 1020 | 740 | 1000 | 850 | 600 |

[a] Local mean dose values for adult cranial CT

EU, is that it works too slow: regular national surveys should be conducted within a reasonable time interval (e.g. 2–3 years), so that the gap between the p 75 and the p 25 level can be reduced more quickly. Therefore, the first quartile levels (P 25) are a better measure for the dose optimization process, especially because it works faster than the proposed p 75-EU DRL policy and it reflects better the new dose reduction possibilities of modern CT scanners (Stamm 2007).

In our country, Belgium, it took nearly 10 years to establish the first national DRL : the Belgian Federal Agency for Nuclear Control (FANC) published the first Belgian DRL in 2007 (Table 1). Because in our department, the mean level of our local cranial CT dose level was quite high in 2006 (mean CTDI vol of 68 mGy - DLP of 1020 mGy.cm), near the national p 75-level, we focused on our national p 25 DRL-level and could reduce, in several steps over a 5-year period (Table 1) and with the introduction of tube current modulation in our head CT protocol, our mean dose level for head CT to a mean of CTDI vol of 34.5 mGy and DLP of 600.4 mGy.cm in 2011, without obvious loss in diagnostic confidence (Fig. 4). This corresponds to a mean effective dose of 1.26 mSv.

In conclusion, to halve the historical EU-DRL, from CTDI of 60 to 30 mGy, seems a good and reasonable objective for dose reduction in head CT today and especially since the introduction of recent iterative reconstruction techniques, whereby noise reduction is possible, achieving this goal should be possible.

### 1.1.4 Dose Modulation Techniques in Head CT:

Tube current or dose modulation techniques were introduced in modern multidetetector CT in the late 1990s and are based on the principle that X-ray attenuation is unevenly distributed in the body (Kalra et al. 2004). Basically, they are based on the measurement of the attenuation by a localizer radiograph, at the start of the examination, and this in the different scan planes: z-axis (longitudinal), angular (x–y plane) or combined (x–y–z axes or 3D).

With the angular modulation technique, the tube current is modulated during the rotation of the scan process, to decrease the X-rays in those projection angles that have less beam attenuation and contribute less to the overall mage noise content. So, the tube current (and dose) can be diminished in non-circular or asymmetric body regions, where some projections have less X-ray attenuation. The most obvious example is the shoulder region, where the attenuation is pronounced in the lateral direction, but much less in other (non-lateral) projections, especially anteroposterior and posteroanterior projections.

In the skull, the lateral diameter is generally smaller than the anteroposterior diameter (angular) and the diameter diminishes gradually up to the vertex (longitudinal).

A recent study showed that with dose modulation substantial dose reduction is possible in different neuroradiology CT protocols (Smith et al. 2008): although the effect of dose modulation on brain CT was uncertain at onset, given that the head is a spheroid structure with quite similar attenuation throughout, which differs from other body parts, a significant reduction of radiation dose was found both in brain CT of adults and children. They found that CTDI vol and DLP were reduced with 60% in adults and 57% in children, using z-axis modulation. With combined (x–y–z) modulation they reached a dose reduction of 50 and 22%, for CTDI vol and DLP, respectively, in unenhanced brain CT in adults.

For cervical spine and cervical and intracranial CT angiography, they got a dose reduction of 37.4 and 37.5% respectively, in terms of DLP, with z-axis dose modulation. With combined (x–y–z) modulation these reductions in DLP were much less, 16.5 and 3.3%, for cervical spine CT and CT angiography of head and cervical spine, respectively.

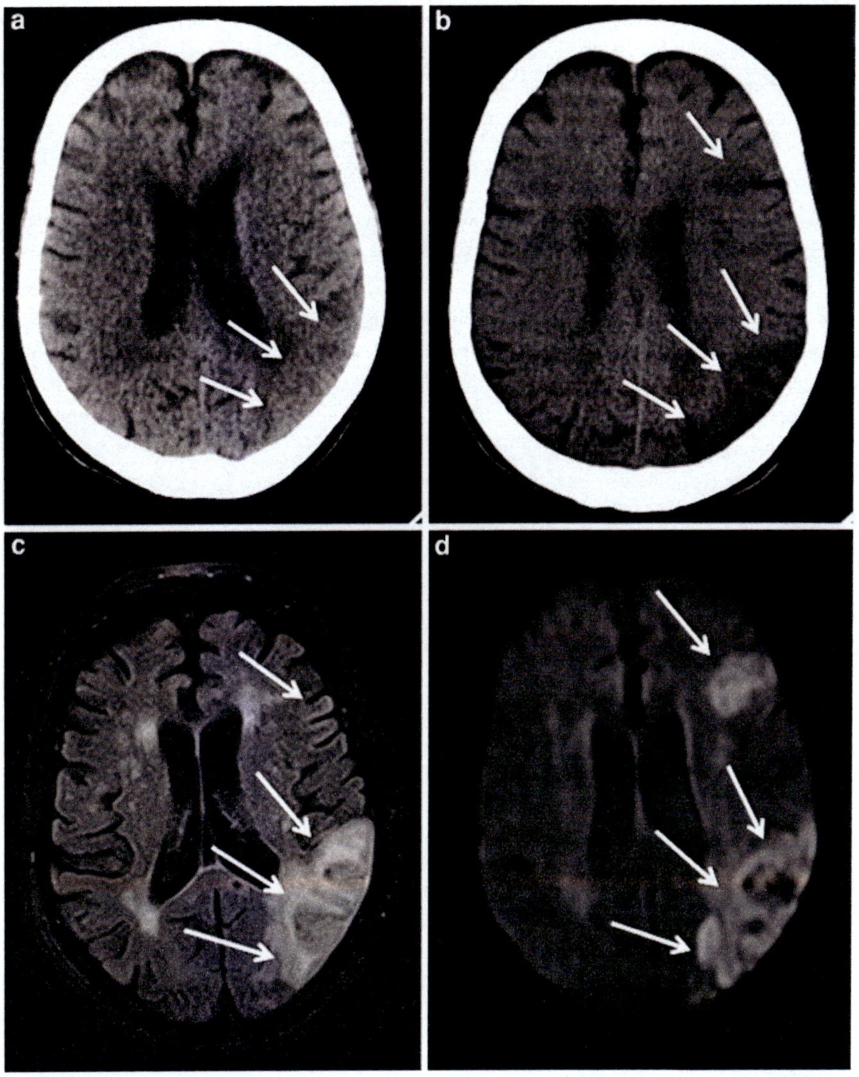


**Fig. 4** Feasibility of lowering dose in cranial CT: evaluation of an 85-year-old woman with recent onset aphasia: (**a**) Axial 5 mm image of 64-MDCT scan with 120 kV and 217 mAs (after modulation) (CTDI vol of 34.3 mGy) is sufficient to visualize subtle area in *left* temporo-occipital region with loss or effacement of normal cortical sulci (*arrows*), suspicious for recent infarction (**b**) Control CT 2 days later with same parameters shows 2 'watershed' infarcts: posteriorly in *left* frontal region (*arrow*) and *left* temporo-occipital region (*arrows*). The calculated effective dose of both CT examinations was 1.14 mSv (**c**) MRI with axial T2-weighted image and (**d**) diffusion image confirmed the CT findings

Another study obtained somewhat less dose reduction than in the previous study by Smith, in brain CT of patients with acute head trauma and stroke, with dose reduction of 35.8 and 35.2% for CTDI vol and DLP, respectively, with z-axis modulation (Zacharia et al. 2011). We got comparable results with implementation of combined (x–y–z) dose modulation in our brain CT protocols, with mean of 28 and 32% dose reduction in CTDI vol on a 64- and 6-MDCT machine, respectively (personal data).

### 1.1.5 Iterative Reconstruction Techniques

Image reconstruction in CT has traditionally been performed with the 'filtered back projection (FBP)' technique: FBP is fast and mathematically simplistic, and thus requires only limited computer power to perform, which was very important in the early days of CT.

However, there is a noise penalty that results from the simplicity of the reconstruction method: in lowering the radiation dose in CT, there is increased image noise, because the FBP technique is not able to generate sufficient diagnostic image quality with reduced tube current (mA) (Leipsic et al. 2010). Iterative reconstruction uses a reconstruction algorithm, whereby image data are corrected using a system of model(s) to improve image noise: the model uses matrix algebra to transform the measured value of each pixel to a new estimate of the pixel value, whereby this estimated value is compared with the ideal value predicted by the (noise) model. This process is repeated in successive 'iterative' steps until the final estimated value and the ideal value converge (Silva et al. 2010). With iterative reconstruction there is a possibility and potential to perform CT studies at reduced dose.

Although in recent years several studies have been published with the use of iterative reconstruction in body CT (abdomen, thorax, cardiac), there is not yet much published about the use of iterative reconstruction in cranial CT. In a recent published study, a dose reduction of 31% was reported in 98 adult head CT examinations with iterative reconstruction, without compromising contrast-to-noise ratio and diagnostic acceptability, whereby mean effective dose was lowered from 2.3 to 1.6 mSv, in comparison with standard dose CT (Kilic et al. 2011). The authors state that 'noise reduction with iterative reconstruction in their study of head CT is less than previously reported in abdomen and chest CT' and they propose less aggressive noise reduction (30%) in head CT to preserve noise at routine level. They found also a minimal loss in image sharpness, because at higher levels of iterative reconstruction the images become smoother.

## 1.2 Dose Reduction in Head CT of Children

Brenner et al 2001 reported an estimated lifetime cancer mortality risk of 0.18% for pediatric abdominal CT and 0.07% for pediatric head CT, both of which were approximately 10 times higher than the same risks for adults. Although these results are debatable (they are estimations) and the fact that the authors stressed that these numbers still represent only a small increase in cancer mortality over the natural cancer background rate, their study indicated the importance to adapt the radiation exposure in CT to a substantially lower level for children and not just apply adult scan parameters in the pediatric population, a method which was common practice until that period (Rogers 2001). Since image quality in CT (e.g., CNR) depends primarily on the detected x-ray fluency, consequently the technique factors used in pediatric CT can and should be reduced in comparison with adult technique factors, because smaller patients attenuate fewer X-rays. Thus, equivalent image quality can (and must) be produced at lower dose levels. Moreover, the values for energy imparted at CT in pediatric patients are generally lower than in adults, but the smaller mass of children (and the longer expected lifetime) causes the corresponding effective dose to be higher in children than in adults undergoing similar CT examinations (Huda et al. 1997).

Even more than in adults, cranial CT is the most common CT examination in children. In neonates and young children, about 25–30% of the active bone marrow is present in the skull, whereby in adults this is only 5–10%. The marrow absorbed dose in a 6-year-old phantom for a pediatric cranial CT has been reported higher than that for chest or abdominal CT (Fearon et al. 1987).

In 1999, a pediatric brain CT study showed that lower tube current can be used for children without difference in image quality (Chan et al. 1999). They compared cranial CT at 120 kV with 200 or 250 mAs (age under or above 5 years; $n = 53$) with 150 or 125 mAs (according to age; $n = 47$) and found no difference in image quality scores at seven different anatomical areas, whereby a dose reduction of 37.5 and 40% was reached (Fig. 5). Similar results were shown by comparing pediatric cranial CT at 140 kV and 180–240 mA (according to age) with lower dose at 90–130 mA (Shah et al. 2005): a 45–50% tube current reduction was possible without any significant effect on image quality and reader confidence in the level of detail available to reach a diagnosis.

Wong et al. proposed to use the maximum antero-posterior diameter (MAPD) of the child's head, measured on a lateral scout view at the start of the examination, as a good criterion for tube current selection (Wong et al. 2001). Another practical proposition is the use of CT technique charts (Boone et al. 2003) where, depending on the child's (head or trunk) diameter or circumference, a tube current reduction factor is given, starting from the tube current used in adults, reducing radiation dose and preserving contrast-to-noise ratio. These factors were calculated based on physically measured data in phantom cylinders of different diameters. Because of the exponential relation between patient thickness and X-ray attenuation, very large dose reductions are proposed in the smallest children (Boone et al. 2003).

Since children have less thick and less dense (less calcified) bones, it seems logical to use lower tube voltage to lower the dose: e.g., lowering the tube voltage from 120 to 80 kV gives a dose reduction of

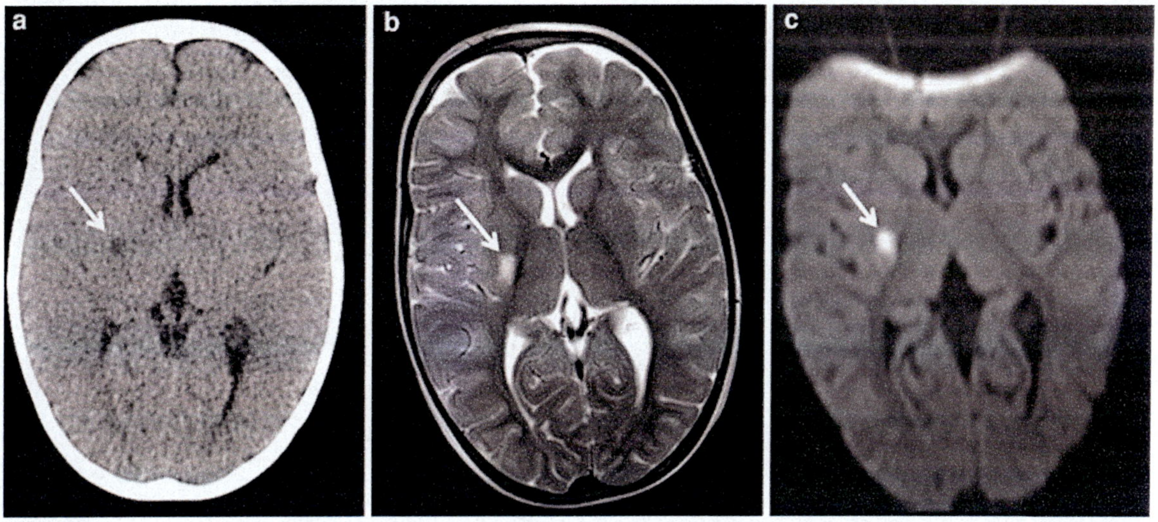


**Fig. 5** A 3-year-old boy with acute neurologic deficit with *right-sided* paresis. **a** Axial 5 mm CT at 120 kV and 108 mAs shows *oval* low density region in *right* capsulo-lenticular region (*arrow*). The CTDI vol of exam was 17 mGy and DLP 312 mGy.cm, which corresponds with a calculated effective dose of 2 mSv. **b** Axial T2-weighted MRI image confirmed the small capsulo-lenticular infarction (*arrow*) **c** Axial diffusion weighted MRI image (B = 1,000) confirms the recent lacunar infarction

**Table 2** Comparison of dose reference levels (DRL) in terms of volume computed tomography dose index (CTDI vol, mGy) for cranial CT in children, in different European countries

| Children | DRL | CT | Head | |
|---|---|---|---|---|
| CTDI vol (mGy) | < 1y | 1–5y | 5–10y | 10–15y |
| Switzerland (2005) | 20 | 30 | 40 | 60 |
| Germany (2006–2007) | 33 | 40 | 50 | 60 |
| UK (2003) | 30 | 45 | 50 | 65 |
| France (2007–2008) | | 31 | 39.5 | 49.5 |
| Belgium (2007–2009) | 35 | 43 | 49 | 50 |
| Local values [a], mean (2010) | 11.3 | 19.1 | 27.4 | 43 |
| Objective dose optimization 2011 | 20 | 25 | 30 | 30–35 |

[a] Local survey in 2010 of cranial CT in children (n = 124), Lier, Belgium

75%. Especially for young children and infants the use of 100 kV as tube voltage in cranial CT seems sufficient (Chan et al. 1999).

Like in adult CT, diagnostic reference levels (DRL) can be used as a tool or 'reference frame' to adjust radiation dose in children, according to age. Recent national surveys of different European countries are now available: see Table 2 (Shrimpton et al. 2005; Galanski et al. 2007; Verdun et al. 2008; Brisse et al. 2009; Buls et al. 2009).

We used these numbers to adapt our scan protocols for children: a level of CTDI vol, according to age, is chosen, whereby the CT technician has to adapt the scan parameters (increasing mAs), starting from the lowest level (child <1 year) in cranial CT of children (Table 2): <1 year: CTDI vol of 20 mGy, 1–5 year: CTDI vol of 25 mGy, 5–10 year: CTDI vol of 30 mGy, 10–15 year: CTDI vol of 35 mGy (comparable with adults).

For pediatric brain CT, additional dose reduction is possible for some indications (Smith et al. 2008): a low-dose protocol can be used for evaluation of hydrocephalus and shunt evaluation or for exclusion of craniosynostosis (Fig. 6)—a standard dose protocol

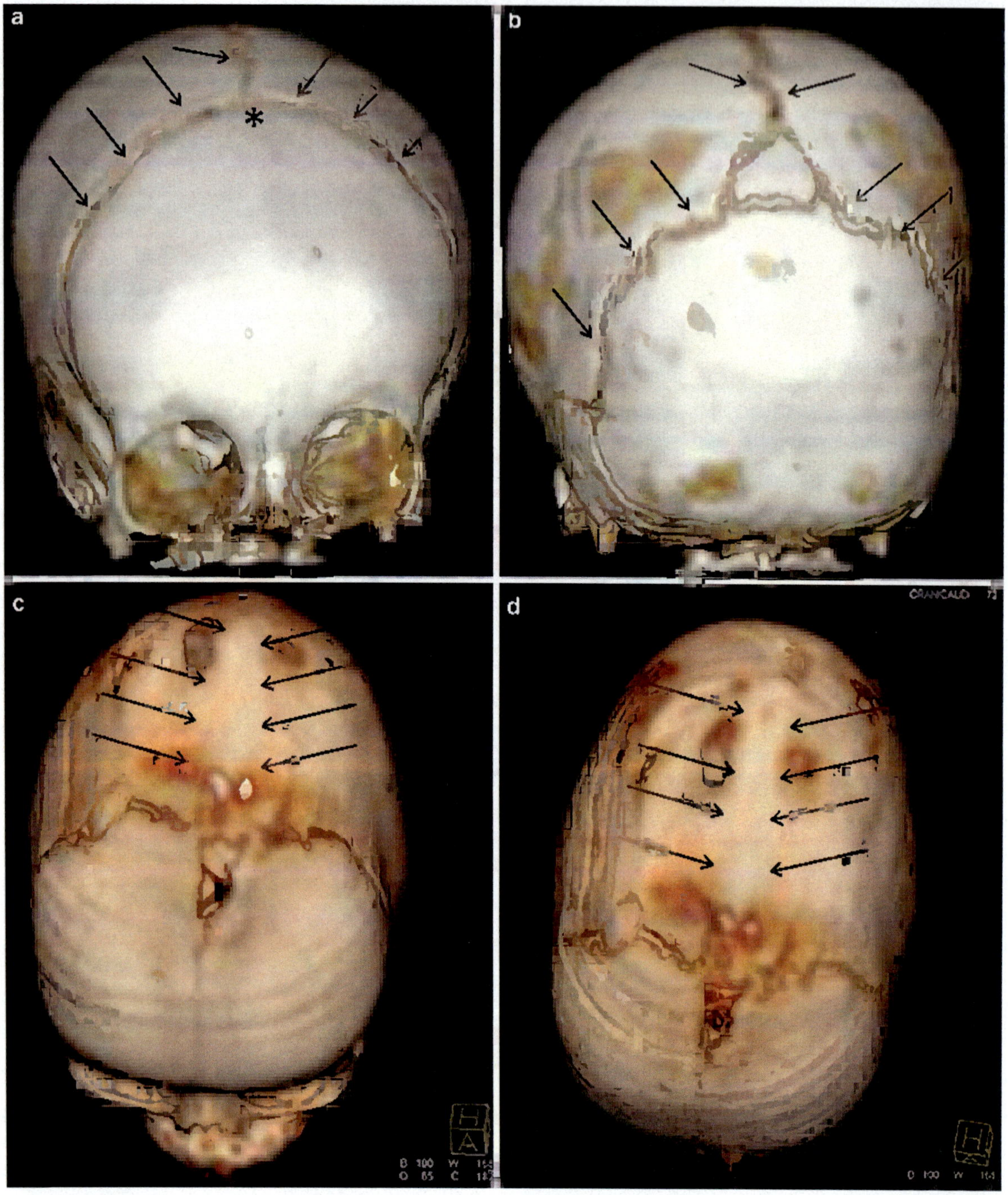


**Fig. 6** Use of a 'low-dose' protocol in cranial CT of children for exclusion of craniosynostosis: Because the primary goal of the CT study is visualization of the skull bone and sutures, lower kV setting at 100 kV or 80 is possible. **a–b** :A 6-month-old girl with clinically small fontanel: Volume rendered, anterior (**a**) and posterior (**b**) CT view of the skull shows absence of anterior fontanel (*asterisk*), but normal cranial sutures (*arrows*) and no evidence for craniosynostosis. CTDI vol of cranial CT exam was 11.4 mm–DLP was 176 mGy, which corresponds with a calculated effective dose of 1.9 mSv **c–d**:A 3-month-old boy with clinical suspicion of craniosynostosis: volume rendered anterior (**c**) and superior (**d**) view confirms the presence of craniosynostosis with a premature closure and bony fusion of the sagittal suture (*arrows*). CTDI vol of cranial CT exam was 11.5 mm–DLP was 181 mGy, which corresponds with a calculated effective dose of 1.98 mSv

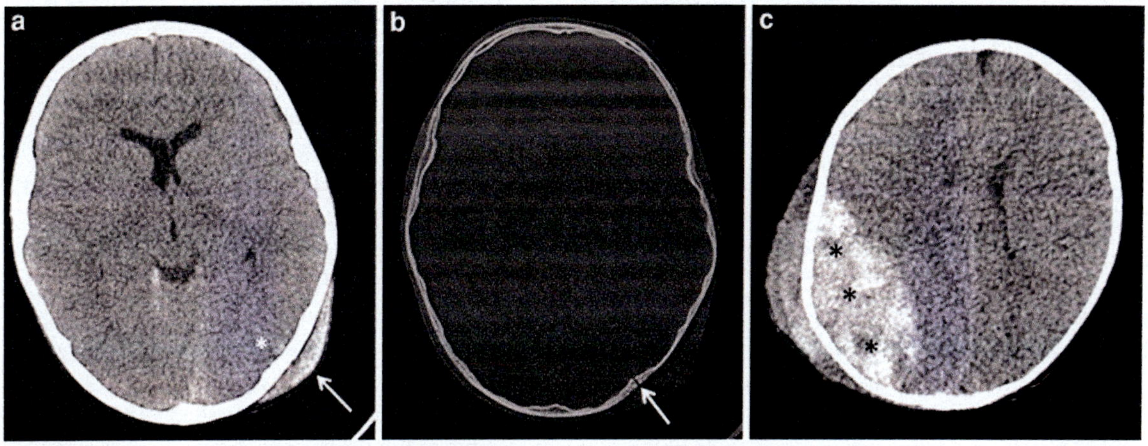


**Fig. 7** Evaluation of craniocerebral trauma in children: **a** A 7-year-old-boy with craniocerebral trauma: axial 5 mm image shows extracranial cephal hematoma *(arrow)* and small parenchymal hemorrhagic contusion *(asterisk)*. **b** Axial 5 mm in bone window shows skull fracture line *(arrow)*. CTDI vol of cranial CT exam was 25.21 mGy and DLP 473 mGy.cm, which corresponds with a calculated effective dose of 1.89 mSv. **c** Severe craniocerebral trauma after motor vehicle accident in a 6-month-old-boy shows extensive right-sided epidural hematoma *(asterisks)*, with mass-effect. At lower age, lower tube potential of 100 kV is sufficient because of less dense bone in small children. CTDI vol of cranial CT exam was 10.4 mGy and DLP of 218 mGy.cm, which corresponds with a calculated effective dose of 2.4 mSv

is used for 'higher dose' indications: trauma, acute neurologic deficit (Fig. 5), seizure, encephalopathy and congenital anomalies.

A local survey of our pediatric cranial CT studies in 2010 (n = 124), gave the following dose data (Table 2): <1 year (n = 14): mean CTDI vol of 11,34 mGy and DLP of 177,86 mGy.cm, 1–5 year (n = 37) : mean CTDI vol of 19,12 mGy and DLP of 330,19 mGy.cm, 5–10 year (n = 31): CTDI vol of 27,37 mGy and DLP of 492,45 mGy.cm, 10–15 year (n = 32): CTDI vol of 43,08 mGy and DLP of 755,48 mGy.cm. With the use of combined (x–y–z) tube current modulation, a mean dose reduction was achieved of 21% in these cranial CT studies in 74 children [personal data].

The large majority of our children were sent for craniocerebral trauma (> 90%) (Fig. 7).

The very low-dose level in our data in children of < 1 year is due to the use of a 'low-dose protocol' for exclusion of craniosynostosis, whereby the main focus of the CT examination is visualization of the bone and cranial sutures, which can be done with the lower tube voltage setting at 80 or 100 kV, in 6 of these 12 children. The higher dose data in the age group 10–15 years is due to the fact that the CT technicians chose erroneously the adult CT protocol in 8 of these 32 children (all 14- and 15-year-olds) and forgot to choose the dedicated pediatric protocol in these 'older' children, although they are well instructed to do otherwise. When the birth date of the patient is introduced at the scan console in CT of children, an automatic blockage of adult scan protocols should be made possible by the software.

### 1.2.1 Conclusion

The goal of radiology is accurate, timely and clinically relevant diagnosis. Reducing patient dose by limiting X-ray exposure has the inevitable consequence of increasing noise in CT images. The key question is to identify the minimum X-ray exposure, i.e. the 'poorest' image quality, required for a given examination and pathology (Britten et al. 2004).

Recent studies have shown the possibility to reduce the radiation in adult cranial CT up to 50%, without significant loss of image quality.

Starting from the historical EU-DRL of 1998, with a CTDI vol of 60 mGy, dose optimization to a level of 30 mGy seems possible for routine standard CT of the brain in adults, especially with the use of tube current modulation and/or iterative reconstruction techniques.

In certain clinical circumstances and patient populations, a tradeoff between reduced radiation dose and image quality is acceptable, without scarifying diagnostic accuracy. 'Low-dose' brain CT may be appropriate when routine follow-up of initial high contrast findings is required (e.g., hydrocephalus or hemorrhage). Also, hospitalized patients who require frequent serial CT scans for neurologic or neurosurgical care may also benefit from this low-dose scanning.

Finally, it is important to lower the dose parameters for pediatric head CT, since children are more sensible to radiation-induced damage. Nowadays, all CT vendors offer specific pediatric scan protocols with adapted lower dose settings and recently, DRL levels of different large national surveys can be used as 'reference frame' to adapt the scan protocols for children to a lower level.

## 2 Dose Optimization and Reduction in CT of Head and Neck Region

### 2.1 Dose Optimization and Reduction in Sinus CT

#### 2.1.1 Introduction

Sinusitis is a frequent disorder. The underlying cause can be viral, bacterial, allergic, vasomotoric or reactive. It can occur as a complication of dental infection or tooth extraction. In acute sinusitis there is generally no need for imaging, except when there is suspicion for complication with intra-orbital or intracranial extension. About one-third of the patients develop a chronic sinusitis. Chronic sinusitis is defined as persistent (acute) inflammation or frequently recurrent episodes of (sub) acute sinusitis. In these patients imaging is indicated: to visualize the grade and extension of the inflammatory sinus pathology, to identify an eventual underlying cause, to describe the site of pathology in the complex anatomy of the maxillofacial region and to guide endoscopic surgery. Better understanding of the physiopathology of sinusitis and the development of functional endoscopic sinus surgery (FESS) have changed the role of imaging: CT has become the 'gold standard' in the evaluation of (chronic) sinusitis, and has largely replaced conventional radiography, as CT is excellent to study key regions of interest, like the osteomeatal complex and anterior ethmoid region (Zinreich et al. 1996; Eggesbö 2006).

Before the advent of helical CT, direct coronal CT was the method of choice for visualization of the sinus-nasal anatomy. Since the introduction of helical and multidetector CT, axial imaging with fine (sub)millimeter collimation and reformations in the axial, coronal and sagittal plane with thin slices has become the method of choice, due to the possibility to get an (nearly) isotropic volume data set. Coronal reformations give equal or even better image quality, due to the absence of dental filling artifacts, which were frequently present in the earlier direct coronal scanning (Eggesbö 2006).

While CT is superior to demonstrate fine bony anatomy, extent and anatomic localization of inflammatory lesions and complications such as sclerotic bone thickening and bone destruction, it has limitations in the differentiation of soft tissue masses, such as distinguishing mucosal thickening from pus-filled areas and inflammatory lesions (like retention cysts, polyps and mucocoeles) from neoplastic processes. MR is superior in soft tissue characterization and has the advantage of using no radiation: MR is useful when in advanced opacification of the sinus-nasal cavities a distinction has to be made between 'simple sinusitis, pyocele, fungal sinusitis and neoplastic disease. It is also excellent to visualize invasion of the orbit or intracranial compartments. If neoplasm or complications of inflammatory processes are to be ruled out, additional imaging with intravenous administered gadolinium is mandatory (Rao and El-Noueam 1998).

#### 2.1.2 Low-Dose CT of the Sinuses

The possibility to use low-dose CT for sinus-nasal imaging has been existing for a long time and introduced, together with low-dose CT of the lungs, the application of low-dose CT in radiology. In 1991, before the introduction of helical CT, two studies already stressed the ability to image the sinuses at a much lower dose than commonly used in clinical practice at that time. Scanning a head phantom with constant tube voltage at 120 kV, six successive sets of axial and coronal examinations were obtained, whereby the mAs setting was consistently reduced by approximately 50% every time (Marmolya et al. 1991): from 451 to 16 mAs in the axial plane and from 503 to 23 mAs in the coronal plane (dose reduction by a factor of 28). The same systematic dose reduction was used in a subsequent prospective study of 60 patients in the same way: divided in to 6 groups of ten patients, each group underwent scanning with one of the six combinations of axial and coronal scanning as in the head phantom study.

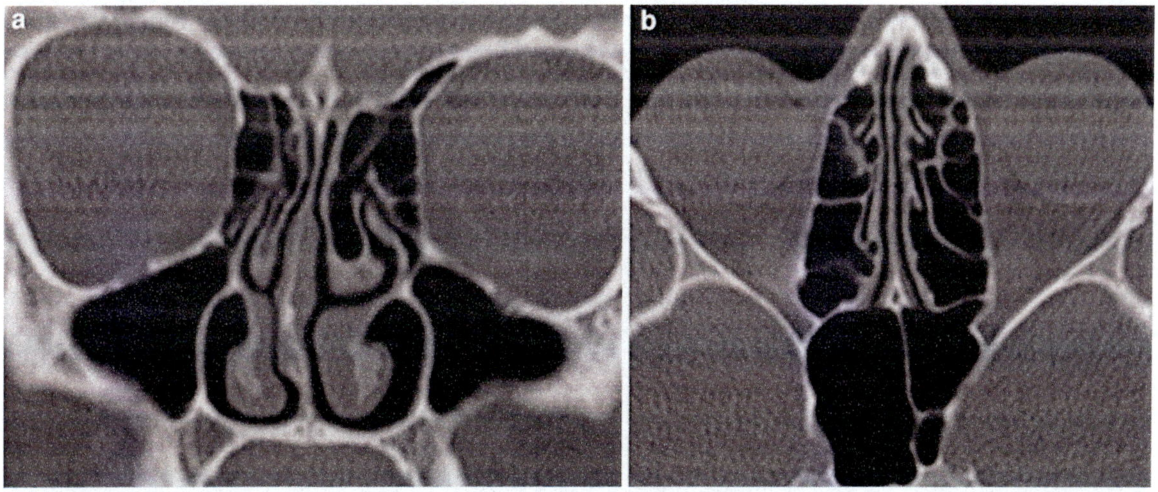


**Fig. 8** Normal anatomy showed in low-dose CT of sinuses: A 24-year-old woman with suspicion of chronic sinusitis. Low-dose 16-MDCT at 120 kV and 25 mAs (CTDI vol of 5.2 mGy) with 2 mm coronal (**a**) and axial (**b**) images show clearly the normal anatomy of the osteomeatal units and infundibulum with clear aeration of both maxillary, ethmoidal and sphenoidal sinuses. Calculated effective dose of CT exam is 0.10 mSv

Additionally, 30 patients received the lowest mAs settings. In both the phantom and patient study the amount of visually perceived noise increased, somewhat more in the axial than in the coronal plane, but all images were considered as of diagnostic image quality: 'On the coronal images of the lowest setting of 23 mAs, the osteomeatal complex was clearly identifiable and presence of air versus soft tissue or fluid could be confidentially diagnosed' (Fig. 8). Another study of the same year recommended a comparable dose reduction: in 44 patients with inflammatory sinus disease, the dose was reduced by lowering the tube current from 390 to 180 mAs , and further to 90 mAs and finally to 60 mAs (Duvoisin et al. 1991). In all cases the exact extent of the disease was correctly assessed on each of the low-dose settings, with no false negatives: 'although the less pleasant appearance to the eyes, the increased noise in the low-dose images seemed not to induce errors of interpretation'. They reported that in cases of extensive sinus disease the thickness and integrity of the fine bony (ethmoid) septa are sometimes difficult to evaluate on low-dose CT images (Fig. 9).

Several more recent studies confirmed these initial observations of the early nineties: both with conventional incremental CT (Czechowski et al. 2001) and single-detector helical CT (Suojanen and Regan 1995; Kearny et al. 1997; Sohaib et al. 2001; Hein et al. 2002; Hagtvedt et al. 2003). They all proposed scan protocols with lower tube current settings of 40 or 50 mAs at 120 kV tube voltage as an alternative of many existing protocols which employed high mAs (up to 200 mAs—in the belief that this necessarily improves scan image quality). However, modern CT scanners are able to deliver excellent image quality at much lower dose levels (Kearny et al. 1997). Also the natural high contrast between the structures of interest (bone, air and soft tissue) in sinus CT gives the possibility to use lower mAs settings and correspondingly lower dose (Sohaib et al. 2001). The problem with these earlier low-dose sinus CT studies is that they did not deliver additional dose descriptors, like CTDI or effective dose, so that comparison between different scanners is difficult: mAs values can vary by a factor of two to three for the same dose with different scanners. Therefore directly comparing mAs values alone, across studies with different scanners, has limitations (Shrimpton et al. 1991).

Tack et al. (2003) calculated the effective dose of these previously reported low-dose CT studies of the sinuses (both incremental and single-detector helical CT studies), by using a commercially available software program on a PC (CT Expo, Hanover, Germany), for a mean scanned region of 12 cm length in their study: they calculated a range of 0.11–0.24 mSv (mean: 0.17 mSv) for men and a range

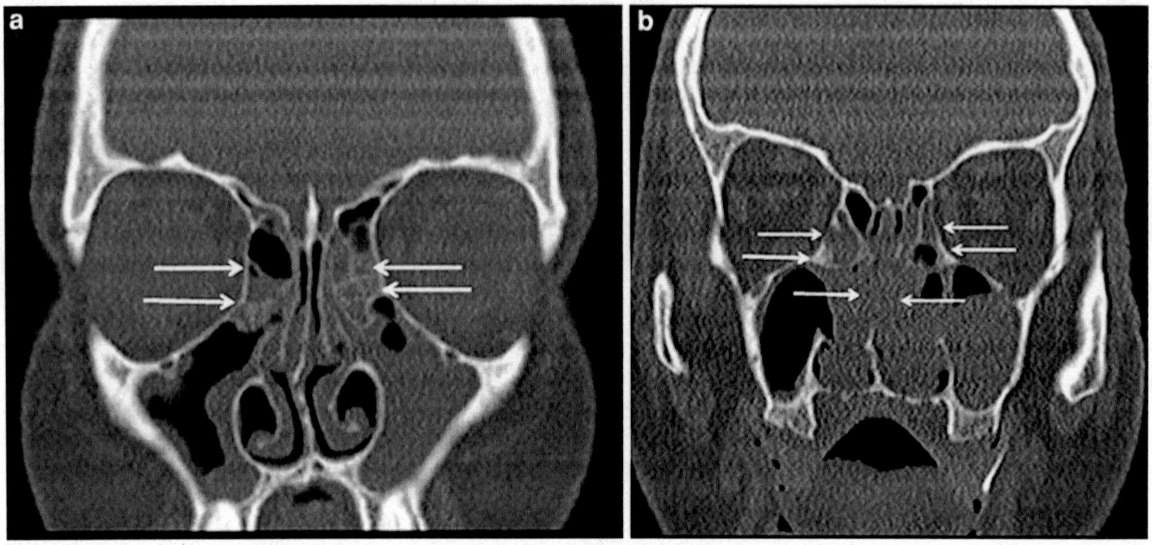


**Fig. 9** In cases of extensive sinus disease it is difficult to evaluate the integrity of the fine bony (ethmoid) septa (*arrows*), especially at low-dose CT. This can be due to bony erosion, partial volume effect or lack of contrast at low-dose. **a** axial 2 mm image of a low-dose 6-MDCT with effective dose of 0.12 mSv in a 18-year-old woman at 80 kV and 52 mAs–CTDI vol of 4.4 mGy and DLP of 50 mGy.cm **b** coronal 2 mm image shows extensive sinus pathology with bony erosions (*arrows*) in another 56-year-old male patient with naso-polyposis. Low-dose CT exam with CTDI vol of 4.42 mGy and DLP of 52 mGy.cm with bony erosion of the ethmoid septa and nasal septum (*arrows*)

of 0.12–0.26 mSv (mean: 0.18 mSv) for women. In their own multidetector CT study, low-dose CT was compared with standard dose CT on a 4-MDCT machine in the same 50 patients, which underwent both protocols. For standard dose CT the scan protocol was 120 kV, 150 mAs, 4 × 1 mm collimation, pitch factor of 0.75 which gave a mean effective dose of 0.70 mSv for men and 0.76 mSv for women. For low-dose CT 120 kV, 10 mAs, 4 × 1 mm collimation and pitch factor of 2 was used, which gave a mean effective dose of 0.047 in men and 0.051 mSv in women, which is comparable with the radiation dose used in a 4-view standard radiographic examination (Tack et al. 2003). They analyzed mucosal abnormalities at eight different sinusnasal anatomic landmarks and two bony abnormalities and found greater variation in analyzing cases of significant discrepancies in observations between three reviewers than between findings obtained at different dose levels: 'in other words, observational variations associated with the decrease in radiation dose (by use of the low-dose protocol) were fewer than those variations than can contribute to the reviewers (radiologists) themselves'. They concluded that low-dose MDCT should be considered the imaging method of choice in the evaluation of chronic sinusitis.

Multidetector CT has the advantage of three-dimensional imaging, whereby all structures are better visualized in one of the three different anatomic planes: e.g. the sphenoethmoidal recess is better visualized in the axial plane and the nasofrontal duct and periodontal spaces are better visualized in the sagittal plane.

Computer-assisted navigation is increasingly used in functional endoscopic surgery (FESS) of the sinuses to prevent injury to vital structures, whereby previous CT scanning is necessary: a recent study showed that low-dose CT is feasible in the pre-operative planning and that no dose dependence on the technical accuracy of the surgeon was found. The only limit for dose reduction in CT before FESS, was the surgeon 's ability to cope with the lower image quality (Nauer et al. 2011).

More recent studies confirmed that low-dose MDCT is now the first imaging technique of choice for evaluation of inflammatory and infectious pathology of the sinuses, with a mean CTDI of 5 mGy and DLP of 50–60 mGy.cm, corresponding with a mean effective dose of 0.1–0.15 mSv: although dual-source high pitch CT imaging or iterative reconstruction was used, they reached similar dose levels as with low-dose MDCT in the previous studies (Schell et al. 2011; Bulla et al. 2011).

Infections of the upper respiratory system are by far the most common cause of illness in infancy and childhood, accounting for approximately 50% of all illness in children younger than 5 years of age, and 30% in children between the ages of 6 and 12 years: the large majority of these upper respiratory infections are viral rhinitis or pharyngitis and are self-limiting diseases, also known as 'common cold'. About 10% of these upper respiratory infections are complicated by sinusitis, which is a common problem in the pediatric population (George and Huges 1990). According to the American College of Radiology, acute sinusitis is a clinical diagnosis that may not need imaging (McAlister et al. 2000). Although the use of radiography is not indicated in these patients and should be discouraged, it is still frequently used for diagnosis: the physical examination alone can give difficulties in the diagnosis of acute bacterial sinusitis, because of the similarity of physical findings in the patient with uncomplicated viral rhinosinusitis. Also the clinical findings of recurrent or chronic sinusitis are often not specific, especially in younger children (McAlister et al. 2000, Kronemer and McAlister 1997). Plain radiography of the sinuses in children is technically demanding and difficult to perform, particularly in very young children, since correct positioning may be difficult to achieve. Therefore the radiographic images may over or underestimate the presence of abnormalities within the sinuses. Furthermore, the interpretation of sinus radiographs in children is difficult: there is a lack of accuracy (low specificity and sensitivity), largely related to the small size of the sinuses, the angulation of the X-ray beam and nasal secretions (McAlister et al. 2000; Kronemer and McAlister 1997).

The American Academy of Pediatrics (2001) therefore advises to reserve the use of imaging of sinusitis for situations in which the patient does not recover or worsens during the course of appropriate antimicrobial therapy or in case of recurrent disease. The use of CT is restricted to children who have very persistent or recurrent sinus infections, not responsive to medical management and whereby surgery is considered an option as a management strategy and to those who present with complications of acute sinusitis. CT scan images give a much better detailed image of the sinus anatomy, and, when taken in conjunction with the clinical findings, remain a useful adjunct to guide (surgical) treatment.

Previous studies already showed the lack of accuracy of sinus radiographs for the diagnosis of sinusitis in children in comparison with CT: in up to 75% of the patients the findings of the radiographs did not correlate with those on CT scans: in about 40% of the patients with normal radiographs, there were signs of pathology on CT scans and vice versa; when there was an abnormality suspected on radiographs in 35% of the patients the CT scan showed normal findings (McAlister et al. 1989). Another disadvantage of sinus radiographs is the great variability in the interpretation of sinus radiographs between radiologists: there is a low interobserver agreement in the evaluation of these radiographs. This interobserver agreement between radiologists is much better with CT (Kronemer and McAlister 1997; McAlister et al. 2000). However, there used to be an important threshold for use of CT in children for sinus evaluation: first of all, the radiation dose of CT is much higher than radiographs and secondly, the use of sedation was frequently necessary (in young children) to perform a good CT exam. With the advent spiral CT and MDCT, CT became the imaging modality of choice for the diagnosis of sinus disease in adults, whereby it is not only possible to lower the radiation dose, but also to shorten the examination time substantially. A study in 125 children showed that the effective dose of low-dose sinus MDCT can be lowered to a level of 0.05 mSv, which was comparable with the level of effective dose measured from standard radiographs in 69 other children (Mulkens et al. 2005a). In a scan protocol with 80 kV and with a mAs range of 15–25 mAs (according to age) on a 6- and 16-MDCT, a CTDI vol of 1.28–2.1 mGy was reached with preservation of diagnostic image quality. (Fig. 10). Scan time was very short with a mean of 2.1 and 9 s (16-and 6-MDCT, respectively), whereby there was no need for sedation for any of the 125 CT exams. Compared to the 'default' examination protocols for sinus CT in children, as proposed by the manufacturer, the radiation using low-dose protocols, expressed in CTDI vol, was 5–7 times lower. The large majority of the children (85%) were referred for CT for evaluation of chronic or recurrent sinus complaints (Fig. 11); only about 15% of the children were referred to CT for evaluation of an acute history with fever, sinus discomfort or headache or for evaluation of fever of unknown origin. This study shows another

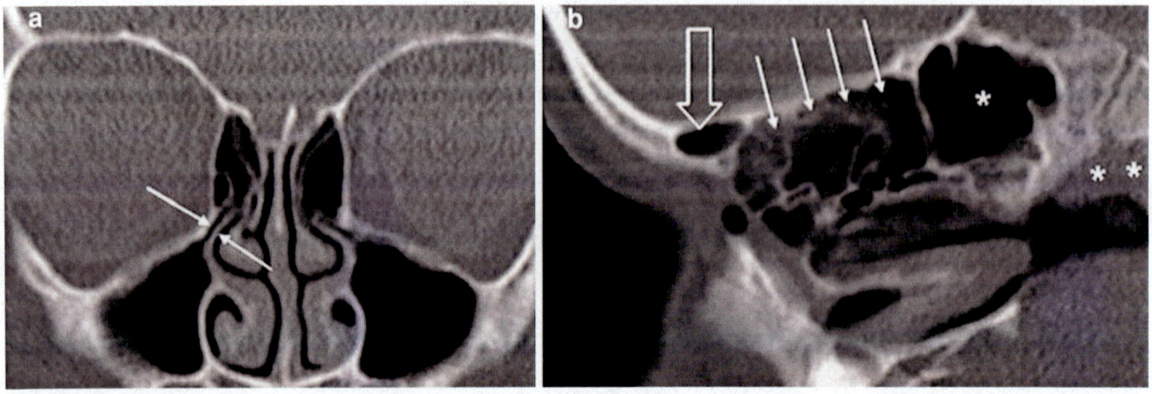


**Fig. 10** Normal findings in low-dose CT exam of the sinuses in a 6-year-old girl (6-MDCT, CTDI vol of 1.68 mGy, effecticve dose of 0.035 mSv). **a** Coronal 2 mm image shows normal maxillary and ethmoidal sinuses with clear depiction of infundibulum, medially bordered by the uncinate process (*arrows*). **b** Sagittal 2 mm image show normal frontal sinus (*open arrow*), ethmoidal cells (*small arrows*), sphenoid sinus (*asterisk*) and adenoids (*double asterisks*)

advantage of the use of low-dose CT in these children: CT permits to visualize in the same time the pharyngeal tonsils (adenoids), middle ear and mastoids, which are displayed in the same scan volume as the sinuses. In this way, CT displays the whole ear -, nose - and throat - region in one examination, which is not possible with radiographs. The presence of adenoid hypertrophy and fluid in the middle ears ('glue ear') and mastoids (Fig. 11) is frequently seen in these children with recurrent upper respiratory infections and this can be accurately diagnosed at the same time with the same low-dose (Mulkens et al. 2005a).

A disadvantage in imaging of sinusitis (both of adults and children) is the high incidence of soft tissue changes found in the sinus cavities in radiographic, CT - and MRI -exams in patients who undergo medical imaging for other reasons and have no clinical evidence of sinus disease. This incidence is reported to be 33–45% (Glasier et al. 1989; Gordts et al. 1997). A common cold or other upper airway infection acutely produces mucosal abnormalities in the sinuses in the majority of adults and children, and this is reflected in imaging, especially in patients who had a 'cold' in the 2 weeks preceding imaging. Therefore, the diagnosis of acute and chronic or recurrent sinusitis should not be made on the imaging findings alone: the diagnosis of acute or chronic sinusitis should be made clinically, with confirmation with laboratory and imaging findings (Gordts et al. 1997; McAlister 2000).

### 2.1.3 Conclusion

With modern multidetector CT, low-dose CT has become the method of choice to evaluate inflammatory pathology of the sinuses, especially in patients with chronic or recurrent sinusitis complaints. In patients with acute sinusitis, there is generally no need for imaging. Both in adults and children, low-dose CT can be done with a mean effective dose which approaches or is comparable with the range of effective doses of standard radiography: 0.05–0.15 mSv. One has to keep in mind that with every imaging technique mucosal abnormalities in the sinus cavities are frequently found in patients referred for other reasons and without clinical signs of sinus pathology. This lack of specificity, together with the lack of soft tissue contrast of low-dose CT is a disadvantage: when there is suspicion of complications of sinus disease with intra-orbital or intracranial extension or of underlying tumor pathology, the use of standard dose CT with I.V. iodine contrast with additional soft window settings or alternatively MRI, should be considered first.

## 2.2 Other Options for CT Dose Optimization in The Head and Neck Region

Since almost all other anatomic structures of interest in the head and neck region are soft tissues (pharynx and larynx, tongue and salivary glands, thyroid and

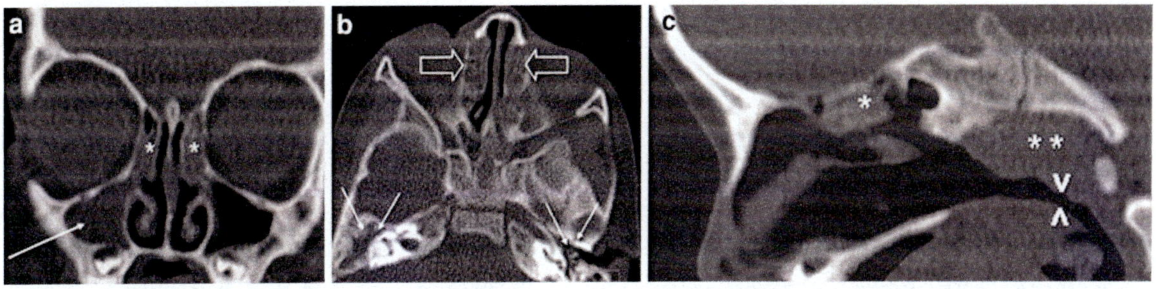


**Fig. 11** A 3-year-old girl with persistent and recurrent upper airway infections, fever, cough and purulent nasal discharge. Low-dose 16-MDCT with CTDI vol of 1.43 mGy and effective dose of 0.036 mSv. A 2 mm coronal image (Fig. 8**a**) shows right maxillary (*arrow*) and bilateral ethmoidal sinusitis (*asterisks*). Axial 2 mm image (Fig. 8**b**) shows bilateral fluid (*arrows*) in the middle ear cavities, additionally. Sagittal 2 mm image (Fig. 8**c**) shows additionally adenoid hypertrophy (*double asterisks*) with narrowing of the nasal airway (*arrowheads*)

parathyroid glands, muscles), the use of low-dose CT is not possible, since sufficient contrast (and dose) is necessary to distinguish between sometimes low contrast lesions and normal soft tissue. Nevertheless, there are some options to optimize the patient's dose and some specific indications whereby low-dose CT can be used.

The use of tube current modulation systems in modern multidetector CT have been shown to optimize and reduce patient's dose with different ranges, depending on the body region examined (McCollough et al. 2006). Automatic tube current modulation in CT is analogous to the automatic exposure control or photo timing technique for automatically terminating radiographic exposure in conventional radiography, once the predetermined radiographic density has been obtained.

Modern modulation systems adjust tube current along the three different scan planes (angularly around the patient and along the long axis of the patient) and this constantly during the time of the scan process and reach a substantial dose reduction with a range of 20% to more than 60%, depending on the anatomic region (Kalra et al. 2004; Mulkens et al. 2005b; McCollough et al. 2006). In the head and neck region, the use of tube current modulation has been shown to reduce the dose with a mean of 20%, both in adults (McCollough et al. 2006) and in children (Greess et al. 2004).

In dental radiology, CT is used in the preoperative planning of dental implant surgery, evaluating the bony anatomy of the mandibula and/or maxilla, measuring bone thickness and evaluating its integrity. Dedicated dental CT software packages are available to visualize the bone in parasagittal and 'panoramic' reconstructions. Several studies have reported the possibility to reduce the dose for dental CT imaging, by reducing the tube current and increasing the pitch, both on single-detector helical CT (Rustemeyer et al. 2004) and multidetector helical CT (Loubele et al. 2005). The dose can hereby be reduced with a factor of eight to nine, with an effective dose in the range of 0.10–0.20 mSv, without scarifying diagnostic image quality:'the dose reduction with acceptable image quality was possible because only the bony anatomy is of interest for indications of maxillofacial surgery and dental implant planning, and not the contrast of the different soft tissues' (Loubele et al. 2005).

In analogy with low-dose CT of the abdomen for detection of urinary lithiasis, low-dose CT of the head and neck region can be used for detection of sialolithiais, i.e. lithiasis of the salivary glands .

In this way the effective dose range was lowered from 1.5 to 2 mSv in our 'standard' head and neck protocol to a range of 0.3–0.5 mSv by using both a lower kV (100 or 110 kV) and lower mAs (50 mAs) on our both 6- and 64-MDCT machines (personal data). We use the same low-dose MDCT protocol for preoperative planning of patients with thyroid surgery: to evaluate the size of the thyroid goiter, its contour and its relationship with the trachea, the great vessels and its extension in the upper mediastinum.

## 2.3 Use of Cone Beam CT in the Head and Neck region

### 2.3.1 Technical Principles

Cone beam CT (CBCT) is a relative recent technique in the growing era of clinical CT technologies: in the past 10 years marketable scanners became available, by parallel advancements in flat-panel-detector (FDP) technology, improved computer power, relative low power requirements of the X-ray tube used in CBCT, so that quite inexpensive and compact office-based head & neck scanners as well as dental imaging scanners became available (Miracle and Mukerji 2008a).

The first clinical application of cone-beam CT in 1982 focused on applications in angiography and intervention (Robb 1982). The rise of the use of CBCT in clinical imaging was more than a decade later with introduction of systems dedicated to head & neck imaging, especially dental imaging (Vandenberghe et al. 2010).

Cone-beam CT uses a conical X-ray beam geometry, between the source (apex) and detector (base) in contrast to the conventional fan-beam geometry in conventional (multidetector) CT, in which the collimator restricts the X-ray beam to approximately 2D geometry. In CBCT, the system uses a 2D FPD and an entire volumetric dataset can be acquired with one single rotation of the gantry, whereby 3D reconstruction algorithms (3D adaptation of the filtered back projection method) creates a 3D volume data set.

A primary technological difference between CBCT and MDCT is the true isotropic nature of the acquisition and reconstruction with very high spatial resolution : it can produce a volumetric data-set with isometric voxels as small as $150 \times 150 \times 150\ \mu m^3$ at the isocentre (up to $75 \times 75 \times 75\ \mu m^3$ for the latest scanners) (Pauwels et al. 2011). MDCT reconstruction produces individual sections, which are then stacked together, generally with $500 \times 500\ \mu m^3$ in-plane and 500–1,000 μm z-axis resolution in modern MDCT machines, although recent high-end MDCT goes up to about 250 μm resolution. CBCT thus improves spatial resolution of CT, with reduced partial volume averaging.

Another obvious advantage of CBCT is its lower susceptibility to metallic artifacts in comparison with standard (MD)CT, which makes it especially attractive for dental imaging (with dental fillings, orthodontic material, metallic implant screws).

Nowadays commercial CBCT scanners, designed for dedicated head & neck imaging have application-specific exposure parameter protocols, with field-of-view (FOV) restricted to a specific (small) area of interest and minimized exposure to adjacent structures.

Less powerful and cheaper X-ray tubes can be used in comparison with MDCT.

In the absence of standardized absorbed dosimetric values, like CTDI in conventional CT, estimations of dose with these CBCT scanners are often evaluated with point-dose measurements generated with thermoluminescent devices (TLD) implanted in anthropomorphic head phantom (Pauwels et al. 2011).

The relatively low patient dose for dedicated dentomaxillofacial scans is a potential attractive feature of CBCT imaging. Effective dose for a head and neck CBCT system in a 16-cm head phantom was calculated to be in the range of 13–82 μSv (Loubele et al. 2009), which was much lower than for MDCT, scanned for the same region: 474–1160 μSv. A recent update on 14 CBCT systems gives an effective dose range of 19–368 μSv, largely depending on the chosen field-of-view (small to large) (Pauwels et al. 2011).

Generally, effective dose of most CBCT scans fall within the 30–80 μSv range, which is low, even in comparison with a standard panoramic radiography view, which delivers around 15 μSv (Miracle and Mukerji 2008a).

In contrast to MDCT, the contrast resolution and temporal resolution of CBCT is lower: the dynamic range of a Si:H FPD is slightly inferior than that of ceramic detectors used in MDCT and they have limited temporal resolution which leads to 'after-glow' or memory effects. Also the low contrast detectability, i.e. the possibility to discriminate differences in tissue attenuation, is lower with CBCT, with soft-tissue contrast discrimination of around 10 HU, where modern MDCT scanners approach 1 HU.

This limited contrast resolution remains a barrier: CBCT cannot be used to evaluate soft tissue and soft tissue pathology, which is a disadvantage in the head & neck region.

### 2.3.2 Clinical Applications of Cone Beam CT

Cone-beam CT is a relatively new CT technique, which has the potential of low-dose cross-sectional and 3D imaging for evaluation of the bony structures of the head and neck region.

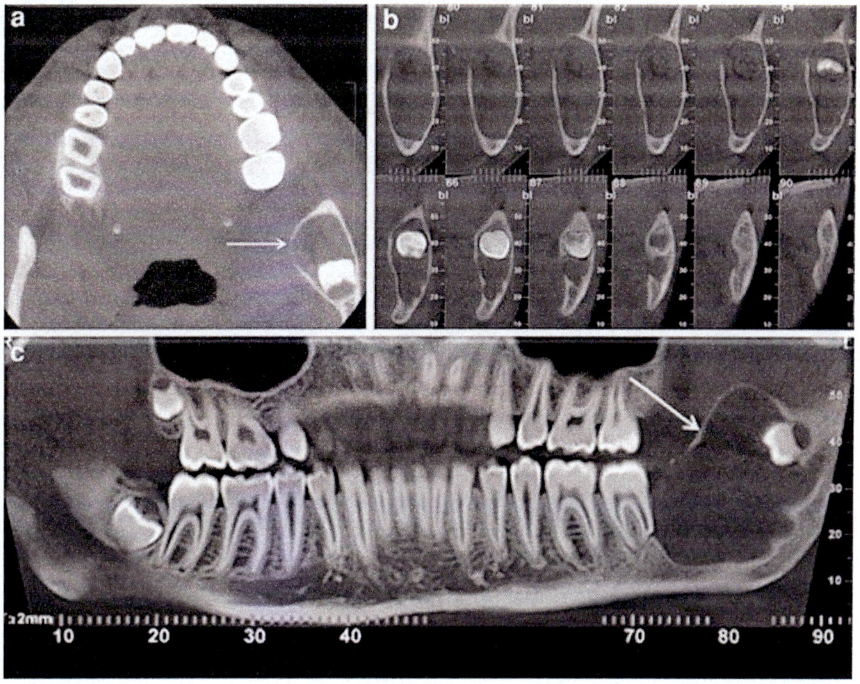


**Fig. 12** Cone-beam CT of the mandibula shows a large follicular cyst in the *left* mandibula (*arrow*) with (**a**) axial image, (**b**) parasagittal views and (**c**) panoramic view. (Courtesy of Casselman and Delanote, Department of Radiology, AZ St. Jan Hospital, Brugge, Belgium)

The earliest dedicated CBCT scanners were used in the field of dentistry and maxillofacial surgery: imaging that was previously done with conventional (MD)CT, now became possible to take place in dental offices. The advanced imaging possibilities of CBCT made it an alternative for diagnostic and treatment-planning evaluation in dentomaxillofacial surgery: endo-osseous implant imaging, orthodontics, evaluation of cysts (Fig. 12) and tumors in the maxialla or mandibula and cranio-facial fractures evaluation.

Preliminary evidence addresses the ability of CBCT imaging to characterize mandibular and maxillar alveolar bone morphology, visualization of the maxillary sinuses, incisive canal, mandibular canal and mental foramina, all structures important in surgical planning of dental implantation. Several studies have shown the geometric 3D accuracy of CBCT imaging in the maxillar and mandibular region (Miracle and Mukherji 2008b; Vandenberghe et al. 2010).

Clear imaging of the complex structural bony anatomy of the maxillofacial region for fracture evaluation (Fig. 13) is a logical application of CBCT: it clearly demonstrates fractures in this region, fluid-levels (patient is mostly in an upright position in contrast to the supine position in MDCT) and is also used in intraoperative planning, surgical navigation, localization of bony fragments and evaluation of screw anchorage, with lower levels of metal artifact than conventional CT.

In orthodontics CBCT is used for overlay-free visualization of structural and anatomical relationships: skeletal growth patterns, dental age estimation, upper airway evaluation, visualization of impacted teeth (Fig. 14) and this at a very low-dose in children (Miracle and Mukerji 2008b; Vandenberghe et al. 2010).

CBCT has been used in endodontics and periodontics: in periradicular surgical planning CBCT have been shown to be superior to radiographs in the characterization of periradicular lucent lesions, sinus involvement and evaluation of periodontitis. (Miracle and Mukerji 2008b; Vandenberghe et al. 2010).

Note that the low-dose requirements and high quality bone definition CBCT can be used to visualize the paranasal sinuses for screening of inflammatory and infectious processes and is foreseen to become in

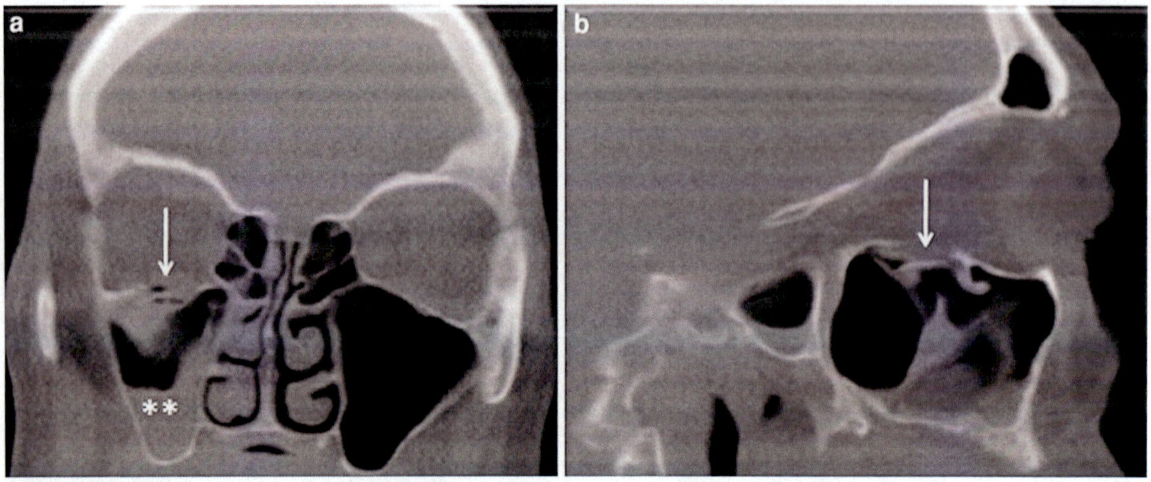


**Fig. 13** Cone-beam CT of young pregnant woman with maxilla-facial trauma shows *right-sided* orbital floor fracture with slight depression of the fracture fragment (*arrow*) and hemosinus with fluid-level (*asterisks*) at low-dose in (**a**) coronal and (**b**) sagittal plane. (Courtesy of Casselman and Delanote, Department of Radiology, AZ St. Jan Hospital, Brugge, Belgium)

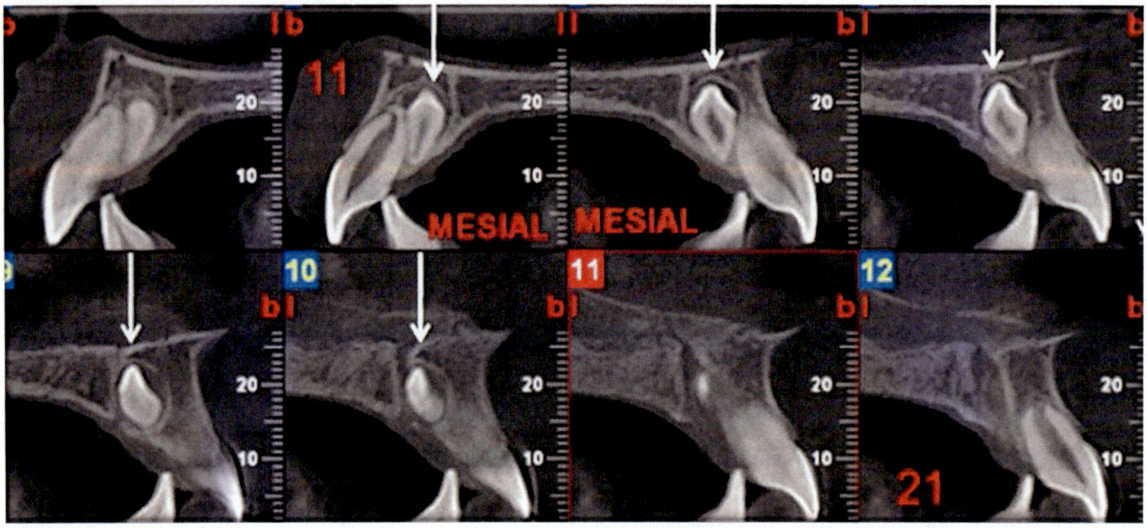


**Fig. 14** Cone-beam CT of the maxilla shows the mesio-dental position of an impacted surnummary tooth in the maxilla (*arrows*) in the sagittal plane (Courtesy of Casselman and Delanote, Department of Radiology, AZ St. Jan Hospital, Brugge, Belgium)

the near future the reference examination in sinus assessment (Hodez et al. 2011).

Recently, the use of CBCT has been very promising in ear pathology evaluation: first applications in chronic otitis, dyplasia and deformity and trauma are encouraging.

Its low-dose and low sensitivity to metallic artifacts makes it the imaging technique of choice for evaluation and follow-up of patients (mainly children) with cochlear implants (Fig. 15) (Hodez et al. 2011; Ruivo et al. 2009): a main disadvantage of conventional CT of the petrous bone is the image degradation by metallic and beam

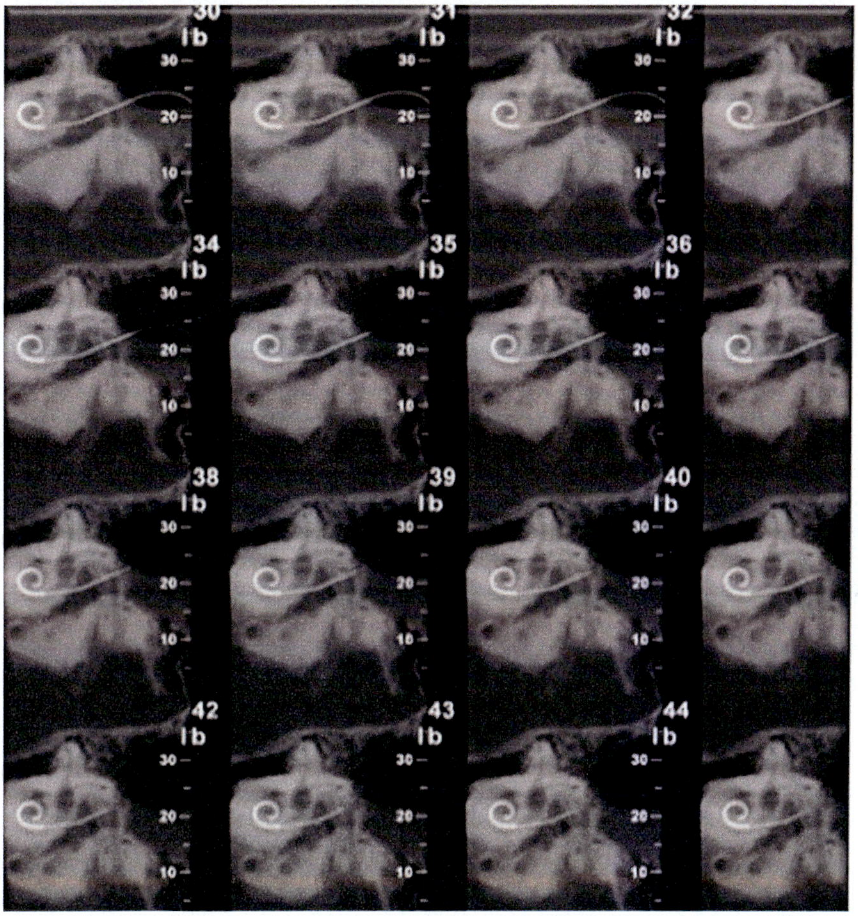

**Fig. 15** Cone-beam CT of the petrous bone shows the exact position in the cochlea of the electrode of the cochlear implant in a child at low-dose in the coronal plane, without metallic artifacts. (Courtesy of Casselman and Delanote, Department of Radiology, AZ St. Jan Hospital, Brugge, Belgium)

hardening artifacts, making it difficult to distinguish the precise intracochlear position of the electrode.

### 2.3.3 Conclusion

Because of its higher spatial resolution at low-dose, cone-beam CT seems a very promising CT technique for dedicated head and neck imaging: the dento-maxillofacial region, sinus imaging and evaluation of the petrous bone and skull base.

But the technique is not without controversy: CBCT has been largely adopted as an office-based service, providing a so-called '1-stop management' with fewer billed services and no radiologist consultation fee. Hereby the images are often performed and interpreted by non-radiologists, often without training, accreditation or license afforded by the radiology community. (Miracle and Mukerji 2008b).

Although constantly growing, most research in the applications of cone-beam CT is still preliminary and further prospective and outcomes-based research is required to make informed recommendations on the appropriate use of CBCT imaging in the head and neck region.

## References

## Brain CT:

American College of Radiology, Appropriateness Criteria for imaging (2011). www.acr.org/SecondaryMainMenuCategories/quality_safety/app_criteria.aspx

Boone JM, Geraghty EM, Seibert JA et al (2003) Dose reduction in pediatric CT: a rational approach. Radiology 228:352–360

Brisse H, Aubert B (2009) CT exposure from pediatric MDCT: results from the 2007–2008 SFIPP/IRSN survey. J Radiol 90:207–215

Britten AJ, Crotty M, Kiremidjian H et al (2004) The addition of computer simulated noise to investigate radiation dose and image quality in images with spatial correlation of statistical noise: an example application to X-ray CT of the brain. Br J Radiol 77:323–328

Brenner DJ, Elliston CD, Hall EJ et al (2001) Estimated risks of radiation-induced fatal cancer from pediatric CT. Am J Roentgenol 176:289–296

Buls N, Bosmans H, Mommaert C et al (2009) Current status on pediatric CT doses: a multicentre study (Belgium). RSNA meeting, Chicago. www.fanc.fgov.be/cws/GED/pop_View.aspx?LG=1&ID=2449

Chan CY, Wong YC, Yu SK et al (1999) Radiation dose reduction in paediatric cranial CT. Pediatr Radiol 29:770–775

Clark J, Cranley K, Robinson J et al (2000) Application of draft European Commission reference levels to a regional CT dose survey. Br J Radiol 73:43–50

Clarke JC, Cranley K, Kelly BE et al (2001) Provision of MRI can significantly reduce CT collective radiation dose. Br J Radiol 74:926–931

Cohnen M, Fisher H, Hamacher J et al (2000) CT of the head by use of reduced current and kilovoltage: relationship between image quality and dose reduction. Am J Neuroradiol 21:1654–1660

European Community (1998) Quality criteria for computed tomography. EC working document EUR 16262, Brussels, EU, 1998

European Commission: Radiation protection 118. Referral guidelines for imaging. Office for Official Publications of the European Communities, Luxembourg, 2008. www.ec.europa.eu/energy/nuclear/radioprotection/publications/doc/118_en.pdf

Fearon T, Vucich J (1987) Normalized pediatric organ-absorbed doses from CT examinations. Am J Roentgenol 148:171–174

Fox AJ (2004) Use of the lowest necessary radiation dose (editorial). Am J Neuroradiol 25:519

Galanski M, Nagel HD, Stamm G (2007) Paediatric CT exposure practice in the federal republic of Germany: results of a nationwide survey in 2005–2006. Medizinische Hochschule, Hannover

Gündogdu S, Mahmutyazicioglu K, Ozdemir H et al (2005) Assessment of image quality of a standard and three dose-reducing protocols in adult cranial CT. Eur Radiol 5:1959–1968

Hart D, Wall BF (2004) UK population dose from medical X-ray examinations. Eur Radiol 50:285–291

Hall EJ, Brenner DJ (2008) Cancer risks from diagnostic radiology. Br J Radiol 81:362–378

Hidajat N, Wolf M, Nunnemann A et al (2001) Survey of conventional and spiral CT doses. Radiology 129:395–401

Hiles PA, Brennen SE, Scott SA et al (2001) A survey of patient dose and image quality for computed tomography in Wales. J Radiol Prot 21:345–354

Huda W, Atherton JV, Ware DA et al (1997) An approach for the estimation of effective radiation dose at CT in pediatric patients. Radiology 203:417–422

International Commission on Radiological Protection (1991) Recommendations of the International Commission on Radiological Protection. ICRP report 60. Annals of the ICRP, 21 (1–3), 1991

Kalra MK, Maher MM, Toth TL et al (2004a) Techniques and applications of automatic tube current modulation. Radiology 233:649–657

Kilic K, Erbas G, Guryldirim M et al (2011) Lowering the dose in head CT using adaptive statistical iterative reconstruction. Am J Neuroradiol, Epub, 11 August 2011, 10.3174/ajnr.A2585

Leipsic J, LaBounty TM, Heilbron B et al (2010) Adaptive statistical iterative reconstruction: assessment of image noise and image quality in coronary CT angiography. Am J Roentgenol 195:649–654

McCrohan JL, Patterson IF, Gagne RM et al (1987) Average radiation doses in standard head examination for 250 CT systems. Radiology 163:263–268

Mullins ME, Lev MH, Bove P et al (2004) Comparison of image quality between conventional and low-dose nonenhanced head CT. Am J Neuroradiol 25:533–538

Oikarinen H, Meriläinen S, Pääkö E et al (2009) Unjustified CT examinations in young patients. Eur Radiol 19:1161–1165

Pantos I, Thalassinou S, Argentos S et al (2011) Adult patient radiation doses from non-cardiac CT examinations: a review of published results. Br J Radiol 84:293–303

Rehani MM, Berry M (2000) Radiation doses in computed tomography. Br Med J 320:593–594

Rogers LF (2001) Taking care of children: check out the parameters used for helical CT (editorial). Am J Roentgenol 176:287

Royal College of Radiologists, UK, Referral guidelines (2011). www.rcr.ac.uk/content.aspx?PageID=955

Shah R, Gupta AK, Rehani MM et al (2005) Effect of reduction in tube current on reader confidence in paediatric computed tomography. Clin Radiol 60:224–231

Shrimpton PC, Jones DG, Hillier MC et al (1991) Survey of CT practice in the UK, NRPB-R249 report. National Radiological Protection Board (NRPB), Chilton, UK

Shrimpton PC, Hillier MC, Lewis MA et al (2005) Dose from CT examination in the UK-2003 review. NRPB-W67 Report. National Radiological Protection Board, Chilton

Silkoset RD, Lysdahl KB, Olerud HM (2010) Variations in doses from CT examinations, presented at: European Congress of Radiology, Vienna

Silva AC, Lawder HJ, Hara A et al (2010) Innovations in CT dose reduction strategy: application of the adaptive statistical iterative reconstruction algorithm. Am J Roentgenol 194:191–199

Smith AB, Dillon WP, Lau BC et al (2008) Radiation dose reduction strategy for CT protocols: successful implementation in neuroradiology section. Radiology 247:499–506

Stamm G (2007) Collective radiation dose from MDCT: critical review of survey studies. In: Radiation dose from adult and pediatric multidetector computed tomography, 1st edn. Springer, Berlin-Heidelberg, pp 81–97

Tsapaki V, Aldrich JE, Sharma R et al (2006) Dose reduction in CT while maintaining diagnostic confidence: Diagnostic reference levels at routine head, chest and abdominal CT–IAEA-coordinated research project. Radiology 240:828–834

Van Unnik J, Broerse JJ, Geleijns J et al (1997) Survey of CT techniques and absorbed dose in various Dutch hospitals. Br J Radiol 70:367–371

Veit R, Guggenberger R, Nosske D et al (2010) Diagnostische referenzwerte für röntgenuntersuchungen. Radiologe 50:907–912

Verdun FR, Gutierrez D, Vader JO et al (2008) CT radiation dose in children: a survey to establish age-based diagnostic reference levels in Switzerland. Eur Radiol 18:1980–1986

Wong ETH, Yu SK, Lai M et al (2001) MAPD–an objective way to select mAs for paediatric brain CT. Br J Radiol 74:932–937

Yeoman LJ, Howarth L, Britten A et al (1992) Gantry angulation in brain CT: dosage implications, effect on posterior fossa artifacts, and current international practice. Radiology 184:113–116

Zacharia TT, Kanekar SG, Nguyen DT et al (2011) Optimization of patient dose and image quality with z-axis dose modulation for computed tomography (CT) in head trauma and stroke. Emerg Radiol 18:103–107

Zwirewich CV, Mayo JR, Müller NL (1991) Low-dose high resolution CT of lung parenchyma. Radiology 180:413–417

## Head and Neck CT

American Academy of Pediatrics (no authors listed) (2001) Subcommittee on management of sinusitis and Committee on quality improvement: clinical practice guideline: management of sinusitis. Pediatrics 108:798–808

Bulla S, Blanke P, Hassepass F et al (2011) Reducing the radiation dose for low-dose CT of the paranasal sinuses using iterative reconstruction: feasibility and image quality. Eur J Radiol, EPub June 8, 2011, doi 10.1016/e.ejrad.2011.05.002

Czechowski J, Janeczek J, Kelly G et al (2001) Radiation dose to the lens in sequential and spiral CT of facial bones and sinuses. Eur Radiol 11:711–713

Duvoisin B, Landry M, Chapuis et al (1991) Low-dose CT and inflammatory disease of the paranasal sinuses. Neuroradiology 33:403–406

Eggesbö HB (2006) Radiological imaging of inflammatory lesions in the nasal cavity and paranasal sinuses. Eur Radiol 16:872–888

George P, Huges J (1990) Respiratory system. In: Summitt (ed) Comprehensive pediatrics, Mosby

Glasier CM, Mallory GB, Steele RW (1989) Significance of opacification of the maxillary and ethmoid sinuses in infants. J Pediatr 114:45–50

Gordts F, Clement PA, Destryker A et al (1997) Prevalence of sinusitis signs on MRI in a non-ENT pediatric population. Rhinology 35:154–157

Greess H, Lutze J, Nomayr A et al (2004) Dose reduction in subsecond multislice spiral CT examination of children by online tube current modulation. Eur Raadiol 14:995–999

Hagtvedt T, Aalokken TM, Notthellen J et al (2003) A new low-dose CT examination compared with standard-dose CT in the diagnosis of acute sinusitis. Eur Radiol 13: 976–980

Hein E, Rogalla P, Klingebiel R et al (2002) Low-dose CT of the paranasal sinuses with eye lens protection: effect on image quality and radiation dose. Eur Radiol 12:1693–1696

Hodez C, Griffaton-Taillandier C, Bensimon I (2011) Cone-beam imaging: applications in ENT. Eur Ann Otorhinolaryngol Head Neck Dis 128:65–78

Kalra MK, Maher MM, Toth TL et al (2004b) Techniques and applications of automatic tube current modulation. Radiology 233:649–657

Kearny SE, Jones P, Meakin K et al (1997) CT scanning of the paranasal sinuses–the effect of reducing mAs. Br J Radiol 70:1071–1074

Kronemer KA, McAlister WH (1997) Sinusitis and its imaging in the pediatric population. Pediatr Radiol 27:837–846

Loubele M, Jacobs R, Maes F et al (2005) Radiation dose vs. image quality for low-dose CT protocols of the head for maxillofacial surgery and oral implant imaging. Radiat Prot Dosimetry 117:211–216

Loubele M, Bogaerts R, Van Dijck E et al (2009) Comparison between effective radiation dose of CBCT and MSCT scanners for dentomaxillofacial applications. Eur J Radiol 71:461–468

Marmolya G, Wiesen EJ, Yagan R et al (1991) Paranasal sinuses: low-dose CT. Radiology 181:689–691

McAlister WH, Lusk R, Muntz HR (1989) Comparison of plain radiographs and coronal CT scan in infants and children. Am J Roentgenol 153:1259–1264

McAlister WH, Parker BR, Kushner DC et al (2000) Sinusitis in the pediatric population. American College of Radiology. ACR Appropriateness Criteria, 1999. Radiology 215: 811–818

McCollough CH, Bruesewitz RT, Kofler JM (2006) CT dose reduction and dose management tools: overview of available options. Radiographics 26:503–512

Miracle AC, Mukerji SK (2008a) Conebeam CT of the head and neck, part 2: clinical applications. Am J Neuroradiol 30:1088–1095

Miracle AC, Mukerji SK (2008b) Conebeam CT of the head and neck, part 2: clinical applications. Am J Neuroradiol 30:1285–1292

Mulkens TH, Broers C, Fieuws S et al (2005a) Comparison of effective doses for low-dose MDCT and radiographic examination of sinuses in children. Am J Roentgenol 184:1611–1618

Mulkens TH, Bellinck P, Baeyaert M et al (2005b) Use of an automatic exposure control mechanism for dose optimization in multidetector-row CT examinations: clinical evaluation. Radiology 237:213–223

Nauer CB, Eichenberger A, Dupach B et al (2011) CT radiation dose for computer-assisted endoscopic sinus surgery: dose survey and determination of dose-reduction limits. Am J Neuroradiol 30:617–622

Pauwels R, Beinsberger J, Collaert B et al (2011) Effective dose range of cone beam computed tomography scanners. Eur J Radiol doi:10.1016/ejrad.2010.11.028

Rao VM, El-Noueam KI (1998) Sinonasal imaging. Anatomy and pathology. Radiol Clin North Am 36:921–939

Robb RA (1982) The dynamic spatial reconstructor: an X-ray video-fluoroscopic CT scanner for dynamic volume imaging of moving organs. IEEE Trans Med Imaging 1:22–33

Ruivo J, Mermuys K, Bacher K et al (2009) Cone beam computed tomography, a low-dose imaging technique in the postoperative assessment of cochlear implantation. Otol Neurotol 30:299–303

Rustemeyer P, Streubuhr U, Suttmoeller J (2004) Low-dose dental computed tomography: significant dose reduction without loss of image quality. Acta Radiol 45:847–853

Schell B, Bauer RW, Lehnert T et al (2011) Low-dose computed tomography of the paranasal sinus and facial skull using a high-pitch dual-source system–fist clinical results. Eur Radiol 21:107–112

Shrimpton PC, Jones DG, Hillier MC et al (1991) Survey of CT practice in the UK, NRPB-R249 report. National Radiological Protection Board (NRPB), Chilton, UK

Sohaib SA, Peppercorn PD, Horrocks JA et al (2001) The effect of decreasing mAs on image quality and patient dose in sinus CT. Br J Radiol 74:157–161

Suojanen JN, Regan F (1995) Spiral CT scanning of the paranasal sinuses. Am J Neuroradiol 16:787–789

Tack D, Widelec J, De Maertelaer V et al (2003) Comparison between low-dose and standard-dose multidetector CT in patients with suspected chronic sinusitis. Am J Roentgenol 181:939–944

Vandenberghe B, Jacobs R, Bosmans H (2010) Modern dental imaging: a review of the current technology and clinical applications in dental practice. Eur Radiol 20:2637–2655

Zinreich SJ, Benson ML, Oliveiro PJ (1996) Sinusonasal cavities: CT normal anatomy, imaging of the osteomeatal complex, and functional endoscopic sinus surgery. In: Harnsberger HR (ed) Head and neck imaging, 3rd edn. St.Louis, Mosby

# Dose Reduction and Optimization in Computed Tomography of the Chest

Pierre Alain Gevenois and Denis Tack

## Contents




**Abstract**

Even if the clinical benefit of multi-detector computed tomography (MDCT) of the chest is expected to be much higher than the potential risks from radiation, reduction and optimization of the radiation dose are highly recommended in accordance with the ALARA principle. As the chest is composed by organs and structures that are characterized by high differences in attenuation values with spontaneously high contrasts, it is well established that MDCT dose can be dramatically reduced. It has been indeed documented that in numerous clinical circumstances, radiation dose cannot be higher than 10 to 20% of the standard doses recommended by the scanner vendors (i.e. $CTDI_{vol}$ from 0.6 to 3 mGy, DLP from 30 to 120 mGy cm, E from 0.6 to 2.5 mSv as compared to 8–14 mSv). This is of particular concern in patients with long life expectancy and can be achieved by automatic exposure control in adjunction to either reduced tube current time product, reduced tube potential, or both. Newly developed dose reduction strategies, in particular iterative reconstructions will enable to obtain CT scans of high quality with a dose close of that delivered for plain film examinations.



P. A. Gevenois (✉)
Department of Radiology, Clinic of Chest Imaging, Hôpital Erasme, Université Libre de Bruxelles, Brussels, Belgium
e-mail: Pierre.Alain.Gevenois@erasme.ulb.ac.be

D. Tack
Department of Radiology, Clinique Louis Caty, RHMS, Rue Louis Caty 136, 7331 Baudour, Belgium


## 1 Introduction

Since the late 1980s, helical computed tomography (CT) revolutionized diagnostic imaging of the chest. Single-detector CT (SDCT) scanners and, more recently, multi-detector CT (MDCT) scanners markedly

D. Tack et al. (eds.), *Radiation Dose from Multidetector CT*, Medical Radiology. Diagnostic Imaging,
DOI: 10.1007/174_2011_419, © Springer-Verlag Berlin Heidelberg 2012

increased the number of indications of CT examinations. As a result, the number of examinations performed increased dramatically as well as the average scanned volume per patient, and the number of acquisitions per examination. The subsequent increase in collective radiation dose has been of concern for radiologists, medical physicists, and governmental regulatory authorities and it has been suggested that the radiation dose delivered by CT was excessive (Rogers 2001a, b).

The radiation dose received by patients undergoing diagnostic CT examinations is generally in the order of 1–24 mSv per examination for adults (Unscear 2000) and 2–6.5 mSv for children (Shrimpton et al. 2003). This effective dose level can be classified as low even though they are invariably greater than those from conventional radiography. Typically, a chest radiographic examination with two views delivers a dose ranging from 0.08 to 0.30 mSv. In contrast, a standard-dose MDCT delivers 4–10 mSv, i.e. a 100-fold risk of death by cancer. In other words, one death by cancer is expected every 250,000 chest X-rays and every 2,500 MDCT examination (Unscear 2000). Most importantly, more than one half of the collective radiation dose delivered for diagnostic imaging procedures is due to CT examinations (Golding and Shrimpton 2002). Consequently, as particular attention has to be paid to dose optimization and reduction, radiologists and medical physicists should be aware of their responsibility in the appropriate balance between image quality necessary for diagnostic purposes and radiation dose delivered to patients (Golding and Shrimpton 2002). In the rapidly evolving field of MDCT, the quest for the highest image quality supposed to lead to the highest diagnostic efficacy has obscured possible issues regarding the radiation dose. In this chapter we review the interactions between image quality, diagnostic performances, and radiation dose. We specifically focus on clinical advances in dose reduction in chest CT.

Although CT is an imaging technique that uses a relatively high radiation dose, it should be noted that it has replaced other techniques—such as pulmonary angiography and bronchography—that delivered even higher doses. Nevertheless, a further step in reducing the radiation dose is needed as CT has become the main source of the radiation delivered by medical diagnostic imaging procedures.

## 2 Unenhanced Chest CT

The concept of reducing the radiation dose in chest CT was first introduced in by Naidich et al. (1990) who reduced the tube current on incremental 10-mm collimation CT and demonstrated that with low tube current settings (i.e. 20 mAs), the image quality is sufficient for assessing the lung parenchyma. While the quality indeed is sufficient for assessing lung parenchyma, the increased noise resulted in marked degradation of the quality of images photographed with mediastinal window settings. Consequently, these authors recommended that such low-dose technique should be most suitable for children and for screening programs. As such, these recommendations have been implemented and further studied in lung cancer screening programs (Henschke et al. 1999; Itoh et al. 2000, Swensen et al. 2002; National Lung Screening Trial Team 2011).

Similar dose reduction strategies have been applied in thin-section CT. No difference in lung parenchyma structures was detectable between low-dose (i.e. 40 mAs) and high-dose (i.e. 400 mAs; Zwirewich et al. 1991; Lee et al. 1994). Although observed differences were not statistically significant, changes in ground-glass opacity were difficult to assess at low-dose CT because of the increased noise. Therefore, it was recommended that 200 mAs should be used for initial thin-section CT and lower doses (i.e. 40–100 mAs) for follow-up examinations. An example of a tree-in bud pattern demonstrated with a dose of 10 mGy ($CTDI_{vol}$) and 1 mGy is shown in Fig. 1.

The relationships between radiation exposure and image quality at mediastinal and pulmonary window settings have been evaluated on conventional 10-mm collimation CT images on a single model of CT scanner with mAs settings ranging from 20 to 400 mAs (Mayo et al. 1987). Although this study showed a consistent increase in image quality with radiation dose, no difference in detection of mediastinal and lung abnormalities could be detected. These findings were confirmed on MDCT by Dinkel et al. (2003) who showed that 90% reduction in dose compared with standard-dose techniques was not associated with impaired detection of suspicious lesions of malignant lymphoma and extrapulmonary tumors.

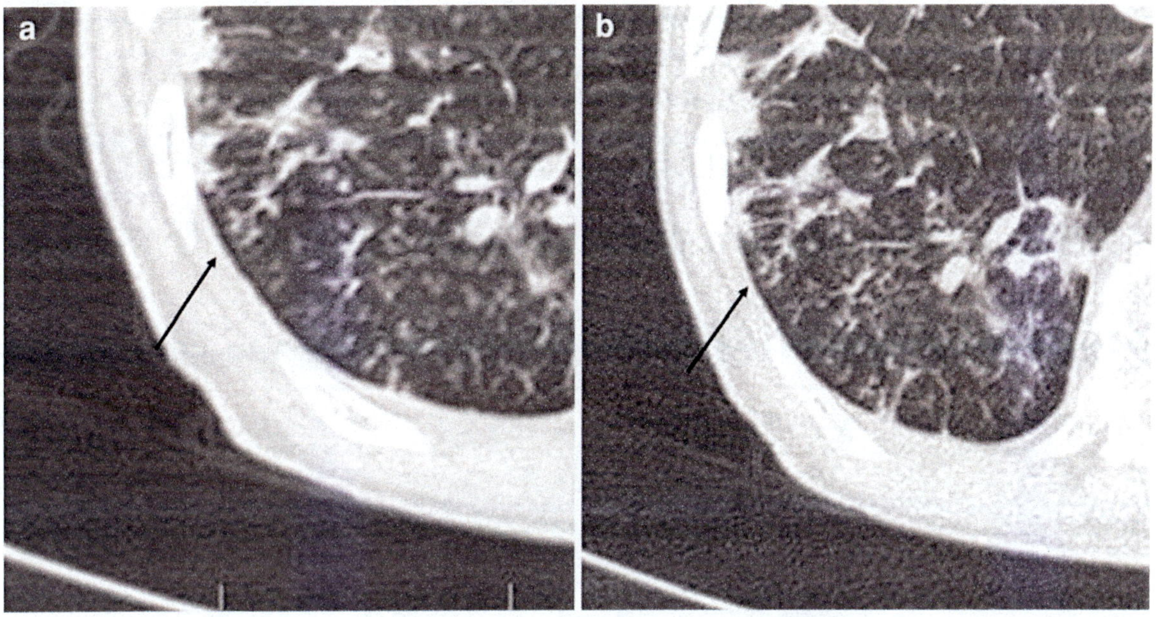


**Fig. 1** High-resolution MDCT performed with a $CTDI_{vol}$ at 10 mGy (**a**) and at 1 mGy (**b**) in a patient with a tuberculous bronchiolitis. A tree-in-bud pattern (*arrow*) is identified in the right lower lobe at both radiation doses

In order to investigate the effect of dose reduction without scanning patients several times at several dose levels, it is now possible to use computed simulated dose reduction by adding random noise to images obtained at standard dose. In a validation trial, it has been shown that experienced chest radiologists were unable to discriminate CT images generated with simulated reduced doses and those really obtained with reduced doses (Mayo et al. 1997). Simulated reduced doses allow investigators to determine the impact of dose reduction by means of tube current reductions on the diagnostic performance without exposing patients to additional radiation and/or injections of iodinated contrast material.

## 3 CT Pulmonary Angiography

The simulated low-dose technique has been used to evaluate the effect of dose reduction on CT pulmonary angiography (CTPA). A group of 21 individuals who showed at least one filling defect within a pulmonary artery were used to simulate CTPA with reduced radiation doses, at 60, 40, 20, and 10 mAs. This study showed that frequencies of positive and inconclusive results, branching order of the most distal artery with a detected filling defect were not changed when tube current–time product was reduced from 90 to 10 mAs. This is illustrated in Fig. 2a–e. On the other hand, the quality of intravascular contrast enhancement dramatically decreased when the tube current–time product setting was lower than 40 mAs. This study suggests thus that the reduction of the tube current–time product setting to 40 mAs to achieve a reduced radiation dose at CTPA appears acceptable (Tack et al. 2005).

Reducing tube potential is an alternative method to reduce the tube current–time product in order to optimize CTPA examinations. Sigal-Cinqualbre et al. (2004) have indeed assessed the feasibility of low-kilovoltage in CTPA protocols and have evaluated the effect of such protocols on image quality. These authors have reduced the tube potential but increased the tube current time product. They have shown that in patients weighting less than 75 kg, 80 kV (and 135 or 180 mAs respectively in patients weighting less than 60 or 75 kg) are sufficient to obtain the same image quality than in patients larger than 75 kg and scanned at 120 kV and 90 mAs. The tube potential of 100 kV was also compared to 140 kV and proved to be superior in terms of vascular enhancement and subjective image quality while reducing the dose by 70%, with $CTDI_{vol}$ values at 10.4 mGy at 140 kV and at 3.4 mGy at 100 kV (Schueller-Weidekamm

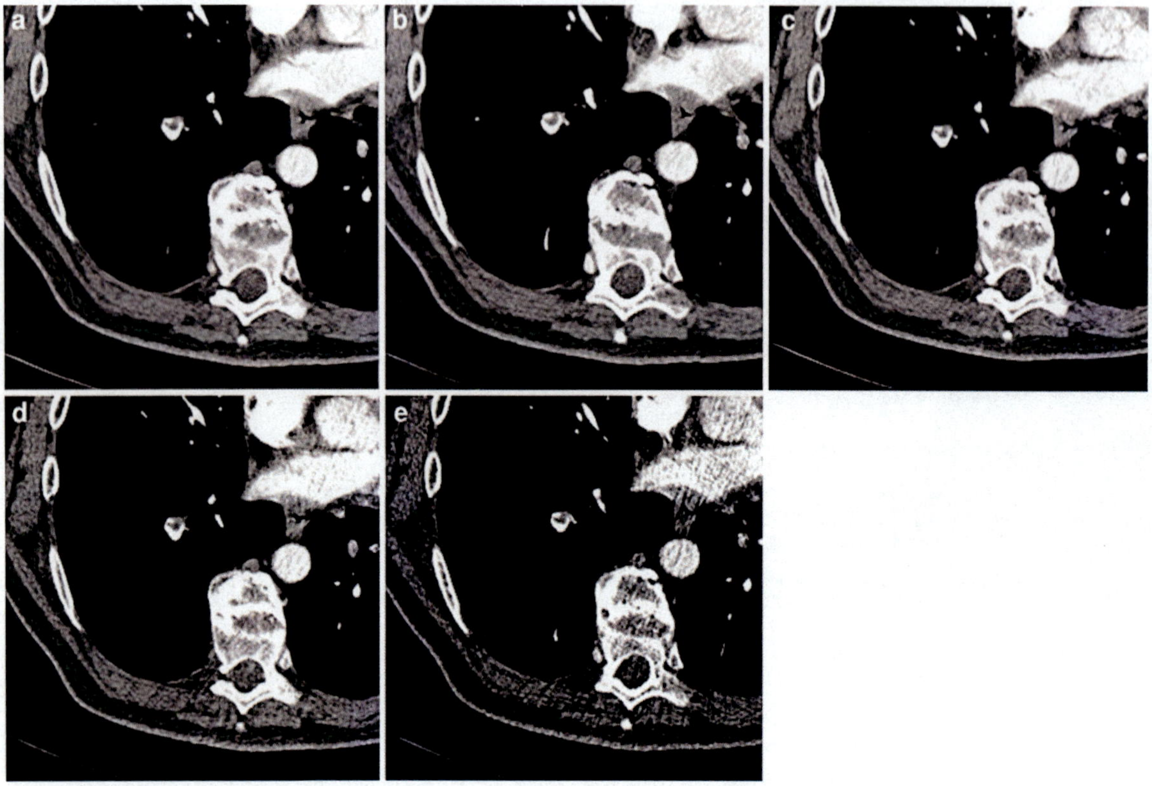


**Fig. 2** CT pulmonary angiography acquired with 120 kV and 90 effective mAs (**a**). Simulated low mAs scans at 60, 40, 20, and 10 effective mAs are shown, respectively, in (**b–e**). An intravascular filling defect corresponding to a pulmonary embolus in a right lower lobe segmental artery is identified. Images reproduced with permission of Denis Tack and the Radiological Society of North America (Tack et al. 2005)

et al. 2006). These results have been confirmed and applied to CTA of the circle of Willis and or of the Aorta (Waaijer et al. 2007; Schindera et al. 2009; Szucs-Farkas et al. 2009). Indeed, the absorption of iodine is much higher at low tube potential such as 80 or 100 kV as compared to 120 or 140 kV. This physical property of iodine that has a high atomic number has to be kept in mind for any vascular CT investigation. An example of a CTPA examination at 80 kV, delivering a DLP of 39 mGy cm corresponding to a sub-millisievert examination is shown in Fig. 11 of "Dose Optimization and Reduction in MDCT of the Abdomen". An acquisition at 100 kV in an obese patient is shown in Fig. 12 of "Dose Optimization and Reduction in MDCT of the Abdomen" illustrating that this low-kV technique can still be used in patients weighting up to 100 kg.

Software is now developed for computer-aided diagnosis (CAD) of pulmonary embolism on CTPA examinations. Such software is sensitive to noise, a higher noise being linked to a higher number of false positives. Owing to this, it is preferable to reduce CTPA radiation dose preferably by reducing the tube potential and not the tube current as the noise related to tube potential reduction is less apparent and can be partly compensated by an increase in tube current (Wittenberg et al. 2011).

## 4 Expiratory CT and Air Trapping

By demonstrating air trapping, expiratory thin-section CT is able to detect some pulmonary disease before the pulmonary functional tests (PFTs; Bankier et al. 2003). This makes this technique an essential part of the diagnosis of bronchiolitis of various origins. As expiratory CT scans are most often obtained after inspiratory CT, this additional acquisition exposes patients to additional radiation dose. This is of concern in patients with bronchiolitis because they can be

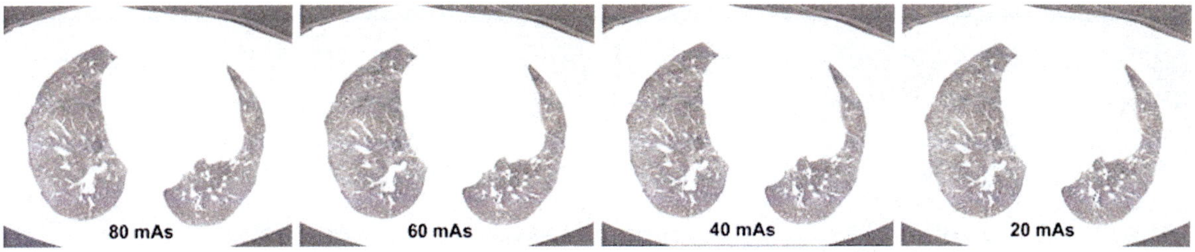


**Fig. 3** Expiratory MDCT 140 kV and 80 effective mAs. Simulated low mAs scans at 60, 40, and 20 effective mAs are shown. Areas of air trapping are equally detectable at each dose. Images are courtesy of Alexander A. Bankier, Boston, MA, USA

young, and despite their relatively favorable prognosis, have a high risk of recurrence resulting in repeated CT follow-up examinations. In order to investigate the possible effect of dose reduction on the visual quantification of air trapping, we considered the "bronchiolitis obliterans syndrome" (BOS) after lung transplantation as a model for bronchiolitis (Bankier et al. 2007). In this model, we applied simulated low-dose techniques on expiratory thin-section CT examinations in patients with possible BOS. In 27 lung transplant recipients, expiratory thin-section CT was performed at 140 kVp and 80 effective mAs. Dose reduction corresponding to 60, 40, and 20 effective mAs was simulated. This study showed that a simulated dose-equivalent to 25% of the standard dose, i.e. 20 mAs, had no substantial effect on the visual quantification of air trapping. An illustrative example is shown in Fig. 3. Because its radiation dose approximates that of incremental thin-section CT with 10 mm section intervals performed with a standard dose, expiratory low-dose MDCT could thus be used in the assessment of air trapping in patients with suspected bronchiolitis. This model could be extended to other origins of bronchiolitis obliterans.

## 5 CT Quantification of Pulmonary Emphysema

Pulmonary emphysema is a chronic obstructive pulmonary disease (COPD) defined as a permanent distal airway enlargement with alveolar wall destruction but without fibrosis (Snider et al. 1985). In the World, COPD is the sixth most common cause of mortality and the twelfth most common cause morbidity (Rennard et al. 2002). The severity of COPD can be, at least in part, assessed by PFTs. These tests are widely available but are not specific. As CT yields densitometric measurements that are highly reproducible and correlated with morphometric measurements of alveolar wall destruction, it can be complementary to PFT in order to assess the extent/severity of pulmonary emphysema. As a result, this technique has been recommended in follow-up studies, particularly in the evaluation of therapeutic interventions (Bae et al. 1997; Gierada et al. 2001; Newell et al. 2004; Dirksen et al. 1999). The recently introduced MDCT is of interest in the quantification of pulmonary emphysema—a heterogeneously distributed disorder—because MDCT is able to image the entire lung parenchyma. On the other hand, as this technique increases the radiation dose by an additional 300% per examination compared to incremental single-detector row CT (Studler et al. 2005), it would be important to reduce the radiation dose as patients with pulmonary emphysema can be young and have a favorable prognosis. The level of radiation that these patients are exposed to with these examinations is compounded with repeated follow-up examinations.

As specific drugs are, respectively, able to stop lung parenchyma destruction or even to restore the lung growth have been elaborated and tested in animal models (Massaro and Massaro 1997), it is of importance that individuals included in clinical trials could be imaged with the lowest possible radiation dose that provides valid measurements. We have investigated the effect of radiation dose on quantitative indexes of MDCT in pulmonary emphysema (Madani et al. 2007). In 70 patients referred for surgical resection of a lung tumor who underwent unenhanced MDCT with 4 × 1mm collimation, 120 kVp, and 20 and 120 effective mAs, we compared relative areas (RA) of lung with attenuation coefficients lower than nine thresholds, and eight percentiles of the distribution of attenuation coefficients with the pathological extent of emphysema measured macroscopically and microscopically. We observed that radiation dose does not substantially

**Table 1** Dose descriptors for standard dose, optimized-dose and low-dose MDCT of the chest

| Technique | Year/quality | Reconstruction technique | Origine references | $CTDI_{vol}$ (mGy) | DLP (mGy cm) |
|---|---|---|---|---|---|
| Helical | Eur 1999 | FBP | Europe DRL (P75) | 35 | 680 |
| Helical | 2010/SD | FBP | Switzerland P75 | 13 | 450 |
| Helical | 2010/SD | FBP | Belgium DRL P75 | NA | 400 |
| Helical | 2010/OD | FBP | Switzerland P25 | 5 | 250 |
| Helical | 2010/OD | FBP | Belgium P25 | 5 | 240 |
| Helical | 2010/OD | FBP | NLST | 3–5 | 120–180 |
| Helical | 2011/OD | FBP | Singh et al. | 3.5 | 120 |
| Helical | 2007/LD | FBP | Bankier et al. | 2 | 70 |
| Helical | 2011/LD | Iterative | Figure 4 | 0.93 | 34 |
| CTPA | 2011/OD | FBP | Pontana et al. | WA | 162 |
| CTPA | 2011/OD | Iterative | Pontana et al. | WA | 104 |
| Helical | 2011/OD | FBP | Bendaoud et al. | WA | 78 |
| Sequential/ children | 2010/LD | FBP | O'Connor et al. | NA | 8–12 |
| Sequential | 2011/OD | FBP | Bendaoud et al. | WA | 16 |

*FBP* reconstruction with filtered back projection algorithms
*WA* weight adapted protocols differing in terms of kV and mAs applied
*SD* standard dose—non-optimized technique—perfect image quality
*OD* optimized dose—result of ALARA process—slightly higher noise as compared to standard dose, but with good to excellent image quality
*LD* low-dose—including higher noise level, but with preserved diagnosis
*DRL* diagnostic reference level corresponding to the 75th percentile of observed dose in surveys
*P25* 25th percentile as observed in a survey study. Considered as reflecting OD at national level

influence the strength of the correlation between RA's (or percentiles) and pathologic references. This suggests that reducing the dose to 20 effective mAs is safe and should be recommended in CT quantification of pulmonary emphysema, especially in patients who face repeated follow-up examinations. Nevertheless, comparisons between examinations, such as in follow-up studies, require that the dose should be kept constant.

## 6 Optimized MDCT Acquisitions Using Automatic Exposure Control

Automatic modulation of the tube current as a function of the patient's absorption is available on modern CT scanners. Differences still exist between vendors regarding the methods used for this modulation, and the dose reductions subsequently achieved. Detailed description, limitations, and results of the different automatic exposure control devices are presented and discussed by Kalra in "Automatic Exposure Control in Multidetector-Row Computed Tomography". The most important feature of these devices is that the radiation dose is adapted to the patient's weight and absorption. Consequently, the role of the CT user is now restricted to select an image quality appropriate to the clinical indication of the CT examination. A reasonable approach for selecting this image quality is presented by Tack in "ALARA Concept for MDCT Optimization: What is Reasonable, what is Achievable?".

## 7 Volumetric Versus Sequential Acquisition For Follow-Up Examinations

The optimized dose of a cohort of COPD patients was reported by Bendaoud et al. (2011) to be as low as 77.7 mGy cm in a series of 63 consecutive patients. For follow-up examinations, this DLP was reduced to 16.1 mGy cm by obtaining sequential 1/10 mm slices instead of helical acquisitions but without loss of

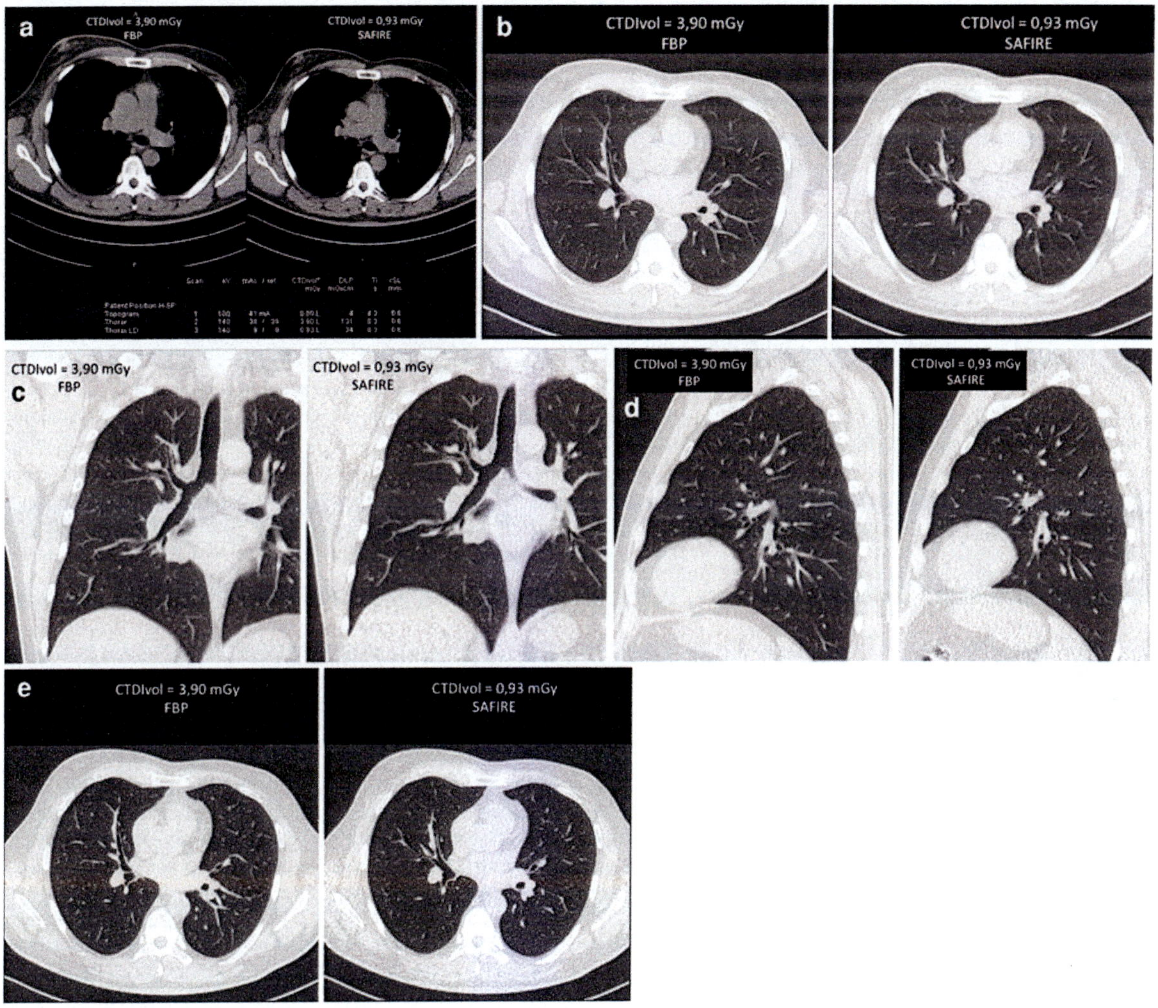


**Fig. 4** Comparison of an optimized-dose (OD) and a low-dose (LD) unenhanced MDCT acquisition in the same patient weighting 70 kg. The $CTDI_{vol}$ of the OD and LD are 3.90 and 0.93 mGy, respectively and the DLP are respectively of 131 and 34 mGy cm, respectively . The LD was reconstructed with the iterative technique (Safire I30 for the mediastinum in **a**, and Safire I50 for the lungs in **b**–**e**). **a**–**d** are in 3 mm thickness whereas (**e**) shows images with 1 mm thickness

diagnostic information. The sequential technique is thus a valuable alternative to helical CT and could be used in patients with cystic fibrosis as in this series.

## 8 Recommendations and Proposals

Recommendations from regulatory authorities such as the European Union are based on a balance between the theoretical radiation risk and the medical benefit expected from CT examinations. In addition, reference values for the upper limits of dose are only based on surveys studies. These values are listed in Table 1. The reference diagnostic level values approximate 14 mGy for the $CTDI_{vol}$ and range between 450 and 650 mGy cm for the dose-length product. Lowering these dose values is mandatory and depending on the patient's weight $CTDI_{vol}$ may be lowered down to 2 mGy. Using modern MDCT scanners, automatic exposure control devices, and reconstructing images with iterative techniques, it is now possible to produce CT images of very high quality with $CTDI_{vol} < 1$–4 mGy and DLP < 40 mGy cm for the entire chest (Singh et al., 2011; Pontana et al. 2011a, b). Examples are given in the image gallery proposed online at the end of this book and in Fig. 4. The corresponding effective dose is lower than 0.8 mGy, very close to that of a plain film examination. Furthermore, low-dose CT images (as for lung cancer screening) can be obtained with doses five to ten times lower than those considered as references (see "Lung Cancer Screening with CT" by Schaeffer).

## 9 Conclusion

Even if the clinical benefit of chest MDCT is expected to be higher than the risks from radiation, reduction and optimization of the radiation dose are recommended in accordance with the ALARA principle. As the chest is composed by organs and structures that are characterized by high differences in attenuation values with a subsequent spontaneously high contrasts, it is expected that radiation dose could be dramatically reduced. It has been indeed documented that in numerous clinical circumstances, dose cannot be higher than 10 to 20% of the standard doses recommended by scanner vendors (i.e., $CTDI_{vol}$ from 0.6 to 3 mGy, DLP from 30 to 120 mGy cm, E from 0.6 to 2.5 mSv as compared to 8–14 mSv). This is of particular concern in patients with long life expectancy and can be achieved by automatic exposure control in adjunction to either reduced tube current time product, reduced tube potential, or both. Newly developed dose reduction strategies, in particular iterative reconstructions, enable to obtain CT scans of high quality with a dose close to that delivered for plain film examinations.

## References


Bae KT, Slone RM, Gierada DS, Yusen RD, Cooper JD (1997) Patients with emphysema: quantitative CT analysis before and after lung volume reduction surgery. Radiology 203:705–714

Bankier AA, Van Muylem A, Scillia P, De Maertelaer V, Estenne M, Gevenois PA (2003) Air trapping in heart–lung transplant recipients: variability of anatomic distribution and extent at sequential expiratory thin-section CT. Radiology 229:737–742

Bankier AA, Schaefer-Prokop C, De Maertelaer V, Tack D, Jaksch P, Klepetko W, Gevenois PA (2007) Air trapping on thin-section CT examinations: comparison of standard-dose and simulated low-dose techniques. Radiology 242: 898–906

Bendaoud S, Remy-Jardin M, Wallaert B et al (2011) Sequential versus volumetric computed tomography in the follow-up of chronic bronchopulmonary diseases: comparison of diagnostic information and radiation dose in 63 adults. J Thorac Imaging 26:190–195

Dinkel HP, Sonnenschein M, Hoppe H, Vock P (2003) Low-dose multislice CT of the thorax in follow-up of malignant lymphoma and extrapulmonary primary tumors. Eur Radiol 13:1241–1249

Dirksen A, Dijkman JH, Madsen F et al (1999) A randomized clinical trial of α1-antitrypsin augmented therapy. Am J Respir Crit Care Med 160:1468–1472

Eur (1999) European guidelines on quality criteria for computed tomography—EUR 16262 EN access on line at http://www.drs.dk/guidelines/ct/quality/htmlindex.htm

Gierada DS, Yusen RD, Pilgram TK et al (2001) Repeatability of quantitative CT indexes of emphysema in patients evaluated for lung volume reduction surgery. Radiology 220:448–454

Golding SJ, Shrimpton PC (2002) Radiation dose in CT: are we meeting the challenge? (commentary). Br J Radiol 75:1–4

Henschke CI, McCauley DI, Yankelevitz DF et al (1999) Early lung cancer action project: overall design and findings from baseline screening. Lancet 354:99–105

Itoh H, Ikeda M, Arahata S et al (2000) Lung cancer screening: minimum tube current required for helical CT. Radiology 215:175–183

Lee KS, Primack SL, Staples CA, Mayo JR, Aldrich JE, Müller NL (1994) Chronic infiltrative lung disease: comparison of diagnostic accuracies of radiography and low- and conventional-dose thin-section CT. Radiology 191:669–673

Madani A, De Maertelaer V, Zanen J, Gevenois PA (2007) Pulmonary emphysema: radiation dose and section thickness at multidetector CT quantification—comparison with macroscopic and microscopic morphometry. Radiology 243:250–257

Massaro GD, Massaro D (1997) Retinoic acid treatment abrogates elastase-induced pulmonary emphysema in rats. Nat Med 3:675–677 (Erratum in: Nat Med 3(7):805, July 1997)

Mayo JR, Webb WR, Gould R et al (1987) High-resolution CT of the lungs: an optimal approach. Radiology 163:507–510

Mayo JR, Whittall KP, Leung AN et al (1997) Simulated dose reduction in conventional chest CT: validation study. Radiology 202:453–457

Naidich DP, Marshall CH, Gribbin C, Arams RS, McCauley DI (1990) Low-dose CT of the lungs: preliminary observations. Radiology 175:729–731

National Lung Screening Trial Team (2011) The national lung screening trial: overview and study design. Radiology 258:243–253

Newell JD, Hogg JC, Snider GL (2004) Report of a workshop: quantitative computed tomography scanning in longitudinal studies of emphysema. Eur Respir J 23:769–775

O'Connor OJ, Vandeleur M, McGarrigle AM, Moore N, McWilliams SR, McSweeney SE, O'Neill M, Ni Chroinin M, Maher MM (2010) Development of low-dose protocols for thin-section CT assessment of cystic fibrosis in pediatric patients. Radiology 257:820–829

Pontana F, Pagniez J, Flohr T et al (2011a) Chest computed tomography using iterative reconstruction versus filtered back projection (part 1): evaluation of image noise reduction in 32 patients. Eur Radiol 21:627–635

Pontana F, Duhamel A, Pagniez J et al (2011b) Chest computed tomography using iterative reconstruction versus filtered back projection (part 2): image quality of low-dose CT examinations in 80 patients. Eur Radiol 21:636–643

Rennard S, Decramer M, Calverley PM, Pride NB, Soriano JB, Vermeire PA, Vestbo J (2002) Impact of COPD in North America and Europe in 2000: subjects' perspective of confronting COPD international survey. Eur Respir J 20:799–805

Rogers L (2001a) Radiation exposure in CT: why so high? Am J Roentgenol 177:277

Rogers LF (2001b) Serious business: radiation safety and radiation protection. Am J Roentgenol 177:1

Schindera ST, Graca P, Patak MA, Abderhalden S, von Allmen G, Vock P, Szucs-Farkas Z (2009) Thoracoabdominal-aortoiliac multidetector-row CT angiography at 80 and 100 kVp: assessment of image quality and radiation dose. Invest Radiol 44:650–655

Schueller-Weidekamm C, Schaefer-Prokop CM, Weber M et al (2006) CT angiography of pulmonary arteries to detect pulmonary embolism: improvement of vascular enhancement with low kilovoltage settings. Radiology 241:899–907

Shrimpton PC, Hillier MC, Lewis MA et al (2003) Data from computed tomography (CT) examinations in the UK—2003 review. NRPB-W67, National Radiological Protection Board, Chilton

Sigal-Cinqualbre AB, Hennequin R, Abada HT, Chen X, Paul JF (2004) Low-kilovoltage multidetector row chest CT in adults: feasability and effect on image quality and iodine dose. Radiology 231:169–174

Singh S, Kalra MK, Gilman MD et al (2011) Adaptive statistical iterative reconstruction technique for radiation dose reduction in chest CT: a pilot study. Radiology 259:565–573

Snider GL, Kleinerman JL, Thurlbeck WM et al (1985) The definition of emphysema: report of a National Heart, Lung, and Blood Institute, Division of Lung Disease workshop. Am Rev Respir Dis 132:182–185

Studler U, Gluecker T, Bongartz G, Roth J, Steinbrich W (2005) Image quality from high-resolution CT of the lung: comparison of axial scans and of sections reconstructed from volumetric data acquired using MDCT. Am J Roentgenol 185:602–607

Swensen SJ, Jett JR, Sloan JA et al (2002) Screening for lung cancer with low-dose spiral computed tomography. Am J Respir Crit Care Med 165:508–513

Szucs-Farkas Z, Schaller C, Bensler S, Patak MA, Vock P, Schindera ST (2009) Detection of pulmonary emboli with CT angiography at reduced radiation exposure and contrast material volume: comparison of 80 and 120 kVp protocols in a matched cohort. Invest Radiol 44:793–799

Tack D, De Maertelaer V, Petit W, Scillia P, Muller P, Suess C, Gevenois PA (2005) Comparisons of standard-dose and simulated low-dose multi-detector-row CT pulmonary angiography. Radiology 236:318–325

Unscear (2000) Sources and effects of ionizing radiation. United Nations scientific committee on the effects of atomic radiation report to the General Assembly. United Nations, New York

Waaijer A, Prokop M, Velthuis BK, Bakker CJ, de Kort GA, van Leeuwen MS (2007) Circle of Willis at CT angiography: dose reduction and image quality–reducing tube voltage and increasing tube current settings. Radiology 242:829–832

Wittenberg R, Peters JF, Sonnemans JJ et al (2011) Impact of image quality on the performance of computer-aided detection of pulmonary embolism. Am J Roentgenol 196:95–101

Zwirewich CV, Mayo JR, Müller NL (1991) Low-dose high-resolution CT of lung parenchyma. Radiology 180:413–417

# Dose Optimization and Reduction in MDCT of the Abdomen

Caroline Keyzer and Denis Tack

## Contents




## Abstract

Computed Tomography (CT) is increasingly used in abdominal imaging with a subsequent increase in the collective radiation dose. This is of particular concern, especially in young patients and in those with chronic diseases who undergo repeated CT studies including treatable cancers. In this chapter, we will first expose the reference radiation levels of abdominal CT and define what can be considered as a low-dose or an optimized dose CT. Second, we will explain the strategies and the technological advances that have been developed to reduce the dose in abdominal CT in conditions characterized by intrinsic high contrast between structures such as ureteral stone, and later in conditions characterized by intrinsic low contrast between structures such as acute appendicitis or acute diverticulitis. Finally, we will provide recommendations for optimizing and reducing the radiation dose in abdominal CT.


## Abbreviations

| | |
|---|---|
| ALARA | As low as reasonably achievable |
| ASIR | Adaptative statistical iterative reconstruction |
| AEC | Automatic exposure control |
| BMI | Body mass index |
| CNR | Contrast-to noise ratio |
| CTA | CT angiography |
| CTDI | Computed tomography dose index |
| CTDIvol | CTDI volume |
| CTDIw | Weighted CTDI |
| DLP | Dose length product |


C. Keyzer (✉)
Department of Radiology, Hôpital Erasme,
Université libre de Bruxelles, Route de Lennik 808,
1070 Brussels, Belgium
e-mail: caroline.keyzer@erasme.ulb.ac.be

D. Tack
Department of Radiology, Clinique Louis Caty,
Hôpital RHMS, Rue Louis Caty 136,
7331 Baudour, Belgium


D. Tack et al. (eds.), *Radiation Dose from Multidetector CT*, Medical Radiology. Diagnostic Imaging,
DOI: 10.1007/174_2011_420, © Springer-Verlag Berlin Heidelberg 2012

| | |
|---|---|
| EU | European union |
| FBP | Filtered back projection |
| IRIS | Iterative reconstruction in image space |
| IVU | Intravenous urography |
| MDCT | Multi-detector row CT |
| MPR | MultiPlanar reconstructions |
| NI | Noise index |
| NRPB | National radiological protection board |
| PICCS | Prior image constrained compressed sensing |
| ROI | Region of interest |
| SD | Standard deviation |
| SDCT | Single-detector row CT |
| SNR | Signal-to-noise ratio |

## 1 Introduction

Since its introduction in the late 1980s, CT has revolutionized imaging of the abdomen. Single-detector row CT (SDCT) and, more recently, multi-detector row CT (MDCT) have substantially increased the number of indications of CT. As a result, the number of performed CT examinations has dramatically increased as well as the average scanned range per patient. The subsequent increase in the collective radiation dose has been of concern for radiologists, medical physicists, as well as for governmental regulatory authorities, and it has been claimed that the radiation dose delivered by CT is excessive (Berrington de Gonzalez et al. 2009; Little et al. 2009; Rogers 2003, 2001).

CT is nowadays widely used in abdominal imaging in various circumstances including acute abdominal pain. This use is explained by its high reproducibility, rapidity, sensitivity, specificity, easiness to perform and little discomfort for the patient (Birnbaum and Wilson 2000; Wise et al. 2001). With MDCT scanners, rapid volume acquisition are now possible and examination of the entire abdomen including pelvis is more and more frequently performed as a screening test in patients suspected of abdominal diseases.

Nevertheless, since the abdomen contains sensitive organs, the radiation dose delivered to patients is of particular concern, especially in young patients and in those with chronic diseases who undergo repeated CT studies including treatable cancers. Strategies to reduce this dose have been developed and clinical investigations have shown that in several abdominal disorders the performance of CT is not decreased by dose reduction. Reducing the dose was has first been investigated in conditions characterized by intrinsic high contrast between structures such as ureteral stone, and later in conditions characterized by intrinsic low contrast between structures such as acute appendicitis or acute diverticulitis. Radiation was first of particular concern in young patients but there is currently also increasing concern about radiation dose optimization in patients who undergo abdomino-pelvic MDCT for the staging and follow-up of cancer (O'Malley et al. 2010; la Fougère et al. 2008; Rodriguez-Vigil et al. 2006; Yamamura et al. 2010).

## 2 Radiation Dose Reference Levels and Definition of Terms Qualifying Dose in Abdominal MDCT

Ideally, the dose delivered to the patient should be at the level below which the image quality would be insufficient to yield an accurate diagnosis and a preserved reader confidence. Practically, the delivered dose should be adapted first to the patient and second to the indication. As evidence-based recommendations based on such an approach do not exist, guidelines have been derived from survey studies reporting the large-scale distribution of the delivered dose. The arbitrary fixed recommended dose threshold corresponds to the third quartile of the distribution observed in these surveys (Shrimpton et al. 2005, 2006), doses higher than the upper third quartile being considered as of unacceptable practice (European Commission 1999). Detailed results of these survey studies are reported and discussed in chapter "Collective Radiation Dose from MDCT: Critical Review of Surveys Studies" by G Stamm.

In 1999, the guidelines established by the Commission of the European Union (EU) have proposed that reference levels for routine abdominal CT examination (from the top of the liver to the aortic bifurcation) should be, respectively for the weighted CT dose index (CTDIw) and dose-length product (DLP), 35 mGy and 780 mGy cm (Dose descriptors are further explained by S Edyvean in chapter "Scanning Parameters Affecting Radiation Dose in CT"). For CT examinations of the liver and the spleen, the corresponding values were 35 mGy and 900 mGy cm. For the pelvis, they were 35 mGy and 570 mGy cm (European Commission 1999). Later on, the National Radiological Protection Board (NRPB) has reported a snapshot of doses delivered in United Kingdom in 2003 (Shrimpton et al. 2005, 2006). In this report, the third quartile value of dose distribution, expressed in DLP, was 559 mGy cm for routine abdominal CT examination obtained with MDCT. The corresponding value for liver examination in patients with possible metastases was 472 mGy cm. These doses are clearly lower than those proposed in 1999 by the Commission of the European Union. This lowering probably reflects the increasing concern in reducing the dose as observed for these last years as well as technological advances in CT technology.

The indication of each examination is important to consider in order to select the required image quality and subsequently the lowest acceptable radiation dose. As an example, the dose delivered for searching metastases or for imaging trauma can be higher than those for imaging acute abdominal pain in non cancer patients.

Furthermore, with MDCT scanners, the ability to rapidly scan large volumes tempts the operator to increase this volume along the Z-axis, and/or to use multiple passes CT instead of single-pass CT. Therefore Z-coverage should be adapted to the clinical indication and to the possible alternative diagnoses. Unjustified screening the entire abdomen because of a "you never know" policy should thus be banished. Such policy is not justified and to be considered as unacceptable in young patients who are at low-risk to have an incidental associated disease. Similarly, repeated acquisitions should not be performed in circumstances where they do not specifically yield additional relevant information.

With the increasing concern in radiation dose, some adjectives are increasingly used to qualify the dose. Terms qualifying radiation dose are not strictly defined. As an example, the dose of a so-called "low-dose" protocol in one institution could correspond to the one of a standard dose in another institution. A confusion of this order can be notably seen in studies investigating the effect of denoising software such as adaptative statistical iterative reconstruction technique (ASIR). The "low-dose" achieved in some of these studies is as high or even higher than that delivered in other studies investigating optimized acquisitions reconstructed with filtered back projection (FBP) technique (see below) (Marin et al. 2009, 2010a, b; Prakash et al. 2010; Allen et al. 2010).

## 2.1 Standard Dose

The term "standard dose" refers to the dose usually recommended by CT manufacturers and often used in routine practice but that could be substantially reduced—to an optimized dose level—without deleterious effect on image quality (and certainly not on diagnostic accuracy). Typically, CTDIvol proposed by manufacturers in Europe range between 11 and 23 mGy in a standard-sized patient. At standard dose, noise in images [Standard Deviation (SD) of attenuation in a region of interest in a homogeneous area, i.e.: aorta] is usually at 12 $\pm$ 3 HU. Standard dose may be considered as an acceptable technique in the work-up of most cancer and in elderly patients. DLP for a standard abdomino-pelvic CT in a standard sized patient should be lower than 800 mGy.cm as detailed by D Tack in "ALARA concept for MDCT Optimization: what is reasonable, what is achievable?".

## 2.2 Optimized Dose

The term "optimized dose" should refer to a dose that provides adequate image quality but not with excessive radiation, and is the practical application of As Low as Reasonably Achievable (ALARA) principle. At optimized dose, noise in images ranges usually from 13 to 22 HU, depending on the image thickness, typically 15 HU in a 3 mm thick slice. Optimized dose is an acceptable technique in young adults (including those with treatable cancer such as lymphoma) and in non-oncology patients. DLP for an abdominal CT in an adult standard sized patient with abdominal pain at optimized dose conditions should range between 200 and 400 mGy cm. Optimization process is per definition a process that eliminates the excess of radiation that does not provide significant increase in image quality. Optimized dose level for a given examination and on a given CT unit is not a priori known, depends on the local radiologist and their PACS equipment, and has to be found out by the local user who is responsible for this process (Golding 2010).

### 2.3 Low-Dose

The term "low-dose" should be restricted to a CT delivered dose not higher than that delivered by a set of plain films investigating the considered condition. At low-dose, image quality is lower but diagnostic accuracy is preserved. At low-dose, noise in images ranges usually from 18 to 30 HU in 3 mm slices [that can be reduced with thick Multiplanar Reconstructions (MPR)]. Low-dose should be the preferred method for scanning young patients and patients with potentially recurring abdominal pain. DLP for an abdominal CT in a young standard sized patient with abdominal pain at low-dose conditions should be around 100 mGy cm and lower than 200 mGy cm. Using a conversion factor of 0.015 mSv/mGy cm (Deak et al. 2010), the corresponding effective dose would be equal or lower than 3 mSv, a limit admitted as that of low-dose abdominal CT.

## 3 Dose Reduction in Abdominal MDCT

### 3.1 High Intrinsic Contrast Between Structures

Radiation dose reduction in abdominal MDCT has been first investigated in diseases and conditions characterized by high intrinsic contrast between structures as in ureteral stones and virtual colonography respectively (Hamm et al. 2002; Tack et al. 2003; van Gelder et al. 2002, 2004). Unenhanced CT has been indeed validated for the diagnosis of ureteral stone, avoiding intravenous administration of iodine contrast material and able to provide information for establishing alternative and/or additional diagnoses (Hamm et al. 2001; Katz et al. 2000; Liu et al. 2000; Smith et al. 1995; Sourtzis et al. 1999). On the other hand, standard dose CT scanning exposes the patient to radiation doses higher than that delivered by intravenous urography (IVU), and patients with ureteral stone may be young, will have repeated control examinations, and are at risk of recurrence.

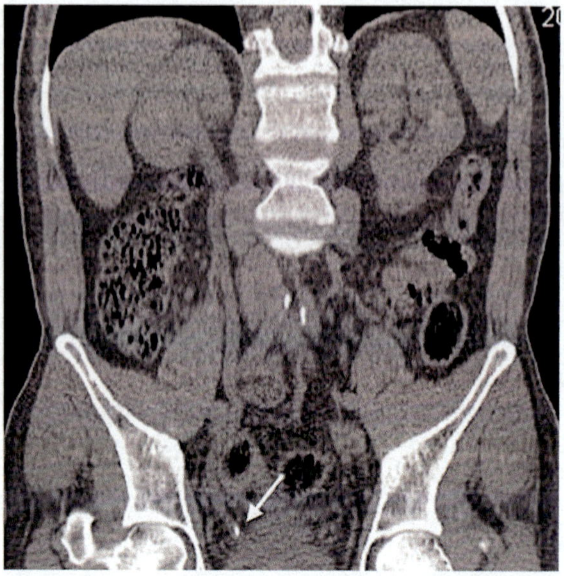

**Fig. 1** Stone in the *right* distal ureter (*arrow*). Three millimeter curved MPR image from a low-dose acquisition performed at 30 effective mAs (4 × 2.5 mm, 120 kVp), without AEC, in a normal weighed patient

Dose reduction can be achieved by increasing the pitch and/or by increasing the X-ray beam width. Even if this modulation provides thicker transverse sections than with standard parameters, the number of ureteral stones missed by using such sections was not substantially higher than that detected by IVU, and ureteral stones smaller than 5 mm in diameter are detected at CT but not at IVU (Liu et al. 2000). However, dose reduction by increasing the pitch was possible on SDCT and MDCT scanners constructed by GE and Toshiba, but not on MDCT scanners by Philips and Siemens. These two manufacturers have introduced the concept of "effective mAs"; the scanner automatically increases the tube current proportionally to the table speed, i.e. the tube current is doubled if the table speed or the pitch doubles. With these scanners, the dose and the slice profile are thus independent from the pitch.

Since MDCT has been equipped with solid state detectors, it has been possible to reduce the tube current as compared to SDCT. Using a MDCT scanner and acquisitions performed with a beam collimation of 4 × 2.5 mm, 120 kVp, and 30 effective mAs, Tack et al. (2003) have reported accuracy higher than 93% and excellent intra- and inter-observer agreements in the detection of ureteral stone. Figures 1, 2, 3 illustrate ureteral stones detected at 30 effective mAs. The mean

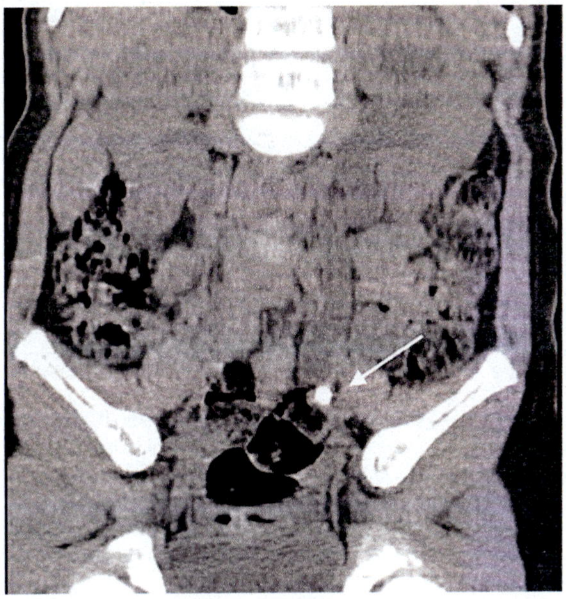

**Fig. 2** Stone in the *left* distal ureter (*arrow*). Three millimeter curved MPR image from a low-dose acquisition performed at 30 effective mAs (4 × 2.5 mm, 120 kVp), without AEC, in a normal weighed patient

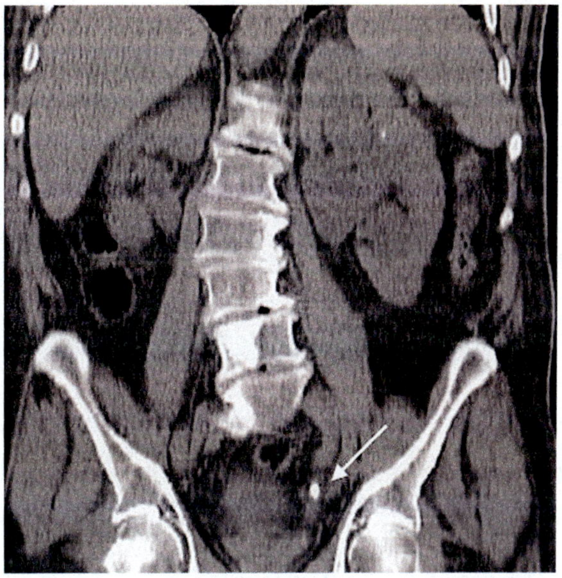

**Fig. 3** Stone in the *left* distal ureter (*arrow*). Five millimeter coronal MPR image (thick MPR) from a low-dose acquisition performed at 30 effective mAs (4 × 2.5 mm, 120 kVp), without AEC, in an obese patient with a BMI of 39.7 kg/m$^2$

effective dose delivered by these authors—1.2 mSv in men, and 1.9 mSv in women—was approximately the same as that delivered by a three-film IVU (approximately 1.5 mSv). However, in this study performed without Automatic Exposure Control (AEC) device, additional images obtained with 60 mAs were required to complement those at 30 mAs. This requirement could be explained by greater image noise in the pelvis than in the abdomen at the same tube current due to the pelvic bones. In such circumstances, the AEC technique, unlike the fixed tube current technique, offers the opportunity to select the desired image quality in order to automatically reduce and increase the tube current following the patient's size ("light" vs. "heavy" patients) and body attenuation (abdomen vs. pelvis).

AEC devices modulate the tube current as a function of the table position along the Z-axis and of the image quality requested by the operator. Such devices reduce the tube current in thin patients and increase it in obese and overweight patients, tending to maintain constant the image quality (Mulkens et al. 2005). Therefore, radiologists using these devices should think in terms of image quality and not of tube current. These devices are extensively described in "Automatic Exposure Control in Multidetector-row Computed Tomography".

Kalra et al. (2005) showed that AEC along the z-axis can be used in patients suspected of urinary stone with 43–66% dose reduction with no compromising stone detectability. Using AEC, the dose delivered to the patient will depend on his body habitus, and as a consequence, the dose will be reduced in thin patients but conversely it will be increased in large and obese patients (Mulkens et al. 2005). AEC systems are the only able to automatically adapt the mA (and the dose) to the patient's absorption. Thus, in abdominal MDCT, these systems should always be activated.

Finally, ultra-low-dose MDCT—120 kVp, 6.9 effective mAs—delivering an effective radiation dose equivalent to one conventional abdominal X-ray view (approximately 0.5 mSv) has been showed to achieve sensitivity and specificity of respectively 97 and 95% for the diagnosis of ureteral stone (Kluner et al. 2006). Furthermore, it has been extensively demonstrated that low-dose unenhanced CT can also provide alternative diagnoses (Tack et al. 2003; Kluner et al. 2006; Dicl et al. 2000; Keyzer et al. 2004). This will be discussed in the following paragraphs.

The effect of dose reduction achieved by decreasing tube voltage is more complex because it affects both image noise by a reduction of photon fluence and contrast by a reduction of the energy of the X-ray

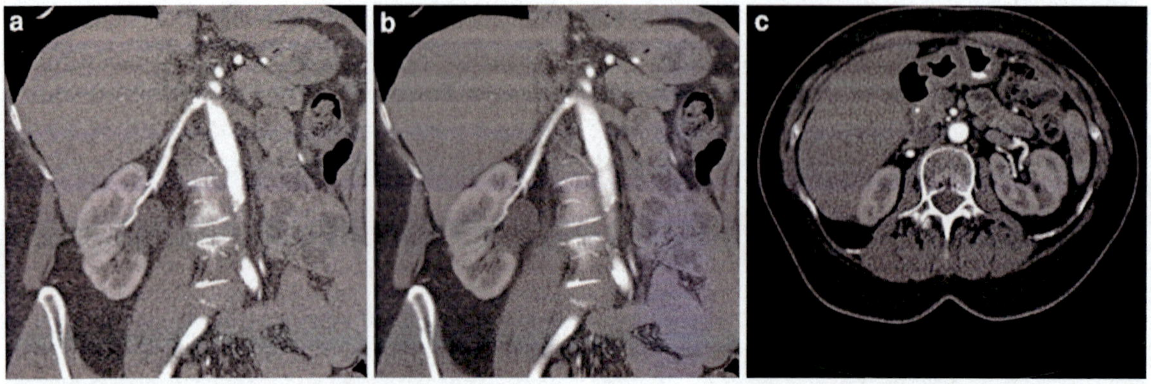


**Fig. 4** CT images of renal arteries obtained at 100 kVp and 87 effective mAs with AEC in a renal donor with a BMI of 20.0 kg/m$^2$ and an abdominal diameter of 30 cm (CTDIvol: 3.90 mGy; DLP:127 mGy cm). **a** 0.75 mm coronal oblique CT image of the *right* renal artery and distal branches. **b** 3 mm CT reformation image of the *right* renal artery and distal branches with reduced noise. **c** Transverse 0.75 mm CT image showing distal branches of *left* renal artery

beam (Kalra et al. 2004a). On the other hand, at IV enhanced CT, a decrease in tube voltage can increase the contrast between vascular and parenchymal structures by increasing X-ray absorption by iodine (Marin et al. 2009). Several studies have validated this technique for MDCT abdominal angiography characterized by a high contrast between the arterial vessels and the poorly enhanced surrounding parenchymas (Sahani et al. 2007; Kalva et al. 2006; Schindera et al. 2009a, b; Wintersperger et al. 2005; Nakayama et al. 2005). The nearer the tube voltage approaches the K-edge of iodine (33.2 keV), the greater the inherent attenuation of the iodinated contrast material (Kalva et al. 2006). Nakayama et al. (2005) showed that scanning at low tube voltage and constant tube current results in degradation of image quality. Dose reduction achieved by decreasing the tube voltage—from 120 to 90 kVp—decreases signal-to-noise ratio, implying that noise has a greater effect on images obtained at 90 kVp than on those at 120 k Vp. Therefore, the use of low-voltage technique alone could be restricted to normal and underweight patients [<80 kg, as reported by Nakayama et al. (2005, 2006)] or compensated by a higher tube current. Sahani et al. (2007) investigated MDCT angiography obtained at different tube potential with the use of AEC in living kidney donors. To avoid a consequent increase of mAs to maintain a constant image noise as set by the operator, they choose an upper limit on the mAs delivered by the tube. These authors showed that, despite a higher image noise, the images were still diagnostically acceptable at 100 kVp with no difference in the visibility of renal arteries and their branches when compared to 120 and 140 kVp, with a significant dose reduction (Sahani et al. 2007). Examples of CT images of renal arteries at 100 kVp are showed in Fig. 4. Furthermore, tube voltage reduction enables to reduce the amount of IV contrast material to be injected in abdominal CT angiography (CTA) (Kalva et al. 2006; Schindera et al. 2009b; Wintersperger et al. 2005; Nakayama et al. 2005, 2006). With the advent of high-output X-ray tubes, it is possible to apply higher tube current-time products to counterbalance greater image noise produced by low tube voltages. Schindera et al. (2009b) showed that with 80 kVp counterbalanced by an increased tube current in comparison of the examination acquired at 100 kVp but with a CTDIvol decreased by about 25%, the image quality of CTA is not compromised. Most importantly, they showed that image quality is still diagnostically acceptable with a contrast medium volume decreased to 45 mL at 80 kVp, which is of great interest in patients with impaired renal function. As the detection of hypervascular liver tumors at IV enhanced MDCT is related to tumor-to-liver contrast, the use of low tube voltage in the late arterial phase could increase the lesion conspicuity and contrast-to-noise ratio (CNR) of these hypervascular lesions at the expense of a higher tube current-time product. Schindera et al. (2008) investigated first this hypothesis on a liver phantom and showed that the CNR and the lesion conspicuity increased with the reduction of tube voltage, associated with 57% of dose reduction as compared to their

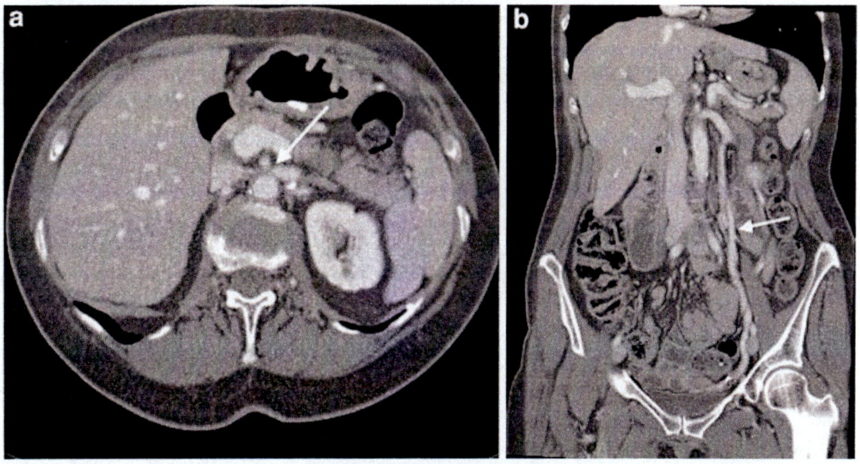


**Fig. 5** Patient with a Nutcracker syndrome (BMI: 20.0 kg/m$^2$). IV enhanced CT obtained at 100 kVp, 95 effective mAs with AEC (CTDI: 4.25 mGy; DLP: 188 mGy cm), at portal venous phase. **a** Transverse CT image showing a stenosis of the left renal vein (*arrow*). **b** Coronal CT image showing the enlargement of the left ovary vein (*arrow*)

standard protocol. Even if the CT parameters of their standard protocol induce a higher radiation dose than that recommended, it is interesting to note that, as illustrated by these authors, the lesion conspicuity increases doubtlessly. This is amazing because, contrarily to what we should have expected, how higher the dose does not mean how higher the image quality in terms of lesion conspicuity. However, these results are obtained on a phantom of smaller diameter than the abdominal diameter of an average adult patient and these results could not be applicable to all patient sizes. In addition, Guimarães et al. (2010) showed recently that the maximum patient diameter for acquiring CT with 80 kV should not exceed 35 cm with the most recently developed CT generation. This indicates that tube voltage as low as 80 kV could be used in children but also in adults. Thus, as long as the patient is not obese, lowered KV settings could be used when imaging the abdomen in both high and low intrinsic contrast conditions. Figures 5, 6, 7, 8 shows abdominal CT images obtained at 100 kVp. Other examples of acquisitions at 100 (in adults) and 80 kVp (in children) are shown in "ALARA concept for MDCT Optimization: what is reasonable, what is achievable?" (see Figs. 18, 23, 25).

### 3.2 Low Intrinsic Contrast Between Structures

Low-dose unenhanced CT with low tube current has been showed to be able to provide alternative diagnoses (Tack et al. 2003; Kluner et al. 2006; Diel et al. 2000; Keyzer et al. 2004, 2009). As periureteric and perinephric fat stranding is still visible at low-dose CT (Heneghan et al. 2003), it can be indeed suggested that any intra-abdominal fat stranding, as in numerous acute abdominal conditions, could also be detectable. These low intrinsic contrast conditions are visible in numerous abdominal acute diseases, as in acute colon diverticulitis and acute appendicitis, as well as in chronic abdominal diseases.

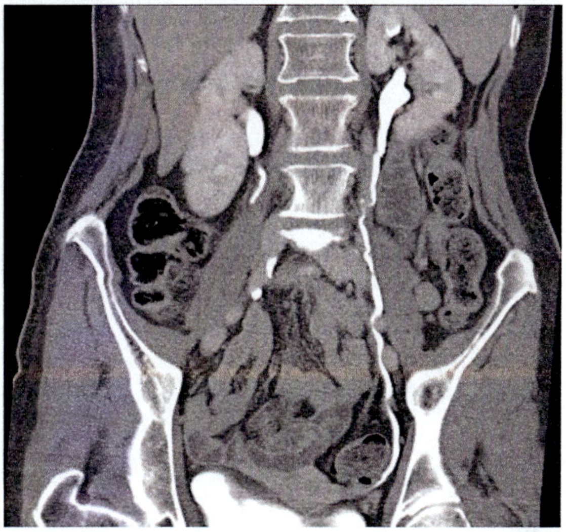

**Fig. 6** Renal donor. Coronal CT urography image obtained at 100 kVp, 101 effective mAs with AEC (CTDI: 4.53 mGy; DLP: 169 mGy cm)

#### 3.2.1 Acute Colon Diverticulitis

Acute diverticulitis can affect young people and is at high risk of recurrence (Ferzoco et al. 1998).

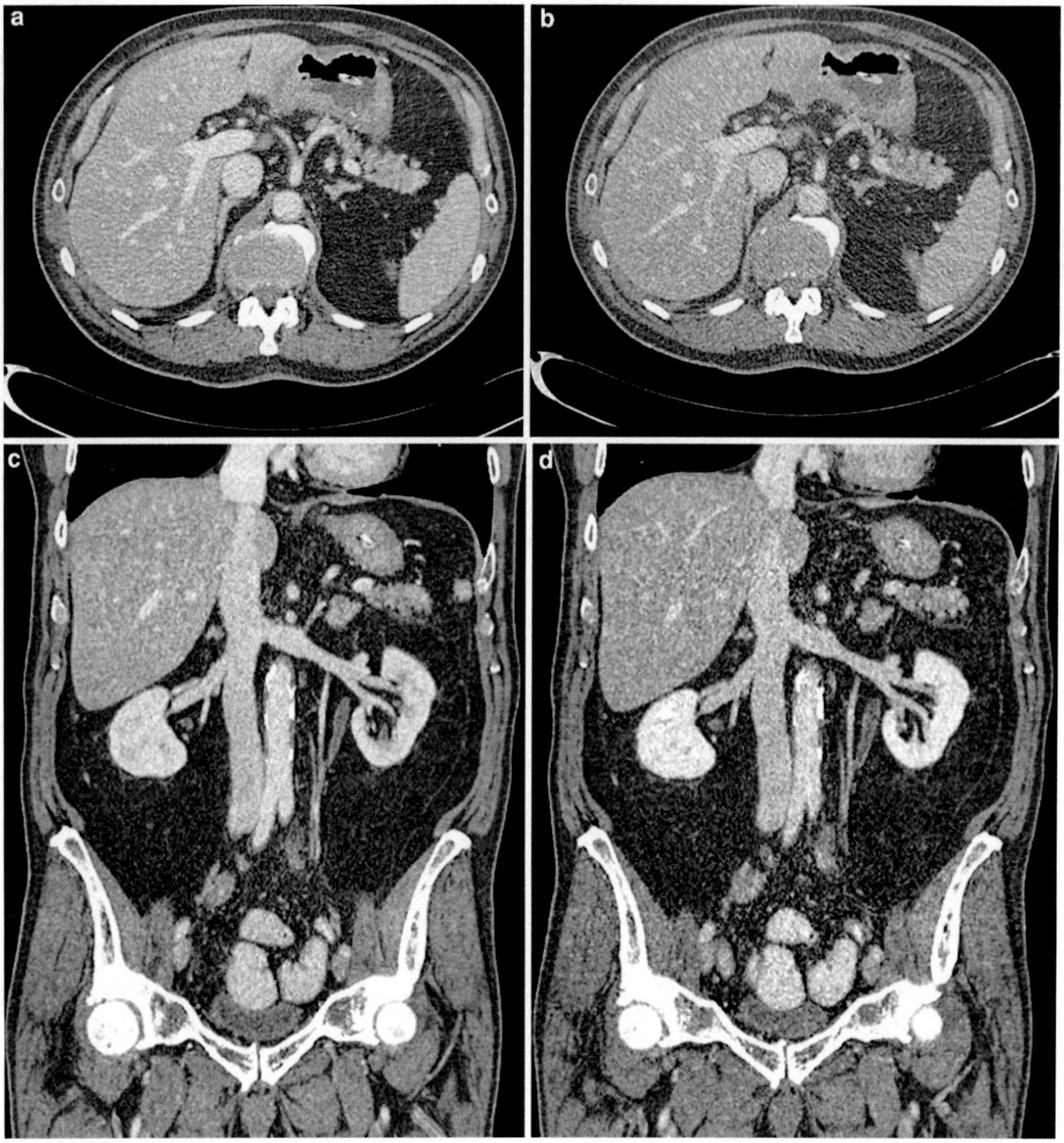


**Fig. 7** Transverse (**a, b**) and coronal (**c, d**) IV enhanced CT images obtained in an 80-year-old-man suspected of small bowel occlusion with a BMI of 26.3 kg/m$^2$. A first acquisition (**a, c**) has been performed at standard-dose CT (120 kVp, 115 effective mAs with AEC; CTDIvol: 8.89 mGy; DLP: 446 mGy cm) directly followed by a low-dose CT (**b, d**) with reduced tube voltage and slightly reduced tube current (100 kVp, 105 effective mAs with AEC; CTDIvol: 4.70 mGy; DLP: 236 mGy cm). Image quality is still acceptable at low-dose CT on transverse image as well as on coronal image with a radiation dose reduced by approximately 50%

Therefore, dose radiation is of particular concern in this disease. Tack et al. (2005) compared unenhanced low-dose MDCT (30 mAs, 120 kVp) and enhanced standard dose MDCT (120 mAs, 120 kVp) in patients suspected of acute diverticulitis. These authors showed that sensitivity and specificity are similar regardless of dose, and that CT has the potential to depict alternative disease. For the diagnosis of acute diverticulitis, sensitivity and specificity of low-dose unenhanced MDCT ranges respectively from 85 to

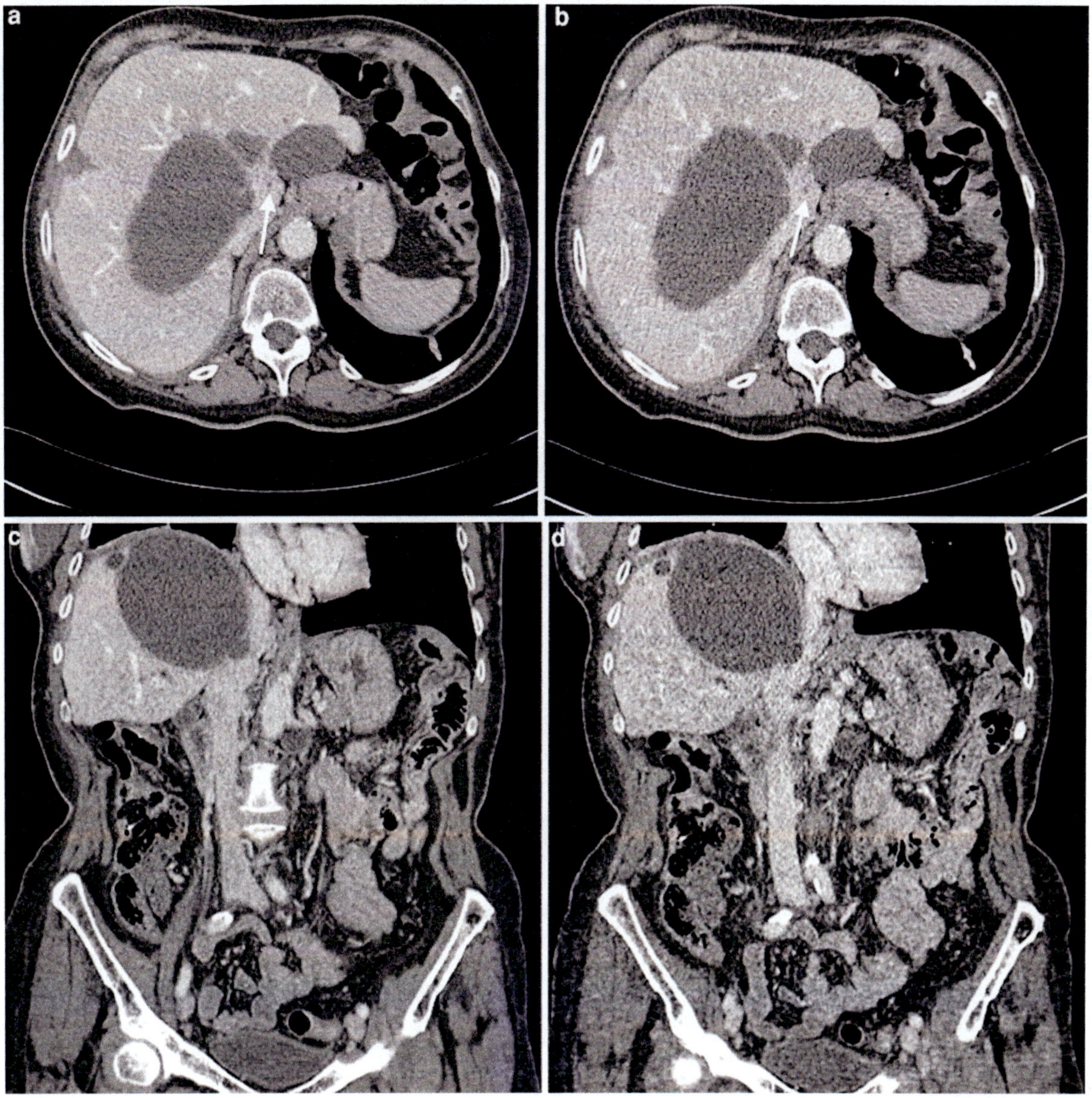

**Fig. 8** Transverse (**a, b**) and coronal (**c, d**) IV enhanced CT images obtained in an 81-year-old-woman with a BMI of 29.3 kg/m$^2$. A first acquisition (**a, c**) has been performed at standard-dose CT (120 kVp, 154 effective mAs with AEC; CTDIvol: 11.8 mGy; DLP: 523 mGy cm) directly followed by a low-dose CT with the same Z-coverage (**b, d**) with reduced tube voltage and slightly reduced tube current (100 kVp, 143 effective mAs with AEC; CTDIvol: 6.38 mGy; DLP: 281 mGy cm. Image quality is still acceptable at low-dose CT on transverse image as well as on coronal image with a radiation dose reduced by approximately 50% in a slightly overweighed patient. Even small hepatic cysts are visible on both acquisitions (*arrow*)

100% and from 92 to 99%, depending on the reader, and are associated with good to excellent reader agreements. In this study, the final diagnosis was achieved without intravenous injection of iodinated contrast medium and with an effective radiation dose corresponding to that of a three-view conventional radiographic examination of the abdomen (Mettler et al. 2008). Indeed, the effective dose of low-dose CT scans obtained with the parameters used by Tack et al. (2005) was calculated at 1.6 mSv in women and 1.2 mSv in men. Fat stranding, known as an excellent sign of acute colon diverticulitis (Kircher et al. 2002),

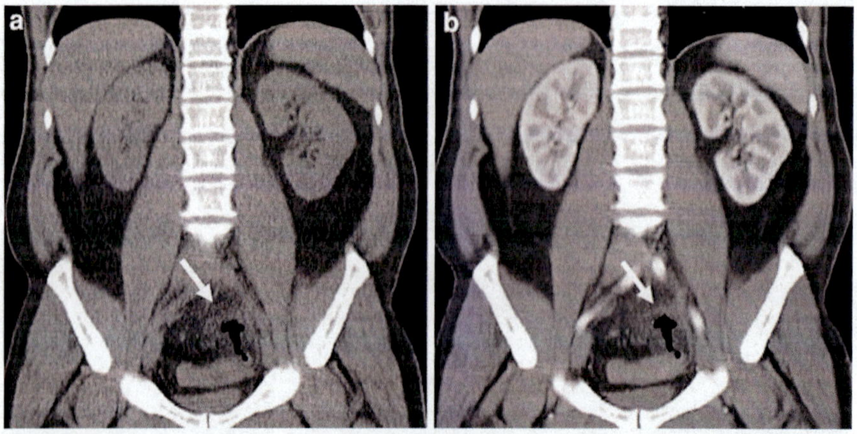


**Fig. 9** Patient with acute sigmoid diverticulitis and gaseous collection (*arrow*). **a** Unenhanced CT performed at 30 effective mAs, 120 kVp, without AEC. **b** IV enhanced CT performed at 120 effective mAs, 120 kVp, without AEC

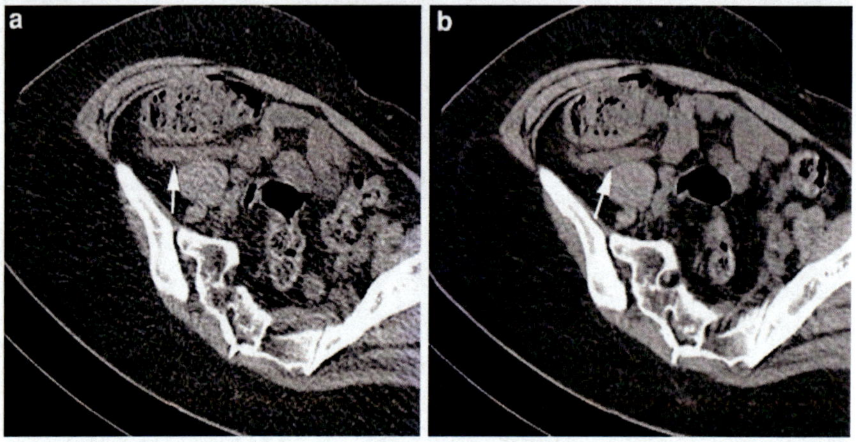


**Fig. 10** Patient with acute appendicitis (*arrow*). **a** Oblique CT image obtained at 30 effective mAs and 120 kVp without AEC and without any contrast material. **b** Oblique CT image obtained at 100 effective mAs and 120 kVp without AEC and without any contrast material

was demonstrated as the most predictive sign for this diagnosis regardless of the dose. In addition, this study revealed that low-dose MDCT enables the correct assessment of the presence of abscess and air collections distant to the colon (Fig. 9; Tack et al. 2005). Subsequently, dose reduction has no effect on the severity grading.

### 3.2.2 Acute Appendicitis

As many individuals suspected of acute appendicitis are young—with a mean age of 30 years (Flum et al. 2001)—the radiation dose should be reduced. Focused CT has the advantage to reduce the radiation dose but with MDCT scanners, rapid volume acquisition became possible and there is a clear trend to scan the entire abdomen and pelvis in all patients suspected of any abdominal disorder (Johnson et al. 2006; O'Malley et al. 2000). In addition, such examinations of the entire abdomen and pelvis are more effective than those focused on the pelvis, because of their ability to detect alternative and/or additional diagnoses (some requiring even urgent surgical treatment) that could otherwise be missed in up to 7% of patients (Kamel et al. 2000).

Another way to reduce the radiation dose is to decrease the tube current-time product and/or the tube potential. Our group compared unenhanced low-dose (30 mAs, 120 kVp) and standard dose (100 mAs, 120 kVp) MDCT in patients with suspected acute appendicitis. The frequency of visualization of the appendix and the diagnostic performance were similar regardless of the radiation dose (Fig. 10). Unenhanced low-dose and standard dose MDCT achieve sensitivity and negative predictive values of 97% or even more. These two characteristics are the most important in patients suspected of acute appendicitis as this condition is potentially life-threatening and can be easily treated by a very efficient surgical procedure (Krieg et al. 1975). Specificity and positive predictive values are lower than sensitivity and negative

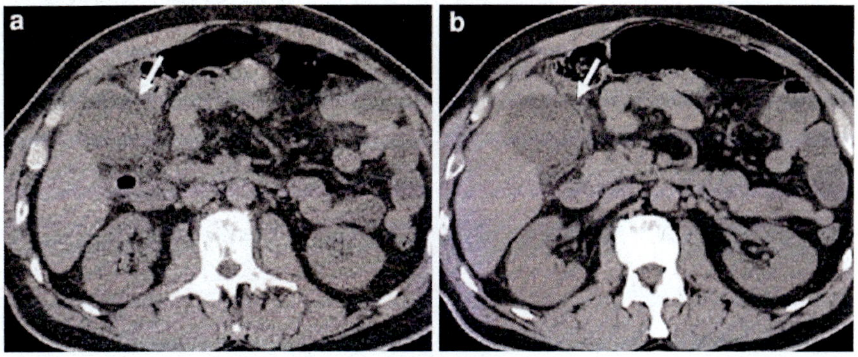


**Fig. 11** Patient with suspected acute appendicitis. Definite diagnosis of acute cholecystitis (*arrow*). **a** Transverse CT image obtained at 30 effective mAs and 120 kVp without AEC and without any contrast material. **b** Transverse CT image obtained at 100 effective mAs and 120 kVp without AEC and without any contrast material

predictive values but they are not different between doses. As in acute colon diverticulitis, fat stranding—i.e. periappendiceal fat stranding—is the most predictive sign of acute appendicitis whatever the dose (Fig. 10; Keyzer et al. 2004). In addition, the ability to propose a correct alternative diagnosis is not influenced by the dose (Fig. 11). Furthermore, in a study based on a technique that simulates dose reduction we also have shown that dose reduction does not affect the correctness of the diagnosis at oral and/or IV enhanced CT as at unenhanced CT (Fig. 12, 13; Keyzer et al. 2009). In these two studies, mAs presets were maintained constant whatever the patient's size. With 30 effective mAs, we showed that for the visualization of the appendix and the diagnosis of acute appendicitis, standard dose and low-dose CT have equivalent diagnostic performance in patients with a BMI greater than 30 kg/m$^2$ (Keyzer et al. 2004, 2009).

Several studies have showed that low-dose CT obtained by decreased tube current-time product (with subsequent effective dose ranging from 1.2 to 4.2 mSv, depending on the study and the patient's gender) has similar diagnostic performance than standard dose CT for the diagnosis of acute appendicitis (Keyzer et al. 2004, 2009; Seo et al. 2009; Platon et al. 2009; Kim et al. 2011). None of these studies has been able to elicit any lower or upper threshold of BMI at which the diagnosis of acute appendicitis or the appendix visualization were hindered at low-dose, with or without the use of AEC (Keyzer et al. 2004, 2009; Seo et al. 2009; Kim et al. 2011). This observation can be explained by the fact that the negative effect of an increase in BMI could be, at least in part, balanced by the accumulation of intra-abdominal fat around the appendix. These observations should however be confirmed by studies focused on patients in extreme BMI categories (underweight and extremely obese patients) as their numbers were low in all these studies.

### 3.2.3 Chronic Abdominal Disorders

In chronic disorders, repeated abdominal CT investigation are performed, even in young patients, in various conditions such as inflammatory bowel disease, pancreatitis, and postoperative complications. Of course, in case of cancer, dose reduction is of lower importance for the patient as he/she is at higher risk of dying of cancer than of developing twenty years later cancer induced by radiation. There is however increasing concern about radiation dose in these patients also and in particular in young patients with treatable neoplasia as lymphoma or testicular carcinoma (O'Malley et al. 2010; la Fougère et al. 2008; Rodriguez-Vigil et al. 2006; Yamamura et al. 2010).

Most of follow-up investigations need the use of intravenous contrast material but there is only few published study that has evaluated the diagnostic performance of enhanced low-dose CT in chronic abdominal disorders or in parenchymal lesion evaluation as in metastasis. Low-contrast detectability is one of most critical issues in hepatic dynamic CT in which detection and characterization of hepatic tumor is a major purpose. Marin et al. used dual energy acquisition at respectively 140 and 80 kVp with an increase in tube current for the lowest energy examination (675 against 385 mA) in patients with known or suspected hypervascular hepatic lesions. They showed that despite an increase in noise for the protocol at 80 kVp—with a subjective lower image quality—the CNR and the tumor detection rate are

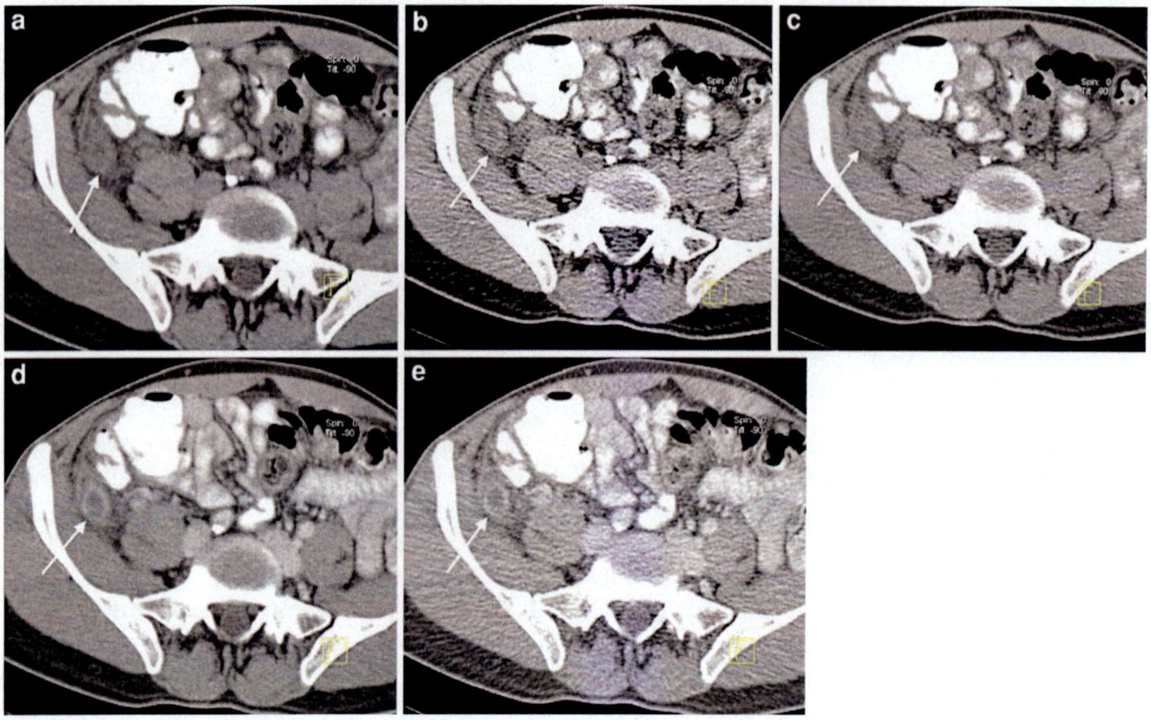


**Fig. 12** Transverse CT images obtained for comparison with firstly oral contrast and secondly IV contrast in a patient (BMI = 22 kg/m$^2$) with acute appendicitis. **a** Transverse CT image obtained with oral contrast at standard dose (100 effective mAs and 120 kVp, without AEC), showing an enlarged, fluid-filled appendix, and moderate periappendiceal fat stranding. **b** Transverse CT image at simulated low-dose (30 effective mAs and 120 kVp, without AEC) with oral contrast showing the same features than (**a**). **c** Thick transverse MPR image (with reduced noise) at simulated low-dose with oral contrast. **d** Transverse CT image obtained at standard dose with oral and IV contrasts showing an enlarged, enhancing, fluid-filled appendix, and moderate periappendiceal fat stranding. **e** Transverse CT image obtained at simulated low-dose with oral and IV contrasts showing the same features than (**d**). The appendix is visible and the diagnosis of acute appendicitis is obvious in all figures from (**a**) to (**e**)

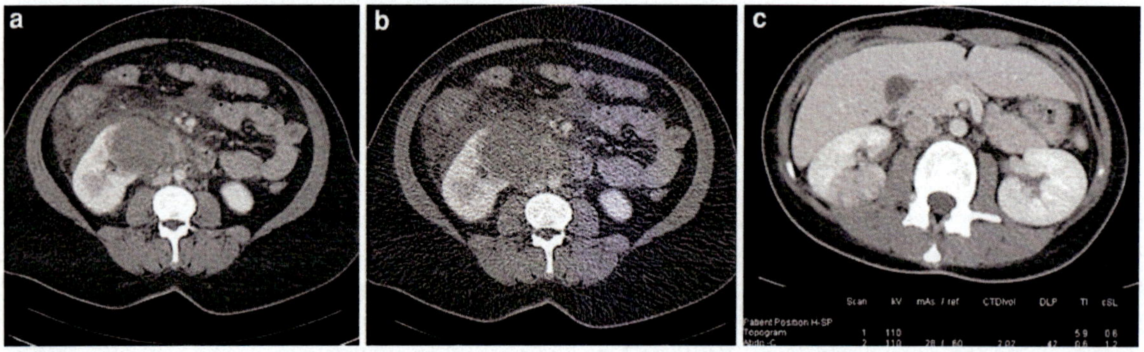


**Fig. 13** Alternative diagnoses: renal abscess and pyelonephritis. Transverse CT images obtained with IV contrast (**a**) at standard dose CT (100 effective mAs and 120 kVp, without AEC) and (**b**) at simulated low-dose CT (simulated 30 effective mAs and 120 kVp, without AEC) in a patient suspected of acute appendicitis with a BMI of 33.6 kg/m$^2$. Renal abscess with marked perirenal and pericolic fat stranding is clearly demonstrated at both doses. **c** Transverse CT image obtained with IV contrast at real low-dose CT (28 effective mAs and 110 kVp, with AEC) for comparison. Pyelonephritis is clearly seen in this patient weighing 50 kg

both increased with a high accuracy in characterization of the tumors with both protocols. However these authors reported an unacceptable high effective dose for the examination performed at 140 kVp and at least just acceptable dose for the acquisition performed at 80 kVp—that we could consider as a standard dose examination as defined previously—(Marin et al. 2009, 2010a, b). It should be noted that, to obtain on one hand higher lesion conspicuity and on the other hand a low-noise image, one would be attracted by using dual energy to scan patients with suspected liver lesion. One should be aware that he would do this at a significant expense of patient radiation dose.

Adaptative noise reduction filters have been developed to decrease noise in images acquired with low-dose CT (Funama et al. 2006; Kalra et al. 2004b; Yanaga et al. 2009). Funama et al. (2006) showed that the use of these filters allows to reduce the radiation dose at abdominal MDCT by approximately 50%, the images obtained at 80 effective mAs with an adaptative reconstruction filter being equivalent to the images obtained at 160 effective mAs without an adaptative reconstruction filter—all other presets being unmodified with a tube voltage of 120 kVp. Image processing with conventional Gaussian filters not only reduces image noise, but also renders the boundaries of structure indistinct (Funama et al. 2006). In their filter technique, the kernel size, smoothing and edge enhancement were changed according to the SD of the CT number in the local region, and the boundaries of each structure could be distinctly preserved. Adaptative noise reduction filters were also reported to reduce noise in low-tube voltage technique in excretory images of MDCT urography. It allows a reduction from 120 to 80 kVp without marked degradation of image quality for the upper collecting system. However, image quality was not sufficient for the pelvis without a compensatory increase in tube current (Yanaga et al. 2009). These filter techniques are further described by Singh and Kalra in "Image filters and radiation dose".

#### 3.2.3.1 Dose Reduction in Crohn's Disease

Crohn's disease is a chronic inflammatory disease characterized by recurrent remissions and relapses, affecting mostly young individuals with a peak incidence in the second and third decades (Loftus et al. 2002). Imaging plays a crucial role in the management of patients with Crohn's disease and MDCT is increasingly used in its follow-up and for identifying complications but also for the primary diagnosis, replacing small-bowel follow-through (Amitai et al. 2008; Desmond et al. 2008; Furukawa et al. 2004). It has been reported that radiation dose of standard MDCT in patients with Crohn's disease, although dependent on various CT parameters, is substantially greater than that of small-bowel follow-through (Desmond et al. 2008; Brenner 2008; Jaffe et al. 2007; Tack and Gevenois 2009). Radiation exposure with CT is therefore of particular concern in these patients, alternative diagnostic imaging such as MRI being associated with other issues as cost and availability. Facing the unreasonable radiation dose delivered in their institution at patients with Crohn's disease, Allen et al. (2010) optimized their MDCT protocol by altering the AEC settings and using a weight-based quality reference mAs. They showed that this dose reduction can be achieved without affecting diagnostic efficacy. They reported a mean CTDIvol of approximately 9 mGy—against 13–16 mGy with the original AEC—corresponding to what we should consider as an optimized-dose but not a low-dose. Interestingly, by comparison with patients with BMI ranging from 25 to 35 kg/m$^2$, thin patients with BMI $< 25$ kg/m$^2$ as well as obese patients with BMI $> 35$ kg/m$^2$ were judged to have a lower quality image in terms of noise. It must be noted that, although weight-based quality reference mAs may be used with all CT scanners, the AEC settings used in this study is specific to Siemens Healthcare MDCT scanners. Noise index (NI) is on the other hand a term specific to scanners manufactured by GE Healthcare for their tube current modulation. It is a measure of image noise on CT inversely proportional to tube current and image quality. The selection of NI gives the user the opportunity to select the level of image noise acceptable for image interpretation. Kambakanone et al. (2010) used a software that generates simulated CT images with various NI levels and assessed the image quality, the reader confidence, and the diagnostic performance in 25 patients (35 MDCT examinations, i.e. baseline and follow-up) with Crohn's disease at 5 NI levels for the simulated CT images (NI at 18, 20, 25, 30, and 35). These authors reported that image quality was acceptable for CT studies with NI between 18 and 25. At NI of 30 and 35, the proportion of CT images considered as acceptable decreased to respectively 88–90% and 74–77%. Reader's confidence decreased with NI at 30 and 35 but

**Table 1** Reported Radiation Dose Measurements for Simulated Low-Dose CT Data Sets (Kambadakone et al (2010))

| CT data sets | Mean CTDI (mGy) | Mean DLP (mGy.cm) | Mean effective dose (mSv) |
|---|---|---|---|
| NI level 18 | 11.04 | 495 | 7.4 |
| NI level 20 | 8.96 | 402 | 6.03 |
| NI level 25 | 5.76 | 259 | 3.88 |
| NI level 30 | 4.00 | 180 | 2.69 |
| NI level 35 | 2.88 | 129 | 1.94 |

agreement between readers for mural and extramural findings was almost perfect at all NI levels. Diagnostic accuracy was reduced with NI levels ≥30. One major drawback of this study was the use of axial images only. Radiation doses for the simulated CT images of this study are given in Table 1. The dose obtained with NI at 25 approaches the dose we should considered as low-dose CT and can certainly be considered as acceptable for investigating patients with Crohn's disease in whom subtle signs can be masked by noise generated by low tube current. Examples of low-dose CT (with reduced tube current and with reduced tube voltage) in patients with Chron's disease are shown in Figs. 14, 15.

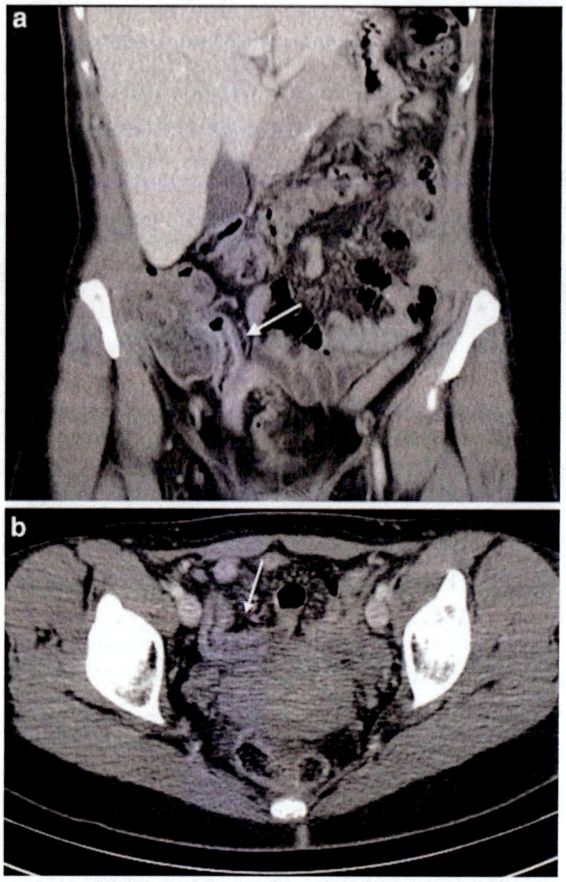

**Fig. 14** Chron's disease. Coronal (**a**) and transverse (**b**) IV-enhanced low-dose CT images obtained in a 35-year-old woman with a BMI of 23.2 kg/m$^2$ with reduced tube current and with AEC (35 effective mAs, 110 kVp; CTDIvol: 2.56 mGy; DLP: 89 mGy cm). Note that the acquisition length has been optimized as well. Images show the mural thickening and enhancement of the terminal ileum (*arrow*)

## 3.3 Dose Reduction in Abdominal MDCT, ASIR and Other Recent Reconstruction Techniques

Traditional CT reconstruction algorithm (FBP reconstruction technique) does not produce consistently diagnostic images if tube current is substantially reduced. Iterative reconstruction is a reconstruction algorithm whereby image data are corrected with an assortment of models. The major drawback of this iterative reconstruction is the long computing time. Therefore a faster iterative reconstruction technique using only one corrective model has been developed and is called Adaptative Statistical Iterative Reconstruction technique (ASIR, GE Healthcare). This reconstruction technique is further detailed in this volume by Singh and Kalra in "Conventional and newer reconstruction techniques in CT". A fully converged 100% ASIR image tends to have a noise-free appearance with homogeneous attenuation that is not appealing to most radiologists as they are used to noisy images inherent to CT. However a mixture of FBP and ASIR can be used and produce an image with reduced noise but that retains a more typical CT appearance (Hara et al. 2009). Abdominal MDCT images obtained with a reduced dose and reconstructed with ASIR (40%) has quantitative and qualitative image noise and quality similar to or even better than those of standard dose CT (Hara et al. 2009). It must be noticed that in these studies, the reported CTDIvol and DLP values for the standard dose are very high (higher than the reference levels proposed by the NRPB), and that those reported for low-dose CT approximates what should be considered as a standard dose CT (Hara et al. 2009).

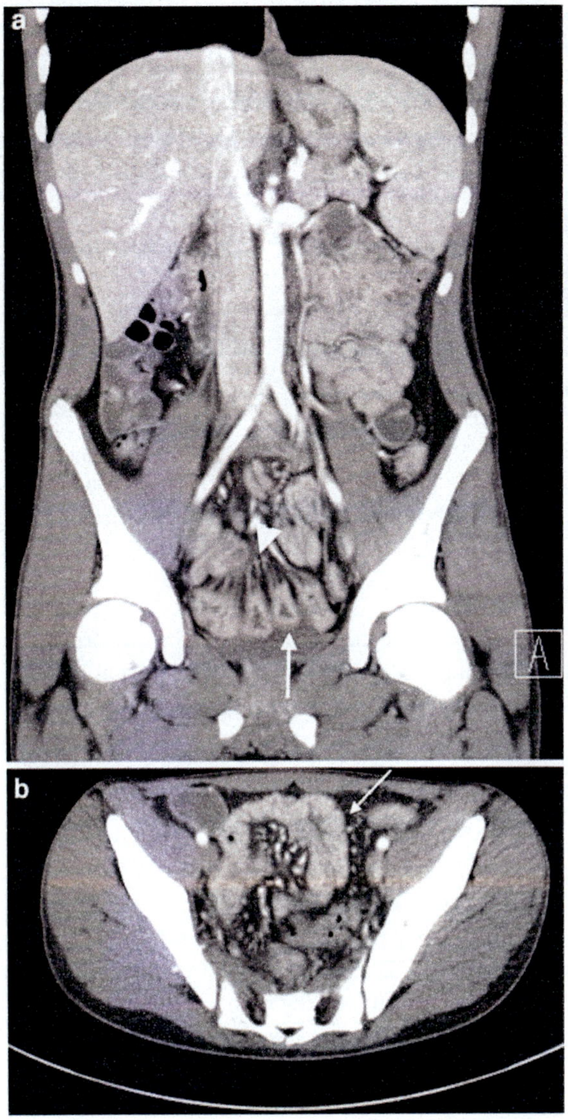


**Fig. 15** Chron's disease. Coronal (**a**) and transverse (**b**) IV-enhanced low-dose CT images obtained in a 19-year-old-man with a BMI of 20.5 kg/m$^2$ with reduced tube voltage and with AEC (69 effective mAs, 100 kVp; CTDIvol: 2.74 mGy; DLP: 126 mGy cm). Images show mural thickening and enhancement of the terminal ileum (*arrow*) and mesenteric manifestation of Chron's disease (*arrowhead*)

Prakash et al. (2010) reported an average 25% dose reduction and lower image noise with the use of ASIR reconstruction compared with FBP in a consecutive series of patients who had abdominal MDCT. However, they reported an overall mean CTDIvol of 11.9 mGy with a mean DLP of 633 mGy cm with ASIR, these values approximating those we expect with a standard dose CT but not with a low-dose CT. These authors did not assess other radiation dose reduction levels for determining whether dose lower than that recommended by the manufacturer could be diagnostically acceptable with ASIR. In a more recent study, Singh et al. (2010) compared image quality and lesion conspicuity on abdominal MDCT acquired with four different tube currents and reconstructed with ASIR and FBP. The four tube currents were 200, 150, 100, and 50 mAs with corresponding CTDIvol of 16.8, 12.6, 8.4, and 4.2 mGy. The latter CTDIvol is a value acceptable for a low-dose CT. These authors showed that ASIR lowers noise, and improves diagnostic confidence and conspicuity of abdominal lesions—at 8.4 mGy with 30% ASIR and at 4.2 mGy with 50 and 70% ASIR in patients weighing 90 kg or less. Images tended to have a blotchy pixilated appearance at higher ASIR proportion. The results of this study need however to be confirmed by further investigation giving their small study sample size (i.e. 22 patients only). In addition, a very recent phantom study has showed that iterative reconstruction algorithm [IRIS (Iterative Reconstruction in Image Space); Siemens Healthcare] allows scanning at 100 kVp (CTDIvol: 5.63 mGy) with similar sensitivity for tumor detection in comparison with a 120 kVp abdominal CT (CTDIvol: 9.35 mGy) reconstructed with FBP technique. Interestingly, these authors reported that the mean CNRs were greater for IRIS data sets at 80 kVp (CTDIvol: 2.78 mGy) than for the FBP data sets at 120 kVp (Schindera et al. 2011). This technique has to be further validated with low-dose abdominal CT obtained with low tube voltage on patients with various abdominal disorders. Examples of low-dose CT with iterative reconstruction are shown in Fig. 16.

Dose reduction has been extensively investigated in CT colonography—as further exposed by J Stoker in "Dose Reduction in Screening Programs: Colon Cancer Screening"—with various techniques: lowering tube current, AEC technique, voltage adjustment, and ASIR technique (van Gelder et al. 2002, 2004; Flicek et al. 2010; Fisichella et al. 2010; Cohnen et al. 2004; Graser et al. 2006; Iannaccone et al. 2003). Recently, Lubner et al. (2011) showed that Prior Image Constrained Compressed Sensing (PICSS) algorithm allows substantial noise reduction as compared with FBP reconstruction technique, without altering attenuation and with an endoluminal image quality equal or even improved (Fig. 17).

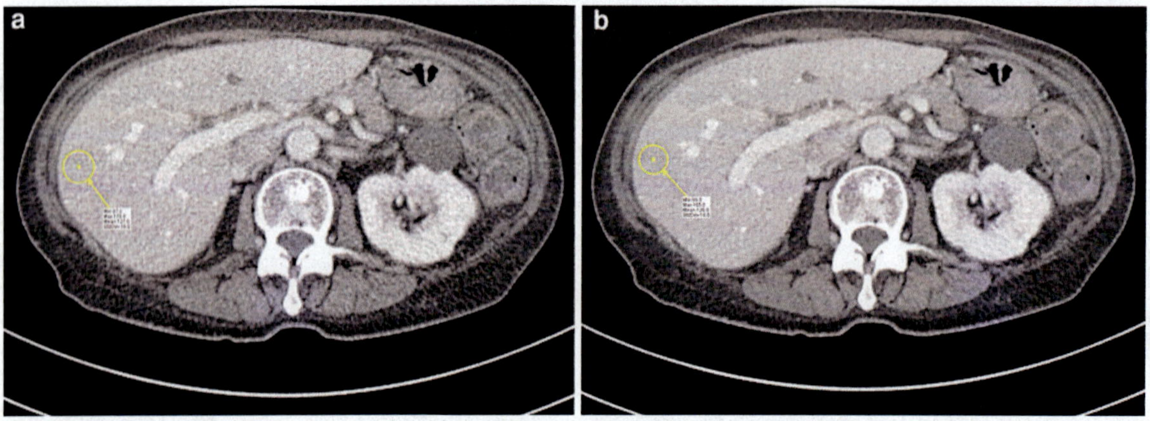


**Fig. 16** Iterative reconstruction. Transverse CT images obtained at 100 kVp and 71 effective mAs (entire abdomen and pelvis at portal phase: DLP = 139 mGy cm) in a 60-year-old woman weighing 60 kg with metrorrhagia. **a** Transverse CT image obtained with FBP reconstruction. Noise measured in the liver is of 16 HU. **b** Transverse CT image obtained with iterative reconstruction. Noise measured in the liver is of 10 HU

This noise reduction is considerably higher than that reported with ASIR (Marin et al. 2010b; Flicek et al. 2010). By adding a denoising algorithm like PICCS, radiation dose could be further reduced while preserving image quality, with little additional cost or time penalty (Lubner et al. 2011).

## 4 Recommendations for Optimizing and Reducing the Radiation Dose in Abdominal MDCT

In this paragraph, recommendations appropriate for abdominal MDCT will be proposed. Such proposals are however still a matter of debate and should be evaluated by further studies.

The presets, Z-axis coverage, and repeated exposure before and after intravenous administration of iodinated contrast material should always be adapted to the suspected diagnosis. For example, in patient suspected of acute appendicitis, the probable ideal acquisition length includes the root of diaphragms, easily seen on the scanogram and being at least 2 cm above the top of the kidneys, to the upper limit of pubic symphysis. Such an acquisition length includes the Douglas pouch and is of 32 cm in standard sized men and 30 cm in standard sized women. Examples of acquisition length optimization are shown in Figs. 14, 18.

Repeated acquisitions should not be performed in circumstances where they do not specifically yield additional information.

The standard presets recommended by the constructors with regard for the guidelines from the Commission of the EU and the NRPB should be only used in patients with suspected neoplasia and/or metastasis, old patients, or severe trauma.

Automatic modulation of the tube current as a function of the patient's absorption is now available on all modern MDCT scanners. Differences still exist between manufacturers regarding the methods used for this modulation and the dose reductions subsequently obtained. The most important feature of these devices is that the radiation dose is adapted to the patient's weight and absorption. Consequently, the role of the CT user is not to adapt the tube current to the patient's weight but more to select appropriate tube potential and image quality to fit with the clinical indication of the CT examination. If the CT equipments includes AEC device, it should be always switched on for abdominal MDCT scans.

It is preferable to use smooth reconstruction algorithms if possible. If the reconstructed images appear too noisy, MPR with increased slice-thickness can be used (Figs. 3, 12).

All available keys of the CT equipment allowing dose reduction (i.e. autokV, ASIR, IRIS, AEC,…) should be used appropriately and "mixed" to obtain a diagnostic image at the lowest possible dose.

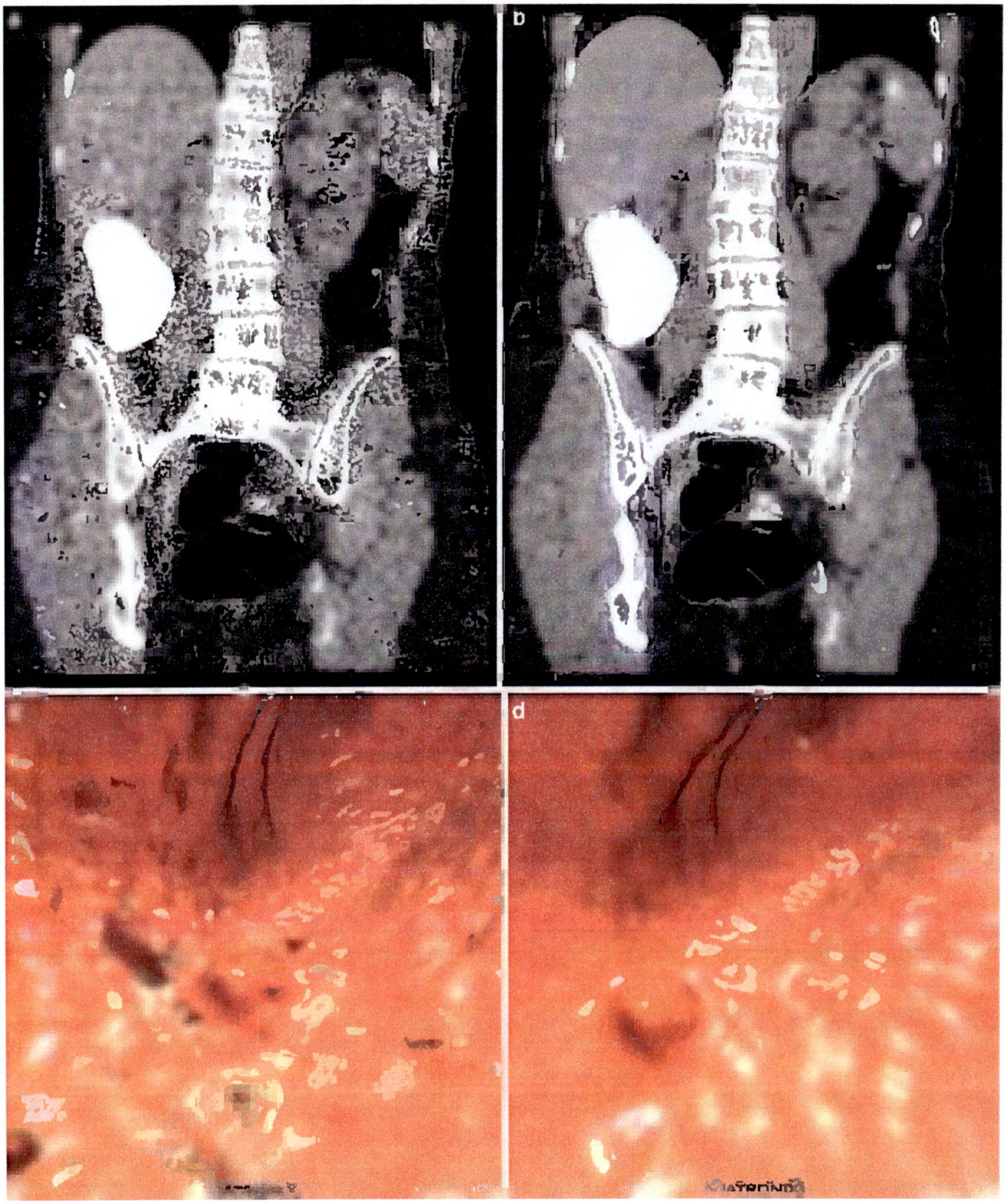


**Fig. 17** Comparison of image quality. **a** Coronal CT colonographic (CTC) two-dimensional image reconstructed with FBP. Note the importance of noise. **b** Coronal CTC two-dimensional image reconstructed with PICCS shows a significant decrease in noise. **c** Three-dimensional endoluminal ultra-low-dose CTC (effective dose: 0.3 mSv) reconstructed with FBP. Polyp is barely visible amongst the noise but is well seen on three-dimensional endoluminal ultra-low-dose CTC reconstructed with PICCS **d**. Images are courtesy of Perry J. Pickhardt and Meghan G. Lubner, University of Wisconsin School of Medicine and Public Health, United States of America

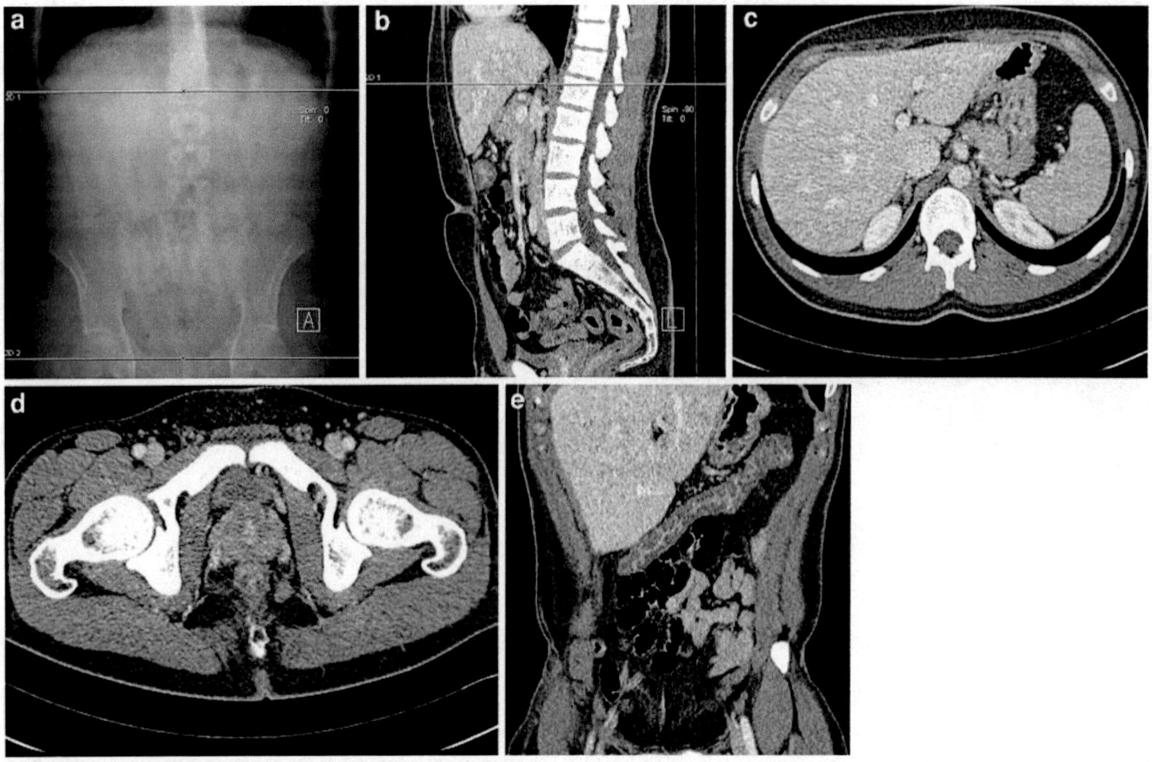


**Fig. 18** Optimization of acquisition-length. **a** Scout-view with lines representing the optimized scanning range (**b**) Sagittal CT image of a entire abdomen and pelvis. Line represents the upper limit of the optimized scanning range (**c**) CT image obtained at the upper limit of the optimized scanning range. Upper pole of kidneys and costophrenic sulci are visible. **d** CT image obtained at the lower limit of the optimized scanning range, at the upper limit of pubic symphysis. **e** Colitis demonstrated in this patient complaining for abdominal pain, detectable on this optimized acquisition length. In this patient, with an optimized acquisition length, dose could have been reduced by 20% with a reduced DLP at163 mGy cm (this examination was acquired at 120 kVp and 78 effective mAs with AEC; DLP: 244 mGy cm; CTDIvol: 6.03 mGy)

## 5 Conclusion

Survey studies have shown that collective doses increased as MDCT replaced SDCT. However, the radiation dose has been optimized during the last decade, mainly through AEC devices and reasonable use of tube current and tube voltage presets. This was achieved thanks to technological improvements and willpower of several study groups to investigate the effect of dose reduction in term of image quality and diagnostic performance. Nevertheless, as both the number of examinations and the number of clinical indications of CT increase, a major effort should be made in order to optimize the radiation dose. In addition, as survey studies have shown that there were still great variations in doses among institutions, a supplementary effort should be made in order to recommend standardized acquisition protocols.

## References

Allen BC, Baker ME, Einstein DM, Remer EM, Herts BR, Achkar JP, Davros WJ, Novak E, Obuchowski NA (2010) Effect of altering automatic exposure control settings and quality reference mAs on radiation dose, image quality, and diagnostic efficacy in MDCT enterography of active inflammatory Crohn's disease. Am J Roentgenol 195:89–100

Amitai MM, razi-Kleinman T, Hertz M, Apter S, Portnoy O, Guranda L, Chowers Y, Avidan B (2008) Multislice CT compared to small bowel follow-through in the evaluation of patients with Crohn disease. Clin Imaging 32:355–361

Berrington de Gonzalez A, Mahesh M, Kim KP, Bhargavan M, Lewis R, Mettler F, Land C (2009) Projected cancer risks from computed tomographic scans performed in the United States in 2007. Arch Intern Med 169:2071–2077

Birnbaum BA, Wilson SR (2000) Appendicitis at the millennium. Radiology 215:337–348

Brenner DJ (2008) Should computed tomography be the modality of choice for imaging Crohn's disease in children? the radiation risk perspective. Gut 57:1489–1490

Cohnen M, Vogt C, Beck A, Andersen K, Heinen W, vom Dahl S, Aurich V, Haeussinger D, Moedder U (2004) Feasibility of MDCT colonography in ultra-low-dose technique in the detection of colorectal lesions: comparison with high-resolution video colonoscopy. Am J Roentgenol 183:1355–1359

Deak PD, Smal Y, Kalender WA (2010) Multisection CT protocols: sex- and age-specific conversion factors used to determine effective dose from dose-length product. Radiology 257:158–166

Desmond AN, O'Regan K, Curran C, McWilliams S, Fitzgerald T, Maher MM, Shanahan F (2008) Crohn's disease: factors associated with exposure to high levels of diagnostic radiation. Gut 57:1524–1529

Diel J, Perlmutter S, Venkataramanan N, Mueller R, Lane MJ, Katz DS (2000) Unenhanced helical CT using increased pitch for suspected renal colic: an effective technique for radiation dose reduction? J Comput Assis Tomogr 24:795–801

European Commission (1999) European guidelines on quality criteria for computed tomography. EUR 16262 EN. Luxembourg, Office for Official Publications of the European Communities. http://www.drs.dk/guidelines/ct/quality/index.htm. Accessed 5 May 2011

Ferzoco LB, Raptopoulos V, Silen W (1998) Acute diverticulitis. N Engl J Med 338:1521–1526

Fisichella VA, Bath M, Allansdotter JA, Jaderling F, Bergsten T, Persson U, Mellingen K, Hellstrom M (2010) Evaluation of image quality and lesion perception by human readers on 3D CT colonography: comparison of standard and low radiation dose. Eur Radiol 20:630–639

Flicek KT, Hara AK, Silva AC, Wu Q, Peter MB, Johnson CD (2010) Reducing the radiation dose for CT colonography using adaptive statistical iterative reconstruction: a pilot study. Am J Roentgenol 195:126–131

Flum DR, Morris A, Koepsell T, Dellinger EP (2001) Has misdiagnosis of appendicitis decreased over time? a population-based analysis. JAMA 286:1748–1753

Funama Y, Awai K, Miyazaki O, Nakayama Y, Goto T, Omi Y, Shimonobo T, Liu D, Yamashita Y, Hori S (2006) Improvement of low-contrast detectability in low-dose hepatic multidetector computed tomography using a novel adaptive filter: evaluation with a computer-simulated liver including tumors. Invest Radiol 41:1–7

Furukawa A, Saotome T, Yamasaki M, Maeda K, Nitta N, Takahashi M, Tsujikawa T, Fujiyama Y, Murata K, Sakamoto T (2004) Cross-sectional imaging in Crohn disease. Radiographics 24:689–702

Golding SJ (2010) Radiation exposure in CT: what is the professionally responsible approach? Radiology 255:683–686

Graser A, Wintersperger BJ, Suess C, Reiser MF, Becker CR (2006) Dose reduction and image quality in MDCT colonography using tube current modulation. Am J Roentgenol 187:695–701

Guimaraes LS, Fletcher JG, Harmsen WS, Yu L, Siddiki H, Melton Z, Huprich JE, Hough D, Hartman R, McCollough CH (2010) Appropriate patient selection at abdominal dual-energy CT using 80 kV: relationship between patient size, image noise, and image quality. Radiology 257:732–742

Hamm M, Wawroschek F, Weckermann D, Knopfle E, Hackel T, Hauser H, Krawczak G, Harzmann R (2001) Unenhanced helical computed tomography in the evaluation of acute flank pain. Eur Urol 39:460–465

Hamm M, Knopfle E, Wartenberg S, Wawroschek F, Weckermann D, Harzmann R (2002) Low dose unenhanced helical computerized tomography for the evaluation of acute flank pain. J Urol 167:1687–1691

Hara AK, Paden RG, Silva AC, Kujak JL, Lawder HJ, Pavlicek W (2009) Iterative reconstruction technique for reducing body radiation dose at CT: feasibility study. Am J Roentgenol 193:764–771

Heneghan JP, McGuire KA, Leder RA, DeLong DM, Yoshizumi T, Nelson RC (2003) Helical CT for nephrolithiasis and ureterolithiasis: comparison of conventional and reduced radiation-dose techniques. Radiology 229:575–580

Iannaccone R, Laghi A, Catalano C, Brink JA, Mangiapane F, Trenna S, Piacentini F, Passariello R (2003) Detection of colorectal lesions: lower-dose multi-detector row helical CT colonography compared with conventional colonoscopy. Radiology 229:775–781

Jaffe TA, Gaca AM, Delaney S, Yoshizumi TT, Toncheva G, Nguyen G, Frush DP (2007) Radiation doses from small-bowel follow-through and abdominopelvic MDCT in Crohn's disease. Am J Roentgenol 189:1015–1022

Johnson PT, Horton KM, Mahesh M, Fishman EK (2006) Multidetector computed tomography for suspected appendicitis: multi-institutional survey of 16-MDCT data acquisition protocols and review of pertinent literature. J Comput Assist Tomogr 30:758–764

Kalra MK, Maher MM, Toth TL, Hamberg LM, Blake MA, Shepard JA, Saini S (2004a) Strategies for CT radiation dose optimization. Radiology 230:619–628

Kalra MK, Maher MM, Blake MA, Lucey BC, Karau K, Toth TL, Avinash G, Halpern EF, Saini S (2004b) Detection and characterization of lesions on low-radiation-dose abdominal CT images postprocessed with noise reduction filters. Radiology 232:791–797

Kalra MK, Maher MM, D'Souza RV, Rizzo S, Halpern EF, Blake MA, Saini S (2005) Detection of urinary tract stones at low-radiation-dose CT with z-axis automatic tube current modulation: phantom and clinical studies. Radiology 235:523–529

Kalva SP, Sahani DV, Hahn PF, Saini S (2006) Using the K-edge to improve contrast conspicuity and to lower radiation dose with a 16-MDCT: a phantom and human study. J Comput Assist Tomogr 30:391–397

Kambadakone AR, Prakash P, Hahn PF, Sahani DV (2010) Low-dose CT examinations in Crohn's disease: impact on image quality, diagnostic performance, and radiation dose. Am J Roentgenol 195:78–88

Kamel IR, Goldberg SN, Keogan MT, Rosen MP, Raptopoulos V (2000) Right lower quadrant pain and suspected appendicitis:

nonfocused appendiceal CT—review of 100 cases. Radiology 217:159–163

Katz DS, Scheer M, Lumerman JH, Mellinger BC, Stillman CA, Lane MJ (2000) Alternative or additional diagnoses on unenhanced helical computed tomography for suspected renal colic: experience with 1000 consecutive examinations. Urology 56:53–57

Keyzer C, Tack D, De Maertelaer V, Bohy P, Gevenois PA, Van Gansbeke D (2004) Acute appendicitis: comparison of low-dose and standard-dose unenhanced multi-detector row CT. Radiology 232:164–172

Keyzer C, Cullus P, Tack D, De Maertelaer V, Bohy P, Gevenois PA (2009) MDCT for suspected acute appendicitis in adults: impact of oral and IV contrast media at standard-dose and simulated low-dose techniques. Am J Roentgenol 193:1272–1281

Kim SY, Lee KH, Kim K, Kim TY, Lee HS, Hwang SS, Song KJ, Kang HS, Kim YH, Rhee JE (2011) Acute appendicitis in young adults: low- versus standard-radiation-dose contrast-enhanced abdominal CT for diagnosis. Radiology 260:437–445

Kircher MF, Rhea JT, Kihiczak D, Novelline RA (2002) Frequency, sensitivity, and specificity of individual signs of diverticulitis on thin-section helical CT with colonic contrast material: experience with 312 cases. Am J Roentgenol 178:1313–1318

Kluner C, Hein PA, Gralla O, Hein E, Hamm B, Romano V, Rogalla P (2006) Does ultra-low-dose CT with a radiation dose equivalent to that of KUB suffice to detect renal and ureteral calculi? J Comput Assist Tomogr 30:44–50

Krieg AF, Gambino R, Galen RS (1975) Why are clinical laboratory tests performed? when are they valid? JAMA 233:76–78

la Fougère C, Pfluger T, Schneider V, Hacker M, Brockel N, Morhard D, Hundt W, Bartenstein P, Becker C, Tiling R (2008) Restaging of patients with lymphoma. Comparison of low dose CT (20 mAs) with contrast enhanced diagnostic CT in combined [18F]-FDG PET/CT. Nuklearmedizin 47:37–42

Little MP, Wakeford R, Tawn EJ, Bouffler SD, Berrington de Gonzalez A (2009) Risks associated with low doses and low dose rates of ionizing radiation: why linearity may be (almost) the best we can do. Radiology 251:6–12

Liu W, Esler SJ, Kenny BJ, Goh RH, Rainbow AJ, Stevenson GW (2000) Low-dose nonenhanced helical CT of renal colic: assessment of ureteric stone detection and measurement of effective dose equivalent. Radiology 215:51–54

Loftus EV Jr, Schoenfeld P, Sandborn WJ (2002) The epidemiology and natural history of Crohn's disease in population-based patient cohorts from North America: a systematic review. Aliment Pharmacol Ther 16:51–60

Lubner MG, Pickhardt PJ, Tang J, Chen GH (2011) Reduced image noise at low-dose multidetector CT of the abdomen with prior image constrained compressed sensing algorithm. Radiology 260:248–256

Marin D, Nelson RC, Samei E, Paulson EK, Ho LM, Boll DT, DeLong DM, Yoshizumi TT, Schindera ST (2009) Hypervascular liver tumors: low tube voltage, high tube current multidetector CT during late hepatic arterial phase for detection—initial clinical experience. Radiology 251:771–779

Marin D, Nelson RC, Barnhart H, Schindera ST, Ho LM, Jaffe TA, Yoshizumi TT, Youngblood R, Samei E (2010a) Detection of pancreatic tumors, image quality, and radiation dose during the pancreatic parenchymal phase: effect of a low-tube-voltage, high-tube-current CT technique—preliminary results. Radiology 256:450–459

Marin D, Nelson RC, Schindera ST, Richard S, Youngblood RS, Yoshizumi TT, Samei E (2010b) Low-tube-voltage, high-tube-current multidetector abdominal CT: improved image quality and decreased radiation dose with adaptive statistical iterative reconstruction algorithm—initial clinical experience. Radiology 254:145–153

Mettler FA Jr, Huda W, Yoshizumi TT, Mahesh M (2008) Effective doses in radiology and diagnostic nuclear medicine: a catalog. Radiology 248:254–263

Mulkens TH, Bellinck P, Baeyaert M, Ghysen D, van Dijck X, Mussen E, Venstermans C, Termote JL (2005) Use of an automatic exposure control mechanism for dose optimization in multi-detector row CT examinations: clinical evaluation. Radiology 237:213–223

Nakayama Y, Awai K, Funama Y, Hatemura M, Imuta M, Nakaura T, Ryu D, Morishita S, Sultana S, Sato N, Yamashita Y (2005) Abdominal CT with low tube voltage: preliminary observations about radiation dose, contrast enhancement, image quality, and noise. Radiology 237:945–951

Nakayama Y, Awai K, Funama Y, Liu D, Nakaura T, Tamura Y, Yamashita Y (2006) Lower tube voltage reduces contrast material and radiation doses on 16-MDCT aortography. Am J Roentgenol 187:W490–W497

O'Malley ME, Halpern E, Mueller PR, Gazelle GS (2000) Helical CT protocols for the abdomen and pelvis: a survey. Am J Roentgenol 175:109–113

O'Malley ME, Chung P, Haider M, Jang HJ, Jhaveri K, Khalili K, Panzarella T, Warde P (2010) Comparison of low dose with standard dose abdominal/pelvic multidetector CT in patients with stage 1 testicular cancer under surveillance. Eur Radiol 20:1624–1630

Platon A, Jlassi H, Rutschmann OT, Becker CD, Verdun FR, Gervaz P, Poletti PA (2009) Evaluation of a low-dose CT protocol with oral contrast for assessment of acute appendicitis. Eur Radiol 19:446–454

Prakash P, Kalra MK, Kambadakone AK, Pien H, Hsieh J, Blake MA, Sahani DV (2010) Reducing abdominal CT radiation dose with adaptive statistical iterative reconstruction technique. Invest Radiol 45:202–210

Rodriguez-Vigil B, Gomez-Leon N, Pinilla I, Hernandez-Maraver D, Coya J, Martin-Curto L, Madero R (2006) PET/CT in lymphoma: prospective study of enhanced full-dose PET/CT versus unenhanced low-dose PET/CT. J Nucl Med 47:1643–1648

Rogers LF (2001) Radiation exposure in CT: why so high? Am J Roentgenol 177:277

Rogers LF (2003) Low-dose CT: how are we doing? Am J Roentgenol 180:303

Sahani DV, Kalva SP, Hahn PF, Saini S (2007) 16-MDCT angiography in living kidney donors at various tube potentials: impact on image quality and radiation dose. Am J Roentgenol 188:115–120

Schindera ST, Nelson RC, Mukundan S Jr, Paulson EK, Jaffe TA, Miller CM, DeLong DM, Kawaji K, Yoshizumi TT, Samei E (2008) Hypervascular liver tumors: low tube voltage, high tube current multi-detector row CT for enhanced detection—phantom study. Radiology 246:125–132

Schindera ST, Nelson RC, Yoshizumi T, Toncheva G, Nguyen G, DeLong DM, Szucs-Farkas Z (2009a) Effect of automatic tube current modulation on radiation dose and image quality for low tube voltage multidetector row CT angiography: phantom study. Acad Radiol 16:997–1002

Schindera ST, Graca P, Patak MA, Abderhalden S, von Allmen G, Vock P, Szucs-Farkas Z (2009b) Thoracoabdominal-aortoiliac multidetector-row CT angiography at 80 and 100 kVp: assessment of image quality and radiation dose. Invest Radiol 44:650–655

Schindera ST, Diedrichsen L, Muller HC, Rusch O, Marin D, Schmidt B, Raupach R, Vock P, Szucs-Farkas Z (2011) Iterative reconstruction algorithm for abdominal multidetector CT at different tube voltages: assessment of diagnostic accuracy, image quality, and radiation dose in a phantom study. Radiology 260:454–462

Seo H, Lee KH, Kim HJ, Kim K, Kang SB, Kim SY, Kim YH (2009) Diagnosis of acute appendicitis with sliding slab ray-sum interpretation of low-dose unenhanced CT and standard-dose i.v. contrast-enhanced CT scans. Am J Roentgenol 193:96–105

Shrimpton PC, Hillier MC, Lewis MA, Dunn M (2005) Doses from computed tomography (CT) examinations in the UK—2003 review. Chilton, NRPB-W67. http://www.hpa.org.uk/Publications/Radiation/NPRBArchive/NRPBWSeriesReports/2005nrpbw067/. Accessed June 2011

Shrimpton PC, Hillier MC, Lewis MA, Dunn M (2006) National survey of doses from CT in the UK: 2003. Br J Radiol 79:968–980

Singh S, Kalra MK, Hsieh J, Licato PE, Do S, Pien HH, Blake MA (2010) Abdominal CT: comparison of adaptive statistical iterative and filtered back projection reconstruction techniques. Radiology 257:373–383

Smith RC, Rosenfield AT, Choe KA, Essenmacher KR, Verga M, Glickman MG, Lange RC (1995) Acute flank pain: comparison of non-contrast-enhanced CT and intravenous urography. Radiology 194:789–794

Sourtzis S, Thibeau JF, Damry N, Raslan A, Vandendris M, Bellemans M (1999) Radiologic investigation of renal colic: unenhanced helical CT compared with excretory urography. Am J Roentgenol 172:1491–1494

Tack D, Gevenois PA (2009) Body MDCT at 140 kV. Am J Roentgenol 192:W139–W140

Tack D, Sourtzis S, Delpierre I, De Maertelaer V, Gevenois PA (2003) Low-dose unenhanced multidetector CT of patients with suspected renal colic. Am J Roentgenol 180:305–311

Tack D, Bohy P, Perlot I, De Maertelaer V, Alkeilani O, Sourtzis S, Gevenois PA (2005) Suspected acute colon diverticulitis: imaging with low-dose unenhanced multidetector row CT. Radiology 237:189–196

van Gelder RE, Venema HW, Serlie IW, Nio CY, Determann RM, Tipker CA, Vos FM, Glas AS, Bartelsman JF, Bossuyt PM, Lameris JS, Stoker J (2002) CT colonography at different radiation dose levels: feasibility of dose reduction. Radiology 224:25–33

van Gelder RE, Venema HW, Florie J, Nio CY, Serlie IW, Schutter MP, van Rijn JC, Vos FM, Glas AS, Bossuyt PM, Bartelsman JF, Lameris JS, Stoker J (2004) CT colonography: feasibility of substantial dose reduction—comparison of medium to very low doses in identical patients. Radiology 232:611–620

Wintersperger B, Jakobs T, Herzog P, Schaller S, Nikolaou K, Suess C, Weber C, Reiser M, Becker C (2005) Aorto-iliac multidetector-row CT angiography with low kV settings: improved vessel enhancement and simultaneous reduction of radiation dose. Eur Radiol 15:334–341

Wise SW, Labuski MR, Kasales CJ, Blebea JS, Meilstrup JW, Holley GP, LaRusso SA, Holliman J, Ruggiero FM, Mauger D (2001) Comparative assessment of CT and sonographic techniques for appendiceal imaging. Am J Roentgenol 176:933–941

Yamamura J, Tornquist K, Buchert R, Wildberger J, Nagel HD, Dichtl D, Adam G, Wedegartner U (2010) Simulated low-dose computed tomography in oncological patients: a feasibility study. J Comput Assist Tomogr 34:302–308

Yanaga Y, Awai K, Funama Y, Nakaura T, Hirai T, Roux S, Yamashita Y (2009) Low-dose MDCT urography: feasibility study of low-tube-voltage technique and adaptive noise reduction filter. Am J Roentgenol 193:W220–W229

# Radiation Dose Optimisation of Cardiac and Vascular MDCT in Adults and Paediatric Patients

Jean François Paul, Caroline Keyzer, Michelle Williams, and Denis Tack

## Contents



J. F. Paul
Department of Radiology,
Marie Lannelongue Surgical Centre,
Plessis-Robinson, France

C. Keyzer
Department of Radiology,
Hôpital Erasme, Université libre de Bruxelles,
Route de Lennik 808,
B 1070 Brussels, Belgium

M. Williams
University of Edinburgh/British Heart Foundation Centre for Cardiovascular Science, Chancellor's Building, 49 Little France Crescent, EH16SU4 Edinburgh, UK

D. Tack (✉)
Department of Radiology,
RHMS Clinique Louis Caty, Rue Louis Caty 136,
B 7331 Baudour, Belgium
e-mail: denis.tack@skynet.be

**Abstract**

CT Angiography (CTA) is now able to provide excellent vascular diagnosis on almost all vessels larger than 1 or 2 mm, including the coronary arteries. The radiation dose from such examinations is of concern because it may be as high as 30 mSv for cardiac CTA (CCTA). Strategies for optimising the radiation dose from CTA and CCTA are various and include the recent developments of new technologies, new software solutions, prospective ECG triggering, strict control of the heart rate, low-tube potential, tube current modulation, adaptive shielding and organ protection device. Effective dose is widely quoted in the literature but the methods used in its calculation are often inadequately documented, and poorly understood. The most common method used to calculate effective dose involves the multiplication of dose length product (DLP) by a conversion factor. However, if a different conversion factor is used this can

D. Tack et al. (eds.), *Radiation Dose from Multidetector CT*, Medical Radiology. Diagnostic Imaging,
DOI: 10.1007/174_2011_509, 

lead to dramatic differences in the effective dose that is presented. The most common conversion factors used are the "chest" CT conversion factors published by the European Commission (0.014 or 0.017). However, these conversion factors do not take into account the 2007 changes in the ICRP tissue weighting factors and underestimate effective dose. Scanner-specific conversion factors have been calculated but are rarely used in the published literature. Here we discuss the factors required to select an appropriate conversion factor in CCTA and the importance of quoting dose length product, conversion factor and effective dose.

**Abbreviations**

| | |
|---|---|
| ASIR | Adaptative statistical iterative reconstruction |
| AEC | Automatic exposure control |
| BMI | Body mass index |
| CNR | Contrast-to-noise ratio |
| CCTA | Cardiac CT angiography |
| CTA | CT angiography |
| CTDI | Computed tomography dose index |
| CTDIvol | CTDI volume |
| CTDIw | Weighted CTDI |
| DE-DS CT | Dual-energy-dual-source CT |
| DLP | Dose length product |
| DSA | Digital subtraction angiography |
| EVAR | Endovascular aneurysm repair |
| FBP | Filtered back projection |
| MDCT | Multi-detector row CT |
| PAOD | Peripheral aortic occlusive disease |
| SNR | Signal-to-noise ratio |
| 1 mm-CT | Image of the abdomen and pelvis |

# 1 Cardiac CT Angiography

## 1.1 CCTA in Adults

### 1.1.1 Introduction

Cardiac CT has acquired the reputation of being a technique involving high radiation doses, particularly following reports of a somewhat disturbing nature (Einstein et al. 2007). With a first-generation 64-slice scanner, the radiation dose is actually between 20 and 30 millisieverts (mSv), depending on the scanner specification and, above all, the usual practices of the technicians (Hausleiter et al. 2009; Huda et al. 2011). The long-term risk of cancer induced by X-rays varies according to the age and sex, and is considered to amount to substantial levels in women under the age of 40 (Einstein et al. 2007). This issue therefore attracts attention and consequently detracts from the non-invasive nature of cardiac CT. If the mean radiation dose is considered to be 15 mSv, this looks to be 2–3 times higher than exposure during coronary angiography but is nevertheless much lower than the fatal risk of the catheterism and than the radiation risk from a thallium scan (30 mSv). In addition, the risk from cardiac CT angiography (CCTA) needs to be put in perspective, by pointing out that it is extrapolated from high level radiation received by atomic bomb survivors, a whole-body exposure that was of a very different nature than that of targeted exposure during medical imaging. The basics of the linear no-threshold model for carcinogenesis and of the DNA double-strand breaks induced by X-rays at low-doses is detailed in Chap. 3 by Chadwick and Leenhouts.

A critical review of the linear no-threshold model (LNT) of carcinogenesis has been addressed by the French Academy of Medicine, as it probably overestimates the true risk. It is worth remembering that no cases of cancer have been definitively attributable to date to diagnostic use of computed tomography (Tubiana 2005). In addition, numerous researches and arguments exist against the linear no-threshold model and even in favour of a protective effect of low-level radiation known as hormesis. These arguments are addressed in Chap. 3 by Cohen. As there is no definite proof of the superiority of one theory on the other (LNT versus hormesis), according to the precautionary principle, radioprotection in the field of medical diagnoses has to be conservative and reduce the radiation level as low as reasonably achievable (ALARA).

Radiation protection has become the leading objective of new developments in CT, and these have been of particular importance for CCTA in the past 5 years. The dose of a CCTA delivered by a 64-detector-row scanner ranged between 8 and 30 mSv and could since be reduced to less than 1 mSv in adults by prospective scanning (Hausleiter et al. 2009), tube

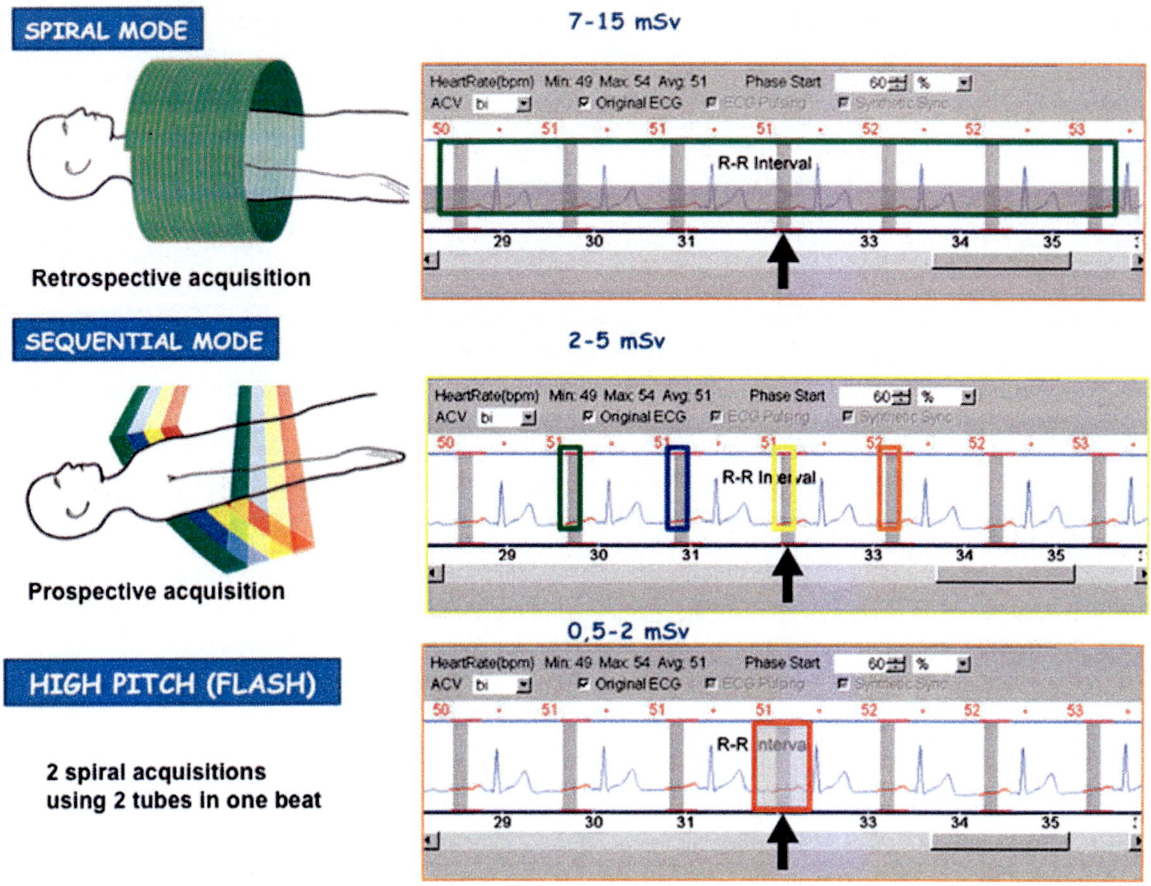


**Fig. 1** Graphic representation of various acquisition modes in ECG-triggered Cardiac CTA. **a** In retrospective mode, exposure time is continuous (*green area*) responsible for high radiation dose. **b** In sequential prospective mode, exposure time in shorter (*green + blue + yellow + orange areas*), responsible for substantially lower radiation dose. **c** Exposition time is even lower in Flash mode (*red area*), due to one beat acquisition

potential adaptations, heart rate control and denoising reconstructions (iterative) algorithms. The first part of this chapter will describe the main techniques for reducing the dose during cardiac CT in adults and children with congenital heart disease.

### 1.1.2 Acquisition in Helical Retrospective Mode

All cardiac CT scanners need to be synchronised with the ECG signal so as to target image acquisition to the different phases of the cardiac cycle, avoiding motion artefacts as much as possible by selecting the phase during which the heart is immobile (Fig. 1). Helical retrospective acquisition involves delivering X-rays throughout the cardiac cycle, whereas the only used the information is that obtained during the phase in which the heart is not moving, usually the diastolic phase. Retrospective acquisition has been the first mode used by MDCT for CCTA on the earliest scanners, four and sixteen detector-row scanners. This mode is associated with the highest radiation dose (Hausleiter et al. 2009). Two main reasons explain the high dose level of CCTA in helical retrospective mode: a low pitch and a continuous radiation exposure, resulting in a long duration of X-ray delivery.

#### 1.1.2.1 Low Pitch

Pitch is defined as the ratio of table feed to detector width. In non-cardiac helical CT, pitch is usually around 1:1. Retrospective cardiac CT generally uses a very low pitch of 0.2 because one needs to acquire sufficient data for each phase of the cardiac cycle. Radiation is delivered at each point in the cardiac cycle so that there are no missing data for an anatomical region at a given cycle time. The very slow table feed results in a prolonged exposure time and thus a higher radiation dose. It is important to point out that on some scanners, pitch may vary according to heart rate (increasing at high heart rates) and the radiation dose then decreases in proportion to the increase in pitch (Paul and Abada 2007).

#### 1.1.2.2 Continuous Acquisition

Uninterrupted, continuous acquisition is the second main reason for the high radiation dose delivered in the retrospective acquisition mode: X-rays are delivered throughout the cardiac cycle whereas the image is reconstructed solely from the phase in which the coronary arteries are fixed, usually in mid-diastole at 60 beat per minute (BPM) cardiac rhythm, or also in end-systole at higher cardiac rhythms (Adler et al. 2010). In the continuous acquisition mode, the useful radiation that is the one used in reconstruction of the CCTA image represents approximately 20% of the total delivered radiation dose only (Paul and Abada 2007).

#### 1.1.2.3 Dose Reduction in the Retrospective Mode: Tube Current Modulation

The main tool for reducing the dose in CCTA in retrospective acquisition mode is to modulate the tube current–time product (expressed in mAs) during the systolic phase, based on the ECG since this phase does not provide diagnostic CCTA images because of its motion artefacts. In practice, if the heart rate is low [<65 beats per minute (BPM)] and regular, the optimum phase is likely to be the mid-diastolic phase, usually at 70–75% of the R–R interval. Thus, the maximum tube current can be restricted to this part of the cycle time and centred at 70–75% of the R–R interval. If the heart rate is higher, the most likely best phase for reconstruction is the end-systolic phase, usually at 40% of the R–R interval (Adler et al. 2010). The maximum tube current period is then prolonged from 40 to 75% of the cardiac cycle, reducing consequently the period of down-modulation of the tube current. The increase in the duration of high tube current at high heart rates not only provides images at both end-systole and end-diastole, but does also increase radiation dose to the patient. It is thus important to optimise the radiation dose by controlling and reducing the heart rate using beta-blockers, a safe procedure if taking into account the recommendations, contraindications (COPD patients) and drug interactions (Torres et al. 2011). The magnitude of dose reduction using ECG-current modulation may vary upon manufacturers. Generally, low-dose phase current is set at 20% of the nominal tube current. Use of ECG-guided mAs modulation with 80% nominal tube current reduction allows a global dose reduction of up to 50% in helical retrospective mode. One of the scanner vendors enables reducing the tube current to 4% of its nominal value, enabling an overall dose reduction by the tube current modulation up to 65% (MinDose—Siemens, Forchheim, Germany) (Pflederer et al. 2010). A drawback of tube current modulation in the R–R interval is the occurrence of arrhythmia because there is a risk that the reconstruction zones differ from one heart cycle to the other, with subsequent motion artefacts. Manual corrections of the reconstruction zones in the R–R interval enable to reduce such artefacts but these are limited to the high exposure period (Cademartiri et al. 2006). Since 2009, all CT manufacturers have provided automatic detection of arrhythmia and immediate prolonged high exposure by disabling the tube current modulation following the arrhythmia. This dose-saving method is effective and would appear to be usable in over 80% of retrospective ECG-triggered CCTA (Paul and Abada 2007).

### 1.1.3 Acquisition in Prospective Mode

Prospective CCTA acquisition mode refers to a mode in which the acquisition is triggered by the ECG signal. The user selects the phase to acquire the images (usually diastole). The related X-ray delivery time is short, approximately 20–25% of the cardiac cycle, and the entire X-ray emission period is used for image reconstruction. Since the absorbed dose of radiation is directly proportional to exposure duration, the dose is reduced by up to 75% as compared to the retrospective mode while the CCTA image quality is preserved (Arnoldi et al. 2009; Shuman et al. 2008).

#### 1.1.3.1 Sequential Prospective Mode: Step-and Shoot-Mode

In sequential prospective mode, also called step-and-shoot mode, the table is fixed during X-ray emission and moves to the next position between two emissions. The number of emission needed to cover the heart that is of approximately 12 cm in height depends on the X-ray beam width. Typically, a $64 \times 0.6$ mm detector array has a width of 40 mm.

The heart may be entirely visualised in three or in four acquisitions. It is to note that with the ICT scanner from Philips, the array has a width of 8 cm (128 × 0.6 mm). With this scanner, the Step-and-Shoot mode can be achieved in two acquisitions. Moreover, using the "Aquilion One" scanner from Toshiba, equipped with a 320 × 0.5 mm detector array of 16 cm width, the entire heart can be acquired in one single rotation, and one heart cycle. In the Step-and-Shoot mode, the emitted radiation is almost entirely used to create an image and, unlike in the retrospective mode, there is no radiation wastage. This mode is characterised by a reduced exposure time as shown in Fig. 1. Compared to the retrospective mode, the exposure time and the dose are reduced by a factor of 4–5 at constant mAs and kVp. Image quality is identical (Efstathopoulos et al. 2009; Blankstein et al. 2009) or even slightly better than that of images provided by the helical retrospective mode (Earls et al. 2008) there is no raw-data interpolation in sequential mode, unlike in helical mode. However, prospective acquisition has one major drawback. It only allows reconstruction of a single phase of the cardiac cycle and therefore provides no information on cardiac dynamics. On the other hand, the ideal phase for reconstruction without movement artefacts needs to be predicted. These requirements explain why the step-and-shoot mode is currently only recommended on single-source scanners with regular heart rates lower than 62 bpm (Earls 2009; Buechel et al. 2011). Using a dual-source scanner (DSCT), the heart rate threshold of 62 bpm can be adjusted to 70 bpm (Sun et al. 2011), thanks to the improved, in agreement with our experience. Arrhythmia contra-indicates the step-and-shoot mode because it is then impossible to predict the appropriate phase for reconstruction. Radiation exposure during cardiac CT in prospective mode varies from 3 to 5 mSv depending on the study, a dose that is lower on average than that reported for coronary angiography (6 mSv) (Blankstein et al. 2009). Prospectively ECG-triggered CCTA images are acquired during a window in diastole. Additional surrounding X-ray beam on time, or padding, is available on some newly developed scanners, can be variably set and the increased padding results in additional available phases for analysis. It is to note that re-radiation dose is linearly increased with the duration of padding. LaBounty et al. (2010) investigated the need and benefit of padding in a prospective multicentre trial. These authors found that with excellent heart rate control, the use of minimal padding was associated with a substantial reduction in radiation dose with preserved image interpretability.

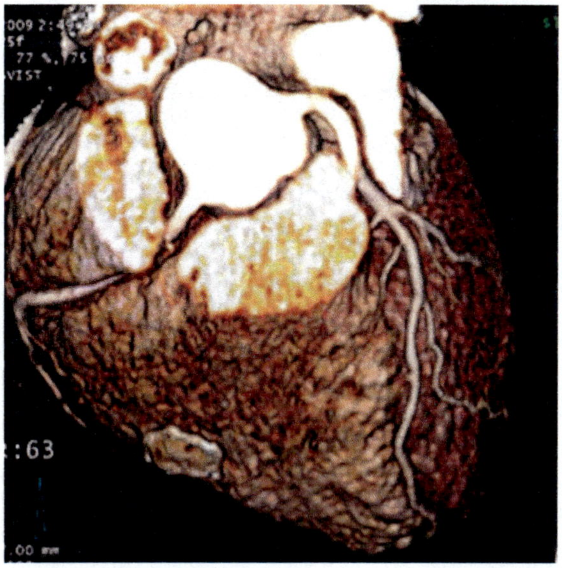


**Fig. 2** 3D VRT representation of a cardiac acquisition in adult patient in flash mode with Pitch 3.2. The coronary arteries were found normal. The tube potential was set at 100 kV and the resulting DLP was 29 mGy.cm

#### 1.1.3.2 High-Pitch Prospective Helical Mode

One particular prospective method is the new high-pitch mode (flash), available on DSCT from Siemens since 2009 and consisting in an ECG-triggered prospective helical mode (Figs. 1, 2). As the entire heart can be covered within 300 ms, the acquisition is obtained during one single heart cycle as it is in the sequential mode with the "Acquillion One" scanner from Toshiba. An image set of the fixed heart is obtained during the diastole, provided a controlled low heart rate of <60 bpm. This latest method would appear to deliver the least radiation of all, with a mean radiation dose below 1 mSv (Achenbach et al. 2010), which is much lower than with all other cardiac imaging techniques using ionising radiation. In a prospective multicentre study, submillisievert CCTA could however only be achieved in standard-sized patients (70–75 kg) with low heart rates (Neefjes et al. 2011). In our experience, however, it requires a very slow heart rate (less than 60 bpm), usually obtained after treatment with beta-blockers. Its very low radiation dose makes it a technique that appears to be highly suitable for screening of coronary lesions in patients who have few, if any, symptoms but are at risk of such lesions.

### 1.1.4 Adjustment of Tube Parameters

#### 1.1.4.1 Tube Potential and Tube Current–Time Product

With preserved and constant image quality, it is now well known that the dose requirements strongly depend on the patients weight or diameter. As an example, a difference of 5 cm in diameter between two patients allows the dose to be reduced by half, without any loss of image quality. The adequate adjustment of the dose in relationship to image quality is thus an important independent factor of radiation dose optimisation of CCTA. Noise is one of the main factors for the perception of image quality. A comprehensive approach to all parameters that influence the image and its quality can be found in "Image Quality in CT: Challenges and Perspectives" by Toth. The level of acceptable noise depends on the radiologist's perception and experience, and we are lacking of guidelines and reference or recommendations. Nevertheless, whoever is performing CCTA examinations is responsible for the adequate selection of tube parameters as they substantially influence the radiation dose. Practically, the dose can be reduced as long as diagnosis is not compromised, and adapted to the patient's body size. As for other CT examinations, default protocols set by the manufacturers are not optimised and may be reduced.

#### 1.1.4.2 Tube Current

On most scanners, the tube current is adapted to the absorption measured from the scout views. Optimisation of the tube current thus consists on adjusting the image quality parameter of the scanner. This parameter is expressed as the "Quality Reference mAs" with Siemens Scanners and, in mAs on the Philips scanner, and as noise index on GE and Toshiba scanners. A comprehensive approach of tube current modulation and its practical application can be found in "Automatic Exposure Control in Multidetector-Row Computed Tomography" by Kalra, and in "ALARA concept for MDCT Optimization: what is reasonable, what is achievable?" by Tack. As a general rule it is not recommended to switch the tube current modulation system off. However, for those who prefer to choose the tube current by themselves, is it possible to determine default mAs settings according to the body weight or to the body mass index. This approach requires, however, the radiographer to be trained in setting up these mAs parameters according to the patient's weight. Adjustment of mAs allows even finer tuning. Optimisation of mAs is dependent on each individual scanner's controls. They can be gradually adjusted as technicians learn from experience (Jung et al. 2003). Adapting radiation settings according to the patient's body mass index (BMI) for coronary CT angiography is relevant (Tatsugami et al. 2009) but may be not optimal because thoracic fat distribution may differ in patients with the same BMI. A pre-contrast image is routinely used to manage contrast delivery in coronary CT, and the noise level of this initial image directly reflects individual X-ray attenuation of the thorax in each patient. It might help selecting appropriate settings, as investigated on a standard 64-slice CT (Paul 2011).

#### 1.1.4.3 Tube Potential

The choice of the correct tube potential is more important for CCTA optimisation than the choice of a noise index. Judicious adjustment of KV is a very effective way of reducing the dose, as the radiation dose is proportional to the square of the kilovoltage. Acquisition at 100 kVp therefore reduces the dose by about a third, at equal mAs, compared with 120 kVp and acquisition at 80 kVp reduces the dose by two-thirds. 100 kVp is usually sufficient for a patient weighing less than 70–75 kg or even up to 80–90 kg if the patient is slim (Sigal-Cinqualbre et al. 2004). Likewise in our experience, 80 kVp is sufficient for most patients weighing less than 60 kg (and consequently for children) (Abada et al. 2006). A low kilovoltage also allows increased contrast attenuation as a result of a better photoelectric effect. This also means that it is possible to reduce the iodine delivery rate needed to obtain good vascular enhancement. This is of importance in particular in patients with impaired renal function or those in whom venous access is difficult (Sigal-Cinqualbre et al. 2004).

#### 1.1.4.4 Breast Shielding and Displacement

According to Foley et al. (2011) the use of a displacement device to avoid direct irradiation of the breast when scanning the heart has been tested with and without adjunction of lead strips on the breast during CCTA. The largest reduction in breast dose surface was obtained with both the displacement device and the lead strip. In addition to the dose reduction to the breast, if the breast is displaced, the mAs applied to the heart can be lowered as well, without impact on image quality or maintained while there will be an improvement of image quality.

#### 1.1.4.5 Coverage in the *z*-Axis

Since the radiation dose is directly proportional to the length of the region exposed to radiation, it is important to adjust the region to be covered to the bare essential (Hausleiter et al. 2006). As a first step, the frontal scout image allows adjustment of the necessary coverage (from the carina to the base of heart). On the frontal scout view, however, the base of the heart may be difficult to locate. This may be solved by a lateral scout view that is not proposed as default on Philips and Siemens scanners but is proposed on the GE and Toshiba systems. The lateral scout view allows a precise location of the inferior aspect of the heart. This is all the more important in which acquisition cannot be stopped once it is in progress with some scanners. It avoids wasted scans where the base of the heart has been cut off, necessitating redo examinations with further radiation exposure and consequently an excessive dose overall. On the other hand, exposure would also be excessive and futile if the scan was to be continued way beyond the heart along the upper abdomen. It should also be pointed out that some very slim patients may have a verticalised heart. In this case, acquisition may start below the carina. An alternative method to the lateral scout view for locating the level of the heart apex is to perform a low-dose calcium scoring. Adjustment of the scan length of CCTA using the images from calcium scoring instead of the scout view is feasible and is associated with a 16% reduction in radiation dose of dual-source CT coronary angiography as reported by Leschka et al. (2010).

### 1.1.5 Iodine Contrast and Dose Optimisation in CCTA

Limitation of radiation exposure during cardiac CT to an ALARA level, while preserving good diagnostic image quality, is mainly dependent on the CT scanner, and on patient's habitus, with some variations according to local radiological practices. Moving heart artefacts are the most determinant of image quality in CCTA. However, contrast-to-noise ratio (CNR) optimization is also of great importance whereas it is somewhat unclear how exactly to optimize it. Contrast level directly influences evaluation of both the lumen and coronary wall. For example, insufficient contrast in the coronary lumen may impair detection of a lesion, and a minimal threshold of 326 Hounsfield units (HU) has been proposed to improve diagnostic accuracy (Cademartiri et al. 2008). However, contrast can also be used as a radioprotection tool. High arterial contrast improves the contrast-to-noise ratio and consequently allows a rise in the "acceptable" noise level threshold for analysis of the coronary system. In CT angiography, for a given tube potential, enhancement is determined by the iodine delivery rate (expressed in grams of iodine per second). The iodine delivery rate is (expressed in mg/s) equal to the iodine concentration of the contrast agent (in mg of iodine per ml) multiplied by the flow rate of the contrast agent (in ml/second). High iodine concentrations and fast injection rates are therefore two levers of vascular enhancement and contrast. If the injection rate is limited by the state of the patient's veins, one can compensate by an increase in iodine concentration in order to maintain the iodine delivery rate. As an example, a concentration of 400 mg/ml allows a reduction of approximately 25% in the injection rate as compared to 300 mg/ml.

### 1.1.6 Iterative Reconstructions

Iterative reconstructions have been recently introduced in the CT technology. This new method for reconstructions of image may substantially reduce noise in images compared to the filtered back projections commonly used to create images form raw data of the CT machines. All main manufacturers have developed these methods claiming its potential for dose reduction. A comprehensive review of the iterative reconstruction techniques and of the related medical literature can be found in "Image Noise Reduction Filters" by Singh et al. Iterative reconstruction technique consists in reducing the image noise. The potential of such denoising algorithms to effectively reduce image noise is no more to demonstrate. However, one should be cautious with its practical application in clinical settings because noise is from far not the unique indicator image quality and image quality is from far not the best warranty for an accurate diagnosis. Studies with endpoint of

**Table 1** Dose from cardiac CTA in adults, according to technical developpments and optimisation methods

| Year of publication | Publication | Study design | Acquisition mode | Tube potential vs heart rate | DLP (mGy.cm) | E (mSv)[a] | Scanner model |
|---|---|---|---|---|---|---|---|
| 2007 | Einstein et al. (2007) | Monte Carlo simulations | Retrospective helical | 120 kV | NA | 20 (6–139) | Siemens 64 [b] |
| 2009 | Hausleiter et al. (2009) | Multicentre observational study | Retrospective helical (>90%) | 120 kV (>90%) | 865 (568–1,259) | 12 | All manufacturers pooled together |
| | | | Helical 77% sequential 23% | 120 kV (>96%) | 1369 (814–1,644) | 19 (11–23) | GE 64 |
| | | | Helical 91% sequential 9% | 120 kV (100%) | 707 (535–913) | 10 (7–13) | Philips 64 |
| | | | Helical 100% | 120 kV (100%) | 622 (522–1,013) | 11 (8–14) | Siemens 64[b] |
| | | | Helical 100% | 120 kV (100%) | 1, 039 (808–1291) | 15 (11–18) | Toshiba 64 |
| 2011 | Fink C et al. (2011a) | Phantom study (averages size—70 kg) | Retrospective Helical | 120 kV | 239 | 5.7 | Siemens definition 64 (single source AS + 128) |
| | | | | 100 kV | 145 | 3.5 | |
| | | | Prospective step and shoot | 120 kV | 166 | 4.0 | |
| | | | | 100 kV | 123 | 3.0 | |
| | | | Retrospective helical | 120 kV | 523 | 9.4 | Siemens definition flasch (dual source) |
| | | | | 100 kV | 296 | 5.3 | |
| | | | Prospective step and shoot | 120 kV | 120 | 5.4 | |
| | | | | 100 kV | 123 | 3.8 | |
| | | | Prospective flash (high pitch) | 120 kV | 136 | 2.5 | |
| | | | | 100 kV | 74 | 1.3 | |
| | | Patient study | Retrospective helical | 120 kV | 554 | 10.0 | |
| | | | | 100 kV | 413 | 7.5 | |
| | | | Prospective step and shoot | 120 kV | 412 | 7.9 | |
| | | | | 100 kV | 279 | 5.5 | |
| | | | Prospective flash (high pitch) | 120 kV | 115 | 2.1 | |
| | | | | 100 kV | 70 | 1.3 | |
| 2011 | Lee et al. (2011) | Patient study | Retrospective | Heart Rate >65 bpm | NA | 22.7 | Toshiba acquillion one |
| | | | Prospective | | NA | 7.3 | |
| | | | Retrospective | Heart Rate <65 bpm | NA | 13.6 | |
| | | | Prospective | | NA | 5.7 | |
| | | | Prospective, using 16 cm beam width (320 × 0.6 mm) | 1 beat/ scan | NA | 9.4 | |
| | | | | 2 beats/ scan | NA | 22.6 | |
| | | | | 3 beats/ scan | NA | 31.25 | |

*Note* [a] Conversion factor used is 0.014 mSv/mGy.cm. According to our recent review of litterature in part 2 of the present chapter, this factor is probably underestimated by a factor of 2–2.5
[b] Single source scanner only
*Abreviations E* effective dose, *DLP* dose length product, *TCM* tube current modulation, *MinDose* TMC at 6% of nominal mAs, *bpm* beats per minute

diagnostic performance are still needed for validating denoising algorithms in clinical settings. In our recent experience of iterative reconstructions in CCTA, it seems that some degree of iterative reconstruction may indeed be useful to improve image quality as compared to filtered back projection at the same radiation level. Indirectly, iterative reconstruction may be thus a tool to lower the radiation dose necessary to achieve the minimal quality level for diagnosis in the future.

### 1.1.7 Summary of Radiation Dose Issue in Adult CCTA

Radiation dose in CCTA strongly depends on the CT technology and latest technological developments. As shown in Table 1, a reduction in DLP from 2,000 to 400 mGy cm can be expected between the 64-detector-row scanners built in 2005 and the actual 2012-scanner generation by scanning in prospective mode. The second most important factor for dose optimisation consists in obtaining the lowest possible heart rate (preferably below 65 bpm). The third determinant factor of dose optimisation is the adequate choice of the tube potential, preferably at 100 kV or even at 80 kV. The acquisition height will also be considered for optimisation, either by adding a lateral scout view (with those scanners that do not require it) or by performing a low-dose calcium score CT (at 20–30 mGy cm). Finally, one should consider displacement devices for the breast, with adjunction of lead shields. Iterative reconstruction could help obtaining further dose reductions, but this has still to be confirmed in prospective clinical studies.

## 1.2 Paediatric Cardiac CTA in Congenital Heart Disease

For the clinical management of patients with complex congenital heart disease (CHD), three-dimensional (3D) accurate evaluation of their morphologic conditions is critical. Three-dimensional imaging should demonstrate the shape and spatial relationships of the great arteries, proximal branch pulmonary arteries and anomalous pulmonary venous or systemic connections and if possible the proximal anatomy of coronary arteries. The 3D extra-cardiac morphologic characteristics may determine the choice and nature of any surgical intervention. Echocardiography is always the first-line imaging modality for CHD patients, due to its simplicity, repeatability and absence of complications. This modality is well established as very effective at describing intra-cardiac anatomy, in real-time mode providing exquisite depiction of cardiac chambers and valves.

In the past ten years, however, multi-detector CT has been proposed as a complementary tool for 3D anatomical visualisation in patients with congenital heart disease. It is increasingly used in many institutions (Gilkeson et al. 2003). MDCT technology, including most recently dual- source CT, provides a volumetric acquisition in a short amount of time, enabling to obtain high quality 3D vascular imaging in neonates. The very short acquisition time of MDCT CCTA has drastically reduced the respiratory artefacts. Cardiac motion may be at least partially resolved by ECG triggering even in babies with very high heart rates. In our paediatric cardiac surgical centre, specialising in CHD, MDCT has become an important complementary imaging technique to US for pre- or post-operative management of children.

### 1.2.1 Non-ECG-Gated Acquisitions

Images of extra-cardiac structures are less sensitive to cardiac motion than the heart itself. ECG-gating may thus be unnecessary for diagnostic purposes, when the clinical question involves extra-cardiac anatomy while in practice, intra-cardiac anatomy is provided by US. Respiratory artefacts are potentially responsible for the most substantial artefacts, that are much more important that those due to cardiac motion. Generally non-ECG-gated acquisitions are acquired faster than ECG-gated acquisitions, thus they might be preferred as the first choice techniques in neonates with CHD. However, new CT scanners with large detector arrays provide very fast ECG-gated acquisitions (ICT 256, Philips, and Acquillion One, Tosgiba).

### 1.2.2 ECG-Gated Acquisitions

When precise visualisation of the coronary artery tree is required, an ECG-gated acquisition may be attempted to improve coronary artery delineation and image quality (Tsai et al. 2007). It is to note that the heart rates in babies are as high as 120 bpm or above. In our experience, CCTA in babies is achievable using MDCT with at least 64-detector-rows, and a temporal resolution of maximum 165 ms. Previous MDCT scanners anterior to 2005 could not reach this performance.

### 1.2.3 Protocols with DSCT

Thanks to improved temporal resolution <100 ms, DSCT has made coronary imaging possible in babies on a routine basis, preferably in the systolic phase because of the high heart rate. This improvement has important clinical implications since CCTA can replace angiography in babies with Tetralogy of Fallot, provide high quality images and reliable 3D depiction of coronary artery course, and can rule out possible coronary anomalies before surgery (Vastel-Amzallag et al. 2011).

#### 1.2.3.1 Retrospective Spiral ECG-Gated Mode

Retrospective gating has been shown to significantly improve coronary visualisation in CHD babies. In a previous full CHD anatomy evaluation strategy, a combination of two acquisitions has been shown to be effective (spiral thoracic scan and ECG-gated cardiac scan) (Ben Saad et al. 2009). The mean radiation dose was 1.8 mSv for both acquisitions, and contrast medium re-injection was required.

#### 1.2.3.2 Prospective Gating Step-and-Shoot

Most studies using prospective gating were conducted successfully in adult patients with stable heart rate, <65 or 70 beats per min. When the heart rate increases beyond this threshold, the diastolic low motion temporal window decreases, with a substantial risk of fuzzy images of the heart. Diastolic acquisition is thus not adapted to high rates that are found in babies, especially in CHD children. Beta-blockers may be insufficient or dangerous in children with CHD. On the other hand, ECG-prospective thoracic DSCT acquisition with systolic acquisition provides excellent thoracic and coronary image quality in babies and infants with CHD, without limitation of cardiac rhythm (Paul et al. 2011). Using the latest version of DSCT with a 4-cm detector, we now scan CHD babies using prospective step-and-shoot mode at end-systole on a routine basis. Prospective step-and-shoot mode with DSCT is appearing to be an interesting alternative to spiral acquisition modes, and may be recommended as a "one-stop-shop" acquisition. The radiation dose is very low (0.26 mSv) using appropriate settings: 80 kVp and 10 mAs/kg up to 6 kg (Fig. 3). This new strategy of acquisition allows a radiation dose reduction of 85% as compared to a previously used two-phase low-dose protocol from our institution when coronary evaluation was

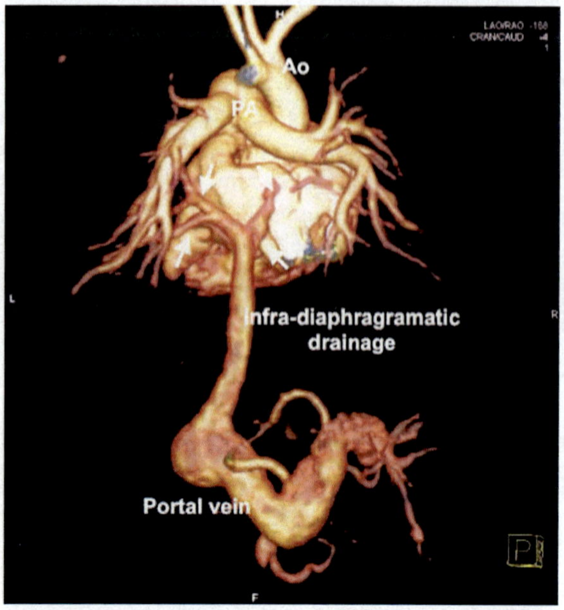


**Fig. 3** 3D-VRT posterior view of a complex malformation of the pulmonary venous drainage into the hepatic and portal veins in a 4.6 kg baby (total infra-diaphragmatic pulmonary venous return). The acquisition is ECG-triggered using sequential mode, at end-systole. The tube potential is set at 80 kV, with 46 mAs. The resulting DLP was 6 mGy.cm

required, making CT safer for these very young children (Ben Saad et al. 2009; Paul et al. 2011). Of note, this prospective ECG-gated protocol is associated with lower radiation dose than those associated with a single spiral thorax CT (0.5 mSv).

Acquisition in prospective mode may be slower than in spiral mode, depending on the number of shoots needed to cover the thorax of a baby. With a 4-cm large detector, only two shots are required to scan the entire thorax of a baby, with a mean acquisition time of 1.3 s. Four X-ray shoots are required using a 2-cm large detector used in the first version of DSCT, responsible for longer acquisition time. Using 2-cm large detector, images acquired in a step-and-shoot mode were also more sensitive to respiratory motion.

Overall, we found that prospective ECG-gated DSCT with end-systolic reconstruction provides good or excellent images of the thorax and coronary arteries in neonates, infants and young children with CHD (Fig. 4). Prospective acquisition at end-systolic phase thus appears to be an efficient alternative to spiral acquisition modes, as it reliably visualises the coronary arteries and thoracic structures for a comprehensive anatomical evaluation.

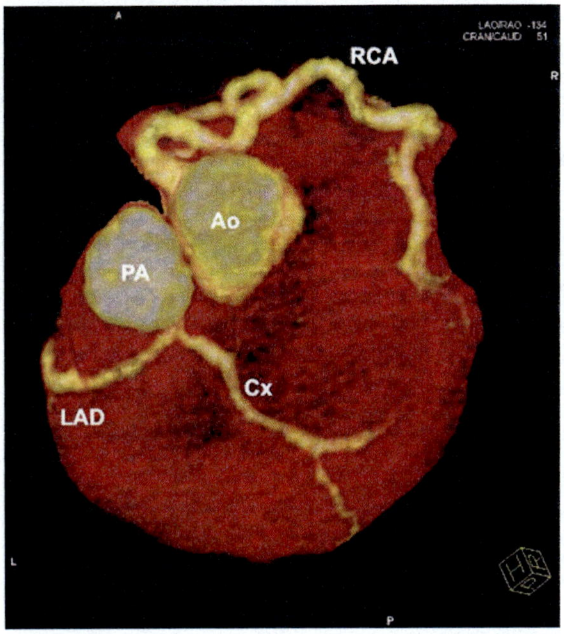


**Fig. 4** CCTA in a 7-year-old infant with anomalous left coronary artery from pulmonary artery (ALCAPA). Acquisition is achieved in sequential mode with ECG-triggering, at systolic phase to visualise coronary arteries despite high heart rate. The tube potential is set at 80 kV, with 90 mAs. The resulting DLP was 22 mGy.cm

#### 1.2.3.3 Flash Spiral Mode

This mode is designed to scan patients using a high-pitch acquisition (pitch value, 3), thanks to a combination of two helical acquisitions, each provided by one of the two tubes. This technique appears suitable to restless babies, due to very low total acquisition time of about 150 ms only for scanning eight centimetres in length.

#### 1.2.3.4 Dose Consideration in Children: New 70 kVp Setting

In our centre, we aimed to apply the ALARA principle as far as possible in neonates and babies with CHD, with the following rules:

1. Systematic use of 80 kV settings (Paul et al. 2004).
2. Adaptation of the mAs to the child's weight.
3. Only one-phase acquisition whenever possible.

Using 80 kV, we use 10 effective mAs per kg of weight up to 6 kg.

These settings are sufficient for good quality images, as far as the mAs is adjusted according to the child's weight.

We choose to link the tube current to the babie's weight. However recent studies recommend to use the body circumference instead of the body weight for fine tube current adaptation (Reid et al. 2010). Using weight-adapted protocol, radiation exposure is estimated to less than 0.5 mSv for a neonate. Half mSv is equivalent to the dose delivered by natural radiation over a 3-month period. Radiation dose due to CT acquisition is less than the radiation dose delivered during conventional angiography (Paul et al. 2010).

For further optimisation of CCTA in children, some manufacturers propose since 2011 new tube potential settings at 70 kV. This new setting is under early evaluation, and it seems to provide adequate images in our first experience in newborns and small children. It is likely to be used in a majority of newborns and could favour further decrease in radiation dose if confirmed in prospective clinical studies.

Anatomical data acquired from CT may be judiciously used to limit the number of views acquired with angiography and sometimes replace conventional angiography (Vastel-Amzallag et al. 2011; Lee et al. 2006). CT may therefore be advantageous in reducing global radiation exposure in CHD patients.

The other advantage of 70 or 80 kVp settings is the potential to reduce the amount of contrast medium required, because attenuation of iodine is more important (iodine has a high atomic number) at lower kVp settings.

### 1.2.4 Contrast Issues in Children with CHD

Contrast medium dose injection must be adapted to the baby's weight. At our institution, we currently use 2 cc per kg of Iopromide (Ultravist, Bayer-Schering Pharmceuticals, Berlin, Germany) at 300 mg/ml of concentration. We did not face any serious adverse reactions over a 10-year period with more than 1,500 contrast-enhanced examinations.

Peripheral venous access is achieved if possible in the paediatric unit. Right arm injection is preferable to avoid possible streaky artefacts on the innominate left brachio-cephalic vein. In some cases, venous connections are congenitally different or surgically modified. This information, when available, is important prior to scanning as it may change the scan injection protocol. Venous visualisation may be realised at first pass, or sometimes later, at the time of venous return. The optimal injection protocol depends on each particular venous anatomy. Catheter permeability is checked before injection. It is essential to avoid any air injection during the scan procedure. All bubbles should be removed when connecting the catheter to the power injector. Because many patients with CHD have a right-to-left shunt, air injection through venous access could cause air systemic embolism, with possible fatal consequences. Extravasation of contrast medium may occur, with an incidence of 1–2% in our centre. These rare complications were treated immediately without any consequence. The main challenge raised by CT in babies lies in the unfavourable contrast dynamics related to patient age and in some cases to impaired flow, which may lead to imaging failure.

Our contrast-related failure rate is about 10%. Imaging failure requires re-imaging and therefore increases the radiation dose and contrast agent dose. Extensive training and experience helps to overcome the difficulties raised by unfavourable contrast dynamics.

#### 1.2.5 Sedation

General anaesthesia is the exception in our experience (three cases in 10 years). In neonates we do not use any sedative drugs: some honey on a pacifier may help. In infants we recommend oral- or intra-rectal sedation (or both) before the CT procedure to prevent baby agitation during the acquisition. This can lead to poor image quality and sometimes the need for repeat examination. Sedation is not always mandatory if the baby is quiet. Experienced technologists are necessary in the CT room for good management of the babies; precise knowledge of infant management and a quiet attitude is of primary importance. With experienced technologists, the mean total examination time in the CT room is generally less than 20 min. Qualified medical monitoring may sometimes be necessary during the examination, depending on the clinical condition of the babies. In all cases, oxygen saturation should be closely monitored.

##### 1.2.5.1 Cardiac CTA: General Conclusion

Although the first generation of 64-slice cardiac scanners delivered fairly high doses of radiation, technological developments have allowed radiation exposure to be significantly reduced to levels below those for coronary angiography and also still well below those for myocardial perfusion scanning. The radiation risk is therefore reduced to an extremely low level under these conditions. This massive reduction in radiation exposure should further increase the development of coronary CT in adults and children with congenital heart disease. However, the choice of dose-reducing acquisition techniques is becoming more complex, and therefore necessitates good technical mastery of these new CT scanners.

## 2 Radiation Dose Optimization in CT Angiography for Aorta and Peripheral Vessels

### 2.1 Introduction

CT Angiography of aorta is increasingly performed not only in patients with aortic diseases but also, iteratively, in patients with endovascular aneurysm repair (EVAR). In addition, CTA of aorta and peripheral vessels is also ordered for screening patients with peripheral aortic occlusive disease (PAOD) but might also be used in younger patients with suspected arteritis, fibrodysplasia, or popliteal entrapment syndrome.

Radiation dose in CTA is of particular concern in these young patients and in patients needing lifelong follow-up CTA examinations after EVAR. Furthermore, PAOD patients undergoing CTA of aorto-iliac and lower extremity arteries are at risk of contrast material-induced nephropathy because many present with impaired renal function. As explained in this chapter, lowering radiation dose by reducing the tube voltage is susceptible to allow a reduction in both the radiation dose and the iodine contrast volume.

Finally, scanning abdominal aorta and lower extremity arteries requires taking into account two different regional body anatomies with different levels of attenuation. An important shift from a region of high attenuation (the abdomen) to a region of low attenuation (lower extremities) leads to consider that a protocol maintaining constant mAs is inappropriate regarding radiation exposure.

Therefore, in this chapter we will address the different approaches contributing to radiation saving and also contrast volume reduction. For CTA, multiple strategies for radiation dose reduction have been considered so far. These include a lowering of tube voltage, automatic exposure control (AEC) with tube current modulation, increased pitch as well as more recent approaches such as iterative reconstruction algorithm and virtual non-enhanced examinations from dual-energy CT.

## 2.2 Low-Tube Voltage

Lowering the tube voltage represents an important dose reduction approach because the radiation varies with the square of tube voltage. A 65% of radiation saving could be attempted if the tube voltage is reduced from 120 to 80 kV with constant tube current. The effect of dose reduction achieved by decreasing tube voltage is complex because it affects both image noise by a reduction of photon fluence and contrast by a reduction of the energy of the X-ray beam (Kalra et al. 2004). On the other hand, at IV-enhanced CT, a decrease in tube voltage can increase the contrast between vascular and parenchymal structures by increasing X-ray absorption by iodine, because the nearer the tube voltage approaches the K-edge of iodine (33.2 keV), the greater the inherent attenuation of the iodinated contrast material (Kalva et al. 2006; Marin et al. 2009).

Several studies have validated this technique for CT angiography characterised by a high contrast between the arterial vessels and the poorly enhanced surrounding parenchymas (Kalva et al. 2006; Sahani et al. 2007; Schindera et al. 2009; Wintersperger et al. 2005; Nakayama et al. 2005). Wintersperger et al. (2005) compared aorto-iliac CTA performed at 120 and 100 kVp with a constant tube current of 200mAs. They showed that contrast-to-noise ratio (CNR), signal-to-noise ratio (SNR) and subjective image quality were similar at 100 kVp as compared to 120 kVp examinations, finding based on the increased iodine attenuation level compensating for increased image noise. Using 100 kVp, they reduced the mean effective dose from approximately 10–6.5 mSv (see Table 2). On the other hand, Nakayama et al. (2005) showed that scanning at low-tube voltage and constant tube current (300mAs) results in degradation of SNR but not in subjective overall image quality. Dose reduction achieved by decreasing the tube voltage from 120 to 90 kVp–decreases SNR, implying that noise has a greater effect on images obtained at 90 kVp than on those at 120 kVp. Therefore, the use of low-voltage technique alone could be restricted to normal and underweight patients [< 80 kg, as reported by Nakayama et al. (2005, 2006)] or compensated by a higher tube current. In addition, Nakayama et al. (2005) reported that images are more highly enhanced when obtained with 90 kVp and an iodine volume reduced by 20% as compared to their standard protocol (120 kVp and 100 ml of contrast material), suggesting that the amount of IV contrast to be injected can be reduced when lowering tube voltage as reported by other authors (Kalva et al. 2006; Schindera et al. 2009; Nakayama et al. 2006).

Sahani et al. (2007) investigated MDCT angiography obtained at different tube potential with the use of AEC in living kidney donors. To avoid a consequent increase of mAs to maintain a constant image noise as set by the operator, they choose an upper limit on the mAs delivered by the tube. These authors showed that, despite a higher image noise, the images were still diagnostically acceptable at 100 kVp with no difference in the visibility of renal arteries and their branches when compared to 120 and 140 kVp, with a significant dose reduction Sahani et al. (2007). With the advent of high-output X-ray tubes, it is possible to apply higher tube current-time products to counterbalance greater image noise produced by low-tube voltages. Schindera et al. (2009) showed that with 80 kVp counterbalanced by an increased tube current in comparison of the examination acquired at 100 kVp but with a CTDIvol decreased by about 25%, the image quality of CTA is not compromised. Most importantly, they showed that image quality is still diagnostically acceptable with a contrast medium volume decreased to 45 ml at 80 kVp, which is of great interest in patients with impaired renal function. Manousaki et al. (2011) evaluated image quality of low-tube voltage CTA for the detection of in-stent restenosis of the renal arteries and compared images obtained at three levels of tube voltage (see Table 2). They conclude that assessment of in-stent restenosis is feasible at 100 kVp with minor loss in image quality with a radiation dose reduced by 45%. In addition, they reported that images obtained at 80 kVp are of unacceptable quality. These results are however based on ten patients only, which is a major limitation of this study, and need to be confirmed on greater patient populations. Furthermore, the body habitus of these patients is not reported in this study (Manousaki et al. 2011).

It is indeed necessary to perform studies that could help us in selecting adequate tube voltage regarding patient physiognomy with consideration of

**Table 2** Reported CT parameters and radiation dose in CTA studies

| Publication | Anatomic region | Tube potential (kVp) | Tube current (mAs) | CTDI vol (mGy)[b] | DLP (mGy.cm) | Effective dose (mSv) [c] | Scanner model |
|---|---|---|---|---|---|---|---|
| Wintersperger et al. (2005) | Abd. aorta | 120 | 200 (w/o AEC) | 15.6 | 675 ± 82 | 10.1 ± 1.2 | Sensation 16, Siemens |
| | | 100 | | 10.0 | 447 ± 30 | 6.7 ± 0.4 | |
| Nakayama et al. (2005) | Abd. aorta | 120 | 300 (w/o AEC) | 13.2[d] | NA | NA | IDT 16, Philips |
| | | 90 | | 5.7[d] | | | |
| Nakayama et al. (2006) | Abd. aorta | 120 | 260–300 (w/oAEC)[a] | 13.4–15.7 | NA | 9.85–11.76 | IDT 16, Philips |
| | | 90 | 405–485 (w/o AEC)[a] | 10.1–12.1 | | 5.90–7.15 | |
| Sahani et al. (2007) | Abd. aorta/renal artery | 140 | Max: 210mAs noise index:15 (AEC) | 25 | NA | NA | Light Speed 16, GE |
| | | 120 | | 17 | | | |
| | | 100 | | 12 | | | |
| Schindera et al. (2009) | Th-Abd. aorta | 100 | 160 (AEC) | 6.8 | 467 ± 74 | NA | Sensation 64, Siemens |
| | | 80 | 260 (AEC) | 5.2 | 358 ± 31 | | |
| Manousaki et al. (2011) | Renal artery | 120 | 160 (w/o AEC) | 12.5 | NA | NA | Sensation 16, Siemens |
| | | 100 | 124–149 (AEC) | 6.9 | | | |
| | | 80 | 98–122 (AEC) | 2.9 | | | |
| Szucs-Farkas et al. (2009) | Abd. aorta (phantom) | 120 | 160 (AEC) | 5.74–20.56[a] | NA | NA | Sensation 64, Siemens |
| | | 100 | 160 (AEC) | 3.57–11.29[a] | | | |
| | | 80 | 260 (AEC) | 2.68–5.18[a] | | | |
| Utsunomyia et al. (2010) | Abd. aorta and peripheral artery | 120 | 182–257 (AEC) | NA | 1,465 ± 209 | 8.1 ± 1.1[e] | Brilliance 64, Philips |
| | | 80 | 583 (w/o AEC) | | 1,024 ± 151 | 5.5 ± 0.9[e] | |
| Schindera et al. (2010) | Th-Abd. aorta | 80 | 260 (AEC) | 4.7–5.3 | NA | NA | Sensation 64, Siemens |
| Fraioli et al. (2006) | Abd. aorta and peripheral artery | 120 | 130 (w/o AEC) | 12.2[d] | NA | 13.7–14.8[f] | Volume Zoom, Siemens |
| | | | 100 (w/o AEC) | 9.4[d] | | 8.2–8.9[f] | |
| | | | 50 (w/o AEC) | 4.7[d] | | 3.7–4.0[f] | |
| Stolzman et al. (2008) | Abd. aorta | 120, SS 3 phases (NE, AP, DP) | 350 | 14.2 | 537.2 ± 116.9 per phase | 9.1 ± 2.0 per phase **27.4** for 3 phases | Definition, Siemens. (DE-DS) |
| | | 80/140 DS DP | 400/95 | 16.9 | 638.1 ± 137.6 | **10.9** ± 2.4 | |
| Chandarana et al. (2008) | Abd. aorta | 120, SS 3 phases (NE, AP, DP) | 200–244 (AEC) | NA | NA | **27.8** | Definition, Siemens. (DE-DS) |
| | | 80/140 DS DP | 370–480/ 56–80 | NA | NA | **11.1** | |

*Note*
[a] In function of patient's weight; in function of phantom size
[b] Reported mean values
[c] Conversion factors used depend on the studies
[d] CTDIw
[e] Estimated on the abdomen only with a conversion factor of 0.012 for the abdomen and 0.016 for the pelvis. Conversion factors for legs are not available
[f] Calculated with WinDose® (Wellhofer Dosimetry, Schwarzenbruck, Germany). Numbers before and after the hyphen are effective doses calculated for men and women, respectively
*DS* dual source, *SS* single source, *NE* nonenhanced, *AP* arterial phase, *DP* delayed phase

the specific-imaged regions. In a phantom study, Szucs-Farkas et al. (2009) investigated low-kilovoltage CT for endoleak detection after endovascular aneurysm repair. They showed that low-kilovoltage CTA protocols have to be tailored not only to patient habitus but also to the size of endoleak to be detected. They indeed reported that tube voltage can be reduced to 80 kVp in small- and intermediate-sized patients and to 100 kVp in large patients with no risk of missing 6-mm endoleaks. If the threshold for leakages demanding treatment is set at 4 mm, 80 kVp can be applied with no limitation in small patients but 100 and 120 kVp would be advisable in intermediate and large patients, respectively. Similarly, in another study investigating aortic attenuation with various tube voltage on phantoms of different sizes, Schindera et al. (2010) reported a higher decrease in aortic attenuation at 120 kVp when the phantom size increased than at 80 and 100 kVp, resulting from a greater beam hardening at higher tube voltage in large phantoms.

Concerning CTA of aorta and peripheral vessels, Utsunomiya et al. (2010) investigated the effect of 80 kVp compared to 120 kVp CTA in patients with PAOD. They used a higher tube current–time product and a lower pitch at 80 kVp to compensate for the increase in image noise (see Table 2). They showed that contrast material volume can be reduced by 30% in 80 kVp protocols (1.2 ml/kg of Iopamiron 300 compared to 1.8 ml/kg at 120 kVP) and that low-tube-voltage CTA may be beneficial in terms of renal protection without impairing arterial attenuation and arterial image quality. The radiation dose levels for 80 kVp protocols are lower than that for 120 kVp but remain relatively standard. Their study sample was however constituted by slim patients (weighing approximately 60 kg with a BMI of 23 kg/m$^2$). An example of CTA of the aorta and arterial vessels of the legs is shown in Fig. 5.

## 2.3 Automatic Exposure Control: Tube Current Modulation

Automatic exposure control devices (AEC) modulate the tube current as a function of the table position along the Z-axis and of the image quality requested by the operator. Such devices reduce the tube current in thin patients and increase it in obese and overweight patients, tending to maintain constant the image quality (Mulkens et al. 2005). Therefore, radiologists using these devices should think in terms of image quality and not of tube current. These devices are extensively described in the "Automatic Exposure Control in Multidetector-row Computed Tomography" by Kalra. These devices are now routinely implemented on most CT scanners for the majority of indications. In imaging aorta and peripheral vessels they are of particular interest because we have to optimize the radiation dose in the abdomen, which represents a region of high attenuation, in contrast with the legs which represent a region of low attenuation.

Before the introduction of automatic techniques, the primary approach to decrease radiation was restricted to the reduction of the tube current. Fraioli et al. (2006) compared image quality and diagnostic performance of CTA of the aorta and peripheral vessels performed at 50, 100 and 130 mAs (without AEC, all other parameters being kept constant) as compared to digital subtraction angiography (DSA), considered as the reference standard. They showed that diagnostic quality of images can be achieved with lower radiation dose. Even in obese patients, while image quality was worse, readers graded the images as adequate for diagnosis. Moreover, they showed comparable sensitivities and specificities for all protocols, with sensitivity and specificity of 96 and 94%, respectively for the detection of all stenosis along the entire vascular tree with the 50-mAs protocol (Fraioli et al. 2006). Similar studies should be performed using AEC devices. In addition, it is important to consider that with lower tube voltages, the AEC devices will automatically increase tube current to maintain a constant image noise. Thus, further studies should be conducted to evaluate the optimal tube current and tube voltage in respect to the body habitus and investigated anatomic region, when using AEC.

## 2.4 Dual-Energy CTA

CT is the imaging method of choice for the detection and classification of endoleaks after endovascular aneurysm repair (EVAR). The optimal CT acquisition is still a matter of debate and a combination of non-enhanced, arterial and delayed CT phases is traditionally proposed (Golzarian et al. 1998;

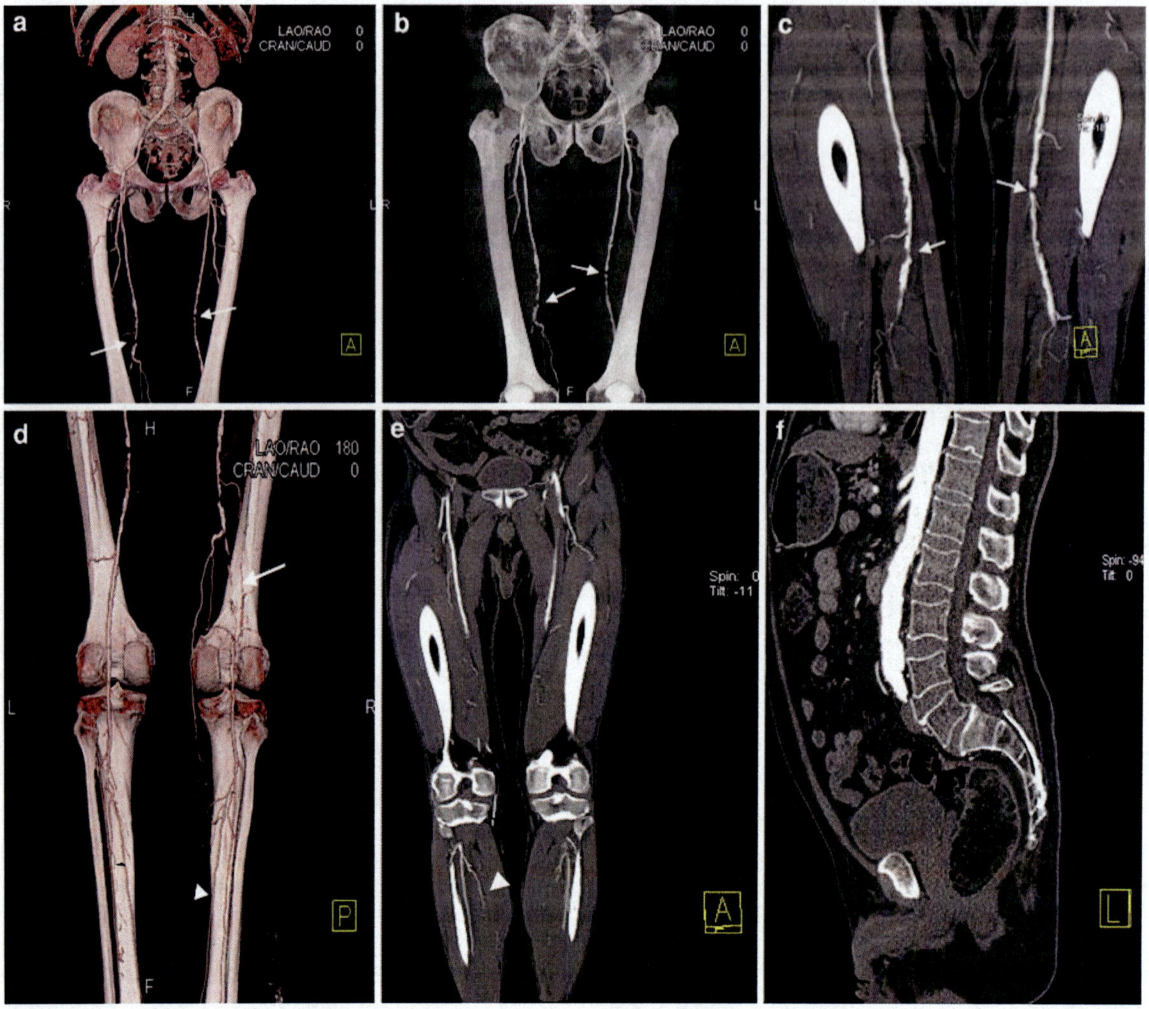


**Fig. 5** CT angiography images of a 74-year-old man with PAOD weighing 80 kg (BMI: 26.1 kg/m$^2$). Acquisition was performed on the abdomen and legs at 100 kVp and 140 effective mAs with AEC (CTDIvol: 4.42 mGy; DLP: 493 mGy.cm). **a** 3D volume rendering clearly the stenosis in the *left* and *right* superficial femoral arteries (*arrows*). **b** Thick maximum intensity projection (MIP) showing clearly the stenosis in the *left* and *right* superficial femoral arteries (*arrows*). **c** Coronal 5 mm-thin MIP of superficial femoral arteries showing the stenosis visible on the 3D (*arrows*). **d** 3D volume rendering showing a right popliteal occlusion (*arrow*). Infragenicular arteries are clearly depicted (*arrowhead*). **e** Coronal 5 mm-thin maximum intensity projection (MIP) with clear depiction of infragenicular arteries. **f** Sagittal

Golzarian and Valenti 2006; Iezzi et al. 2006; Sawhney et al. 2001). Patients who undergo EVAR are to be followed up for a long time and are exposed to large cumulative radiation doses. Macari et al. (2006) reported that arterial CT phase could be skipped and proposed only standard non-enhanced and delayed phase images for endoleak detection.

Dual-energy CTA can be obtained with various methods, by all CT manufacturers. Among them, the dual-source CT method consists in two X-ray tubes and two corresponding detectors arrays that are arranged on the gantry with an angular offset of 90°. When both tubes are working at different tube voltages, data from the two X-ray spectra that may improve tissue characterisation are obtained. Acquisition of dual-energy data enables the reconstruction of virtual non-enhanced images, on which the iodine content of contrast-enhanced dual-energy dual-source (DE-DS) CT images has been subtracted. Stolzmann et al. (2008) have showed in patients with EVAR that virtual non-enhanced CT can be reconstructed from DE-DS CT images obtained during the delayed phase

CT after contrast injection. In their study, they reported that the combination of delayed phase and virtual nonenhanced CT reconstructed both from a single DE-DS CT enable an accurate diagnosis of endoleak as compared to the standard triple-phase protocol (nonenhanced, arterial phase and delayed phase) (Stolzmann et al. 2008). As compared to the standard protocol, the one DE-DS CT scan resulted in a 61% decrease in radiation dose (see Table 2). The mean CTDIvol reported for their DE-DS CT scan is approximately 17 mGy with a corresponding calculated effective dose of 11 mSv which is relatively high. With a similar study design, Chandarana et al. (2008) reported very similar results, also in terms of radiation dose with a mean effective dose as high as in Stolzman's study (i.e., 11, 1 mSv with DE-DS). However, these results are encouraging and further studies should be conducted to evaluate lowering in radiation dose with DE-DS CT.

## 2.5 Post-Processing Approaches for Dose Reduction

Several post-processing algorithms have been recently developed allowing lowering of radiation dose based on reduced image noise. Szucs-Farkas et al. assessed the effect of a nonlinear noise filter on the image quality and the detection rate of simulated endoleaks in an abdominal aortic aneurysm phantom scanned at low kVp CTA. They reported an increase in CNR with the application of noise filter in simulated intermediate-sized and large patients. The noise filter improved the subjective image quality at 80 and 100 kVp in simulated intermediate-sized patients and at 100 kVp in simulated large patients, with a higher detection of endoleaks on the filtered 100 kVp images than on the non-filtered 100 kVp images in simulated large patients (Szucs-Farkas et al. 2011). Filter techniques are further described in "Image Noise Reduction Filters" by Singh and Kalra.

Traditional CT reconstruction algorithm (FBP reconstruction technique) does not produce consistently diagnostic images if tube current is substantially reduced. Iterative reconstruction is a reconstruction algorithm whereby image data are corrected with an assortment of models. The major drawback of this iterative reconstruction is the long computing time. Therefore a faster iterative reconstruction technique using only one corrective model has been developed and is called Adaptative Statistical Iterative Reconstruction technique (ASIR). This reconstruction technique is further detailed in "Conventional and Newer Reconstruction Techniques in CT" by Singh and Kalra. A fully converged 100% ASIR image tends to have a noise-free appearance with homogeneous attenuation that is not appealing to most radiologists as they are used to noisy images inherent to CT. However a mixture of FBP and ASIR can be used and produce an image with reduced noise but that retains a more typical CT appearance (Hara et al. 2009).

Unfortunately, clinical applications of this technique for CTA studies have not been reported so far.

## 2.6 Recommendations for Optimising and Reducing the Radiation Dose in CTA

The indication of each examination is important to consider in order selecting the required image quality and subsequently the lowest acceptable radiation dose. As an example, dose delivered in old patients suspected of PAOD can be higher than in young patients suspected of popliteal entrapment. However, dose reduction by lowering tube voltage can be of particular value in older patients suspected of PAOD because it enables to reduce the volume of contrast to be injected, which is an important issue in these patients having frequently an impaired renal function.

Furthermore, in patients who are subject to continued imaging surveillance as in patients after EVAR, multiphase acquisitions should not be performed in circumstances where they do not specifically yield additional relevant information, in particular in the long-term follow-up. As in all CT examinations, the ability to rapidly scan large volumes with MDCT tempts the operator to increase this volume along the Z-axis. Therefore Z-coverage should be adapted strictly to the clinical indication.

Automatic modulation of the tube current as a function of the patient's absorption is now available on all modern MDCT scanners. Differences still exist between manufacturers regarding the methods used for this modulation and the dose reductions subsequently obtained. The most important feature of these devices is that the radiation dose is adapted to the patient's weight and absorption. Consequently, the role of the CT user is not to adapt the tube current to the patient's weight but more to select appropriate tube potential and image quality to fit with the clinical indication of the CT examination. If the CT equipments includes AEC device, it should be always switched on for CTA.

All available keys of the CT equipment allowing dose reduction (i.e. autokV, ASIR, AEC, ...) should be used appropriately and "mixed" to obtain a diagnostic image at the lowest possible dose. When DECT is available, CT examination could be restricted to one delayed acquisition after contrast injection with reconstruction of virtual non-enhanced CT in patients followed after EVAR.

## 3 Conclusion to CTA Optimisation

Various techniques exist to lower the radiation dose of CTA studies of the body. Low-tube voltage CTA with 80 or 100 kVp represents the most commonly applied technique for radiation dose reduction. The subsequent increased contrast between the arterial system and surrounding parenchymal structures offsets the greater image noise, and allows a reduction in contrast volume to be injected. Another radiation saving approach during CTA is lowering or modulating the tube current. However, the optimal combination and tube voltage in respect to the body habitus and investigated anatomic region has not yet been determined, in particular when using AEC.

Dual-energy CTA with reconstruction of virtual non-enhanced images is valuable in patients requiring non-enhanced CT, in particular in post-EVAR patients.

Post-processing algorithms such as noise filters or iterative reconstructions are promising strategies to reduce radiation dose in CTA.

## 4 Conversion Factors Specific to CCTA

### 4.1 Introduction

The effective dose of cardiac CT is widely quoted in the radiology and cardiology literature. However, the methods used to calculate effective dose are often inadequately documented, and poorly understood. The radiation dose of cardiac investigations is an important consideration as cardiac imaging is responsible for up to 30% of population radiation exposure due to diagnostic imaging (Fazel et al. 2009). Computed tomography of the heart is likely to become an increasing component of the radiation exposure due to cardiac investigations. Advances in multidetector CT technology and reconstruction algorithms mean that CCTA is now possible at lower radiation doses and there is an increasing volume of research into radiation dose reduction techniques. It is important to understand how such research studies calculate effective dose in order to facilitate comparisons between studies and the translation of new techniques into clinical practice. The "gold-standard" method for the calculation of effective dose is based on organ-dose estimates. However, a simpler method involving the multiplication of dose length product (DLP) by a conversion factor is widely used. The choice of conversion factor can lead to the calculation of dramatically different effective doses. Here we discuss the issues that should be considered in selecting an appropriate conversion factor for cardiac CT.

### 4.2 Calculation of Effective Dose

Effective dose was proposed in 1975 as a concept for the combination of organ doses based on the principles of radiation risk and the corresponding health detriment to the exposed person (Jacobi 1975). It estimates the whole-body radiation dose that would be required to produce the same stochastic risk as the partial-body dose delivered during the CT scan. This takes into account the fact that our estimates of radiation risk such as carcinogenesis are based on whole-body irradiation, whereas medical imaging only exposes a small area (Goldman 2007). Effective dose is calculated by summing the absorbed doses to individual organs weighted for their radiation sensitivity. It is measured in millisieverts (mSv). The "gold-standard" method for the estimation of effective dose uses Monte Carlo simulations in anthropomorphic phantoms (Christner et al. 2010). This can be time consuming and requires access to specialist software. A complete review of such software can be found in "Software for Calculating Dose and Risk" by Georg Stamm. Thus a more simple method to calculate effective dose is widely used. This involves the multiplication of dose length product

(DLP) by a conversion factor. DLP is a measure of the radiation delivered to a patient during the CT scan and is presented on the console of most modern scanners. It is measured in units of milligray-centimetre (mGy.cm). DLP is the product of the volume CT dose index (CTDIvol) and the scan length. CTDIvol is derived from phantom measurements and the pitch value of the scan. Thus the calculation of effective dose using DLP and a conversion factor is a multistage process (see Fig. 6).

### 4.3 ICRP Tissue Weighting Factors

The conversion factors used to calculate effective dose from DLP are based on tissue weighting factors defined by the International Commission on Radiological Protection. The ICRP is an independent international organisation that was established in 1928 to advance the science of radiological protection. Since 1977 the ICRP have published three sets of tissue weighting factors (see Table 3). ICRP 26 was published in 1977, ICRP 60 in 1991 and ICRP 103 in 2007 (ICRP 1977, 1990, 2007). The role and objectives of ICRP are described in "ICRP role in CT radiation dose" by Rehani. These tissue weighting factors are based on statistical analysis of available data on radiation risk and the expert opinion of the committee. The risks that are considered are cancer incidence, cancer mortality, life shortening and hereditary risk (Roobottom et al. 2010). The majority of the information available on radiation risk is derived from the long-term study of Japanese atomic bomb survivors in the Life Span Study cohort (Pierce and Preston 2000). This is supplemented with details of radiation workers and other populations that have experienced a high radiation exposure (Cardis et al. 2007). Thus the data that the ICRP tissue weighting factors are based on includes information from both sexes and all ages (Christner et al. 2010).

### 4.4 Changes in the ICRP Tissue Weighting Factors

The ICRP tissue weighting factors have changed since their initial publication in 1977 as further information on the risk of radiation exposures has become available. In the most recent update in 2007

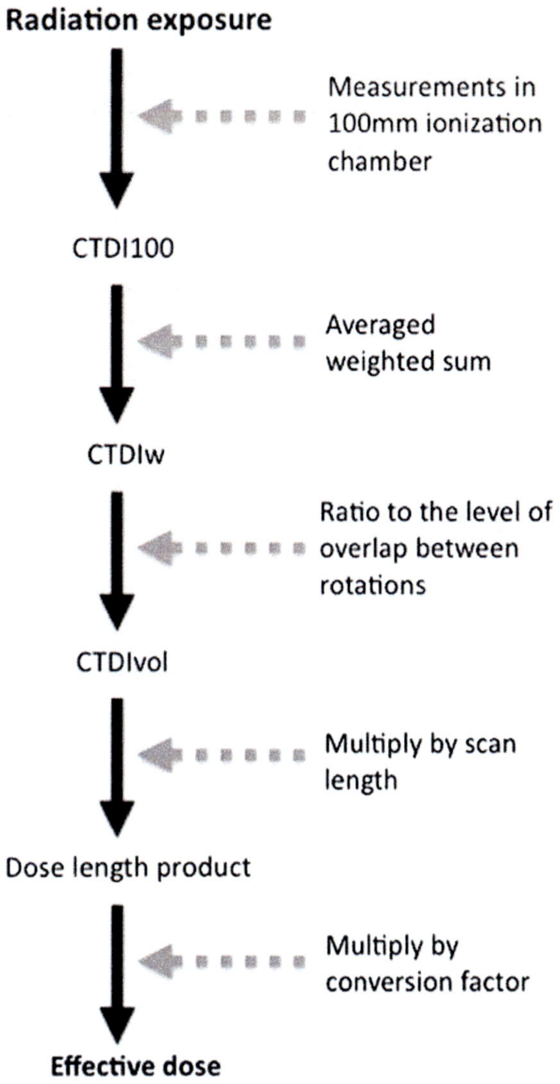


**Fig. 6** Calculation of effective dose using the conversion factor method. (CTDI100, computed tomography dose index measured in an 100 mm ionisation chamber; CTDIw, weighted computed tomography dose index; CTDIvol, volume computed tomography dose index)

there were a number of changes of particular importance to cardiac CT.

In ICRP 103 the tissue weighting factor for breast tissue was increased from 0.05 to 0.12. The reason for this increase was new data from the Japanese Life Span Study cohort. Breast cancer was found to account for 18% of the radiation-associated solid cancers averaged over males and females compared with 11% in the previous assessment

**Table 3** ICRP tissue weighting factors in 1977, 1991 and 2007 (ICRP 1977, 1990, 2007)

| Tissue | | ICRP publication | | |
|---|---|---|---|---|
| | | 26 | 60 | 103 |
| | | 1977 | 1991 | 2007 |
| Gonads | | 0.25 | 0.2 | 0.08 |
| Red bone marrow | | 0.12 | 0.12 | 0.12 |
| Colon | | – | 0.12 | 0.12 |
| Lung | | 0.12 | 0.12 | 0.12 |
| Stomach | | – | 0.12 | 0.12 |
| Bladder | | – | 0.05 | 0.04 |
| Liver | | – | 0.05 | 0.04 |
| Oesophagus | | – | 0.05 | 0.04 |
| Thyroid | | 0.03 | 0.05 | 0.04 |
| Breast | | 0.15 | 0.05 | 0.12 |
| Bone surface | | 0.03 | 0.01 | 0.01 |
| Skin | | – | 0.01 | 0.01 |
| Brain | | – | Remainder organ | 0.01 |
| Salivary glands | | – | – | 0.01 |
| Remainder organs | | 0.03 | 0.05 | 0.12 |
| | Adrenals | – | 0.005 | 0.0086 |
| | Kidneys | – | 0.005 | 0.0086 |
| | Muscle | – | 0.005 | 0.0086 |
| | Pancreas | – | 0.005 | 0.0086 |
| | Small intestine | – | 0.005 | 0.0086 |
| | Spleen | – | 0.005 | 0.0086 |
| | Thymus | – | 0.005 | 0.0086 |
| | Uterus and cervix | – | 0.005 | 0.0086 |
| | Brain | – | 0.05 | See above |
| | Upper large intestine | – | 0.005 | – |
| | Extrathoracic region | – | – | 0.0086 |
| | Gallbladder | – | – | 0.0086 |
| | Heart | – | – | 0.0086 |
| | Lymphatic nodes | – | – | 0.0086 |
| | Oral mucosa | – | – | 0.0086 |
| | Prostate | – | – | 0.0086 |
| Total | | 1 | 1 | 1 |

(Preston et al. 2007). The proposed increase in the breast tissue weighting factor is actually larger than the mean risk in both males and females, in order to avoid underestimation of risk in women (Martin 2007). Breast tissue is a major constituent of the area scanned during cardiac CT therefore this change in the breast tissue weighting factor is particularly important to the calculation of effective dose in CCTA.

The tissue weighting factor for the "remainder organs" was also increased in ICRP 103 from 0.05 to 0.12 and the definition of the "remainder organs" was changed to include the heart. The effect of these changes on the calculation of effective dose in CCTA

**Table 4** Published conversion factors for anatomical regions of common CT scans (mSv $mGy^{-1}$ $cm^{-1}$) (Shrimpton 2004; Ka et al. 1999; Bongartz et al. 2000, 2004)

| Body area | Publication | | | |
|---|---|---|---|---|
| | Jessen 1999 | European Commission 2000 | European Commission Appendix B 2004 | European Commission Appendix C 2004 |
| Head | 0.0021 | 0.0023 | 0.0023 | 0.0021 |
| Neck | 0.0048 | 0.0054 | – | 0.0059 |
| Head and neck | – | – | – | 0.031 |
| Chest | 0.014 | 0.017 | 0.018 | 0.014 |
| Abdomen | 0.012 | 0.015 | 0.017 | – |
| Abdomen and pelvis | – | – | – | 0.015 |
| Pelvis | 0.016 | 0.019 | 0.017 | – |
| Trunk | – | – | – | 0.015 |

is smaller than the effect of the change in the breast tissue weighting factor, but nevertheless these alterations do contribute to the overall difference between calculations made with ICRP 60 and ICRP 103 tissue weighting factors.

These changes in tissue weighting factors mean that effective doses calculated using ICRP 103 rather than ICRP 60 are up to a 40% higher (Christner et al. 2010; Einstein et al. 2010; Fink et al. 2011). It also means that differences between scanners and protocols become more important due to the differential exposure of breast tissue (Fink et al. 2011). It is important to remember when making comparisons between imaging modalities, such as between invasive coronary angiography, nuclear medicine and cardiac CT, that the tissue weighting factors used in each calculation should be the same.

## 4.5 Body Region-Specific Conversion Factors

In 2000 and 2004 the European Commission published generic conversion factors for the anatomical body areas of common CT scans (see Table 4). The conversion factor for chest CT was 0.017 in the 2000 publication and 0.014 in the 2004 publication. However, neither of these conversion factors are appropriate for use in cardiac CT.

Firstly, both of these European Commission publications are based on the old ICRP 60 tissue weighting factors. Secondly, these generic "chest" conversion factors were not calculated for the scan range of cardiac CT. Cardiac CT uses a smaller scan range than chest CT. The cardiac CT scan range covers mainly the lower chest and upper abdomen. This region contains an increased proportion of radiosensitive tissue, such as breast, as compared to the chest CT scan range (Geleijns et al. 2011).

Thus both of these generic "chest" conversion factors underestimate the radiation dose of cardiac CT (Huda et al. 2010). When compared to organ-dose calculations using the ICRP 103 tissue weighting factors the 0.014 conversion factor underestimates effective dose by 53% and the 0.017 conversion factor underestimates effective dose by 43% (Geleijns et al. 2011). Despite this, the current Society of Cardiovascular Computed Tomography *"Guidelines on radiation dose and dose-optimisation strategies in cardiovascular CT"* published in 2011 recommends the use of the 0.014 conversion factor (Halliburton et al. 2011). However, the guidelines do acknowledge that this conversion factor will underestimate effective dose and is likely to change in the future as further data on the risk of radiation exposure becomes available.

## 4.6 Considerations Required for the Calculation of CCTA Conversion Factors

A more accurate conversion factor for the calculation of effective dose in cardiac CT must take into account the new ICRP 103 tissue weighting factors.

However, in order to calculate the most accurate conversion factor additional factors should be considered such as patient size and shape, scan range, tube voltage, gantry position, and scanner type.

As has previously been discussed, the scan range for cardiac CT is smaller than that for chest CT. However, different types of cardiac examinations require different z-axis coverage. For example CT scans to obtain details of coronary arteries, pulmonary vessels, ascending aorta or bypass grafts all require different scan lengths. Tailoring the scan length to the size of the heart leads to substantial reductions in radiation dose (Khan et al. 2011). However, shorter scan lengths contain a higher proportion of radiosensitive tissue such as the breast. Thus for shorter scan lengths the conversion factor may be higher (Deak et al. 2010). In addition, the importance of breast tissue in the calculation of the radiation risk of CCTA may mean that effective dose is underestimated in women (Faletra et al. 2010).

Published conversion factors assume a standard-sized patient. However, many of the patients who undergo cardiac CT are obese. In our institution the average body mass index of patients undergoing CCTA is 30 kg/m$^2$. Adipose tissue attenuates the radiation dose received by deeper radiosensitive tissues and thus standard conversion factors would overestimate radiation risk (McCollough et al. 2011). The conversion factor used to calculate effective dose should decrease as the size of a patient increases. Differences in patient size lead to an uncertainty in the calculation of effective dose with conversion factors of ±15–20% (Martin 2007).

Effective dose is age independent, whereas the risk of radiation is highly age dependent (Faletra et al. 2010). The tissue weighting factors are averaged over age and sex so estimated cancer risk may be a factor of 3 higher or lower when applied to a reference patient, and varies even further when applied to an individual (Roobottom et al. 2010). Radiation-induced malignancies have a biological latency of 10–40 years, and are less likely to present in older individuals (Budoff and Gupta 2010). In addition the radiosensitivity of many tissues, including breast tissue, decreases with age (Roobottom et al. 2010). Thus the risk to different age groups for a uniform whole-body exposure varies by a factor of 4–5 between the ages of 5 and 75 years (Martin 2007).

The tube voltage alters the X-ray beam penetration and therefore the relative radiation dose to deeper lying organs. At a higher tube voltage, the energy and mean free path of scattered X-ray photons also increases (Huda et al. 2010). This means that the radiation dose to organs such as the lung, stomach and red bone marrow increases with a higher tube voltage, and that the conversion factor should increase as the tube voltage increases (see Table 5). The variation in adult subjects caused by changes in tube voltage is small, about 2.6% across all body regions (Deak et al. 2010). For cardiac CT a 4% increase in the conversion factor is required for each 10 kV increase in tube voltage (Huda and Mettler 2011). However, the effect of tube voltage is more significant in paediatric patients where lower tube voltages are used (Deak et al. 2010).

Many modern CT scanners do not require the X-ray beam to be switched on for the full gantry rotation. Instead radiation exposure is during a half-gantry rotation, and this reduces the radiation dose of the scan. However, the location of the X-ray tube during the exposure is important for the calculation of effective dose. For example, if the exposure is anteroposterior then the breast tissue will receive a higher radiation dose than if the exposure was posteroanterior. With current generations of CT scanners it is difficult to determine the location of the gantry during exposure. However, the incorporation of gantry position into the calculation of conversion factors would lead to a more accurate calculation of effective dose (Roobottom et al. 2010).

A wide variety of radiation dose reduction techniques have been developed for cardiac CT. However, as these change the pattern of radiation exposure, different conversion factors must be developed (Gosling et al. 2010). Tube current modulation in chest CT would be expected to reduce the conversion factor by 8% (Huda et al. 2010). Axial scanning techniques using wide volumes, such as 256 and 320 MDCT scanners, have a beam width that is larger than the 100 mm long ionisation chamber that is used to calculate CTDI. Thus a scaling factor must be incorporated into effective dose calculations in wide volume scanning to take account of the extended coverage and peak voltage (Mori et al. 2006). A new parameter, the extended DLP (DLPe), is quoted on such scanner consoles and can be used to calculate effective dose.

**Table 5** Average values of effective dose per unit dose length product at different tube voltages (Huda et al. 2010)

| Tube voltage (kV) | Average E/DLP ± standard deviation mSv $mGy^{-1}$ $cm^{-1}$ |
|---|---|
| 80 | 0.0231 ± 0.0036 |
| 100 | 0.0264 ± 0.003 |
| 120 | 0.0264 ± 0.002 |
| 140 | 0.0271 ± 0.009 |

## 4.7 Paediatric Considerations

Dose metrics designed to estimate effective dose in an adult population will underestimate the dose in paediatric patients (McCollough et al. 2011). In addition to the importance of age on the risk of radiation exposures, the smaller patient size and lower tube voltages must be considered when calculating effective dose in paediatric patients. The smaller patient size leads to lower attenuation of the X-ray beam and thus higher organ doses (Berrington de González et al. 2009). As discussed previously, lowering the tube voltage leads to a small reduction in the conversion factor (Huda et al. 2010). In Appendix C of the 2004 European Commission report the body region-specific conversion factors were extended to cover phantoms of 0, 1, 5 and 10 years (Shrimpton 2004). Thus there are published conversion factors for "chest" CT in paediatric patients. However, as with the "chest" conversion factors for adult patients these conversion factors will underestimate the effective dose. It is important for paediatric patients that an appropriate conversion factor is used that takes into account the considerations discussed for adult patients, the difference in radiation risk for paediatric patients and the size of the patient being scanned (Huda et al. 2008).

## 4.8 Scanner-Specific Conversion Factors

The 0.014 conversion factor underestimates radiation dose because it is independent of the scanner type, scanner mode, patient size and patient sex (Halliburton et al. 2011). A variety of scanner specific conversion factors have been calculated for cardiac CT (see Table 6). These conversion factors vary between 0.018 and 0.04 depending on the scanner type and protocol used.

## 4.9 Current Application of Conversion Factors in Cardiac CT

Despite the publication of scanner-specific conversion factors these are applied in less than 3% of the current cardiac CT literature (Williams et al. 2012). The most common conversion factors used in papers that discuss the radiation dose of cardiac CT are 0.014 and 0.017. There is a trend towards the increasing use of the 0.014 conversion factor, and thus the underestimation of the radiation dose of cardiac CT in the contemporary literature as illustrated in Fig. 7 (Williams et al. 2012). In addition, 13% published papers that discuss effective dose do not document the conversion factor used to calculate these doses. This means that comparisons cannot be drawn between the radiation dose reduction techniques used in these and other research papers.

## 4.10 Uncertainties in the Calculation of Conversion Factors

The calculation of effective dose is a multistage process and at each stage of the calculation there are uncertainties. Conversion factors are often quoted to two or three significant figures but the approximations used in their calculation are rarely considered (Martin 2007). This means that more certainty is attributed to effective dose than the calculation actually permits. When used to quantify an individual medical exposure the level of uncertainty is ±40% due to both the inherent uncertainties in the calculation and the fact that conversion factors are averaged across age and sex (Halliburton et al. 2011).

The tissue weighting factors published by the ICRP are grossly rounded for ease of use and do not indicate the underlying approximations. For example, uncertainties in the Japanese Life Span Study include how the diagnosis of cancer was made, the individual dose

**Table 6** Scanner- and protocol-specific conversion factors calculated for cardiac CT using ICRP 103 or ICRP 60 tissue weighting factors (Einstein et al. 2010; Fink et al. 2011; Geleijns et al. 2011; Huda et al. 2010; Gosling et al. 2010; Goetti et al. 2011; Matsubara et al. 2009)

| | CT scanner | | Protocol | ICRP 60 | ICRP 103 |
|---|---|---|---|---|---|
| Matsubara et al. (2009) | GE LightSpeed VCT | 64 MDCT | ECG-gated cardiac CT 120 kV | 0.03 | 0.040 |
| Einstein et al. (2010) | Toshiba Aquilion One | 320 MDCT | Helical cardiac CT | 0.022 | 0.029 |
| | | | Helical cardiac CT, ECG-gated tube current modulation | 0.02 | 0.027 |
| | | | Prospective helical cardiac CT | 0.02 | 0.027 |
| | | | Volume cardiac CT with standard exposure time | 0.021 | 0.029 |
| | | | Volume cardiac CT with optimised exposure time | 0.022 | 0.031 |
| | | | Volume cardiac CT with optimised exposure time, 100 kV | 0.024 | 0.034 |
| | | | Bolus tracking | 0.014 | 0.017 |
| Huda et al. (2010) | GE LightSpeed VCT | 64 MDCT | ECG-gated cardiac CT 100 kV | – | 0.0263 |
| | | | ECG-gated cardiac CT 120 kV | – | 0.0263 |
| | Siemens Somatom Sensation | 64 MDCT | ECG-gated cardiac CT 100 kV | – | 0.0262 |
| | | | ECG-gated cardiac CT 120 kV | – | 0.0265 |
| | Siemens Somatom Definition AS | 64 MDCT | ECG-gated cardiac CT 100 kV | – | 0.0268 |
| | | | ECG-gated cardiac CT 120 kV | – | 0.0262 |
| Gosling et al. (2010) | GE Lightspeed VCT HD750 | 64 MDCT | Prospective ECG-gated cardiac CT (100 or 120 kV) | – | 0.028 |
| Goetti et al. (2011) | Siemens Somatom Definition Flash | Dual- Source 128 MDCT | Retrospective and prospective ECG-gated cardiac CT (100 or 120 kV) | 0.028 | 0.034 |
| Geleijns et al. (2011) | Toshiba Aquilion 64 MDCT | 64 MDCT | ECG-gated cardiac CT 120 kV | 0.024 (range 0.017–0.03) | 0.030 (range 0.019–0.043) |
| Fink et al. (2011) | Siemens Somatom Definition AS | 64 MDCT | Retrospective and prospective ECG-gated cardiac CT (100 or 120 kV) | 0.032 | 0.024 |
| | Siemens Somaton Definition | 64 MDCT | | 0.028 | 0.021 |
| | Siemens Somatom Definition Flash | Dual- Source 128 MDCT | | 0.023 | 0.018 |

*kV* tube voltage, *MDCT* multidetector computed tomography

reconstructions, statistical variations in the genetic make-up and size of individuals, the type of risk model use, the extrapolation from high to low dose risk, the models used to predict cancer risk as a function of age and the time since exposure (Martin 2007). The differences between ICRP 60 and ICRP 103 also reflect differences in the type of data used. For example, cancer mortality was used in ICRP 60 and cancer incidence was used in ICRP 103 (Brenner 2008). In addition, these tissue weighting factors are derived from entirely different types of exposure than which occurs during medical imaging.

The conversion factor method of calculating effective dose has a deviation of ±15% compared to the gold-standard organ-dose-based technique (Christner et al. 2010). Uncertainties are present in the calculation of effective dose at every stage in the calculation (see Table 7). For example, CTDI-based

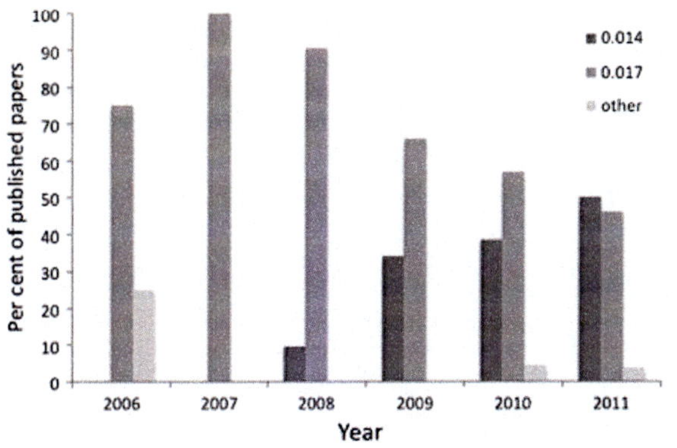


**Fig. 7** The use of conversion factors in papers discussing the radiation dose of cardiac CT

dosimetry may underestimate exposures by 20–30% for 64 MDCT scanners and more for wide beam scanners (Perisinakis et al. 2010).

## 4.11 Alternatives to the Calculation of Effective Dose

Effective dose was designed to reflect overall risk, averaged over all ages and both sexes for a reference patient (Christner et al. 2010). It reflects a combination of the risk of carcinogenesis, life shortening and hereditary effects. It was developed for use in occupational radiation protection and is not specific to an individual's age, sex or shape. Thus, a variety of alternatives to effective dose have been proposed. An appropriate alternative would reflect differences in age, gender and body habitus, would be less dependent on committee derived conversion factors, would be less prone to uncertainties during its calculation and would be simple to interpret (Brenner 2008).

One such proposal replaces the tissue weighting factors with the best estimates of organ-specific lifetime attributable risk of cancer. These risk coefficients are taken from the Biological Effects of Ionising radiation VII report (Nuclear Regulatory Commission 2006). This parameter, named effective risk (Brenner 2008) or risk index (Li et al. 2011), includes only the biological risk of cancer and can be age, sex and gender specific. It is thus particularly useful for assessment of paediatric risk (Li et al. 2011). However, these risk-based calculations are also a multistage process, which can feature inherent uncertainties.

Dose length product itself is not an indicator of risk as it does not take account of the radiosensitivity of the irradiated tissues (Goldman 2007). DLP is a quantitative measure of the total amount of radiation incident on a patient (Huda et al. 2010). It is useful for comparisons between CT protocols and is particularly helpful when comparing research studies (Goetti et al. 2011). There is an increasing trend towards the presentation of DLP in research studies, either alone, or in combination with effective dose (Williams et al. 2012). It is particularly important that while estimates of effective dose may change with time as new conversion factors are developed and applied, the dose length product will remain consistent. Therefore, in order to facilitate straightforward comparisons between research studies it is important to quote dose length product, alone or in addition to effective dose and the conversion factor.

## 4.12 Conclusion

Effective dose is a useful parameter that provides an estimation of the health risk of radiation exposures and allows comparisons between different imaging modalities. However, the inherent uncertainties in its calculation mean that more confidence is often attributed to values of effective dose than is appropriate. The calculation of effective dose in the cardiac CT is often performed using the DLP and a conversion factor. However, the calculation and application of these conversion factors is often poorly understood. Changes in the tissue weighting factors produced by the ICRP in 2007 have significant implications for the calculation of effective dose in cardiac CT. Generic "chest" conversion factors are widely used in the cardiac CT literature, leading to underestimations of the effective dose. It is important that the conversion factors used to calculate effective dose for CCTA include the most recent tissue weighting factors and are appropriate for the anatomical region scanned. Scanner-specific conversion factors have been calculated for a variety of protocols, but are rarely used in the contemporary CT literature. The appropriate conversion factor for 64 MDCT electrocardiogram-gated cardiac CT varies from 0.021 to 0.040. If different conversion factors are used then dramatically different effective doses will be calculated.

**Table 7** Estimates of standard error in quantities used to evaluate effective dose in CCTA (Martin 2007)

| Quantity | | Standard error (%) |
|---|---|---|
| Uncertainties in measurement of dose variables | Local X-ray dose calibration | ±10 |
| | Calibration of X-ray dose standards | ±5 |
| | Making measurement of X-ray dose | ±10 |
| | Uncertainty in radiology measurement | ±15 |
| Uncertainties in organ-dose conversion coefficients | Radiology tissue attenuations | ±2 |
| | Radiology tissue density composition | ±10 |
| | Systematic error for radiography and computerised tomography | ±10 |
| | Statistical error in Monte Carlo simulations | ±5 |
| | Radiology shape and geometry for organs almost entirely in beam | ±15 |
| | Radiology shape and geometry for organs partially in or outside beam | ±40 |
| Uncertainties in tissue weighting factors | | Determined by body region |

Tissue weighting factors will continue to change as further epidemiological data and models of cancer risk become available. Thus it is important that when presenting effective dose the parameters used to calculate this should be stated, including the dose length product and the conversion factor.

## References

### Part 1: Cardiac CT Angiography

Abada HT, Larchez C, Daoud B, Sigal-Cinqualbre A, Paul JF (2006) MDCT of the coronary arteries: feasibility of low-dose CT with ECG-pulsed tube current modulation to reduce radiation dose. AJR 186(6 Suppl 2):S387–S390

Achenbach S, Marwan M, Ropers D et al (2010) Coronary computed tomography angiography with a consistent dose below 1 mSv using prospectively electrocardiogram-triggered high-pitch spiral acquisition. Eur Heart J 31(3):340–346

Adler G, Meille L, Rohnean A, Sigal-Cinqualbre A, Capderou A, Paul JF (2010) Robustness of end-systolic reconstructions in coronary dual-source CT angiography for high heart rate patients. Eur Radiol 20:1118–1123

Arnoldi E, Johnson TR, Rist C et al (2009) Adequate image quality with reduced radiation dose in prospectively triggered coronary CTA compared with retrospective techniques. Eur Radiol 19(9):2147–2155

Ben Saad M, Rohnean A, Sigal-Cinqualbre A, Adler G, Paul JF (2009) Evaluation of image quality and radiation dose of thoracic and coronary dual-source CT in 110 infants with congenital heart disease. Pediatr Radiol 39(7):668–676

Blankstein R, Shah A, Pale R et al (2009) Radiation dose and image quality of prospective triggering with dual-source cardiac computed tomography. Am J Cardiol 103(8):1168–1173

Buechel RR, Husmann L, Herzog BA et al (2011) Low-dose computed tomography coronary angiography with prospective electrocardiogram triggering feasibility in a large population. J Am Coll Cardiol 57(3):332–336

Cademartiri F, Mollet NR, Runza G et al (2006) Improving diagnostic accuracy of MDCT coronary angiography in patients with mild heart rhythm irregularities using ECG editing. AJR 186(3):634–638

Cademartiri F, Maffei E, Palumbo AA et al (2008) Influence of intra-coronary enhancement on diagnostic accuracy with 64-slice CT coronary angiography. Eur Radiol 18(3):576–583

Earls JP (2009) How to use a prospective gated technique for cardiac CT. J Cardiovasc Comput Tomogr 3(1):45–51

Earls JP, Berman EL, Urban BA et al (2008) Prospectively gated transverse coronary CT angiography versus retrospectively gated helical technique: improved image quality and reduced radiation dose. Radiology 246(3):742–753

Efstathopoulos EP, Kelekis NL, Pantos I et al (2009) Reduction of the estimated radiation dose and associated patient risk with prospective ECG-gated 256-slice CT coronary angiography. Phys Med Biol 54(17):5209–5222

Einstein AJ, Henzlova MJ, Rajagopalan S (2007) Estimating risk of cancer associated with radiation exposure from 64-slice computed tomography coronary angiography. JAMA 298(3): 317–323

Fink C, Krissak R, Henzler T, Lechel U, Brix G, Takx RA, Nance JW, Abro JA, Schoenberg SO, Schoepf UJ (2011a) Radiation dose at coronary CT angiography: second-generation dual-source CT versus single-source 64-MDCT and first-generation dual-source CT. Am J Roentgenol 196(5): W550–W557

Foley SJ, McEntee MF, Achenbach S, Brennan PC, Rainford LS, Dodd JD (2011) Breast surface radiation dose during coronary CT angiography: reduction by breast displacement and lead shielding. AJR 197:367–373

Gilkeson RC, Ciancibello L, Zahka K (2003) Pictorial essay multidetector CT evaluation of congenital heart disease in pediatric and adult patients. AJR 180(4):973–980

Hausleiter J, Meyer T, Hadamitzky M et al (2006) Radiation dose estimates from cardiac multislice computed tomography in daily practice: impact of different scanning protocols on effective dose estimates. Circulation 113(10):1305–1310

Hausleiter J, Meyer T, Hermann F et al (2009) Estimated radiation dose associated with cardiac CT angiography. JAMA 301(5):500–507

Huda W, Shoepf UJ, Abro JA, Mah E, Costello P (2011) Radiation-related cancer risks in a clinical patient population undergoing cardiac CT. AJR 196:W159–W165

Jung B, Mahnken AH, Stargardt A et al (2003) Individually weight-adapted examination protocol in retrospectively ECG-gated MSCT of the heart. Eur Radiol 13(12):2560–2566

Labounty TM, Leipsic J, Min JK, Heilbron B, Mancini GB, Lin FY, Earls JP (2010) Effect of padding duration on radiation dose and image interpretation in prospectively ECG-triggered coronary CT angiography. AJR 194:933–937

Lee T, Tsai IC, Fu YC et al (2006) Using multidetector-row CT in neonates with complex congenital heart disease to replace diagnostic cardiac catheterization for anatomical investigation: initial experiences in technical and clinical feasibility. Pediatr Radiol 36(12):1273–1282

Lee AB, Nandurkar D, Schneider-Kolsky ME, Crossett M, Seneviratne SK, Cameron JD, Troupis JM (2011) Coronary image quality of 320-MDCT in patients with heart rates above 65 beats per minute: preliminary experience. Am J Roentgenol 196(6):W729–W735 Jun

Leschka S, Kim CH, Baumueller S, Stolzmann P, Scheffel H, Marincek B, Alkadhi H (2010) Scan length adjustment of CT coronary angiography using the calcium scoring scan: effect on radiation dose. AJR 194:W272–W277

Neefjes LA, Dharampal AS, Rossi A, Nieman K, Weustink AC, Dijkshoorn ML, Ten Kate GJ, Dedic A, Papadopoulou SL, van Straten M, Cademartiri F, Krestin GP, de Feyter PJ, Mollet NR (2011) Image quality and radiation exposure using different low-dose scan protocols in dual-source CT coronary angiography: randomized study. Radiology 261:779–786

Paul JF (2011) Individually adapted coronary 64-slice CT angiography based on precontrast attenuation values, using different kVp and tube current settings: evaluation of image quality. Int J Cardiovasc Imag 21:165–176

Paul JF, Abada HT (2007) Strategies for reduction of radiation dose in cardiac multislice CT. Eur Radiol 17(8):2028–2037

Paul JF, Abada HT, Sigal-Cinqualbre A (2004) Should low-kilovoltage chest CT protocols be the rule for pediatric patients? AJR 183(4):1172; author reply

Paul JF, Rohnean A, Sigal-Cinqualbre A (2010) Multidetector CT for congenital heart patients: what a paediatric radiologist should know. Pediatr Radiol 40(6):869–875

Paul JF, Rohnean A, Elfassy E, Sigal-Cinqualbre A (2011) Radiation dose for thoracic and coronary step-and-shoot CT using a 128-slice dual-source machine in infants and small children with congenital heart disease. Pediatr Radiol 41: 244–249

Pflederer T, Jakstat J, Marwan M et al (2010) Radiation exposure and image quality in staged low-dose protocols for coronary dual-source CT angiography: a randomized comparison. Eur Radiol 20(5):1197–1206

Reid J, Gamberoni J, Dong F, Davros W (2010) Optimization of kVp and mAs for pediatric low-dose simulated abdominal CT: is it best to base parameter selection on object circumference? AJR 195(4):1015–1020

Shuman WP, Branch KR, May JM, Mitsumori LM, Lockhart DW, Dubinsky TJ, Warren BH, Caldwell JH (2008) Prospective versus retrospective ECG gating for 64-detector CT of the coronary arteries: comparison of image quality and patient radiation dose. Radiology 248:431–437

Sigal-Cinqualbre AB, Hennequin R, Abada HT, Chen X, Paul JF (2004) Low-kilovoltage multi-detector row chest CT in adults: feasibility and effect on image quality and iodine dose. Radiology 231(1):169–174

Sun ML, Lu B, Wu RZ et al (2011) Diagnostic accuracy of dual-source CT coronary angiography with prospective ECG-triggering on different heart rate patients. Eur Radiol 21(8):1635–1642

Tatsugami F, Husmann L, Herzog BA et al (2009) Evaluation of a body mass index-adapted protocol for low-dose 64-MDCT coronary angiography with prospective ECG triggering. AJR 192(3):635–638

Torres FS, Jeddiyan S, Jiménez-Juan L, Nguyen ET (2011) Beta-blockers to control heart rate during coronary CT angiography. Radiology 259(2):615–616. May 2011, author reply 616–617

Tsai IC, Lee T, Chen MC et al (2007) Visualization of neonatal coronary arteries on multidetector row CT: ECG-gated versus non-ECG-gated technique. Pediatr Radiol 37: 818–825

Tubiana M (2005) Dose-effect relationship and estimation of the carcinogenic effects of low doses of ionizing radiation: the joint report of the Academie des Sciences (Paris) and of the Academie Nationale de Medecine. Int J Radiat Oncol Biol Phys 63(2):317–319

Vastel-Amzallag C, Le Bret E, Paul JF et al (2011) Diagnostic accuracy of dual-source multislice computed tomographic analysis for the preoperative detection of coronary artery anomalies in 100 patients with tetralogy of fallot. J Thor Cardiovasc Surg 142(1):120–126

## Part 2: Radiation Dose Optimization in CT Angiography (CTA) for Aorta And Peripheral Vessels

Chandarana H, Godoy MC, Vlahos I, Graser A, Babb J, Leidecker C, Macari M (2008) Abdominal aorta: evaluation with dual-source dual-energy multidetector CT after endovascular repair of aneurysms–initial observations. Radiology 249:692–700

Fraioli F, Catalano C, Napoli A, Francone M, Venditti F, Danti M, Pediconi F, Passariello R (2006) Low-dose multidetector-row CT angiography of the infra-renal aorta and lower extremity vessels: image quality and diagnostic accuracy in comparison with standard DSA. Eur Radiol 16:137–146

Golzarian J, Valenti D (2006) Endoleakage after endovascular treatment of abdominal aortic aneurysms: diagnosis, significance and treatment. Eur Radiol 16:2849–2857

Golzarian J, Dussaussois L, Abada HT, Gevenois PA, Van Gansbeke D, Ferreira J, Struyven J (1998) Helical CT of aorta after endoluminal stent-graft therapy: value of biphasic acquisition. Am J Roentgenol 171:329–331

Hara AK, Paden RG, Silva AC, Kujak JL, Lawder HJ, Pavlicek W (2009) Iterative reconstruction technique for reducing body radiation dose at CT: feasibility study. Am J Roentgenol 193:764–771

Iezzi R, Cotroneo AR, Filippone A, Di Fabio F, Quinto F, Colosimo C, Bonomo L (2006) Multidetector CT in abdominal aortic aneurysm treated with endovascular repair: are unenhanced and delayed phase enhanced images effective for endoleak detection? Radiology 241:915–921

Kalra MK, Maher MM, Toth TL, Hamberg LM, Blake MA, Shepard JA, Saini S (2004) Strategies for CT radiation dose optimization. Radiology 230:619–628

Kalva SP, Sahani DV, Hahn PF, Saini S (2006) Using the K-edge to improve contrast conspicuity and to lower radiation dose with a 16-MDCT: a phantom and human study. J Comput Assist Tomogr 30:391–397

Macari M, Chandarana H, Schmidt B, Lee J, Lamparello P, Babb J (2006) Abdominal aortic aneurysm: can the arterial phase at CT evaluation after endovascular repair be eliminated to reduce radiation dose? Radiology 241:908–914

Manousaki E, Perisinakis K, Karantanas A, Tsetis D (2011) MDCT angiography assessment of renal artery in-stent restenosis: can we reduce the radiation exposure burden? A feasibility study. Eur J Radiol 79:224–231

Marin D, Nelson RC, Samei E, Paulson EK, Ho LM, Boll DT, DeLong DM, Yoshizumi TT, Schindera ST (2009) Hypervascular liver tumors: low tube voltage, high tube current multidetector CT during late hepatic arterial phase for detection–initial clinical experience. Radiology 251:771–779

Mulkens TH, Bellinck P, Baeyaert M, Ghysen D, Van Dijck X, Mussen E, Venstermans C, Termote JL (2005) Use of an automatic exposure control mechanism for dose optimization in multi-detector row CT examinations: clinical evaluation. Radiology 237:213–223

Nakayama Y, Awai K, Funama Y, Hatemura M, Imuta M, Nakaura T, Ryu D, Morishita S, Sultana S, Sato N, Yamashita Y (2005) Abdominal CT with low tube voltage: preliminary observations about radiation dose, contrast enhancement, image quality, and noise. Radiology 237:945–951

Nakayama Y, Awai K, Funama Y, Liu D, Nakaura T, Tamura Y, Yamashita Y (2006) Lower tube voltage reduces contrast material and radiation doses on 16-MDCT aortography. Am J Roentgenol 187:W490–W497

Sahani DV, Kalva SP, Hahn PF, Saini S (2007) 16-MDCT angiography in living kidney donors at various tube potentials: impact on image quality and radiation dose. Am J Roentgenol 188:115–120

Sawhney R, Kerlan RK, Wall SD, Chuter TA, Ruiz DE, Canto CJ, Laberge JM, Reilly LM, Yee J, Wilson MW, Jean-Claude J, Faruqi RM, Gordon RL (2001) Analysis of initial CT findings after endovascular repair of abdominal aortic aneurysm. Radiology 220:157–160

Schindera ST, Nelson RC, Yoshizumi T, Toncheva G, Nguyen G, DeLong DM, Szucs-Farkas Z (2009a) Effect of automatic tube current modulation on radiation dose and image quality for low tube voltage multidetector row CT angiography: phantom study. Acad Radiol 16:997–1002

Schindera ST, Graca P, Patak MA, Abderhalden S, von Allmen G, Vock P, Szucs-Farkas Z (2009b) Thoracoabdominal-aortoiliac multidetector-row CT angiography at 80 and 100 kVp: assessment of image quality and radiation dose. Invest Radiol 44:650–655

Schindera ST, Tock I, Marin D, Nelson RC, Raupach R, Hagemeister M, von Allmen G, Vock P, Szucs-Farkas Z (2010) Effect of beam hardening on arterial enhancement in thoracoabdominal CT angiography with increasing patient size: an in vitro and in vivo study. Radiology 256:528–535

Stolzmann P, Frauenfelder T, Pfammatter T, Peter N, Scheffel H, Lachat M, Schmidt B, Marincek B, Alkadhi H, Schertler T (2008) Endoleaks after endovascular abdominal aortic aneurysm repair: detection with dual-energy dual-source CT. Radiology 249:682–691

Szucs-Farkas Z, Semadeni M, Bensler S, Patak MA, von Allmen G, Vock P, Schindera ST (2009) Endoleak detection with CT angiography in an abdominal aortic aneurysm phantom: effect of tube energy, simulated patient size, and physical properties of endoleaks. Radiology 251:590–598

Szucs-Farkas Z, Bensler S, Torrente JC, Cullmann JL, Vock P, Schindera ST (2011) Nonlinear three-dimensional noise filter with low-dose CT angiography: effect on the detection of small high-contrast objects in a phantom model. Radiology 258:261–269

Utsunomiya D, Oda S, Funama Y, Awai K, Nakaura T, Yanaga Y, Hirai T, Yamashita Y (2010) Comparison of standard- and low-tube voltage MDCT angiography in patients with peripheral arterial disease. Eur Radiol 20:2758–2765

Wintersperger B, Jakobs T, Herzog P, Schaller S, Nikolaou K, Suess C, Weber C, Reiser M, Becker C (2005) Aorto-iliac multidetector-row CT angiography with low kV settings: improved vessel enhancement and simultaneous reduction of radiation dose. Eur Radiol 15:334–341


## Part 3: Conversion Factors Specific to CCTA


Berrington de González A, Mahesh M, Kim K-P, Bhargavan M, Lewis R, Mettler F et al (2009) Projected cancer risks from computed tomographic scans performed in the United States in 2007. Arch Intern Med 169(22):2071–2017

Bongartz G, Golding S, Jurik A, Leonardi M, van Meerten E v P, Geleijns J et al (2000) European guidelines on quality criteria for computed tomography. EUR 16262. Luxembourg

Bongartz G, Golding SJ, Jurik AG, Leonardi M, van Persijn van Meerten E, Rodríguez R et al (2004) European field survey of the clinical application of CT with a focus on the evaluation of CT protocols and assessment of patient dose.

In: European guidelines for multislice computed tomography funded by the European Commission 2004: contract number FIGMCT2000-20078-CT-TIP. European Commission, Brussels
Brenner DJ (2008) Effective dose: a flawed concept that could and should be replaced. British J Radiol 81(967):521–523
Budoff MJ, Gupta M (2010) Radiation exposure from cardiac imaging procedures: do the risks outweigh the benefits? J Am Coll Cardiol 56(9):712–714
Cardis E, Vrijheid M, Blettner M, Gilbert E, Hakama M, Hill C et al (2007) The 15-country collaborative study of cancer risk among radiation workers in the nuclear industry: estimates of radiation-related cancer risks. Radiat Res 167(4):396–416
Christner J, Kofler JM, McCollough CH (2010) Estimating effective dose for CT using dose-length product compared with using organ doses: consequences of adopting International Commission on Radiological Protection publication 103 or dual-energy scanning. AJR 194(4):881–889
Deak PD, Smal Y, Kalender WA (2010) Multisection CT protocols: sex- and age-specific conversion factors used to determine effectve dose from dose-length product. Radiology 257(1):158–166
Einstein AJ, Elliston CD, Arai AE, Chen MY, Mather R, N. PGD et al (2010) Radiation dose from single-heartbeat coronary CT angiography performed with a 320-detector row volume scanner. Radiology 254(3):698–706
Faletra FF, D'Angeli I, Klersy C, Averaimo M, Klimusina J, Pasotti E et al (2010) Estimates of lifetime attributable risk of cancer after a single radiation exposure from 64-slice computed tomographic coronary angiography. Heart 96(12):927–932
Fazel R, Krumholz HM, Wang Y, Ross JS, Chen J, Ting HH et al (2009) Exposure to low-dose ionizing radiation from medical imaging procedures. N Engl J Med 361(9):849–857
Fink C, Krissak R, Henzler T, Lechel U, Brix G, Takx RAP et al (2011b) Radiation dose at coronary CT angiography: second-generation dual-source CT versus single-source 64-MDCT and first generation dual-source CT. AJR 196(5):550–557
Geleijns J, Joemai RMS, Dewey M, de Roos A, Zankl M, Cantera AC et al (2011) Radiation exposure to patients in a multicenter coronary angiography trial (CORE 64). AJR 196(5):1126–1132
Goetti R, Leschka S, Boschung M, Mayer S, Wyss C, Stolzmann P et al (2011) Radiation doses from phantom measurements at high-pitch dual-source computed tomography coronary angiography. Eur J Radiol. [Epub ahead of print]
Goldman LW (2007) Principles of CT: radiation dose and image quality. J Nucl Med Technol 35(4):213–225, 226–228
Gosling O, Loader R, Venables P, Rowles N, Morgan-hughes G, Cardiac RC (2010) CT, are we underestimating the dose? A radiation dose study utilizing the 2007 ICRP tissue weighting factors and a cardiac specific scan volume. Clin Radiol 65(12):1013–1017
Halliburton SS, Abbara S, Chen MY, Gentry R, Mahesh M, Raff GL et al (2011) SCCT guidelines on radiation dose and dose-optimization strategies in cardiovascular CT. J Cardiovasc Comput Tomogr 5(4):198–224
Huda W, Mettler FA (2011) Volume CT dose index and dose-length product displayed during CT: what good are they? Radiation 258:236–242
Huda W, Ogden KM, Khorasani MR (2008) Converting dose-length product to effective dose at CT. Radiology 248(3):995–1003
Huda W, Tipnis S, Sterzik A, Schoepf UJ (2010) Computing effective dose in cardiac CT. Phys Med Biol 55(13): 3675–3684
ICRP (1977) Recommendations of the ICRP. ICRP Publication 26. Ann. ICRP. 1(3)
ICRP (1990) Recommendations of the International Commission on Radiological Protection. ICRP Publication 60. Ann. ICRP 1991. 21(1–3):1–201
ICRP (2007) The 2007 Recommendations of the International Commission on Radiological Protection. Ann. ICRP 37(2–4): 1–332
Jacobi W (1975) The concept of the effective dose—a proposal for the combination of organ doses. Radiat Environ Biophys 12(2):101–109
Ka J, Shrimpton PC, Geleijns J, Panzer W, Tosi G (1999) Dosimetry for optimisation of patient protection in computed tomography. Appl Radiat Isotopes 50(1):165–172
Khan A, Nasir K, Khosa F, Saghir A, Sarwar S, Clouse ME (2011) Prospective gating with 320-MDCT angiography: effect of volume scan length on radiation dose. AJR 196(2):407–411
Li X, Samei E, Segars WP, Sturgeon GM, Colsher JG, Frush DP (2011) Patient-specific radiation dose and cancer risk for pediatric chest CT. Radiology 259(3):862–874
Martin CJ (2007) Effective dose: how should it be applied to medical exposures? Br J Radiol 80(956):639–647
Matsubara K, Koshida K, Suzuki M, Shimono T, Yamamoto T, Matsui O (2009) Effective dose evaluation of multidetector CT examinations: influence of the ICRP recommendation in 2007. Eur Radiol 19(12):2855–2861
McCollough CH, Leng S, Yu L, Cody DD, Boone JM, Mcnitt-gray MF (2011) CT dose index and patient dose: they are not the same thing. Radiology 259(2):311–316
Mori S, Nishizawa K, Ohno M, Endo M (2006) Conversion factor for CT dosimetry to assess patient dose using a 256-slice CT scanner. British J Radiol 79(947):888–892
Nuclear Regulatory Commission (2006) Beir VII : health risks from exposure to low levels of ionizing radiation. National Academies Press, Washington DC
Perisinakis K, Seimenis I, Tzedakis A, Papadakis AE, Damilakis J (2010) Individualized assessment of radiation dose in patients undergoing coronary computed tomographic angiography with 256-slice scanning. Circulation 122(23):2394–2402
Pierce DA, Preston DL (2000) Radiation-related cancer risks at low doses among atomic bomb survivors. Radiat Res 154(2):178–186
Preston DL, Ron E, Tokuoka S, Funamoto S, Nishi N, Soda M et al (2007) Solid cancer incidence in atomic bomb survivors: 1958–1998. Radiat Res 168(1):1–64
Roobottom CA, Mitchell G, Morgan-Hughes G (2010) Radiation-reduction strategies in cardiac computed tomographic angiography. Clin Radiol 65(11):859–867
Shrimpton P (2004) Assessment of patient dose in CT. In: European guidelines for multislice computed tomography funded by the European Commission, contract number FIGMCT2000-20078-CT-TIP. European Commission, Luxembourg, p 2004
Williams MC, Maclachlan DS, Misradraee S, Newby DE, Weir NW (2012) Computed tomography coronary angiography (CTCA) radiation dose: a systematic review of the application of conversion factors. Abstract B-0399. European Congress of Radiology

# Dose Optimization and Reduction in Musculoskeletal CT Including the Spine

A. Gervaise, P. Teixeira, N. Villani, S. Lecocq, M. Louis, and A. Blum

## Contents




**Abstract**

Due to improvements in temporal and spatial resolution, and despite its radiating character, CT is still indicated for the assessment of many musculoskeletal disorders. New exploration techniques, such as dynamic CT of the joints and bone perfusion imaging, are now available in musculoskeletal imaging. However, they require the repetition of many phases and lead to an increase in dose. For these new applications and for spine and proximal joint imaging in the vicinity of radiosensitive organs, optimization and dose reduction are critical. In this chapter, we report the typical doses delivered in musculoskeletal CT examinations and discuss several options for allowing dose optimization and reduction, depending on behavioral and technical factors. Among them, tube current and tube potential optimization are still critical and must be adapted to the type of exploration and the body habitus of each patient. Recent technical factors can also help to reduce the doses such as automatic tube current modulation, active collimation or new CT iterative reconstructions. Although these technical factors allow for an important reduction of the doses, behavioral factors such as respecting the indications and limitations of the scan coverage remain essential. Finally, we will also indicate how to optimize and reduce the doses in particular applications of musculoskeletal imaging, such as dynamic CT, bone and soft tissue perfusion CT and dual-energy CT.



A. Gervaise · P. Teixeira · S. Lecocq · M. Louis · A. Blum
Guilloz Imaging Department, Hôpital Central, CHU Nancy, 29 avenue du Maréchal de Lattre de Tassigny, 54035 Nancy Cedex, France

A. Gervaise (✉)
Medical Imaging Department, Hôpital d'Instruction des Armées Legouest, 27 avenue de Plantières, BP 90001, 57077 Metz Cedex 3, France
e-mail: alban.gervaise@hotmail.fr

N. Villani
Medical Radiophysics Unit, CRAN UMR 7039 CNRS, Centre Alexis Vautrin, Avenue de Bourgogne, 54511 Vandoeuvre-les-Nancy, France


D. Tack et al. (eds.), *Radiation Dose from Multidetector CT*, Medical Radiology. Diagnostic Imaging,
DOI: 10.1007/174_2011_500, 

## 1 Introduction

Since its introduction in the 1970s, computed tomography (CT) has played an important role in the diagnosis of musculoskeletal disorders. It quickly became the method of choice for the diagnosis of traumatic, degenerative or developmental lesions. Although image quality is altered by streak artifacts of medical devices, CT is still indicated in post-operative imaging (Blum et al. 2000; Cotten et al. 2002; Fayad et al. 2005). Today, CT is also widely used in interventional imaging (i.e., guided injection, biopsy, vertebroplasty, etc.) (West et al. 2009).

The diagnostic performance of CT is however limited by the low-contrast resolution, which leads to a poor analysis of soft tissues when compared with magnetic resonance imaging (MRI). The analysis of intra-articular lesions is also very difficult in the absence of intra-articular contrast. CT studies may also be an important source of ionizing radiation. This may help explain the prominent role of MRI in the evaluation of musculoskeletal disorders.

With multi-detector computed tomography (MDCT), wide-range detectors and a significant reduction in radiation exposure, CT has regained its former importance in the evaluation of the musculoskeletal system. Spatial and temporal resolutions were considerably increased. Submillimetric isotropic acquisition allows multiplanar and volume rendering (VR) three-dimensional (3D) reformations, improving the diagnosis and preoperative planning of bone and soft tissues disorders (Iochum et al. 2001). Improvements in temporal resolution limit motion artifacts especially in large-volume explorations, which are particularly suitable for the evaluation of polytraumatized patients with musculoskeletal injuries (Fig. 1). Additionally, high temporal resolution allows dynamic imaging of joints. Novel CT techniques, such as dual-energy and CT perfusion are also available for musculoskeletal imaging. Dual-energy CT is based on image acquisition with a beam with variable kilovoltage allowing not only a better characterization of tissues, but also a reduction in metal artifacts. Bone and contrast media can also be subtracted with this technique (Karcaaltincaba and Aktas 2011). With CT perfusion, multiple and successive phases are acquired allowing an optimal analysis of the contrast bolus. This technique provides a functional evaluation of bone and soft tissues' tumors with the advantages of being more reproducible and easier to analyze than MRI (Oldrini et al. 2009; Goh and Padhani 2006). Other benefits of CT scanning include a lower cost, better availability, fewer contraindications and the possibility to image post-operative or unstable patients (Semelka et al. 2007; West et al. 2009).

Finally, advances in CT technology helps to reduce the radiation exposure. After a review of the typical doses used in musculoskeletal CT examinations, we will discuss in detail the various methods of dose reduction in the field of musculoskeletal imaging, with a special emphasis on both behavioral and technical factors.

## 2 Typical Doses Used in Musculoskeletal CT Examinations

The International Commission on Radiological Protection (1991) advocates the establishment of recommended doses for CT examinations. When greater exposure is proposed, the need for it, and the implications of its use, should be examined. The Council Directive of June 30, 1997, requests each Member State of the European Union to establish and enforce the use of reference levels of diagnostic radiation exposure that should not be exceeded during standard procedures (European Community 1997). The European Commission proposes reference values of weighted CT Dose Index (CTDIw) and Dose Length Product (DLP) for various types of CT studies (European Commission 1999).

For the lumbar spine, the proposed reference levels are a CTDIw of 35 mGy and a DLP of 800 mGy cm. For the pelvic girdle (i.e., hip, sacroiliac), the proposed reference levels are a CTDIw of 25 mGy and a DLP of 520 mGy cm. For the exploration of a traumatic spine, the proposed values are a CTDIw of 70 mGy and a DLP of 460 mGy cm (European Commission 1999). These reference doses are, however, based on survey data from the late 1980s and early 1990s, prior to the widespread introduction of spiral CT and MDCT (Shrimpton and Edyvean 1998; Hidajat et al. 2001). Since then, MDCT has dramatically changed clinical practice, and the guidelines should be reviewed accordingly (Hidajat et al. 2001; Bongartz et al. 2004).

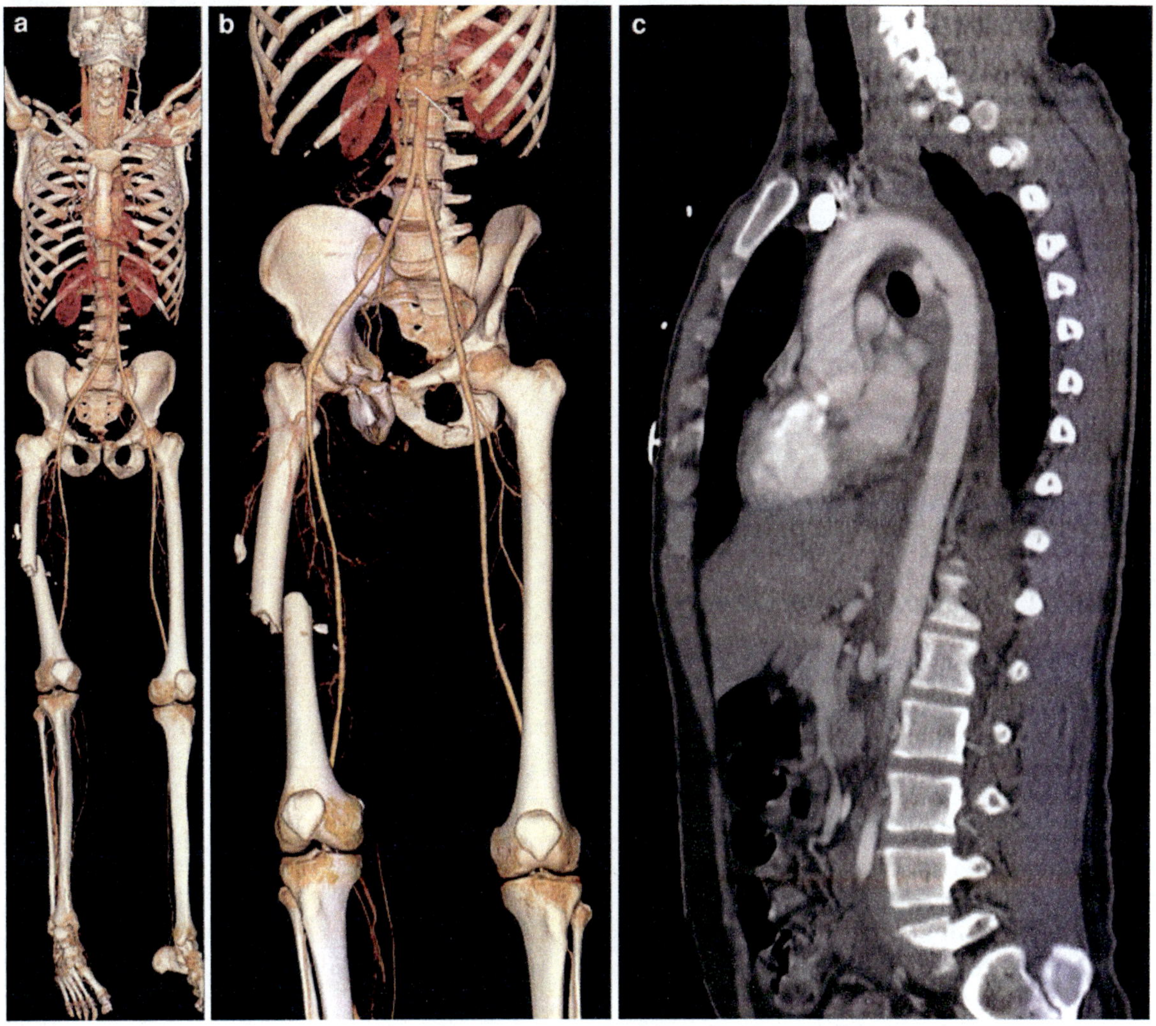


**Fig. 1** Whole-body CT-scan of a 28-year-old man for assessment of bike on car polytrauma. Arterial acquisition with 3D reformations in VR of the whole body (**a**) then centered on the right femoral fracture (**b**) and sagittal oblique reformation of the thoracic aorta (**c**). The acquisition was performed with a 64-detector row CT covering the whole body, representing a 180 cm acquisition in 34 s (64 × 0.5 mm, rotation time 0.5, pitch 0.828, 120 kV, current tube modulation with mAs range 50–145 mAs, DLP = 2,090 mGy cm). This acquisition was performed at the arterial phase with thin slices, allowing for 3D VR vascular reformation. This reformation allows for a better analysis of the ratio between the diaphyseal fracture of the right femur and the superficial femoral artery and to assist in preoperative assessment. Note also the bilateral fracture of the obturator rings and the rupture of the aortic isthmus

For example, it is interesting to note that these guidelines recommend a nominal slice thickness of 2–5 mm for a lumbar spine CT, while most MDCT acquisitions today are systematically performed with submillimetric slice thicknesses. Moreover, due to the improvement of MDCT acquisition speed, it is now possible to obtain a wide *z*-axis coverage, which leads to new indications, such as whole-body bone CT for the assessment of a myeloma (Horger et al. 2005; Gleeson et al. 2009) or whole-spine CT for the assessment of osteoporosis (Damilakis et al. 2010). The new techniques made possible by the developments in CT technology, such as dynamic imaging, perfusion and dual-energy still do not have established dose reference levels. Finally, the dose exposure of CT studies in some parts of the musculoskeletal system (such as peripheral joints) either has not yet been evaluated or has no reference dose values determined (i.e., shoulder).

**Table 1** Spine CT scan doses from a literature review (Pantos et al. 2011)

| Spine segment | CTDIw[a] (mGy) | DLP[a] (mGy cm) | Effective Dose[a] (mSv) |
|---|---|---|---|
| Cervical | 44.3 (5.3–103.2) | 324 (56–1,275) | 2.6 (0.3–7.5) |
| Thoracic | NA | 253 (66–515) | 4.6 (1.0–9.8) |
| Lumbar | 30.3 (10.6–59.7) | 302 (49–870)[b] | 5.2 (0.8–15.7) |

*NA* not available

[a] Values are given as the median, and range values are in parentheses

[b] Note the differences between lumbar spine CT doses given by Pantos et al. (2011) and Biswas et al. (2009) in Table 2. This differences can be principally explained by the increase in dose between single detector CT and MDCT [Pantos et al. (2011) mainly refers to surveys performed on single detector CT while Biswas et al. (2009) performed its study on MDCT] and also reflect the increase in *z*-axis coverage supported by faster acquisitions with MDCT

In the literature, publications addressing CT scan radiation doses are still rare, and the results described are variable. In a literature review from 2008, Mettler et al. (2008) reported an average effective dose of 6 mSv for spine CTs, with values ranging from 1.5 to 10 mSv. In a more recent literature review, Pantos et al. (2011) reported an even higher range, from 0.8 to 15.7 mSv for a lumbar spine CT, with a median dose of 5.2 mSv (Table 1). On the other hand, a study focusing on musculoskeletal CT doses, Biswas et al. (2009) revealed an average dose of 19.15 mSv in their institution for the acquisition of lumbar spine CT (Table 2). This large dose variability can mainly be explained by the difference in the *z*-axis coverage between these studies. For example, Galanski et al. (2001) reported an average dose of 2.7 mSv with an average coverage of only 5.8 cm with a single-slice CT scanner. Biswas et al. (2009) on the other hand reported an average dose of 19.15 mSv, for an average coverage of 25.5 cm, with a 16-detector row CT scanner. These differences in the delivered radiation dose are more related to the CT acquisition protocol used, rather than a difference in the number of detectors rows. Although the change from single-slice CT to MDCT implied in an increase of the delivered dose (Thomton et al. 2003), the switch from 4 to 16 or 64-detector row CT did not. The technical improvements that accompanied the increase of detector rows keep the delivered dose relatively stable (Mori et al. 2006; Jaffe et al. 2009; Fuji et al. 2009). In fact, the increase in the overall number of CT scans performed (Brenner and Hall 2007) as well as the increase in *z*-axis coverage supported by faster acquisitions lead to increased radiation exposure (Mettler et al. 2008; Richards et al. 2010). Furthermore, within a single institution, significant variations regarding CTDI and DLP are also observed (Tables 2 and 3). This can be explained by the adjustment of exposure parameters according to patient size and CT indication. For example, tube output parameters are kept low for the evaluation of bony structures, whereas for a focused soft tissue evaluation it is necessary that the tube output has to be increased. Implementation of new dose reduction techniques, such as iterative reconstruction, also influences the dose delivered during CT-scan (Table 3).

Very few studies report CT exposure levels on peripheral joints. To our knowledge, the only study analyzing all the doses delivered in musculoskeletal CT, including peripheral joints, was performed by Biswas et al. (2009). Their results showed that with respect to the radiation exposure on CT the farther from trunk the lower the effective dose, which was almost negligible for wrist studies (Table 2). This is due to the fact that peripheral joints are small in size, so tube output parameters and *z*-axis coverage can be shortened. In addition, the tissue weight coefficient used to calculate the effective dose is very small in view of the absence of nearby radiosensitive organs. Table 4 summarizes the values of the tissue weights used by Biswas et al. (2009) to estimate the effective dose in musculoskeletal CT in various anatomic locations.

## 3 Modalities for Dose Reduction in Musculoskeletal CT

The rational for CT dose reduction arises from three major principles of radioprotection: justification, optimization and substitution (International Commission on Radiological Protection 1977). These principles have notably been included in the European directive Euratom 97/43 (European Community 1997)

**Table 2** Upper and lower extremity joint and spine exposure data for computerized tomography (Biswas et al. 2009)

| Joint scan | CTDIvol[a] (mGy) | DLP[a] (mGy cm) | Effective dose[a] (mSv) |
|---|---|---|---|
| Wrist and hand | 14.41 ± 15.52 | 137 ± 134 | 0.03 ± 0.03 |
| Elbow[b] | 21.52 ± 23.83 | 293 ± 311 | 0.14 ± 0.22 |
| Shoulder | 19.49 ± 13.77 | 316 ± 211 | 2.06 ± 1.52 |
| Hip | 19.83 ± 7.67 | 422 ± 174 | 3.09 ± 1.37 |
| Knee | 18.39 ± 14.43 | 360 ± 288 | 0.16 ± 0.12 |
| Ankle and foot[c] | 17.88 ± 13.39 | 310 ± 210 | 0.07 ± 0.05 |
| Cervical spine | 64.17 ± 29.04 | 1,414 ± 831 | 4.36 ± 2.03 |
| Thoracic spine | 64.39 ± 22.23 | 2,171 ± 805 | 17.99 ± 6.12 |
| Lumbar spine | 66.53 ± 21.56 | 1,701 ± 689 | 19.15 ± 5.63 |

[a] The values are given as the mean ± the standard deviation
[b] Arm only (arm above the head)
[c] Unilateral

**Table 3** Lumbar spine CT and shoulder CT-arthrography doses in the present authors' institution before and after implementation of iterative reconstructions Adaptive Iterative Dose Reduction 3D (AIDR 3D, second version of Toshiba CT iterative reconstruction)

| | CTDIvol[a] (mGy) | DLP[a] (mGy cm) | Effective dose[a] (mSv) |
|---|---|---|---|
| Lumbar spine CT | | | |
| Before iterative reconstruction[b] | 40.2 ± 11.4 | 1,094 ± 309 | 12.32 ± 3.5 |
| With AIDR 3D | 25.5 ± 11.9 | 695 ± 338 | 7.83 ± 3.8 |
| Shoulder CT-arthrography | | | |
| Before iterative reconstruction[b] | 43.9 ± 15.9 | 611 ± 260 | 3.98 ± 1.7 |
| With AIDR 3D | 16.1 ± 4.3 | 205 ± 82 | 1.34 ± 0.5 |

[a] The values are given as the mean ± standard deviation
[b] CT-scans performed in Filtered Back Projection with Quantum Denoising System (Toshiba)

**Table 4** Dose conversion factors used to estimate effective doses for different musculoskeletal CT-scan examinations calculated by Biswas et al. (2009)

| Joint and spine CT scan | Dose conversion factors[a] (μSv/mGy cm) |
|---|---|
| Shoulder | 6.52 |
| Elbow[b] | 0.48 |
| Wrist and hand | 0.22 |
| Hip | 7.31 |
| Knee | 0.44 |
| Ankle and foot[c] | 0.23 |
| Cervical spine | 3.08 |
| Thoracic spine | 8.29 |
| Lumbar spine | 11.26 |

[a] Dose conversion factors are calculated by dividing the effective dose by the dose length product given by the study of Biswas et al. (2009). Note that Biswas et al. calculated these factors with IMPACT dosimetry calculator software according to ICRP 60. New factors should be used to take into account the ICRP 103 values
[b] Arm only (arm above the head)
[c] Unilateral

and in the precautionary principle As Low As Reasonably Achievable (ALARA). The ALARA principles have been widely and repetitively discussed in the literature (Kalra et al. 2004; Semelka et al. 2007; McCollough et al. 2009; Lee and Chhem 2010; Singh et al. 2011; Dougeni et al. 2011). We are going to approach each of these principles successively demonstrating their behavioral implications, technological fundaments and focusing on their application in musculoskeletal CT.

## 3.1 Behavioral Factors

**Awareness and education**. First, as in any other field, the level of education and awareness among radiologists and technologists are important elements in the process of dose reduction. Wallace et al. (2010) showed that after educating a physician, it was possible to reduce, by 29%, the lumbar spine CT doses used within several institutions.

**Justification and substitution**. Justification and substitution are also two important elements, particularly in musculoskeletal CT, where the substitution with imaging methods without ionizing radiation, such as ultrasound or MRI are often possible (Semelka et al. 2007; West et al. 2009; Borgen et al. 2006). For instance, Oikarinen et al. (2009) showed in their study on 30 lumbar spine CT performed on patients younger than 35 years that in only seven (23%) of them the indication could be justified. Among these studies, 20 could have been replaced by MRI, and three patients needed no imaging at all. Clarke et al. (2001) also showed that 90% of lumbar spine CT could have been replaced by MRI. MRI, however, is not always feasible because of patient claustrophobia, incompatible implants, pacemakers or critical medical conditions (Semelka et al. 2007). The performance of CT is, nonetheless superior to that of MRI in some settings (West et al. 2009). In spine imaging, CT shows a better sensitivity for the detection of early infection-related bone changes (Tins et al. 2007). CT is also better than MRI for the characterization of gas and calcifications. Because of its high spatial resolution, CT also allows a better visualization of scaphoid cortical fractures (Memarsadeghi et al. 2006), a better analysis of wrist ligaments lesions when combined with arthrography (Moser et al. 2007) and a better detection of some osteoid osteomas with respect to MRI (Liu et al. 2003). Finally, CT-angiography is sometimes better than MR-angiography for the assessment of vascular invasion from bone and soft tissue tumors (Argin et al. 2009; Thévenin et al. 2010). In our institutions, CT is indicated in the following situations: complex fracture, fracture with vascular impairment, fracture-dislocations, occult fractures (other than hip and scaphoid), bone and soft tissue tumors, postoperative follow-up, bone dysplasia, intervertebral disc herniations and joint evaluation. CT arthrography can be performed in almost any joint and offers a better evaluation of superficial cartilage lesions and multiplanar reformations which can be useful in the preoperative evaluation (Omoumi et al. 2009; Wyler et al. 2009).

**Scan coverage and number of phases**. During the realization of a scan, the dose can be mastered by reducing the number of acquisitions (i.e., phases) and the length of acquisition in the *z*-axis (Rehani et al. 2000). The coverage must be limited to the zone of interest, previously identified by the scout views. As mentioned above, it is one of the major reasons for dose differences between various examinations ("The smaller the exposed area, the smaller the dose"). In musculoskeletal CT most examinations consist of a single-phase non enhanced acquisition. With the development of interventional, dynamic and perfusion CT, multiple acquisitions are performed in the same area making the limitation of the number of phases important for dose reduction.

**Position and centering**. A precise centering of the anatomical zone to be scanned in the isocenter of the CT gantry provides optimal image quality and delivered dose (Kalra and Toth 2007). Spatial resolution is better in the isocenter of the gantry because more interpolations of the data are performed than at the periphery (Li et al. 2007). With the increase of the width of the beams, and particularly with 64 or 320-MDCT, cone beams generate more artifacts (Mahesh 2009). These artifacts are less severe in the isocenter of the gantry and are not noticed in practice with a good centering. Moreover, a good centering is particularly important with the use of the automatic dose modulation because the calculations are made considering the patient to be in the isocenter of the gantry. Improper centering can increase the dose significantly (Mahesh 2009). The width of the scanned volume should also be as narrow as possible to limit scattered radiation and beam-hardening artifacts. Therefore, shoulder girdles should be placed on different levels when exploring the shoulder. During acquisitions on the lower limb (i.e., foot, ankle, knee), the contralateral limb should be flexed out of the scanning field when possible. Additionally peripheral joints should be scanned as far as possible from the trunk of the patient in order to decrease the dose received in radiosensitive organs. Biswas et al. (2009) showed that the acquisition of an elbow alongside the body as compared to above the head was the source of a considerable increase of the effective dose (8.35 vs. 0.14 mSv, respectively).

## 3.2 Technical Factors

**Scan modes**. While with the spread of MDCT the helical mode lead to a replacement of the sequential acquisition mode, the development of wide-detector area CT scanners lead to its come back. 320-detector row CT scanners now allow the acquisition of a 16 cm volume, covering the entire length of most joints with a single tube rotation (i.e., shoulder, wrist and hand, hip, sacroiliac, knee, ankle and foot). This scanning mode considerably reduces acquisition time (up to 0.24 s for the acquisition of a 16 cm volume, with no gaps), and hence motion artifacts. Moreover it allows a significant dose reduction with respect to the conventional helical mode. With wide-detector area CT, overbeaming is proportionately less important, compared to 16- or 64-detector row CT scanners (Perisinakis et al. 2009; Mori et al. 2008). In addition, the use of volume mode suppresses the overranging which is characteristic of the helical mode (Gervaise et al. 2010). In helical mode, the additional radiation dose due to overranging increases with the number of detectors and is also proportionally more important for the acquisition of smaller volume lengths (van der Molen and Geleijns 2007), as is the case of peripheral joint acquisitions. Thus, when evaluating small parts with a 16- or 64-detector row CT scanner, some authors suggest using the sequential or step-and-shoot acquisition mode to avoid the additional dose exposure due to overranging (Schilham et al. 2010; Kalra et al. 2004).

**Tube potential**. Reduction of the tube kilovoltage (kV) accounts for an important dose reduction (for example, keeping other parameters constant, a kilovoltage decrease from 120 to 80 kV reduces the delivered dose by a factor of 2.2 (Mahesh 2009), but it is also responsible for considerable increase in image noise (Kalender et al. 2009). In practice, the increase in noise is not detrimental to the analysis of bone structure, thanks to its high natural contrast. It is therefore possible to image peripheral joints at 80 kV (i.e., wrist, knee, ankle, foot) (Figs. 2, 3). For large proximal joints (i.e., shoulder, hip, sacroiliac, spine), the kV must be adapted to the body habitus of the patient: 120 kV for a standard patient, 100 kV for thin patients, and 135–140 kV for patients with excess weight to maintain adequate image quality. For proximal joint CT-arthrography, it is better to use a maximal kilovoltage of 120 because the density of the iodine at 120 is higher than at 140 kV, which can improve the contrast-to-noise ratio (Subhas et al. 2010). During vascular or perfusion examinations, a lower kV of 100 or even 80, depending on the thickness of the anatomical zone to cover, is possible (Nakaura et al. 2011). Some teams also proposed low-dose acquisitions at 100 kV for spinal traumas (Mulkens et al. 2007) or myeloma (Kröpil et al. 2008) assessment. Acquisitions with kV as low as 80 have been advocated for scoliosis (Abul-Kasim et al. 2008) or osteoporosis assessment (Damilakis et al. 2010).

**Tube current and mAs**. The reduction in milli-Amperage (mA) causes a proportional decrease of the delivered dose, but also an increase in image noise. This can be deleterious to the interpretation of the CT-scans which require a good contrast-to-noise ratio, as is the case for discoradicular pathologies. In their study on lumbar spine CT, Bohy et al. (2005) showed that a mAs reduction beyond 35% of the standard settings lead to a decrease in the diagnostic performance of lumbar spine CT. Today, the development of automatic dose modulation allows the adaptation of the mA to the patient's body habitus (McCollough et al. 2006). Van Straten et al. (2009) showed that this type of modulation was particularly interesting in some anatomical regions such as shoulders and pelvis, where it accounted for an effective dose reduction of 11 and 17%, respectively. Its use is also interesting to adapt the mA to the variations in the patient's body habitus when long body segments are imaged (e.g. lumbar spine) while keeping a homogeneous image quality. Mulkens et al. (2005) showed that the use of automatic dose modulation in three-dimension (3D-AEC) allowed for a dose reduction of 37% in lumbar spine CT studies. Mastora et al. (2001) also found that online tube current modulation resulted in a 35% reduction in the product of mean tube current and time with no loss in image quality when exploring the thoracic outlet for

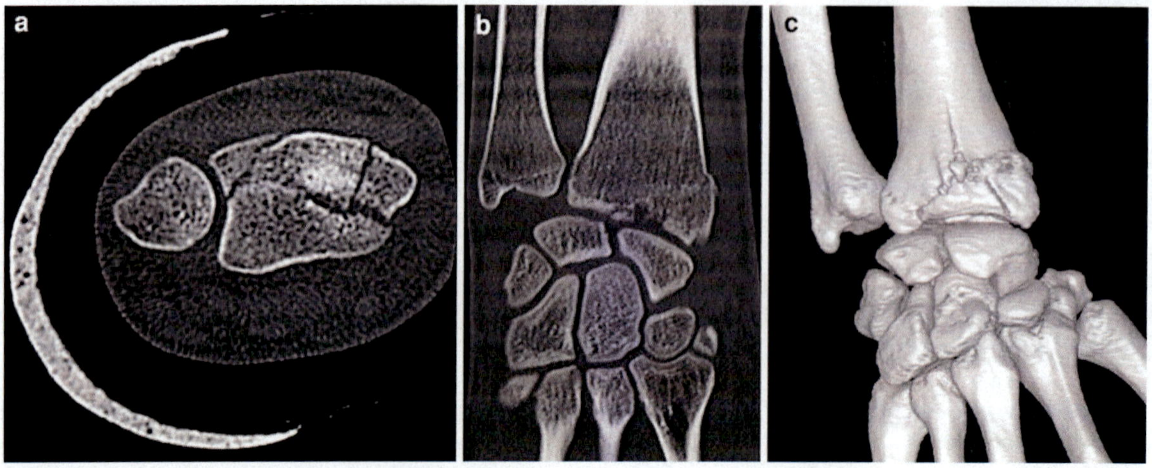


**Fig. 2** CT-scan of the right wrist of a 20-year-old man during the preoperative assessment of a parachute trauma with 0.5 mm axial slices in bone window centered on the distal extremity of the radius (**a**), coronal reformation in bone window in 1.5 mm slice (**b**), and 3D reformation in VR (**c**). Note the good analysis of the bone structures thanks to coronal and 3D reformations in spite of the important reduction of the acquisition parameters (volume acquisition in 200 × 0.5 mm, 80 kV, 50 mAs, rotation time 0.5 s) and scan dose (DLP = 39.3 mGy cm and effective dose = 0.008 mSv). In comparison, this CT dose is only 21 times more than a standard wrist radiographic examination (0.38 μSv) (Noel et al. 2011)

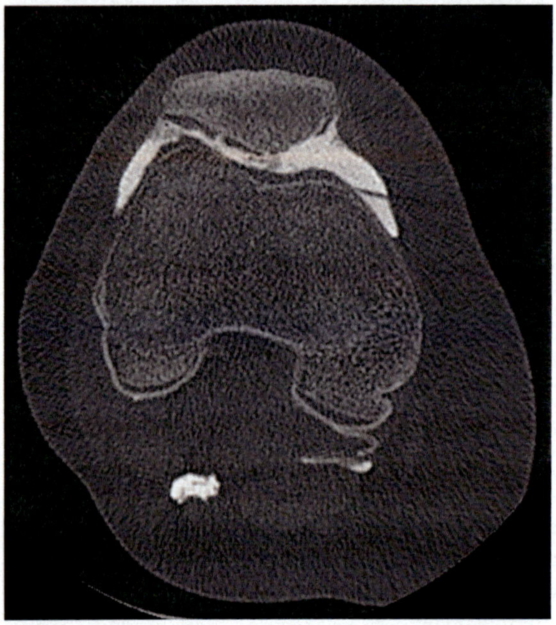

**Fig. 3** CT-arthrography of the right knee of a 64-year-old woman presenting with post-traumatic pain by rupture of a popliteal cyst. Axial slice centered on the patellofemoral joint acquired in volumic scan mode with 80 kV, 50 mAs, rotation time 0.5 s and with DLP = 15.3 mGy cm. Note the good visualization of the patellofemoral chondropathy in spite of the important reduction of the acquisition parameters

suspected thoracic outlet syndrome. Moreover, some authors proposed low-dose protocols with low mA. Horger et al. (2005) showed that whole-body low-dose MDCT is appropriate for the diagnosis of lytic bone lesions and for the assessment of fracture risk in multiple myeloma patients. In their study, a 16 × 1.5 mm collimation was used with a tube voltage of 120 kV and a tube current time product ranging from 40 to 70 mAs. The effective dose of MDCT calculated with a tube current time product of 40 mAs was only 1.7-fold higher than the mean radiation dose associated with whole-body conventional X-ray (4.1 vs. 2.4 mSv) (Horger et al. 2005).

**Pitch**. With some current MDCT using the concept of effective mAs (mAs/pitch), pitch modification has no influence on the dose because it is automatically adapted to mA (Nagel 2007). A high pitch, of about 1.5, is preferred to reduce the acquisition time and motion artifacts (for example, during the exploration of a polytraumatized patient). The pitch should, however, remain lower than 2 to keep an optimal quality of multi-planar reformations (Nagel 2007) and to avoid helical artifacts (Kalra et al. 2004). In contrast, a small pitch is preferred to reduce metal hardware-related artifacts (Stradiotti et al. 2009).

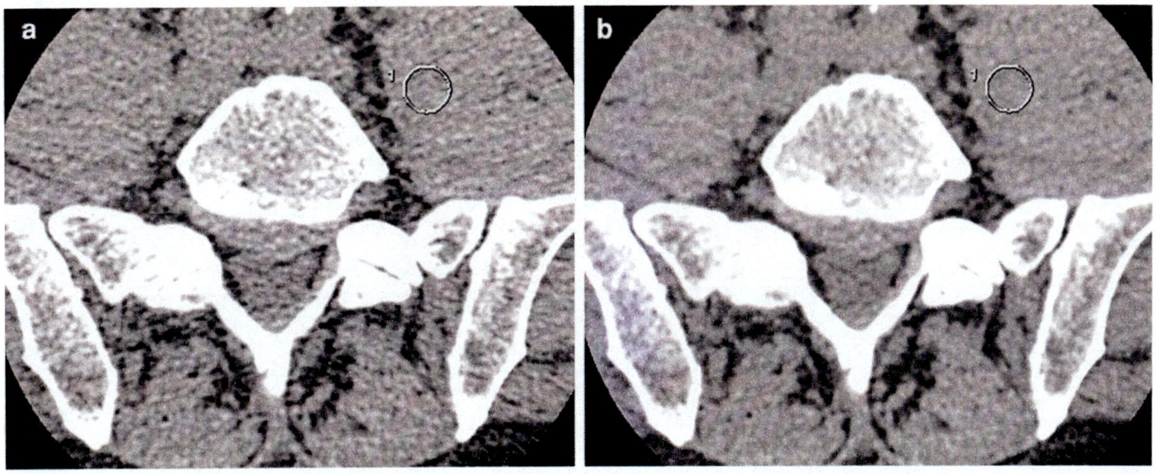


**Fig. 4** Transverse lumbar spine CT images reconstructed with standard filtered back projection (FBP) (**a**) and Adaptive Iterative Dose Reduction 3D (AIDR 3D) (**b**) in a 56-year-old man (1 mm slices, 135 kV, tube current modulation with noise index set at 8, DLP = 347 mGy cm). Note the noise reduction with AIDR 3D compared to FBP, without any significant change in image pattern (standard deviation values of the ROIs placed in left psoas muscles are 27.94 HU with FBP and 18.39 HU with AIDR 3D, which corresponds to a noise reduction of 34%)

**Slice thickness**. In general, acquisitions are performed with thin slices (0.5–1 mm) required for bone structure analysis and reconstructed in thicker slices (2–5 mm) for soft tissues analysis. Submillimetric slices improve spatial resolution, reduce partial volume effects and allow the reconstruction in a quasi-isotropic volume (von Falck et al. 2010). On the other hand, thin slice acquisition can lead to an increased radiation dose to the patient (McNitt-Gray 2002). In case of excessive mA reduction, the acquisition in thin slices engenders an increase in image noise. So, whereas the acquisition is made in submillimetric slices, the soft tissues analysis is performed on thick slices with a better signal-to-noise ratio (von Falck et al. 2010).

**Iterative reconstruction**. The use of iterative reconstruction is a considerable advance in terms of CT dose reduction (Table 3). The first result showed a dose reduction of at least 50%, while keeping an equivalent image quality (Hara et al. 2009; Silva et al. 2009). Few studies have focused on the evaluation of the benefits of iterative reconstruction in musculoskeletal imaging. In our institution, we conducted a study on 15 lumbar spine CT acquired in volume mode with a 320-detector row CT scanner. The images acquired using iterative reconstruction (Adaptive Iterative Dose Reduction—AIDR, first version of Toshiba CT iterative reconstruction) were compared to those acquired using standard filtered back projection (FBP) (Gervaise et al. 2011). Image noise and signal-to-noise ratio (SNR) were quantified, measuring the values of the regions of interest (ROI) placed in similar anatomic regions on both AIDR and FBP series. A subjective analysis of the image quality was performed by two radiologists. Our results showed a significant reduction of 31% (24–37%) of the mean image noise with AIDR, compared with FBP images and an improvement of 47% (33–63%) of the mean SNR. The qualitative evaluation also showed a significant improvement of the image quality on the AIDR series when compared with FBP images. Despite the image noise reduction, there was no modification of spatial resolution. Finally, our study showed a mean potential dose reduction of 52% with AIDR compared to FBP. These preliminary results are promising, and even more so, as iterative reconstructions continue to quickly evolve (Fig. 4).

Whereas iterative reconstruction is particularly interesting to reduce the dose of examinations maintaining a good SNR, it is less useful in cases directed primarily to bone analysis, for example in search of a fracture. The high natural contrast of bone structures allows low-dose acquisitions sometimes noisy, but with no affect on the interpretation. However, one of the other main advantages of iterative reconstruction is the reduction of artifacts associated with beam hardening and FBP (Boas and Fleischmann 2011) (Fig. 5). It is thus particularly interesting for bone and soft tissues analysis when metal hardware is present. Traditionally,

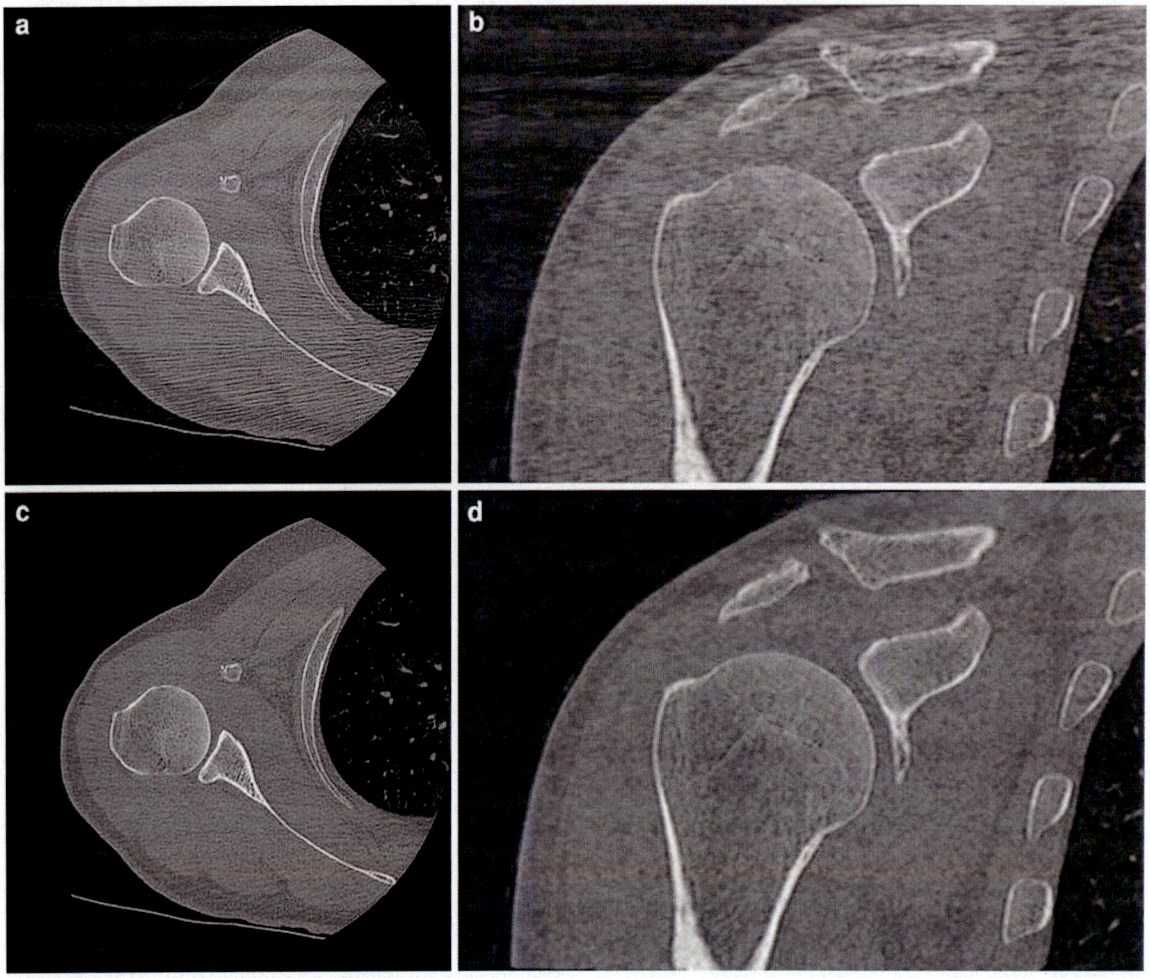

**Fig. 5** Shoulder CT images reconstructed with standard filtered back projection (FBP) (**a**, **b**) and Adaptive Iterative Dose Reduction 3D (AIDR 3D) (**c**, **d**) in a 59-year-old man. 0.5 mm axial slices (**a**, **c**) and 0.5 sagittal reformations (**b**, **d**) in bone windowing. Note the noise reduction with AIDR 3D compared to FBP associated with a reduction of streak artifacts (volume acquisition in 240 × 0.5 mm, 120 kV, 150 mAs, rotation time 0.75 s, DLP = 151 mGy cm and effective dose = 1 mSv)

a better visualization of metallic materials requires the increase of parameters such as the kVp and the mAs, as well as a low pitch and a thin collimation. All these parametric changes are a source of dose increase. Iterative reconstruction reduces the metal and the streak artifacts while avoiding a dose increase due to the optimization of the acquisition parameters.

**Noise reduction filter**. The improvement of the SNR necessary for the analysis of soft tissue, particularly in discoradicular pathology, can also be made by the use of noise reduction filters with a post-processing software. The application of these filters is performed on already-reconstructed images, and can be used with any CT image and even 3D reformations. Contrary to filters used during the process of image reconstruction, some of these noise reduction filters seem to smoothen the image without altering spatial resolution. However, studies should be performed to confirm the benefits of these new post-treatment software packages.

**Overranging shield**. These shields reduce the overranging by using an active collimation in the *z*-axis at the beginning and at the end of the helical CT scan (Stierstorfer et al. 2007). They are particularly interesting for the study of small length body parts with a 16- or 64-detector row CT when overranging is an important factor affecting the radiation dose delivered to the patient. Christner et al. (2010) showed that with a 64-detector row CT, with a pitch of 1, a total nominal beam width of 38.4 mm and an acquisition length of 15 cm, the dose reduction with a shield reached up 16% of the total dose delivered. On the other hand, for acquisitions with a coverage of more than 300 mm in a 64-detector row CT scanner, overranging represented less than 3% of the total dose, whichever pitch was used (Christner et al. 2010). In musculoskeletal CT, this active collimation is thus particularly efficient to reduce the dose during the acquisition with a 16- or 64-detector CT-scan of the shoulders and hips, considering the short coverage and the proximity of radiosensitive organs (i.e., the thyroid and gonads).

## 4 Dynamic Studies of Joint Motion

A study of motion can be performed by the mean of multiple static acquisitions at different joint position or as a continuous dynamic acquisition. This latter must be privileged during motion studies of joints (Wolfe et al. 2000; Moojen et al. 2003; Foumani et al. 2009) not only because the constraints are different between a moving and a static system but also because the phenomenon of hysteresis can influence the position of various anatomical structures (Berdia et al. 2006; Short et al. 1997). The improvement of the temporal resolution of MDCT and the development of wide-detector area CT scanners allow dynamic studies of peripheral joints (Hristova et al. 2009; Blum et al. 2009). The adaptation of the acquisition parameters, as well as the application of recent methods of dose reduction help to maintain a low radiation dose. Thus, CT becomes a functional analysis tool, improving the analysis of in vivo articular motion and joint dysfunction.

A dynamic motion study is possible in helical mode with a 64-detector row CT scanner. Tay et al. (2007) showed in an experimental study that it was possible to perform the motion acquisition of a wrist in four phases with a very low pitch (0.1) by using a protocol with retrospective gating. This technique, however, creates many motion and band artifacts as well as an important increase in radiation dose (Tay et al. 2007), making it a lot less efficient than volume acquisitions with wide-detector CT scanners.

In our institution, we study the motion of joints with a 320-detector row CT, allowing the acquisition of volumes up to 16 cm in length. A tube rotation speed of 0.35 s combined with a partial reconstruction technique of the data warrants a temporal resolution as low as 0.24 s. This volume acquisition mode also presents some advantages: reduction of the dose compared to the helical mode (Gervaise et al. 2010) and the temporal uniformity of the acquired volume (every single voxel acquired at the same time with no table movement and no gaps). Using this technique, we are able to evaluate joint motion in several clinical settings: wrist occult instabilities, patellofemoral pain syndromes, posterior impingement of the ankle and subtalar joint motion analysis (Fig. 6).

These motion studies require the repetition of several acquisitions, which leads to increased radiation dose. On a peripheral joint however, performing low-dose acquisition with an effective dose lower than 1 mSv without compromise to the interpretation of the motion is possible (Snel et al. 2000). For the flexion/extension study of the wrist with an acquisition in volume mode of eight phases (80 kV, 17 mAs, rotation time of 0.35 s, scan length of 10 cm), the DLP is only 133 mGy cm, corresponding to an effective dose of 0.1 mSv (Fig. 7). Thanks to this low effective dose, it is possible to study several types of movements (i.e., flexion/extension, clenching the fist, ulnar and radial deviations), while keeping a total effective dose largely below 1 mSv.

For the dynamic exploration of the hip or the shoulder, it is important to reduce radiation dose by optimizing the scan parameters. If the motion study concerns only the bone segments, the high natural contrast of the bone allows for considerable reduction in kV and mAs (Gurung et al. 2005). It is also important to reduce and center the zone of interest. Even though Hristova et al. (2009) showed improvement of the image quality by continuous acquisition of data, the intermittent acquisition mode is preferred. In this mode the number of phases are generally limited to 12 allowing the reduction in radiation dose by reducing the exposure time. On the pelvis, the radiation dose can be maintained under 10 mSv, which corresponds to that of a standard multiphasic abdominopelvic CT.

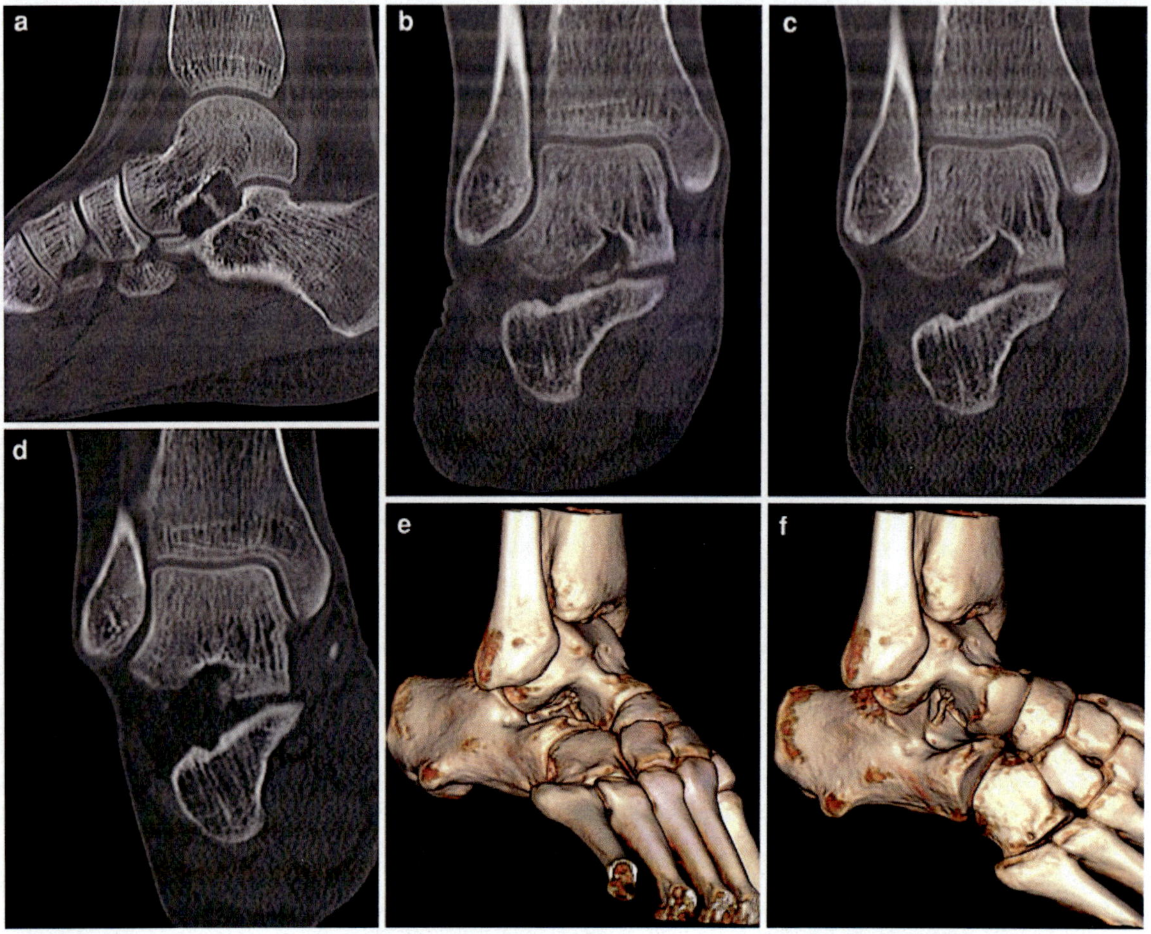


**Fig. 6** Dynamic CT scan of the subtalar joint of the right ankle of a 39-year-old woman presenting with a calcification of cervical ligament of the sinus tarsi. Examination performed with a 320-detector row CT with acquisition of seven dynamic phases during eversion/inversion motion of the ankle (120 kV, 75 mAs, rotation time 0.5 s, DLP = 811 mGy cm, corresponding to an effective dose of 0.6 mSv). Sagittal reformation on the subtalar joint shows the ligament calcification (**a**). Coronal reformations focused on the subtalar joint during the eversion/inversion motion of the ankle (**b–d**) and 3D VR reformations in eversion (**e**) and inversion (**f**) showing the range of motion of the right ankle. In spite of the ligament calcification, this dynamic study shows a conservation of the articular range of motion

## 5 Perfusion Studies

The tumor perfusion with CT-scan was described several years ago (Levine and Neff 1983). Similar to dynamic examinations, CT perfusion of bone and soft tissue tumors are possible due to the improvement of the MDCTs' temporal resolution and the development of wide-detector area CT scanners. CT perfusion studies provide data comparable to that of an MRI on tumoral vascularity, with a better visualization of bone reactive changes (periosteal apposition, cortical fracture, osteolysis) and tumoral neovascularization. The quantification of the enhancement is also easier on CT perfusion when compared to MRI perfusion (Miles et al. 2001). Perfusion studies can be performed in helical mode with MDCT scanners with bidirectional scanning (Ketelsen et al. 2010) or in volume mode with a wide-detector area CT scanners. Tumor perfusion in volume mode, without table movement, can reduce motion artifacts and improve the quality of the reconstructions and perfusion curves. This technique also allows the use of the first acquisition as a bone subtraction mask, thus

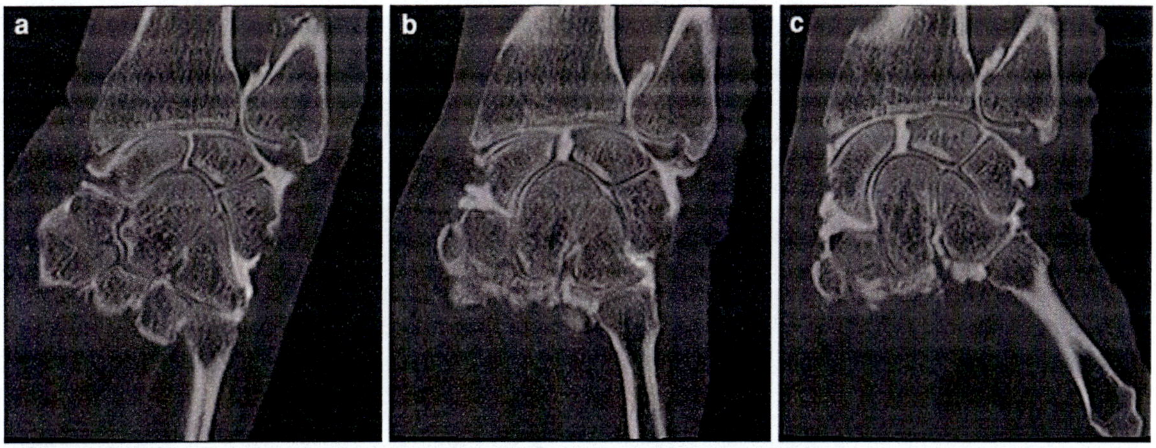

**Fig. 7** Dynamic CT-arthrography of the left wrist of a 57-year-old man presenting with scapholunate and luno-triquetral ligament tears. Examination performed with a 320-detector row CT during a radio-ulnar deviation motion with successive acquisitions of eight volumes (scan length of 10 cm, 80 kV, 17 mAs, rotation time of 0.35 s, corresponding to an acquisition time of 2.8 s, DLP = 133 mGy cm and an effective dose of approximately 0.1 mSv). Frontal reformations in 1.5 mm slices: in radial deviation (phase 1: **a**), in neutral position (phase 3: **b**) and in ulnar deviation (phase 5: **c**). Note the increase of the scapho-lunate gap with the ulnar deviation of the wrist

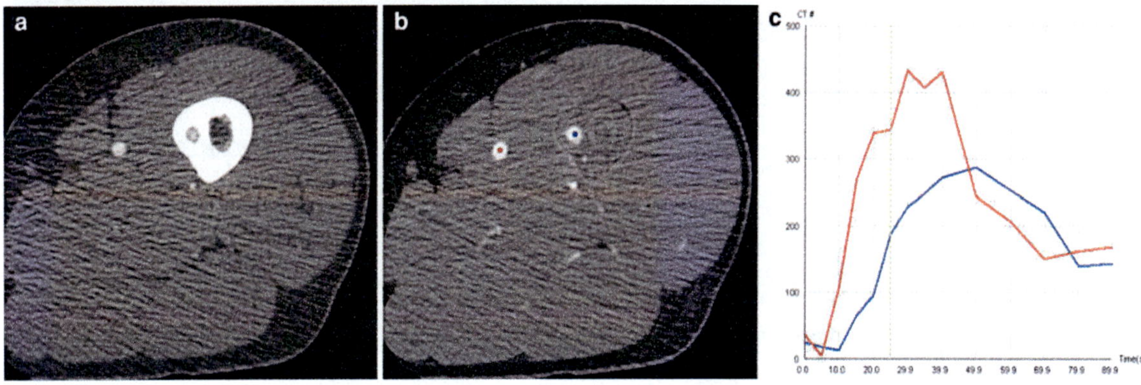

**Fig. 8** Tumor perfusion CT of an osteoid osteoma in the left femoral diaphysis of a 38-year-old patient, with 0.5 mm axial slice after contrast injection at the arterial phase, without (**a**) and with bone subtraction (**b**). Perfusion curves of the left superficial femoral artery (*red*) and of the nidus (*blue*) (**c**). The acquisition was performed with a 320-detector row CT with a 16 cm coverage, with 15 phases (first phase without injection, then nine phases every 5 s and five phases every 10 s), 120 kV, 75 mAs and rotation time of 0.5 s, DLP = 495 mGy cm. Note the good visualization of the nidus thanks to the bone subtraction images, confirming the early arterial contrast enhancement also shown by the CT tumor perfusion curve

improving the detection and characterization of intra-osseous abnormalities. However, these perfusion studies lead to an important increase in radiation dose (Ketelsen et al. 2010). The protocol optimization should be performed by adapting the parameters of acquisition (reduction of the kV and the mAs), by reducing the coverage of the scanned area and by limiting the number of acquisition phases.

In our institution, for example, we studied the benefits of CT perfusion for the diagnosis and the follow-up of osteoid osteomas (Heck et al. 2010). A pathology in which MRI findings may be misleading (Liu et al. 2003), and for which CT can facilitate the diagnosis by showing the bone reaction around a small nidus. In addition to characterization of the lesion, the CT perfusion highlights the hypervascularization of the

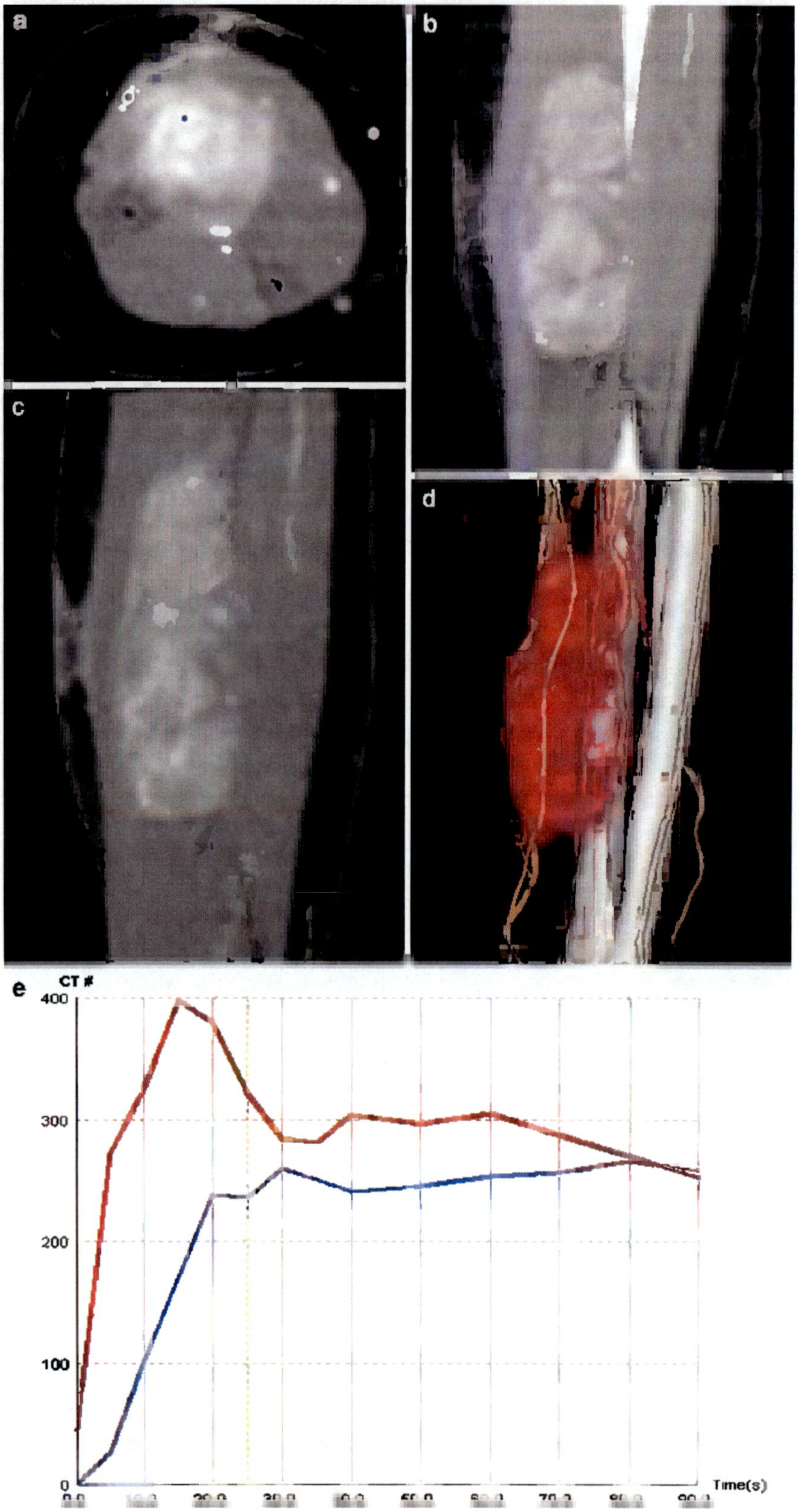


**Fig. 9** Tumor perfusion CT-scan of a schwannoma of the forearm in a 51-year-old woman. 0.5 mm axial slice, at the arterial phase (**a**), sagittal reformation without (**b**) and with bone subtraction (**c**), 3D reformation in VR (**d**) and analysis of the perfusion curves by post-processing software (**e**). The acquisition was performed with a 320-detector row CT in volume mode with 240 × 0.5 mm, 12 cm coverage, 80 kV, 50 mAs and rotation time of 0.5 s, acquisition of a first phase without injection, then an intermittent acquisition of nine phases every 5 s, then of five phases every 10 s. The total DLP for 15 phases is 590 mGy cm. The vascular reformations allow for a better analysis of the ratio between the tumor and the vessels and to assist in preoperative planning. The perfusion curves allow for a better analysis of the tumor angiogenesis

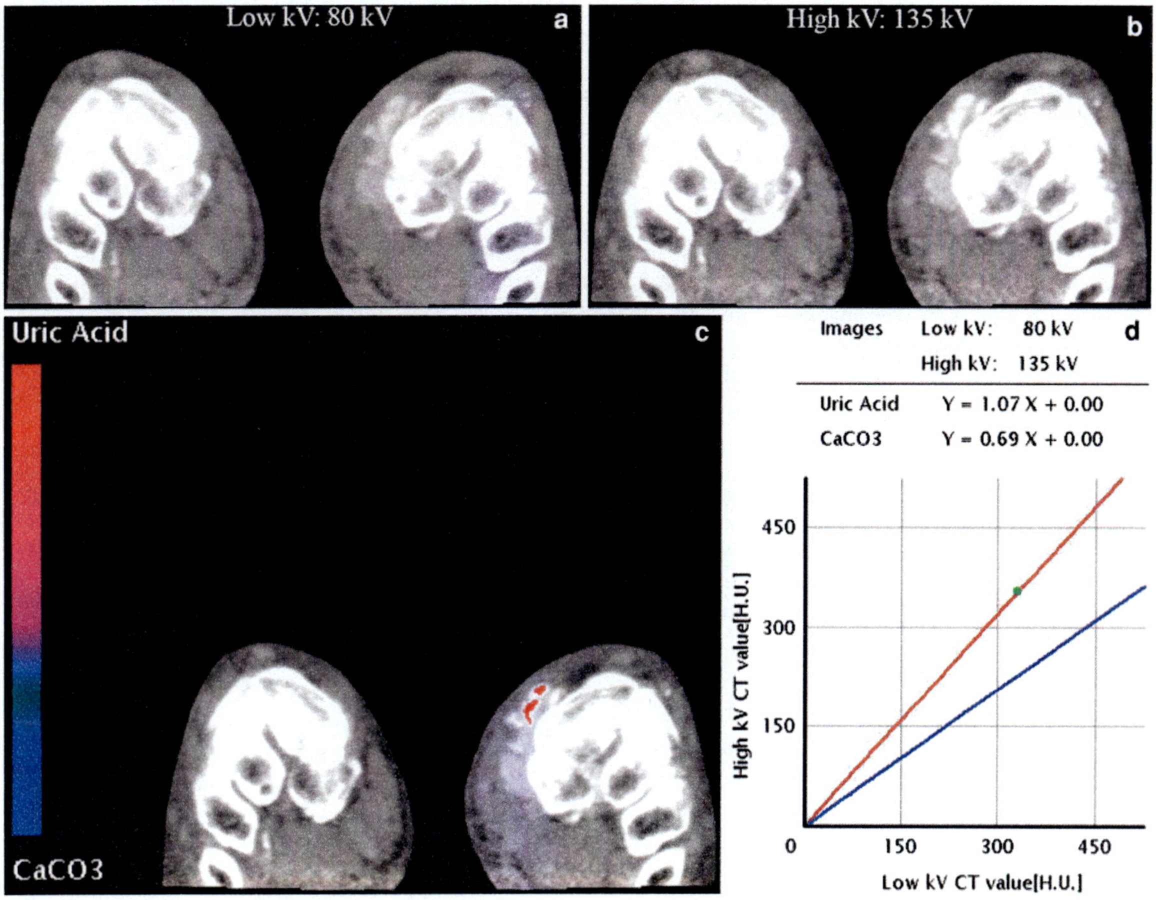


**Fig. 10** Dual-energy CT of a 66-year-old man with tophaceous gout of the feet. Examination performed with a 320-detector row CT with acquisition of two successive volumes of 16 cm focusing on feet/ankles and hands/wrists in 80 kV/217 mAs (**a**) and 135 kV/37 mAs (**b**) (collimation of 320 × 0.5 mm, rotation time of 0.75 s). The total dose is 397 mGy cm, corresponding to an effective dose of 0.09 mSv. Post-processing (**c** and **d**) allows for the characterization of the urate deposits by differentiating them from calcifications, thus confirming the diagnosis of tophaceous gout

nidus. A precontrast mask volume can be subtracted from the subsequent injected volumes removing cortical and trabecular bone and helping to demonstrate bone medullary edema-like changes around the nidus. Thus, this additional information, usually provided by MRI, is now accessible through CT scans. To control the radiation dose, we limit the coverage area of the scanner to the zone of interest (approximately 4–8 cm). Moreover, kV and mAs are adapted to the body habitus of the patient and to the anatomical zone. The number of phases is also limited to 15, with an acquisition interval of 5 s for the first nine phases (arterial phase), and then of 10 s for the latter phases. All these measures provide a perfusion study with a total DLP usually between 500 and 800 mGy cm (Figs. 8 and 9).

## 6 Dual-Energy CT

All manufacturers provide dual energy acquisition on their CT scanners. The techniques used among them are however, quite different. This might have an influence on the results and on the clinical applications of these techniques. Dual-energy CT has several potential applications in the evaluation of musculoskeletal disorders but further studies are still necessary to fully assess its performance (Karcaaltincaba and Aktas 2011).

One application concerns the detection and characterization of urate deposits in gout (Choi et al. 2009). An initial study by Nicolaou et al. (2010) with a dual-source CT scanner showed that the acquisition of all peripheral joints (elbows, wrists, hands, knees, ankles and feet) provides a good sensitivity and specificity for the detection and the location of tophaceous gout with a total effective dose that varied between 2 and 3 mSv. With the 320-detector row CT, a dual-energy technique is obtained from the successive acquisition of two volumes at different kVp acquired without table feed (the first acquisition with a high kilovoltage and a low milliamperage and the opposite for the second). Thanks to post-treatment software, this method differentiates the deposits of gout from simple calcium deposits, while keeping a low total effective dose (Fig. 10).

Another application of dual-energy CT is bone removal during reconstruction, allowing the identification of bone marrow edema. Pache et al. (2010) showed that it is possible to see a post-traumatic bone marrow edema on knee dual-energy CT, with an increase of the radiation of approximately 28% compared with single-energy CT.

Finally, Subhas et al. (2010) showed that compared to a single-energy acquisition dual-energy CT provides a better signal-to-noise ratio relationship on CT-arthrography of the shoulder with an equivalent dose.

## 7 Conclusion

CT is an ever evolving imaging modality that remains an important tool for the evaluation of musculoskeletal disorders. Although further studies are still necessary to ascertain the optimal delivered dose, the developments in CT technology lead to a major reduction of patient exposure. The dose reduction techniques discussed, not only allow the acquisition of high quality images with minimal dose, but also open the possibility for new CT applications. Novel techniques such as dual energy CT or CT perfusion often requires extended volume exploration and/or multiphasic acquisitions not feasible previously due to radiation exposure limitations in clinical examinations.

## References


Abul-Kasim K, Gunnarsson M, Maly P, Ohlin A, Sundgren PC (2008) Radiation dose optimization in CT planning of corrective scoliosis surgery: a phantom study. Neuroradiol J 21:374–382

Argin M, Isayev H, Kececi B, Arkun R, Sabah D (2009) Multidetector-row computed tomographic angiography findings of musculoskeletal tumors: retrospective analysis and correlation with surgical findings. Acta Radiol 50: 1150–1159

Berdia S, Short WH, Wermer FW, Green JK, Panjabi M (2006) The hysteresis effect in carpal kinematics. J Hand Surg Am 31:594–600

Biswas D, Bible JE, Bohan M, Simpson AK, Whang PG, Grauer JN (2009) Radiation exposure from musculoskeletal computerized tomographic scans. J Bone Joint Surg Am 91:1882–1889

Blum A, Lecocq S, Roch D, Louis M, Batch T, Dap F, Dautel G (2009) Etude cinématique du poignet en 3D et 4D avec un scanner 320 canaux. In: SIMS Opus XXXVI. Poignet et main, éd Sauramps médical, Montpellier, pp 375–389

Blum A, Walter F, Ludig T, Zhu X, Roland J (2000) Multislice CT: principles and new CT-scan applications. J Radiol 81:1597–1614

Boas FE, Fleischmann D (2011) Evaluation of two iterative techniques for reducing metal artifacts in computed tomography. Radiology 259:894–902

Bohy P, de Maertelaer V, Roquigny A, Keyzer C, Tack D, Genevois PA (2005) Multidetector CT in patients suspected of having lumbar disk herniation: comparison of standard-dose and simulated low-dose techniques. Radiology 244:524–531

Bongartz G, Golding SJ, Jurik AG et al (2004) European guidelines for multislice computed tomography. Funded by the European Commission (Contract number FIG-MCT2000- 20078-CT-TIP), Mar 2004

Borgen L, Ostense H, Stranden E, Olerud HM, Gudmundsen TE (2006) Shift in imaging modalities of the spine through 25 years and its impact on patient ionizing radiation doses. Eur J Radiol 60:115–119

Brenner DJ, Hall EJ (2007) Computed tomography an increasing source of radiation exposure. N Engl J Med 357:2277–2284

Choi HK, Al-Arfaj AM, Eftekhari A, Munk PL, Shojania K, Reid G, Nicolaou S (2009) Dual energy computed tomography in tophaceous gout. Ann Rheum Dis 68:1609–1612

Christner JA, Zavaletta VA, Eusemann CD, Walz-Flannigan AI, McCollough CH (2010) Dose reduction in helical CT: dynamically adjustable z-axis X-ray beam collimation. Am J Roentgenol 194:W49–W55

Clarke JC, Cranley K, Kelly BE, Bell K, Smith PH (2001) Provision of MRI can significantly reduce CT collective dose. Br J Radiol 74:926–931

Cotten A, Iochum S, Blum A (2002) 3D imaging in musculoskeletal system. In: Baert AL, Caramella D, Bartolozzi C (eds) 3D image processing: techniques and clinical applications. Springer, Berlin, pp 247–255

Damilakis J, Adams JE, Guglielmi G, Link TM (2010) Radiation exposure in X-ray-based imaging techniques used in osteoporosis. Eur Radiol 20:2707–2714

Dougeni E, Faulkner K, Panayiotakis G (2011) A review of patient dose and optimization methods in adult and paediatric CT scanning. Eur J Radiol [Epub ahead of print]

European Commission (1999) European guidelines on quality criteria for computed tomography. Report EUR 16262, Luxembourg

European Community (1997) Council directive 97/43/EURATOM, 30 June 1997, on health protection of individuals against the dangers of ionizing radiation in relation to medical exposure (repealing directive 84/466/Euratom). Off J Eur Commun L180 40:22–27
Fayad LM, Bluemke DA, Fishman EK (2005) Musculoskeletal imaging with computed tomography and magnetic resonance imaging: when is computed tomography the study of choice? Curr Probl Diagn Radiol 34:220–237
Foumani M, Strackee SD, Jonges R, Blankevoort L, Zwinderman AH, Carelsen B, Streekstra GJ (2009) In vivo three-dimensional carpal bone kinematics during flexion-extension and radio-ulnar deviation of the wrist: dynamic motion versus step-wise static wrist positions. J Biomech 42:2664–2671
Fuji K, Aoyama T, Yamauchi-Kawaura C, Koyama S, Yamauchi M, Akahane K, Nishizawa K (2009) Radiation dose evaluation in 64-slice CT examinations with adult and paediatric anthropomorphic phantoms. Br J Radiol 82: 1010–1018
Galanski M, Nagel HD, Stamm G (2001) CT radiation exposure risk in Germany. Rofo 173:R1–R66
Gervaise A, Louis M, Batch T, Loeuille D, Noel A, Guillemin F, Blum A (2010) Réduction de dose dans l'exploration du rachis lombaire grâce au scanner 320-détecteurs: étude initiale. J Radiol 91:779–785
Gervaise A, Osemont B, Lecocq S, Micard E, Noel A, Felblinger J, Blum A (2011) CT image quality improvement using adaptive iterative dose reduction with wide-volume acquisition on 320-detector CT. Eur Radiol [Epub ahead of print]
Gleeson TG, Morirty J, Shortt CP, Gleeson JP, Fitzpatrick P, Byrne B, McHugh J, O'Connell M, O'Gorman P, Eustace SJ (2009) Accuracy of whole-body low-dose multidetector CT (WBLDCT) versus skeletal survey in the detection of myelomatous lesions, and correlation of disease distribution with whole-body MRI (WBMRI). Skelet Radiol 38: 225–236
Goh V, Padhani AR (2006) Imaging tumor angiogenesis: functional assessment using MDCT or MRI? Abdom Imaging 31:194–199
Gurung J, Khan MF, Maataoui A, Herzog C, Bux R, Ackermann H, Vogl TJ (2005) Multislice CT of the pelvis: dose reduction with regard to image quality using 16-row CT. Eur Radiol 15:1898–1905
Hara AK, Paden RG, Silva AC, Kujak JL, Lawder HJ, Pavlicek W (2009) Iterative reconstruction technique for reducing body radiation dose at CT: feasibility study. Am J Roentgenol 193:764–771
Heck O, Louis M, Wassel J, Lecocq S, Gondim-Teixeira P, Moisei A, Blum A (2010) Apport du scanner volumique dynamique dans le diagnostic d'ostéome ostéoïde. Journées Françaises de Radiologie, Paris
Hidajat N, Wolf M, Nunnemann A, Liersch P, Gebauer B, Teichgraber U, Schroder RJ, Felix R (2001) Survey of conventional and spiral CT doses. Radiology 218:395–401
Horger M, Claussen CD, Bross-Bach U, Vonthein R, Trabold T, Heuschmid M, Pfannenberg C (2005) Whole-body lowdose multidetector row-CT in the diagnosis of multiple myeloma: an alternative to conventional radiography. Eur J Radiol 54:289–297
Hristova L, Batch T, Blum A (2009) Analyse des artéfacts de mouvement de l'exploration dynamique et volumique au scanner 320 barettes (abstract). J Radiol 90(10):1583
International Commission on Radiological Protection (1977) Recommendations of the International Commission on Radiological Protection, ICRP publication 26. Pergamon, Oxford
International Commission on Radiological Protection (1991) Recommendations of the International Commission on Radiological Protection. ICRP Publication 60. Pergamon, Oxford
Iochum S, Ludig T, Walter F, Fuchs A, Henrot P, Blum A (2001) Value of volume rendering in musculo-skeletal disorders. J Radiol 82:221–230
Jaffe TA, Yoshizumi TT, Toncheva G, Anderson-Evans C, Lowry C, Miller CM, Nelson RC, Ravin CE (2009) Radiation dose for body CT protocols: variability of scanners at one institution. Am J Roentgenol 193:1141–1147
Kalender WA, Deak P, Kellermeier M, van Straten M, Vollmar SV (2009) Application and patient size-dependent optimization of X-ray spectra for CT. Med Phys 36: 993–1007
Kalra MK, Maher MM, Toth TL, Hamberg LM, Blake MA, Shepard JA, Saini S (2004) Strategies for CT radiation dose optimization. Radiology 230:619–628
Kalra MK, Toth TL (2007) Patient centering in MDCT: dose effects. In: Tack D, Genevois PA (eds) Radiation dose from adult and pediatric multidetector computed tomography. Springer, Berlin, pp 129–132
Karcaaltincaba M, Aktas A (2011) Dual-energy CT revisited with multidetector CT: review of principles and clinical applications. Diagn Interv Radiol 17:181–194
Ketelsen D, Horger M, Buchgeister M, Fenchel M, Thomas C, Boehringer N, Schulze M, Tsiflikas I, Claussen CD, Heuschmid M (2010) Estimation of radiation exposure of 128-slice 4D-perfusion CT for the assessment of tumor vascularity. Korean J Radiol 11:547–552
Kröpil P, Fenk R, Fritz LB, Blondin D, Kobbe G, Mödder U, Cohnen M (2008) Comparison of whole-body 64-slice multidetector computed tomography and conventional radiography in staging of multiple myeloma. Eur Radiol 18:51–58
Lee TY, Chhem RK (2010) Impact of new technologies on dose reduction in CT. Eur J Radiol 76:28–35
Levine E, Neff JR (1983) Dynamic computed tomography scanning of benign bone lesions: preliminary results. Skelet Radiol 9:238–245
Li J, Udayasankar UK, Toth TL, Seamans J, Small WC, Kalra MK (2007) Automatic patient centering for MDCT: effect on radiation dose. Am J Roentgenol 188:547–552
Liu PT, Chivers FS, Roberts CC, Schultz CJ, Beauchamp CP (2003) Imaging of osteoid osteoma with dynamic gadolinium-enhanced MR imaging. Radiology 227:691–700
McNitt-Gray MF (2002) AAPM/RSNA physics tutorial for residents: topics in CT radiation dose in CT. Radiographics 22:1541 1553
Mahesh M (2009) Scan parameters and image quality in MDCT. In: Mahesh M (ed) MDCT physics: The basics—technology, image quality and radiation dose. Lippincott Williams & Wilkins, Philadelphia, pp 47–78

Mastora I, Rémy-Jardin M, Seuss C, Scherf C, Guillot JP, Rémy J (2001) Dose reduction in spiral CT angiography of thoracic outlet syndrome by anatomically adapted tube current modulation. Eur Radiol 11:590–596
McCollough CH, Bruesewitz MR, Kofler JM (2006) CT dose reduction and dose management tools: overview of available options. Radiographics 26:503–512
McCollough CH, Primak AN, Braun N, Kofler J, Yu L, Christner J (2009) Strategies for reducing radiation dose in CT. Radiol Clin North Am 47:27–40
Memarsadeghi M, Breitenseher M, Schaefer-Prokop C, Weber M, Aldrian S, Gäbler C, Prokop M (2006) Occult scaphoid fractures: CT versus MR imaging. Radiology 240: 169–176
Mettler FA, Huda W, Yoshizumi TT, Mahesh M (2008) Effective doses in radiology and diagnostic nuclear medicine: a catalog. Radiology 248:254–263
Miles KA, Charnsangavej C, Lee F, Fishman E, Horton K, Lee TY (2001) Application of CT in the investigation of angiogenesis in oncology. Acad Radiol 7:840–850
Moojen TM, Snel JG, Ritt MJ, Venema HW, Kauer JM, Bos KE (2003) In vivo analysis of carpal kinematics and comparative review of the literature. J Hand Surg Am 28: 81–87
Mori S, Endo M, Nishizawa K, Murase K, Fujiwara H, Tanada S (2006) Comparison of patient doses in 256-slice CT and 16-slice CT scanners. Br J Radiol 79:56–61
Mori S, Nishizawa K, Kondo C, Ohno M, Akahane K, Endo M (2008) Effective doses in subjects undergoing computed tomography cardiac imaging with the 256-multislice CT scanner. Eur J Radiol 65:442–448
Moser T, Dosch JC, Moussaoui A, Dietemann JL (2007) Wrist ligament tears: evaluation of MRI and combined MDCT and MR arthrography. Am J Roentgenol 188:1278–1286
Mulkens TH, Bellinck P, Baeyaert M, Ghysen D, Van Dijck X, Mussen E, Venstermans C, Termote JL (2005) Use of an automatic exposure control mechanism for dose optimization in multi-detector row CT examinations: clinical evaluation. Radiology 237:213–223
Mulkens TH, Marchal P, Daineffe S, Salgado R, Bellinck P, te Rijdt B, Kegelaers B, Termote JL (2007) Comparison of low-dose with standard-dose multidetector CT in cervical spine trauma. Am J Neuroradiol 28:1444–1450
Nagel HD (2007) CT parameters that influence the radiation dose. In: Tack D, Genevois PA (eds) Radiation dose from adult and pediatric multidetector computed tomography. Springer, Berlin, pp 51–79
Nakaura T, Awai K, Oda S, Yanaga Y, Namimoto T, Harada K, Uemura S, Yamashita Y (2011) A low-kilovolt (peak) high tube current technique improves venous enhancement and reduces the radiation dose at indirect multidetector-row CT venography: initial experience. J Comput Assist Tomogr 35:141–147
Nicolaou S, Yong-Hing CJ, Galea-Soler S, Hou DJ, Louis L, Munk P (2010) Dual-energy CT as a potential new diagnostic tool in the management of gout in the acute setting. Am J Roentgenol 194:1072–1078
Noel A, Ottenin MA, Germain C, Soler M, Villani N, Grosprêtre O, Blum A (2011) Comparison of irradiation for tomosynthesis and CT of the wrist. J Radiol 92:32–39
Oikarinen H, Meriläinen S, Pääkkö E, Karttunen A, Nieminen MT, Tervonen O (2009) Unjustified CT examinations in young patients. Eur Radiol 19:1161–1165
Oldrini G, Lombard V, Roch D, Detreille R, Lecocq S, Louis M, Wassel J, Batch T, Blum A (2009) Courbes de rehaussement des tumeurs osseuses et des parties molles: comparaison entre scanner et IRM (abstract). J Radiol 90:1578
Omoumi P, Mercier GA, Lecouvet F, Simoni P, Vande Berg BC (2009) CT arthrography, MR arthrography, PET, and scintigraphy in osteoarthritis. Radiol Clin North Am 47: 595–615
Pache G, Krauss B, Strohm P, Saueressig U, Blanke P, Bulla S, Schäfer O, Helwig P, Kotter E, Langer M, Baumann T (2010) Dual-energy CT virtual noncalcium technique: detecting posttraumatic bone marrow lesions- feasibility study. Radiology 256:617–624
Pantos I, Thalassinou S, Argentos S, Kelekis NL, Panayiotakis G, Efstathopoulos EP (2011) Adult patient radiation doses from non-cardiac CT examinations: a review of published results. Br J Radiol 84:293–303
Perisinakis K, Papadakis AE, Damilakis J (2009) The effect of X-ray beam quality and geometry on radiation utilization efficiency in multidetector CT imaging. Med Phys 36:1258–1266
Rehani MM, Bongartz G, Kalender W et al (2000) Managing X-ray dose in computed tomography: ICRP special task force report. Ann ICRP 30:7–45
Richards PJ, George J, Metelko M, Brown M (2010) Spine computed tomography doses and cancer induction. Spine 35:430–433
Schilham A, van der Molen AJ, Prokop M, Jong HW (2010) Overranging at multi-section CT: an underestimated source of excess radiation exposure. Radiographics 30: 1057–1067
Semelka RC, Armao DM, Elias J, Huda W (2007) Imaging strategies to reduce the risk of radiation in CT studies, including selective substitution with MRI. JMRI 25:900–909
Short WH, Werner FW, Fortino MD, Mann KA (1997) Analysis of the kinematics of the scaphoid and lunate in the intact wrist joint. Hand Clin 13:93–108
Shrimpton PC, Edyvean S (1998) CT scanner dosimetry. Br J Radiol 71:1–3
Silva A, Lawder H, Hara A, Kujak J, Pavlicek W (2009) Innovations in CT dose reduction strategy: application of the adaptive statistical iterative reconstruction algorithm. Am J Roentgenol 194:191–199
Singh S, Kalra MK, Thrall JH, Mahesh M (2011) CT radiation dose reduction by modifying primary factors. J Am Coll Radiol 8:369–372
Snel JG, Venema HW, Moojen TM, Ritt JP, Grimbergen CA, den Heeten GJ (2000) Quantitative in vivo analysis of the kinematics of carpal bones from three-dimensional CT images using a deformable surface model and a three-dimensional matching technique. Med Phys 27:2037–2047
Stierstorfer K, Kuhn U, Wolf H, Petersilka M, Suess C, Flohr T (2007) Principle and performance of a dynamic collimation technique for spiral CT (abstract). In: Radiological society of North America scientific assembly and annual meeting

program. Radiological Society of North America, Oak Brook, SSA16-04

Stradiotti P, Curti A, Castellazzi G, Zerbi A (2009) Metal-related artifacts in instrumented spine: techniques for reducing artifacts in CT and MRI: state of the art. Eur Spine J 18:S102–S108

Subhas N, Freire M, Primak AN, Polster JM, Recht MP, Davros WJ, Winalski CS (2010) CT arthrography: in vitro evaluation of single and dual energy for optimization of technique. Skelet Radiol 39:1025–1031

Tay SC, Pimak AN, Fletcher JG, Schmidt B, Amrami KK, Berger RA, Mc Collough CH (2007) Four-dimensional computed tomographic imaging in the wrist: proof of feasibility in a cadaveric model. Skelet Radiol 36: 1163–1169

Thévenin FS, Drapé JL, Biau D, Campagna R, Richarme D, Guerini H, Chevrot A, Larousserie F, Babinet A, Anract P, Feydy A (2010) Assessment of vascular invasion by bone and soft tissue tumors of the limbs: usefulness of MDCT angiography. Eur Radiol 20:1524–1531

Thomton FJ, Paulson EK, Yoshizumi TT, Frush DP, Nelson RC (2003) Single versus multi-detector row CT: comparison of radiation doses and dose profiles. Acad Radiol 10:379–385

Tins BJ, Cassar-Pullicino VN, Lalam RK (2007) Magnetic resonance imaging of spinal infection. Top Magn Reson Imaging 18(3):213–222

van der Molen AJ, Geleijns J (2007) Overranging in multisection CT: quantification and relative contribution to dose—comparison of four 16-section CT scanners. Radiology 242:208–216

van Straten M, Deak P, Shrimpton PC, Kalender WA (2009) The effect of angular and longitudinal tube current modulations on the estimation of organ and effective doses in X-ray computed tomography. Med Phys 36(11):4881–4889

von Falck C, Galanski M, Shin H (2010) Sliding-thin-slab averaging for improved depiction of low-contrast lesions with radiation dose savings at thin-section CT. Radiographics 30:317–326

Wallace AB, Goergen SK, Schick D, Soblusky T, Jolley D (2010) Multidetector CT dose: clincal pratice improvement strategies from a successful optimization program. J Am Coll Radiol 7:614–624

West ATH, Marshall TJ, Bearcroft PW (2009) CT of the musculoskeletal system: what is left is the days of MRI? Eur Radiol 19:152–164

Wolfe SW, Neu C, Crisco JJ (2000) In vivo scaphoid, lunate and capitate kinematics in flexion and in extension. J Hand Surg Am 25:860–869

Wyler A, Bousson V, Bergot C, Polivka M, Leveque E, Vicaut E, Laredo JD (2009) Comparison of MR-arthrography and CT-arthrography in hyaline cartilage-thickness measurement in radiographically normal cadaver hips with anatomy as gold standard. Osteoarthr Cartil 17:19–25

# Dose Reduction in CT Fluoroscopy

N. Buls, F. Vandenbroucke, and J. de Mey

## Contents




**Abstract**

CT Fluoroscopy (CTF) is a technique that requires adequate radiation protection management for both patient and staff. Since the scanning plane is kept constant during the entire procedure, the same skin area is repeatedly exposed and cumulative patient skin doses can be substantial. Whereas, with conventional fluoroscopy the 2 Gy threshold dose for tissue reactions is reached after 100–200 min of fluoroscopy, it can be reached in CTF only after 3–10 min of scanning when a high tube current is applied. In contrast to diagnostic CT where the operator is protected behind the lead screen of the console, CTF procedures require the presence of the staff in the examination room. For the physician, particularly the doses to the lens of 'the eyes and the hands are of concern. Doses to the eyes can be anywhere in the range of 0.01–0.2 mGy per procedure. If protection is not used, there can be a substantial risk of lens opacity for procedures that require long fluoroscopy times and with several procedures per day, such as in busy department. Effective protection can be used to reduce the probability of cataract to a negligible level. Operators need to be aware of different methods of CTF guidance and the factors that determine radiation exposure of both patient and staff. This becomes more important as the spectrum of CTF procedures might expand to more complex procedures that may require longer fluoroscopy times.



N. Buls (✉) · F. Vandenbroucke · J. de Mey
UZ Brussel, Laarbeeklaan 101, 1090 Brussel, Belgium
e-mail: Nico.Buls@uzbrussel.be



D. Tack et al. (eds.), *Radiation Dose from Multidetector CT*, Medical Radiology. Diagnostic Imaging,
DOI: 10.1007/174_2011_453, © Springer-Verlag Berlin Heidelberg 2012

## 1 Introduction

Computed Tomography Fluoroscopy (CTF) is a technique that provides the physician immediate feedback due to the real-time reconstruction and display of CT images as in ultrasound and conventional fluoroscopy. It matches the advantages of the quality of CT images with the speed of fluoroscopic guidance. CTF images have (1) a wide dynamic range for imaging air, soft tissue and bone (2) they do not superimpose anatomical structures as does conventional fluoroscopy (3) and provide acceptable image quality less affected by patient breathing and motion (Kato et al. 1996; Froelich et al. 1998; Nickoloff et al. 2000). These characteristics allow immediate correction for depth and direction of a needle during a percutaneous procedure. The obvious benefits of obtaining CT images in real time has made CTF a popular image-guiding tool for various types of non-vascular and therapeutic interventions. Reported procedures with CTF guidance are, among others, core biopsies, fluid collection aspirations, catheter insertion and drainage, local drug injections, radio-frequency (RF) ablation procedures, placement of marking coils before stereotactic radiotherapy, lumbar nerve root blocks, vertebroplasty, jejunostomy tube insertion, arthrodesis of the spine and arthrography. The term "fluoroscopy" in CTF is only used by analogy with its conventional radiology counterpart; the only common thing is that both techniques are based on X-ray imaging giving the impression of a real-time imaging display. In this chapter, the use of real-time CT is referred to as CT fluoroscopy.

### 1.1 Radiation Risk

A drawback of CTF is the potential for significantly high patient and staff doses. This is reported by several authors and also by competent bodies such as the UNSCEAR in their 2000 report and the ICRP in their report "managing patient dose in CT" (ICRP 2000). The interventional nature of CTF requires specific radiation protection considerations compared to conventional CT.

First of all, the patient skin dose is of concern. Since the scanning plane is kept constant during the entire procedure, the same skin area is repeatedly exposed and cumulative patient skin doses can be substantial and may reach thresholds for radiation injuries. 'Maximum patient skin dose' is therefore the risk-related quantity of concern, rather than the 'effective dose of the patient'. Effective dose from CTF is usually from the same order of magnitude as doses from diagnostic CT scans due to the small-irradiated patient volume. With CTF, the user can select high exposure settings in terms of high tube potentials (120 kVp) and high tube currents (90 mA). These are high values when compared to the exposure factors used in, for example, vascular interventional radiology (IR). Furthermore, prolonged CT-scanning times can be necessary in cases of small and lesions with difficult accessibility. This results in substantial skin doses.

In contrast to conventional CT where the operator is protected behind the lead screen of the console, CTF procedures require the presence of the staff in the examination room during CT scanning (Fig. 1a). As a result, the operator is exposed to an intense scatter radiation field. For such IR procedures it is standard practice for the medical staff to protect themselves by wearing a lead apron. A lead apron efficiently shields most important organs, reducing the effective dose of the individual. However, surface doses to the parts of the body that are not shielded by the apron can be substantial. These are in particular the doses to both hands and to the head eyes. Furthermore, information of these doses is often unavailable, as they are not monitored routinely. The dose to the hands is of concern due to its proximity to the scanning plane, and although it is unacceptable to scan with the hands in the primary beam and every effort must be made to keep out of the primary beam, the risk exists and it has been reported (Fig. 1b). The dose to the eyes may need to be monitored to ensure that it does not approach the level at which lens opacities might occur. Recent epidemiological studies show increased sensitivity to radiation than previously considered (ICRP 2011). Ideally, a CT room should be as well equipped regarding radiation protection devices when compared to X-ray equipment that is used in, for example, a vascular interventional radiology suite with mobile lead shields or other barriers. As in many IR procedures, specialists other

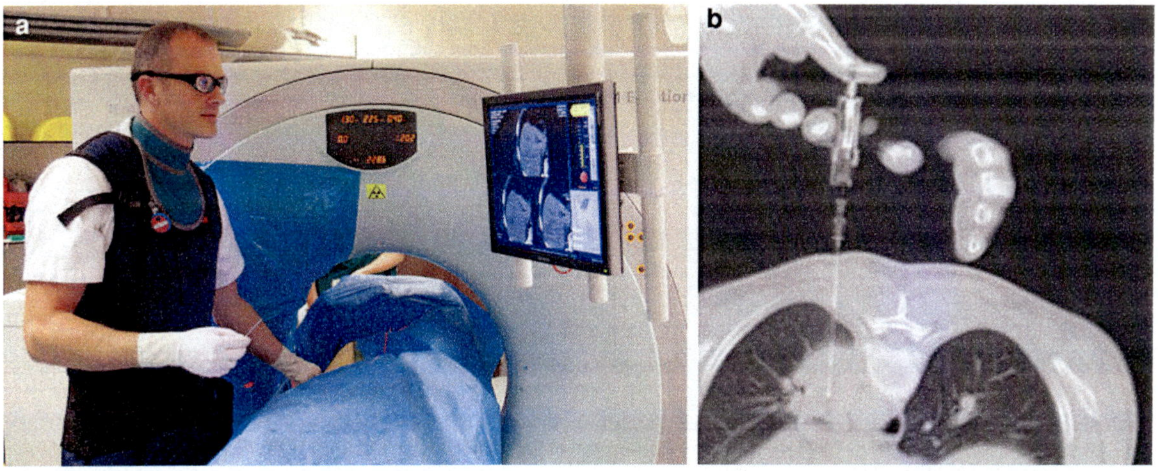

**Fig. 1** **a, b** The presence of staff in the examination room during CT scanning can lead to their exposure to an intense scatter radiation field, especially of body parts not protected by the lead apron. Particular concern is for hands and eyes

than radiologists could be involved. Although it is a requirement of the Euratom 97/43 directive (Euratom 1997) that staff performing practical aspects of a medical exposure should have received adequate training in radiation protection, a non-radiologist (e.g. pneumonologist) may have not had in-depth training in radiation management using diverse forms of fluoroscopic equipment such as CTF. The learning process involved with an ever evolving technology such as CTF has a profound impact on both patient and staff doses. It is clear that CTF is another advancement in radiology with additional challenges in radiation management (Wagner 2000).

## 2 Technical Development

Since its introduction in radiology about 40 years ago, CT has been used as a guidance tool for various percutaneous interventions in both adults (Haaga and Alfidi 1976; Moran et al. 1979) and children (Baran et al. 1984). During the past 35 years, CT technology has made rapid progress with the development of slip ring technology, X-ray tubes with improved heat capacity, sub-second rotation times, fast array processors, and the development of partial reconstruction algorithms. These advantages contributed to the development of a CTF system (or real-time CT scanning system) that was introduced by Katada et al. (1994). They modified a third generation CT scanner by adding a high-speed array processor (real-time reconstruction unit) to increase the image reconstruction speed (Katada et al. 1996) of the CT images. The first image is created from the initial 360° of raw data acquired during scanning. Subsequently, the corresponding data of the next 60° scanning are processed by the real-time reconstruction unit and replace the first 60° data set of the previous image. This technique of synchronous addition of new and subtraction of old 60° data sets allows updating of the image at a rate of six frames per second and provides the operator a nearly real-time display of CT images. The system used a reduced image matrix of $256 \times 256$ in order to achieve a higher response rate that resulted in a delay time of only 0.17 s.

Figure 1a shows the configuration of a typical CTF system. The physician can operate the equipment entirely from in-room controls, being able to manage the procedure alongside the table, similar to an angiography suite. The obtained real-time images are displayed on an in-room monitor located next to the scan. A joystick attached to the couch can be used for controlling the patient position.

Recent multi-detector row CT scanners can often acquire multiple sections (usually three) that are displayed simultaneously on multiple monitors at increased frame rates (between 6 and 13 frames/second). Multiple-image CT fluoroscopy has the potential to increase the likelihood of localizing the tip of the needle in the z-direction during a single shot

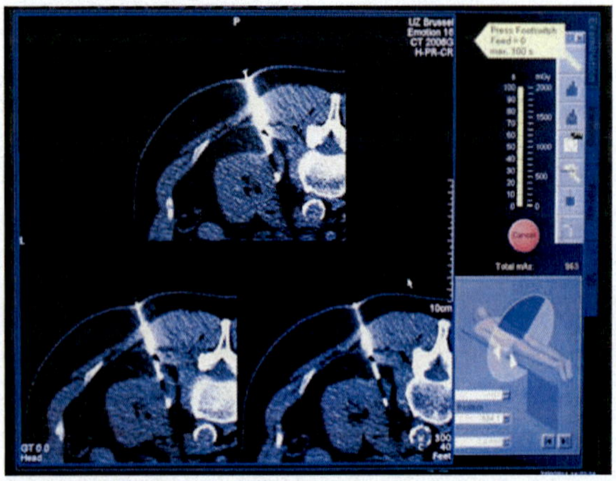

**Fig. 2** Multiple-image CT fluoroscopy

exposure due to the larger coverage (Kataoka et al. 2006). This could be especially helpful in angulated access routes (Fig. 2). Today, also 3D interventional modules with real-time coronal, sagittal and oblique reconstructions are available, allowing safer and faster interventions. Automatic needle detection and path planning applications give a more accurate overview of the needle position and easier needle navigation.

Today, CTF is available from most CT manufacturers. The CTF packages are usually sold as upgrade options, usually consisting of an exposure foot pedal, tabletop control mechanism, in-room monitor(s) and sometimes including hardware to enable rapid image reconstruction (Keat 2001).

## 2.1 Scanning Techniques: Real-Time Method and Quick-Check Method

There are two common CT fluoroscopic guidance methods: the initial real-time (continuous) method and the quick-check (intermittent) method developed by Silverman et al. (1999). The distinction between both is whether the system is operated continuously in real time during needle manipulation or whether it is operated intermittently between interventional actions. Real-time CTF shows the exact needle trajectory during advancement or manipulation and requires the use of a standoff needle holder in order to increase distance to the scanning plane. With the quick-check method single fluoroscopic spot images are acquired to check needle location after manipulation and to confirm alignment with the puncture tract. During these spot images, the physician can retract his hands from the scanning plane. This reduces scatter exposure to the hands due to the increased distance of the manipulators hands to the scanning plane, and also prevents exposing his hands to the primary beam (Fig. 1b). It is well acknowledged that the quick-check method reduces CT scanning time, and thus both patient and staff exposure. It is advocated to be used whenever possible, reserving the use of the real-time mode only in selected cases in which respiratory motion is a problem or in cases when passing 'dangerous' structures (Carlson et al. 2001; Silverman et al. 1999; Paulson et al. 2001; Buls et al. 2003; Brennan et al. 2003).

# 3 Interventional Techniques: Clinical Procedures

Non-vascular diagnostic and therapeutic interventions with CT fluoroscopy are becoming more and more important in patients workup. This evolution is seen despite the improving performance of diagnostic imaging (CT, MR, ultrasound and nuclear medicine) and the improvement of surgical techniques. There are four main reasons for the shift to a more invasive diagnostic and therapeutic approach in radiology.

First, due to the technical evolution, CT fluoroscopy proves to be an accurate, safe and fast technique in guiding interventional procedures. Besides the evolution in imaging techniques, the development of new biopsy needles made it possible to obtain core biopsies under image guiding in an accurate way. New drainage catheters and new ablation techniques opened a broad spectrum of therapeutical options in non-vascular interventional radiology. A second reason is the evolution in oncology. A few decades ago major surgery was often the only option in oncology and it was obvious that a percutaneous biopsy before surgery was not useful in the patient workup. During the last decades a broad spectrum of new therapeutical options were developed in radiotherapy, oncology and surgery. Optimal morphological tumor staging (TNM classification), anatomopathological staging (cancer type) in combination with biological tumor staging (receptors, etc.) is indispensable in modern oncological treatment. A third reason is the general trend toward a less invasive treatment. Percutaneous abscess drainage, pleural fluid drainage, RF ablation and percutaneous hepatobiliary interventions can sometimes avoid open surgery. Fourthly, percutaneous techniques are also economically attractive. A percutaneous biopsy of a suspected mass can often be done without the need for hospitalization. It is the fastest way to get information about the cancer type, without the need of complex and time-consuming procedures to characterize the primary tumor. A percutaneous abscess drainage can be performed without the supplementary costs of a general anesthesia.

### 3.1 Diagnostic Percutaneous Biopsy

Image-guided biopsy can be performed with fine needles or with cutting core biopsy needles. CT-guided fine needle aspiration or core biopsy is generally regarded as a safe procedure with limited morbidity and extremely rare mortality even in difficult interventions (Zech et al. 2002). Even in children it is reported as a safe and accurate procedure that obviates open surgical biopsy in most patients (Cahill et al. 2004). Fine needle aspiration biopsy is sensitive in the detection of tumoral lesions (90%) but often does not allow adequate sub-typing of carcinoma and seldom yields specific pathologic diagnosis in cases of benign disease.

Pneumothorax remains the most frequent complication in lung biopsies with tube thoracostomy sometimes required. The use of fine needles (>19 G) reduces bleeding complications and pneumothorax rate (Geraghty et al. 2003).

In difficult lesion localization gantry tilt, angulated needle placement or an alternative approach (transsternal, through an iatrogenic pneumothorax, transcaval or transaortic) can be valuable options. Salinisation, the injection of a saline solution through a small needle, can open a window for the bigger biopsy needle or drainage catheter (Klose 1993). A coaxial biopsy technique is an extra manipulation, but has the advantage of more needle stability and gives the possibility to take additional biopsies without the need of multiple skin passages. Even in lung biopsies this coaxial technique is reported to be safe (Laurent et al. 1999).

The assistance of an in-room anatomopathologist can be an aid to be sure that the biopsy sample is accurate for a correct diagnosis. However this is still time consuming, and would have a major impact on workflow, since image-guided biopsy has become a routine procedure with short in-room times (around 15 min).

In most cases diagnostic interventional procedures are performed under local anesthesia with lidoca and require no sedation. In nearly all the recent studies diagnostic biopsy is performed on an outpatient basis. In some cases the patient needs close observation for a short period.

### 3.2 Therapeutic Percutaneous Interventions

Percutaneous drainage of fluid collections (abscess, bilioma, urinoma, seroma and hematoma), tissue ablation, nerve block and lesion marking before surgery with image guidance are well-established methods developed during the last decades.

Percutaneous drainage of various fluid collections has been performed under ultrasound and CT guidance for more than 35 years. This technique has proven to be highly effective, with low morbidity. CT fluoroscopy on the other hand has shown to be a practical clinical tool, especially in the more complex and difficult cases (Meyer et al. 1998). Percutaneous biliary drainage procedures are often performed with fluoroscopic monitoring since the combination of CTF and C-arm fluoroscopy can be an advantage (Laufer et al. 2001). Percutaneous catheter biliary or abscess drainage may require dilatation through the abdominal and back musculature and often results in placement of large catheters (>10F), these interventions are more painful and higher levels of sedation or even general anesthesia can be necessary. In guiding a peripheral nerve block, CT fluoroscopy offers the major advantage not only as real-time viewing during needle progression but also to evaluate the diffusion of the injected solution if contrast agent is added to the solution. Even a transaortic approach with small 21 gauge needles has proven to be save (Lee 2000).

Strategies to obtain tissue ablation include chemical or thermal ablation. Tissue instillation with agents such as ethanol has become less popular since the development of thermal ablation possibilities. Thermal ablation techniques such as radiofrequency ablation, laser ablation, microwave ablation, ultrasound ablation and cryoablation use a large number of potential energy sources. A lot of different strategies are used for applications under different image-guiding modalities. Radiofrequency ablation under CT or ultrasound guidance is the most often used technique in the last decade and proved to be an effective and safe method (Rosenthal et al. 2003). Lately, microwave ablation plays a growing role in the destruction of larger lesions (Li et al. 2011).

## 3.3 Typical CTF Procedure

The following section describes the course of a typical CTF biopsy procedure (Fig. 3a–c). A CT scan prior to the CTF procedure can be taken over the region of the concerned area to make a decision about the ideal trajectory to follow. A control scan at the slice of entry of the needle is taken and the patient is exactly positioned to where the physician can insert the needle, usually indicated by a laser marker. The CTF procedure starts with the selection of the technical scan parameters by the operator. The applied tube current depends on the scan region and patient size (see Tables 1, 2, 3, 4 and 5) and should be selected as low as possible to allow an adequate image quality. In some cases contrast medium is administered to opacify vessels or to retrieve a better delineation of soft tissue lesions (liver, kidneys and pancreas). After sterile preparation of skin and draping, local anesthesia is applied from the skin to the lesion or to the capsule of the organ it lies in (e.g. liver capsule). The anesthetics syringe needle can be bended (Fig. 3, top) to avoid the radiologist's hand being in the scanning plane. CT fluoroscopy is performed to check the anesthetic needle tract. After local anesthesia, a guiding needle can be placed through the skin just before the lesion (Fig. 3, mid) under CTF guidance.

A needle holder can be used to increase the distance of the operators' hands to the scanning plane. Finally, a biopsy needle is placed through the guiding needle and it is advanced through the lesion (Fig. 3, bottom) by applying fluoroscopy. Due to the guiding needle, there is less resistance through the skin during the needle introduction and the biopsy itself. It also provides support for the biopsy needle, allowing the hands to be removed from the scan plane during fluoroscopy. When the biopsy needle is positioned into the lesion, a control fluoroscopy is necessary. Final CTF is applied after the technical procedure to check for bleeding, pneumothorax or other related complications.

Drainage of collections is performed following the same general technique. In more difficult procedures a short guiding needle can be applied (Seldinger technique). A guide-wire is then slided through the guiding needle into the collection, followed by dilatation of the tract and finally placement of a drainage catheter. For larger lesions, direct puncture with a drainage catheter can be performed. Minimal table movements make it possible to follow the tip of the drainage catheter during placement.

## 3.4 Some Clinical Cases

The main advantage of doing interventional procedures under CTF is the possibility of constant needle or catheter tract monitoring. Some clinical examples in diagnostic and therapeutic procedures are discussed in the following cases. The choice of technical material and the choice of the puncture tract can differ; monitoring the needle during the intervention however stays indispensable.

1. To guarantee accurate lung nodule biopsy it is necessary to view and follow the needle tip going into the lesion. Figure 4 shows a lesion adjacent to the anterior pleural wall. After pushing out the biopsy needle, the small lesion is displaced centrally. Without CTF imaging during the procedure this would result in a non-diagnostic biopsy (Fig. 4 right).
2. Access in a non-axial plane or changing the patient position are possible solutions to increasing accessability of lesions in difficult locations like a lung lesion adjacent to the rib (Fig. 5).
3. Almost every mediastinal mass or lymph node can be accessed under CTF guidance. Paravertebral access is possible in combination with salinisation of the paravertebral subpleural space (Fig. 6, up left and right). Anterior access is possible parasternal (Fig. 6, bottom left) or even transsternaly. Access to a lymph node anterior to the trachea can be done through an intentionally created pneumothorax and transtracheal puncture (Fig. 6, bottom right).
4. Vertebral biopsy can be done either through a transpedicular (Fig. 7, left) or a lateral approach (Fig. 7, right).
5. Access of an adrenal mass is possible by liver passage (Fig. 8, left) or costodiaphragmatic sinus

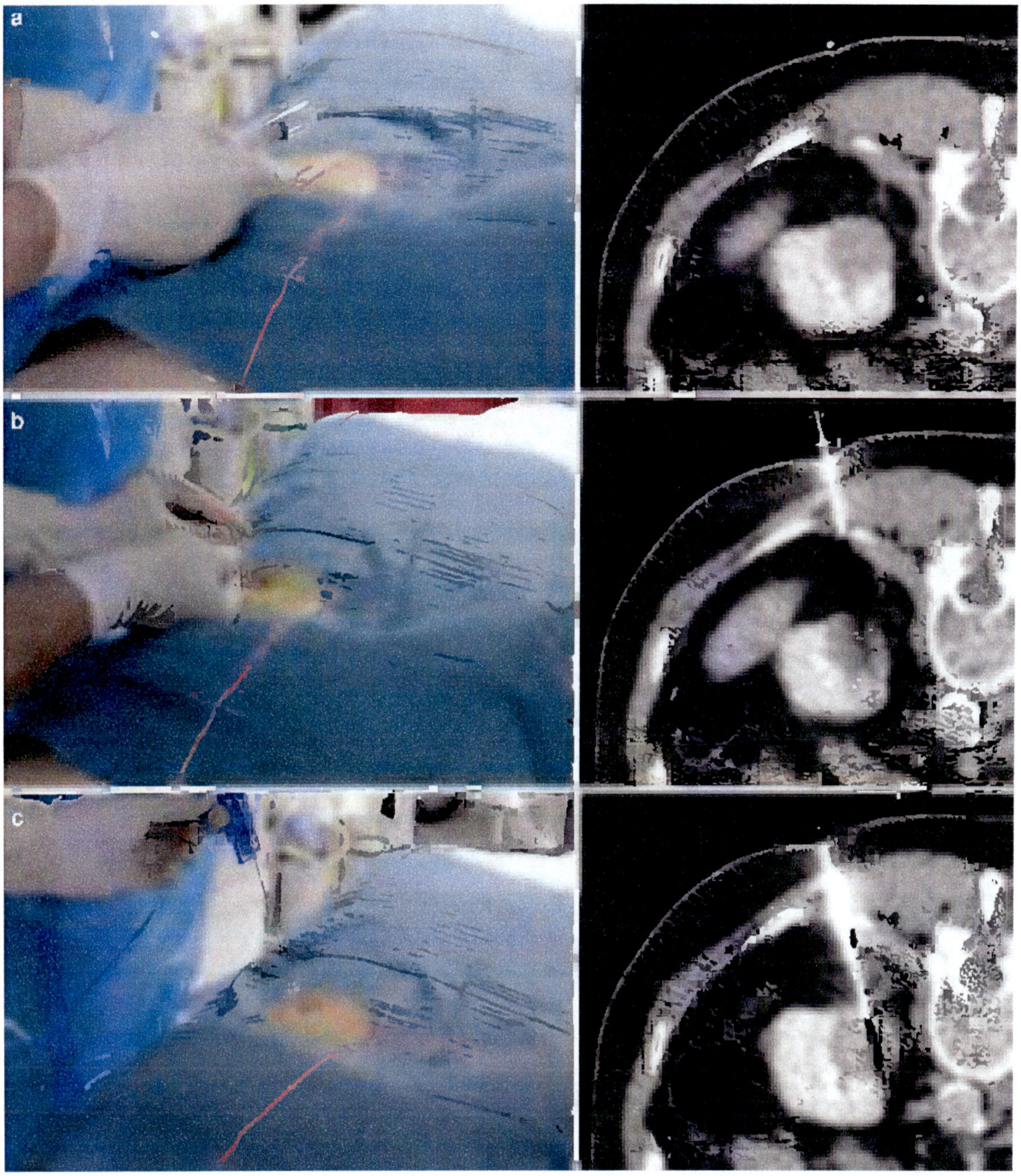


**Fig. 3** **a–c** The course of a typical biopsy procedure

passage (Fig. 8, right). Passage through the costodiaphragmatic sinus of the lung is safe if lung passage is limited to ±2 cm.

6. Abdominal collection in a postoperative patient (a). Salinisation with fine needle insertion (b) was performed to create a safe passage (c) for the locked drainage catheter (d). (Fig. 9).
7. RF ablation is mostly used for liver lesions and can be done under ultrasound or CT fluoroscopy guidance. In case of ablation of smaller bone

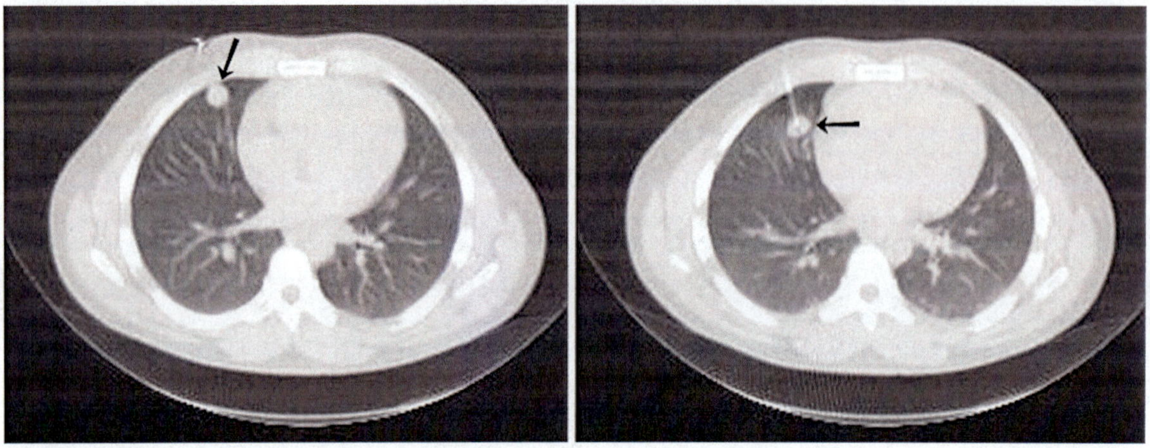

**Fig. 4** *Case* 1 lung nodule pushed away during biopsy

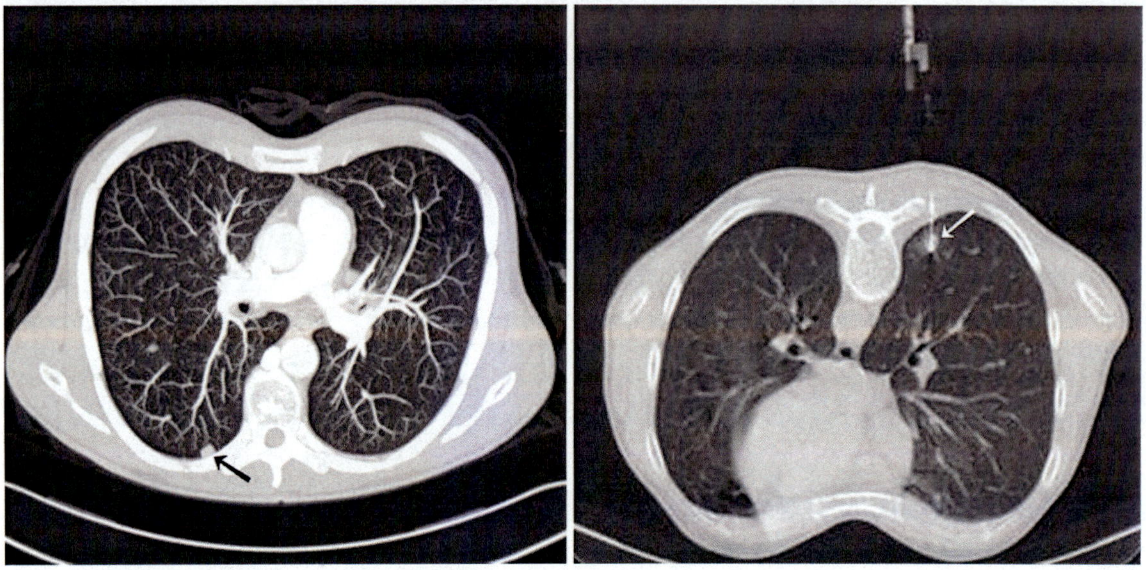

**Fig. 5** *Case* 2 lung nodule biopsy in difficult accessible locations

lesions CT fluoroscopy is needed (ablation of osteoid osteoma Fig. 10, up left and right). CT fluoroscopy guidance is also necessary for ablation of lesions in the lung (Fig. 10, bottom left, ablation and Fig. 10, bottom right control 3 weeks after ablation).

8. A coeliac block under CT fluoroscopy guidance, with anterior approach is demonstrated in Fig. 11, up left and right. Another possibility to performing a coeliac block is the posterior approach, shown in Fig. 11, bottom left paravertebral and Fig. 11, bottom right with passage through the aorta. Aortic passage is safe with smaller needles, in this case 20 Gauge needle.
9. Lung lesions can be marked to optimize radiotherapy. This is shown in Fig. 12, where a small vascular platinum coil is placed in a lung nodule adjacent to the mediastinum.

## 4 Dose to the Patient

Since the scanning plane is mostly kept constant during a CTF procedure, the same skin area is repeatedly exposed and cumulative patient skin doses can be substantial. Maximum patient skin dose is therefore the risk-related quantity of concern in CTF.

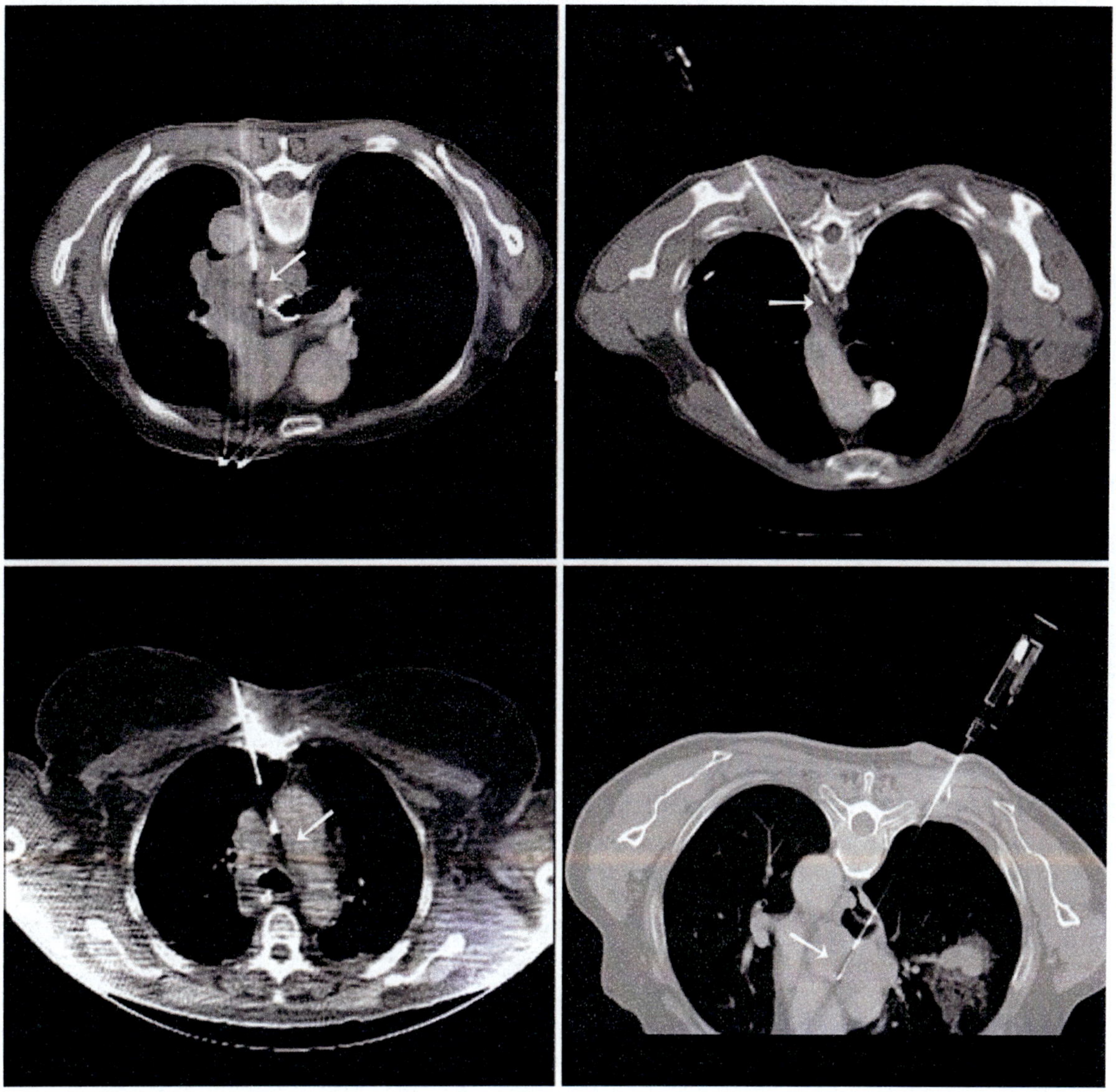

**Fig. 6** *Case* 3 biopsy of mediastinal mass by paravertebral access (*up left* and *right*), anterior access (*bottom left*) and transtracheal with intentionally created pneumothorax (*bottom right*)

## 4.1 Tissue Reactions

In the field of interventional radiology (IR), specific concern exists for radiation-induced skin injuries. Skin changes such as erythema, ulcers, telangiectasia and dermal atrophy are potential tissue reactions (Koenig et al. 2001; Wagner 2007; Balter et al. 2010). Already in 1994, the United States Food and Drug Administration issued a public health advisory concerning the avoidance of induced skin injuries during fluoroscopically guided procedures (US FDA 1994). Also, the United Nations Scientific Committee on Effects of Atomic Radiation specifically expresses their concern about the potential for high patient and staff doses with CTF in their 2000 report (UNSCEAR 2000).

Fluoroscopy-induced injuries can be recognized by the location of the injury as being congruent to the entrance of the X-ray beam. The injury often shows well-defined borders and it may occur on any part of a patient's body. Its appearance and severity depends on the circumstances surrounding the radiation event

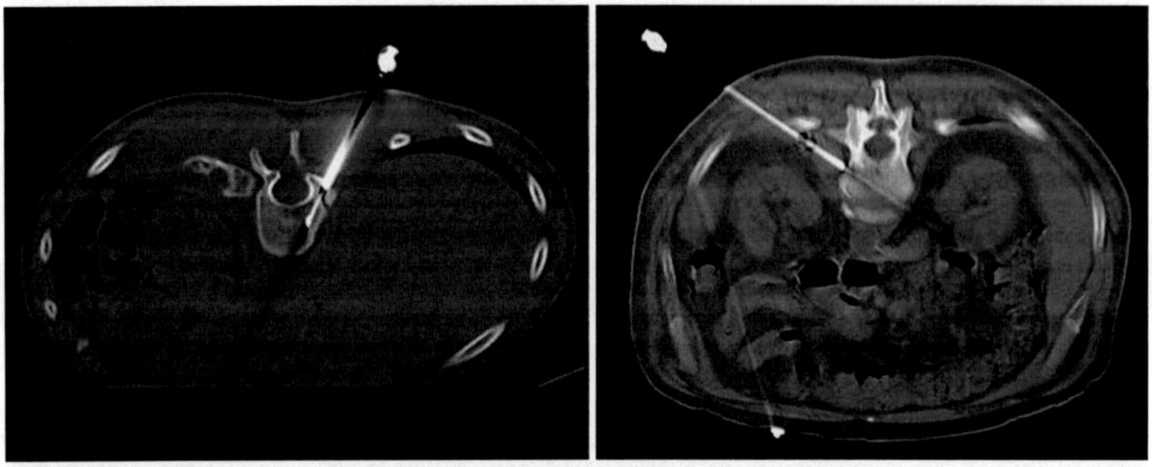

**Fig. 7** *Case* 4 vertebral biopsy in transpedicular (*left*) and lateral (*right*) way

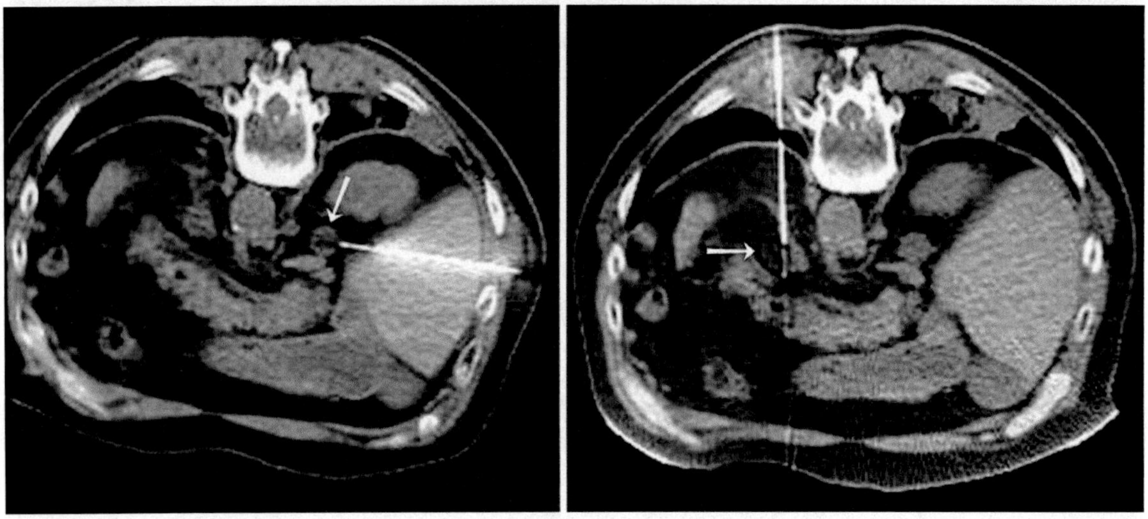

**Fig. 8** *Case* 5 surrenal biopsy by liver passage (*left*) and costodiaphragmatic sinus passage (*right*)

and patient-specific factors such as smoking, poor nutrition, disorders of immune system (such as with cancer, or treatment of cancer or chronic infections), obesity and the presence of skin folds. Therefore, the preexisting condition of the patient and the skin prior to irradiation is of great importance. Skin that is previously compromised from previous irradiation, chemotherapy, steroid use or surgery is more prone to radiation injury. Different parts of the skin also demonstrate different levels of sensitivity to radiation. The skin on the anterior surface of the neck is the most sensitive region. Other sensitive body parts are (in descending order of sensitivity): flexor surfaces (the "front" of the forearms or upper arms for example) of the extremities, the trunk, the back, the extensor surfaces ("back" of the forearm or upper arm for example) of the extremities, the nape of the neck, the scalp, the palms of the hands and the soles of the feet (Balter et al. 2010). Radiation skin injury occurs only when the radiation dose exceeds a certain threshold, and their severity increases rapidly with dose. Skin reactions depend on numerous patient specific parameters that are difficult to predict with high accuracy. For this reason, the minimum dose that might cause a skin change should not be expressed as a single threshold dose, but preferably as a threshold

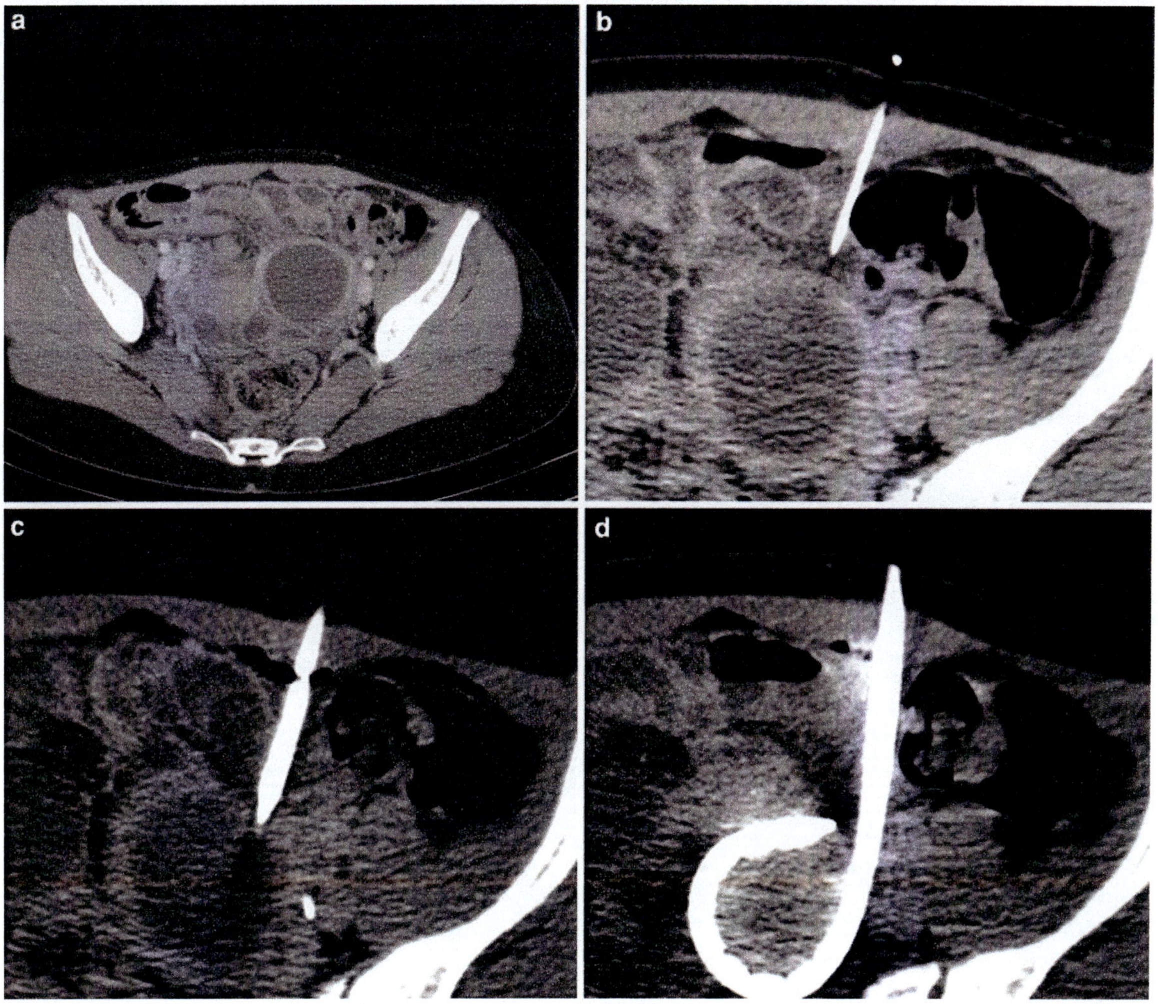


**Fig. 9** **a–d** *Case* 6 drainage of abdominal collection

that includes a range of doses (Balter et al. 2010). At skin doses up to approximately 2 Gy, no harmful effects are expected to be observed unless there has been prior irradiation of the skin. In the dose band of 2–5 Gy transient erythema may be a prompt reaction to radiation exposure. Epilation (hair loss) that heals in the midterm may also be observed. Between 5 and 10 Gy epilation appears as an early reaction. For doses at the upper band limit, permanent partial epilation may be observed in the midterm. Long-term dermal atrophy or induration is also possible. At doses between 10 and 15 Gy, dry or moist desquamation (skin loss) may develop as an early symptom. Prolonged erythema and permanent epilation in the midterm may be followed by telangiectasia (an abnormal collection of small blood vessels), dermal atrophy or induration in the long term. For doses exceeding 15 Gy, edema (skin swelling) and acute ulceration may appear as prompt reactions. Epilation and moist desquamation occur early after irradiation. In the midterm, if desquamation does not heal, a secondary ulceration may occur. Dermal necrosis that requires surgical intervention appears at higher doses. In the long term, telangiectasia, dermal atrophy or induration and secondary skin breakdown are probable. Surgical treatment may be required if a persistent wound progresses into a deeper lesion. In most cases there is a delay between the induction of the injury and the recognition of symptoms (Wagner 2007). Typically about two to three weeks' time is required

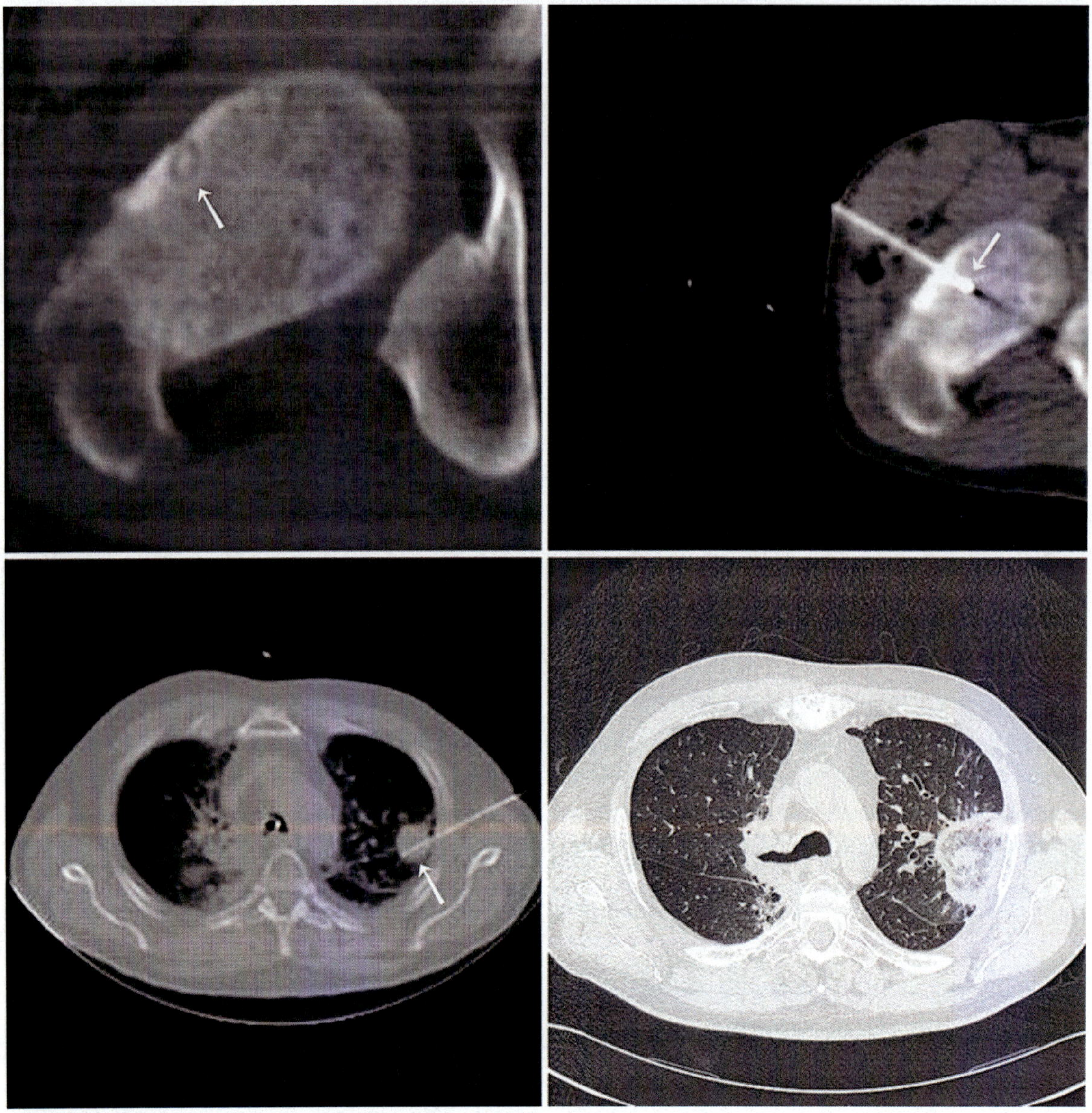

**Fig. 10** *Case* 7 radiofrequency ablation of osteoid osteoma (*up left* and *right*) and lung nodule (*bottom left*) with control image 3 weeks after ablation (*bottom right*)

before symptoms emerge, and three to four weeks before the symptoms are sufficiently irritating for the patient to see a doctor. Thus, if not informed in advance, physicians and patients do not usually associate the skin reaction with a radiological procedure. Patients who are suspected to have received doses high enough to cause skin injuries should be followed-up. The Society of Interventional Radiology guidelines for patient radiation dose management recommend a 2-week skin check when the procedure involves a peak skin dose of 3 Gy or higher (Stecker et al. 2009).

## 4.2 Skin Dose Characteristic in CT

The main determinants of patient skin dose in CT are not only the technical exposure factors (beam width, tube potential and tube current), but also the location of the patient inside the gantry.

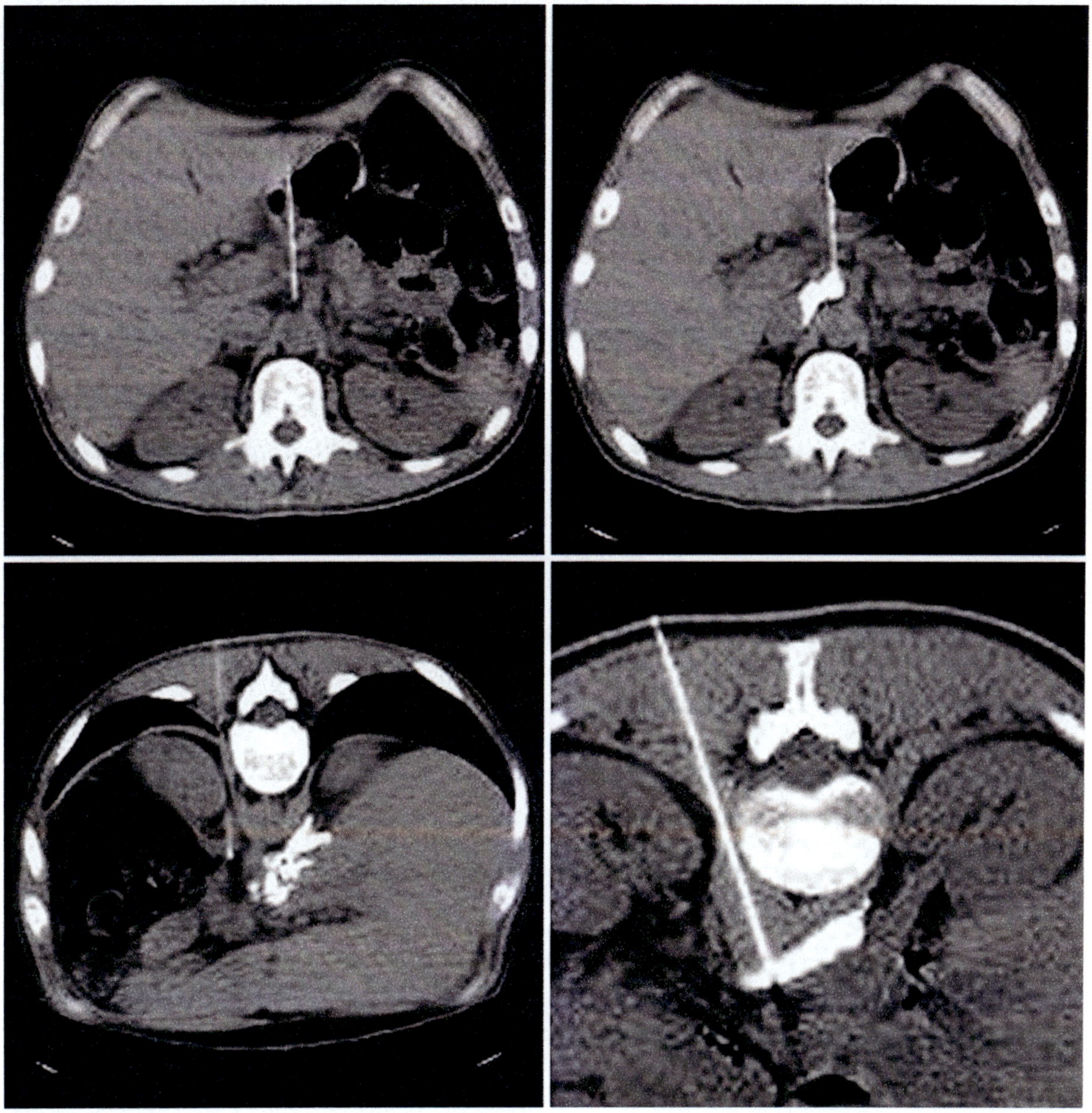

**Fig. 11** *Case* 8 coeliac block with anterior approach (*up left* and *right*) and posterior approach paravertebral (*bottom left*) and with passage through the aorta (*bottom right*)

### 4.2.1 Influence of Patient Size and Position Inside the Gantry

Avilés et al. (2001, 2004) studied extensively the relation between skin dose in CT and both the position and size of the patient. They found that, for phantoms simulating adult patients, the skin dose is independent of phantom size and varies mainly with phantom position along the vertical axis of the CT plane. The maximum surface dose is reached at the isocenter of the scanner and decreases as the surface moves vertically away. The design of the bow-tie filter determines the shape of this variation. This effect of patient position on skin dose is illustrated by Fig. 13, which shows the normalized peak surface dose in function of the vertical position in the gantry for two phantom sizes. The data was obtained by measuring the surface dose with thermoluminescent dosimeters (TLD) on the surface of both 32 cm and 16 cm diameter phantoms for various vertical positions in the gantry of a Siemens Somatom Emotion

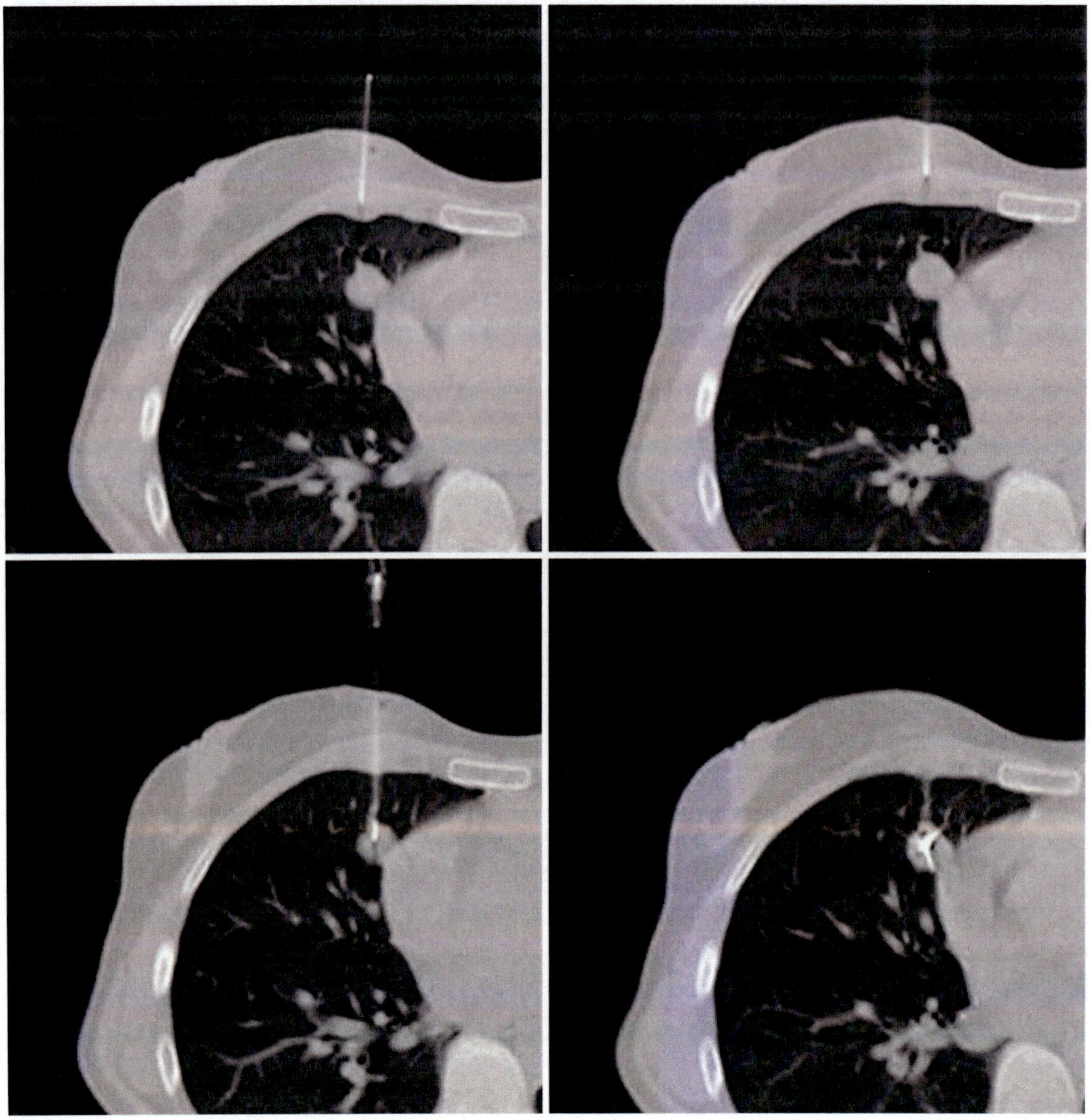

**Fig. 12** *Case* 9 coil (*marker*) placement in lung lesions to optimize radiotherapy

Duo scanner (Siemens Medical Systems, Erlangen, Germany). As can be observed, surface doses are independent of phantom size. However, patient size has an indirect effect on skin dose because it determines the location of the patient surface in the gantry. As a consequence, skin doses will be higher for smaller patients (smaller equivalent diameter), for children, and also for patients where the table is placed in the lowest position inside the gantry. In this position, the shortest distance between isocenter and anterior skin surface is likely to be reached. The data of Fig. 13 shows that, when both phantoms are placed in isocenter, the skin dose rate is almost doubled for the 16 cm phantom compared to the 32 cm phantom, and the skin dose rate at isocenter is almost three times as high as the skin dose rate at a distance of 16 cm from the isocenter. The strong effect of patient size and position warrants the knowledge of both when estimating patient skin dose in CT, especially when using phantoms.

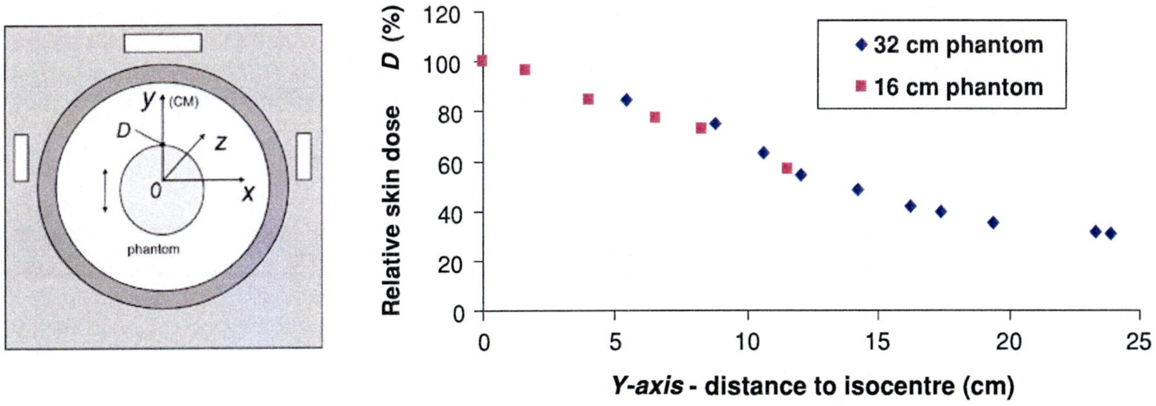


**Fig. 13** Relative skin dose in function of its distance to the isocenter, for two phantom sizes (after Avilés et al. 2001)

### 4.2.2 Influence of Technical Scan Settings: Dose Optimization

With CTF, the operator can select tube potential (kVp), tube current (mA), tube rotation time (s) and slice thickness (mm). Scanner technique settings play an important role in both patient and staff dose since the relative X-ray tube output is roughly proportional to the product of the tube current (mA) with the square of the tube potential ($kVp^2$) and the exposure time (s). A low kVp-mA-s technique will thus result in a significant decrease in patient and staff dose. Reported scan parameters for CTF vary depending on the used scanner type and model. Tube potential can typically range between 80 and 130 kVp, but is often reported fixed at 120 kVp for CTF as in conventional CT. Reported tube current settings usually vary between 20 and 90 mA. Slice thickness should be sufficiently wide to monitor the puncture tract and is usually set at 5–10 mm or less.

The most important adjustable parameter in CTF that affects dose is the tube current. CTF does not apply automatic tube current modulation as recent systems do in conventional CT. Tube current has to be intentionally adapted by the user according to the size of the anatomical region of interest. Equally to conventional CT, there is a linear relationship between tube current (mA) or tube current–time product (mAs) and dose, and an inverse proportional relationship between image noise and the square root of dose. Within the ALARA concept, the lowest possible tube current values should be used that allow an adequate image quality in the anatomical region of interest. As CTF procedures require less diagnostic image quality, tube currents can be drastically reduced when compared to conventional CT. Also, procedures in low attenuating regions such as the thorax allow a tube current reduction in comparison to higher attenuating regions such as the abdomen. Table 1 shows technical CTF settings that are reported in the literature. Tube currents normally range from 10 to 90 mA, and are often set at 50 mA.

Up to now, no real guidelines exist for tube current settings, as is the case with conventional CT. A study by Carlson et al. (2001), from data on 203 consecutive CTF procedures reported following typical applied tube current values: 10 mA for pediatric patients, 10–40 mA for chest cases, 40–50 mA for abdominal cases and 30–50 mA for bone cases. A further reduction could be obtained by using even lower current values when possible, particularly when lesions are large, fluid or cystic (good inherent contrast), superficial or easily accessible. This encourages greater radiologist involvement in setting up the scan so the lowest current value is used.

It should be noted, however, that tube current settings that are established with one specific CT scanner model might not be applied generally. Often, *dose* in CT is characterized by tube current due to their linear relationship, but tube output (mGy/mA) might differ a lot depending on CT scanner hardware components such as the X-ray tube and beam shape filtration. Selected dose values should be specified in physical measurable dose quantities such as $CTDI_w$ and $CTDI_{vol}$, rather than as mA values.

**Table 1** Technical CTF scan settings that are reported in the literature

| Author | Scanner model | Tube potential (kVp) | Tube current (mA) | Slice thickness (mm) |
|---|---|---|---|---|
| Buls et al. (2003) | Siemens Somatom plus 4 | 120 | 90 | 8 |
| Buls et al. (2004) | Siemens Emotion duo | 120 | 38 | 5 |
| Kataoka et al. (2006) | GE HiSpeed CT/I | 120 | 30–80 | 7 |
| Kataoka et al. (2006) | Toshiba Aquilion 16 | 120 | 30–80 | 8 |
| Brennan et al. (2003) | N.a. | 120 | 80 | 5 |
| Hohl et al. (2008) | Siemens Somatom Sensation 64 | 120 | 60 | 14.4 |
| Trumm et al. (2008) | Siemens Somatom plus 4 | 120 | 15–25 | 10 |
| Stoeckelhuber et al. (2005) | Toshiba Aquilion multi | 120 | 50 | N.a. |
| Meleka et al. (2005) | Toshiba Aquilion 16 | 120 | 50 | N.a. |
| Yamagami et al. (2003) | Toshiba X Vigor Laudator | 120 | 30–50 | 3 |
| Gianfelice et al. (2000) | GE Prospeed | 120 | 50 | 10 |
| Froelich et al. (1998) | Siemens Somatom plus 4 | 120 | 50 | N. a. |
| Paulson et al. (2001) | GE HiSpeed CT/I | 140 | 13 | 5 |
| Silverman et al. (1999) | Siemens Somatom plus 4 | 120 | 50–90 | 10 |

## 4.3 Reported Patient Doses From CTF

Comparing reported patient doses from CTF is not straightforward as several variables should be taken into account such as types of included procedures (biopsies, aspirations, etc.), type of scanner, exposure settings (kVp, mA and collimation), exposure time, CTF technique (intermittent or continious) and patient's position inside the gantry. Also, the applied method of patient skin dose estimation might vary. Some authors use the periphery CTDI of the standard ∅32 cm dosimetric body phantom as a metric for patient surface dose (Nickoloff et al. 2000; Teeuwisse et al. 2001), others apply a correction factor to convert periphery CTDI to skin dose (Nawfel et al. 2000), and also, humanoid Alderson phantoms (The Phantom Laboratory, New York) are used to measure surface dose rate (Paulson et al. 2001; Hohl et al. 2008). With phantoms, patient size is standardized, which allows the investigation of the influence of parameters such as tube current, beam collimation independently. Usually, the measured surface dose rate data are extrapolated according to the exposure length of the CTF procedure. A drawback of such a method is that it may not include important factors that influence skin dose such as the movement of the patient in relation to the thin beam slice, and the influence of patient position (and size) in the gantry. These factors are included when in vivo skin dose monitoring is applied (Buls et al. 2003).

### 4.3.1 Reported Patient Skin Dose Rates

Reported patient surface dose rates that are measured by phantom are shown in Table 2. For comparison, the surface dose rate that is observed for typical conventional angiography equipment is also included. The last column estimates the exposure time that is required to reach the 2 Gy threshold dose for radiation skin effects.

Depending on technical settings, reported surface dose rates might vary from 10 cGy/min up to about 60 cGy/min. For equal technical settings, reported surface doses tend to be higher for smaller phantom sizes (data expressed per mAs). This is in congruence with the fact that surface dose decreases as the surface moves further away from the isocenter, as discussed in Sect. 4.2.1. With a dose rate of 62.4 cGy/min, the 2 Gy threshold skin dose for transient erythema would be already reached after 3.2 min of scanning. Such scanning times could be reached for one patient when difficult procedures are involved. Mean reported exposure times are usually below 1 min (Table 3), but maximum CT scanning times for one case of 9.1 min

**Table 2** Reported patient skin dose rates in CTF, determined by phantom measurements

| Method | Author | Tube potential (KVp) | Tube current (mA) | Dose rate (cGy/min) | Exposure time (min) required to reach 2 Gy threshold |
|---|---|---|---|---|---|
| Periphery CTDI of ∅32 cm PMMA phantom | | | | | |
| | Nickoloff et al. (2000) | 120 | 30 | 23.9 | 8.4 |
| | Teeuwisse et al. (2001) | 120 | 25 | 12.6 | 15.9 |
| | Teeuwisse et al. (2001) | 140 | 25 | 17.4 | 11.4 |
| | Nawfel et al. (2000) | 80 | 135 | 27.6 | 7.2 |
| | Nawfel et al. (2000) | 120 | 50 | 32.4 | 6.2 |
| | Nawfel et al. (2000) | 120 | 90 | 62.4 | 3.2 |
| Periphery CTDI of ∅20 cm PMMA phantom | | | | | |
| | Silverman et al. (1999) | Varying | Varying | 18.6–82.8 | 10.8–2.4 |
| Periphery CTDI of ∅16 cm PMMA phantom | | | | | |
| | Nickoloff et al. (2000) | 120 | 30 | 46.3 | 4.3 |
| | Teeuwisse et al. (2001) | 120 | 25 | 20.4 | 9.8 |
| | Teeuwisse et al. (2001) | 140 | 25 | 28.2 | 7.1 |
| TLD on Alderson Humanoid phantom | | | | | |
| | Paulson et al. (2001) | 140 | 10 | 10.8 | 18.5 |
| Typical conventional fluoroscopy: TLD on 20 cm PMMA | | | | | |
| | Angiography abd | 80 | 3 | Typ. 1.0–2.0 | 200–100 |

(Silverman et al. 1999) and 13.6 min (Buls et al. 2003) are also reported. Such exposure times could clearly result in skin doses above 2 Gy when high exposure settings are used.

As stated before, tube current has a nearly linear relationship with dose under equal exposure conditions. This is illustrated by the data of Nawfel et al. (2000) who reported a dose rate of 32.4 cGy/min with 50 mA, compared to 62.4 cGy/min with 90 mA. Paulson et al. (2001) intentionally applied a low tube current of 10 mA, which resulted in a surface dose rate of only 10.8 cGy/min.

Surface dose rates from CTF can also be compared to the observed skin dose rates for conventional fluoroscopy. For a C-arm angiography X-ray equipment the surface dose rate measured on a 20 cm PMMA phantom is typically below 2 cGy/min during fluoroscopy. This is roughly a factor 30 less than the surface dose rate observed during CTF with maximal exposure settings of 120 kVp and 90 mA. In consequence, patient skin doses accumulate very rapidly in CTF compared to conventional fluoroscopy. Whereas with conventional fluoroscopy the 2 Gy threshold dose is reached after 100–200 min of fluoroscopy, it can be reached in CTF after only 3–10 min of scanning.

### 4.3.2 Reported Skin Doses

Table 3 shows reported patient skin doses from CTF for various types of CTF procedures, together with their respective scan settings and applied CTF technique. Doses are expressed per procedure and vary from about 30 up to 800 mGy. For comparison, reported skin doses from typical conventional fluoroscopy angiography and IR procedures are also included.

**Table 3** Reported patient entrance skin doses per procedure during CTF

| Author | Procedures | CTF technique | Technical settings (kVp)/(mA) | Exposure time (s) | Skin dose (mGy) |
|---|---|---|---|---|---|
| Silverman et al. (1999) | Biopsies (61), aspirations/drainages (34) | Quick-check (19) Real-time (71) | 120/50–90 | 79 | 740 |
| Paulson et al. (2001) | Biopsies (85), aspirations/drainages (78), injections (57) | Quick-check (87) Real-time (2) Combination (11) | 140/10 | 18 | 32 |
| Teeuwisse et al. (2001) | Biopsies (35) | Quick-check | 120–140/25 | 28 | 130 |
| Nickoloff et al. (2000) | Biopsies (78) | N.a. | 120/30 | 97 | 400 |
| Buls et al. (2003) | Biopsies (46), aspirations/drainages (22), ablations (14) | Quick-check | 120/90 | 151 | 346 |
| Buls et al. (2004) | Biopsies (48) | Quick-check | 120/38 | 73 | 111 |
| Carlson et al. (2001) | Biopsies (146), aspirations/drainages (57) | Quick-check (97) Combination (3) | 120/10–50 | 21 | 43 |
| Carlson et al. (2005) | Biopsies (56) bellows | Quick-check | 120/10–50 | 16 | 38 |
| | Biopsies (57) | Quick-check | 120/10–50 | 22 | 51 |
| Nawfel et al. (2000) | Biopsies | | 120/90 | 80 | 832 |
| Typical IR conventional fluoroscopy | | | | | |
| McParland (1998) | Hepatic angiography | | | | 340 |
| McParland (1998) | Renal angiography | | | | 100 |
| Miller et al. (2003) | Carotid stent | | | | 597 |
| Miller et al. (2003) | Renal PTA with stent | | | | 1,812 |

The reported mean exposure times from CTF vary from 15 to 150 s and are usually below 60 s. Some authors reported very short exposure times that were achieved for various types of procedures. Paulson et al. (2001) reported a mean exposure time of only 18 s for 189 various procedures. Also, Carlson et al. (2001, 2005) reported very short exposure times for various types of procedures with median values in the range of 16–22 s.

The combination of such short exposure times with a low tube current technique results in strongly reduced patient doses. Paulson et al. (2001) and Carlson et al. (2001) and reported skin doses of only 32 and 43 mGy per procedure, respectively. The fact that these values were reported for various types of CTF procedures shows that a low tube current—exposure time technique can be achieved in clinical routine.

## 5 Dose to the Staff

Unlike diagnostic CT, the physician enters the room during CTF scanning and stands near the X-ray source while manipulating the interventional device.

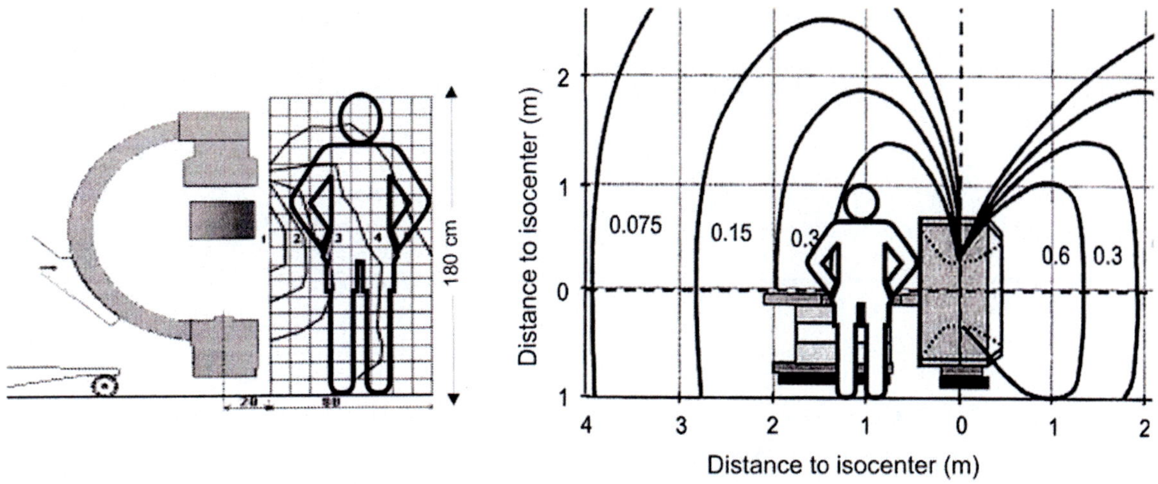


**Fig. 14** Isoexposure contours of a conventional fluoroscopy C-arm equipment and a CT scanner (*left image* from Philips Medical Systems, *right image* from Bushberg et al. 2002)

Also other staff members such as, for example, nurses or anesthesiologists can be present in the room during scanning and are as well subjected to scattered radiation. Radiation protection for the staff should be not only optimized for whole body exposures (e.g. with a lead apron), but also for exposures to specific tissues such as the lens of the eye and the hands as they are usually unshielded. Particularly the dose to the lens of the eyes is of concern as recent epidemiological evidence indicates that the threshold dose for detectable lens opacities is almost tenfold lower than previously considered. The lens of the eye is one of the radiosensitive tissues in the body a number of studies suggest there may be significant risk of lens opacities in populations exposed to low doses of ionizing radiation (ICRP 2011). These observations will have clear implications for those working with X-rays in interventional rooms such as with CTF.

## 5.1 Scattered Radiation

The main source of radiation to the radiologist is the scattered radiation that exits the patient. For all radiographic procedures except mammography, most photon interactions in soft tissue produce scattered X-ray photons. Scattered photons are detrimental in radiographic imaging because they violate the basic geometric premise that photons travel in straight lines (Bushberg et al. 2002). Compton scattering (also called inelastic scattering) is the predominant interaction of X-ray photons in the diagnostic energy range. Compton scattering results in the ionization of an atom and a division of the incident photon energy between the scattered photon and an ejected electron. The Compton scattered photon may traverse the medium (patient) without interaction or may undergo subsequent interactions. The majority of the incident photon energy (120 $keV_p$) is transferred to the scattered photon, which results in scattered photons with relatively high energies and about equal penetrability as the primary beam.

The scatter interaction fraction is proportional to the primary photon fraction and the probability of interaction increases as the incident photon energy increases. In general, the scatter radiation field per unit of time around a CT scanner is more intense and energetic than the scatter field encountered in conventional fluoroscopy (e.g. angiography room). This is due to the use of both more intense (due to increased mA and kVp) and higher energy (increased kVp) beams in CTF. Interventional procedures with conventional fluoroscopy usually operate with beam energies at around 80 kVp and tube currents between 1 and 10 mA, compared to 120 kVp and 30–90 mA with CTF. These elevated scatter radiation fields involved with CTF result in an elevated risk for the operator and require adequate radiation protection management.

**Table 4** Reported scattered dose rates from CTF, determined by measuring ambient dose rates from phantoms

| Method | Author | Technical settings (kVp)/(mA) | Scattered dose rate at the level of the | | | |
|---|---|---|---|---|---|---|
| | | | Hand (μGy/s) @ (cm) from plane | | Body-Head (μGy/s) @ (cm) from plane | |
| Scattered exposure from ∅32 cm PMMA phantom | | | | | | |
| | Nickoloff et al. (2000) | 120/30 | 17 | 20 | 0.93 | 100 |
| | Kato et al. (1996) | 80/30 | 1,140 | 0 | | |
| | Kato et al. (1996) | 80/30 | 19 | 4 | | |
| Scattered exposure from ∅20 cm PMMA phantom | | | | | | |
| | Silverman et al. (1999) | 120/50 | 29.5 | 10 | 0.97 | 100 |
| | Nawfel et al. (2000) | 120/50 | 23.6 | 10 | | |
| Scattered exposure from Alderson humanoid phantom | | | | | | |
| | Hohl et al. (2008) | 120/60 | 110 | 10 | | |
| | Stoeckelhuber et al. (2005) | 120/50 | 39.5 | 15 | | |
| | Paulson et al. (2001) | 140/10 | 0.06 | 25 | 0.03 | 60 |
| Scattered exposure, not specified | | | | | | |
| | Gianfelice et al. (2000) | 120/50 | 18 | 10 | | |
| Scattered exposure from Alderson humanoid phantom with a lead drape | | | | | | |
| | Stoeckelhuber et al. (2005) | 120/50 | 3.2 | 15 | | |
| Scattered exposure from Alderson humanoid phantom with 30 cm needle holder | | | | | | |
| | Stoeckelhuber et al. (2005) | 120/50 | 13.2 | 30 | | |
| Scattered exposure from Alderson humanoid phantom with angular beam modulation | | | | | | |
| | Hohl et al. (2008) | 120/60 | 80 | 10 | | |
| Scattered exposure from ∅20 cm PMMA phantom with a lead drape | | | | | | |
| | Nawfel et al. (2000) | 120/50 | 6.8 | 10 | | |

Another concern in CTF is the direction of the scattered radiation field. In radiography, the direction of scattered radiation is mainly directed back toward the X-ray tube. This is a well-known effect and it is already reported by several authors (Trout and Kelley 1972) and reports (ICRP 2001). For this reason, an under-table X-ray tube geometry is generally applied in interventional radiology (IR), which directs the scatter radiation toward the floor, and prevents that the upper body of the worker (head and neck) receives a large fraction of scattered radiation. With CTF, the operator cannot control the scatter direction as in IR due to the continuous rotation of the X-ray beam around the patient. The scatter field in CT is nearly symmetrical in both horizontal and vertical directions, apart from absorption of nearby components such as the gantry or the table stand. Figure 14 shows the scatter radiation direction of a conventional fluoroscopy C-arm X-ray system and a CT scanner system. The under-table tube geometry of the C-arm system causes the scattered radiation to be directed toward the floor, reducing operator exposure. Such dose-reducing method is not possible with CTF. As a result, optimization is more difficult.

## 5.2 Personal Protection–Radiation Dose Monitoring

For CTF, it is standard practice that the medical staff protects themselves from scattered radiation by wearing a lead apron. An apron with 0.5 mm lead equivalent efficiently shields most radiosensitive organs (lungs, red bone marrow, stomach, gonads, colon, etc.), limiting the effective dose of the individual. For interventions where scattered radiation is directed toward the upper part of the body, such as with CTF, it is also recommended to use additional

**Table 5** Reported staff doses per procedure from CTF

| Author | Method of dose measurement | CTF technique/method | Technical settings (kVp)/(mA) | Exposure time (s) | Dose at the level of | |
|---|---|---|---|---|---|---|
| | | | | | Hand (mGy) | Head/eyes (mGy) |
| Nickoloff et al. (2000) | Indirect (20–100 cm) | 20 cm needle holder | 120/30 | 100 | 1.70 | 0.09 |
| [a]Kato et al. (1996) | Indirect (4 cm) | 4 cm needle holder | 80/30 | 59 | 1.50 | |
| Nawfel et al. (2000) | Indirect (10–100 cm) | | 120/50 | 80 | 2.2 | 0.1 |
| [a]Paulson et al. (2001) | Indirect (25–60 cm) | | 140/13 | 18 | 0.001 | 0.0006 |
| Gianfelice et al. (2000) | Indirect (10 cm) | 10 cm needle holder | 120/50 | 50 | 0.90 | |
| Gianfelice et al. (2000) | Indirect (10 cm) | 10 cm needle holder | 120/50 | 26 | 0.46 | |
| Nawfel et al. (2000) | Direct by TLD | | 120/50 | N.a. | 1.70 | |
| [a]Irie et al. (2001a) | Direct by TLD | 7 cm needle holder | 120/30 | 38 | 0.76 | |
| [a]Irie et al. (2001a) | Direct by TLD | 7 cm needle holder and lead plate | 120/30 | 50 | 0.41 | |
| [a]Irie et al. (2001a) | Direct by TLD | 15 cm needle holder and lead plate | 120/30 | 41 | 0.06 | |
| [a]Brennan et al. (2003) | Direct by TLD | | 120/80 | N.a. | | 0.20 |
| Buls et al. (2003) | Direct by TLD | | 120/90 | 151 | 0.70 | 0.21 |
| Buls et al. (2004) | Direct by TLD | Under-table tube exposure | 120/38 | 73 | 0.29 | 0.14 |

[a] Data expressed as dose equivalent (mSv)

lead collar protection. The use of an additional collar results in high organ dose reductions for all organs at risk in the neck region (thyroid, esophagus). Especially the dose to the thyroid is of interest as it presents a significant contribution (5%) to the effective dose. Appropriate personal protection limits the effective dose to the worker, however, surface doses to unshielded parts of the body can be substantial.

According to legislation, classified radiation workers are subjected to annual dose limits and they should be monitored by a radiation badge accordingly. For workers who systematically wear a lead apron as in CTF, the use of two radiation badges is recommended (ICRP 1982). One dosimeter should be worn under the apron (shielded) and a second one should be worn outside (unshielded) the apron. A single dosimeter worn under the apron will underestimate the effective dose of the worker as it does not take into account the dose to the unshielded parts of the body, and it also does not provide information of the dose to the eyes, which is of special interest in CTF.

## 5.3 Reported Scattered Dose Rates From CTF

Several authors evaluated scattered exposure rates from a phantom during CTF by measuring ambient dose rates at various distances with dose-monitoring equipment. The dose to the operator during CTF can be estimated from these data by multiplying the dose rate that is observed at a specific distance by the time the operator spends at that location during scanning. Usually, the dose rates at two distances to the scanning plane are considered: the level of the hand (5–25 cm) and the level of the body/head ($\sim$100 cm).

Such data often provide useful information concerning the influence of several parameters (e.g. distance, tube current, etc.) on scatter dose rate but they do not include the actual variation of the position of the staff during the procedure. Table 4 shows reported scattered dose rates at two positions from the scanning plane: the considered position of the hand and the body of the operator. As with patient dose rates, several phantoms sizes are used. The second part of the table shows reported scattered dose rates when radiation protection methods are applied, such as using a lead drape or prolonged standoff needle devices.

Reported scatter dose rates at the level of the hand of the operator usually vary between 20 and 40 $\mu$Gy/s, depending on the scanner type, technical scan settings and the distance to the scanning plane of the measurement. Lower dose rates can be achieved by (1) reducing exposure settings (2) increasing distance to the scanning plane with the use of needle holders or (3) by using a lead barrier. The dose rate inside the primary beam itself can be over 1,000 $\mu$Gy/s, even with reduced scan settings. Entering the primary beam leads to unacceptable high doses.

At the level of the head (eyes), dose rates are reduced due to the increased distance to the area where the primary beam enters the patient. For the dose at the level of the head, two authors reported a similar dose rate of about 1 $\mu$Gy/s at a distance of 100 cm.

## 5.4 Reported Doses to the Staff From CTF

The actual dose to the operator will depend on the time that he spends at specific distances to the scatter source during the CTF procedure. Besides estimated doses that are derived from ambient dose rate data (indirect measurements), doses are also reported from direct in vivo measurements that are performed during CTF procedures. Direct measurements tend to be more accurate as they include the actual variation of individual staff positioning during each CTF procedure. They are usually performed with personalized ring badges containing thermoluminescent dosimeters (TLDs). Table 5 shows reported doses to the operator, both from indirect and direct measurements. The first part of the table shows reported doses from indirect measurements based on ambient dose rates, the second part shows data from direct in vivo measurements by using TLDs. Reported doses to the hands from the literature are partly given as radiation doses, expressed in Gy, and partly as the superficial dose equivalent $H_s(0.07)$ in soft tissue, expressed in Sv. For exposures with X-rays of the diagnostic energy range, both unities yield comparable values. For CT X-ray energies, a conversion factor of 1.1 can be applied to transfer dose (Gy) to dose equivalent (Sv) in soft tissue. The data in Table 5 are expressed as radiation doses (mGy) unless stated otherwise.

When no specific radiation protection methods are applied, reported doses to the dominant hand in CTF vary between 0.46 and 2.2 mGy per procedure, depending on the technical settings, the exposure time and the method of dose estimation. Doses to the eyes can be anywhere in the range of <0.01 and 0.2 mGy per procedure.

## 5.5 Staff Effective Dose

When appropriate personal protection is used, the effective dose to the worker remains limited in CTF. Teeuwisse et al. (2001) evaluated effective doses ($E$) to both the physician and the assisting radiographer by placing electronic personal dosimeters (EPD) outside the lead apron (unshielded). They estimated that the average dose per CTF procedure to the radiologist was well below 10 μSv and the average dose to the assisting radiographer was below 1 μSv. Actual effective dose values would be even lower as the attenuation of the lead apron is not included in the above data. For a radiologist performing 70% of the CTF procedures at their hospital, they estimated an annual effective dose less than 0.1 mSv. Also, Paulson et al. (2001) measured a limited mean effective dose to the physician of 25 μSv per procedure.

# 6 Reducing Dose to the Staff

## 6.1 By Reducing Patient Dose

The main source of radiation to the radiologist is the scattered radiation that exits the patient. Decreasing patient dose will decrease scatter radiation, as is true with other radiological procedures. In radiology, both tube current and exposure time have a linear relationship with patient and staff dose. Reducing the exposure to the patient by controlling the tube current and exposure time results in an equal reduction of the dose to the staff. Paulson et al. (2001) reported a negligible dose to the operator by applying a low tube current—exposure time technique (Tables 4 and 5). Also slice thickness influences scatter radiation. A reduction in slice thickness from 10 to 5 or 2 mm can result in personnel exposure reductions of 50–80% (Nawfel et al. 2000).

## 6.2 Distance

Distance is a very efficient and costless radiation protection tool. The exposure rate from a point source of radiation decreases by the square of the distance to the source. For example, the dose rate from a source would be four times lower when the distance is doubled. This *inverse square law* is the result of the geometric relationship between the surface area and the radius of a sphere (Bushberg et al. 2002). This relationship is only valid for point sources (i.e. sources whose dimensions are small with respect to the distance from the source). Thus, the *inverse square law* would not be strictly valid in CTF where the radiation source size (patient) is large with respect to the distance between staff member and patient. However, experimental data from Nawfel et al. (2000) shows that scatter exposure rate is approximated by the inverse square law at distances greater than 30 cm from the scanning plane.

## 6.3 Needle Holders—Robotically Driven Interventions

Since the introduction of CTF, standoff needle devices have been developed to increase the distance of the physician's hand to the scanning plane (Kato et al. 1996; Irie et al. 2001b; Daly et al. 1998). Figure 3 mid and bottom shows a picture of an abdominal CTF procedure with a 15 cm needle holder. Besides reducing the scatter radiation level to the hand due to the larger distance, they also prevent entering the primary beam directly. They should always be used when the real-time scanning method is applied. Irie et al. (2001a) developed three devices 7, 10 and 15 cm in length that yielded markedly reduced doses to the physician's hand (see Table 5). Stoeckelhuber et al. (2005) reported a scatter dose rate reduction from 39.5 to 13.2 $\mu$Gy/s by using a 35 cm needle holder compared to a 15 cm needle holder (Table 4). Besides dedicated tools, less expensive but sometimes also less efficient objects such as sponge forceps or towel clamps are also applied (Daly et al. 1998; Paulson et al. 2001). Although it has been shown that needle holders reduce the dose to the hand, there are some reported drawbacks due to a reduced tactile feedback. Although Kato et al. (1996) and Irie et al. (2001a) concluded that dedicated needle holders did not cause any artifacts that interfered with the biopsy procedure, Carlson et al. (2001) did not advocate the use of holders due to their decreased tactile feedback and difficulties when penetrating resistant tissue planes. Also, Silverman et al. (1999) reported that there were times when the needle became dislodged from the holder, and at other times it was difficult to exert sufficient inward force. The use of needle holders requires training in order to prevent a prolonged exposure time due to reduced tactile feedback.

The ultimate way of reducing staff exposure is a CTF procedure that does not require the staff members to be present in the CT room. Solomon et al. (2002) developed a robot that could hold, orient and advance a needle, with CTF guidance. This robot could be either computer or joystick controlled. In an evaluation with twenty-three biopsy interventions no complications were encountered and dose to the physician was eliminated. Although they do not report fluoroscopic screening times in their study, they claim that patient exposure could also be reduced since the computer can advance the robot's needle to the target without the need of continuous imaging. The main drawbacks of such system are the extra preparation time to install the robot and the cost prize. Solomon et al. (2002) estimated that a commercial unit might cost in the range of $20,000.

## 6.4 Using a Lead Drape

An efficient and easy to use method of reducing scatter exposure is placing a lead drape on the patient caudal from the cutaneous access side, adjacent to the scanning plane (Fig. 15). This lead barrier absorbs scattered photons that leave the patients body directed toward the operator and reduces scatter dose considerably (see also Table 4). Several authors have

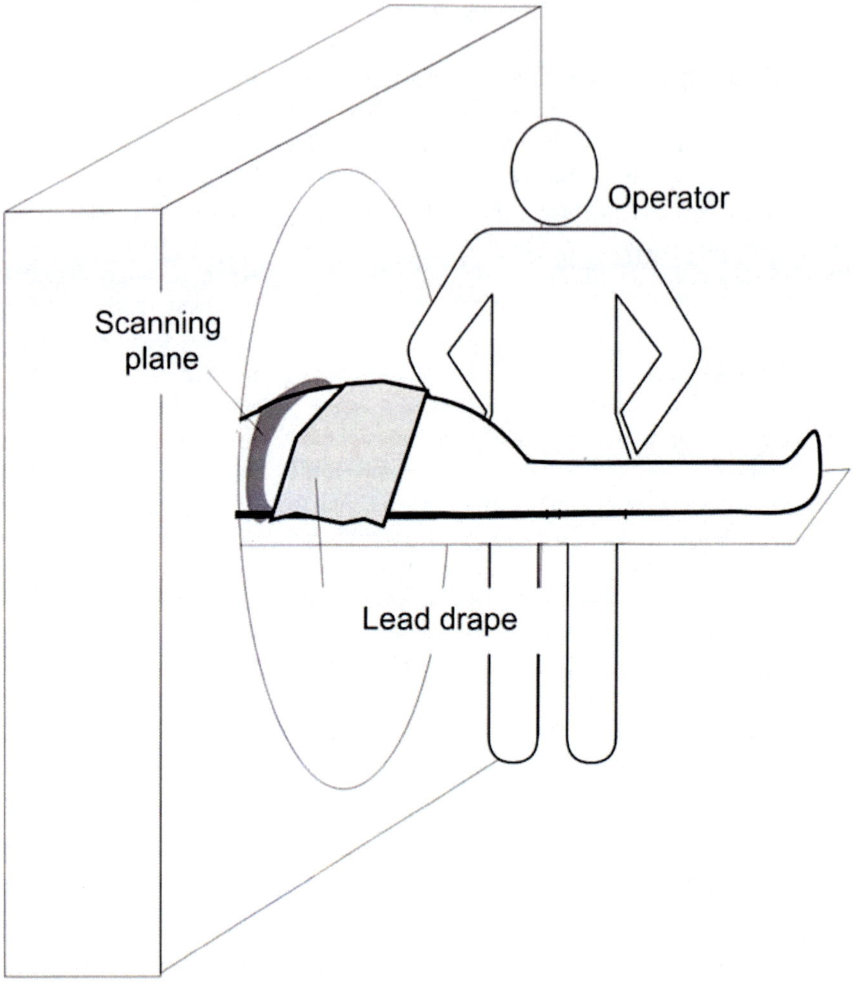


**Fig. 15** A lead drape placed caudal from the scanning plane reduces scattered radiation towards the operator

reported the use of a lead drape (Nawfel et al. 2000; Silverman et al. 1999; Stoeckelhuber et al. 2005; Irie et al. 2000). Nawfel et al. 2000 investigated scatter exposure to the hand by measuring ambient dose rates at specific distances to a phantom. According to their results, a 0.5 mm lead drape reduced the scattered exposure by approximately 70% at a distance of 10 cm from the scanning plane. Irie et al. (2001a) conducted a similar study by placing a small lead plate directly under the hand of the physician. They measured a hand dose of 0.41 mSv per case with the lead plate compared to 0.76 mSv per case without the lead plate (Table 5). The small lead plate was easy to sterilize and caused little discomfort for the patients. Also, scatter dose reductions up to 97% are reported by using two lead drapes; one placed above and one placed below the patient (Stoeckelhuber et al. 2005). Neeman et al. 2006 reported a 20–35% dose reduction to the hand by placing fenestrated shielded drapes at the entrance of the CT gantry.

## 6.5 Leaded Gloves

Using leaded gloves can also protect the hands of the operator. However, the lead equivalent of gloves that are thin enough to permit an adequate sense of touch is often limited with high energy X-rays beams that are used with CTF (120 kVp). Nickoloff et al. (2000) evaluated the protection of three different types of thin leaded gloves, which permitted an adequate sense of touch to direct biopsy needles. The leaded gloves provided only a 15–33% reduction to the radiation dose to the hands at a tube potential of 120 kVp. This is low compared to the protection of a lead drape (95%), which has more lead content.

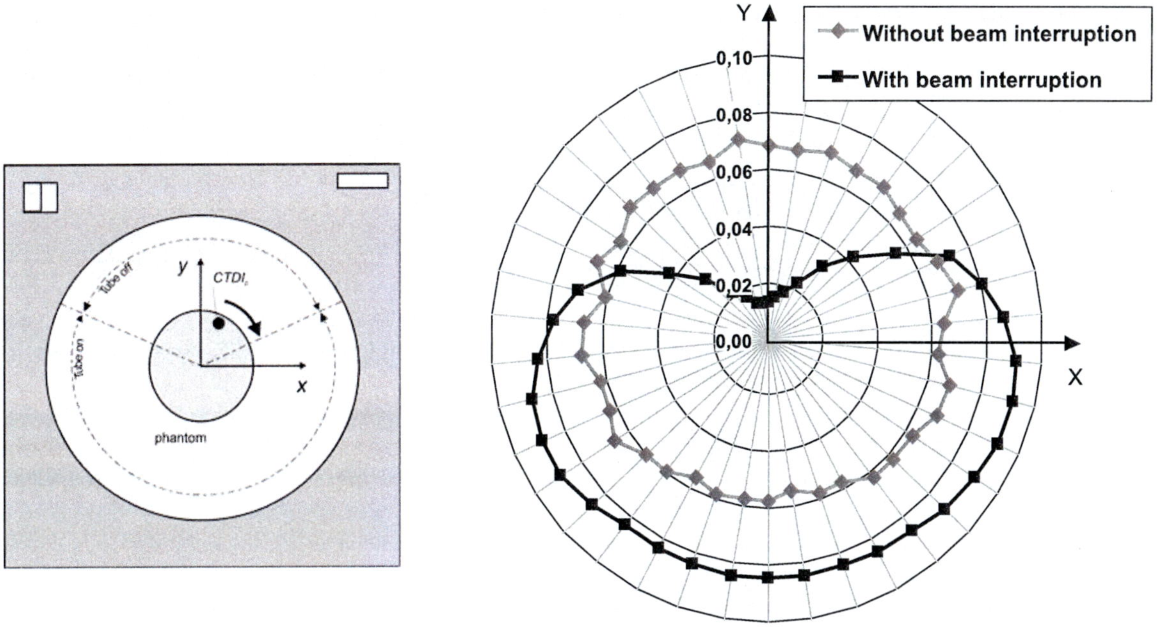


**Fig. 16** Patient surface dose distribution, with and without a beam interruption CTF device. *Right image* shows relative periphery CTDI for different angular positions

## 6.6 Angular Beam Modulation: Simulating the Under-Table Tube Geometry

When performing interventions that require fluoroscopy it is common to use X-ray systems with the tube positioned under the table. Such an under-table setup reduces the amount of backscatter radiation that is directed toward the upper body part of the staff that is standing next to the patient (see Sect. 5.1). In CT fluoroscopy, this principle is applied by one manufacturer (HandCARE$^{TM}$ option, Siemens, Erlangen, Germany). This angular beam modulation system reduces the scattered radiation exposure to the physician by interrupting X-ray exposure when the tube rotates above the patient (within a 120° angle sector), while maintaining the integrated mAs per rotation. As a result, the scatter radiation that leaves the anterior part of the patient will be limited, thus reducing the exposure that is directed toward the operator. A patient study demonstrated that the dose to the operator's hand could be halved by using such system (Buls et al. 2004), and a recent phantom study demonstrated a dose reduction of 27% (Hohl et al. 2008).

However, while reducing exposure to the staff, such systems can increase patient's peak skin doses as the same dose is delivered to a smaller skin area in comparison to 360° CT-scanning. Figure 16 shows the relative patient dose distribution with and without a CTF system that interrupts exposure. The data is obtained by measuring the normalized periphery *CTDI* in a 32 cm phantom for various angular positions with a 10-degree increment (Buls et al. 2004). With continuous scanning, the surface dose is more or less equally distributed around the patient whereas with the beam interruption device, the surface dose is concentrated in the posterior part of the patient. As a result, the peak skin dose rate is about 1.5 times increased in that part compared to continuous scanning.

## 6.7 Learning Curve

With acquisition of any new image-guided interventional apparatus, there is inevitably a period of time during which learning is necessary to acquire expertise and perform the procedures efficiently (Gianfelice et al. 2000). This becomes more important as the spectrum of CTF procedures expands to complex types of interventions, which may require longer exposure times due to the lack of expertise. Gianfelice et al. (2000) studied the effect of the learning process for biopsy procedures on exposure times. They observed a significant reduction from 50.3 to 25.8 s per patient after a 2-year period or 250 consecutive patients. The learning process associated with CTF technology impacts procedure parameters by decreasing both mean procedure and fluoroscopy times, thereby increasing patient turnover and decreasing radiation exposure to the patient and the operator.

Also other methods could be used to decrease exposure time. A study by Carlson et al. (2005) reported a mean exposure time reduction from 18.0 to 12.6 s by using a breath-hold monitoring and feedback system with biopsies of the lung and the upper abdomen.

## 7 Regulatory Dose Limits and Risk of Cataract Occurence

In most countries, the annual regulatory dose limits for classified workers are: 20 mSv for the effective (total body) dose, 500 mSv for the equivalent dose to the skin and 150 mSv for the equivalent dose to the eyes (ICRP 2007). However, in April 2011, the ICRP published a statement that recommends a dose limit to the eyes of only 20 mSv (ICRP 2011). This is almost an 8-fold reduction and is based on recent studies that demonstrated increased sensitivity of the eye lens to radiation. The ICRP reviewed epidemiological evidence suggesting that there are some tissue reaction effects, particularly those with very late manifestation, where threshold doses are or might be lower than previously considered. Consequently, for occupational exposure in planned exposure situations the Commission now recommends an equivalent dose limit for the lens of the eye of 20 mSv per year (previously 150 mSv), averaged over defined periods of 5 years, with no single year exceeding 50 mSv.

For the staff in CTF, the dose to the hands or the eyes will be the critical factor with regard to regulatory dose limits, not the effective dose. The number of CTF procedures before exceeding regulatory dose limits can be estimated from the data in Table 5. In order not to exceed the dose limit of 20 mSv to the eyes, about 100 CTF procedures would be allowed when using the highest reported dose of 0.2 mGy per procedure (Buls et al. 2003; Brennan et al. 2003). At a maximal permissible dose of 500 mSv to the hands per year, about 230 CTF procedures would be allowed when using the highest reported dose of 2.2 mGy per procedure (Nawfel et al. 2000). These numbers increase rapidly when more dose-saving CTF methods are applied by either using reduced exposure settings, or by using standoff needle devices or other methods to reduce the scattered dose to the eyes and hands. For example, using the reported data of Gianfelice et al. (2000) with 120 kVp, 30 mA and 26 s exposure time, over 1,000 CTF procedures could be performed before exceeding dose limits to the hands. The combination with using a lead drape could increase this number even further up to over 8,000 procedures. Sufficient protection of the eye lens can be achieved by using a lead barrier or wearing lead glass eye wear.

For patients, no legal dose limits apply but it is mandatory to respect Diagnostic Reference Levels (DRLs). DRLs are dose levels in diagnostic practices for typical examinations that are expected not to be exceeded for standard procedures when good practice is applied (Euratom 1997). In contrast to standard CT examinations where DRLs are well established in terms of *CTDI* and *DLP*, they do not exist for CTF up to now. In strict sense, CTF is not a diagnostic investigation so DRLs would not apply. However, typical dose levels for interventional procedures using conventional fluoroscopy do exist. These are usually expressed as Dose Area Product (DAP) values. DRLs for CTF could indicate whether the levels of patient dose are unusually high for a specific procedure. If so, a local review should be initiated to determine whether protection has been adequately optimized or whether corrective action is required.

## 8 Conclusions

Non-vascular diagnostic and therapeutic interventions are becoming more and more important in patient workup. This shift to a more invasive diagnostic and therapeutic approach in radiology is seen in spite of the improving performance of imaging techniques and the improvement of surgical techniques. CT fluoroscopy (CTF) has proven to be an effective modality for guiding diagnostic and therapeutic radiological interventions. With CTF, the physician can follow the exact trajectory of needle placement from the skin surface to the targeted

**Table 6** Factors that affect both patient and staff doses in CTF

| Parameter | Potential risk | Measures |
|---|---|---|
| Compared to conventional CT, the position of the scan plane stays constant with CTF | The same patient skin area is repeatedly exposed, resulting in high-accumulated skin doses that may reach 2 Gy. Risk for radiation induced skin injuries | Operators must be aware of the potential for skin injuries and recognize the characteristics of skin doses in CTF |
| Compared to conventional fluoroscopy, CTF allows high exposure settings in terms of tube current (mA) and tube potential (kVp). Automated tube current modulation is not available with CTF | As a result, patient surface (skin) dose rates are much higher in CTF. They can vary from 10 up to 60 cGy/min. Also, scattered radiation dose rates toward the operator are much more intense and energetic | The lowest possible tube current values should be used that allow an adequate image quality in the anatomical region of interest. Reported values are typically between 10 and 30 mA for chest cases, and between 30 and 50 mA for abdominal cases. Tube currents above 50 mA should be avoided |
| Exposure time or CT-scanning time (s) | Prolonged exposure times can be necessary in cases of small and difficult accessible lesions or cases with increased patient motion. Both patient skin dose rate and scatter dose rate increase linearly with exposure time | Limit exposure time as much as possible by using the quick-check method. Typical reported exposure times are below 60 s per procedure. Very short exposure times, in the range of 20 s, are also reported in clinical routine for various types of procedures |
| CTF-technique: real-time method or quick-check method | Real-time method increases exposure time considerably and therefore also patient and staff doses | Avoid real-time scanning. Use the standard quick-check method and reserve real-time method only for limited cases with increased patient motion |
| Patient size and children | Skin dose rate increases for smaller patients due to the shorter distance between skin and isocenter | Give special attention to tube current reduction for smaller patients. For pediatric patients typical tube current values of 10 mA are reported |
| Position of the patient inside gantry | Surface dose rate decreases when the surface moves away from isocentre. The maximal skin dose rate is reached at the isocenter | Position the center of the patient in the isocentre, thus maximizing the distance between skin surface and isocentre for minimizing skin dose. Avoid the patient surface being positioned at isocenter |
| In contrast to conventional CT, the operator stands next to X-ray source during CT scanning | The operator is exposed to scattered radiation | Staff members should always wear appropriate lead aprons complemented with a thyroid collar. Simultaneous dose monitoring by two radiation badges (over and under the apron) is recommended. Particular attention is required to the protection of the lens of the eyes and the hands |
| The CT tube rotates continuously around the patient during exposure | The direction of the scattered radiation field is nearly symmetric and is not as controllable as in conventional fluoroscopy (e.g. angiography). It also is more intense as in conventional fluoroscopy | See below |
| Slice thickness (mm) | Both patient skin dose and scattered exposure increases with slice thickness | Select the smallest possible slice thickness in function of the puncture access route. Usually between 5 and 10 mm. A too small selected slice thickness may influence CTF efficiency and may increase exposure time |

(continued)

**Table 6** (continued)

| Parameter | Potential risk | Measures |
|---|---|---|
| Standoff needle device | These have usually a length between 10 and 30 cm. They prevent entering the primary beam with the hands and reduce scatter dose at the level of the hand due to the larger distance to scanning plane | Should be always used during real-time scanning. Is not required when the quick-check method is applied. Could result in reduced tactile feedback and, hence, may influence CTF efficiency and exposure time |
| Lead drape placed on the patient caudal from scanning plane | A 0.5 mm lead equivalent drape reduces scattered exposure to the hands (up to 95%) and upper part of operator's body | Lead drapes are reported to be very efficient and very easy to use. They should be always applied with CTF |
| Thin leaded gloves | Reduces scattered exposure to hands | Dose reduction not as significant as a lead drape. May reduce tactile feedback |
| Lead glass eye wear | Reduces scattered exposure to lens of the eyes | Recent studies show increased sensitivity of the eye lens to radiation and thus protection of the eye using lead glass eye wear is very important |
| Angular beam modulation: interruption of CT exposure when tube rotates above table | Reduces scattered exposure considerably to hands and upper part of operator's body, but can increase patient skin dose rate by 1.5 | Should be only used with reduced tube current settings to limit patient skin dose |
| Physicians of various specialties perform CTF procedures | Non-radiologist operators may have not had in-depth training in radiation management. Risk of using non-optimized exposure settings or increased exposure times | Provide dedicated training for all CTF operators |
| Several staff members can be present in CT room | Several staff members are exposed to scattered radiation | Limit number of staff personnel in CT room, provide dedicated training and clear guidelines. Increase distance to patient as much as possible |
| CTF is a relatively new technique and its spectrum could expand to more complex interventions | Risk of prolonged exposure times due to learning curve | Provide dedicated training |

lesion due to the display of CT images in real time, and it can be applied in soft tissue, fluid- and air-filled cavities and bones. CTF-guided procedures are particularly challenging in uncooperative patients or in organs that are prone to respiratory motion such as the lung or liver.

A drawback of CTF remains the potential for significantly high patient and staff doses. For the patient, the same skin area is repeatedly exposed and the physician is exposed to scattered radiation as he enters the CT room while scanning. If CTF is used improperly by a combination of a high current and prolonged exposure times, it has a potential for patient skin injuries. Whereas with conventional fluoroscopy the 2-Gy threshold dose for tissue reactions is reached after 100–200 min of fluoroscopy, it can be reached in CTF after only 3–10 min of scanning when a high tube current is applied. For the physician, particularly the doses to the lens of the eyes and the hands are of concern. Doses to the hands have been reported up to 2.2 mGy per procedure and dose rates at the level of the hands may vary between 20 and 40 $\mu$Gy/s when no radiation protection measures are applied. Doses to the eyes can be anywhere in the range of <0.01–0.2 mGy per procedure. If protection is not used, there can be a substantial risk of lens opacity for procedures that require long fluoroscopy times and with several procedures per day, such as in busy department. However, even in these situations, one can use effective protection to reduce the probability of cataract to a negligible level. Operators need to be aware of different methods of CTF guidance and the factors that determine radiation exposure of both patient and staff. This becomes more important as the spectrum of CTF procedures might expand to more complex procedures that may require longer fluoroscopy times.

Table 6 summarizes the factors that affect patient and staff doses in CTF, their risk potential and proposes measures to be taken for dose optimization.

Although CT Fluoroscopy has the potential to deliver high doses to both patient and staff, radiation doses can be reduced to acceptable levels. This can be achieved by adequate personal protection by a lead apron, a thyroid collar and lead glass eye wear, and proper radiation management that uses a combination of manually selecting low tube currents and by using the quick-check or intermittent CTF method that limits fluoroscopy time as much as possible. Literature data indicates that such a method can be easily applied in clinical routine.

## References


Avilés LP, Castellano IA, Dance DR, Vañò E (2001) Analysis of surface dose variation in CT procedures. Br J Radiol 74:1128–1136

Avilés LP, Dance DR, Castellano IA, Vañò E (2004) Monte Carlo simulations in CT for the study of the surface air kerma and energy imparted to phantoms of varying size and position. Phys Med Biol 49:1439–1454

Balter S, Hopewell JW, Miller DL, Wagner LK, Zelefsky MJ (2010) Fluoroscopically guided interventional procedures: a review of radiation effects on patients' skin and hair. Radiology 254:327–341

Baran GW, Haaga JR, Shurin SB, Alfidi RJ (1984) CT-guided percutaneous biopsies in pediatric patients. Pediatr Radiol 14:161–164

Brennan SB, Byrne B, Shortt M, Gilligan P, Kenny P, Fenlon HM (2003) Evaluation of staff radiation doses from 'Quick-Check' CT for CT-guided interventional procedures. Ir J Med Sci 172(4):1–16

Buls N, Pages J, de Mey J, Osteaux M (2003) Evaluation of patient and staff doses during various CT Fluoroscopy guided interventions. Health Phys 85(2):165–173

Buls N, de Mey J, Vandenbroucke F, Vanderdood K, Osteaux M (2004) Dose reduction in CT fluoroscopy. 16th European Congress of Radiology 5–9 March 2004, Vienna. Abstract proceedings Eur Radiol

Bushberg JT, Seibert JA, Leidholdt EM, Boone JM (2002) The essential physics of medical imaging. Lippincott Williams & Wilkins, Philadelphia

Cahill AM, Baskin KM, Kaye RD, Fitz CR, Towbin RB (2004) CT-guided percutaneous lung biopsy in children. J Vasc Interv Radiol 15:955–960

Carlson SK, Bender CE, Classic KL, Zink FE, Quam JP, Ward EM, Oberg AL (2001) Benefits and safety of CT fluoroscopy in interventional radiologic procedures. Radiology 219:515–520

Carlson SK, Felmlee JP, Bender CE, Ehman RL, Classic KL, Hoskin TL, Harmsen WS, Hu HH (2005) CT Fluoroscopy-guided biopsy of the lung or upper abdomen with a breath-hold monitoring and feedback system: a prospective randomized controlled clinical trial. Radiology 237:701–708

Council directive 97/43/Euratom on health protection of individuals against the dangers of ionising radiation in relation to medical exposure (1997) Official J Eur Community L180:22

Daly B, Templeton Krebs TL, Carroll K, Wong-You-Cheong JJ (1998) Evaluation of biopsy needles and prototypic needle guide devices with CT fluoroscopic guidance in simulated organ tissue. Radiology 209:850–855

Froelich JJ, Saar B, Hoppe M, Ishaque N, Walthers EM, Regn J, Klose KJ (1998) Real-time CT-fluoroscopy for guidance of percutaneous drainage procedures. J Vasc Interv Radiol 9(5):735–740

Geraghty PR, Kee ST, McFarlane G, Razavi MK, Sze DY, Dake MD (2003) CT-guided transthoracic needle aspiration biopsy of pulmonary nodules: needle size and pneumothorax rate. Radiology 229:475–481

Gianfelice D, Lepanto L, Perreault P, Chartrand-Lefebvre C, Milette PC (2000) Effect of the learning process on procedure times and radiation exposure for CT fluoroscopy-guided percutaneous biopsy procedures. J Vasc Interv Radiol 11:1217–1221

Haaga JR, Alfidi RJ (1976) Precise biopsy localisation by computed tomography. Radiology 118:603

Hohl C, Suess C, Wildberger JE, Honnef D, Das M, Mühlenbruch G, Schaller A, Günther RW, Mahnken AH (2008) Dose reduction during CT fluoroscopy: phantom study of angular beam modulation. Radiology 246(2):519–525

International Commission on Radiation Protection (1982) General principles of monitoring for radiation protection of workers ICRP Publication, p. 35

International Commission on Radiological Protection (2000) Managing patient dose in Computed Tomography ICRP Publication 87. Ann. ICRP 30(4):1–43

International Commission on Radiological Protection (2001) Avoidance of Radiation Injuries from Medical Interventional Procedures ICRP Publication 85: Ann ICRP 30(2)

International Commission on Radiological Protection (2007) Recommendations of the ICRP, Pergamon Press; ICRP Publication, Oxford, p. 103

International Commission on Radiological Protection (2011) Statement on tissue reactions. ICRP ref 4825-3093-1464. Approved by the Commission on 21 April 2011

Irie T, Kajitani M, Yoshioka H, Matsueda K, Inaba Y, Arai Y, Nakajima K, Nozawa K, Itai Y (2000) CT fluoroscopy for lung nodule biopsy: a new device for needle placement and phantom study. J Vasc Interv Radiol 11:359–364

Irie T, Kajitani M, Matsueda K, Arai Y, Inaba Y, Kujiraoka Y, Itai Y (2001a) Biopsy of lung nodules with use of I–I device under intermittent CT fluoroscopy guidance: preliminary clinical study. J Vasc Interv Radiol 12:215–219

Irie T, Kajitani M, Itai Y (2001b) CT fluoroscopy-guided intervention: Marked reduction of scattered radiation dose to the physician's hand by use of a lead plate and an improved I–I device. J Vasc Interv Radiol 12:1417–1421

Katada K, Anno H, Koga S (1994) Initial trial with CT fluoroscopy. Radiology 190:662

Katada K, Kato R, Anno H, Ogura Y, Koga S, Ida Y, Sato M, Nonomura K (1996) Guidance with real-time CT fluoroscopy: early clinical experience. Radiology 200:851–856

Kataoka ML, Raptopoulos VD, Lin PJ, Siewert B, Goldberg SN, Kruskal J (2006) Multiple-image in-room CT imaging guidance for interventional procedures. Radiology 239:863–868

Kato R, Katada K, Anno H, Suzuki S, Ida Y, Koga S (1996) Radiation dosimetry at CT fluoroscopy: physician's hand dose and development of needle holders. Radiology 201:576–578

Keat N (2001) Real-time CT and CT fluoroscopy. Br J Radiol 74:1088–1090

Klose KC (1993) CT-guided large-bore biopsy: extrapleural injection of saline for safe transpleural access to pulmonary lesions. Cardiovasc Intervent Radiol 16:259–261

Koenig TR, Wolff D, Mettler FA, Wagner LK (2001) Skin injuries from fluoroscopically guided procedures: part 1, characteristics of radiation injury. AJR 177:3–11

Laufer U, Kirchner J, Kickuth R, Adams S, Jendreck M, Liermann D (2001) A comparative study of CT fluoroscopy combined with fluoroscopy versus fluoroscopy alone for percutaneous transhepatic biliary drainage. Cardiovasc Intervent Radiol 24:240–244

Laurent F, Michel P, Latrabe V, Tunon de Lara M, Marthan R (1999) Pneumothoraces and chest tube placement after CT-guided transthoracic lung biopsy using a coaxial technique: incidence and risk factors. Am J Roentgenol 172:1049–1053

Lee JM (2000) CT-guided celiac plexus block for intractable abdominal pain. J Korean Med Sci 15:173–178

Li X, Fan W, Zhang L, Zhao M, Huang Z, Li W, Gu Y, Gao F, Huang J, Li C, Zhang F, Wu P (2011) CT-guided percutaneous microwave ablation of adrenal malignant carcinoma: Preliminary Results. Cancer. doi: 10.1002/cncr.26128. [Epub ahead of print]

Mcparland BJ (1998) Entrance skin dose estimates derived from dose-area product measurements in interventional radiological procedures. Br J Radiol 71:1288–1295

Meleka S, Patra A, Minkoff E, Murphy K (2005) Value of CT fluoroscopy for lumbar facet blocks. Am J Neuroradiol 26:1001–1003

Meyer CA, White CS, Wu J, Futterer SF, Templeton PA (1998) Real-time CT fluoroscopy: usefulness in thoracic drainage. Am J Roentgenol 171:1097–1101

Miller DL, Balter S, Cole PE, Lu HT et al (2003) Radiation doses in interventional radiology procedures: the RAD-IR study. J Vasc Interv Radiol 14:977–990

Moran CJ, Naidich TP, Gado MH, Marchosky JA (1979) Central nervous system lesions biopsied or treated by CT-guided needle placement. Radiology 131:681–686

Nawfel RD, Philip F, Judy PF, Silverman SG, Hooton S, Tuncali K, Adams DF (2000) Patient and personnel exposure during CT fluoroscopy-guided interventional procedures. Radiology 216:180–184

Neeman Z, Dromi SA, Sarin S, Wood BJ (2006) CT fluoroscopy shielding: decreases in scattered radiation for the patient and operator. J Vasc Interv Radiol 17(12):1999–2004

Nickoloff EL, Khandji A, Dutta A (2000) Radiation doses during CT fluoroscopy. Health Phys 79(6):675–681

Paulson EK, Sheafor DH, Enterline DS, McAdams HP, Yoshizumi T (2001) CT fluoroscopy-guided interventional procedures: techniques and radiation dose to radiologists. Radiology 220:161–167

Rosenthal DI, Hornicek FJ, Torriani M, Gebhardt MC, Mankin HJ (2003) Osteoid osteoma: percutaneous treatment with radiofrequency energy. Radiology 229:171–175

Silverman SG, Tuncali K, Adams DF, Nawfel RD, Zou KH, Judy PF (1999) CT fluoroscopy-guided abdominal interventions: techniques, results and radiation exposure. Radiology 212:673–681

Solomon SB, Patriciu A, Bohlman ME, Kavoussi LR, Stoianovici D (2002) Robotically driven interventions: a method of using CT fluoroscopy without radiation exposure to the physician. Radiology 225:277–282

Stecker MS, Balter S, Towbin RB, Miller DL, Vañó E, Bartal G, Angle JF et al (2009) Guidelines for patient radiation dose management. J Vasc Interv Radiol 20:S263–S273

Stoeckelhuber BM, Leibecke T, Schulz E, Melchert UH, Bergmann-Koester CU, Helmberger T, Gelissen J (2005) Radiation dose to the radiologist's hand during continuous CT Fluoroscopy-guided interventions. Cardiovasc Intervent Radiol 28:589–594

Teeuwisse WM, Geleijns J, Broerse JJ, Obermann WR, Van Persijn Van Meerten EL (2001) Patient and staff dose during CT guided biopsy, drainage and coagulation. Br J Radiol 74:720–726

Trout ED, Kelley JP (1972) Scattered radiation from a tissue equivalent phantom for X-rays from 50 to 300 kVp. Radiology 104:161–169

Trumm CG, Jakobs TF, Zech CJ, Helmberger TK, Reiser MF, Hoffmann RT (2008) CT fluoroscopy-guided percutaneous vertebroplasty for the treatment of osteolytic breast cancer metastases: results in 62 sessions with 86 vertebrae treated. J Vasc Interv Radiol 19(11):1596–1606

United Nations Scientific Committee on the Effects of Atomic Radiation (2000) Sources and effects of ionizing radiation. New York: United Nations: vol 1 Sources

United States Food and Drug Administration (1994) Public health advisory. Avoidance of serious X-ray-induced skin injuries to patients during fluoroscopically-guided procedures. Rockville, MD, Center for devices and radiological health, United States Food and Drug Administration, September 30

Wagner LK (2000) CT fluoroscopy: another advancement with additional challenges in radiation management. Radiology 216:9–10

Wagner LK (2007) Radiation injury is a potentially serious complication to fluoroscopically-guided complex interventions. Biomed Imaging Interv J32:e22

Yamagami T, Iida S, Kato T, Tanaka O, Nishimura T (2003) Combining fine-needle aspiration and core biopsy under CT fluoroscopy guidance: a better way to treat patients with lung nodules? Am J Roentgenol 180:811–815

Zech CJ, Helmberger T, Wichmann MW, Holzknecht N, Diebold J, Reiser MF (2002) Large core biopsy of the pancreas under CT fluoroscopy control: results and complications. J Comput Assist Tomogr 26:743–749

# Dose Optimization and Reduction in CT of Children

Peter Vock, Enno Stranzinger, and Rainer Wolf

## Contents



P. Vock (✉) · E. Stranzinger · R. Wolf
Department of Diagnostic,
Interventional and Pediatric Radiology,
University Hospital, Inselspital,
3010 Bern, Switzerland
e-mail: peter.vock@insel.ch

**Abstract**

Children differ from adult patients in that they vary tremendously in their small size—which mandates adaptation of physical scan parameters—but also in their elevated susceptibility to ionizing radiation, and the different pathology during childhood. While the many technical innovations in CT during the last decade have impacted the entire field of clinical applications, faster scanning in children often makes the difference by eliminating motion artifacts; a number of new features contribute to reducing radiation exposure of children, most importantly iterative reconstruction and adaptive dose shielding. Limited cooperation of children often influences image quality more significantly than the choice of scanning parameters. Decreasing anxiety, avoiding pain, exercising cooperation before the scan, and avoiding artifacts by eliminating foreign bodies from the scan field are measures of high importance; a child-friendly atmosphere and staff further contribute to a successful scan. Choosing appropriate pediatric protocols means using each feature of a specific scanner to the best of the individual child, often accepting noise, scanning the minimal length and avoiding repeat/multiphase scans of the same volume. It is suggested to start with a scanner-optimized adult abdominal or head scan protocol and to reduce mAs according to tables available in the internet. In addition, lowering tube voltage is an excellent tool for high-contrast organs and CT angiography in children. Radiation risks based on biology and physics have been covered in previous chapters and are, of course, also valid for children.

D. Tack et al. (eds.), *Radiation Dose from Multidetector CT*, Medical Radiology. Diagnostic Imaging,
DOI: 10.1007/174_2011_527, 

Similarly, clinical approaches to dose optimization and reduction are similar in pediatric and adult CT examinations (Huda et al., Pediatr Radiol 32:272–279, 2000). This chapter will concentrate on the fact that children are not just adults with smaller dimensions, thus it will point out what is special in children.

## 1 Why Dose Optimization and Reduction in CT is Even More Important in Children

Several independent arguments clearly justify an even more careful use of the "as low as reasonably achievable" (ALARA) principle in children than in adults (Frush et al. 2003; Vock 2002) (Table 1):

- Children are indeed—depending on their stage of growth—*smaller* than adults, and this means that the physical laws of radiation interaction and absorption have to be respected during protocol definition (Boone et al. 2003; Huda 2002). Usually, a decreased number of photons is required which translates into a lower tube output (mAs). Often the use of a lower X-ray energy (kV) is appropriate as well in children. These facts—though known over decades for radiography—were not realised for CT by many radiologists until 2001 (Paterson et al. 2001).
- At the same physical energy exposure of ionizing radiation, the *biological effects* are *more severe* in children (Brenner et al. 2001; 2003; Brenner 2002; Frush et al. 2003; Pierce and Preston 2000); the risk of lethal cancer is multiplied by a factor of 2.5 on average, as compared to adult people, starting at around 10 in neonates and approaching adult values during adolescence. This is mostly explained by the fact that *proliferating tissues* are more vulnerable to the effects of radiation and that proliferation is much more active during the growth period than later in life. Furthermore, the distribution of tissues is different in childhood: e.g., red bone marrow will hardly be irradiated during a CT extremity exam in adults, whereas it will partly be included in the volume of primary radiation exposure in a child.
- Children have a *longer life expectancy* than the average adult population studied by CT. Their natural lifetime left at the moment of CT scanning is in the range of 70 years, whereas it is more often 10–20 years than 30–40 years in the adult CT population. Of course, since it is likely that the risk of radiation-induced carcinogenesis persists during the entire life span and since the delay of cancer manifestation is more often decades than years, more children than adults will be alive at the end of the latency period of radiation-induced cancers, and a significant percentage among them will die from cancer.
- Children usually have *less fatty tissue* between visceral organs than adults. To keep the contrast needed to differentiate structures with only tiny fatty layers in between, the signal-to-noise ratio (S/N) and, thus, the dose has to be increased, or the contrast has to be improved by other modifications of the protocol, such as by using a lower X-ray energy (kV). Furthermore, the axial cross-section of a child tends to be more rounded than in adults, with nearly equal x and y diameters, a less attractive prerequisite for dose modulation in the xy-plane
- *Cooperation* is not as easy for children as it is for adults. This means that the combined contributions of trained personnel, patient preparation, the atmosphere in the examination room and sometimes the presence of a parent are all needed to reach an optimal result using minimal radiation exposure. Of course, cooperation is easier the shorter the time of measurement: it becomes

**Table 1** Why children need specific CT planning

| Difference | Cause, consequence |
|---|---|
| Smaller dimensions | Adapt protocol according to decreased absorption |
| Higher biologic sensitivity | Growth, cell proliferation, tissue distribution |
| Long life expectancy | Increased risk of tumor manifestation despite long latency |
| Less fatty tissue | Adapt protocol to maintain contrast |
| Cooperation may not be possible | Prepare patient, immobilize, scan fast (high pitch) |
| Alternative imaging test is more often equivalent or better | Consider ultrasound, MRI |
| Different pathology in children | Requires different justification/approach/knowledge |

slightly less important but stays critical with modern faster measurement techniques.

- *Alternatives* to CT exist in children—in contrast to multiple applications in adults. Children are excellent candidates for *ultrasound* imaging, and—other than in adults—many more details in more regions of the body can be shown. Cerebral ultrasound in the neonate is just one prominent example. Similarly, *MRI,* another alternative to CT without ionizing radiation, has an excellent accuracy in children; most contraindications to MRI, such as cardiac pacemakers, neurostimulators, ferromagnetic foreign bodies, or claustrophobia, are rarely a problem in children.
- *Pathology is different* in children than in adults. While congenital and inflammatory disorders are more frequently seen, degenerative and neoplastic diseases are clearly less abundant during the growth period. A different spectrum of pathology means a different diagnostic approach. Above all, justification follows the specific pathology and does not just ask for the best technical method for one organ but rather for weighing the advantages and risks of all methods in the specific situation.

## 2 Impact of New CT Scanners on Pediatric Patients

A number of significant technical innovations have been introduced to CT scanners over the years: the most important steps have been the spiral/helical scanning mode, multichannel-multidetector-units, two- and three-dimensional dose modulation, adaptive shielding, and iterative reconstruction. As medical aspects and the biologic impact of CT scanning are different in children and in adults, the impact of this recent development is special in children and asks for some consideration (Table 2). These obvious advantages have to be balanced with the disadvantages that are often tightly combined. In a phase of fast development, there are major differences between the scanners of different manufacturers. Because these will level out mostly within some years, we will concentrate on the issues that most multi-row detector scanners have in common.

- *Faster Scanning*. This is obviously the single most important factor for the growing number of applications of CT in pediatrics (Mettler et al. 2000; Nickoloff and Alderson 2001; Nickoloff 2002). Children no longer need to stay immobile during 10–15 min, and often CT scanning is possible without sedation or with sedation instead of intubation anesthesia on several higher end multidetector scanners at fast scanning modes. On these scanners and using these scanning modes, motion artifacts have substantially disappeared, and the body volume studied during one session is no longer limited by the maximal period of cooperation of a child. In particular, faster scanning is made possible with wider detector configuration scanners (≥4 cm) and/or combinations of high non-overlapping pitch and faster table speed with faster gantry rotation times. Vascular applications of CT in children have only become available with modern scanners, thanks to the fact that the first or second pass of contrast agents can be used to get a high intravascular contrast before diffusion to the

**Table 2** Impact of modern CT scanners on pediatric CT

| Technical feature of modern CT | Consequence |
|---|---|
| Faster scanning | Less cooperation/ immobilization needed, new applications (e.g. vascular, multi-phasic), larger volume covered per time |
| Better z-axis resolution | Isotropic geometric resolution, noise |
| Slice thickness | Correct slice profile, more noise on thin slices (or increased radiation exposure) |
| Dose shaping (bow tie) filters | Useful for object with small dimensions |
| Dose modulation | Constant S/N, dose reduction (if used appropriately) |
| Geometric detector efficiency | Z-axis overbeaming (collimation), non-active detector area (element spacing) |
| Overscanning in spiral mode | Additional dose outside planned volume |
| Adaptive dose shielding (to overcome overscanning) | Use this option if it is available on your scanner |
| Iterative reconstruction | Similar image noise at lower dose; this feature is still undergoing clinical tests; however it likely will reduce exposure to a higher degree than most other options |

interstitial space occurs. Similarly, multiphasic examinations essentially have only been introduced with the arrival of the modern generation of CT scanners. New medical applications indeed are the most important reason for an important rise of the number of CT examinations performed in children during the last 12 years. Cardiac CT deserves special mention among these: prospective ECG gating of the tube is combined with a fast scan during a few cardiac cycles; with the top scanners, the diastolic period of just one cycle is used to get all data needed and to further reduce exposure based on either a very broad detector of up to 256–320 z-axis elements (although in neonates and infants, even 128 z-axis elements might be adequate) or on a dual-source scanner with two tube-detector arrays gathering the information at a very high pitch (Han et al. 2011). High-pitch scanning has similarly been shown to be robust in chest CT even in non-cooperative children (Lell et al. 2011).

- *Better z-axis resolution.* The smaller dimensions of children basically require a high geometric resolution, with ideally isotropic voxels. The z-axis size of a voxel, a major problem with single-detector rows, can be reduced to submillimetric dimensions on scanners with multiple detector rows, without compromising the volume coverage of the scan. This is a major advantage, particularly to avoid partial volume effects and secondarily for multiplanar 2D reformations and for 3D analysis of data.
- *Slice thickness.* Thinner collimation in multi-row detector CT scanners produces raw data of an intrinsically high geometric resolution. However, the smaller submillimetric voxel volume necessarily causes a major signal drop and, thus, a drop of the S/N unless the X-ray flux is increased proportionally. This phenomenon has impacted the clinical application of four detector-row scanners, where radiation exposure has increased in relation to single-row scanners due to lower radiation dose efficiency of earlier generations of four detector-row scanners. Subsequent scanners (especially $\geq$16 detector rows) however, have equal or better radiation dose efficiency for acquisition of submillimetric slice volumes. To handle this physical fact, most experts now suggest to scan at a thin collimation and a low dose but then to reconstruct thicker images of 3–6 mm with a much better S/N for diagnosis. Thus, thin noisy slices are just consulted in case of partial volume problems, and they are used for post-processing. In conclusion, it is useful to have the submillimetric slices available but to rely mostly on thicker ones for routine work, even in children. Another problem with slice thickness has occurred on single-row scanners: using an elevated pitch (1.5–3), as needed for faster scanning and for dose reduction, has caused a major widening of the slice profile (which may still achieve up to 30% at a pitch greater or equal to 1.3 on some $\leq$16 row scanners). With most modern state-of-the-art multirow scanners—thanks to more data available for interpolation—the slice profile is close to the nominal value, and the pitch factor has lost most of its critical influence.
- *Beam shaping filters (bow tie or dose shaping filters).* Beam shaping filters are used to adapt the X-ray profile. Obviously, objects with a diameter much less than the diameter of the gantry do not require the same X-ray flux in the periphery of the field of view as thick objects do. Specific filters are used by most manufacturers to adapt the beam profile to the smaller dimension of an adult head, an extremity or a child, and they help to control radiation exposure. Unfortunately, the user usually does not know the type of filter used with specific protocols and also cannot choose from different specific filters when preparing an examination. Appropriate functioning of the dose shaping filters requires appropriate centering of the patients. Since most modern multi-row detectors are equipped with these filters, it is imperative that children should be centered appropriately in the gantry isocenter for both acquisition of localizer radiograph and actual cross-sectional images.
- *Dose modulation.* The introduction of advanced dose modulation techniques in CT practically provides automatic exposure control (AEC), as used in fluoroscopy systems to keep the S/N at the detector constant during an examination. Body areas with smaller diameters and moderate bony components do not require the same X-ray flux as thick areas with a lot of bony structures. Dose modulation in the xy-plane and the z-axis is therefore a major step forward that should be used generally. However, let us keep in mind that it is not perfect at all: in small children the x and y diameters often do not differ a lot; depending on the modulation rules used by the manufacturer, modulation may even increase

exposure beyond the nominal value, e.g. when the scan starts at a level with a thin body diameter, or when local organ shielding is used for the thyroid or the breast gland. The degree of adaptation of exposure to the local physical absorption (in order to maintain a constant S/N at the detector) also depends on the relation between the length of the detector and the length of the scan. When a scan covers only a small distance, as appropriate in scanning one anatomical region of a child, and when the detector—due to many rows (e.g. 64)—becomes long in the z-axis, the best modulation of tube output will fit the needs of the central detector elements whereas the elements above and below may receive too many or too few photons. In other words, the efficacy of dose modulation intrinsically decreases with an increasing number of detector rows. This is true independent of the type of modulation, whether based on absorption measurements from localizer scans or interactively based on the data on the previous rotation.

- *Geometric detector efficiency*. Geometric efficiency of modern CT scanners is mostly determined by two factors, the z-axis geometric efficiency and the detector array geometric efficiency. To avoid penumbral effects in the outer portions of the detector array, collimation of the X-ray beam is usually set wider than the length of the detector array in multirow scanners; this means a decreased *z-axis geometric efficiency* and, consecutively, an increase in exposure due to X-rays that will not hit the detector. The effect is most severe with four row scanners and with narrow submillimetric slices; in this extreme condition, dose may be doubled whereas the increase is rather in the range of 5–20% with 8–64 row scanners. As for dose modulation, this phenomenon is physically the same in children and in adults but again—due to the small dimension of a child's body—the effects beyond the planned and properly detected proportion of X-rays may easily extend to critical organs not to be studied in children, such as the thyroid in chest exams or the testes in abdominal exams. *Detector array geometric efficiency* is defined by the proportion of the overall detector area that contains active detector material. The proportional area of septa between active elements generally increases with the number of detector elements in the xy-plane and as well with the number of rows in the z-axis. Again this effect is not unique in children but has to be considered in pediatric CT.

  *Detector materials* have been improved over time, and still there is a search for more sensitive detectors that would also contribute to lower the exposure.

  *Modern multidetector row scanners are now equipped with collimator cams positioned near the X-ray tube, which collimate some of the unused beam falling beyond the detector* edge, and these cams help improve the radiation dose efficiency.
- *Additional rotations for interpolation in spiral mode (overscanning)*. Projections outside the reconstructed z-axis range are needed in spiral (helical) mode at each end of the scan. Since spiral scanning has become the standard in most CT applications, this phenomenon must not be forgotten. The relative contribution to radiation exposure is usually around 5–25% and is more important the shorter the scan length is. In multi-slice scanners it also increases with the number of detector rows since this usually causes a larger total beam width (collimation, i.e. the sum of all detector elements in the z-axis). Again, in pediatric CT we have to be especially aware of radiation exposure beyond the planned scan range: e.g. with 64 rows of 0.6 mm of detector length, half an additional rotation at pitch 1 will cover nearly 2 more centimetres both at the top and the bottom, whereas with a full additional rotation twice nearly 4 cm of the body will be scanned outside the volume of interest at the ends. As for z-axis geometric efficiency, important organs outside our scanning volume might be exposed to direct instead of scattered radiation and receive a significant dose. This major disadvantage has been overcome by the manufacturers in their most recent scanner generation: adaptive dose shields absorb the photons outside the z-axis range needed to reconstruct the defined volume. Therefore, they have no disadvantage and can always be used when they are available in a specific scanner.
- *Iterative reconstruction*. During the first decades of clinical CT, filtered back-projection (FBP) was the only mathematical technique used for image reconstruction, due to the limited power of computers. Iterative reconstruction (IR) has become possible in consequence to the technical development of very fast computers; it essentially means more computation per image than using FBP but

also less image noise at a given exposure. In other words, IR—if appropriately used—allows for a lower exposure than FBP to get an identical image noise level. Technically, different modifications of IR have been proposed, based on raw data and/or image data as well as on different number of iterations. Early successful pediatric experience has been reported for the abdomen (Vorona et al. 2011) and the heart (Miéville et al. 2011); it seems to be similarly effective as IR in adult patients, and experts anticipate a dose reduction of 30–40%. Ongoing clinical application and further maturation of IR will prove how far one can go with IR in children, and this will likely depend on the body area as well as on the clinical question.

## 3 Justification

The "as low as reasonably achievable" (ALARA) principle may mean that an imaging study using ionising radiation has to be cancelled when there is an equivalent test available that does not need radiation exposure: the global sum of its advantages has to be greater than the sum of its disadvantages in order to justify a specific test. Indeed, justification is the single most effective step in radiation protection. No other step discussed later will reduce exposure by 100%, and even when a CT exam is replaced by another X-ray study, this usually means a major reduction of exposure since most other X-ray examinations cause a much smaller effective dose than CT studies do (Shrimpton et al. 2005). However, justification is also the most difficult step since the risk of immediately not doing the examination cannot be directly compared to the long-time risk of inducing cancer (Vock 2005). What may be good for an elderly patient in internal medicine may not be an appropriate approach for a pediatric patient. Imaging studies not only involve ionising radiation but also a number of other risks and chances, and they are often quite expensive. Depending on the specific medical infrastructure of a country, there is still a lack of high-tech equipment, and doing the study on the wrong patient may exclude another patient from getting the same CT examination that may be critical for his treatment or even the survival.

Slovis (2002) estimated around 40% of all pediatric CT examinations as not clearly indicated. All these reasons together underscore the importance of justification. Several countries have developed guidelines in using imaging procedures: in the US, the appropriateness criteria defined by a panel of experts (using a score of 1–9) have been introduced by the American College of Radiology (2011). For instance, appropriateness of CT of the brain in suspected physical child abuse will be low (2, mostly inappropriate) or very high (9, most appropriate), depending on the age, the results of physical examination and laboratory exams. The Royal College of Radiologists (RCR Referral Guidelines 2007) has issued *referral guidelines* that have been adapted periodically. Pediatrics makes up an entire section of the guidelines that is further classified by anatomical areas and, within each area, by important clinical entities. Except for trauma, CT is rarely mentioned and the conditions for its use are further commented. It is obvious that major efforts are still needed to differentiate the diagnostic decision trees in specific clinical situations, including the age of the child, the habitus, the pathology, the body region as well as the urgency, and the availability of alternative diagnostic tools.

Head trauma is also an example for clinical criteria helping to decide about the individual need for CT evaluation (Oman et al. 2006) Hardly ever is medical diagnostic imaging justified just for demonstrating morphology, as true for any other diagnostic tests it is expected to detect disease, to differentiate between different pathologies, to stage disease or to provide information about the effects of treatment; however, all this information is not helpful unless it helps in the further management of the patient and is obtained with an appropriate "cost." Cost clearly includes both the financial cost of the examination and its medical risk. In pediatric CT, although there are risks with anesthesia and intravenous contrast medium injection, the main two risks usually are the inaccuracy of the test (false negative, false positive findings) and the risk of radiation exposure, which is more important than in adult patients, even at the same nominal effective dose.

Before any imaging examination with X-rays is considered, alternatives must therefore be evaluated: ultrasound is the first line-imaging test in children since the slim body usually favors the access even to deep organs without any radiation exposure, combining morphologic with real-time motional and even flow information. In experienced hands, it can provide a lot of essential information, thus avoiding CT. When ultrasound and radiography are unlikely to answer—or have not answered—the specific medical question, the choice is often between MRI and CT. In this situation the severity of suspected disease, the duration of the examination, radiation exposure, side effects of contrast agents and anesthesia, the volume of interest and the specific information required have to be considered in addition to the availability of the method. While there is no general answer, a disease concentrated in one organ or one limited region of the body, a situation requiring detailed information about soft tissues, the nervous system, the cardiovascular system, or the bone marrow are often best approached by MRI. On the other hand, a large volume of the body, time and anesthetic restrictions and emergency conditions, such as multiple trauma, the need for information about cortical bone and calcification, or the combination with image-guided intervention favor CT. Malignant disease with a poor prognosis will decrease the weight of radiation exposure; however, with an increasing chance of curative treatment—e.g. in malignant lymphoma—the added risk of many follow-up studies under and after treatment must be considered.

Follow-up CT scans are often performed too early, e.g. at a moment when the biology of the disease does not allow yet any treatment effects to be visible. Justification has to be as restrictive as for the first examination, and alternatives may be adequate to observe known manifestations of disease. Justification as the first step of diagnostic imaging means a close cooperation between the referring doctor and the radiologist since it cannot be done by the clinician alone nor by the radiologist alone. Both need education to adequately perform this important task; it is obvious that sub specialised pediatric radiologists will have a significant advantage of knowledge and experience in the pathology of a child and/or a specific diseased organ.

## 4 Patient Preparation

Patient preparation for CT of adult patients usually means obtaining informed consent, checking the renal function and, for the gastrointestinal tract, instructing the patient about oral bowel contrast application or contrast enema. In children, preparation is usually more complex and is an important prerequisite for a successful examination (Table 3). Older children often want to be considered as individuals whereas in young children the preparation—beyond the patient herself/himself—often involves the physician, the nurse, and the parents. They usually have a better approach to the child and are essential in convincing the child about the need for the examination, in informing about the procedure and its possible discomfort but also in staying with the child during the examination, or in calming by hand contact or conversation. Specially trained staff will put the intravenous line well in advance, will address the children properly, and make them feel comfortable; an environment without machine and noise may meet the child's perceptions of the world and trigger trust. All actions avoiding pain and excitement and, thus, motion artifacts or even repeated scans should be considered to improve the quality of the examination and to control radiation exposure. Depending on the individual, medication, fixation for painless positioning, sedation, anesthetic supervision or general anesthesia may be appropriate. Many specialized centers, ours included, prefer propofol as medication;

**Table 3** Patient preparation for pediatric CT

| | |
|---|---|
| Decrease anxiety | Inform where appropriate<br>Have an accompanying person in room<br>Provide calm neighborhood |
| Avoid pain | Put i.v. line well in advance<br>Immobilize<br>Sedate/anaesthetise/(intubate) |
| Exercise cooperation | In scanner, without radiation, exercise respiration and any specific cooperation expected; under intubation, use hyper-ventilation against pulmonary atelectasis before scanning |
| Put local protection device | Outside scanned volume (thyroid, breast, testes, lenses)<br>Organ protection within scanned volume (lenses, thyroid, breast, testes) |
| Avoid artifacts by external and internal radiodense foreign bodies | If justifiable, position wires/electrodes, cannulas, metallic devices outside the scan plane momentarily |

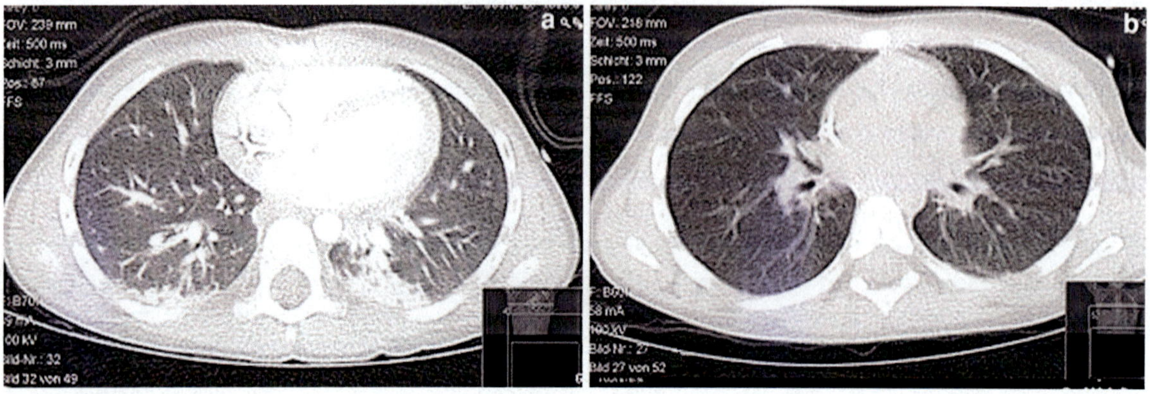


**Fig. 1** Influence of hypoventilation on scan quality in a child of 15 kg. **a** CT scan performed immediately after an MRI examination under general anesthesia. There is lung collapse in the dependent parts of the lung, and focal lung disease cannot be ruled out there. **b** Follow-up examination without previous MRI examination showing full lung inflation

to avoid local pain at the injection site, it has to be preceeded by injection of another local anesthetic drug. General anesthesia, while still used for young, retarded, or handicapped children, is nowadays tolerated well; when imaging the chest, it is wise to hyperventilate the child immediately before the scan in order to avoid lung collapse. Similarly, it is not advisable to plan a CT scan after an MRI examination in general anesthesia (Fig. 1). General anesthesia can more and more be avoided thanks to the speed of modern scanners. Exercising the cooperation and respiratory apnea within the scanner but without radiation is a useful, risk-free procedure to avoid repeated scans. Apnea can mostly be achieved at the age of 5–7 years, and elder children can even cooperate with inspiratory apnea. Below 5 years it is often wise to accept superficial continuous respiration. The test before the use of radiation will allow for an individual adaptation of these age limits. And even in the same patient, depending on the mood and the atmosphere, cooperation may be possible one time and no longer be achieved the next time.

Local superficial protective absorbing devices deserve special mention. They are available for the lenses of the eyes, the thyroid gland, the breast glands, the testes, and they are an efficient shield against external scatter radiation when the organ is outside the scanned area of the body (Beaconsfield et al. 1998; Brnic et al. 2003; Hidajat et al. 1996; Hohl et al. 2005; Price et al. 1999); of course, internal scatter will hardly be affected. Protecting organs located superficially within the area scanned is an alternative approach and must be used carefully since it might cause artifacts and lower the diagnostic quality (Fricke et al. 2003); Hopper et al. 1997). In our own experience, breast protection in adult women has not been as effective as suggested initially by Hopper. The group of Fricke has reported better success in girls, keeping the absorbing material at a distance of around 2–3 cm from the skin by interposing a layer of foam, thus avoiding severe degradation of image quality. Testicular capsules are highly appropriate in shielding from indirect and direct exposure, and usually important information is not lost at the level of the testes. In contrast, the deep location of the ovaries basically excludes any local protection by an absorbing material.

Finally, it is worthwhile to take *radiodense foreign bodies* out of the scanning plane whenever this is possible. Often, major artifacts can be avoided by just choosing the ideal position of the device. Since scanning takes only a few seconds, one may be able to drop the ECG wires just during the scan. Of course, this decision has to be taken together with the clinician or the anesthesiologist.

## 5 Principles of Pediatric Protocol Definition

### 5.1 Accept Noise as Long as the Scan is Diagnostic

A referring doctor as well as a radiologist basically wants the best for the patient. Since images at higher dose look nicer than those obtained at low dose,

**Table 4** Protocol definition for dose reduction in CT of children

| | |
|---|---|
| 1 | Accept noise as long as the scan is diagnostic for the specific clinical question |
| | Realise that in digital X ray imaging noise reduction requires higher exposure<br>Reduce mAs (and possibly kV)<br>Reconstruct additional thick noise-reduced slices without increase of exposure<br>Use iterative reconstruction to keep noise tolerable at even lower exposure |
| 2 | Optimise scan parameters within the axial plane for your specific child |
| | Center the child to the very center of the gantry to avoid asymmetrical exposure<br>Use posteroanterior rather than anteroposterior localizer (scout) view at low kV<br>Increase tube filtration (if available)<br>Use maximal slice thickness appropriate for specific diagnosis (often done by scanning thin sections but analyzing thicker ones)<br>Decrease kVp for thin objects and for CT angiography<br>Use shortest rotation time available (only few exceptions in children)<br>Decrease baseline mA (CTDI) according to body diameter and composition<br>Use xy-plane dose modulation to minimize CTDI |
| 3 | Optimize scan parameters for volume coverage in your specific child |
| | Use representative volume sample when entire volume is not needed (by sequential scans with gaps) to reduce DLP<br>Use spiral scan with pitch > 1 (e.g. 1.5) to reduce DLP<br>Use thicker collimation with overlapping reconstruction when thin slices are not needed<br>Use z-axis dose modulation to decrease DLP<br>Use noise-defined 3D automatic exposure control |
| 4 | Scan minimal length |
| | Be restrictive in defining uppermost and lowermost limits to keep DLP low<br>Use localizing projection scan extending just minimally beyond scan limits |
| 5 | Minimize repeated scanning of identical area |
| | Avoid major overlap when scanning adjacent areas with different protocols<br>Avoid non-enhanced scans unless specifically justified (e.g. for densitometry)<br>Optimize the protocol to obtain all the information requested during one scan (e.g. contiguous 5 mm images and 1 mm HRCT images every 10 mm)<br>Minimize number of scans in multiphase scanning to decrease DLP<br>In case of multiphase scanning, use shorter scan length for additional scans<br>Use lower CTDI for non-enhanced or repeat scans unless high quality is needed<br>Use minimal number of additional sequential functional scans to keep DLP low<br>Minimize length of scans and fluoroscopy time in interventional applications<br>Replace test bolus/bolus triggering by standard scan delay unless timing is very critical |

equalling a nice and good one tends to prefer the beautiful higher dose images. This mechanism has favored higher dose practice over many years. Nowadays, radiologists and clinicians have to realize that *image quality cannot be the only criterion* when biological facts tell us that ionizing radiation may indeed induce cancer at a dose very close to the dose of one CT scan (in around 1‰ of small children). Unfortunately, it is not easy to balance an actual medical need with a rare statistical (stochastic) risk evident only within decades. Since we cannot easily quantify the risk, we should at least try to diminish it. Bringing the dose down to 50% mostly will not affect the diagnosis although the images will be slightly inhomogeneous. Often—of course depending on the organ and the medical question—a greater dose reduction will be tolerable. It is the radiologist's important task to go to the limits, i.e. to accept as much noise as the specific medical task allows for (Ravenel et al. 2001; Cody et al. 2004; Shah et al. 2005; Vock 2005). The practical ways of simultaneously achieving dose reduction and *controlling the noise level* will be discussed under points 2 and 3 (Table 4). The acceptable noise level can be defined by guidelines on the *quality criteria* for specific medical imaging tasks, as initiated by the European Commission (European Commission 2000). Whether post-processing using noise-reducing filters can be used in this situation without loss of sensitivity, is still an open question (Kalra et al. 2004).

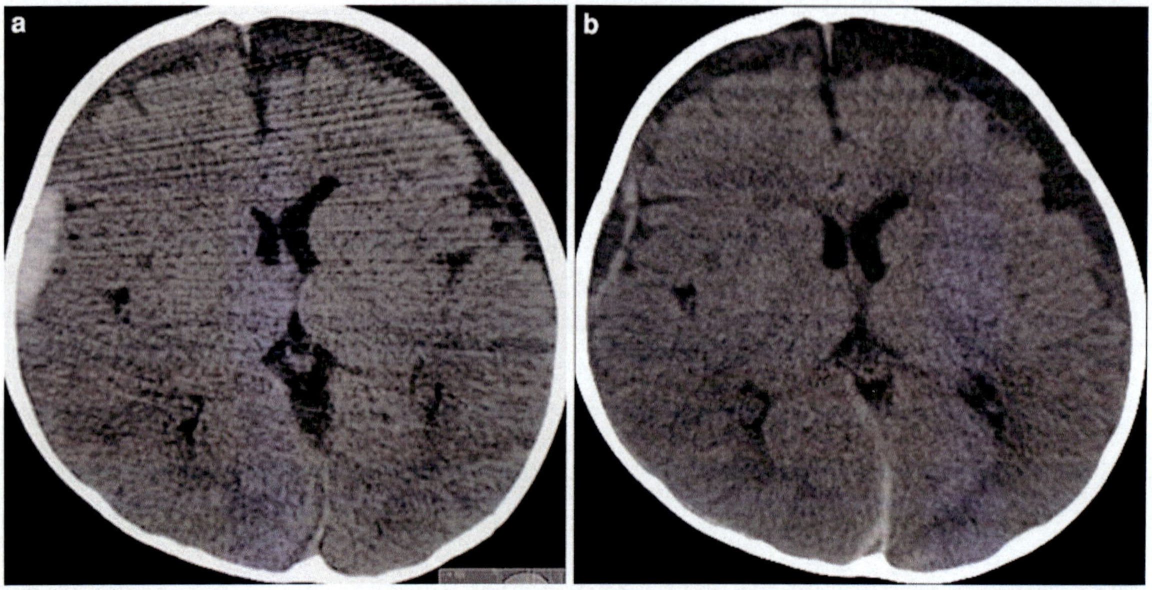


**Fig. 2** Influence of decreasing the voltage on the quality of a brain CT in a 1-year-old child with subdural hematomas of variable age. **a** Scan at 120 kV, 250 mAs, $CTDI_{Vol}$ of 45 mGy, DLP of 688 mGy cm, estimated effective dose of 4.8 mSv. **b** Scan 2 days later at 100 kV, 330 mAs, $CTDI_{Vol}$ of 43 mGy, DLP of 613 mGy cm, estimated effective dose of 4.3 mSv. Note the markedly improved contrast in this follow-up scan despite a slightly lower effective dose

There is another way of reducing the dose and still maintaining the signal-to-noise ratio (SNR) by post-processing: with modern scanners, while one usually does not want to lose z-axis resolution by prospectively scanning thicker slices, one can easily *acquire noisy thin slices* of 0.5–1.5 mm but simultaneously reconstruct *thicker images* of 2–6 mm, *used primarily for interpretation*. The thicker images have a better SNR; the thin images still are used to look at critical details and to get 2D reformation and 3D analysis.

Despite the lack of widespread pediatric experience, *iterative reconstruction* very likely will become the routine technique of image reconstruction (Vorona et al. 2011; Miéville et al. 2011). While it might be used to improve image quality at constant radiation exposure, more likely it will serve to obtain low-dose CT protocols in children at a constant acceptable noise level.

## 5.2 Optimize Scan Parameters within the Axial Plane

Prior to optimizing scan parameters the child has to be positioned carefully in the center of the aperture which really is needed for a symmetrical dose distribution without peaks, especially with beam shaping filters (see Sect. 2).

Also, it has been suggested to use the *posteroanterior projection* for the *scan projection radiograph* (localizer radiograph, scout view, or topogram or surview) in order to minimize exposure to the lenses, the thyroid, and the breast glands. At the time of writing of this manuscript, there are some unpublished reports that acquisition of PA projection radiograph increases radiation dose with AEC techniques compared to AP radiograph-based AEC (personal communication: Mannudeep Kalra, MD, Massachusetts General Hospital). Therefore, we recommend users to exercise caution when switching to PA projection radiograph instead of AP projection radiograph when using longitudinal or combined modulation type of AEC. Radiation dose increment with AEC based on PA projection radiograph alone may be higher than minimal dose savings with acquisition of PA projection over AP projection radiograph.

Different scanners have different geometry, tube filtration, and slightly differing efficiencies of the detectors and the data acquisition system, factors that usually cannot be influenced by the radiologist or technician. It is likely that the market competition will minimize these differences within the next few years.

**Table 5** Suggested pediatric CT protocols (64 rows, 0.6 mm detector width, 1.5 mm + 5 mm slice thickness)

| Age (y) | Newborn | 1 y | 5 y | 10 y | 15 y | Small adult | Medium adult | Large adult |
|---|---|---|---|---|---|---|---|---|
| Weight (kg) | 3–4 | 7 | 20 | 30 | 55 | 65 | 75 | 100 |
| PA Thickness (cm) | 9 | 12 | 14 | 16 | 19 | 22 | 25 | 31 |
| Chest | | | | | | | | |
| *Author's preference* | | | | | | | | |
| kVp | 100(80*) | 100(80*) | 100(80*) | 100(80*) | 100(80*) | 100(80*) | 120(100*) | 120(120*) |
| mAs | 30 | 30 | 40 | 40 | 50 | 70 | 70 | 90 |
| $CTDI_{vol}$ | 1.18(.54) | 1.18(.54) | 1.57(.72) | 1.57(.72) | 1.96(.90) | 2.75(1.26) | 4.74(2.75) | 6.08(6.08) |
| *EK Fishman* | | | | | | | | |
| kVp | 120 | 120 | 120 | 120 | 120 | 120 | 120 | |
| mAs | 17 | 17 | 30 | 40 | 90 | 130 | 170 | |
| *Image Gently* | | | | | | | | |
| kVp | B | B | B | B | B | B | B | B |
| mAs | 0.42a | 0.49a | 0.57a | 0.64a | 0.73a | 0.82a | 0.91a | 1–16a |
| Abdomen | | | | | | | | |
| *Author's preference* | | | | | | | | |
| kVp | 100 | 100 | 100 | 100 | 100 | 100 | 120 | 120(-140) |
| mAs | 40 | 45 | 50 | 55 | 75 | 100 | 90 | 110 |
| $CTDI_{vol}$ | 1.57 | 1.77 | 1.97 | 2.16 | 2.95 | 3.93 | 6.08 | 7.43(11.55) |
| *EK Fishman* | | | | | | | | |
| kVp | 120 | 120 | 120 | 120 | 120 | 120 | 120 | |
| mAs | 30 | 40 | 60 | 75 | 130 | 180 | 276 | |
| *Image Gently* | | | | | | | | |
| kVp | B | B | B | B | B | B | Base B | B |
| mAs | 0.43a | 0.51a | 0.59a | 0.66a | 0.76a | 0.90a | a | 1.27a |

* 80 kV: for vascular malformation, bronchial tree
Author's preference: values used for Siemens Somatom Sensation Cardiac, 64 row-detector
Fishman (2011)
Image Gently (2007): based on optimized medium adult abdominal protocol [B kVp, a mAs], tube voltage is kept identical and mAs adapted to the PA thickness of the child for chest and abdomen examinations

It is also probable that *additional filtration* will be available for thin patients, decreasing the range of photon energies and therefore reducing the proportion of low-energy photons absorbed almost completely in the body, similar to the current experience made in radiography and fluoroscopy. On the other side, we are free to choose the kVp, the rotation time, and mA. The kVp value needed goes with the diameter of the patient (Frush et al. 2002), and pediatric protocols provided by the manufacturer may suggest the appropriate kVp, mostly following the arguments discussed under section 1 above. Figure 2 demonstrates that lower tube voltage often allows to improve image quality at the same or a lower dose. The shortest *rotation time* is mostly appropriate in pediatric CT; since with small objects the capacity of the tube and the acquisition system are not critical this serves to minimize motion artifacts. Exceptions requiring slower rotation are the same as in adult patients but should be used restrictively. Defining the *tube current* (*mA*) needed is clearly the most critical and difficult choice. Again, general physical rules apply, and—often scanner-specific—protocols for different regions and ages have been proposed (Table 5). Figure 3 illustrates the significant impact of a combined application of reduction of both kV and

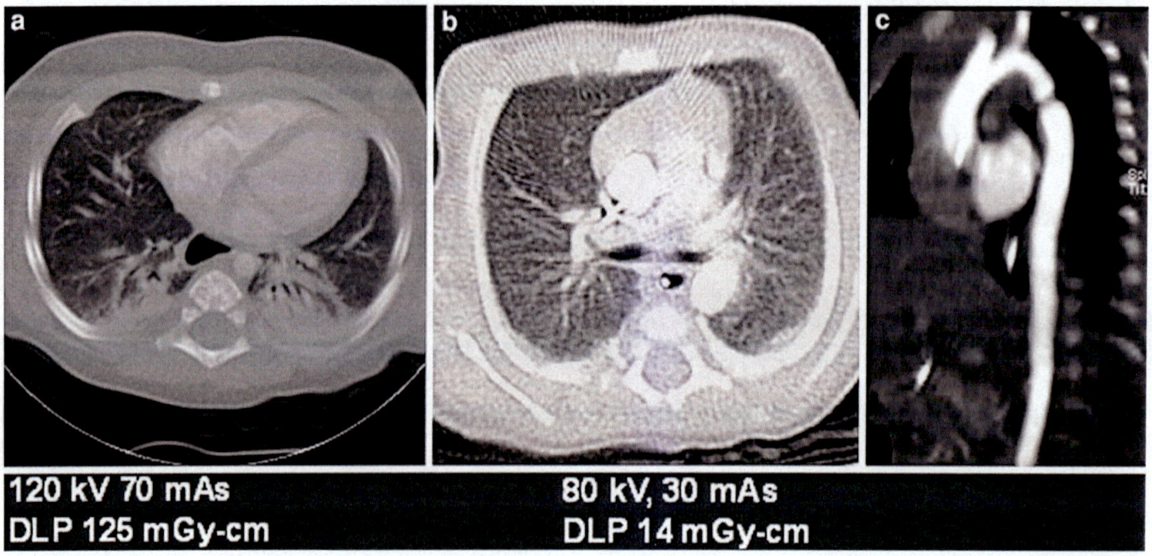


**Fig. 3** Two newborn babies showing the impact of kV and mAs on quality and on radiation exposure. **a** 120 kV, 70 mAs, DLP 125 mGy cm, estimated effective dose 4.8 mSv. **b** 80 kV, 30 mAs, DLP 14 mGy cm, estimated effective dose 0.5 mSv. **c** reformation from scan in **b**, showing aortic coarctation. While noise in the lung is much higher at **b** than at **a**, the radiation exposure has been decreased by roughly 90% without compromising the vascular diagnosis

mA. In practical work it is important to realize that for every reduction of the patient diameter by 3.5 cm there is roughly 50% less absorption, and the current can be reduced accordingly in children. Furthermore, based on the minimal risk of modern contrast agents, it might be appropriate in children to replace a native scan by a contrast-enhanced scan, using lower mAs in view of the improved contrast. Unfortunately, no standards of *acceptable noise* with a specific reconstruction algorithm needed in different medical indications have yet been described. Definition of the desired noise level will facilitate scan protocol selection in the near future thanks to interactive *dose modulation* mechanisms that are currently used in their first generation; since these options for automatic dose reduction are mostly effective in spiral volumetric scanning they will be discussed below with the approach to volume coverage.

$CTDI_w$, the CTDI weighted for central and peripheral locations, is the entity reflecting the selection of parameters during one rotation, such as used in sequential axial scanning, but also one of the most important parameters in spiral scanning. It is most helpful for comparing the relative exposure by different protocols. However, it is clearly based on a round phantom and neither respects the diameter, the shape nor the composition of the individual patient.

## 5.3 Optimize Scan Parameters for Volume Coverage

The way we scan the volume to be studied is the single most important determinant of radiation exposure in CT protocol definition. The term used to characterize volume exposure is the *dose-length product* (*DLP*), a parameter directly derived from the product of the $CTDI_w$ and the length of the scan. DLP has the same restrictions as $CTDI_w$ of being a physical parameter not adapted to the individual patient body. But DLP and $CTDI_w$ have the important advantage of being measurable and, thus, offered by the scanner at the end of a study or even earlier for prospective planning. Since the literature gives factors to translate average DLP values into effective dose (Chapple et al. 2002; Shrimpton et al. 2005), DLP as the only practical risk parameter must be checked regularly by both the radiologist and the technician; CT doses can therefore be estimated both for the individual patient (Table 6) and for the population (Pages et al. 2003).

Historically, with *sequential CT* contiguous slices were usually measured, giving a more or less homogeneous dose distribution that we define as 100%. To improve z-axis resolution, one had to use some overlap; an overlap of 20% (e.g. slice 5 mm, distance

**Table 6** Size-specific dose estimates (SSDE): conversion factors to adapt CTDI to individual patients

| 32 cm PMMA phantom | Conversion Factor | 16 cm PMMA phantom |
|---|---|---|
| lat + ap [cm] | | lat + ap [cm] |
| 16 | 2.79 | |
| 20 | 2.59 | |
| 24 | 2.41 | |
| 28 | 2.24 | |
| 32 | 2.08 | |
| 36 | 1.94 | |
| 40 | 1.80 | |
| 44 | 1.67 | |
| 48 | 1.56 | |
| 52 | 1.45 | 13.7 |
| 56 | 1.35 | 17.5 |
| 60 | 1.25 | 21.5 |
| 64 | 1.16 | 25.5 |
| 68 | 1.08 | 29 |
| 72 | 1.01 | 32.5 |
| 76 | 0.94 | 36.5 |
| 82 | 0.84 | 42 |
| 86 | 0.78 | 46 |
| 90 | 0.72 | 50 |
| | 0.64 | 56 |
| | 0.57 | 62 |
| | 0.49 | 70 |

Modified and simplified from AAPM Report No. 204 (2011)
This table provides conversion factors based on 32 cm/16 cm diameter PMMA phantoms
lat + ap is the sum of the lateral and the anteroposterior dimensions of the patient, as obtained by physical measurement, from the CT projection radiographs or—retrospectively—from the CT image. This parameter best reflects the effective diameter; the original publication also shows size-specific conversion factors for the lateral dimension and for the anteroposterior dimension
Individual patient's CTDI: $CTDI_{vol[pat]} = CTDI_{vol[phantom]} \times$ conversion factor

between slices 4 mm) increased exposure to 120%. On the other side, for HRCT in diffuse interstitial disease of the lung, scanning a sample of 10% of the organ (1 mm slice, distance between slices 10 mm), as often considered adequate, reduces exposure to 10%. The introduction of *spiral CT scanning* with a *single row of detectors* avoided overlapping scanning, leaving exposure at 100% in the example cited, even when images were reconstructed at smaller distances of 1–4 mm; of course, this was only true with identical parameters and when table movement during one rotation was exactly the value of the slice collimation; this basic condition was defined as a *pitch* of 1 and, in consequence, a movement of twice the collimation was called a pitch of 2. For this type of scanner, it was therefore attractive to increase the pitch in order to reduce radiation exposure (Donnelly et al. 2001), with the only restriction that high pitch values caused a major thickening of the resulting slice above the collimation. Although not important for long z-axis volume scans, spiral scanning means a small additional exposure outside the defined volume during the first and the last rotation of the gantry since data are incomplete and have to be discarded partially.

Current *multi-row detector scanners* have increased the options for protocols enormously but also share a disadvantage in performing the HRCT protocol of the lung and other applications where partial sampling of a volume would be medically adequate. They may have to scan two or four slices instead of the single one needed, and collimation at the detector may cause a loss of signal. Apart from this restriction, however, they are mostly used in the spiral mode and have enhanced the speed and the resolution of CT scanning, avoiding the problem of tube heating and offering real *isotropic data* for 3D analysis. The new scan geometry needs more complex image calculation to correct for the diverging beam of the outer detectors but the operator does not have to take care of this modification. Also, the pitch factor has become less important since the increased speed offers other ways to cover a large volume and still to control exposure; similarly, combining the information about different detector rows for the reconstruction of one image has overcome the problem of slice thickening, as seen with early spiral scanners and higher pitch factors.

The increased power of modern scanners has mostly eliminated hardware restrictions of older generations and made it easy to define protocols with a high radiation exposure, reaching the range of complex angiographic or fluoroscopic studies. This has increased the pressure of using any solution available to reduce radiation exposure. Current CT scanners offer one or several of the following options: **XY-plane dose modulation:** this option was introduced to overcome the physical problem that the human body is neither round nor of homogeneous density (Greess et al. 2004). To achieve the same SNR, less radiation is required in the direction of the smaller diameter (anteroposterior at the level of the shoulders, y-axis) than in the direction of the larger diameter (left to right at the same level, x-axis), and this difference is exaggerated by the presence of more bony mass in the x-axis. Modulation reduces the nominal mAs by around 20–40%, depending on the body region, and it is generally appropriate to use it. Specific new applications of xy-dose modulation are used for the heart and other organs, such as the breast gland. This means prospectively ECG-gated mA modulation with nearly no current during the phases of the heart that are not used for reconstruction and diagnostic mA during important phases, such as the mid-to-late diastoly. A similar approach might be used to decrease the radiation exposure of the breast gland in chest CT of young women by decreasing mA when the tube is located in front and—for compensation—by increasing mA when the tube is in the back of the patient.

**Z-axis dose modulation:** as for the axial plane, physically in the longitudinal axis of the body (z-axis), the radiation needed for an adequate SNR will vary with the diameter and density of the patient. For e.g., in cervicothoracic scanning, the cervical area and the lower chest require much less dose for a given image quality than the thoracic inlet and shoulder area. Similarly, until recently, one had to interrupt scanning at a level between physically different adjacent body areas; e.g., to use a lower radiation exposure for the upper than the lower abdomen one had to stop the upper scan at the pelvic rim and to start another scan with modified parameters for the pelvis, often with a significant technical delay. Modern scanners allow for adapting the tube output during one single scan in this and other clinical applications. The option of z-axis dependent dose modulation is steered again either from the localizing view or interactively; it is clearly welcome to reduce radiation exposure and should be used generally (Tack et al. 2003).

Nowadays dose modulation is often three-dimensional, providing *noise-defined automatic exposure control* (*AEC*) . The solutions implemented in specific scanners may have rules for adaptation not easily understood by the user; one therefore has to be careful not to run into dose augmentation, e.g. by starting the scan at a level with low dose requirement at a nominal mAs value selected for the thickest scan level to be covered. Software tools can simplify the choice, e.g. by offering a selection of images with different noise.

*High-pitch scanning* is another tool contributing to a fast volume coverage at minimal dose; while it requires top-end hardware, it additionally avoids most motion artifacts and is ideal in many children (Han et al. 2011; Miéville et al. 2011).

Control of noise in the image is one approach whereas observation of the DLP per examination is another practical approach: since in CT examinations the DLP is a good representative of effective dose to a specific area of the body, *diagnostic reference levels* (*DRL*) indicating an upper DLP not to be exceeded in typical clinical tasks are the practical solution (Shrimpton and Wall 2000; Wall 2001). DRLs correspond to the third quartile (75% lower values obtained from a population with the same examination). They do not represent an absolute barrier; however, they should be defined for specific body areas, according to the weight and the medical task. Since the DLP is available immediately during the study, each radiologist can prospectively plan the DLP to stay within the specific DRL or, exceptionally and with an appropriate justification, to exceed it for a concrete reason.

## 5.4 Scan Minimal Length

This rule applies both for the scout view and the rotational scan since there is really no value in going beyond the tissue volume where pathology is suspected. It has to be followed at two levels: the referring physician and the radiologist have to find a compromise about the minimal *body areas to be investigated*; the radiologist and the technician have to fine-tune the *upper and lower ends of the examination* (Donnelly et al. 2001). In a lung scan, there is no reason to include the entire thoracic inlet with the thyroid gland as well as the upper half of the abdomen with multiple radiosensitive organs (Campbell et al. 2005). In a pelvic scan of a boy, there is hardly ever a medical reason to include the testes. Independent of the organs included, any increase in scan length will proportionally increase energy deposition and the biological effects of ionising radiation. While other rules are the primary responsibility of the radiologist, the technician and her/his experience are most critical for this rule. In routine scanning, it is simply not justified to extend the length beyond the minimum required. For e.g., a chest scan has to cover the lowest part of the costophrenic sulcus and—in neoplastic disease—the adrenal glands; any inclusion of more abdominal structures will induce non-justified radiation exposure to sensitive organs.

For two reasons, the rule should be used less strictly for the localizing than for the sectional scan. First, radiation exposure—although often neglected in dose estimation—is small during a localizing projectional view, usually contributing a very low percentage to the global exposure. Second, the localizer has to include the starting and ending levels of the spiral scan and is a prerequisite for properly limiting the scan length to the minimum needed in the specific medical situation.

## 5.5 Avoid Non-Justified Multiple Scans of the Same Area

Numerous opportunities exist with the current powerful scanners to scan the same volume of the body twice or even several times. Since there is no longer a technical restriction, multiphase studies can be performed without tube heating or data overflow.

Perhaps the most frequent neglection of this rule happens when two adjacent body areas are scanned with different protocols and a large overlap. The obvious example for this may be cervicothoracic scanning in malignant lymphoma; while the head and neck scan is planned on a lateral localiser, the scan of the trunk is planned on an anteroposterior localizer, and large overlaps at the thoracic inlet often cause multiple scanning of sensitive organs, such as the thyroid gland.

A number of *medical reasons* may require different types of repeat scans of the same area:

- Correct timing of scans, using a test bolus or repetitive scanning of one plane at low dose for bolus triggering of the proper diagnostic scan,
- dynamic enhancement studies including arterial, parenchymal, venous and/or excretion phases of organs, such as the kidney or liver [urinary excretion may often be checked by a simple low-dose ap radiograph or localizer instead of a repeated CT scan],
- functional lung scans to detect air trapping in inspiration and expiration; in young children unable to cooperate this may also be achieved by scanning in right and left lateral decubitus position with the dependent lung in expiration and the non-dependent lung in inspiration,
- supine and prone scans for demonstrating positional gravitational effects,
- CT-guided intervention, with or without fluoroscopy,
- screening with thick slices and subsequent detailed analysis with thin slices,
- exceptionally in childhood: native and contrast-enhanced scan after intravenous bolus injection.

Some but by far not all of these technical possibilities are justified in medical problem solving, and it is probably the most difficult task of the resident in radiology to think of all these potential options but not to overuse them in view of radiation exposure. For e.g., renal CT may often be adequately performed with a single scan after a two-phasic injection of the contrast agent, showing both the parenchyma and the pelvicalyceal systems. It is quite clear that *double scanning* means *twice the radiation exposure* as long as the same parameters are used, and even more scans will increase exposure proportionally. Apart from medical experience, a few general guidelines may help to appropriately select the number of scans. First of all and again, the individual *situation of the current patient* must be checked: will any of the repeat scans help this patient? Will it influence the management or even the outcome? Is it cost-efficient when we add radiation exposure to the financial cost? Second, *repeat scans* can often be *limited to a smaller volume* or performed at *lower dose* that will not hide the additional information expected. Third, fixed standard scan timing can often replace individual triggering or test bolus unless cardiovascular disease is present and timing is very critical. Fourth, while CT fluoroscopy is a very helpful tool in case of a difficult access, other biopsies or drainages can often be done under CT image control or even under ultrasound guidance. Fifth, in the lung one single scan can usually be used to obtain all the information needed: using thin detector rows of around 1 mm will allow to calculate both thin HRCT sections at any z-axis level and thick 5 mm scans, as needed for tumor search or mediastinal analysis; for reformations and 3D post-processing, continuous and overlapping images can be prepared from the same raw data.

## 5.6 Specific Protocols

Be aware that specific parameters often depend on the specific scanner used. This is why the Society of Pediatric Radiology and the *Image Gently* (Image gently 2007) campaign suggest an approach of first optimizing adult abdomen and head CT protocols, using all tools and arguments discussed above and consulting a qualified medical physicist experienced in diagnostic radiology. Due to the greater volume of adult scans, it is easier to optimize adult protocols first. The second step then is to modify the adult protocol according to the individual child's pa diameter or age, leaving the kVp and the pitch unchanged as all other parameters except for the mAs (Table 5) (Image gently 2007). For e.g., for a thoracic/abdominal scan, the correction factor will be 0.42/0.43 for newborns, 0.57/0.59 at the age of 5 years, and 0.73/0.76 at 15 years respectively. For head examinations, the factor will increase from 0.74 at birth to 0.93 at 5 years and soon reach adult values. *AAPM Report No. 204* has worked on size-specific dose estimates (SSDE) and, based on different phantom measurements and Montecarlo simulations, has brought this approach to perfection: simple patient diameters serve to find the individual $CTDI_{vol}$ conversion factor (Table 6) that covers important tube voltages and different CT brands (AAPM Report No. 204, 2011).

This approach becomes less useful if one wants to change the tube voltage, the pitch or the slice collimation. When scanning children, we often decrease the tube tension from 120 kV to 100 kV, in specific situations even to 80 kV (Table 5). Indeed, protocols have to be adapted to the scanner (manufacturer, number of rows, scanner functions) which is well illustrated by Fishman on his web site (Fishman 2011); some of his typical and frequently used protocols are also shown in Table 5. For the head, Fishman suggests 120 kV and 90/150/220 mAs at the ages of <6 months/6 months–3 years/3–6 years respectively (Fishman 2011). Special indications, such as the temporal bone, again can be done at much lower kV and mAs (Nauer et al. 2011).

## 5.7 Estimation of Effective Dose

Effective dose is a global surrogate of the stochastic risk due to ionizing radiation, primarily created for epidemiologic population purposes. It is a mathematical value obtained by integrating the products of organ doses and the respective organ weighting factors, as defined by the International Commission on Radiological Protection. An approximate estimation based on the DLP has been suggested by several authors (Table 7). However, it should be kept in mind that the effective dose does not intend to reflect the individual risk and, thus, should not be used to assess the individual probability of cancer induction by CT.

**Table 7** Effective dose estimated from dose-length product

| Age | Head | Neck | Chest | Abdomen/pelvis |
|---|---|---|---|---|
| 0 year | .011/.027 | .017/- | .039/.034 | .049/.040 |
| 1 year | .007/.008 | .012/- | .026/.021 | .030/.024 |
| 5 year | .004/.004 | .011/- | .018/.014 | .020/.016 |
| 10 year | .003/.003 | .008/- | .013/.011 | .015/.014 |
| 15 year | | | -/.015 | .015/.009 |
| Adult | .002/.003 | .006/- | .014/.009 | .015/- |

Numbers give normalized effective dose per dose-length product (mSv per mGy cm)
First number from Shrimpton et al. (2005)/second number from Chapple et al. (2002)

In conclusion, CT is characterized by a significantly higher radiation exposure than radiography. Based on its excellent diagnostic potential in a range of medical situations its use has significantly increased in children. However, due to the increased biologic impact of radiation exposure in children, pediatric CT examinations should follow a strict justification and optimization by careful selection of protocol parameters as well as the range. Patient preparation becomes as important as optimization of parameters in pediatric CT. The steps discussed above help the radiologist to apply the "as low as reasonably achievable" (ALARA) principle when scanning children (Slovis 2003).

**Acknowledgments** The authors thank Barbara Le Blanc for typing the manuscript and Mannudeep Kalra for contributing important suggestions on protocol definition.

## References

AAPM Report No. 204 (2011) Size-specific dose estimates (SSDE) in pediatric and adult body CT examinations. American Association of Physicists in Medicine, ISBN: 978-1-936366-08-8. http://www.aapm.org/pubs/reports/ RPT_204.pdf Accessed 12 December 2011

American College of Radiology (2011) ACR appropriateness criteria, diagnostic imaging topics. http://www.acr.org/SecondaryMainMenuCategories/quality_safety/app_criteria.aspx. Accessed 15 November 2011

Beaconsfield T, Nicholson R, Thornton A, Al-Kutoubi A (1998) Would thyroid and breast shielding be beneficial in CT of the head? Eur Radiol 8:664–667

Boone JM, Geraghty EM, Seibert JA, Wootton-Gorges SL (2003) Dose reduction in pediatric CT: a rational approach. Radiology 228:352–360

Brenner DJ (2002) Estimating cancer risks from pediatric CT: going from the qualitative to the quantitative. Pediatr Radiol 32:228–231

Brenner DJ, Elliston CD, Hall EJ, Berdon WE (2001) Estimated risks of radiation—induced fatal cancer from pediatric CT. AJR Am J Roentgenol 176:289–296

Brenner DJ, Doll R, Goodhead DT, Hall EJ, Land CE, Little JB, Lubin JH, Preston DL, Preston RJ, Puskin JS, Ron E, Sachs RK, Samet JM, Setlow RB, Zaider M (2003) Cancer risks attributable to low doses of ionizing radiation: assessing what we really know. Proc Natl Acad Sci U S A 100:13761–13766

Brnic Z, Vekic B, Hebrang A, Anic P (2003) Efficacy of breast shielding during CT of the head. Eur Radiol 13:2436–2440

Campbell J, Kaira MK, Rizzo S, Maher MM, Shepard JA (2005) Scanning beyond anatomic limits of the thorax in chest CT: findings, radiation dose, and automatic tube current modulation. J Roentgenol AJR 185:1525–1530

Chapple CL, Willis S, Frame J (2002) Effective dose in paediatric computed tomography. Phys Med Biol 47:107–115

Cody DD, Moxley DM, Krugh KT, O'Daniel JC, Wagner LK, Eftekhari F (2004) Strategies for formulating appropriate MDCT techniques when imaging the chest, abdomen, and pelvis in pediatric patients. Am J Roentgenol AJR 182: 849–859

Donnelly LF, Emery KH, Brody AS, Laor T, Gylys-Morin VM, Anton GA, Thomas SR, Frush DP (2001) Minimizing radiation dose for pediatric body applications of single-detector helical CT: strategies at a large children's hospital. AJR Am J Roentgenol 176:303–306

European Commission (2000) European guidelines on quality criteria for computed tomography, EUR 16262EN. Office for Official Publications of the European Communities, Luxembourg. www.drs.dk/guidelines/ct/quality/index.htm. Accessed 15 Nov 2011

Fishman EK (2011) CTisus, Pediatric protocols. http://www.ctisus.org/protocols/pediatric Accessed 15 November 2011

Fricke BL, Donnelly LF, Frush DP, Yoshizumi T, Varchena V, Poe SA, Lucaya J (2003) In-plane bismuth breast shields for pediatric CT: effects on radiation dose and image quality using experimental and clinical data. Am J Roentgenol AJR 180:407–411

Frush DP, Soden B, Frush KS, Lowry C (2002) Improved pediatric multidetector CT using a size-based color-coded format. AJR Am J Roentgenol 178:721–726

Frush DP, Donnelly LF, Rosen NS (2003) Computed tomography and radiation risks: what pediatric health care providers should know. Pediatrics 112:951–957

Greess H, Lutze J, Nömayr A, Wolf H, Hothorn T, Kalender WA, Bautz W (2004) Dose reduction in subsecond multislice spiral CT examination of children by online tube current modulation. Eur Radiol 14:995–999

Han BK, Lindberg J, Grant K, Schwartz RS, Lesser JR (2011) Accuracy and safety of high pitch computed tomography imaging in young children with complex congenital heart disease. Am J Cardiol 107:1541–1546

Hidajat N, Schroder RJ, Vogl T, Schedel H, Felix R (1996) The efficacy of lead shielding in patient dosage reduction in computed tomography (German). Rofo 165:462–465

Hohl C, Mahnken AH, Klotz E, Das M, Stargardt A, Mühlenbruch G, Schmidt T, Günther RW, Wildberger JE (2005) Radiation dose reduction to the male gonads during MDCT: the effectiveness of a lead shield. Am J Roentgenol AJR 184:128–130

Hopper KD, King SH, Lobell ME, TenHave TR, Weyver JS (1997) Rhe breast: in-plane X-ray protection during diagnostic thoracic CT—shielding with bismuth radioprotective garments. Radiology 205:853–858

Huda W (2002) Effective dose to adult and pediatric patients. Pediatr Radiol 32:272–279

Huda W, Scalzetti EM, Levin G (2000) Technique factors and image quality as functions of patient weight at abdominal CT. Radiology 217:430–435

Image gently (2007) The alliance for radiation safety in pediatric imaging. Pediatric CT Protocol Guidance. http://www.pedrad.org/associations/5364/ig/?page=598. Accessed 15 Nov 2011

Kalra MK, Maher MM, Blake MA, Lucey BC, Karau K, Toth TL, Gopal A, Halpern EF, Saini S (2004) Detection and characterization of lesions on low-radition-dose abdominal CT images postprocessed with noise reduction filters. Radiology 232:791–797

Lell MM, May M, Deak P, Alibek S, Kuefner M, Kuettner A, Köhler H, Achenbach S, Uder M, Radkow T (2011) High-pitch spiral computed tomography: effect on image quality and radiation does in pediatric chest computed tomography. Invest Radiol 46:116–123

Mettler FA, Wiest PW, Locken JA, Kelsey CA (2000) CT scanning: patterns of use and dose. J Radiol Prot 20:353–359

Miéville FA, Gudinchet F, Rizzo E, Ou P, Brunelle F, Bochud FO, Verdun FR (2011) Paediatric cardiac CT examinations: impact of the iterative reconstruction method ASIR on image quality—preliminary findings. Pediatr Radiol 41: 1154–1164

Nauer CB, Rieke A, Zubler C, Candreia C, Arnold A, Senn P (2011) Low-dose temporal bone CT in infants and young children: effective dose and image quality. AJNR Am J Neuroradiol 32(8):1375–1380

Nickoloff E (2002) Current adult and pediatric CT doses. Pediatr Radiol 32:250–260

Nickoloff EL, Alderson PO (2001) Radiation exposures to patients from CT. Reality, public perception, and policy. AJR Am J Roentgenol 177:285–287

Oman JA, Cooper RJ, Holmes JF, Viccellio P, Nyce A, Ross SE et al (2006) for the NEXUS II investigators, Performance of a decision rule to predict need for Computed tomography among children with blunt head trauma. Pediatrics 117: 238–246

Pages J, Buls N, Osteaux M (2003) CT doses in children: a multicentre study. Brit J Radiol 76:803–811

Paterson A, Frush DP, Donnelly LF (2001) Helical CT of the body: are settings adjusted for pediatric patients? AJR 176: 297–301

Pierce DA, Preston DL (2000) Radiation-related cancer risks at low doses among atomic bomb survivors. Radiat Res 154: 178–186

Price R, Halson P, Sampson M (1999) Dose reduction during CT scanning in an anthropomorphic phantom by the use of a male gonad shield. Br J Radiol 72:489–494

Ravenel JG, Scalzetti EM, Huda W, Garrisi W (2001) Radiation exposure and image quality in chest CT examinations. AJR 177:279–284

RCR Referral guidelines (2007) Making the best use of clinical radiology, 7th edn. MBUR7. http://www.rcr.ac.uk/content.aspx?PageID=995. 15 Nov 2011

Shah R, Gupta AK, Rehani MM, Pandey AK, Mukhopadhyay S (2005) Effect of reduction in tube current on reader confidence in paediatric computed tomography. Clin Radiol 60:224–231

Shrimpton PC, Wall BF (2000) Reference doses for paediatric computed tomography. Radiat Prot Dosim 90:249–252

Shrimpton PC, Hillier MC, Lewis MA, Dunn M (2005) Doses from computed tomography (CT) examinations in the UK—2003 review. UK Health protection agency, NRPB-W67

Slovis TL (2002) The ALARA (as low as reasonably achievable) concept in pediatric CT intelligent dose reduction, ALARA conference proceedings. Pediatr Radiol 32:219–220

Slovis TL (2003) Children, computed tomography radiation dose, and the As low as reasonably achievable (ALARA) concept. Pediatrics 112:971–972

Tack D, De Maertelaer V, Gevenois PA (2003) Dose reduction in multidetector CT using attenuation-based online tube current modulation. Am J Roentgenol AJR 181:331–334

Vock P (2002) CT radiation exposure in children: consequences of the American discussion for Europe (German). Radiologe 42:697–702

Vock P (2005) CT dose reduction in children. Eur Radiol 15:2330–2340

Vorona GA, Ceschin RC, Clayton BL, Sutcavage T, Tadros SS, Panigrahy A (2011) Reducing abdominal CT radiation dose with the adaptive statistical iterative reconstruction technique in children: a feasibility study. Pediatr Radiol 41: 1174–1182

Wall BF (2001) Diagnostic reference levels—the way forward, commentary. Brit J Radiol 74:785–788

# CT Scanning in Pregnancy

D. E. Litmanovich and A. A. Bankier

## Contents




### Abstract

CT evaluation of pregnant patients with medical conditions not related to pregnancy is a valuable and reliable tool, but poses a recurring dilemma on the other hand due to radiation exposure concern for both mother and fetus. Maternal exposure is substantial including the exposure of breast tissue, highly sensitive during radiation, with a potential to increase relative risk for breast cancer over lifetime. Fetal exposure may theoretically lead to congenital malformations, and despite no known risks for development of congenital malformations or mental retardation in a fetus exposed to ionizing radiation at the MDCT levels typically used for diagnostic imaging, there is still a theoretical risk of carcinogenesis. An understanding of fetal and maternal effects of ionizing radiation by different CT protocols at different stages of gestation is essential for proper administration of the CT examinations in patients with non-obstetric conditions. Understanding of basic principles of maternal and fetal dosimetry is also essential for quality assurance. The approach to the informed consent and administration of iodinated intravenous contrast are also essential and discussed in this chapter. Available MDCT protocols and effective methods for radiation dose reduction are discussed for specific clinical conditions such as: pulmonary embolism, acute appendicitis, urolithiasis, and trauma.



D. E. Litmanovich (✉) · A. A. Bankier
Department of Radiology,
Beth Israel Deaconess Medical Center,
330 Brookline Ave, Boston, MA 02215, USA
e-mail: dlitmano@bidmc.harvard.edu


D. Tack et al. (eds.), *Radiation Dose from Multidetector CT*, Medical Radiology. Diagnostic Imaging,
DOI: 10.1007/174_2011_521, 

# 1 Introduction

Imaging of pregnant patients presents an exceptional challenge to radiologists and clinicians due to an array of unique aspects seen in pregnancy. The main challenge is the "2 in 1" imaging, i.e., the simultaneous imaging of mother and fetus, as imaging techniques optimal for the mother may be harmful for the fetus and vice versa. At the same time, physiologic changes during pregnancy such as increased plasma volume, cardiac output, and heart rate, in conjunction with Virchow's triad (hypercoagulability, venous stasis and vascular damage), create altered hemodynamics (Toglia and Weg 1996).

Heightened general awareness of diagnostic imaging radiation exposure (caused by dramatic increase in CT utilization in the last decade) mainly addresses the relationship between radiation exposure and the associated lifetime attributable risk of cancer in the general population (Smith-Bindman et al. 2009; Brenner and Hall 2007). Several publications have addressed specific concerns related to radiation of young females, citing an increase in cancer risk of up to 0.8% for a 20 y/o woman undergoing chest CTA and potential increase in relative risk for breast cancer of up to 4.2% per single cardiothoracic CTA (Smith-Bindman et al. 2009; Hurwitz et al. 2007). Unfortunately, there is a lower than desirable level of awareness of radiation risk aspects associated with imaging during pregnancy in both the radiology and non-radiology communities (Patel et al. 2007; Groves et al. 2006; Ratnapalan et al. 2004; Wieseler et al. 2010; El-Khoury et al. 2003; Lazarus et al. 2009).

With the general concern for CT radiation exposure on one side and increasing imaging of pregnant patients for non-obstetric conditions on the other, this chapter covers the need for evidence-based imaging guidelines that address the following main issues: risk of CT radiation exposure to the mother, risk of direct and indirect CT radiation exposure to the fetus, approach to CT imaging of pregnant patients in typical clinical scenarios, and the currently available options for CT radiation dose reduction. Certain aspects such as safety of iodinated contrast administration and the importance of informed consent will be discussed as well.

## 1.1 Radiation Exposure

While addressing radiation exposure in pregnant patients, its crucial to acknowledge that two patients are exposed at the same time: mother and fetus, and the intensity of the exposure, as well as potential consequences vary substantially between the two.

### 1.1.1 Fetal Radiation Exposure

Fetal radiation is of concern because of stochastic and deterministic (non-stochastic) effects.

*Stochastic effect* is a result of ionizing radiation producing cellular damage via chemical and/or physical processes. Those processes can lead to nuclear DNA changes resulting in genetic mutations or carcinogenesis. The linear or no threshold approach to stochastic effect postulates that it may occur with any amount of radiation exposure and its severity is independent of the radiation dose (Protection ICoR 2000, 2003; American College of Radiology 2008). It has been based on probability calculations that exposure of 50 mGy (5 rad) is required for doubling of baseline risk of childhood carcinogenesis from 0.1 to 0.2% (Protection ICoR 2000). Despite recent wide use of CT scanning, no documented radiation effect has been reported at this level.

In 2008 The American College of Radiology published practice guidelines for imaging pregnant patients including estimated fetal risk based on gestational age and magnitude of radiation exposure (Table 1) (American College of Radiology 2008). These estimates are based on extrapolation from animal studies, atomic bomb survivors' epidemiologic studies, and studies of groups exposed to medical radiation (Lee and Chew 2009). All the estimated risks are unlikely at exposure levels less than 100 mGy (10 rad) (American College of Radiology 2008)

*Non-stochastic (deterministic) effect also known as teratogenesis* or the threshold effect is caused by radiation at higher doses. The effects are predictable and a result of physical and/or chemical processes leading to either cellular death resulting in morphologic changes, or changes in nuclear DNA leading to carcinogenesis, chromosomal aberrations and genetic mutations. Presence of a threshold following linear progression is the main difference compared to the stochastic effect, increasing in frequency and severity with the increase of the exposure dose (Brent 2009). The threshold for considerable deterministic effect is

**Table 1** Summary of potential deterministic effects on the embryo and fetus from radiation exposure (modified from American College of Radiology 2008)

| Gestational age (weeks) | | | |
|---|---|---|---|
| Potential effect of radiation exposure | | | |
| | <50 mGy | 50–100 mGy | >100 mGy |
| 0–2 (before implantation) | No effect | No effect | No effect |
| 3–4 (organogenesis) | No effect | Probably none | Possible spontaneous abortion |
| 5–10 (organogenesis) | No effect | Uncertain | Possible malformations |
| 11–17 (fetal period) | No effect | Uncertain | Possible IQ deficit or MR |
| 18–27 (fetal period) | No effect | No effect | IQ deficit not detectable at diagnostic doses |
| >27 (fetal period) | No effect | No effect | No effect applicable to diagnostic medicine |

*MR* mental retardation

**Table 2** Potential teratogenesis effects of different amounts of radiation exposure at different stages of pregnancy (modified from Patel et al. 2007)

| Gestational age (weeks) | Potential effect of radiation exposure | Estimated threshold dose (mGy) |
|---|---|---|
| 0–2 | All (death of embryo) or none | 50–100 |
| 3–8 | Congenital multisystem anomalies | 200 |
| | Growth retardation | 200–250 |
| 8–15 | Severe MR (High risk)[a] | 60–310 |
| | IQ deficit | 25 IQ point loss per 1 Gy |
| | Microcephaly | 200 |
| 16–25 | Severe mental retardation (low risk) | 250–280 |

*MR* mental retardation, data based on results of animal studies, epidemiologic studies of atomic bomb survivors, and studies of groups exposed to radiation for medical reasons
[a] Period of rapid neuronal development and migration

considered 150 mGy (15 rad) such that, if reached, might require termination of pregnancy (Martin et al. 1990). Table 2 summarizes the potential effects of different amounts of radiation exposure at different stages of pregnancy, with an emphasis on timing of exposure, in particular for brain-related consequences.

### 1.1.2 Diagnostic Radiation Fetal Exposure

The average direct exposure of the fetus from single or sometimes combined diagnostic studies at all stages of pregnancy is usually substantially less than 50 mGy (Wieseler et al. 2010). Evidently the extent of exposure mainly depends on the character of the exposure: direct such as CT abdomen or pelvis vs. indirect: CT of the head, neck, chest, or extremities.

The dose to the individual conceptus varies with the proximity of the uterus to the anatomic location of the scan plane, the thickness of the patient, the depth of the conceptus, and X-ray technique factors. The conceptus dose can vary by a factor of two to four for a specific examination with a spectrum of values from 0 mGy (CT head) to 34 mGy (CTA of aorta including chest, abdomen, and pelvis). In addition, these values may vary because of the imaging techniques required to produce the desired image quality for each type of examination, the required anatomic coverage, or both (McCollough et al. 2007).

Automated exposure control capabilities that provide real-time X-ray tube current modulation based on tissue attenuation help minimize the radiation dose delivered to a patient with a small body habitus, and hence to the conceptus, by preventing unnecessarily high tube current settings. The radiation dose is increased to ensure adequate image quality in large patients, but substantial amount of the additional X-ray dose is absorbed by the additional adipose tissue with doses to internal organs being increased not in a direct proportion to increases in tube current settings (McCollough et al. 2007). Monte Carlo simulations indicate that an increase of the scanner output by a factor of two in very large patients (weight, approximately 100 kg; lateral thickness, 50 cm or less) results in an increase of only 25% in the effective dose. This is because the effective dose is strongly dependent on the dose delivered to internal organs (McCollough et al. 2007; Schmidt 2001; Schmidt and Kalender 2002). CT projection radiography (scout view) delivers a minimal radiation dose to the conceptus; and the benefits of its use for accurate localization of the CT scan enabling automatic exposure control outweigh the small radiation risk.

#### 1.1.2.1 Direct Fetal Exposure

With 16 slice MDCT scanner, early pregnancy average fetal dose range received from different CT abdomen protocols was from 1.5 to 3.8 mGy (Jaffe et al. 2008) with kVp of 140 and mA ranging from 10 to 380 due to applied dose modulation. With appendix CT protocol (140 kVp, 340 mA) the average dose of 15.2–16.8 mGY at 0 months and 20–40 mGy at 3 months have been shown. Renal stone evaluating protocol (140 kVp, 160 mA) has delivered doses between 8 and 12 mGy and 4 and 7 mGy, respectively (Hurwitz et al. 2006a). Dr. Jaffe and colleagues have also compared different vendors, GE Healthcare VCT 64-MDCT scanner and Siemens Healthcare Scanners, for the radiation dose delivered to the uterus. The measurements, made using both an anthropomorphic female phantom and a metal oxide semiconductor field effect transistor (MOSFET) dosimeter placed in the expected uterine location, as well as the CTDI vol obtained from the scanner console, showed a range of 9–37.7 mGy using 120 and 130 kVp settings (Jaffe et al. 2009). Dr. Angel and colleagues have shown that fetal radiation dose is inversely proportional to patient perimeter (size), to an extent exceeding the correlation with age of the pregnancy (Angel et al. 2008), with average dose from the abdominal CT being 10.8 mGy/100 mAs. Dr. McCollough and colleagues report estimated conceptus doses from single CT acquisition of abdomen and pelvis of 25 mGy (McCollough et al. 2007). Retrospective evaluation of 86 abdomino-pelvic examinations in pregnant patients have demonstrated a calculated average fetal dose of 24.8 mGy (Goldberg-Stein et al. 2011). Thus, even with direct radiation exposure, fetal radiation dose has not been shown to exceed 40 mGy.

With this data in mind, it would be unreasonable to reject, delay, or substitute a necessary CT scan due to concern for fetal radiation exposure.

#### 1.1.2.2 Indirect Fetal Exposure

The scale of indirect radiation exposure such as CT head, neck, or chest is several magnitudes less than 0.5 mGy (Hurwitz et al. 2006a, 2007; Jaffe et al. 2008, 2009; Litmanovich et al. 2011). Based on Dr. Winer-Muram's Monte Carlo-based assessment of fetal radiation dose from CTPA, calculated fetal dose of up to 0.2 mGy has been show in first trimester, increasing up to 0.8 mGy in second and 1.3 mGy in the last trimester, when kVp of 120 and mA of 100 was used (Winer-Muram et al. 2002). Doshi et al. have shown, based on phantom assessment, that the calculated fetal dose in late pregnancy received from CTPA is in the range of 0.6–2.3 mGy (Doshi et al. 2008). Dr. Hurwitz has reported even lower doses to the fetus regardless of gestation age from CTPA protocol: 0.24–0.47 mGy and approximately 0.6 mGy at 0 and 3 months of pregnancy, respectively with scan parameters of 140 kVp and 340 mA (Hurwitz et al. 2006a).

### 1.1.3 Maternal Exposure

Understandably, radiation exposure of a pregnant woman is of even higher concern than an age-matched non-pregnant female due to increased sensitivity of glandular breast tissue (Smith-Bindman et al. 2009). Thus, radiation exposure to the breast is an increasingly important consideration when planning thoracic and abdomino-pelvic CT examinations (Hurwitz et al. 2006b, 2007). As with the fetal radiation dose, breast radiation is directly influenced by direct vs. indirect exposure. Reported direct breast dose during thoracic examinations varies depending on the protocol used (Litmanovich et al. 2011; Hurwitz et al. 2006b). Dose range from 43 to 90 mGy (on coronary CTA protocols, rarely used during pregnancy) were shown (Hurwitz et al. 2006b, 2007) with kVp ranging from 120 to 140 and mA from 300 kVp to 645 used. More modern protocols with automatic exposure deliver a dose between 10 and

15 mGy with the potential for further reduction as will be explained later (Litmanovich et al. 2011). Not enough data exists on assessing indirect breast radiation, with the reported values of 2–4 mGy for CT appendicitis protocol and less than 1.5 mGy for renal calculus protocol (Hurwitz et al. 2006b).

## 1.2 Informed Consent

Despite the widely established role of CT examinations in pregnant patients, radiologists should be aware that such imaging involves potential medico-legal risk (Berlin 1996). To minimize this potential, certain guidelines for imaging pregnant patients with ionizing radiation should be followed. These include: (1) Established process for evaluating pregnant patients in a radiological facility, (2) Radiologist knowledgeable about MRI/CT exposure effects accessible to patients and referring physicians, (3) Documenting in the radiology report all discussions with patients about the risks/benefits of a specific CT examination. While obtaining informed consent, radiologist should explain the need for imaging and the importance of the diagnosis for the patient's care as well as a brief explanation of the ordered imaging test. While summarizing the estimated risk to mother and fetus, radiologist would have a chance to confirm patient's comprehension of the risks and benefits as well as alternative options prior to consenting (Pahade et al. 2009). The emphasis on a low risk of harm to the fetus by CT scanning compared to the known 15% risk for spontaneous abortion and 1–3% risk for major malformation is extremely important.

## 1.3 Maternal and Fetal Dosimetry

Multiple studies have demonstrated successful assessment of radiation dose using variety of dosimetry techniques (Hurwitz et al. 2006a, b, 2007; Litmanovich et al. 2011) such as thermoluminescent dosimeters (TLDs), metal oxide semiconductor field effect transistor (MOSFET technology or both with an anthropomorphic phantom. MOSFET technology was first used in 1989 to measure patient skin entrance doses (Peet and Pryor 1999). Radiologist and physicist together can estimate fetal or breast dose, although if the patient undergoes head or neck scanning or if the study is done in the first two weeks of the pregnancy, no such estimate is required (Wagner et al. 1997). In the first case scenario, the scattered radiation is miniscule and in the second, there is an all or nothing response (American College of Radiology 2008).

In the vast majority of cases, dose estimation is done in a retrospective manner. In a retrospective case scenario, average dose to the uterus can be estimated by a medical physicist, usually based on widely described methods of fetal dose calculations (McCollough et al. 2007; Angel et al. 2008; Wagner et al. 1997). If the fetal dose is below 50 mGy (threshold level), dose information is entered in the dosimetry report. If the dose estimation exceeds 50 mGy, detailed dosimetry assessment might be required including fetal depth and patient size (Wieseler et al. 2010; Angel et al. 2008) and the dosimetry report is placed in the patient's chart.

When a prospective assessment of fetal dose is planned, MOSFET or TLD technology should be involved. Detectors can be placed on the surface of the patient over an appropriate area corresponding to the center of the fetus (based on gestation age), and obstetrics and gynecology specialists might need to be consulted. Fetal dose is estimated to be about one-third of the entrance dose of the average patient (Huda 2009). Again, if the estimated dose is above 50 mGy, detailed dosimetry report might be needed. Assessment of the breast, lung, and thyroid doses can be obtained with similar approach (Wieseler et al. 2010; Angel et al. 2009; Parker et al. 2005; Vollmar and Kalender 2008).

## 1.4 Intravenous Iodine Contrast Administration

Iodine contrast agents are hydrophilic and of moderate molecular weight, thus they can cross the placenta by passive diffusion eventually excreted by fetal kidneys (Lee and Chew 2009). Although there is a potential to induce neonatal hypothyroidism by maternal use of iodine-containing medications, no such effect has ever been reported with clinical doses of iodinated contrast media (Atwell et al. 2008). A 2008 ACR report states that iodinated contrast media may be given to the pregnant patient if needed (American College of Radiology 2008). However, because of the theoretic concern that fetal thyroid function may be affected, neonates of all mothers exposed to iodinated contrast media during pregnancy should be screened for hypothyroidism (Webb et al. 2005; American College of Radiology 2004).

In cases when a nursing patient undergoing CT examination involving IV iodinated contrast agent, interruption of nursing is often suggested for varying amounts of time, usually 12–24 h. However, estimated amount of iodinated contrast agent absorbed through infants' bowel is approximately 0.01% of the contrast agent administered to the mother, which is less than 1% of the permitted infant dose of 2 ml/kg. Thus, no interruption of lactation is required (Webb et al. 2005; Bona et al. 1992; Halvorsen 2008; Ito 2000).

## 1.5 Dose Reduction Techniques for CT Scanning in Pregnant Patients: General Concept

Approach to dose reduction in pregnant patients is similar to general population with particular emphasis on the following: Protocols should be tailored for each patient with no use of standard protocols. Adjusting kVp for small-size patients and use of automatic tube current modulation are obligatory. When appropriate, low kilovoltage setting for contrast opacification improvement should be applied. Pitch of more than one can be used in the vast majority of CT examinations without compromising diagnostic accuracy. Single scout view and no direct imaging of the fetus for planning purposes contributes to limiting radiation exposure. Limiting the field of view as well as limiting the length of the examination (Z-axis) appropriately is important. Incorporation of novel reconstruction algorithms to reduce imaging noise and allow reduction in milliamperage as well as increase in the noise index when appropriate can substantially affect radiation dose. Imaging in multiple phases should be avoided. Internal barium shielding with oral 30% barium sulfate solution neutralizes the internal scattered radiation from thoracic CT examinations. Overall control of appropriateness criteria, CT protocols, and radiation dose should be established on each clinical practice basis.

## 1.6 Dose Reduction Techniques for CT Scanning in Pregnant Patients: Specific Clinical Scenarios

Doubling of the number of CT examinations in pregnant patients has been observed in the period between 1997 and 2006 as demonstrated by a retrospective study of Lazarus and colleagues with the average estimated fetal radiation exposure per examination of 4.3 mGy (range, 0.01–43.9 mGy) (Lazarus et al. 2009). Although a substantial number of examinations were head and neck scans (37%), 32% were of the abdomen and pelvis and 27% were pulmonary CT angiograms. Another study (Goldberg-Stein et al. 2011) has also shown overall increase in CT utilization in pregnancy between 1998 and 2005, with the two most frequent indications being suspected pulmonary embolism and appendicitis. These trends require that the radiological community be not only aware of the radiation exposure to mother and fetus, but be trained in adaptation of existing protocol to pregnant patients and prepared to modify scanning parameters for maximum radiation dose saving to solidify an evidence-based departmental policy (El-Khoury et al. 2003). In the next paragraphs we will focus on detailed discussion of specific CT examinations during pregnancy.

### 1.6.1 Head and Neck

#### 1.6.1.1 CT Head and Neck

Since no fetal exposure is documented for these examinations, regular radiation dose reduction measures and protocol optimization approach are sufficient.

### 1.6.2 Thorax

1. *CT pulmonary embolism*

Pulmonary embolism is one of the leading non-obstetric causes of maternal mortality with the rate as high as 2–3 per 10,000 pregnancies (Bourjeily et al. 2009). The main reason for this predisposition is pregnancy-related Virchow's triad: hypercoagulability, venous stasis, and vascular damage.

Diagnosis of pulmonary embolism in pregnant patients is problematic due to a variety of reasons: sensitivity and specificity of clinical findings are decreased since normal physiologic changes may mimic pulmonary embolism and D-dimer assay is used mainly for its negative predictive value (Patel et al. 2007; Pahade et al. 2009). First-line imaging tests such as chest radiograph and US of lower extremities if the patient has symptoms attributable to deep vein thrombosis should be done first (Pahade et al. 2009). If the results of these examinations are negative or equivocal, second-line imaging such as CT pulmonary angiography (CTPA) or ventilation-perfusion imaging (V/Q) should be obtained. The choice between CTPA and V/Q might be difficult since both studies have demonstrated similar high sensitivity, specificity, and accuracy (Revel et al. 2011). In addition, a recent study has shown that negative CTPA in pregnant patients safely excludes clinically significant pulmonary embolism (Bourjeily et al. 2011). Recently published guidelines for imaging pregnant patients with suspected pulmonary embolism stratify the approach with the use of V/Q scan as a modality of choice in patients with normal chest radiographs (Leung et al. 2011).

Fetal radiation exposure is similarly low with these two modalities, both less than 1 mGy, with the tendency for the lower CTPA doses at the early stages of pregnancy (Jaffe et al. 2009; Litmanovich et al. 2011; Hurwitz et al. 2006b; Cook and Kyriou 2005). The major disadvantage of CTPA is substantially higher breast radiation dose compared to V/Q scan, 10–90 mGy opposed to 0.28 mGy, respectively (Cook and Kyriou 2005). The choice between the modalities is based on availability, local expertise, necessity to exclude alternative diagnosis (done with CTPA), and radiation exposure consideration.

Discussion regarding V/Q scan is beyond the scope of this chapter. The following focuses on the overall decrease of the radiation dose and methods to improve image quality of CTPA in pregnancy.

#### 1.6.2.1 Strategies to Decrease CT Radiation Dose

The majority of methods used to decrease radiation dose in CTPA being used in the general population can be applied in pregnant patients, with some modifications:

1. CT venography to evaluate pelvic veins for the presence of deep vein thrombosis is contraindicated in pregnancy.
2. Optimization of scan coverage: Z-axis is required. By keeping the superior margin of the study 1 cm above the aortic arch and the inferior margin at the level of diaphragm, delivered dose can be decreased by up to 40% (Kallen et al. 2009).
3. Obligatory use of automatic exposure control with relatively high noise index (16 or higher) with the maximum available mA of 200 is suitable in the vast majority of patients (Litmanovich et al. 2009).
4. Multiple studies have shown the advantages of low kilovoltage for improved opacification of the vascular tree, in particular pulmonary arteries (Schueller-Weidekamm et al. 2006; Heyer et al. 2007; Sigal-Cinqualbre et al. 2004; Tack et al. 2005; Bankier and Tack 2010). The advantage in dose saving with lower kVp is dramatic given the exponential relationship between kVp and radiation dose. A study comparing image quality in a group of 26 pregnant patients with suspected pulmonary embolism imaged with 100 kVp and restricted (up to 200 mA) setting with a control group of 26 age-matched non-pregnant patients demonstrated diagnostic quality images in all the patients (Fig. 1) (Litmanovich et al. 2009) while decreasing the CTDI vol, DLP, and calculated effective dose by a factor of 4. CTDI vol of less than 5 were routinely achieved as well as DLP values not exceeding 150 mGy-cm (Table 3). To verify radiation dose delivered by the modified pregnancy CTPA protocol estimated by scanner software, organ doses were measured in an anthropomorphic phantom (Litmanovich et al. 2011). Breast organ dose in the range of 4–6 mGy was measured, substantially lower than previously published. Fetal dose less than 0.1 mGy was documented, reflecting the scattered nature of pelvic radiation with CTPA. Lung radiation dose of less than 8.1 mGy was recorded (Litmanovich et al. 2011).
5. Routine use of pitch of greater than 1 (preferably 1.5–2) is suggested, as well as an increase in collimation (1.5 mm).
6. Application of novel reconstructing algorithms such as ASIR. Since decrease in kVp and mA leads to increased image noise, reduction of noise with the variety of currently available reconstruction algorithms allows us to decrease these parameters even further. In our institution 30% blend is routinely used for pregnant CTPA.
7. Shielding of the breast tissue and fetus should be considered.

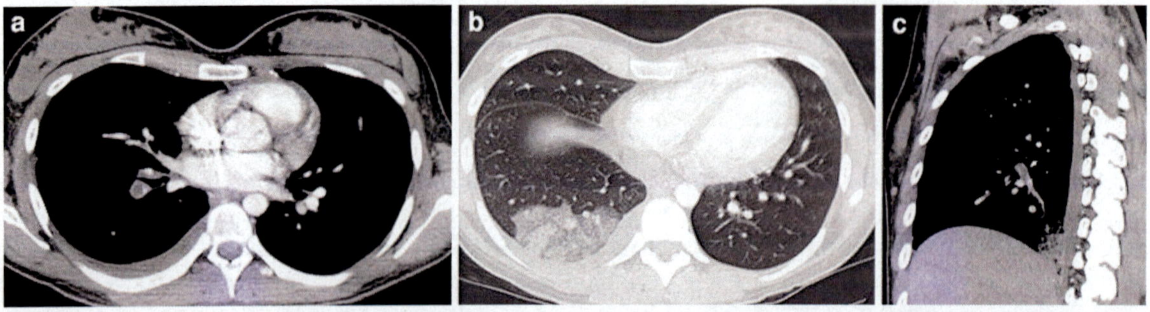

**Fig. 1** Pulmonary embolism in 19-year-old woman at 18 weeks gestation who presented with pleuritic chest pain (**a**, **b**, **c**). CT pulmonary angiography images obtained with 100 kVp and max mA of 200 demonstrate acute thrombus within the right lower lobe posterior-basal segmental artery (**a**) and peripheral consolidation suggestive of infarction (**b**). Oblique maximum intensity projection images (**c**) demonstrate both thrombus and corresponding infarct. Dose lengh product for that study was 144 mGy-cm

**Table 3** CTPA acquisition parameters for pregnant patients (modified from Litmanovich et al. 2009)

| | |
|---|---|
| kVp | 100 |
| mA | Up to 200 |
| Scan range | 1 cm above aortic arch—dome of the diaphragm |
| Injection parameters | Automatic triggering (threshold, 150 HU; ROI in the main pulmonary artery) |

(a) Fetal shielding can be internal and external. Internal shielding is provided by oral administration of 30% barium sulfate 20–30 min before the CT examination. By distributing in the stomach, duodenum and proximal small bowel, barium suspension serves as an internal shield from scattered radiation inside the maternal body (Yousefzadeh et al. 2006). External shielding, given the miniscule dose delivered to the fetus, is not necessary but may provide the patient more reassurance than actual risk reduction (McCollough et al. 2007).

(b) Breast shielding still remains debatable. Extensive discussion of this topic can be found in chaper "CT and Shielding" of this volume. As in the regular population, despite substantial dose reduction achieved with breast shielding (up to 30–50% depending on the study), beam hardening artifacts and increased image noise remain a problem even more substantial for the pregnant population. This is related to lower than usual kVp and mA settings in pregnant CTPA protocol. Thus the reduction in radiation dose could be achieved more efficiently by a reduction of tube output (Hartmann et al. 2010).

#### 1.6.2.2 Methods to Improve Image Quality

Recent studies have shown that there is a high risk of a suboptimal CTPA image quality during pregnancy when standard CTA acquisition protocols are used (Andreou et al. 2008; King-IM et al. 2008; Ridge et al. 2009). The reason for this is a combination of decreased vascular contrast enhancement in a hyperdynamic circulation and a change in breathing pattern in pregnant women with an increased risk for Valsalva maneuvers. To improve image quality and to keep radiation as low as possible, an adaptation of the protocol is necessary: (Pahade et al. 2009; Hartmann et al. 2010; Ridge et al. 2011; Schaefer-Prokop and Prokop 2008). The modifications needed are summarized in (Table 4).

2. *CT chest*

CT chest with an indication other than suspected pulmonary embolism is rarely performed during pregnancy (Goldberg-Stein et al. 2011), although with the increasing average age of the pregnant population, it might become more common. If undertaken, the usual indication is a mass suspected on chest radiograph. All the modifications discussed for CTPA are relevant for chest CT with the caveat that entire chest should be included, but the lower margin of the scan should be at the level of the diaphragm to avoid primary beam radiation of the fetus.

In calculating CT dose to women, most previous studies were not based on dedicated thoracic CT

**Table 4** Strategies to improve contrast opacification of pulmonary arteries and image quality for CTPA in pregnant patients (modified from Hartman et al. 2010)

| |
|---|
| Short scan duration (faster scanners, preferably 64-slices or more) |
| High iodine influx (increased flow > 5 cc/min, high iodine concentration > 350 iodium/ml, or both) |
| Suspended respiration |

protocols but instead relied on indirect calculations of the potential radiation exposure to the breast and fetus from whole-body vascular CT examinations (Jaffe et al. 2008; Hurwitz et al. 2006a). With few exceptions (Jaffe et al. 2009; Hurwitz et al. 2009) many of these studies were performed with examination protocols using tube settings of 140 kV often without the use of dose modulation (Hurwitz et al. 2006a, b, 2007). In addition, significant variation in organ dose between those derived from direct detector organ measurements and those calculated by applying Monte Carlo simulation has been observed, emphasizing the importance of actual dose measurements (Lechel et al. 2009). We measured the organ doses delivered in an anthropomorphic phantom by five CT protocols to the breast, the lung, and the pelvis using current dose reduction methods for routine CT 64-MDCT imaging. The breast and lung doses were substantially less than previously published: 11–15 mGy for the breast and 18 mGy for the lungs, using the current standard clinical chest CT protocol used at our institution. The protocol operates at 120 kVp and uses automatic dose modulation, ranging from 120 to 320 mA, noise index of 11.57 and pitch of 0.984. We attribute this dose reduction to the systematic use of tube settings of 120 kV or less and to the use of an automatic dose modulation algorithm provided by the manufacturer. Increasing the pitch above 1 (for Example 1.3) would substantially drop the radiation dose without scarifying image quality and should be obtained when applied in pregnancy.

Breast radiation, although, still higher than measured with dedicated PE pregnancy protocol, is lower than previously reported by different investigators (Hurwitz et al. 2006b, 2009; Angel et al. 2009) by at least 50%.

Our study also shows that the average radiation dose delivered to the phantom lung parenchyma was consistently higher than the doses delivered to the breast and the pelvis, respectively, which is consistent with the dose reported by Angel et al. with Monte Carlo simulation (Angel et al. 2009). This was true for both the standard-dose and reduced-dose protocols of our study (120 kVp, automatic dose modulation, ranging from 60 to 200 mA, a noise index of 26.00, and pitch of 0.984). Even though the reduced-dose protocols could decrease the average radiation to the lung, its relative role as the primary radiation recipient of the organs investigated in this study remains unchanged. This finding suggests that irradiation of the lung should be carefully considered when planning examination protocols and ordering CT studies given the increasing numbers of younger patients referred for CT, including pregnant women, and the subsequent increased cumulative risk for radiation-induced lung injury (Brenner and Hall 2007; Mayo et al. 2003; Tack and Gevenois 2009).

As with multiple previous phantom-based dosimetry results, fetal dose obtained with this protocol was less than 0.2 mGy (Litmanovich et al. 2011). Interestingly, the phantom doses to the upper and lower pelvis were lower than those previously reported for ventilation-perfusion scintigraphy performed in pregnant patients with suspected pulmonary embolism (Cook and Kyriou 2005). On the other hand, the doses were not zero. This finding could contradict the assumption from the CTDIvol measurement methods that any body part or organ located more than 5 cm from the lowest tube position along the *Z*-axis, corresponding to the lowest CT slice position and the average slice thickness × 0.5 × pitch, receives no radiation. The length in the *Z*-axis of a CTDIvol measurement is 10 cm, but the X-ray beam is in the center of this 10-cm segment. Thus, the distance at which the dose is considered as 0 is 10/2 = 5 cm along the X-ray beam. The minimal distance between the end of anatomic CT coverage and the pelvic detectors used in our measurements was 20 cm. Although the risk for fetal abnormalities is considered to be negligible at or below 50 mGy (Patel et al. 2007), our findings indicate the potential presence of a stochastic risk that should be considered when designing examination protocols according to the ALARA (as low as reasonably achievable) principle.

### 1.6.3 Abdomen:

1. *CT of suspected appendicitis*

Appendicitis is by far the most common cause of surgical abdomen in pregnancy, associated with premature labor, fetal morbidity and mortality, and a higher rate of complications (Tracey and Fletcher 2000). Since surgery is associated with preterm labor, fetal loss, and decreased birth weight, exact diagnosis before the surgery is crucial (Guttman et al. 2004). Obviously, non-ionizing modalities such as US and MRI should be the modalities of choice (Angel et al. 2009; Pedrosa et al. 2006; Vu et al. 2009; Lim et al. 1992; Cobben et al. 2004). If these modalities are unavailable or inconclusive (US), or if there is lack of expertise (MRI), given the importance of timely diagnosis in pregnant patients overweighing the potential risk of developing radiation-induced childhood cancer, CT evaluation should be considered.

High sensitivity and specificity of CT in pregnant patients with suspected appendicitis have been shown (Ames Castro et al. 2001; Lazarus et al. 2007). Intravenous contrast should be administered unless specific non-pregnancy-related contraindications exist (Patel et al. 2007). Oral contrast, although not considered part of routine CT examination in some practices, should be administered in pregnant patients to improve visualization of the appendix.

Estimated fetal CT radiation exposure for CT appendicitis varies by protocol, with a range of 10–40 mGy (Hurwitz et al. 2006a). Applying the following modifications will bring the fetal dose to the lower end of the spectrum:

1. Single phase scanning
2. Limited length of examination (Z-axis)
3. Lower edge of kVP—not more than 120 kVP in the vast majority of cases
4. Automatic exposure control in all cases
5. Higher noise index allowed

In every case of such a CT examination, fetal dose should be estimated (using retrospective or prospective approach) and documented appropriately, with more detailed dose assessment if the estimated dose exceeds 50 mGy (on rare occasions).

2. *CT of suspected urolithiasis*

Urolithiasis is the most common painful non-obstetric condition and most common non-obstetric reason for hospitalization in pregnant patients (McAleer and Loughlin 2004; Parulkar et al. 1998). The prevalence of disease is up to 5 per 1,000 pregnancies (Wieseler et al. 2010). Up to 75% of the calculi pass spontaneously (Evans and Wollin 2001), but in up to one-third of patients, diagnosis of renal colic can be mistaken for appendicitis, diverticulitis or placental abruption (Stothers and Lee 1992). On the other hand, normal changes during pregnancy such as physiologic dilatation of the collecting system can be mistaken for hydronephrosis and vice versa.

If not addressed appropriately, urolithiasis can lead to premature labor, in most of the cases due to pyelonephritis (Parulkar et al. 1998).

Ultrasound is a modality of choice for diagnosis of urolithiasis in pregnancy, but might present difficulty, in particular starting from the second trimester. MR urography should be considered as second-line test when US fails to establish diagnosis but symptoms persist, given its high sensitivity for detection of urinary tract dilatation and identification site of obstruction (Roy et al. 1996).

If both US and MR urography fail to diagnose the problem (or if MR urography is not available), other ionizing radiation modalities such as nuclear studies, intravenous urography and CT might be considered. While discussion of the first two modalities is beyond the scope of this chapter, we will however focus on CT examination for diagnosis of urolithiasis.

Mean estimated fetal dose from regular CT abdomen and pelvis is 33 mGy (8 and 25 mGy respectively) (Patel et al. 2007). These figures correspond to kvP of 130–140 and also will depend on the presence of automatic exposure control.

Low-dose CT for detection of calculi has been validated for general population (Katz et al. 2003). CT is more effective than excretory urography for the detection of ureteral calculi with sensitivity and specificity ranging between 92 and 99% (Smith et al. 1995; Ripolles et al. 2004). CT also is better than urography for diagnosing the complications of stone disease. Low-dose CT also allows identification of abnormalities outside of the urinary tract as well as alternative causes of flank pain (Patel et al. 2007; McCollough et al. 2007; Jaffe et al. 2008; Hurwitz et al. 2006a; Pedrosa et al. 2007; Lameris et al. 2009). Unlike excretory urography, CT performed by using a stone detection protocol does not necessitate the injection of an intravenous contrast medium.

Modified technique of low-dose CT for detection of calculi allows substantial reduction of fetal dose to 4–7.2 mGy at the very first weeks of pregnancy and 8.5–11.7 mGy at 3 months of gestation (Hurwitz et al. 2006a). The protocol parameters used were kVp of 140 and mA of 160, using 16-row multidetector scanner.

With the multidetector scans currently available, a combination of lower kVp (120) as well as automatic exposure control may decrease the dose even further.

When automatic exposure control is applied, as patient size changes, the change in CT scanner technique factors varies by a relatively small amount compared to radiographic studies such as IVP. In small patients, for whom the CT scanner output would be decreased, peripheral attenuation also would be decreased, causing an increase in internal doses in relation to the scanner output. In large patients, for whom the scanner output is increased, the peripheral attenuation also is increased, with a resultant decrease in the internal doses in relation to the scanner output (Schmidt 2001; Schmidt and Kalender 2002). The result is relatively constant organ doses when scanner output is adjusted for patient size. Automated exposure control systems are particularly beneficial in that they adjust the scanner output on the basis of patient attenuation in a relatively consistent manner (McCollough et al. 2007). McCollough and colleagues estimated that the fetal radiation dose from CT is approximately 10 mGy which is lower than that from limited IVP for a patient with an antero-posterior thickness of 25 cm or greater.

3. *CT in trauma*

Trauma is one of the leading non-obstetric causes of maternal and fetal death (Baerga-Varela et al. 2000; Grossman 2004) and affects up to 7% of pregnant patients. Most common cause of trauma in pregnancy is motor vehicle collisions (up to two-thirds of cases) and trauma more commonly occurs in the third trimester (McCollough et al. 2007; Baerga-Varela et al. 2000; Grossman 2004; Esposito et al. 1991). Fetal death can occur with both minor and major trauma (Baerga-Varela et al. 2000). The reported rate of fetal mortality after blunt trauma ranges from 3.4% to 38%, secondary to placental abruption, maternal death, or shock (Grossman 2004). Physiologic changes in pregnancy can mask the severity of maternal condition.

The cardinal principle in the management of trauma in pregnancy is that there can be no fetal survival without maternal survival. Therefore in pregnant trauma patients priority is given to maternal survival. The possible exception is third-trimester trauma in which the prognosis for maternal survival is poor. In this situation, immediate cesarean section may be necessary to save the fetus.

The International Commission on Radiological Protection (Protection ICoR 2003) has issued the following guidelines for radiologic examination of pregnant patients:

> When pregnant women require… radiological examinations, in which the primary beam irradiates the foetus, care must be taken to ascertain that the examination is indeed indicated. Sometimes the risk of irradiating the foetus is much less than that of not making a necessary diagnosis.… In such cases,… minimize the number of views and… absorbed dose per view. However, these alterations of technique should not be done to the undue detriment of the diagnostic value

Thus, concerns about fetal radiation exposure should neither deter nor delay radiologic evaluation, and after initial stabilization of the mother, assessment of maternal injuries should be done. However, imaging technical parameters should be appropriately modified.

*Indirect fetal radiation* As discussed earlier, the principal difference is if the fetus is in the primary beam of radiation or not. Examination that does not involve direct exposure to the maternal abdomen (e.g, head, neck, or chest CT) should be performed without concerns for fetal radiation effects.

*Direct fetal radiation* With blunt abdominal trauma, there is a role for initial evaluation with abdominal ultrasound, in particular in patients with low level trauma and low likelihood of injury. Study showed that in patients with negative US results, 96% did not need additional testing that used ionizing radiation, and US was therefore recommended as an accurate screening tool (Brown et al. 2005). Ultrasound is also more suited for the rapid triage of patients in unstable condition. On the other hand, if the severity of the maternal situation is at least moderate, but the mother is in stable condition, any delay in diagnosis could be crucial. In this case CT of the abdomen would be the initial modality of choice (Rhea et al. 2004; Lowdermilk et al. 1999; Goldman and Wagner 1999; Steffer and ICoR 2007).

CT is more sensitive than US for detection of small amounts of fluid, retroperitoneal hemorrhage, and organ injury (Lowdermilk et al. 1999; Goldman and Wagner 1999) as well as pancreatic injury. Also significant perfusion defects in the placenta at CT may be a significant negative prognosticator of fetal survival even if US scans appear normal (Goldman and Wagner 1999).

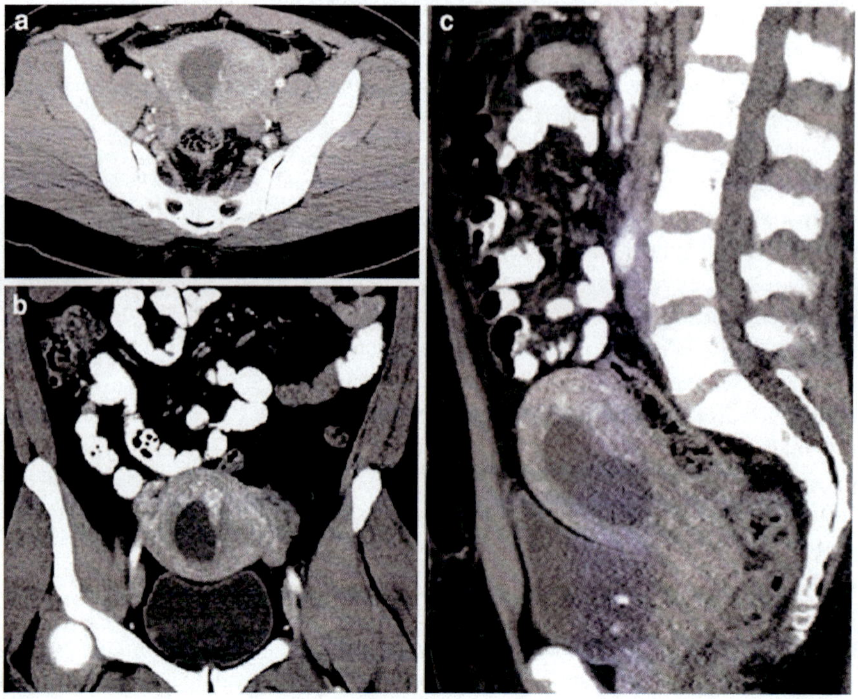


**Fig. 2** 24-year-old woman at 8 weeks gestation who was involved in motor vehicle accident. Axial (**a**), coronal (**b**), and saggital (**c**) CT abdomen images demonstrate enlargement of the uterus and enhancing placenta consistent with early stages of pregnancy. This study was sufficient to exclude clinically suspected accident-related complications

CT scanning, when properly performed with modern equipment, should be reasonably safe (Fig. 2). The dose from CT becomes a more important issue when multiple passes through the fetus are involved. Previously discussed modifications of CT abdomen should be applied in cases of trauma with the following modification:

1. Pitch > 1
2. For CT of the mid abdomen in early pregnancy, when the conceptus will not be directly irradiated, we suggest imaging in the nephrographic or cortico-medullary phase followed by delayed imaging to exclude active bleeding.
3. For later stages of pregnancy, we suggest only late-phase imaging with the same technique.
4. Pelvic evaluation is performed to investigate peritoneal fluid or skeletal injuries. If CT of the pelvis is required, pitch of 1.5 or more is suggested. In cases where CT evaluation of complex bone injury is needed, the technique will be governed by the imaging detail required, but the examination should be confined to the appropriate area of interest.
5. Patients with gross hematuria and a pelvic fracture are at risk for bladder rupture and require cystography. Although CT cystography would expose the fetus to direct radiation regardless of the stage of pregnancy, it can be obtained at low dose (kVp 120, automatic exposure control, mA not exceeding 200), but the advantages of cross-sectional information and higher sensitivity and specificity are apparent. CT acquisition should be done after filling the bladder with at least 300–350 mL of contrast material. There is no need for additional scanning after draining of the bladder.

## 2 Summary

Despite ionizing radiation, CT remains a crucial modality of choice in a variety of potential clinical scenarios during pregnancy. Combined efforts of a referring clinician and radiologist are essential for providing the best practice. When an acute problem is identified by a clinician and the pregnant patient is referred to imaging with a specific question, it is the radiologist's role to decide if the diagnostic question can be answered with a non-ionizing modality such as US or MRI. If CT is the modality of choice based on feasibility and/or specific questions asked, it is the radiologist's role to estimate fetal and maternal risk from known radiation dose in each specific case as well as to structure the examination to achieve minimal radiation exposure without compromising diagnostic accuracy. (Maglinte et al. 2003). The most frequently asked questions that might require CT examination are pulmonary embolism, aortic dissection, appendicitis, urolithiasis, and trauma with the latter being unequivocally evaluated by CT in the vast majority of cases (Lazarus et al. 2009; Rhea et al. 2004; Lowdermilk et al. 1999).

The best practice for imaging of pregnant or potentially pregnant patients with ionizing radiation is as follows: "To maintain a high standard of safety, particularly when imaging potentially pregnant patients, imaging radiation must be applied at as low as reasonably achievable levels (ALARA), while the degree of medical benefit must counterbalance the well-managed levels of risk" (American College of Radiology 2008; Maglinte et al. 2003). Both American College of Radiology and American Congress of Obstetricians and Gynecologists agree that the necessary imaging examination should be performed after clinical work-up, and the radiation level should be kept as low as reasonably achievable (American College of Radiology 2008; Chen et al. 2008) and the patient should give informed consent before the procedure.

Radiation dose to the fetus from a single CT examination is far below the dose that can potentially result in fetal anomalies (Brent 2009). Concern may be raised if multiple consecutive studies are expected or have been performed and the cumulative dose approaches undesired thresholds (Wieseler et al. 2010). In both case scenarios, radiation dose from CT scan can be substantially decreased when proper CT parameters are used, including all the currently available dose reduction tools such as automatic exposure control and adaptive statistical iterative reconstruction algorithms.

## References

American College of Radiology (2004) Committee on Drugs and Contrast Media. Manual on contrast media, 6th ed. Reston, VA, pp 61–66

American College of Radiology (2008) ACR practice guideline for imaging pregnant or potentially pregnant adolescents and women with ionizing radiation. American College of Radiology, Reston

Ames Castro M, Shipp TD, Castro EE, Ouzounian J, Rao P (2001) The use of helical computed tomography in pregnancy for the diagnosis of acute appendicitis. Am J Obstet Gynecol 184:954–957

Andreou AK, Curtin JJ, Wilde S, Clark A (2008) Does pregnancy affect vascular enhancement in patients undergoing CT pulmonary angiography? Eur Radiol 18:2716–2722

Angel E, Wellnitz CV, Goodsitt MM et al (2008) Radiation dose to the fetus for pregnant patients undergoing multidetector CT imaging: Monte Carlo simulations estimating fetal dose for a range of gestational age and patient size. Radiology 249:220–227

Angel E, Yaghmai N, Jude CM et al (2009a) Monte Carlo simulations to assess the effects of tube current modulation on breast dose for multidetector CT. Phys Med Biol 54: 497–512

Angel E, Yaghmai N, Jude CM et al (2009b) Dose to radiosensitive organs during routine chest CT: effects of tube current modulation. AJR 193:1340–1345

Atwell TD, Lteif AN, Brown DL, McCann M, Townsend JE, Leroy AJ (2008) Neonatal thyroid function after administration of IV iodinated contrast agent to 21 pregnant patients. AJR 191:268–271

Baerga-Varela Y, Zietlow SP, Bannon MP, Harmsen WS, Ilstrup DM (2000) Trauma in pregnancy. Mayo Clin Proc 75:1243–1248

Bankier AA, Tack D (2010) Dose reduction strategies for thoracic multidetector computed tomography: background, current issues, and recommendations. J Thorac Imaging 25: 278–288

Berlin L (1996) Radiation exposure and the pregnant patient. AJR 167:1377–1379

Bona G, Zaffaroni M, Defilippi C, Gallina MR, Mostert M (1992) Effects of iopamidol on neonatal thyroid function. Eur J Radiol 14:22–25

Bourjeily G, Paidas M, Khalil H, Rosene-Montella K, Rodger M (2009) Pulmonary embolism in pregnancy. Lancet 375: 500–512

Bourjeily G, Khalil H, Raker C et al (2011) Outcomes of negative multidetector computed tomography with pulmonary angiography in pregnant women suspected of pulmonary embolism. Lung 19(5):267–274

Brenner DJ, Hall EJ (2007) Computed tomography—an increasing source of radiation exposure. N Engl J Med 357: 2277–2284

Brent RL (2009) Saving lives and changing family histories: appropriate counseling of pregnant women and men and women of reproductive age, concerning the risk of diagnostic radiation exposures during and before pregnancy. Am J Obstet Gynecol 200:4–24

Brown MA, Sirlin CB, Farahmand N, Hoyt DB, Casola G (2005) Screening sonography in pregnant patients with blunt abdominal trauma. J Ultrasound Med 24:175–181, quiz 183–184

Chen MM, Coakley FV, Kaimal A, Laros RK Jr (2008) Guidelines for computed tomography and magnetic resonance imaging use during pregnancy and lactation. Obstet Gynecol 112:333–340

Cobben LP, Groot I, Haans L, Blickman JG, Puylaert J (2004) MRI for clinically suspected appendicitis during pregnancy. AJR 183:671–675

Cook JV, Kyriou J (2005) Radiation from CT and perfusion scanning in pregnancy. BMJ 331:350
Doshi SK, Negus IS, Oduko JM (2008) Fetal radiation dose from CT pulmonary angiography in late pregnancy: a phantom study. Br J Radiol 81:653–658
El-Khoury GY, Madsen MT, Blake ME, Yankowitz J (2003) A new pregnancy policy for a new era. AJR 181:335–340
Esposito TJ, Gens DR, Smith LG, Scorpio R, Buchman T (1991) Trauma during pregnancy. A review of 79 cases. Arch Surg 126:1073–1078
Evans HJ, Wollin TA (2001) The management of urinary calculi in pregnancy. Curr Opin Urol 11:379–384
Goldberg-Stein S, Liu B, Hahn PF, Lee SI (2011) Body CT during pregnancy: utilization trends, examination indications, and fetal radiation doses. AJR 196:146–151
Goldman SM, Wagner LK (1999) Radiologic ABCs of maternal and fetal survival after trauma: when minutes may count. Radiographics 19:1349–1357
Grossman NB (2004) Blunt trauma in pregnancy. Am Fam Physician 70:1303–1310
Groves AM, Yates SJ, Win T et al (2006) CT pulmonary angiography versus ventilation-perfusion scintigraphy in pregnancy: implications from a UK survey of doctors' knowledge of radiation exposure. Radiology 240:765–770
Guttman R, Goldman RD, Koren G (2004) Appendicitis during pregnancy. Can Fam Physician 50:355–357
Halvorsen RA (2008) Which study when? Iodinated contrast-enhanced CT versus gadolinium-enhanced MR imaging. Radiology 249:9–15
Hartmann IJ, Wittenberg R, Schaefer-Prokop C (2010) Imaging of acute pulmonary embolism using multi-detector CT angiography: an update on imaging technique and interpretation. Eur J Radiol 74:40–49
Heyer CM, Mohr PS, Lemburg SP, Peters SA, Nicolas V (2007) Image quality and radiation exposure at pulmonary CT angiography with 100- or 120-kVp protocol: prospective randomized study. Radiology 245:577–583
Huda WSR (2009) Review of radiologic physics, 3rd edn. Lippinkott Wiliams & Wilkins, Philadelphia
Hurwitz LM, Yoshizumi T, Reiman RE et al (2006a) Radiation dose to the fetus from body MDCT during early gestation. AJR 186:871–876
Hurwitz LM, Yoshizumi TT, Reiman RE et al (2006b) Radiation dose to the female breast from 16-MDCT body protocols. AJR 186:1718–1722
Hurwitz LM, Reiman RE, Yoshizumi TT et al (2007) Radiation dose from contemporary cardiothoracic multidetector CT protocols with an anthropomorphic female phantom: implications for cancer induction. Radiology 245:742–750
Hurwitz LM, Yoshizumi TT, Goodman PC et al (2009) Radiation dose savings for adult pulmonary embolus 64-MDCT using bismuth breast shields, lower peak kilovoltage, and automatic tube current modulation. AJR 192: 244–253
Ito S (2000) Drug therapy for breast-feeding women. N Engl J Med 343:118–126
Jaffe TA, Yoshizumi TT, Toncheva GI, Nguyen G, Hurwitz LM, Nelson RC (2008) Early first-trimester fetal radiation dose estimation in 16-MDCT without and with automated tube current modulation. AJR 190:860–864
Jaffe TA, Yoshizumi TT, Toncheva G et al (2009a) Radiation dose for body CT protocols: variability of scanners at one institution. AJR 193:1141–1147
Jaffe TA, Neville AM, Anderson-Evans C et al (2009b) Early first trimester fetal dose estimation method in a multivendor study of 16- and 64-MDCT scanners and low-dose imaging protocols. AJR 193:1019–1024
Kallen JA, Coughlin BF, O'Loughlin MT, Stein B (2009) Reduced Z-axis coverage multidetector CT angiography for suspected acute pulmonary embolism could decrease dose and maintain diagnostic accuracy. Emerg Radiol 17:31–35
Katz DS, Venkataramanan N, Napel S, Sommer FG (2003) Can low-dose unenhanced multidetector CT be used for routine evaluation of suspected renal colic? AJR 180:313–315
King-IM JU, Freeman SJ, Boylan T, Cheow HK (2008) Quality of CT pulmonary angiography for suspected pulmonary embolus in pregnancy. Eur Radiol 18:2709–2715
Lameris W, van Randen A, van Es HW et al (2009) Imaging strategies for detection of urgent conditions in patients with acute abdominal pain: diagnostic accuracy study. BMJ 338:b2431
Lazarus E, Mayo-Smith WW, Mainiero MB, Spencer PK (2007) CT in the evaluation of nontraumatic abdominal pain in pregnant women. Radiology 244:784–790
Lazarus E, Debenedectis C, North D, Spencer PK, Mayo-Smith WW (2009) Utilization of imaging in pregnant patients: 10-year review of 5270 examinations in 3285 patients–1997–2006. Radiology 251:517–524
Lechel U, Becker C, Langenfeld-Jager G, Brix G (2009) Dose reduction by automatic exposure control in multidetector computed tomography: comparison between measurement and calculation. Eur Radiol 19:1027–1034
Lee I, Chew FS (2009) Use of IV iodinated and gadolinium contrast media in the pregnant or lactating patient: self-assessment module. AJR 193:S70–S73
Leung AN, Bull TM, Jaeschke R et al (2011) An official American thoracic society/society of thoracic radiology clinical practice guideline: evaluation of suspected pulmonary embolism in pregnancy. Am J Respir Crit Care Med 184:1200–1208
Lim HK, Bae SH, Seo GS (1992) Diagnosis of acute appendicitis in pregnant women: value of sonography. AJR 159:539–542
Litmanovich D, Boiselle PM, Bankier AA, Kataoka ML, Pianykh O, Raptopoulos V (2009) Dose reduction in computed tomographic angiography of pregnant patients with suspected acute pulmonary embolism. J Comput Assist Tomogr 33:961–966
Litmanovich D, Tack D, Lin PJ, Boiselle PM, Raptopoulos V, Bankier AA (2011) Female breast, lung, and pelvic organ radiation from dose-reduced 64-MDCT thoracic examination protocols: a phantom study. AJR 197:929–934
Lowdermilk C, Gavant ML, Qaisi W, West OC, Goldman SM (1999) Screening helical CT for evaluation of blunt traumatic injury in the pregnant patient. Radiographics 19:S243–S255, discussion S256–S248
Maglinte DD, Gourtsoyiannis N, Rex D, Howard TJ, Kelvin FM (2003) Classification of small bowel Crohn's subtypes based on multimodality imaging. Radiol Clin North Am 41:285–303
Martin JN Jr, Ridgway LE 3rd, Connors JJ, Sessums JK, Martin RW, Morrison JC (1990) Angiographic arterial embolization and computed tomography-directed drainage for the management of hemorrhage and infection with abdominal pregnancy. Obstet Gynecol 76:941–945

Mayo JR, Aldrich J, Muller NL (2003) Radiation exposure at chest CT: a statement of the Fleischner Society. Radiology 228:15–21
McAleer SJ, Loughlin KR (2004) Nephrolithiasis and pregnancy. Curr Opin Urol 14:123–127
McCollough CH, Schueler BA, Atwell TD et al (2007) Radiation exposure and pregnancy: when should we be concerned? Radiographics 27:909–917, discussion 917–918
Pahade JK, Litmanovich D, Pedrosa I, Romero J, Bankier AA, Boiselle PM (2009) Quality initiatives: imaging pregnant patients with suspected pulmonary embolism: what the radiologist needs to know. Radiographics 29:639–654
Parker MS, Hui FK, Camacho MA, Chung JK, Broga DW, Sethi NN (2005) Female breast radiation exposure during CT pulmonary angiography. AJR 185:1228–1233
Parulkar BG, Hopkins TB, Wollin MR, Howard PJ Jr, Lal A (1998) Renal colic during pregnancy: a case for conservative treatment. J Urol 159:365–368
Patel SJ, Reede DL, Katz DS, Subramaniam R, Amorosa JK (2007) Imaging the pregnant patient for nonobstetric conditions: algorithms and radiation dose considerations. Radiographics 27:1705–1722
Pedrosa I, Levine D, Eyvazzadeh AD, Siewert B, Ngo L, Rofsky NM (2006) MR imaging evaluation of acute appendicitis in pregnancy. Radiology 238:891–899
Pedrosa I, Zeikus EA, Levine D, Rofsky NM (2007) MR imaging of acute right lower quadrant pain in pregnant and nonpregnant patients. Radiographics 27:721–743, discussion 743–753
Peet DJ, Pryor MD (1999) Evaluation of a MOSFET radiation sensor for the measurement of entrance surface dose in diagnostic radiology. Br J Radiol 72:562–568
Protection ICoR (2000) Pregnancy and medical radiation. Ann ICRP 30:iii–viii, 1–43
Protection ICoR (2003) Biological effects after prenatal irradiation (embryo and fetus). ICRP publication no 90, New York, pp 7–8
Ratnapalan S, Bona N, Chandra K, Koren G (2004) Physicians' perceptions of teratogenic risk associated with radiography and CT during early pregnancy. AJR 182:1107–1109
Revel MP, Cohen S, Sanchez O et al (2011) Pulmonary embolism during pregnancy: diagnosis with lung scintigraphy or CT angiography? Radiology 258:590–598
Rhea JT, Garza DH, Novelline RA (2004) Controversies in emergency radiology. CT versus ultrasound in the evaluation of blunt abdominal trauma. Emerg Radiol 10:289–295
Ridge CA, McDermott S, Freyne BJ, Brennan DJ, Collins CD, Skehan SJ (2009) Pulmonary embolism in pregnancy: comparison of pulmonary CT angiography and lung scintigraphy. AJR 193:1223–1227
Ridge CA, Mhuircheartaigh JN, Dodd JD, Skehan SJ (2011) Pulmonary CT angiography protocol adapted to the hemodynamic effects of pregnancy. AJR 197:1058–1063
Ripolles T, Errando J, Agramunt M, Martinez MJ (2004) Ureteral colic: US versus CT. Abdom Imaging 29:263–266
Roy C, Saussine C, LeBras Y et al (1996) Assessment of painful ureterohydronephrosis during pregnancy by MR urography. Eur Radiol 6:334–338
Schaefer-Prokop C, Prokop M (2008) CTPA for the diagnosis of acute pulmonary embolism during pregnancy. Eur Radiol 18:2705–2708
Schmidt B (2001) Dose calculations for computed tomography. Reports from the Institute of Medical Physics. Shaker, Aachen
Schmidt B, Kalender W (2002) A fast voxel-based Monte Carlo method for scanner-abd patient-specific dose calculations in computed tomography. In: Guerra AD (ed) Physica medica: European journal of medical physics. Instituti Editoriali e Politgrafici Internzionali, Pisa, pp 43–53
Schueller-Weidekamm C, Schaefer-Prokop CM, Weber M, Herold CJ, Prokop M (2006) CT angiography of pulmonary arteries to detect pulmonary embolism: improvement of vascular enhancement with low kilovoltage settings. Radiology 241:899–907
Sigal-Cinqualbre AB, Hennequin R, Abada HT, Chen X, Paul JF (2004) Low-kilovoltage multi-detector row chest CT in adults: feasibility and effect on image quality and iodine dose. Radiology 231:169–174
Smith RC, Rosenfield AT, Choe KA et al (1995) Acute flank pain: comparison of non-contrast-enhanced CT and intravenous urography. Radiology 194:789–794
Smith-Bindman R, Lipson J, Marcus R et al (2009) Radiation dose associated with common computed tomography examinations and the associated lifetime attributable risk of cancer. Arch Intern Med 169:2078–2086
Steffer C, Protection ICoR (2007) The ICRP 2007 recommendations. Radiat Prot Dosimetry 127:2–7
Stothers L, Lee LM (1992) Renal colic in pregnancy. J Urol 148:1383–1387
Tack D, Gevenois PA (2009) Body MDCT at 140 kV. AJR 192:W139–W140, author reply W141–W135
Tack D, De Maertelaer V, Petit W et al (2005) Multi-detector row CT pulmonary angiography: comparison of standard-dose and simulated low-dose techniques. Radiology 236:318–325
Toglia MR, Weg JG (1996) Venous thromboembolism during pregnancy. N Engl J Med 335:108–114
Tracey M, Fletcher HS (2000) Appendicitis in pregnancy. Am Surg 66:555–559, discussion 559–560
Vollmar SV, Kalender WA (2008) Reduction of dose to the female breast in thoracic CT: a comparison of standard-protocol, bismuth-shielded, partial and tube-current-modulated CT examinations. Eur Radiol 18:1674–1682
Vu L, Ambrose D, Vos P, Tiwari P, Rosengarten M, Wiseman S (2009) Evaluation of MRI for the diagnosis of appendicitis during pregnancy when ultrasound is inconclusive. J Surg Res 156:145–149
Wagner LK, Lester RG, Saldana LR (1997) Exposure of the pregnant patient to diagnostic radiation: a guide to medical management. Medical Physics, Madison
Webb JA, Thomsen HS, Morcos SK (2005) The use of iodinated and gadolinium contrast media during pregnancy and lactation. Eur Radiol 15:1234–1240
Wieseler KM, Bhargava P, Kanal KM, Vaidya S, Stewart BK, Dighe MK (2010) Imaging in pregnant patients: examination appropriateness. Radiographics 30:1215–1229, discussion 1230–1213
Winer-Muram HT, Boone JM, Brown HL, Jennings SG, Mabie WC, Lombardo GT (2002) Pulmonary embolism in pregnant patients: fetal radiation dose with helical CT. Radiology 224:487–492
Yousefzadeh DK, Ward MB, Reft C (2006) Internal barium shielding to minimize fetal irradiation in spiral chest CT: a phantom simulation experiment. Radiology 239:751–758

# Part IV

# Radiation Risk Management in Low Dose MDCT Screening Programs

# Radiation Risk Associated with Lung Cancer Screening

Cornelia Schaefer-Prokop, Krijn van Muiswinkel, and Mathias Prokop

## Contents



C. Schaefer-Prokop (✉) · K. van Muiswinkel
Department of Radiology,
Meander Medical Center Amersfoort,
Utrechtseweg 160, 3800 BM,
Amersfoort, The Netherlands
e-mail: cornelia.schaeferprokop@gmail.com

C. Schaefer-Prokop
Department of Radiology,
Diagnostic Image Analysis Group,
University Hospital Nijmegen, St Radboud,
6500 HB, Nijmegen, The Netherlands

M. Prokop
Department of Radiology,
University Hospital Nijmegen, St Radboud,
6500 HB, Nijmegen, The Netherlands

**Abstract**

Computed tomographic (CT) cancer screening has seen a steady increase in interest with the introduction of multislice CT scanners. The recent publication of the US National lung screening trial has proven a statistically significant reduction of cancer-related mortality and has boosted the discussion about the usefulness of introducing population-wide screening for lung cancer. While the potential benefits of screening are obvious, radiation dose may pose a long-term risk for the screened individual. This article describes the basis for radiation risk estimation and discusses the current dose controversy with special emphasis on CT screening for lung cancer. While there is no and probably never will be epidemiologic evidence for cancer induction in the dose range used for a single lung cancer screening examination, a non-negligible population risk cannot be ruled out considering the current evidence. Precise predictions of cancer risks are difficult because they depend heavily on the underlying statistical or radiobiologic model. While the risk of most radiation-induced cancers decreases with age, the relative risk of radiation-induced lung cancer peaks in the time interval between 40 and 70 years of age. However, if performed in a dose-conscious fashion, individual risks of lung cancer screening are very small and far outweighed by the published benefits of screening.

D. Tack et al. (eds.), *Radiation Dose from Multidetector CT*, Medical Radiology. Diagnostic Imaging,
DOI: 10.1007/174_2011_491, 

# 1 Introduction

It is estimated that about 570,000 Americans will die from cancer in 2011, corresponding to more than 1,500 deaths per day (http://www.cancer.gov/statistics). For both, men and women, lung carcinoma is the number one cause of cancer-related deaths. Lung cancer surpasses prostate and colorectal cancer in men, and breast and colorectal cancer in women. These four cancers account for almost half of total cancer deaths.

There is a strong relationship between tumor size at time of diagnosis and the survival rate. This correlation is reflected by the new classification of the T denominator in the seventh edition of the TNM classification (Detterbeck et al. 2009) and is also the motivation for the efforts to detect the tumor in an early and potentially treatable stage by screening asymptomatic patients at increased risk for cancer.

The discussion of whether and how to screen for lung cancer is decades old. Screening trials utilizing chest X-ray and sputum cytology conducted more than 20 years ago were not able to show any decrease in cancer mortality. The introduction of spiral CT made it technically possible to obtain volumetric data with a lower radiation dose than normally used for diagnostic purposes. This started a heated discussion about the usefulness of screening using low-dose CT. First studies (see Table 1) yielded encouraging results but were not designed as a prospective randomized trial that could prove that screening using low dose CT (LDCT) would result in significant reduction of cancer-related mortality.

In the August issue of the 2011 NEJM, the results of the multicenter North-American National Lung cancer Screening Trial (NLST) were published. This trial had been designed to have a more than 90% power to find a 20% decrease of mortality rate (NEJM 2011). Results were able to prove a 20.3% decrease in mortality ($p = 0.0004$) from lung cancer in the low dose CT group as compared to the radiography group (National Lung Screening Trial Research Team 2011). Thus, for the first time a trial provided statistical support that screening with LDCT is not only able to detect more lung tumors at an earlier stage compared to radiography but also that LDCT screening significantly reduces lung cancer-related mortality.

Apart from the risks associated with the workup or treatment of false-positive or of indeterminate findings, the risk from radiation-induced cancer has been discussed controversially in the literature. Brenner, in particular, has calculated risk estimates for various screening applications of CT, such as lung cancer, colon cancer and full-body CT screening (Brenner 2004; Brenner and Georgsson 2005; Brenner and Elliston 2004). For lung cancer, for example, the lifetime risk of a cancer that is induced by the CT screening examination has been calculated to amount up to 0.85% under unfavorable conditions with an upper 95% confidence interval of as much as 5.5% (Brenner 2004). These numbers have to be weighed against the incidence of screening detected cancers and—more importantly—the actual decrease of cancer-related mortality due to screening.

The following chapter will discuss the basis for radiation risk estimation and give an overview of the current dose controversy in CT screening for lung cancer.

## 1.1 Results of Lung Cancer Screening Trials: What did We Learn So Far?

Early detection trials with chest radiography and sputum cytology in the 1970s were ineffective in decreasing lung cancer mortality despite the higher proportion of early-stage cancers identified by screening (Melamad et al. 1984). A 25-year follow-up of this Mayo trial even yielded a higher mortality in the CXR arm compared to the standard-care arm, indicating the inefficiency of CXR screening and pointing toward the problem of overdiagnosis (Marcus et al. 2006).

The first American screening study, the Early Lung Cancer Action Project (ELCAP) was published in 1999. The investigators found that CT had a six-times higher accuracy than CXR for identifying small lung tumors (56% of cases were <1 cm). Reported resectability rate was 96% with a frequency of stage 1 neoplasms of 85% (McCauley et al. 1999).

In the following years a multitude of observational studies and randomized controlled trials were conducted in total including more than 90,000 subjects. At baseline the overall frequency of participants with suspicious non-calcified solid lesions was 20% (range 7–53%), the lung cancer detection rate was 15 (range 0.4–2.7) and the proportion of Stage 1 lung cancers was on average 81% (range 50–100%) (Pastorino 2010, Table 1).

The NLST trial compared LDCT with CXR in the control arm. A total of 53,454 individuals were included between 2002 and 2004. Analysis in October 2010 revealed 356 deaths in the LDCT arm versus 443 deaths in the CXR arm, corresponding to 247 and 309 per 100,000 person-years, respectively, and a 20.3% reduction in lung-cancer specific mortality (National Lung Screening Trial Research Team 2011).

Table 1 summarizes CT protocols, age and size of study group and the number of CT screening rounds. Low dose protocols are usually based on choosing lower mAs than for clinical routine. Typical exposure parameters are 120 kV and 30–60 mAs. In the Nelson trial, the voltage was increased to 140 kV (at 30 mAs) for patients with a body weight above 80 kg (Xu et al. 2006). The mAs setting, however, is no good parameter to indicate the exposure because $CTDI_{vol}$ per 100 mAs varies substantially between scanner manufacturers and increases with higher kV settings. Differences of up to a factor of 2 are possible for identical kV and mAs settings. For this reason $CTDI_{vol}$ should be provided instead of mAs. In case adaptive dose modulation is used, CTDI values can no longer be provided on a population basis but need to be reported individually. CTDI values used for lung cancer screening can vary between less than 1 mGy and more than 5 mGy. Most studies used 2–4 mGy.

Most lung cancer screening studies planned 3–5 CT screening rounds for patients with no actionable or indeterminate nodule. In patients with nodules requiring short-term follow-up, additional follow up CTs were obtained 6 weeks to 6 months after the scan on which the nodule was detected to prove or exclude nodule growth.

## 1.2 Estimation of Radiation-Induced Cancer Risk

The estimation of radiation-induced cancer risk is difficult. The risk estimates of inducing malignancy through ionizing radiation have mainly been gathered from the atomic bomb blasts in Japan. However, it is not clear whether these estimates represent real risk at low dose (Jett 2005).

The largest source of data comes from the Life Span Study (LSS) cohort consisting of about 120,000 survivors of the atomic bombings in Hiroshima and Nagasaki in 1945. The LSS cohort compares survivors who were within 2.5 km of the hypocenters of the bombings to a similar size sample of survivors who were between 3 and 10 km from the hypocenters and whose radiation doses were considered negligible, which was defined as below 5 mSv. The cohort is well characterized with respect to radiation dose and cancer incidence and mortality. It still serves as the most important source for risk estimation of radiation, even at low doses because a large proportion of the cohort received radiation doses between 5 and 50 mSv. In addition to the atomic bomb survivors, cohorts of individuals exposed for medical reasons have been used to further evaluate the age-dependence, especially age at exposure and time since exposure (Little 1999; National Research Council Committee on the Biological Effects of Ionizing Radiations 2005; Brenner et al. 2003). These further studies generally confirm the findings that were derived from the A-bomb survivor cohort but provide additional information about modifying factors in different cohorts.

An excess risk of ionizing radiation has been proven for doses above 100 mSv. Below that level, proof of excess risk exists for certain conditions like fetal exposure. Among approximately 30,000 individuals in the cancer incidence cohort of atomic bomb survivors who received doses between 5 and 100 mSv (mean 29 mSv), there was a statistically significant increase in cancer risk compared to that in the control group (77 excess cancers, $P < 0.05$) (Pierce and Preston 2000). For doses below 20 mSv, the radiation risk is so low that the population that needs to be studied to obtain significant results is substantially larger than all existing cohorts. Assuming that the excess risk is proportional to the radiation dose, the sample size needed to determine a significant effect of radiation increases by a approximate factor of 100 if the radiation dose is reduced by a factor of 10 (e.g. 100–10 mSv) (Brenner et al. 2003). Statistical proof of risks at low radiation dose therefore requires an excessive size of the study population. In practice, this makes it highly improbable that an excess risk below 10 mSv can ever be proven by epidemiological studies.

For this reason, the risk of ionizing radiation at very low doses has to be based on assumptions that can be derived from radiobiological models or from fitting curves to existing risk data (National Research Council Committee on the Biological Effects of Ionizing Radiations 2005). Most discussion in the past decade, however, has solely focused on such extrapolation of data and is usually based on the so-called linear no threshold theory, which is considered the best available theory that can describe the overall cancer risk (National Research Council Committee on the Biological Effects of Ionizing Radiations 2005). This theory is currently used for calculation of risk of radiation-induced cancer, even below the 5 mSv threshold used in the LSS cohort from Japan. Contradicting data from radiobiological models that support a more complex interaction have been almost completely neglected in the current public discussion (Tubiana et al. 2009).

The linear non-threshold theory (LNT) is based on the assumption that a single photon can cause damage (cancer) and that this damage is proportionally increased as more photons cross a tissue (see also Risks from Ionising Radiation by Chadwick in this book). This mechanistic approach of interaction of radiation, or more precisely, interaction of secondary electrons with the cell nuclei, may be too simplistic because it does not take other factors, such as cellular repair mechanisms into account. It also does not explain why organisms with many cells do not develop a higher cancer rate: in fact, radiation-induced cancer rates in humans and mice do not differ by a factor that accounts for the different number of cells (see also "The Cancer Risk from Low Level Radiation" by Cohen in this book). However, the LNT can be fitted to the existing data and provides a simple model for risk calculations.

Apart from the LNT, there are various other models that extrapolate the risk toward low doses that often fit the current data better than the LNT. The *decreasing slope model* predicts a higher risk at low dose. This model fits well with the current cancer incidence data and can be explained by a highly sensitive subpopulation that might be genetically more susceptible to radiation damage (Brenner et al. 2003). The increasing slope theory is used to explain current leukemia data (Pierce and Preston 2000).

A *threshold model* predicts a negligible risk below a threshold dose. The 95% confidence interval for a threshold level includes a range between 0 and 60 mSv (Pierce and Preston 2000). This model fits current sarcoma data (Preston et al. 2007).

Finally, the *hormesis model* predicts protective effects below a threshold dose, even for non-cancer deaths (Feinendegen 2005). It has been shown that low-dose radiation can increase the production of enzymes that repair DNA damage, can stimulate apoptosis (= the suicide) of damaged cells, stimulate human T killer lymphocytes and stimulate scavenging processes of corrosive chemicals out of cells. The absolute amount of these positive effects, however, is controversial, and hormesis is currently not considered for risk estimations of low dose exposures (National Research Council Committee on the Biological Effects of Ionizing Radiations 2005; Brenner et al. 2003).

Because it is probably more prudent to overestimate the radiation-induced risk than to underestimate it, most authors to date have opted for the LNT for risk estimation.

No risk has been proven epidemiologically for the CT dose range <20 mSv. To be more precise: radiation dose <5 mSv was considered negligible in the LSS data. However, an increased cancer risk even at low radiation is extremely likely, at least for a more radiation-sensitive subpopulation (Hendrick 2010). Estimates of cancer risk are regularly updated and released by the US National Academy of Sciences on Biological Effects of Ionizing Radiation (BEIR VII group) and the International Commission on Radiation Protection (IRCP). While the 2007 ICRP risk estimates used sex- and age-averaged data, the most recent BEIR VII report also includes the age-dependence of radiation-induced cancer incidence and mortality (National Research Council of the National Academics 2006). The BEIR VII stated that "low dose induced genetic risks are very small when compared to baseline risks in the population" meaning that genetic risks can be neglected when considering a CT screening setting. The BEIR VII also stated that knowledge based on the epidemiologic, animal and mechanistic studies so far tends to favor a simple proportionate relationship at low doses between radiation dose and cancer risk (National Research Council of the National Academics 2006).

## 2 Risk Estimates

Radiation risk is expressed as excess relative risk (ERR) or excess absolute risk (EAR). Given a baseline cancer risk (incidence or mortality) of $\lambda$, the risk after exposure to a certain radiation dose D can be expressed as

**Table 1** List of lung cancer screening trials with details about acquisition parameters and number of follow-up CT

| | | | | | Inclusion | | | Definition LDCT | Rounds of FU | Length of FU (years) | Detected lungcancer |
|---|---|---|---|---|---|---|---|---|---|---|---|
| | Study | Trial period | Study type | No. of participants | Age (years) | Pack years | KV | mA | | | |
| Hitachi employee's health insurance | Nawa et al. (2002) | 1998–2000 | Non randomized, | 7,956 | 50–70 | Smoking history | 120 | 50 | | | 41 (0.44%) |
| | | | Cohort | | | | | | | | |
| Local (Milano) | Pastorino et al. (2003) | | Non randomized, | 1,035 | >50 | >20 | 140 | 40 | 1, 2, 3, 4, 5 | 5 | 440 (29%) |
| | | | Cohort | | | | | | | | |
| | Gohagan et al. (2004) | 2000–2001 | RCT | 3,318 | 55–74 | >30 | 120/140 | 60 | | | 30 (2%) |
| | | | LDCT vs CXR | | | | | | | | 7 (0.4%) |
| | Diederich et al. (2004) | | Non randomized, | 817 | >40 | >20 | 120 | 50 | 1, 2, 3 | 3 | 10 (1.2%) |
| | | | Cohort | | | | | | | | |
| | Swensen et al. (2005) | 1999–2003 | Non randomized, | 1,520 | >50 | >20 | 120 | 40 | 1, 2, 3, 4, 5 | 5 | 68 (4.5%) |
| | | | Cohort | | | | | | | | |
| Local (Turin) | Cardinale et al. (2005) | 2001–2003 | Non randomized, | 519 | >55 | Smoking history | | | 1, 2, 3, 4, 5 | 5 | 6 (1.2%) |
| | | | Cohort | | | | | | | | |
| | Chong et al. (2005) | 1999–2003 | Non randomized, | 6,406 | >45 | >20 | 120 | 40/50 | | | 23 (0.36%) |
| | | | Cohort | | | | | | | | |
| | MacRedmond et al. (2006) | | Non randomized, | 449 | >45 | >10 | | 50 | 1, 2 | 2 | 6 (1.3%) |
| | | | Cohort | | | | | | | | |
| ELCAP | NY ELCAP (2007) | 2000–2003 | Non randomized, | 6,295 | >60 | >10 | 120 | 40 | | | 124 (1.9%) |
| | | | Cohort | | | | | | | | |

(continued)

**Table 1** (continued)

| | | | | | Inclusion | | | Definition LDCT | Rounds of FU | Length of FU (years) | Detected lungcancer |
|---|---|---|---|---|---|---|---|---|---|---|---|
| | Study | Trial period | Study type | No. of participants | Age (years) | Pack years | KV | mA | | | |
| Depiscan | Blanchon et al. (2007) | 2002–2004 | RCT | 765 | 50–75 | >20 | 100–140 | 20–100 | 1, 2, 3, 4, 5 | 2 | 8 (2.4%) |
| | | | LDCT vs CXR | | | | | | | | 1 (0.4%) |
| COSMOS | Veronesi et al. (2008) | 2004–2006 | Non randomized, | 5,201 | 50–8 | >20 | | | 1, 2, 3, 4, 5 | 1 | 79 (1.5%) |
| | | | Cohort | | | | | | | | |
| ITALUNG | Lopes Pegna et al. (2009) | | RCT | 3,206 | 55–69 | >20 | 120 | 50 | 1, 2, 3, 4 | 4 | 21 (1.5%) |
| | | | LDCT vs no screening | | | | | | | | |
| DANTE | Infante et al. (2009) | 2001–2006 | RCT | 2,472 | 60–75 | >20 | 140 | 40 | 1, 2, 3, 4, 5 | 4 | 60 (4.7%) |
| | | | LDCT vs no screening | | | | | | | | 34 (2.8%) |
| DLCST | Pedersen et al. (2009) | 2004–2008 | RCT | 4,104 | | >20 | 120 | 40 | 1, 2, 3, 4, 5 | 5 | 17 (0.8%) |
| | | | LDCT vs no screening | | | | | | | | |
| | Menezes et al. (2010) | 2003–2007 | Non randomized, | 3,352 | >50 | >10 | 120 | 40/60 | | | 62 (1.8%) |
| | | | Cohort | | | | | | | | |
| NLST | NLST (2011) | 2002–2009 | RCT | 53,454 | 55–74 | >30 | 120–140 | 40/80 | 1, 2, 3 | 3 | 1,060 (4%) |
| | | | LDCT vs CXR | | | | | | | | 941 (3.4%) |
| UK | Baldwin et al. (2011) | 2011–current | RCT | | 50–75 | | 90–140 | | 1 | | |
| | | | LDCT vs usual care | | | | | | | | |

(continued)

**Table 1** (continued)

| | Study | Trial period | Study type | No. of participants | Inclusion Age (years) | Pack years | KV | Definition LDCT mA | Rounds of FU | Length of FU (years) | Detected lungcancer |
|---|---|---|---|---|---|---|---|---|---|---|---|
| LUSI (germany) | Becker et al. (2008) | 2007–curent | RCT | 4,000 | 50–69 | >40 | | | 1, 2, 3, 4, 5 | 5 | |
| | | | LDCT vs usual care | | | | | | | | |
| MILD Italy | Pastorino et al. (2006) | 2005–current | RCT | 4,479 | 49–75 | | 120–140 | 20–60 | Yearly of every 2 years | 10 | |
| | | | LDCT vs usual care | | | | | | | | |
| Nelson | van Klaveren et al. (2009) | 2003–2006 | RCT | 15,822 | 50–74 | >15–18.75 | 80–140 | 20 | 1, 2, 4 | 5 | |
| | | | LDCT vs no screening | | | | | | | | |

$$\lambda(D) = \lambda[1 + \text{ERR}(D)] = \lambda + \text{EAR}(D)$$

In general, baseline cancer risk ($\lambda$) depends on age and sex of an individual as well as on population-specific factors (such as smoking status). The cancer risk after exposure to ionizing radiation depends on the age at exposure to radiation, the radiation dose as well as sex and current age of the individual. Excess relative risk (ERR) gives a multiplicative risk while excess absolute risk (EAR) provides an absolute risk.

The lifetime attributable risk (LAR) estimates the probability that an individual will develop or die from a cancer associated with the exposure. The LAR is calculated by summing the ERR for each age (a) from age of exposure (e) to 100 years, weighted by the age- and sex-specific cancer rates [$\lambda$(a)] and the probability of survival S(a) to each age:

$$\text{LAR} = \Sigma\, \text{ERR}\ (D,\ e,\ a)\ \lambda\ (a)\ S(a)/S(e)$$

It has to be noted that LAR has been calculated for the general population but not for a population with reduced probability of survival. Radiation risks in clinical patients with a serious illness therefore would have a lower LAR than the general population. Similarly, heavy smokers do have a reduced probability of survival, not only due to higher lung cancer risks but also due to COPD and cardiovascular as well as many other smoking-induced illnesses. The LAR therefore poses an *upper limit* for radiation-induced cancer risk in smokers.

The age-dependence of cancer risks has been revised numerous times (Pastorino 2010; National Research Council Committee on the Biological Effects of Ionizing Radiations 2005; Brenner et al. 2003). It also strongly depends on the mathematical models used to predict ERR. Models are based on epidemiologic, animal and mechanistic studies and may vary substantially with respect to the resulting ERR and LAR. As a consequence, there may be substantial errors that have to be taken into account when interpreting actual risk calculations. All estimates demonstrate substantial increase in cancer incidence and mortality for young individuals exposed at an age below 30. For a screening population with an age above 50, the cancer incidence is much lower than for the general population. However, some predictions show a continuous decrease of risk at all ages, others demonstrate a relative plateau in the age range between 30 and 60 years that is mainly

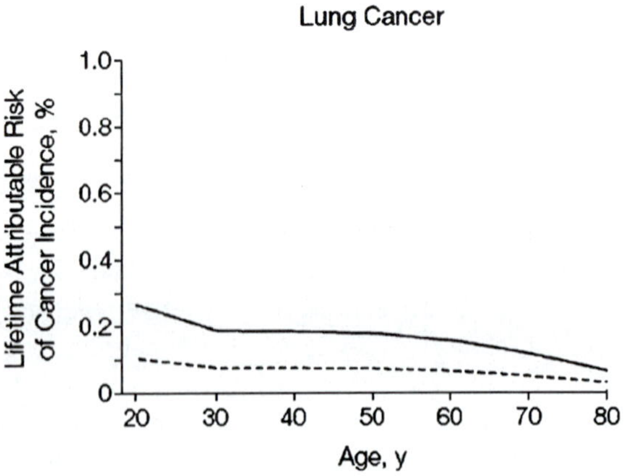


**Fig. 1** Dependence of lifetime attributable risk of cancer incidence and age: note that the risk for lung cancer remains almost constant for the ages of 40–70 (modified from Einstein A, Jama, 2007; 298(3) 317, Fig. 2)

caused by the increasing risk for developing lung cancer at that age range (Brenner 2004).

Most types of cancer have the highest excess cancer mortality when the exposure happened at a young age. Lung cancer, however, has the highest excess cancer mortality in the age range between 40 and 70, which makes it the dominant cause for cancer induction in the older age group (National Research Council 1990; Thompson et al. 1994). In the context of risk estimations for CT lung screening therefore two additional aspects have to be considered: there is a near multiplicative interaction or at best an intermediate interaction (between additive and multiplicative) between the increased background cancer risk and the risk from radiation [Br (Gilbert et al. 2003; Ford et al. 2003; Tokarskaya et al. 2002)]. Further on, the risk for females is substantially higher than for males (Fig. 1).

Table 1 summarizes the lifetime cancer risks (LAR) for an unselected population that has similar characteristics as the general US population and was exposed to 100 mSv at age 50, derived from the preliminary BEIR VII risk tables. These risk estimates are compared to the baseline risk for the same population.

## 3 Individual Risk Versus Population Risk

Various recent studies have used the LNT to estimate radiation-induced cancer rates in the general population. All the limitations of the LNT apply. In addition, little attention has been paid to the individual mortality risks of the examined population: many of the exposed individuals suffer from serious illnesses such as cancer or cardiovascular disease, which carry a substantial mortality in themselves.

A report from Oxford estimated that cancers induced by diagnostic X-rays contributed to as much as 3.2% of all cancers in Japan, causing 7,587 cases per year (Berrington de Gonzalez and Darby 2004). Numbers were considerable smaller in the United Kingdom or in Germany (2,049 cases, 0.6% attributable risk in the UK and 2,049 cases, 1.5% attributable risk in Germany). Radiation from CT scans was responsible for the largest number of cases of the nine listed cancers in that statistical analysis.

For diagnostic tests the immediate risk of not performing a test must be compared to the small individual risk of side effects from the test itself. In a clinical setting the advantages clearly outperform the risk. Take the risk for pulmonary embolism, for example: the mortality risk may be up to 30% if untreated, the diagnosis may be delayed or missed without imaging in up to 70% of cases. Recurrent embolism rates are <1% if CT is negative (Goodman et al. 2000). Radiation dose is 1–7 mSv, depending on the examination technique. The calculated LAR for cancer incidence at that dose, averaged over the age range of the US population, is in the range of 0.01–0.1%, depending on gender and the chosen dose settings for the scan. For elderly patients the risk is substantially less.

The individual risk to the patient caused by radiation exposure induced by screening is very small compared to the baseline risk of developing a specific type of cancer (Table 2). However, when looking at large groups of people exposed to ionizing radiation, this population effect may no longer be negligible. A small excess mortality risk (LAR) of 0.05% for an individual translates into 50 radiation-induced deaths per 100,000 population exposed. Such a risk is in the order of magnitude of a single abdominal CT exam with an effective dose of 10 mSv.

In a screening population, a number of special considerations have to be made: the subjects are usually of older age and have a higher prevalence and incidence of a certain disease (e.g. lung cancer, COPD and cardiovascular disease in smokers). When calculating risk, a linear model is usually applied and the effective dose can be used as a good starting point to derive risks from data such as those given in Table 1. However, the

**Table 2** Lifetime attributable cancer risk (LAR) for the general US population (1999) exposed at age 50 to a radiation dose of 100 mSv

| | | Incident | | Mortality | |
|---|---|---|---|---|---|
| | | Men | Women | Men | Women |
| All cancers | Baseline risk | 46,330 | 37,490 | 22,810 | 18,030 |
| All cancers | LAR | 594 | 742 | 361 | 474 |
| Leukemia | Baseline risk | 830 | 590 | 710 | 530 |
| Leukemia | LAR | 84 | 62 | 71 | 54 |
| Solid cancers | Baseline risk | 45,500 | 36,900 | 22,100 | 17,500 |
| Solid cancers | LAR | 510 | 680 | 290 | 420 |
| Lung cancer | Baseline risk | 7,700 | 5,400 | 7,700 | 4,600 |
| Lung cancer | LAR | 140 | 300 | 140 | 270 |

Incidence and mortality data are provided per 100,000 individuals exposed. For comparison the baseline risk for the same population is provided as well. Data adapted from the BEIR VII report (Pastorino 2010)

temporal profile of the dose exposure is different: protracted exposures are associated with lower risks of cancer than those of an acute exposure to the same total dose (Brenner 2004). In addition, the latent period between radiation exposure and cancer death increases with decreasing exposure and it is possible that for low doses the latent period exceeds the normal life span (Cohen 2002).

This has to be weighted against the fact that radiation risk for lung cancer peaks at 40–70 years of age and that screening exams have to be repeated at certain time intervals. While radiation-induced cancer rates generally decrease with advancing age, the relative risk of radiation-induced lung cancer peaks at the age of 50–60, which leads to a plateau of LAR for exposures between age 40 and 60 (Brenner 2004). For lung cancer screening, radiation-induced lung cancer becomes the dominant risk in the relevant age group (Brenner 2004). This leads to a discrepancy between risk estimates derived from effective exposure and risk estimates derived from organ exposures. The risk model and the model of risk transport strongly affect the outcome of such calculations and lead to substantial error margins (up to a factor of three and more) (Brenner 2004).

## 4 Risk–Benefit Analysis

As a consequence of what said so far, the population risk, given as calculated number of deaths from radiation-induced cancer per 100,000 subjects exposed to CT screening, may not be negligible. The radiation-induced risk of CT cancer screening depends on age, sex, organ system, dose per examination, number of examinations and time interval between examinations (National Research Council Committee on the Biological Effects of Ionizing Radiations 2005). This has to be weighed against the spontaneous risk for developing a cancer, which varies from organ to organ and is also sex-dependent. For lung cancer, the risk is additionally influenced by smoking status: when a the relative risk of developing lung cancer is assumed to be 1.0 for current smokers, this risk decreases in ex-smokers (0.089 in men and 0.37 in women) and never smokers (0.042 in men and 0.196 in women) (Crispo et al. 2004). This dependence on smoking status is stronger in males than in females, indicating that cancer risk in never smoking males is more than 20 times smaller than in currently smoking males, while the corresponding risk reduction in females is only a factor of five.

Inclusion of nonsmokers therefore has an impact on risk–benefit analysis because the percentage of screening-detected cancers should be lower if nonsmokers are included. This is in accordance with reported cancer rates in studies that included non-smokers: instead of a cancer detection rates of 1–5% if only smokers are included, rates for mixed studies have reported cancer rates of $0.4 = -0.5\%$ (Chong et al. 2005, Japan).

Brenner provided estimates for lung cancer, colon cancer and full body CT screening that were based on published doses per examination as well as some estimates about start of screening and frequency of screening examinations (Brenner 2004; Brenner and

Georgsson 2005; Brenner and Elliston 2004). The overall results were more favorable for colon cancer screening than for lung cancer screening.

For 50-year-old female current smoker, Brenner estimated the Lifetime Attributable Risk (LAR) for a single lung cancer screening exam with a lung dose of approximately 5 mGy to be 0.055% ca. 1 in 1,800 screened subjects in a 50-year-old female smoker, and for a 50-year-old male former smoker to be ca. 0.012% (ca. 1 in 8,300 screened subjects) (Brenner 2004). These risks fell below 0.01% for a female smoker at age 70 and well below 0.005% for a former male smoker of the same age.

Although these risks compare favorably with those from a pair of prone and supine CT colonography examinations (0.14% at age 50 and 0.07% at age 70), the number of scans advised for lung cancer screening will probably be much higher than for colon cancer screening. Lung cancer screening is usually performed every 1–2 years (http://www.cancer.gov/statistics; Detterbeck et al. 2009; National Lung Screening Trial Research Team 2011) while colon cancer screening examinatios are performed every 3–5 years because of a substantially longer lead time before a colonic polyp will develop into a cancer. When starting at age 50 and ending at age 75, a person entering a colon cancer screening program will incur an excess cancer risk of approximately 0.14% (Melamad et al. 1984). A person entering a lung cancer screening program at age 50 and ending at age 75 can expect to receive 12–25 scans (not to mention those required to assess growth of nodules found at screening) while a person in a CT colonography program will receive between 5 and 8 scans.

As a result, Brenner estimated a LAR for a 50-year-old female smoker entering a yearly lung cancer screening program to amount up to 0.85% (ca. 1 in 120 screened subjects). This number is still substantially lower than the estimated background lung cancer risk of 16.9% in such a person, but it becomes a relevant issue for the effectiveness of such screening programs (Brenner 2004). If 50% of all current and former smokers in the US population aged 50–75 years received annual screening, the estimated number of lung cancers associated with radiation from screening would amount to 36,000. This means a 1.8% increase over the otherwise expected number with 95% intervals of 0.5–5.5%. Brenner therefore postulated that the mortality benefit of a screening program has to be substantially higher than 5% to outweigh the potential radiation risk. Given the mortality reduction of 20% found in the NLST trial, this condition would be fulfilled.

It also has to be noted that the assumptions made by Brenner are on the conservative side. His calculations were based on a single low-dose CT of the chest with a dose of 2.5–9 mGy (mean 5 mGy) with correspondingly increased total doses for repeat examinations ranging between 25 and 90 mGy (mean of 50 mGy for 10 repeat examinations). Reducing the exposure to below 1 mGy per examination, a number that is within reach with modern scanners and iterative reconstruction techniques, the calculated cancer risks would be reduced by a factor of five to an LAR of 0.17% for a 50-year-old female smoker. One has to also keep in mind that the radiation dose would then be well below the 5 mSv threshold used in the A-bomb survivor data and well below the average effective dose of about 3 mSv per year from natural background radiation in the United States (Mettler et al. 2009).

For the Italung-CT trial (one of three screening trails in Italy) a risk–benefit analysis of X-ray exposure associated with lung cancer screening was published (Mascalchi et al. 2006). The cumulative effective dose using MDCT was calculated to be 3.3 mSv (120 kV, 20 mAs, 1.1–1.2 mSv per examination). Calculation included the baseline CT and a certain number of CT follow up examinations for nodules >5 mm seen during the baseline examination taking the incidence data from the ELCAP study into account and assuming a 4-year screening program. Potential fatal cancers induced by radiation exposure were calculated to be 0.11 per 1,000 subjects, which is 10–100 times lower than the number of expected lives saved by screening assuming a 20–30% lung cancer-specific mortality reduction in current smokers. Noteworthy is that the risk–benefit ratio, however, was less favorable for never-smokers or former smokers, assuming a 10% efficacy of screening and a similar magnitude of lives at risk and lives saved by screening.

An advantageous risk–benefit ratio is well documented for digital screening mammography: a two-view digital mammogram involves an average mean glandular radiation dose of 3.7 mGy that is associated with a LAR of fatal breast cancer of 1.3 per 100,000 women aged 40 years at exposure and less than one case per one million women aged 80 years at exposure. Annual screening in women aged 40–80 years is associated with a LAR of fatal breast cancer of 20–25 cases in 100,000. These numbers by far outweigh a cancer detection rate that was estimated to be around 30% per 1,000 (Vaino H Bianchini 2002).

## 5 Dose Containment

When performing CT screening examinations, it is obvious that dose containment is mandatory. Low-dose scanning is possible for the lungs and the colon because of high contrast between gas and soft tissues. Nodule detection decreases only slightly when very low dose is used and nodule volumetry appears to be stable even at high noise levels. Doses as low as 0.12 mSv have been suggested (Gergely et al. 2005), which would reduce cancer risks by more than a factor of 20.

Some radiologists, especially in a litigation-prone environment, will prefer less radical measures because interpretation of images containing a lot of image noise may be difficult. Recent technical advances in CT have made it possible to obtain a predefined image quality at reduced dose levels. These developments include improved efficiency of the detector systems (detector material as well as collimation and electronics), adaptive dose modulation in the xy-plane and z-direction, dose adaptation to patient size, and adaptive noise reducing filters and iterative image reconstruction that work on raw and image data.

Dose modulation in the scan plane (XY modulation) varies the tube current as the X-ray tube rotates around the body: in regions with a reduced diameter, for example the AP direction in the shoulder region, the tube current is reduced, while in regions with an increased diameter, for example the lateral direction in the shoulder region, the tube current is increased. The technique reduces streak artifacts and can reduce radiation dose by an average of approximately 20% without affecting signal-to-noise ratios (Kalender et al. 1999).

Dose modulation in the Z-direction (Z-modulation) varies the tube current as the scan progresses along the patient axis: in regions with reduced absorption, for example the neck or the mid-chest, tube current is reduced, while in regions with high absorption, for example, the shoulders or the pelvis, tube current is increased. The technique ensures constant image quality independent of the body region and can reduce radiation dose by more than 50% in low-absorption areas such as the lung (Kalra et al. 2005). It can contribute to a reduction in organ dose to the lungs that is more pronounced than that indicated by the dose-length product (DLP) or the average $CTDI_{vol}$ of the examination.

Adaptation of the dose to patient size (automated exposure control) adjusts the general setting of the tube current to the size of the patient. The technique ensures constant image quality independent of patient size (Mulkens et al. 2005). Individual dose adaptation is essential at low doses because rapid loss of quality may occur if the dose chosen is too low. In addition, individual adaptation of dose avoids overdosing thin patients and underdosing obese patients. In general one should use the lowest possible dose level to achieve the desired tasks. However, there are few guidelines as to how high the noise and thus, how low the dose can be without loosing diagnostic information.

Adaptive filtering of the raw data can also reduce streak artifacts and can ensure more homogeneous image quality. The technique locally averages raw data for high absorption, and therefore, high-noise projections, that way substantially improving the signal-to-noise ratio in the resulting image. It works best in regions with substantial differences in local absorption such as the shoulders or the pelvis (Kachelriess et al. 2001). Post-processing filters work on reconstructed image data and use edge-preserving algorithms to locally reduce image noise without excessively blurring the image (Hu et al. 2011; Honda et al. 2011; Pontana et al. 2011). Iterative image reconstruction techniques further improve image quality at low dose. They allow for substantially reducing radiation exposure. An effective dose of well below 1 mSv becomes possible for lung cancer screening with modern CT equipment.

Combinations of these techniques are now available for most vendors and should help improve image quality even at low radiation doses. For full-body screening, dose containment will remain problematic but lung and colon cancer screening will be possible at dose levels that are more than five times below the ones that have been used in the calculation of cancer risks in screening cohorts (Brenner 2004; Brenner and Georgsson 2005; Brenner and Elliston 2004).

## 6 Summary

If performed in a dose-conscious fashion, individual risks with lung cancer screening are very small. While there is no and probably never will be epidemiologic evidence for cancer induction in the dose range used for a single lung cancer screening examination, a non-negligible population risk may be postulated considering current evidence. Precise predictions of cancer risks are difficult because they depend heavily on the used mathematical model. Lung cancer plays a special role for the cancer risk in a typical screening population because its relative risk peaks in the time interval between 40 and 70 years of age.

When basing risk assessment on organ dose and the LNT, risks for lung cancer development caused by yearly screening CT examinations may be substantial if screening is performed over long periods of time at doses currently discussed in the literature. This is especially important for long-term follow-up in patients with slow-growing subsolid nodules that are likely to represent indolent tumors (Godoy and Naidich 2009).

On the other hand, most recent technical advances in dose saving strategies have not yet been considered in the publications on radiation-induced cancer risks. There is the potential for substantial dose reduction up to a factor of 5–20, which would make risk—benefit estimates more attractive. As the radiation exposure is reduced to below 1 mSv, the risk estimates from A-bomb survivors have too large an error rate to be of scientific value. Radiobiological models indicate that risks at such very low levels of radiation may not be correctly estimated using the LNT.

In the future, CT lung cancer screening may evolve into chest screening and also assesses cardiovascular risk, COPD, or osteoporosis. This will further tilt the balance of risk and benefits toward the benefits of screening. At the same time, very low dose techniques may reduce risk below levels that can be scientifically assessed.

## References

Baldwin DR, Duffy SW, Wald NJ, Page R, Hansell DM, Field JK (2011) UK lung screen (UKLS) nodule management protocol: modelling of a single screen randomised controlled trial of low-dose CT screening for lung cancer. Thorax 66(4):308–313

Becker N, Delorme S, Kauczor HU (2008) LUSI: the German component of the European trial on the efficacy of multislice-CT for the early detection of lung cancer. Onkologie 31:PO320

Berrington de Gonzalez A, Darby S (2004) Risk of cancer from diagnostic X-rays: estimates for the UK and 14 other countries. Lancet 363:345–351 Oxford

Blanchon T, Bréchot JM, Grenier PA, Ferretti GR, Lemarié E, Milleron B, Chagué D, Laurent F, Martinet Y, Beigelman-Aubry C, Blanchon F, Revel MP, Friard S, Rémy-Jardin M, Vasile M, Santelmo N, Lecalier A, Lefébure P, Moro-Sibilot D, Breton JL, Carette MF, Brambilla C, Fournel F, Kieffer A, Frija G, Flahault A, Dépiscan Group (2007) Baseline results of the depiscan study: a French randomized pilot trial of lung cancer screening comparing low dose CT scan (LDCT) and chest X-ray (CXR). Lung Cancer 58(1): 50–58

Brenner DJ (2004) Radiation risks potentially associated with low-dose CT screening of adult smokers for lung cancer. Radiology 231:440–445

Brenner DJ, Elliston CD (2004) Estimated radiation risks potentially associated with full-body CT screening. Radiology 232:735–738

Brenner DJ, Georgsson MA (2005) Mass screening with CT colonography: should the radiation exposure be of concern? Gastroenterology 129:328–337

Brenner DJ, Doll R, Goodhead DT, Hall EJ, Land CE, Little JB, Lubin JH, Preston DL, Preston RJ, Puskin JS, Ron E, Sachs RK, Samet JM, Setlow RB, Zaider M (2003) Cancer risks attributable to low doses of ionizing radiation: assessing what we really know. Proc Natl Acad Sci (PNAS) 100:13761–13766

Cardinale L, Cortese G, Borasio P, Dogliotti L, Ferraris F, Novello S, Perotto F, Scagliotti G, Fava C (2005) Low dose CT in early lung cancer diagnosis: prevalence data. Radiol Med 110(5–6):532–543

Chong S, Lee KS, Chung MJ, Kim TS et al (2005) Lung cancer screening with low-dose helical CT in Korea: experiences at the samsung medical center. J Korean Med Sci 20(3): 402–408

Cohen BI (2002) Cancer risk from low level radiation. AJR 179:1137–1143

Crispo A, Brennan P, Jöckel KH et al (2004) The cumulative risk of lung cancer among current, ex- and never-smokers in European men. Br J Cancer 91(7):1280–1286

Detterbeck FC, Boffa DJ, Tanoue LT (2009) The new lung cancer staging system. Chest 136:260–271

Diederich S, Thomas M, Semik M, Lenzen H, Roos N, Weber A, Heindel W, Wormanns D (2004) Screening for early lung cancer with low-dose spiral computed tomography: results of annual follow-up examinations in asymptomatic smokers. Eur Radiol 14(4):691–702

Feinendegen LE (2005) Evidence for beneficial low level radiation effects and radiation hormesis. Br J Radiol 78(925): 3–7

Ford MB, Sigurdson AJ, petrulis ES et al (2003) Effect of smoking and radiotherapy on lung carcinoma in breast cancer survivors. Cancer 98:1457–1464

Gergely I, Neumann C, Reiger F, Dorffner R (2005) Lung nodule detection with ultra-low-dose CT in routine follow-up of cancer patients. Rofo 177(8):1077–1083

Gilbert ES, Stovall M, Gospodarowicz M et al (2003) Lung cancer after treatment for Hofgkin's disease: focus on radiation effects. Radiat Res 159:151–173

Godoy MC, Naidich DP (2009) Subsolid pulmonary nodules and the spectrum of peripheral adenocarcinomas of the lung: recommended interim guidelines for assessment and management. Radiology 253(3):606–622, Review

Gohagan J, Marcus P, Fagerstrom R, Pinsky P, Kramer B, Prorok P, Writing Committee, Lung Screening Study Research Group (2004) Baseline findings of a randomized feasibility trial of lung cancer screening with spiral CT scan vs chest radiograph: the lung screening study of the national cancer institute. Chest 126(1):114–121

Goodman LR, Lipchik RJ, Kuzo RS, Liu Y, McAuliffe TL, O'Brien DJ (2000) Subsequent pulmonary embolism: risk after a negative helical CT pulmonary angiogram—prospective comparison with scintigraphy. Radiology 215: 535–542

Hendrick RE (2010) Radiation doses and cancer risks from breast imaging studies. Radiology 257:246–253

Henschke CI, McCauley DI, Yankelevitz DF et al (1999) Early lung cancer action project: overall design and findings from baseline screening. Lancet 354:99–105

Honda O, Yanagawa M, Inoue A et al (2011) Image quality of multiplanar reconstruction of pulmonary CT scans using adaptive statistical iterative reconstruction. Br J Radiol 84(1000):335–341

Hu XH, Ding XF, Wu RZ, Zhang MM (2011) Radiation dose of non-enhanced chest CT can be reduced 40% by using iterative reconstruction in image space. Clin Radiol 66(11): 1023–1029

Infante M, Cavuto S, Lutman FR, Brambilla G, Chiesa G, Ceresoli G, Passera E, Angeli E, Chiarenza M, Aranzulla G, Cariboni U, Errico V, Inzirillo F, Bottoni E, Voulaz E, Alloisio M, Destro A, Roncalli M, Santoro A, Ravasi G, DANTE Study Group (2009) A randomized study of lung cancer screening with spiral computed tomography: three-year results from the DANTE trial. Am J Respir Crit Care Med 180(5):445–453

Jett RJ (2005) Limitations of screening for lung cancer with low-dose spiral computed tomography. Clin Cancer Res 11:4988s–4992s

Kachelriess M, Watzke O, Kalender WA (2001) Generalized multi-dimensional adaptive filtering for conventional and spiral single-slice, multi-slice, and cone-beam CT. Med Phys 28:475–490

Kalender WA, Wolf H, Suess C, Gies M, Greess H, Bautz WA (1999) Dose reduction in CT by on-line tube current control: principles and validation on phantoms and cadavers. Eur Radiol 9(2):323–328

Kalra MK, Rizzo S, Maher MM, Halpern EF, Toth TL, Shepard JA, Aquino SL (2005) Chest CT performed with Z-axis modulation: scanning protocol and radiation dose. Radiology 237:303–308

Kramer BS, Berg CD, Aberle DR, Prorok PC (2011) Lung cancer screening with low-dose helical CT: results from the national lung screening trial (NLST). J Med Screen 18(3): 109–111

Little JB (1999) Induction of genetic instability by ionizing radiation. C R Acad Sci III 322:127–134

Lopes Pegna A, Picozzi G, Mascalchi M, Maria Carozzi F, Carrozzi L, Comin C, Spinelli C, Falaschi F, Grazzini M, Innocenti F, Ronchi C, Paci E, ITALUNG Study Research Group (2009) Design, recruitment and baseline results of the ITALUNG trial for lung cancer screening with low-dose CT. Lung Cancer 64(1):34–40

MacRedmond R, McVey G, Lee M, Costello RW, Kenny D, Foley C, Logan PM (2006) Screening for lung cancer using low dose CT scanning: results of 2 year follow up. Thorax 61(1):54–56

Marcus PM, Bergstralh EJ, Zweig MH et al (2006) Extended lung cancer incidence follow-up in the Mayo lung project and overdiagnosis. J Nat Cancer Inst 98:748–756

Mascalchi M, Belli G, Zappa M et al (2006) Risk-Benefit analysis of X-ray exposure associated with lung cancer screening in the ITALUNG CT trial. AJR 187:421–429

Melamad MR, Flehinger BJ, Zaman MB et al (1984) Screening for lung cancer; results of the Memorial Sloan Kettering study in New York. Chest 86:44–53

Menezes RJ, Roberts HC, Paul NS, McGregor M, Chung TB, Patsios D, Weisbrod G, Herman S, Pereira A, McGregor A, Dong Z, Sitartchouk I, Boerner S, Tsao MS, Keshavjee S, Shepherd FA (2010) Lung cancer screening using low-dose computed tomography in at-risk individuals: the Toronto experience. Lung Cancer 7(2):177–183

Mettler FA, Bhargavan M, Faulkner K et al (2009) Radiologic and nuclear medicine studies in the United States and worldwide: frequency, radiation dose and comparison with other radiation sources—1950–2007. Radiology 253:520–531

Mulkens TH, Bellinck P, Baeyaert M, Ghysen D, Van Dijck X, Mussen E, Venstermans C, Termote JL (2005) Use of an automatic exposure control mechanism for dose optimization in multi-detector row CT examinations: clinical evaluation. Radiology 237(1):213–223

National Lung Screening Trial Research Team (2011) The national lung screening trial: overview and study design. Radiology 258:243–253

National Research Council (1990) Committee on the biological effects of ionizing radiations. Health effects of exposure to low levels of ionizing radiation: BEIR V. National Academy Press, Washington, DC

National Research Council Committee on the Biological Effects of Ionizing Radiations (2005) Health effects of exposure to low levels of ionizing radiation: BEIR VII. National Academy Press, Washington, DC

National Research Council of the National Academics (2006) Health risks from exposure to low levels of ionizing radiation. BEIR VII, phase 2—Committee to assess health risks from exposure to low levels of ionizing radiation. National Academic Press, Washington, DC

Nawa T, Nakagawa T, Kusano S, Kawasaki Y, Sugawara Y, Nakata H (2002) Lung cancer screening using low-dose spiral CT: results of baseline and 1-year follow-up studies. Chest 122(1):15–20

New York Early Lung Cancer Action Project Investigators (2007) CT screening for lung cancer: diagnoses resulting from the New York early lung cancer action project. Radiology 243(1):239–249

Pastorino U (2010) Lung cancer screening (mini review). Br J Cancer 102:1681–1686

Pastorino U, Bellomi M, Landoni C, De Fiori E, Arnaldi P, Picchio M, Pelosi G, Boyle P, Fazio F (2003) Early lung-cancer detection with spiral CT and positron emission tomography in heavy smokers: 2-year results. Lancet 362(9384):593–597

Pastorino U (2006) Early detection of lung cancer. Respiration 73(1):5–13

Pedersen JH, Ashraf H, Dirksen A, Bach K, Hansen H, Toennesen P, Thorsen H, Brodersen J, Skov BG, Døssing M, Mortensen J, Richter K, Clementsen P, Seersholm N (2009) The Danish randomized lung cancer CT screening trial—overall design and results of the prevalence round. J Thorac Oncol 4(5):608–614

Pierce DA, Preston DL (2000) Radiation-related cancer risks at low doses among atomic bomb survivors. Radiat Res 154: 178–186

Pontana F, Pagniez J, Flohr T et al (2011) Chest computed tomography using iterative reconstruction vs filtered back projection (Part 1): evaluation of image noise reduction in 32 patients. Eur Radiol 21(3):627–635

Preston DL, Ron E, Tokuoka S, Funamoto S, Nishi N, Soda M, Mabuchi K, Kodama K (2007) Solid cancer incidence in atomic bomb survivors: 1958–1998. Radiat Res 168(1): 1–64

Reduced lung-cancer mortality with low-dose computed tomographic screening (2011) The national lung screening trial research team. NEJM 365:395–409

Swensen SJ, Jett JR, Hartman TE, Midthun DE, Mandrekar SJ, Hillman SL, Sykes AM, Aughenbaugh GL, Bungum AO, Allen KL (2005) CT screening for lung cancer: five-year prospective experience. Radiology 235(1):259–265

Thompson DE, Mabuchi K, Ron E et al (1994) Cancer incidence in atomiv bomb survivors. Part II. Solid tumors, 1958–1987. Rad Res 137(suppl 2):S17–S67

Tokarskaya ZB, Scott BR, Zhuntova GV et al (2002) Interaction of radiation and smoking in lung cancer induction among workers at the Mayak nuclear enterprise. Health Phys 83:833–846

Tubiana M, Feinendegen LE, Yang C, Kamisnki JM (2009) The linear no-threshold is inconsistent with radiation biologic and experimental data. Radiology 251:13–22

Vaino H, Bianchini F (eds) (2002) International agency for the research on Cancer. Breast cancer screening handbook of cancer prevention, vol 7. International Agency for the Research on Cancer, Lyon, pp 91–107

van Klaveren RJ, Oudkerk M, Prokop M, Scholten ET, Nackaerts K, Vernhout R, van Iersel CA, van den Bergh KA, van 't Westeinde S, van der Aalst C, Thunnissen E, Xu DM, Wang Y, Zhao Y, Gietema HA, de Hoop BJ, Groen HJ, de Bock GH, van Ooijen P, Weenink C, Verschakelen J, Lammers JW, Timens W, Willebrand D, Vink A, Mali W, de Koning HJ (2009) Management of lung nodules detected by volume CT scanning. N Engl J Med 361(23):2221–2229

Veronesi G, Bellomi M, Mulshine JL, Pelosi G, Scanagatta P, Paganelli G, Maisonneuve P, Preda L, Leo F, Bertolotti R, Solli P, Spaggiari L (2008) Lung cancer screening with low-dose computed tomography: a non-invasive diagnostic protocol for baseline lung nodules. Lung Cancer 61(3):340–349

Xu DM, Gietema H, de Koning H et al (2006) Nodule management protocol of the Nelson randomized lung cancer screening trial. Lung Cancer 54:177–184

# Dose Reduction in Screening Programs: Colon Cancer Screening

Thierry N. Boellaard, Henk W. Venema, and Jaap Stoker

## Contents



T. N. Boellaard (✉) · J. Stoker
Department of Radiology, Academic Medical Center,
University of Amsterdam, P.O. Box 22660,
1100 DD Amsterdam, The Netherlands
e-mail: t.n.boellaard@amc.uva.nl

H. W. Venema
Departments of Radiology and Medical Physics,
Academic Medical Center, University of Amsterdam,
P.O. Box 22660, 1100 DD Amsterdam, The Netherlands

**Abstract**

Colorectal cancer is one of the most common causes of cancer-related death in the Western world and screening is the most feasible option to reduce this mortality. Screening is performed by detection of the precursor lesions (adenoma) and early colorectal cancer, followed by appropriate treatment. CT colonography is a multi-detector-row CT technique with high accuracy for the detection of adenomas and colorectal cancer and is therefore an option for screening. It has replaced barium enema as the preferred imaging technique for screening. Although CT colonography has several advantages compared to other screening options, ionizing radiation remains an important drawback. Dose reduction is important to prevent unnecessary radiation exposure and thereby improves the benefit-risk ratio and acceptance of CT colonography as a screening tool. Whether dose reduction is possible depends on several factors, including subject characteristics, the target lesions (intracolonic/extracolonic) and type of oral bowel preparation. Dose reduction can be achieved by adjusting the CT scanner parameters (tube current, tube voltage, pitch and rotation time). Additionally, technical specifications of the CT scanner affect the radiation dose (e.g. number of


DOI: 10.1007/174_2011_483, 

detector rows and filter type). Newer functionality such as automatic current selection, advanced noise reduction filters and improved reconstruction techniques even enable radiation dose reduction without visual loss of image quality. This chapter gives an overview of CT colonography, factors that influence radiation dose and reviews the current literature on dose reduction in CT colonography.

**Abbreviations**

| | |
|---|---|
| ASIR | Adaptive statistical iterative reconstruction |
| CAD | Computer-aided detection |
| C-RADS | CT Colonography Reporting and Data System |
| PICCS | Prior image constrained compressed sensing |
| kV | Kilo voltage |
| mA | Milliampere |
| mAs | Milliampere-second |
| MDCT | Multi-detector-row CT |
| MPR | Multiplanar reformatting |
| mSv | MilliSieverts |

# 1 Colorectal Cancer Screening

## 1.1 Disease Prevalence

Colorectal cancer is one of the leading causes of cancer-related mortality. It is estimated that in developed countries in 2008, 727,400 individuals were diagnosed with colorectal cancer and 320,100 died as a consequence of this disease (Jemal et al. 2011). Most colorectal cancers are thought to develop from adenomas through the so-called adenoma-carcinoma sequence. Adenomas and especially advanced adenomas have a risk of developing into cancer. An advanced adenoma is defined as an adenoma $\geq$10 mm, with villous histology ($\geq$25% villous) or with high grade dysplasia. Advanced adenomas and carcinomas together are known as advanced neoplasia. Despite improvements in treatment of colorectal cancer, mortality has not decreased to a considerable extent. The most important reason is the presence of extensive disease at the time of diagnosis. Early detection of colorectal cancer and prevention by removing the precursors of colorectal cancer (adenomatous polyps) by screening is possible and at this moment seems to be the most feasible solution to substantially reduce incidence and mortality of colorectal cancer (Cunningham et al. 2010).

## 1.2 Screening Tests

Currently, screening for colorectal cancer is performed in several countries and considered in others. Several screening techniques are available, including fecal occult blood test, sigmoidoscopy, double-contrast barium enema and colonoscopy. Although fecal occult blood test has a proven impact on disease-related mortality (Hewitson et al. 2008), it has a limited sensitivity and specificity for the detection of colorectal cancer and is even more limited for assessment of adenomatous polyps. Sigmoidoscopy is not a full colon examination, although the results for detection of colorectal cancer and polyps are considerably better than for the fecal occult blood test. Importantly, screening with sigmoidoscopy has proven to reduce colorectal cancer mortality to a greater extent than with fecal occult blood test (Atkin et al. 2010). Barium enema has been studied as a screening test, but it has considerable limitations in sensitivity and specificity and is, therefore, surpassed by other techniques. Colonoscopy has the highest sensitivity and specificity, and offers the opportunity of instant polyp removal or histological biopsy in tumors. On the other hand colonoscopy is a burdensome procedure and is not without complications, which limits acceptance by participants. Burden is primarily caused by an extensive bowel preparation, the burden of the examination itself has decreased by the widespread use of conscious sedation during the examination. Computed tomography (CT) colonography (also known as virtual colonoscopy) using MDCT technique is considered as a valuable alternative for colorectal cancer screening. CT colonography is an abdominal CT scan aimed to detect colorectal cancer and/or polyps. CT colonography is now preferred over barium enemas as imaging technique for the detection of colorectal polyps and cancer (Sosna et al. 2008).

## 2 CT Colonography Procedure

CT colonography is performed after bowel preparation as otherwise colorectal cancer and polyps will be obscured by stool. Adequate bowel distension is a prerequisite for good visualization of the bowel surface and prevents collapsed bowel from mimicking colorectal cancer.

### 2.1 Bowel Preparation

The first CT colonography examinations were performed after cathartic bowel preparation as used in colonoscopy. Many centers still use these preparations in clinical practice because these have been extensively studied and demonstrated to enable good accuracy for detection of colorectal cancer and adenomas. These preparations are combined with either iodine or barium for tagging. Tagging causes large contrast between bowel content and colonic lesions because it increases the CT value of the fluid or stool. The use of tagging is considered the best practice by all recent guidelines (Burling 2010; ACR 2009).

However, such extensive bowel preparations cause excessive diarrhea and consequently considerable burden. Therefore, moderate purgative and even minimal bowel preparations are now increasingly being used. These preparations have been shown to improve the patient comfort, which is very important for the acceptance of CT colonography as a screening tool. These types of preparations have become possible by the introduction of stool and fluid tagging which makes full cleansing superfluous. Not only low-fiber diet is important to reduce the chance of having untagged feces (Liedenbaum et al. 2010b), but also stool softeners may be used for better homogeneity. In several studies minimal bowel preparations did not seem to have negative influence on sensitivity for $\geq$10 mm polyps (Liedenbaum et al. 2010a; Nagata et al. 2009; Iannaccone et al. 2004), however, both sensitivity and specificity vary substantially between studies, which have been performed with a small number of subjects (Mahgerefteh et al. 2009). These type of bowel preparations have not yet been validated in large studies. There is a large variety of minimal bowel preparation schemes and the optimal bowel preparation scheme remains to be determined.

In general no intravenous contrast medium is administered as it is not mandatory for colonic lesion detection. It might even be detrimental as reduced contrast between contrast-enhanced lesions and tagged stool may reduce the conspicuity of polyps and cancers. In symptomatic individuals often intravenous contrast medium will be used in one position to detect possible metastatic disease.

### 2.2 Procedure

CT colonography is preferably performed in both supine and prone position. As an alternative for prone position, a decubitus position may be used (e.g. in elderly people with breathing difficulties or severe osteoarthritis). Dual positioning leads to an increased polyp sensitivity and more adequately distended segments. A collapsed segment in one position is often well distended in the other position. Thereby, movement of residual fluid and stool between both positions facilitates evaluation of otherwise obscured bowel surface and polyps submerged in possible untagged fluid and stool. Although not a firm criterion, it might also help to differentiate between polyps. In general the position of polyps is not influenced by the direction of the gravity, although pedunculated polyps and mobile segments can be pitfalls. The colon is insufflated, preferably using carbon dioxide with an automated insufflator, but room air can be used as an alternative. CT scan parameters will be discussed in Sect. 4.

### 2.3 Evaluation and Computer-Aided Detection

CT colonography examinations are read using a combination of two-dimensional (2D) reading, including multiplanar reformatting (MPR) and three-dimensional (3D) reading. There is consensus that either a primary 2D reading method (3D only used for problem solving) or a primary 3D reading method (2D only used for problem solving) should be used. There seems to be no major differences in performance of both reading strategies.

When limited bowel preparation is used in combination with fecal tagging and the images are evaluated with 3D reading, it is necessary to remove the tagged substances from the image beforehand. Otherwise polyps that are covered by fluid or stool remain invisible while stool might be read as a polyp or cancer at 3D. The removal of tagged material is done by a procedure usually known as electronic cleansing (Zalis et al. 2004; Franaszek et al. 2006). In minimal bowel preparation CT colonography, however, adequate cleansing can be difficult with current cleansing algorithms and artifacts prevent adequate readability.

Colorectal cancer can present as an obstructing mass or as a sessile (polypoid) or flat lesion. Sessile polyps are recognized as focal elevations of the colonic wall. Some polyps have another morphology: pedunculated or flat. Flat lesions are more difficult to identify than sessile or pedunculated polyps as flat lesions concern slight elevations or (less frequently) depressions of the colonic surface. Rarely flat lesions do not have an elevated or depressed morphology and are in plane with the colonic mucosa. These latter lesions cannot be identified at CT colonography and are often even hard to identify at colonoscopy without specific measures (e.g. dye spray facilitating identification of disturbance of normal colonic surface pattern by a flat lesion).

Differentiation between polyp and untagged stool is done primarily by the lack of contrast within a polyp (in contrast to stool) and by evaluating the internal structure of the lesion: polyps have a homogeneous morphology while stool is heterogeneous and can have air inside the lesion. Helpful but a less reliable feature is the lack of change of relative position of a potential lesion between the two scans. This feature is indicative for a polyp, although bowel segments are mobile and especially pedunculated polyps can change position. The opposite may occur as well, as sticky stool can be adherent to the colonic wall without being influenced by the effect of gravity.

Computer-aided detection (CAD) has been introduced in CT colonography to reduce reader variability and possibly increase sensitivity. Based on shape features and internal characteristics colorectal cancer and polyps are identified. Computer-aided detection schemes have been designed for application in situations where extensive bowel preparation has been applied, as well as for tagged examinations (Summers et al. 2005a, b). There are several CAD reading strategies: first read (the observer only evaluates CAD hits), concurrent read (CAD hits are shown while the observer is reading the exam) and second read (CAD hits are shown to the observer after reading the complete exam). The first read strategy may have the advantage of having a shorter reading time. However, second read may result in improved detection rates. The U.S. Food and Drug Administration (FDA) has recently approved CAD systems (iCAD,VeraLook and Medicsight, ColonCAD API) for second read strategy, which is an important step for further development of CAD techniques for CT colonography.

## 3 CT Colonography Performance

CT colonography can identify colorectal cancer and polyps. However, adenomatous polyps—precursors of colorectal cancer—cannot be differentiated from other polypoid lesions at CT colonography (e.g. hyperplastic polyps). Since large polyps other than adenomas are rare, polyp size (diameter) is the most important criterion for the differentiation between types of polyps. In screening colonoscopy, the cancer risk in different polyp size categories is as follows: for $\geq$10 mm polyps the cancer risk is 2.6% (with increasing chance of cancer with increasing size), for 6–9 mm 0.2% and <6 mm 0%. Additionally, there is a chance of polyps containing advanced histology, which is 30.6%, 6.6% and 1.7% for the three size categories, respectively (Lieberman et al. 2008). Polyps with advanced histology have an increased risk of developing into colorectal cancer. Due to the very low advanced histology/cancer risk, small polyps (<6 mm) can be disregarded.

CT colonography should have a good performance for the detection of colorectal cancer and for polyps with a diameter $\geq$10 mm. Individuals with these lesions will be referred for colonoscopy. Additionally, polyps in the intermediate size range 6–9 mm cannot be neglected. These polyps might be removed by colonoscopy, although in screening a possible strategy for handling 6–9 mm polyps is a surveillance CT colonography (e.g. re-examination after three years), before a possible referral for colonoscopy.

As CT colonography will be used to select patients for colonoscopy, the test characteristics (i.e. sensitivity, specificity and predictive values) *per patient* are of primary importance. This as patients will be selected for colonoscopy based on the presence of at least one relevant lesion and therefore the number of lesions is less important. Colonoscopy will be performed for polyp removal by biopsy with subsequent histopathology of the lesion. In colorectal cancer biopsy is performed for histopathology. The per polyp test characteristics are therefore less relevant than the per patient characteristics.

### 3.1 Detection of Colorectal Cancer and Polyps

Diagnostic performance of CT colonography for colorectal cancer has recently been studied in a meta-analysis (Pickhardt et al. 2011). Sensitivity of CT colonography was 96.1% compared to 94.7% for optical colonoscopy. In systematic reviews of the literature, CT colonography has been shown to have good test characteristics: detection of participants with colorectal cancer and large (often adenomatous) polyps (diameter ≥10 mm). These systematic reviews primarily concern studies in symptomatic populations. For larger polyps (diameter ≥10 mm) per patient sensitivity is 82–93% and specificity 92–97% (Sosna et al. 2003, 2008; Mulhall et al. 2005; Halligan et al. 2005; Chaparro et al. 2009). For polyps ≥6 mm per patient sensitivity is 86%, with a specificity of 86% (Halligan et al. 2005).

Several CT colonography studies in asymptomatic screening populations have been performed. A large study by Kim et al. (N = 3,120 and 3,163 for CT colonography and optical colonoscopy, respectively) compared the yield of CT colonography and colonoscopy. In this study the yield was similar for both modalities: 3.2 vs. 3.4% patients with advanced adenomas (Kim et al. 2007). The diagnostic performance in screening has recently been summarized in a meta-analysis (N = 4,086) (de Haan et al. 2011). This meta-analysis combined results of five studies. The estimated sensitivities per patient were: 82.9% for ≥6 mm and 87.9% for ≥10 mm adenomas. Corresponding specificities were 91.4 and 97.6%, respectively.

More research in larger screening populations is necessary to determine the cost-effectiveness of CT colonography as a screening technique and its effect on mortality.

CAD performance has been studied in both small datasets with high lesion prevalence as well as in large screening populations. No systematic review has been performed, probably due to the high variety in data reporting (Robinson et al. 2008). Initial sensitivities in high prevalence studies have been confirmed in large screening cohorts. For example Summers et al. (N = 792) showed a good per polyp and per patient sensitivity of computer-aided detection for adenomas were: both 89.3% with 2.1 false positive per patient (Summers et al. 2005b). In a large stand-alone CAD trial in an asymptomatic screening population (N = 3,077), per patient CAD sensitivities were 93.8 and 96.5% for ≥6 mm and ≥10 mm polyps. Per polyp sensitivities were 90.1 and 96% for ≥6 mm and ≥10 mm polyps. The mean and median false-positive rates were 9.4 and 6 per patient (prone and supine combined) (Lawrence et al. 2010).

### 3.2 Extracolonic Findings

Apart from colorectal lesions, extracolonic findings may be present. These findings are currently classified by the C-RADS classification (Zalis et al. 2005). This classification is a step toward more uniform reporting. The frequency and relevance greatly depends on the population studied. In symptomatic populations the chance of extracolonic findings will be highest. A systematic review of the literature showed that in almost 40% of individuals with symptoms of colorectal cancer, extracolonic findings were observed (Xiong et al. 2005). In 10.5% of all patients an important finding was found, including extracolonic cancer in 2.7% of the patients. In some of the patients these relevant findings were already known prior to the CT colonography examination.

In a screening setting the number of extracolonic findings is considerably lower than in symptomatic individuals. In a large screening trial, 10.7% had possibly or probably important findings, 7.7% of the participants needed further workup, and ultimately a relevant lesion was found in 2.5% of all participants (Kim et al. 2007). Extracolonic malignancies were detected in approximately 0.35% of screening participants (Pickhardt et al. 2010). The most common types of cancers found at screening CT colonography were renal cell carcinoma, lung cancer and non-Hodgkin lymphoma. More than half of these cancers are being detected in clinical stage I (Pickhardt et al. 2010). Other common important findings include: aortoiliac aneurysms, adrenal lesions and ovarian cysts. These facts emphasize that extracolonic information resulting from CT colonography screening will have considerable consequences. Some authors suggest that detecting important extracolonic finding may add to the benefit of CT colonography. However, they may cause unnecessary workup and procedures and add substantially to the total CT colonography costs and burden. For example, ovarian masses are frequently found and additional imaging studies and surgical procedures cause burden and costs while the masses rarely concern cancer. Estimations for costs resulting from workup for extracolonic findings vary substantially and may add tens to hundreds of dollars per participant screened.

At this moment, there are no guidelines for the management of extracolonic findings. Clear guidelines for incidental findings tailored to an asymptomatic population may reduce the number of unnecessary workups and therefore may be beneficial for cost-effectiveness and acceptance. Today, the benefits and burden of extracolonic findings are not clear enough and for an important advisory committee on colorectal cancer screening, this was an important reason to refrain from advising CT colonography for colorectal cancer screening yet (USPSTF 2008).

The frequency of extracolonic findings also depends on the dose level of the CT colonography examination, as will be discussed later.

The encouraging results make CT colonography a potential valuable screening method for colorectal cancer. However, while further studies are performed to more extensively study CT colonography as screening method, an important drawback of CT should be considered. The use of ionizing radiation—with the risk of induction of cancer and genetic damage—has to be weighed against the potential benefits of screening with CT colonography.

# 4 Possibilities for Dose Reduction in CT Colonography

The choice of CT colonography scan parameters has a direct effect on radiation exposure. First an overview is given of the factors influencing radiation dose and image quality at CT colonography. This is followed by a discussion on the possibilities of the adjustment of the tube current to the posture of the patient and tube current modulation, possibilities for noise reduction by the use of noise reduction filters and iterative reconstruction techniques, dual-energy CT, a survey on the CT colonography scan parameters that are used by different groups, a section on experimental studies in dose reduction using simulation methods and phantoms, and finally the results of some clinical studies using reduced radiation dose CT protocols.

## 4.1 Scan Parameters and CT Colonography

CT colonography scan parameters were initially based on clinical abdominal CT protocols, and later on were adjusted to lower dose settings. Dose reduction was possible because essential differences exist between the two examinations with regard to the kind of details that have to be visualized. In clinical abdominal CT subtle contrasts between the different soft tissues are important and may be obscured when the images are too noisy. Therefore, a relatively high dose is required in order to reduce the noise. In CT colonography examinations, on the other hand, target lesions (colorectal cancer and adenomatous polyps) remain visible in much noisier images. This is due to the large contrast between the bowel wall and intraluminal air. This provides the opportunity to reduce the radiation exposure.

It is obvious that tagging necessitates a higher dose than that required for examinations where the colon is perfectly clean. After all, in this last situation the contrast between polyps and surroundings may be considerably reduced. More on this topic in Sect. 4.3.2.

## 4.2 Factors Influencing CT Radiation Dose

The effective dose of a CT examination is a measure of the radiation risk associated with the examination. It depends in the first place on the amount of radiation used in the examination, which is directly related to the effective mAs level: the tube current (in mA) multiplied by the rotation time (in s) divided by the pitch, and the tube voltage (kV) of the examination. It also depends on the construction of the CT scanner (geometry, amount of filtration of the X-ray beam, presence or absence of a shaped filter), the number of detector rows and the collimation, as discussed hereafter.

Reduction of radiation exposure at CT can be achieved in several ways. The simplest approach is to reduce the effective mAs level—by reducing the tube current or the rotation time or by increasing the pitch—which leads to a proportional decrease in radiation dose. The choice of the tube voltage is also an important factor. A tube voltage of 120 kV is generally used, although the use of higher tube voltages (140 kV), or lower ones (80 or 100 kV) can be considered in specific situations. The choice of the tube voltage has a marked effect on the effective dose: compared with the 120 kV situation, the use of 140 kV leads to an increase in effective dose with a factor in the order of 1.3 to 1.6, the use of 100 kV to a reduction in dose of a factor 1.5 to 1.7, and the use of 80 kV even to reduction in the order of a factor 3 to 4. All these figures depend somewhat on the type of CT scanner used in the examination. The reduction of radiation dose leads to a reduction of the radiation used in the imaging process, and therefore to an increase in noise and a decrease in image quality (see Sect. 4.3).

The introduction of MDCT scanners initially produced a slight increase in effective dose because of a reduced efficiency of the use of ionizing radiation compared with single-detector-row scanners, due to the penumbra effect, also called *overbeaming*. This is especially the case in four-detector-row scanners, for which typical increases of 10–30% in effective dose have been reported for the same protocols (Kalender 2005). For modern scanners with 16 to 64 or more detector rows this effect is of less importance (Kalender 2005; Cody and Mahesh 2007; Rogalla et al. 2009). Another source of dose inefficiency is the fact that in spiral CT an additional layer of tissue is irradiated adjacent to the volume to be depicted because the reconstruction of the first and last slices requires data beyond the boundaries of this volume, a phenomenon known as *overranging* (Tzedakis et al. 2005; van der Molen and Geleijns 2007; Schilham et al. 2010). This effect of overranging is most pronounced for CT scanners with a large beam collimation, for example in 128-detector-row CT scanners, where the total beam width can be up to 80 mm. The latest generation of CT scanners with a large number of detector rows is equipped with dynamic collimators, which reduce the additional dose due to overranging with up to 50% (Schilham et al. 2010).

At the moment of writing (September 2011) one type of CT scanner is equipped with 320 detector rows (Toshiba Aquilion One). Helical scanning for this scanner is restricted to 160 detector rows, and the additional dose due to overranging is for this scanner also reduced by application of above-mentioned dynamic collimators.

## 4.3 Image Quality of CT Colonography: Noise, Contrast, Sharpness

Image quality of a CT colonography examination is determined by noise, contrast and sharpness.

### 4.3.1 Noise

The noise in a CT colonography examination is primarily dependent on the amount of radiation, or the number and energy of the photons, that is used in the CT scan. As discussed in 1.4.2, the number of photons depends on the effective mAs level and the tube voltage of the scan. Reduction of the effective mAs level with a factor four doubles the noise in the CT images.

At a lower tube voltage less photons are produced, and these photons will have less penetrating power due to their decreased energy. Therefore, the noise will increase with decreasing kV. However, the detrimental effect of an increase in noise is counteracted by an increase in contrast, as discussed below. An increase in kV leads to the opposite effect.

Because the number of photons that reach the detectors of the CT scanner is the decisive factor for the noise level in the CT colonography images, it is clear that—other things being equal—the size of the patient is a very important factor as well, and the noise level may become extremely high in scans of very obese persons. This point is addressed in Sect. 4.4.

### 4.3.2 Contrast

The important contrast in a CT colonography examination is the contrast between the lesions in the colon wall and their surroundings. In a perfectly cleansed colon the lumen is filled with air, but with the use of tagging the lesions may be immersed in tagged material (Fig. 1). In this situation the contrast may be reduced considerably; in the example shown in Fig. 1 with nearly a factor of 3. This reduction of contrast will impair the visibility of these polyps when the lowest

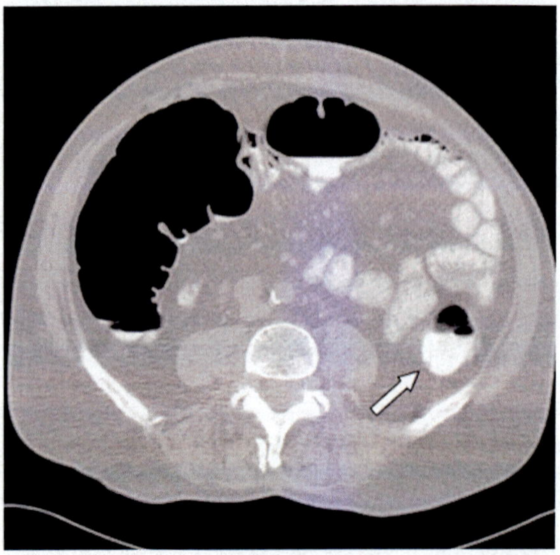

**Fig. 1** Example of a polyp (*arrow*) at CT colonography (level-100, window 1,200) submerged in tagged fluid. The CT value of soft tissue is in the order of 30 HU; in the tagged fluid the CT value is in the order of 400 HU. Therefore the contrast is only 370 HU, considerably less than in the situation that the polyp is surrounded by air or carbon dioxide. In that case the contrast is 1,030 HU, or nearly a factor of 3 higher

mAs values are used. Consider, for example, the polyp in Fig. 1 with a CT number of 30 HU, surrounded by tagged material with a CT number of 400 HU. When we compare this situation with the same polyp surrounded by air (−1,000 HU), the mAs value has to be increased in the order of a factor of nearly 8 ($1{,}030^2/370^2$) to obtain the same image quality. This example stresses the importance of using a bowel preparation scheme that produces tagging with sufficient contrast. When tagging is used the contrast between a lesion and its surrounding will depend on the tube voltage that is used in the CT colonography examination. For lower tube voltages, the contrast between tissue and the materials with high atomic numbers that are used in tagging, such as iodine ($Z = 53$) and barium ($Z = 56$), will increase. This phenomenon counteracts the increase in noise that also occurs at lower tube voltages. Thus for the same dose, reduction in kV may give a better contrast-to-noise ratio (Fig. 2).

Recently, Kalender et al. showed that for the imaging of iodine/soft tissue contrast the optimal tube voltage is in the order of 80 kV or even less, depending on the size of the patient (Kalender et al. 2009). For the imaging of density differences (e.g. polyps in air), 120 kV appears to be nearly optimal. In this case, however, the sensitivity of polyp detection on tube voltage is not strongly dependent on the exact choice of tube voltage, as it is for iodine-soft tissue contrast. Clearly the choice of an optimal tube voltage for CT colonography needs further investigation.

### 4.3.3 Sharpness

Irrespective of whether a primary 3D or a primary 2D reading method is used (Sect. 2.3), it is clear that an optimal visualization of the lesions in 3D is of utmost importance. This optimal visualization is achieved when the images that are used have an isotropic resolution, i.e. the *same* resolution in all directions, and preferentially, of course, the same *high* resolution in all directions. This was not the case in the early years of CT colonography. The in-plane resolution for the CT colonography images, by which we mean the full-width-at-half-maximum of the point spread function is customary in the order of 1 mm or slightly less, depending on the scanner mode and the kernel used in the reconstruction, whereas in the early years values of the full-width-at-half-maximum of the point spread function in the longitudinal direction (equivalent to the slice thickness) of 5 or 3 mm were used, due to limitations of the CT scanners at that time. With the widespread use of MDCT scanners the slice thickness has dropped substantially, and reconstructions can be made now of submillimeter slices. An important point is that the noise in the images increases with the reciprocal of the square root of the slice thickness. This can be counteracted by reconstructing (somewhat noisy) images with a thin slice thickness, so that an isotropic resolution is obtained, and by viewing multiplanar reconstruction (MPR) images with a somewhat increased thickness in the viewing direction, where the unsharpness matters least. Also for 3D viewing isotropic resolution is advantageous.

## 4.4 Tube Current Adaptations to Posture; Tube Current Modulation

In the first years of CT colonography nearly always the same CT protocols were applied to all patients and care was taken that a good image quality was

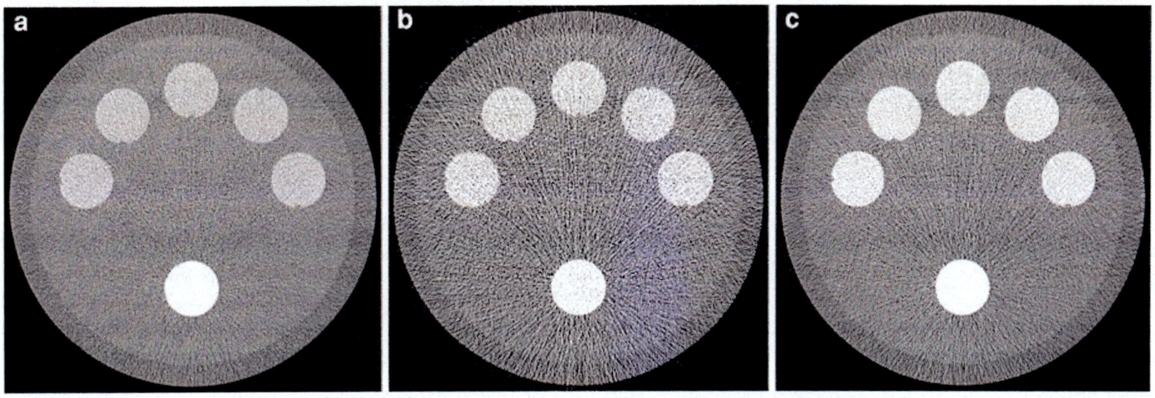

**Fig. 2** Simulated CT images (level 0, window 1,600) of a mathematical phantom mimicking an abdominal cross-section (diameter 34 cm) containing 5 cross-sections of the colon, each one containing a 6 mm polyp, and a stylized vertebra in the *lower* part of the image. The colon is filled with iodine-tagged water. The simulation at the *left* (**a**), was made with 120 kV, 25 mAs, in the *middle* (**b**), with 80 kV, 25 mAs and at the *right* (**c**), with 80 kV, 75 mAs. The slice thickness for all images is 2.5 mm. This simulation shows the effect of reduction of the tube voltage from 120 to 80 kV on the contrast and the noise level. The dose of the simulated CT scan at the *right* (**c**) is slightly lower than of the simulated CT scan at the *left* (**a**), yet the signal to noise ratio (and the visibility of the polyps) is better

obtained in (almost) all these patients. Although this is understandable from a pragmatic point of view, it inevitably leads to more than necessary radiation exposure in slim or average posture individuals. Moreover in very obese patients the CT settings might be insufficient for an adequate diagnostic quality because of the very high noise level. More recently, automatic tube current selection based on measurements of the attenuation in the body has become available. Nowadays nearly all CT scanners have the possibility of tube current modulation. In this last option the tube current is continuously changed during the rotation of the X-ray tube, reducing the tube current in areas where the patient is relatively transparent for the X-rays, and using higher mA values in the regions of high attenuation, in order to reduce the noise (Greess et al. 1999; Kalra et al. 2004). Optimal noise reduction is obtained by combining angular modulation, i.e. the adaptation of tube current while the X-ray tube rotates around the patient, and longitudinal modulation, while the patient moves through the X-ray beam and different anatomical regions are scanned (McCollough et al. 2006). A substantial dose reduction can be obtained, while retaining (or even improving) the image quality (Graser et al. 2006).

More information on tube current modulation can be found in "Automatic Exposure Control in Multidetector-row CT".

## 4.5 Noise Reduction Filters

CT images are inevitably noisy because in the CT scan transmission measurements are made using X-ray beams which contain only finite numbers of photons. Especially when a low tube current is used, and/or the attenuation of the patient is high, the noise in the reconstructed images can be severe. The noise can be reduced by filtering, which can be applied both to the X-ray transmission measurements (*the raw data*), and on the images after reconstruction. Noise reduction can be obtained by linear and nonlinear procedures. When linear procedures are used, the noise is reduced by smoothing, but the edges in the image, that may have clinical significance, are smoothed as well. Therefore, nonlinear procedures have been the most popular ones, as these procedures attempt to leave the relevant features of the images intact, while reducing the noise level.

Raw data filtering exploits the fact that the noise is mainly caused by noise in the raw data for which the X-ray beam is highly attenuated. By using proper smoothing techniques the noise may be reduced considerably while the sharpness of the reconstructed image is only marginally reduced (Hsieh 1998; Kachelriess et al. 2001; La Riviere 2005). In a study in which MDCT scans were made of the pelvis of fifty patients with rectal or bladder cancer, the image quality improved considerably by

**Table 1** Daily practice protocols in different institutions with median values of scan parameters and effective dose per protocol in 2007

| | Number of simultaneously acquired slices | | | | |
|---|---|---|---|---|---|
| | 64 | 40 | 16 | 4 | 1 |
| Number of protocols | 21 | 1 | 11 | 4 | 2 |
| Tube voltage (kV) | 120 | 120 | 120 | 120 | 120 |
| Rotation time (s) | 0.5 | 0.4 | 0.5 | 0.5 | 0.75 |
| Collimation (mm) | 0.625 | 0.625 | 1.25 | 1.875 | 5 |
| Effective mAs | 58/50[a] | 113 | 62/56[a] | 83.5/30.5[a] | 55 |
| Dose modulation | 12 | 1 | 2 | – | – |
| Effective dose (mSv) | 9.1 | 13.7 | 11.5 | 9.1 | 4.2 |

Effective dose calculations were performed for an adult hermaphrodite of 170 cm and 70 kg

[a] Results for median values of effective mAs for supine and prone positions (supine/prone)

Liedenbaum et al. Radiation dose in CT colonography–trends in time and differences between daily practice and screening protocols. European Radiology 2008 18 (10):2222–2230. With kind permission of Springer Science + Business Media

use of this technique (Baum et al. 2003). In a feasibility study in which the image quality was compared with CT colonography images that were reconstructed after raw data filtering and conventionally reconstructed images, a dose reduction of a factor 2 was possible without loss of image quality (Manduca et al. 2009).

Nonlinear 3D filtering of the reconstructed images was assessed in low-dose CT of the abdomen in a general setting (Rizzo et al. 2005). The authors concluded that nonlinear filtering can reduce image noise without affecting image contrast, lesion conspicuity or lesion detection with low-dose CT of the abdomen and pelvis.

For the very low (simulated) dose settings that were used in the study of van Gelder and colleagues the use of a Gaussian (linear) filter was advantageous (van Gelder et al. 2004).

Nonlinear filtering techniques were applied in a clinical CT colonography study in which 115 patients were examined at 10 mAs and presumably 120 kV (Cohnen et al. 2004; Vogt et al. 2004). They concluded that with this technique the sensitivity and specificity for the detection of polyps 5 mm or greater in size were excellent (94 and 84%, respectively).

## 4.6 Iterative Reconstruction

Traditionally, the reconstruction in CT is performed using filtered back projection (Kalender 2005). Recently, iterative techniques have been introduced for the reconstruction of CT images. This technique makes it possible to correct for the differences in accuracy of the raw data and has the potential to reconstruct images with less noise, or with the same diagnostic quality at a lower dose. Although an iterative technique was already used in the first CT scanner (Hounsfield 1973), application has been frustrated by very long reconstruction times. The development of vastly improved hardware and of new iterative reconstruction techniques has made the introduction of iterative reconstruction for CT feasible (Hara et al. 2009). An iterative reconstruction technique (ASIR) was compared with filtered backprojection in a CT colonography study which involved both a colon phantom and 18 patients (Flicek et al. 2010). The authors found that the dose could be reduced by 50% without affecting the image quality as judged by observers. Another iterative technique (PICCS) was applied as post-processing method to standard filtered backprojection images of CT colonography examinations of 20 patients, but findings beyond the colon were assessed (Lubner et al. 2011). A noise reduction by a factor of 3 was obtained, without apparent loss of spatial resolution. Still other iterative reconstruction techniques have been described, with promising results (Winklehner et al. 2011; Renker et al. 2011). Most studies show preliminary results, however, and more extensive studies are needed, however, to establish the performance of iterative reconstruction techniques relative to conventional reconstruction methods unambiguously.

### 4.7 Dual-Energy CT

Dual-energy is not a new technique, but since a few years simultaneous acquisition of low- and high-voltage scans (e.g. 80 or 100 and 140 kV) is possible (Johnson et al. 2007). The information that is thus obtained enables more accurate differentiation between tissues types with different effective atomic numbers. Dual-energy CT has the ability to differentiate iodine or barium very well from other tissues or materials with lower atomic numbers.

One dual-energy CT colonography study has evaluated the feasibility of characterizing lesions by their uptake of intravenous iodine contrast (Karcaaltincaba et al. 2009). Enhancement of the polyps or cancers allowed differentiation from (non-tagged) stool. Other studies used dual-energy CT colonography in attempt to improve the performance of electronic cleansing algorithms to remove tagged stool from the images (Carmi et al. 2008, 2011). Unfortunately, the differentiation of tissues according to their effective atomic numbers makes the images relatively noisy (Johnson et al. 2007). Therefore the doses for dual-energy CT colonography scans must be relatively high. Dual-energy scanners can however be equipped with latest dose reducing functionality (e.g. iterative reconstruction). Effective dose of dual-energy CT can therefore approximate the doses used in single-energy CT without latest dose reducing functionality.

### 4.8 Survey of CT Colonography Scan Parameters

For CT colonography different scan protocols have been used with a wide range in the resulting dose. In 2008 a paper was published reporting on the scan parameters collected by an international inventory from CT colonography centers. Effective radiation doses were calculated by means of the ImPACT CT Patient Dosimetry Calculator (Jones and Shrimpton 1991). The relative accuracy of these figures is in the order of 10–20%. As the effective dose values were determined using a mathematical androgynous phantom, these are mean values for men and woman.

This inventory showed that the median effective dose in 2007 for a clinical CT colonography examination was 5.2 mSv for supine and 3.0 for prone position (Liedenbaum et al. 2008), resulting in a median effective dose per institution of 9.1 mSv (range 2.8–22 mSv) (see Table 1). An earlier inventory indicated that the median effective radiation dose was 11.0 mSv in 2004 (Jensch et al. 2006). The reduction from 11.0 to 9.1 mSv, however, was not significant. Protocols for screening CT colonography used significantly less radiation, with a median effective dose of 5.6 mSv (2.8 mSv for supine and 2.5 mSv for prone series)(see Fig. 3 and Tables 1 and 2).

### 4.9 Experimental Studies in Dose Reduction: Simulation

Experimental dose reduction studies have demonstrated that dose reduction is possible beyond the common radiation doses used in 2007. The mAs setting is the major factor influencing radiation exposure for the commonly used tube voltage of 120 kV.

Initially, tube current reduction from 100 to 30 mAs was shown to be possible without detrimental effect on polyp detection (van Gelder et al. 2002). This study concerned 50 individuals examined with 100 mAs CT colonography where 50 and 30 mAs CT colonographic examinations were simulated by modifying the raw data. Although image quality decreased, sensitivity and specificity were not affected. A further experimental study of the same group showed that dose reduction might be possible beyond the setting of 10 mAs that is the lowest setting of most CT scanners at present (van Gelder et al. 2004). CT colonography examinations of 15 patients at 100 mAs were modified to scans at 25, 6.3, 1.6, and 0.4 mAs using the same technique described earlier, corresponding to effective doses of 3, 0.8, 0.2, and 0.05 mSv for the two positions combined. For the lowest three mAs levels a Gaussian kernel was used to reduce the noise, which was mandatory for the primary 3D visualization that was used in this study. Detection of polyps $\geq 5$ mm was undisturbed down to 1.6 mAs (0.2 mSv for two positions) (Figs. 4 and 5).

The same simulation method was used in a study on the effect of the use of low mAs values on computer-aided detection (de Vries et al. 2005). Twenty CT colonography examinations after extensive bowel preparation, made with 120 kV and 25–100 mAs, depending on the size of the patient, were used. These patients had at least one colonoscopically proven polyp larger than 5 mm. Simulated low-dose

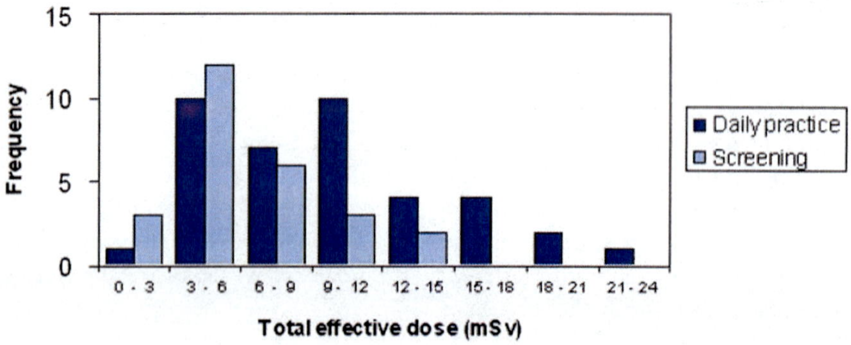


**Fig. 3** Histogram of effective dose in daily practice and screening protocols Liedenbaum et al. Radiation dose in CT colonography–trends in time and differences between daily practice and screening protocols. European Radiology 2008 18 (10):2222–2230. With kind permission of Springer Science + Business Media

**Table 2** Screening protocols in different institutions with median values of scan parameters and effective dose per protocol in 2007

| | Number of simultaneously acquired slices | | | |
|---|---|---|---|---|
| | 64 | 16 | 4 | 1 |
| Number of protocols | 13 | 9 | 2 | 1 |
| Tube voltage (kV) | 120 | 120 | 120 | 120 |
| Rotation time (s) | 0.5 | 0.5 | 0.5 | 0.50 |
| Collimation (mm) | 0.6 | 1.125 | 1.125 | 5 |
| Effective mAs | 50/36[a] | 40/32[a] | 44 | 57 |
| Dose modulation | 7 | 5 | – | – |
| Effective dose (mSv) | 5.8 | 5.6 | 7.8 | 4.3 |

Effective dose calculations were performed for an adult hermaphrodite of 170 cm and 70 kg

[a] Results for median value of effective mAs for supine and prone (supine/prone)

Liedenbaum et al. Radiation dose in CT colonography–trends in time and differences between daily practice and screening protocols. European Radiology 2008 18 (10):2222–2230. With kind permission of Springer Science + Business Media

scans were made at 6.25 mAs. CAD on the simulated low-dose data was feasible at the cost of only a slight increase in number of false positives or a small drop in sensitivity as compared to normal dose data. At a sensitivity of 90% a median number of six false positives were detected at normal dose and nine false positives at low-dose. When the operating point of the algorithm was moved to obtain six false positives at the low-dose setting the sensitivity dropped from 90 to 87%.

## 4.10 Experimental Dose Reduction Studies: Phantoms and Specimens

Phantom and specimen studies have been performed to study optimal CT settings including tube current. A study of a colectomy specimen with 177 polyps demonstrated that tube current (50, 100 and 150 mA; effective dose 1.4–10.0 mSv per position, also depending on pitch and collimation) had no effect on polyp detection except for polyps <5 mm (Taylor et al. 2003). A study using an anthropomorphic colon phantom showed that in the range of 10–140 mAs (effective dose for one position 0.7–11.6 mSv), tube current had no effect on the detection of polyps ≥8 mm irrespective of slice thickness and detector collimation studied (Wessling et al. 2003). Depiction of smaller polyps (6 and 2 mm) was less, but results improved with a collimation of 1 mm instead of 2.5 mm, and were only slightly influenced by the reduction in tube current.

A study with a glass colon phantom containing 140 polyps (size 5–12 mm) that was scanned for a large range of mAs values (5–308 mAs) and a collimation of 1.25, 2.5 and 5 mm, showed that all polyps could

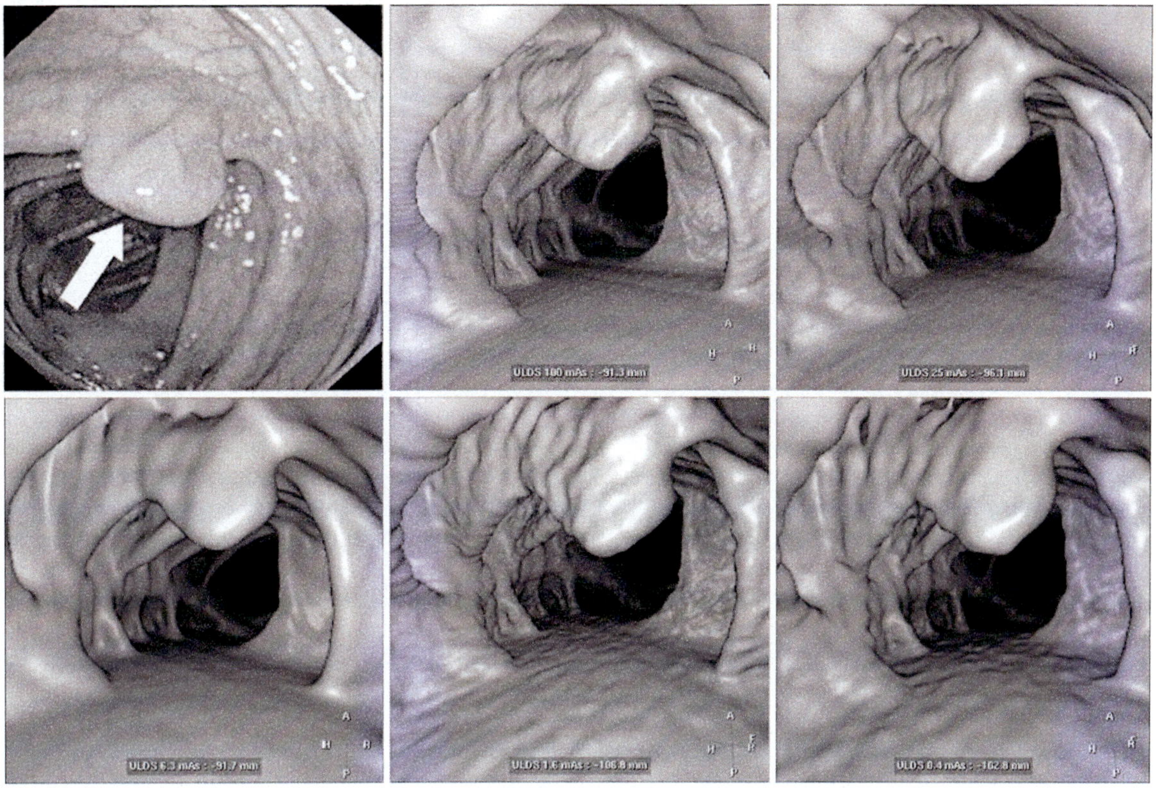


**Fig. 4** Images of a 15 mm polyp in a 60-year-old male patient at colonoscopy and at CT colonography with five doses. *Top row*: Left: Colonoscopic image shows 15 mm polyp in ascending colon (*arrow*). *Middle*: CT colonographic image obtained at 100 mAs. *Right*: CT colonographic image simulated at 25 mAs. *Bottom row*: *Left*: CT colonographic image simulated at 6.3 mAs. *Middle*: CT colonographic image simulated at 1.6 mAs. *Right*: CT colonographic image simulated at 0.4 mAs. Although the image quality decreases, polyp visibility is unimpaired. (permission for reprint provided by the RSNA; van Gelder et al. CT colonography: Feasibility of substantial dose reduction—comparison of medium to very low doses in identical patients. *Radiology* 2004;232:611–620)

be identified, except for five of the presumably 35 polyps of 5 mm in the 5 mAs scan with a collimation of 1.25 mm (Johnson et al. 2004).

A number of other phantom studies have been published with comparable findings on the influence of dose on polyp visibility (Laghi et al. 2003; Sundaram et al. 2003; Luz et al. 2004). Most studies agree on the fact that the use of thinner collimation helps in the visualization, especially for smaller polyps. Noticeable is also that polyp visibility appears to be better in the longitudinal than in the transverse direction of the colon (Johnson et al. 2004; Luz et al. 2004).

Kim and colleagues (Kim et al. 2008) studied the influence of slice thickness and tube current on polyp detectability using a CAD system in a number of pig colon phantoms with artificial polyps. Polyp detection increased for smaller slice thickness, although the number of false positives also increased. The detectability was independent of the dose, down to the lowest mAs level (10 mAs).

In all these studies phantoms were used that contained polyps in air, thus with a very high contrast. In a phantom study by de Vries et al. the visibility of polyps covered by tagging was addressed. The influence of the density of the tagging on the detectibility of simulated 6 mm sessile polyps was studied for different mAs values, at 120 kV. As expected (see Sect. 4.3.2), the sensitivity of detection of polyps covered by tagging depended strongly on the density of the tagging material. While for polyps in air the sensitivity was 100% at the lowest mAs values used (10 mAs), for polyps covered by tagging much higher mAs values had to be used to obtain sensitivities in the order of 90–100%, for example 40 mAs for a contrast between polyp and tagging of approximately 500 HU (de Vries et al. 2008).

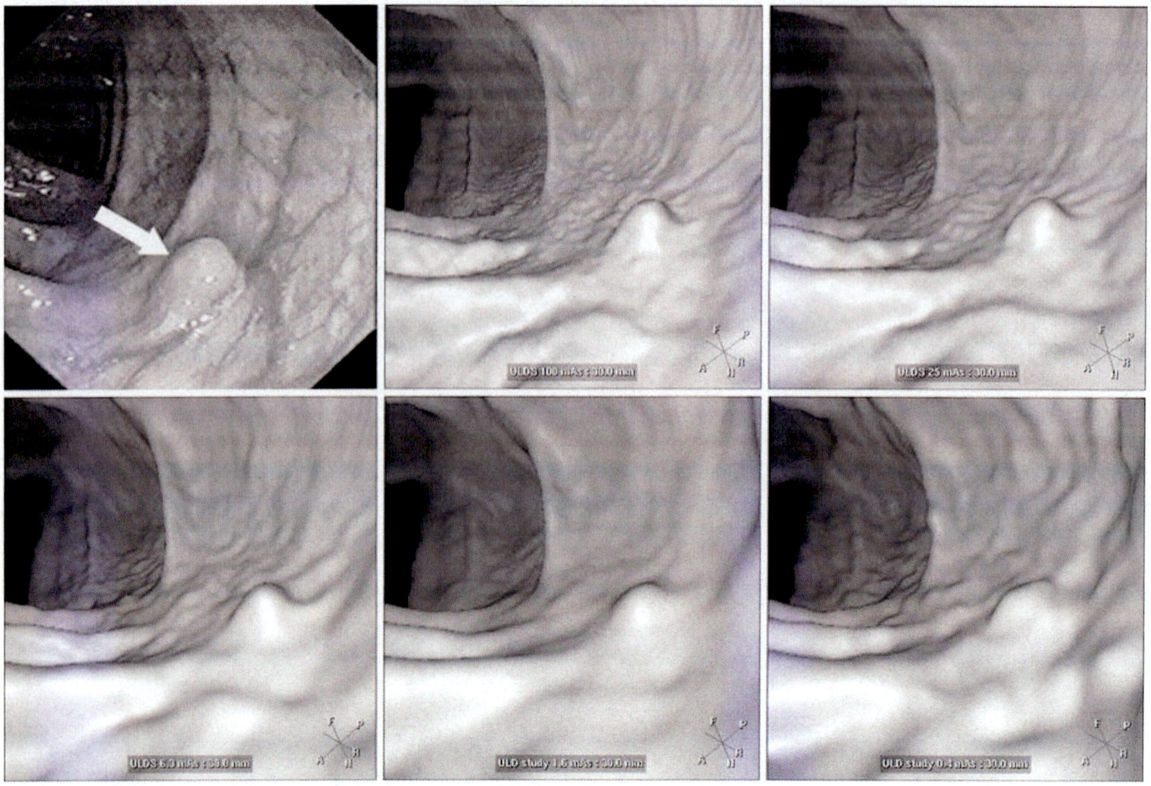


**Fig. 5** Images of a 5 mm polyp in a 57-year-old male patient at colonoscopy and at CT colonography with five doses. *Top row*: *Left*: Colonoscopic image shows 5 mm polyp (*arrow*) in transverse colon. *Middle*: CT colonographic image obtained at 100 mAs. *Right*: CT colonographic image at simulated 25 mAs. *Bottom row*: *Left*: CT colonographic image simulated at at 6.3 mAs. *Middle*: CT colonographic image simulated at 1.6 mAs. *Right*: CT colonographic image simulated at 0.4 mAs. The image quality decreases and polyp visibility is affected at lowest doses as a result of increased image noise and smoothing. (permission for reprint provided by the RSNA; van Gelder et al. CT colonography: feasibility of substantial dose reduction—comparison of medium to very low doses in identical patients. *Radiology* 2004;232:611–620)

It can be concluded that the sensitivity for the detection of polyps of 6 mm or larger in air is hardly influenced by the choice of the mAs level, and that thus very low-dose scans can be used without loss of sensitivity. It is possible, however, that at the lowest dose settings some polyps covered by tagging may remain undetected, especially when the CT number of the tagging is low.

## 4.11 Clinical Decreased Radiation Dose Studies

Several clinical studies have reported on the use of low-dose scanning. In an initial study with extensive bowel preparation, 105 patients were studied using 120 kV, 50 mAs (effective dose for two positions 5.0 mSv for men and 7.8 for women) using $4 \times 1$ mm section collimation (Macari et al. 2002). Per polyp sensitivity for polyps >10 mm was 93% (13/14), for 6–9 mm polyps it was 70%. Another study reported on 27 patients using supine and prone 10 mAs CT colonography [effective dose for two positions combined were 1.7 mSv (for men) and 2.3 mSv (for women)] (Iannaccone et al. 2003). In this study all colorectal cancers (9/9) and all polyps $\geq$6 mm (6/6) were detected. Two studies have reported on low-dose CT colonography in children (Anupindi et al. 2005; Capunay et al. 2005).

In a series of 137 patients with extensive bowel cleansing CT colonography was performed at 120 kV, 10 mAs (supine position only; effective doses 0.7 mSv for men and 1.2 mSv for women), 1.25 mm slice width; nonlinear Gaussian filters were used for noise reduction (Cohnen et al. 2004). Combined 2D MPR and 3D endoluminal views were used. CT colonography detected 23 (82%) of 28 polyps ≥5 mm: 11 (78.6%) of 14 large polyps (>10 mm) and 12 (85.7%) of 14 medium polyps (9.9–5 mm). On a patient-by-patient basis, overall sensitivity was 70.3% and specificity 80.8%. Fisicella and colleagues compared the sensitivity of a low-dose protocol 1.03 ± 0.4 mSv (range 0.4–1.9 mSv) with their standard dose protocol 3.9 ± 1.3 (SD) mSv (range 1.6–6.8 mSv). Although more artifacts were present at low-dose acquisitions, no significant difference in sensitivity between the dose levels was found for polyps ≥6 mm (Fisichella et al. 2010). These results are in the range of previous studies using higher tube current settings.

With the introduction of tagging, the contrast between polyp and bowel content is reduced in case the polyp is surrounded by the tagged material instead of air. This impairs the visibility of these polyps when the lowest mAs settings are used, as discussed above (1.4.3). Florie et al. performed an experimental study with dose reduction in limited bowel preparation CT colonography (Florie et al. 2007). Lower dose levels were simulated using controlled addition of noise to raw transmission measurements. In this study diagnostic accuracy was compared between the original CT colonography examination (5.8–8.2 mSv) and simulated 2.3 and 0.7 mSv dose levels. Dose reduction down to 0.7 mSv was not associated with significant changes in diagnostic value (polyps ≥10 mm). The use of limited bowel preparation and tagging (diatrizoate meglumine and diatrizoate sodium) at low dose (140 kV, 10 mAs; effective dose for two positions 1.8 mSv for men and 2.4 mSv for women) has also been studied in 203 patients (Iannaccone et al. 2004). Using 3 mm slice thickness with primary 2D reading, CT colonography had an average sensitivity of 95.5% for the identification of colorectal polyps ≥8 mm. Per patient average sensitivity for all polyps was high: 89.9% and average specificity of 92.2% and for lesions ≥10 mm sensitivity and specificity were 100%. This study shows that good results are achievable with low-dose scanning in limited bowel prepped CT colonography examinations.

The fact that the results of this low-dose study are quite good, notwithstanding the problems pointed out earlier (Sect. 4.3.2), may have several explanations. In the first place it appears from the studies quoted earlier that in the cleansed situation virtually all polyps are seen, even at very low effective dose levels so that the polyps remain visible even if the image quality is somewhat more deteriorated. Secondly, only part of the polyps is surrounded by tagged material, so that possible reduced visibility for these polyps will lead to a much lower overall reduction in visibility. The use of both supine and prone position further increases the likelihood that a lesion in at least one position will not be covered by tagged material.

## 5 Discussion

The need to reduce the radiation dose of CT colonography examinations, especially when used in a screening setting, is dictated by the possible detrimental effects of X-rays on the human body. Unfortunately there is still controversy on the magnitude of the risks involved, and it is not very probable that these controversies will soon be resolved. Nevertheless, reduction of dose remains important. However, this must not be at the expense of the effectiveness of CT colonography as a screening tool. An adjunct of the reduction of radiation dose will be that visualization of extracolonic findings will be affected. These issues will be discussed in this section. Most important is the effect on the detection of colorectal cancer and polyps, not only by human observers, but also by algorithms that are used in computer-aided detection schemes.

### 5.1 Detection of Colorectal Cancer and Polyps

Both experimental and clinical studies (vide supra) have shown that radiation exposure can be reduced substantially without detrimental effect on the detection of clinically relevant polyps (6 mm or larger) in air; this most likely also applies to colorectal cancer although there are no data specific for colorectal cancer. Present protocols often use settings of in the order of 50 mAs at 120 kV (Liedenbaum et al. 2008). Reduction seems to be possible to approximately 10 mAs, which is close to the lowest mAs setting for most CT scanners. Experimental studies have demonstrated the feasibility of CT colonography with even much lower radiation exposure. With simulated

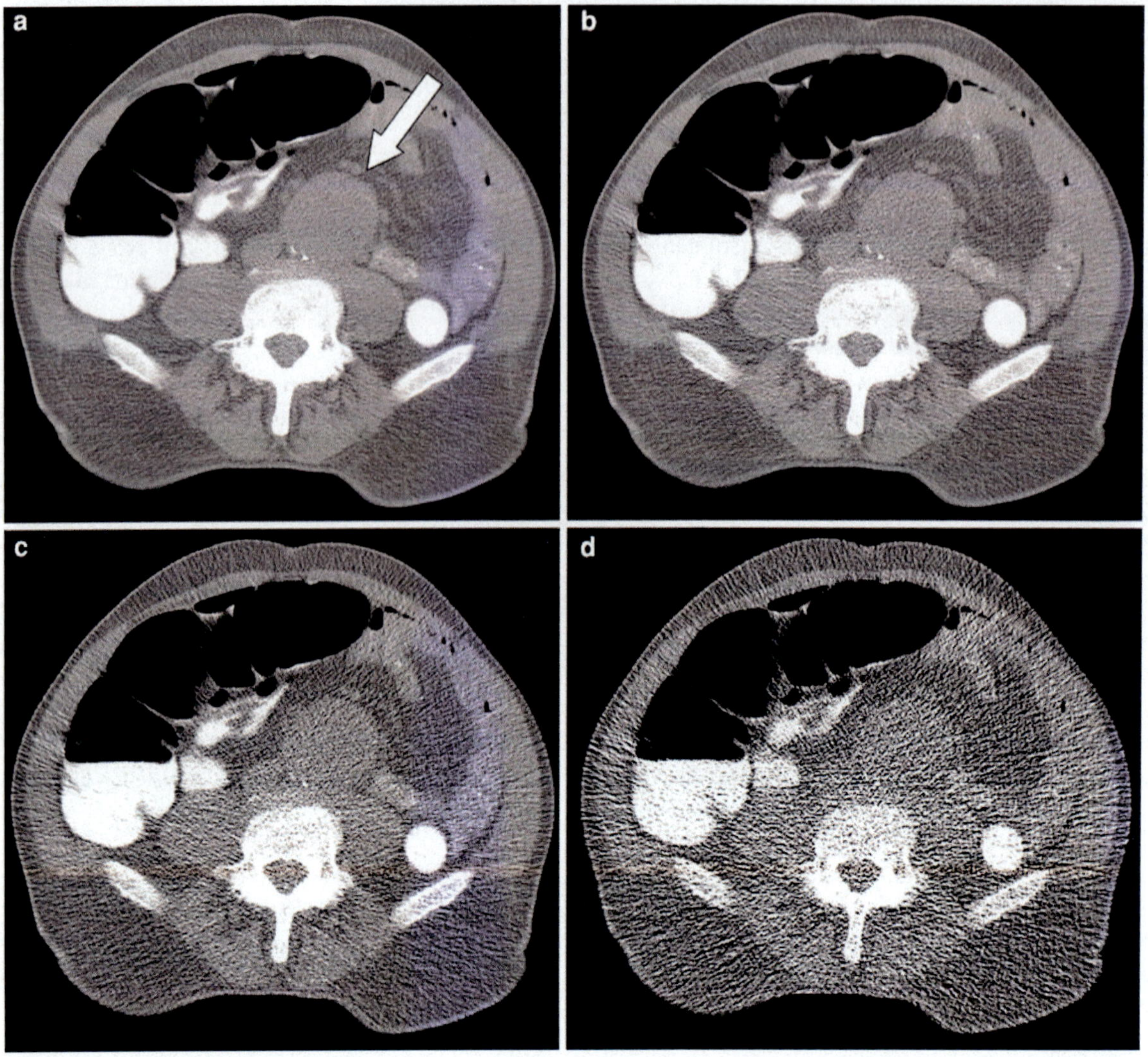


**Fig. 6** CT colonography in supine position after extensive bowel preparation and tagging with iodine in a 76-year-old man. *Left upper panel* CT colonographic image obtained at 50 mAs; *right upper panel* CT colonographic image simulated at 25 mAs; *left lower panel* CT colonographic image simulated at 6.3 mAs; *right lower panel* CT colonographic image simulated at 1.6 mAs. The examination was performed for surveillance for colorectal cancer. As incidental finding a 4.7 cm aneurysm of the distal abdominal aorta was found, which was however already known prior to the examination. The aneurysm is still identifiable at the lowest dose

ultra-low-dose CT colonography detection of larger polyps (≥10 mm) was unimpaired at a setting of 1.6 mAs, corresponding with effective doses of 0.2 mSv for two positions (van Gelder et al. 2004). However, this setting is an order of magnitude lower than what can be realized with present-day scanners, and it is improbable that such an extremely low mAs setting will soon be realized.

A substantial lower dose *can* be obtained with present-day scanners by using a lower tube voltage. Most CT scanners nowadays have a lowest setting of 80 kV, and in comparison with the tube voltage that is customarily used of 120 kV, the choice of this lower tube voltage results in a dose reduction by a factor 3 or 4 (see Sect. 4.2). The performance of ultra-low-dose CT achieved with this low tube voltage in combination with a low mAs setting should be verified in clinical practice.

In practice, the situation is more complicated because nowadays fecal tagging is almost always used. The possibilities of ultra-low-dose CT in this situation are more limited because of the reduced contrast of the polyps relative to their surroundings (see Sect. 4.3.2). It is important that a bowel preparation scheme is used that produces tagging with sufficient contrast. The choice of a lower tube voltage than the customary setting of 120 kV could be advantageous for CT colonography examinations with limited bowel preparation and fecal tagging. In these examinations one could chose a tube voltage of 80 or 90 kV, and a somewhat higher mAs level, as at these lower tube voltages the contrast-to-noise ratio for polyps embedded in material of higher atomic numbers, such as the tagging agents iodine and barium, will be increased for the same dose. The magnitude of this effect will, however, also depends on the size (girth) of the patient. As mentioned earlier, even in a situation of limited bowel preparation only a small portion of polyps will be covered by tagging material, and it is conceivable that one should be prepared to accept a slightly decreased visibility of these polyps, as long as the overall performance is not impaired to a significant degree. Clearly, further study is needed with respect to this point.

Nowadays the availability of CT scanners with a large number of detector rows of small width, with an accompanying slice width of 1 mm or less is advantageous for the visualization of polyps, especially of small polyps. Although the clinical relevance of detecting these small polyps (5 mm or less) is low, the increased spatial resolution might be important for detection of flat lesions. Whether (sub-) millimeter slice width leads to substantial benefits for sensitivity and specificity has yet to be determined, but some beneficial effects can be expected. A truly isotropic resolution is advantageous for reconstructions and for computer-aided detection because of the inherent 3D nature of the depicted volume of interest.

Of course, when the slice width is reduced without adjusting the other scan parameters, the noise in each image will increase. This does not have to be a problem, as this increase can be counteracted by viewing MPR images with a slightly increased thickness (Prokop 2003). For computer-aided detection (CAD) truly isotropic resolution will be advantageous as well, both for electronic cleansing of tagged examinations (see Sect. 2.3) and the detection of the polyps.

It is clear that all available means to obtain an optimal image quality for a given dose should be utilized. Thus, tube current adaptation to the body size, and/or tube current modulation should be used, as the posture of a patient, and the shape of the cross-section (e.g. of the pelvis) influence image noise to a large extent. By using these measures, the differences in noise level in different parts of the patient, and between different patients, will be considerably reduced. Application of noise reduction filters and/or iterative reconstruction techniques appears to be promising to reduce the dose of CTC examinations without affecting the image quality. As mentioned earlier, more extensive studies are needed to establish the value of these techniques in a clinical context.

## 5.2 Extracolonic Findings

Extracolonic findings are relatively common at regular-dose CT colonography in symptomatic patients. Almost 40% of individuals with symptoms of colorectal cancer have extracolonic findings, although the prevalence of new, relevant findings is relatively low (Xiong et al. 2005). In a screening setting the number of relevant findings is even substantially lower (Kim et al. 2007).

Although some consider extracolonic findings a beneficial part of CT colonography—total body screening, this potentially is not the case. Many extracolonic findings are not relevant or already known and some relevant new findings may concern untreatable disease (Figs. 6 and 7). The anxiety of participants, additional diagnostic workup and possible treatment and use of resources are major disadvantages. Since many guidelines for incidental findings are based on symptomatic patients, additional workup most likely is advised too often in the asymptomatic screening population. Future guidelines, specified for an asymptomatic population may reduce the amount of workup and therefore lower burden and costs, while increasing the acceptance. Extracolonic findings may be an important factor determining whether CT colonography is a cost-effective screening method. Therefore, low radiation dose CT colonography may also be considered a boon in this respect as this will impair the detection of extracolonic findings (Figs. 6 and 7).

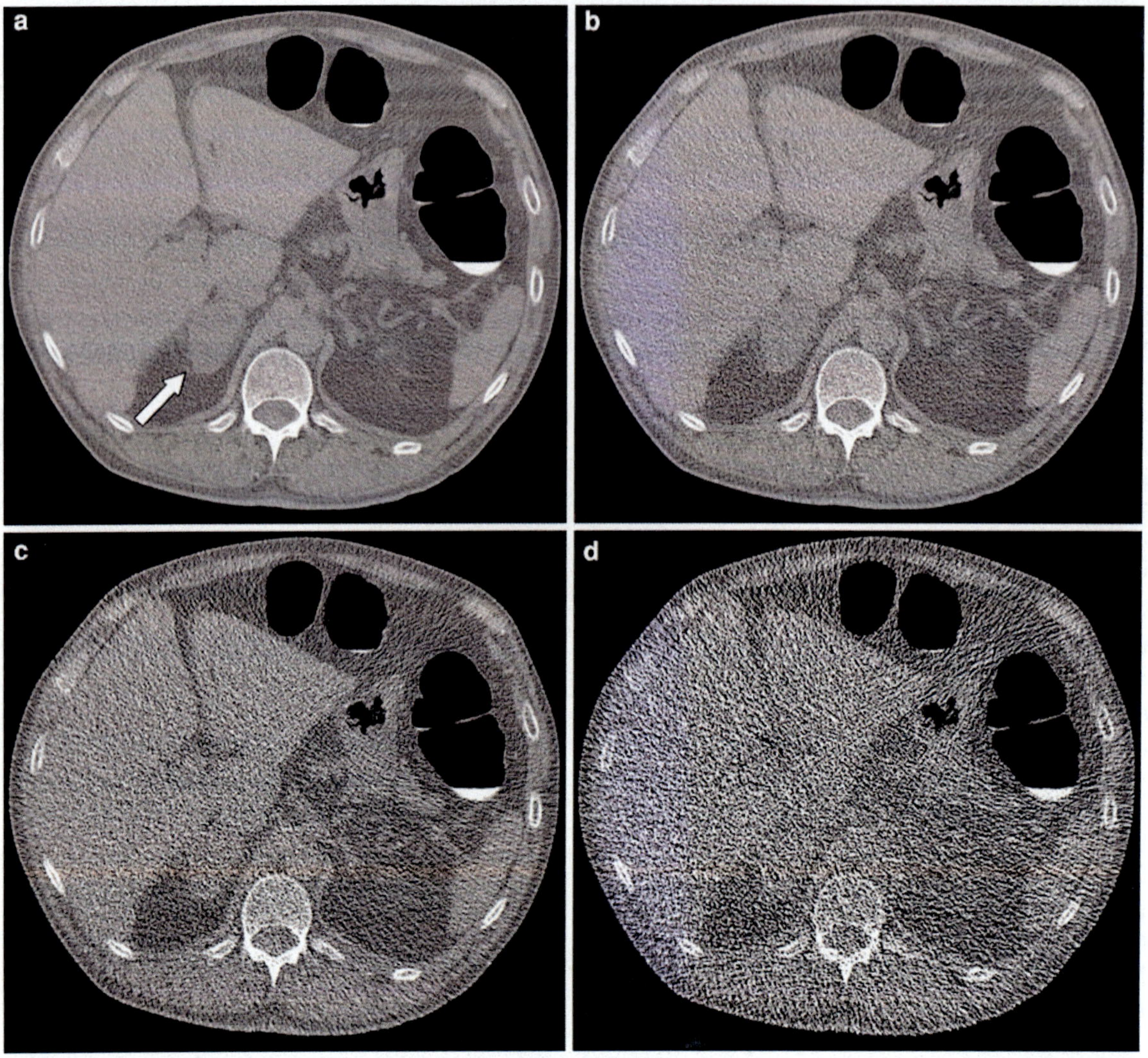


**Fig. 7** CT colonography in supine position after extensive bowel preparation and tagging with iodine contrast medium in a 57-year-old woman. *Left upper panel* CT colonographic image obtained at 70 mAs; *right upper panel* CT colonographic image simulated at 25 mAs; *left lower panel* CT colonographic image simulated at 6.3 mAs; *right lower panel* CT colonographic image simulated at 1.6 mAs. The examination was performed for surveillance for colorectal cancer. As incidental finding an enlarged right adrenal is visible with CT features (size, density) suggestive for a metastasis. This finding was not known prior to the CT colonography and prompted further workup. The patient proved to have lung cancer with a metastasis in the *right* adrenal gland. The enlarged *right* adrenal is not identifiable at the lowest simulated dose

## 5.3 Risk Versus Benefit

The risks of a CT colonography examination (apart from rare complications such as perforation) are difficult to assess with certainty, as already mentioned in the introduction to this discussion. In a recent study on radiation-related cancer risks Berrington de González and colleagues estimated that for effective doses of 7 to 8 mSv for a CT colonography examination, which they calculated for the participants of the ACRIN National Colonography trial, the risk of induction of cancer is 0.06% for a 50-year-old person (de González et al. 2011). For a screening CT colonography examination with lower dose the risk will of course be proportionally less. The above-mentioned risk is less than the risk of 0.14% calculated earlier by

Brenner and Georgsson for a similar effective dose (Brenner and Georgsson 2005). This is due to the fact that in more recent study data from the most recent BEIR report were used (Brenner and Georgsson 2005; BEIR VII 2006).

In assessing these risks it is of course also important to realize that a radiation-induced cancer may become manifest only after a long latent period, possibly tens of years. When individuals are to be examined more than once, the risk will increase proportionally. However, the risk on a fatal cancer will reduce with an increase of age. Furthermore there is an ongoing discussion on the statistical evidence for the estimates depend heavily on the assumptions made (Brenner and Georgsson 2005; Brenner and Sachs 2006; Prokop 2005; Friedl and Ruhm 2006; Tubiana et al. 2006, 2009; Little et al. 2009). Nevertheless, it is prudent to assume that exposure to the amount of radiation used in a CT colonography examination is accompanied with a small risk of induction of cancer, and that this risk becomes smaller when the dose is reduced.

Berrington de González and colleagues also attempted to determine the benefit-risk ratio of CT colonography for colorectal cancer screening (de González et al. 2011). The calculated benefit-risk ratio ranged from 24:1 (95% uncertainty interval, 13:1–45:1) to 35:1 (95% uncertainty interval, 19:1–65:1) depending on the model used.

The benefit of CT colonography is the detection of colorectal cancer and advanced adenoma (advanced neoplasia). Data on colorectal cancer detection in screening CT colonography is limited due to the low prevalence in screening studies. The patient sensitivity for advanced adenomas of $\geq$6 and $\geq$10 mm is good (75.9 and 83.3%) and specificity is even better (94.6 and 98.7% respectively) (de Haan et al. 2011). More studies are necessary on participation of CT colonography screening, cost-effectiveness (influenced among others by extracolonic findings) and effect on mortality. Cost-effectiveness has been studied by modeling studies only, in which results depend on the model used and multiple assumptions. In a recent study it was concluded that CT colonography was not yet cost-effective for screening, as compared to FOBT and colonoscopy (Lansdorp-Vogelaar et al. 2011). Further studies should concentrate on the evaluation the cost-effectiveness of low-dose CTC screening programs in combination with fecal tagging.

## 6 Conclusions

For CT colonography to be considered as screening tool the benefit of its use must outweigh the risks/disadvantages. CT colonography has been demonstrated to have a high accuracy for the lesions important in screening. The benefit of CT colonography for reducing mortality and morbidity for colorectal cancer has not been determined yet, although present data on accuracy are encouraging. The risks and disadvantages include the possibility of the induction of cancer, as well as other factors such as false positives, extracolonic findings and costs. With regard to the induction of cancer, with the scan parameters used until now the risk seems to be relatively small, but cannot be completely neglected. Moreover, the risk will increase with the number of examinations performed. Although the frequency of screening for colon cancer with CT colonography most likely will be less than, for instance, for lung cancer or breast cancer, further reduction in radiation exposure of CT colonography is desirable. Apart from reducing the risk of cancer induction, reduction in radiation exposure may also be valuable for patient acceptance and adherence by reducing the fear for radiation exposure. Decreased radiation exposure will result in noisier images that at a certain level will preclude the evaluation of extracolonic findings. This might be an advantage when extracolonic findings might prove to be detrimental for cost-effective screening of colorectal cancer with CT colonography.

Low radiation dose CT colonography with acceptable to good sensitivity and specificity is feasible, even in combination with limited bowel preparation and tagging. Efforts should be made to further study the limits and pros and cons of low radiation dose CT colonography.

**Acknowledgment** Thierry Boellaard and Jaap Stoker pay tribute to our co-author Henk Venema who deceased after finalizing this chapter. Henk Venema was pivotal for this work and to our work in general on radiation dose in CT colonography.

## References


ACR (2009) ACR practice guideline for the performance of computed tomography (CT) colonography in adults. ACR practice guideline. Am Coll Radiol pp 1–10

Anupindi S, Perumpillichira J, Jaramillo D, Zalis ME, Israel EJ (2005) Low-dose CT colonography in children: initial experience, technical feasibility, and utility. Pediatr Radiol 35(5):518–524. doi:10.1007/s00247-004-1394-2

Atkin WS, Edwards R, Kralj-Hans I, Wooldrage K, Hart AR, Northover JM, Parkin DM, Wardle J, Duffy SW, Cuzick J (2010) Once-only flexible sigmoidoscopy screening in prevention of colorectal cancer: a multicentre randomised controlled trial. Lancet 375(9726):1624–1633. doi:10.1016/S0140-6736(10)60551-X

Baum U, Noemayr A, Reissig A, Lell M, Cavallaro A, Kachelriess M, Riedel T, Kalender WA, Bautz W (2003) Improvement of the image quality of MSCT of the pelvis with a raw data-based, multidimensional filter. Rofo 175(11):1572–1576. doi:10.1055/s-2003-43401

BEIR VII (2006) Committee to assess health risks from exposure to low levels of ionizing radiation, board on radiation effects research, division of earth and life studies, national research council of the national academies. Health risks from exposure to low levels of ionizing radiation: BEIR VII phase 2. National Academies Press, Washington

Brenner DJ, Georgsson MA (2005) Mass screening with CT colonography: should the radiation exposure be of concern? Gastroenterology 129(1):328–337

Brenner DJ, Sachs RK (2006) Estimating radiation-induced cancer risks at very low doses: rationale for using a linear no-threshold approach. Radiat Environ Biophys 44(4):253–256. doi:10.1007/s00411-006-0029-4

Burling D (2010) CT colonography standards. Clin Radiol 65(6):474–480. doi:10.1016/j.crad.2009.12.003

Cai W, Lee JG, Zalis ME, Yoshida H (2011) Mosaic decomposition: an electronic cleansing method for inhomogeneously tagged regions in noncathartic CT colonography. IEEE Trans Med Imaging 30(3):559–574. doi:10.1109/TMI.2010.2087389

Capunay CM, Carrascosa PM, Bou-Khair A, Castagnino N, Ninomiya I, Carrascosa JM (2005) Low radiation dose multislice CT colonography in children: experience after 100 studies. Eur J Radiol 56(3):398–402. doi:10.1016/j.ejrad.2005.06.002

Carmi R, Kafri G, Goshen L, Amin-Spector S, Altman A, Sosna J (2008) A unique noncathartic CT colonography approach by using two-layer dual-energy MDCT and a special algorithmic colon cleansing method. IEEE Nucl Sci Symp Conf Record

Chaparro M, Gisbert JP, Del Campo L, Cantero J, Mate J (2009) Accuracy of computed tomographic colonography for the detection of polyps and colorectal tumors: a systematic review and meta-analysis. Digestion 80(1):1–17. doi:10.1159/000215387

Cody DD, Mahesh M (2007) AAPM/RSNA physics tutorial for residents: technologic advances in multidetector CT with a focus on cardiac imaging. Radiographics: a review publication of the radiological society of North America, Inc 27 (6):1829–1837. doi: 10.1148/rg.276075120

Cohnen M, Vogt C, Beck A, Andersen K, Heinen W, vom Dahl S, Aurich V, Haeussinger D, Moedder U (2004) Feasibility of MDCT colonography in ultra-low-dose technique in the detection of colorectal lesions: comparison with high-resolution video colonoscopy. AJR Am J Roentgenol 183(5):1355–1359

Cunningham D, Atkin W, Lenz HJ, Lynch HT, Minsky B, Nordlinger B, Starling N (2010) Colorectal cancer. Lancet 375(9719):1030–1047. doi:10.1016/S0140-6736(10)60353-4

de González AB, Kim KP, Knudsen AB, Lansdorp-Vogelaar I, Rutter CM, Smith-Bindman R, Yee J, Kuntz KM, van Ballegooijen M, Zauber AG, Berg CD (2011) Radiation-related cancer risks from CT colonography screening: a risk-benefit analysis. AJR Am J Roentgenol 196(4):816–823. doi:10.2214/AJR.10.4907

de Haan MC, van Gelder RE, Graser A, Bipat S, Stoker J (2011) Diagnostic value of CT-colonography as compared to colonoscopy in an asymptomatic screening population: a meta-analysis. Eur Radiol 21(8):1747–1763. doi:10.1007/s00330-011-2104-8

de Vries A, Schoonenberg G, Venema H, Grigorescu S, Peters J, Stoker J (2005) Feasibility of automated detection of colon polyps on simulated ultra low dose CTC datasets. In: Proceedings 91st scientifi c assembly and annual meeting radiological society of North America, Oak Brook, USA, 2005

de Vries AH, Venema HW, Florie J, Nio CY, Stoker J (2008) Influence of tagged fecal material on detectability of colorectal polyps at CT: phantom study. AJR Am J Roentgenol 191(4):1101. doi:10.2214/AJR.07.3740

Fisichella VA, Bath M, Allansdotter Johnsson A, Jaderling F, Bergsten T, Persson U, Mellingen K, Hellstrom M (2010) Evaluation of image quality and lesion perception by human readers on 3D CT colonography: comparison of standard and low radiation dose. Eur Radiol 20(3):630–639. doi: 10.1007/s00330-009-1601-5

Flicek KT, Hara AK, Silva AC, Wu Q, Peter MB, Johnson CD (2010) Reducing the radiation dose for CT colonography using adaptive statistical iterative reconstruction: a pilot study. AJR Am J Roentgenol 195(1):126–131. doi:10.2214/AJR.09.3855

Florie J, van Gelder RE, Schutter MP, van Randen A, Venema HW, de Jager S, van der Hulst VP, Prent A, Bipat S, Bossuyt PM, Baak LC, Stoker J (2007) Feasibility study of computed tomography colonography using limited bowel preparation at normal and low-dose levels study. Eur Radiol 17(12):3112–3122. doi:10.1007/s00330-007-0668-0

Franaszek M, Summers RM, Pickhardt PJ, Choi JR (2006) Hybrid segmentation of colon filled with air and opacified fluid for CT colonography. IEEE Trans Med Imaging 25(3):358–368. doi:10.1109/TMI.2005.863836

Friedl AA, Ruhm W (2006) LNT: a never-ending story. Radiat Environ Biophys 44(4):241–244. doi:10.1007/s00411-006-0028-5

Graser A, Wintersperger BJ, Suess C, Reiser MF, Becker CR (2006) Dose reduction and image quality in MDCT colonography using tube current modulation. AJR Am J Roentgenol 187(3):695–701. doi:10.2214/AJR.05.0662

Greess H, Wolf H, Baum U, Kalender WA, Bautz W (1999) Dosage reduction in computed tomography by anatomy-oriented attenuation-based tube-current modulation: the first clinical results. Rofo 170(3):246–250. doi:10.1055/s-2007-1011035

Halligan S, Altman DG, Taylor SA, Mallett S, Deeks JJ, Bartram CI, Atkin W (2005) CT colonography in the detection of colorectal polyps and cancer: systematic review, meta-analysis, and proposed minimum data set for study level reporting. Radiology 237(3):893–904. doi: 10.1148/radiol.2373050176

Hara AK, Paden RG, Silva AC, Kujak JL, Lawder HJ, Pavlicek W (2009) Iterative reconstruction technique for reducing body radiation dose at CT: feasibility study. AJR Am J Roentgenol 193(3):764–771. doi:10.2214/AJR.09.2397

Hewitson P, Glasziou P, Watson E, Towler B, Irwig L (2008) Cochrane systematic review of colorectal cancer screening using the fecal occult blood test (hemoccult): an update. Am J Gastroenterol 103(6):1541–1549. doi:10.1111/j.1572-0241.2008.01875.x

Hounsfield GN (1973) Computerized transverse axial scanning (tomography) 1 description of system. Br J Radiol 46(552): 1016–1022

Hsieh J (1998) Adaptive streak artifact reduction in computed tomography resulting from excessive X-ray photon noise. Med Phys 25(11):2139–2147

Iannaccone R, Laghi A, Catalano C, Mangiapane F, Piacentini F, Passariello R (2003) Feasibility of ultra-low-dose multislice CT colonography for the detection of colorectal lesions: preliminary experience. Eur Radiol 13(6):1297–1302. doi:10.1007/s00330-002-1704-8

Iannaccone R, Laghi A, Catalano C, Mangiapane F, Lamazza A, Schillaci A, Sinibaldi G, Murakami T, Sammartino P, Hori M, Piacentini F, Nofroni I, Stipa V, Passariello R (2004) Computed tomographic colonography without cathartic preparation for the detection of colorectal polyps. Gastroenterology 127(5):1300–1311

Jemal A, Bray F, Center MM, Ferlay J, Ward E, Forman D (2011) Global cancer statistics. CA Cancer J Clin 61(2):69–90. doi:10.3322/caac.20107

Jensch S, van Gelder RE, Venema HW, Reitsma JB, Bossuyt PM, Lameris JS, Stoker J (2006) Effective radiation doses in CT colonography: results of an inventory among research institutions. Eur Radiol 16(5):981–987. doi:10.1007/s00330-005-0047-7

Johnson KT, Johnson CD, Anderson SM, Bruesewitz MR, McCollough CH (2004) CT colonography: determination of optimal CT technique using a novel colon phantom. Abdom Imaging 29(2):173–176. doi:10.1007/s00261-003-0069-z

Johnson TR, Krauss B, Sedlmair M, Grasruck M, Bruder H, Morhard D, Fink C, Weckbach S, Lenhard M, Schmidt B, Flohr T, Reiser MF, Becker CR (2007) Material differentiation by dual energy CT: initial experience. Eur Radiol 17(6):1510–1517. doi:10.1007/s00330-006-0517-6

Jones DG, Shrimpton PC (1991) Survey of CT practice in the UK: normalised organ doses for X-ray computed tomography calculated using Monte Carlo techniques. National Radiological Protection Board, Harwell. Available at: www.impactscan.org/ctdosimetry.htm

Kachelriess M, Watzke O, Kalender WA (2001) Generalized multi-dimensional adaptive filtering for conventional and spiral single-slice, multi-slice, and cone-beam CT. Med Phys 28(4):475–490

Kalender WA (2005) Computed tomography fundamentals, system technology, image quality, applications. 2nd revised and enlarged edition. Publicis MCD Verlag, Munich

Kalender WA, Deak P, Kellermeier M, van Straten M, Vollmar SV (2009) Application- and patient size-dependent optimization of X-ray spectra for CT. Med Phys 36(3):993–1007

Kalra MK, Maher MM, Toth TL, Schmidt B, Westerman BL, Morgan HT, Saini S (2004) Techniques and applications of automatic tube current modulation for CT. Radiology 233(3):649–657. doi:10.1148/radiol.2333031150

Karcaaltincaba M, Karaosmanoglu D, Akata D, Senturk S, Ozmen M, Alibek S (2009) Dual energy virtual CT colonoscopy with dual source computed tomography: initial experience. Rofo 181(9):859–862. doi:10.1055/s-0028-1109569

Kim DH, Pickhardt PJ, Taylor AJ, Leung WK, Winter TC, Hinshaw JL, Gopal DV, Reichelderfer M, Hsu RH, Pfau PR (2007) CT colonography versus colonoscopy for the detection of advanced neoplasia. N Engl J Med 357(14): 1403–1412. doi:10.1056/NEJMoa070543

Kim SH, Lee JM, Shin CI, Kim HC, Lee JG, Kim JH, Choi JY, Eun HW, Han JK, Lee JY, Choi BI (2008) Effects of spatial resolution and tube current on computer-aided detection of polyps on CT colonographic images: phantom study. Radiology 248(2):492–503. doi:10.1148/radiol.2482071025

La Riviere PJ (2005) Penalized-likelihood sinogram smoothing for low-dose CT. Med Phys 32(6):1676–1683

Laghi A, Iannaccone R, Mangiapane F, Piacentini F, Iori S, Passariello R (2003) Experimental colonic phantom for the evaluation of the optimal scanning technique for CT colonography using a multidetector spiral CT equipment. Eur Radiol 13(3):459–466. doi:10.1007/s00330-002-1671-0

Lansdorp-Vogelaar I, Knudsen AB, Brenner H (2011) Cost-effectiveness of colorectal cancer screening. Epidemiol Rev 33(1):88–100. doi:10.1093/epirev/mxr004

Lawrence EM, Pickhardt PJ, Kim DH, Robbins JB (2010) Colorectal polyps: stand-alone performance of computer-aided detection in a large asymptomatic screening population. Radiology 256(3):791–798. doi:10.1148/radiol.10092292

Lieberman D, Moravec M, Holub J, Michaels L, Eisen G (2008) Polyp size and advanced histology in patients undergoing colonoscopy screening: implications for CT colonography. Gastroenterology 135(4):1100–1105. doi: 10.1053/j.gastro.2008.06.083

Liedenbaum MH, Venema HW, Stoker J (2008) Radiation dose in CT colonography–trends in time and differences between daily practice and screening protocols. Eur Radiol 18(10):2222–2230. doi:10.1007/s00330-008-0994-x

Liedenbaum MH, de Vries AH, Gouw CI, van Rijn AF, Bipat S, Dekker E, Stoker J (2010a) CT colonography with minimal bowel preparation: evaluation of tagging quality, patient acceptance and diagnostic accuracy in two iodine-based preparation schemes. Eur Radiol 20(2):367–376. doi: 10.1007/s00330-009-1570-8

Liedenbaum MH, Denters MJ, de Vries AH, van Ravesteijn VF, Bipat S, Vos FM, Dekker E, Stoker J (2010b) Low-fiber diet in limited bowel preparation for CT colonography: influence on image quality and patient acceptance. AJR Am J Roentgenol 195(1):W31–W37. doi:10.2214/AJR.09.3572

Little MP, Wakeford R, Tawn EJ, Bouffler SD, Berrington de González A (2009) Risks associated with low doses and low dose rates of ionizing radiation: why linearity may be (almost) the best we can do. Radiology 251(1):6–12. doi: 10.1148/radiol.2511081686

Lubner MG, Pickhardt PJ, Tang J, Chen GH (2011) Reduced image noise at low-dose multidetector CT of the abdomen with prior image constrained compressed sensing algorithm. Radiology 260(1):248–256. doi:10.1148/radiol.11101380

Luz O, Schafer J, Dammann F, Vonthein R, Heuschmid M, Claussen CD (2004) Evaluation of different 16-row CT colonography protocols using a porcine model. Rofo 176(10):1493–1500. doi:10.1055/s-2004-813407

Macari M, Bini EJ, Xue X, Milano A, Katz SS, Resnick D, Chandarana H, Krinsky G, Klingenbeck K, Marshall CH, Megibow AJ (2002) Colorectal neoplasms: prospective comparison of thin-section low-dose multi-detector row CT colonography and conventional colonoscopy for detection. Radiology 224(2):383–392

Mahgerefteh S, Fraifeld S, Blachar A, Sosna J (2009) CT colonography with decreased purgation: balancing preparation, performance, and patient acceptance. AJR Am J Roentgenol 193(6):1531–1539. doi:10.2214/AJR.09.2342

Manduca A, Yu L, Trzasko JD, Khaylova N, Kofler JM, McCollough CM, Fletcher JG (2009) Projection space denoising with bilateral filtering and CT noise modeling for dose reduction in CT. Med Phys 36(11):4911–4919

McCollough CH, Bruesewitz MR, Kofler Jr. JM (2006) CT dose reduction and dose management tools: overview of available options. Radiographics : a review publication of the radiological society of North America, Inc 26 (2):503–512. doi: 10.1148/rg.262055138

Mulhall BP, Veerappan GR, Jackson JL (2005) Meta-analysis: computed tomographic colonography. Ann Intern Med 142(8):635–650

Nagata K, Okawa T, Honma A, Endo S, Kudo SE, Yoshida H (2009) Full-laxative versus minimum-laxative fecal-tagging CT colonography using 64-detector row CT: prospective blinded comparison of diagnostic performance, tagging quality, and patient acceptance. Academic Radiol 16(7):780–789. doi:10.1016/j.acra.2008.12.027

Pickhardt PJ, Kim DH, Meiners RJ, Wyatt KS, Hanson ME, Barlow DS, Cullen PA, Remtulla RA, Cash BD (2010) Colorectal and extracolonic cancers detected at screening CT colonography in 10, 286 asymptomatic adults. Radiology 255(1):83–88. doi:10.1148/radiol.09090939

Pickhardt PJ, Hassan C, Halligan S, Marmo R (2011) Colorectal cancer: CT colonography and colonoscopy for detection–systematic review and meta-analysis. Radiology 259(2):393–405. doi:10.1148/radiol.11101887

Prokop M (2003) General principles of MDCT. Eur J Radiol 45(Suppl1):S4–S10

Prokop M (2005) New challenges in MDCT. Eur Radiol 15(Suppl 5):E35–E45

Renker M, Nance JW Jr, Schoepf UJ, O'Brien TX, Zwerner PL, Meyer M, Kerl JM, Bauer RW, Fink C, Vogl TJ, Henzler T (2011) Evaluation of heavily calcified vessels with coronary CT angiography: comparison of iterative and filtered back projection image reconstruction. Radiology 260(2):390–399. doi:10.1148/radiol.11103574

Rizzo SM, Kalra MK, Schmidt B, Raupach R, Maher MM, Blake MA, Saini S (2005) CT images of abdomen and pelvis: effect of nonlinear three-dimensional optimized reconstruction algorithm on image quality and lesion characteristics. Radiology 237(1):309–315. doi:10.1148/radiol.2371041879

Robinson C, Halligan S, Taylor SA, Mallett S, Altman DG (2008) CT colonography: a systematic review of standard of reporting for studies of computer-aided detection. Radiology 246(2):426–433. doi:10.1148/radiol.2461070121

Rogalla P, Kloeters C, Hein PA (2009) CT technology overview: 64-slice and beyond. Radiol Clin North Am 47(1):1–11. doi:10.1016/j.rcl.2008.10.004

Schilham A, van der Molen AJ, Prokop M, de Jong HW (2010) Overranging at multisection CT: an underestimated source of excess radiation exposure. Radiographics : a review publication of the radiological society of North America, Inc 30 (4):1057–1067. doi: 10.1148/rg.304095167

Sosna J, Morrin MM, Kruskal JB, Lavin PT, Rosen MP, Raptopoulos V (2003) CT colonography of colorectal polyps: a metaanalysis. AJR Am J Roentgenol 181(6): 1593–1598

Sosna J, Sella T, Sy O, Lavin PT, Eliahou R, Fraifeld S, Libson E (2008) Critical analysis of the performance of double-contrast barium enema for detecting colorectal polyps > or = 6 mm in the era of CT colonography. AJR Am J Roentgenol 190(2):374–385. doi:10.2214/AJR.07.2099

Summers RM, Franaszek M, Miller MT, Pickhardt PJ, Choi JR, Schindler WR (2005a) Computer-aided detection of polyps on oral contrast-enhanced CT colonography. AJR Am J Roentgenol 184(1):105–108

Summers RM, Yao J, Pickhardt PJ, Franaszek M, Bitter I, Brickman D, Krishna V, Choi JR (2005b) Computed tomographic virtual colonoscopy computer-aided polyp detection in a screening population. Gastroenterology 129(6):1832–1844. doi:10.1053/j.gastro.2005.08.054

Sundaram P, Beaulieu CF, Paik DS, Schraedley-Desmond P, Napel S (2003) CT colonography: does improved z resolution help computer-aided polyp detection? Med Phys 30(10):2663–2674

Taylor SA, Halligan S, Bartram CI, Morgan PR, Talbot IC, Fry N, Saunders BP, Khosraviani K, Atkin W (2003) Multi-detector row CT colonography: effect of collimation, pitch, and orientation on polyp detection in a human colectomy specimen. Radiology 229(1):109–118. doi:10.1148/radiol.2291020561

Tubiana M, Aurengo A, Averbeck D, Masse R (2006) Recent reports on the effect of low doses of ionizing radiation and its dose-effect relationship. Radiat Environ Biophys 44(4):245–251. doi:10.1007/s00411-006-0032-9

Tubiana M, Feinendegen LE, Yang C, Kaminski JM (2009) The linear no-threshold relationship is inconsistent with radiation biologic and experimental data. Radiology 251(1):13–22. doi:10.1148/radiol.2511080671

Tzedakis A, Damilakis J, Perisinakis K, Stratakis J, Gourtsoyiannis N (2005) The effect of z overscanning on patient effective dose from multidetector helical computed tomography examinations. Med Phys 32(6):1621–1629

USPSTF (2008) Screening for colorectal cancer: U.S. preventive services task force recommendation statement. Ann Intern Med 149(9):627–637 van der Molen AJ, Geleijns J (2007) Overranging in multisection CT: quantification and relative contribution to dose–comparison of four 16-section CT scanners. Radiology 242(1):208–216. doi:10.1148/radiol.2421051350

van Gelder RE, Venema HW, Serlie IW, Nio CY, Determann RM, Tipker CA, Vos FM, Glas AS, Bartelsman JF, Bossuyt PM, Lameris JS, Stoker J (2002) CT colonography at different radiation dose levels: feasibility of dose reduction. Radiology 224(1):25–33

van Gelder RE, Venema HW, Florie J, Nio CY, Serlie IW, Schutter MP, van Rijn JC, Vos FM, Glas AS, Bossuyt PM, Bartelsman JF, Lameris JS, Stoker J (2004) CT colonography: feasibility of substantial dose reduction–comparison of medium to very low doses in identical patients. Radiology 232(2):611–620. doi:10.1148/radiol.2322031069

Vogt C, Cohnen M, Beck A, vom Dahl S, Aurich V, Modder U, Haussinger D (2004) Detection of colorectal polyps by multislice CT colonography with ultra-low-dose technique: comparison with high-resolution videocolonoscopy. Gastrointest Endosc 60(2):201–209

Wessling J, Fischbach R, Meier N, Allkemper T, Klusmeier J, Ludwig K, Heindel W (2003) CT colonography: protocol optimization with multi-detector row CT–study in an anthropomorphic colon phantom. Radiology 228(3):753–759. doi:10.1148/radiol.2283020928

Winklehner A, Karlo C, Puippe G, Schmidt B, Flohr T, Goetti R, Pfammatter T, Frauenfelder T, Alkadhi H (2011) Raw data-based iterative reconstruction in body CTA: evaluation of radiation dose saving potential. Eur Radiol. doi:10.1007/s00330-011-2227-y

Xiong T, Richardson M, Woodroffe R, Halligan S, Morton D, Lilford RJ (2005) Incidental lesions found on CT colonography: their nature and frequency. Br J Radiol 78(925):22–29

Zalis ME, Perumpillichira J, Hahn PF (2004) Digital subtraction bowel cleansing for CT colonography using morphological and linear filtration methods. IEEE Trans Med Imaging 23(11):1335–1343. doi:10.1109/TMI.2004.826050

Zalis ME, Barish MA, Choi JR, Dachman AH, Fenlon HM, Ferrucci JT, Glick SN, Laghi A, Macari M, McFarland EG, Morrin MM, Pickhardt PJ, Soto J, Yee J (2005) CT colonography reporting and data system: a consensus proposal. Radiology 236(1):3–9. doi:236/1/3[pii]10.1148/radiol.2361041926

# Part V

# Initiatives for Dose Reduction

# CT Dose Perspectives and Initiatives of the IAEA

Madan M. Rehani and Olivera Ciraj-Bjelac

## Contents




**Abstract**

The International Atomic Energy Agency initiated a program in 2001 on Radiation Protection of Patients which included many actions to reduce patient doses in computed tomography without compromising image quality. The hallmark has been international cooperation under the International Action Plan for the Radiological Protection of Patients. Specific actions included a survey of practice in developing countries in terms of justification and optimisation in CT, frequency of adult and pediatric CT examinations, availability and use of imaging protocols, dose tracking initiative, development and dissemination of training materials and activities in the area of radiation protection in new computed tomography-based imaging modalities, all on a global scale. The achievements of the International Action Plan, which include harmonised training material, guidance documents, a number of publications, a website on radiation protection of patients (http://rpop.iaea.org) and a series of actions in developing countries that have shown positive impacts on patient protection, are summarised in this chapter. Such large-scale multi-national studies are the first of its kind and provide good insight into the situation and opportunities for improvement.



M. M. Rehani (✉)
International Atomic Energy Agency,
Vienna International Centre,
1400 Vienna, Austria
e-mail: M.M.Rehani@iaea.org

O. Ciraj-Bjelac
Vinca Institute of Nuclear Sciences,
M.P. Alasa 12-14, Vinca, Belgrade, Serbia


## 1 Introduction

The International Atomic Energy Agency (IAEA) is the world's centre of cooperation in the nuclear field. It was set up in 1957 as the world's "Atoms for Peace" organization within the United Nations


D. Tack et al. (eds.), *Radiation Dose from Multidetector CT*, Medical Radiology. Diagnostic Imaging,
DOI: 10.1007/174_2011_487, © Springer-Verlag Berlin Heidelberg 2012

family. The IAEA works with its Member States and multiple partners worldwide to promote safe, secure and peaceful nuclear technologies.

The IAEA Secretariat is composed of a team of 2300 multi-disciplinary professional and support staff from more than 100 countries. However, there are a handful of professionals (normally 4) who are actively involved with radiation protection in radiology located in 2 separate functional units—radiation safety and in dosimetry and medical radiation physics section.

The IAEA's mission is guided by the interests and needs of Member States, strategic plans and the vision embodied in the IAEA Statute. Three main pillars—or areas of work—underpin the IAEA's mission: Safety and Security; Science and Technology and Safeguards and Verification. The mission with a direct link to radiation safety is "To establish or adopt, standards of safety for protection of health and minimization of danger to life and property, and to provide for the application of these standards". The United Nations Scientific Committee on Effects of Atomic Radiation (UNSCEAR) has the responsibility to provide data on usage of radiation in the world and radiation effects whereas the International Commission on Radiological Protection (ICRP) provides principles of radiological protection and recommendations. There is a global acceptance of concepts and principles of radiation protection as developed by the ICRP such as justification, optimisation and dose limitation. In radiation protection of patients, there is a universal agreement that there should be no dose limits and that the concept of diagnostic reference levels should be used with flexibility. The IAEA takes into account information provided by UNSCEAR and ICRP and forms radiation safety standards.

## 2 IAEA Safety Standards

The standard applicable for radiation safety in radiology is the International Basic Safety Standards for Protection against Ionizing Radiation and for the Safety of Radiation Sources (BSS). It provides "requirements" and thus has a regulatory tone. The purpose is to provide a harmonized regulatory framework that countries can use to adapt it for framing national regulations. The currently available BSS was published as IAEA Safety Series No. 115 (IAEA 1996). The BSS is undergoing revision and the revised BSS is expected to be published in 2012–2013, but the interim version shall be available in late 2011 or early 2012. The BSS is jointly sponsored by the Food and Agriculture Organization of the United Nations (FAO), the IAEA, the International Labour Office (ILO), the Organisation for Economic Co-operation and Development/Nuclear Energy Agency (OECD/NEA), the Pan American Health Organization (PAHO) and the World Health Organization (WHO). The BSS is a part of the IAEA's regulatory related publications called IAEA Safety Standards Series.

The IAEA has published a Safety Report (IAEA 2002a) and a Safety Guide (IAEA 2006) to assist regulatory authorities in monitoring compliance with the BSS (or equivalent national regulations). Further, a number of safety reports have been published in specific areas like PET/CT (IAEA 2008a), cardiac CT (IAEA 2008b), CT colonography (IAEA 2008c) and also on establishing guidance levels in X ray guided medical interventional procedures (IAEA 2009b). There are other publications in the family of TECDOCs (IAEA 2009a) and an international code of practice on dosimetry in diagnostic radiology (IAEA 2007).

The IAEA not only uses a top-down approach through provision of "requirements" and guidance to meet these requirements, but also a bottom-up approach to assess ground realities in Member States and develop guidance (Rehani and Tsapaki 2011). These activities, which are described later in this chapter, are aimed at building capacities in many developing countries in patient dose management in diagnostic and interventional radiology (Muhogora et al. 2008, 2009, 2010; Ciraj-Bjelac et al. 2011; Tsapaki et al. 2009).

## 3 International Action Plan Radiation Protection of Patients

Realising that the major part of radiation protection efforts had been directed for over half a century at radiation protection of workers, and that there are major issues in relation to medical exposure, which is by far the largest dose contributor to the global population from man-made radiation sources, the IAEA established an International Action Plan (IAP) in 2002 in cooperation with international organisations and professional bodies (IAEA 2002b). These include WHO, PAHO, UNSCEAR, ICRP, European Commission (EC), International Electrotechnical

Commission (IEC), International Organization for Standardization (ISO) and professional societies in the field of radiology (ISR: International Society of Radiology), medical physics (IOMP: International Organization for Medical Physics), nuclear medicine (WFNMB: World Federation of Nuclear Medicine and Biology), radiographers (ISRRT: International Society of Radiographers and Radiological Technologists) and radiation oncology (ESTRO: European Society for Radiotherapy and Oncology).

The vision of the IAP was to coordinate international efforts, and to provide guidance, on the radiation protection of patients and the overall objective is to make progress in radiation protection of the patient as a whole.

International actions are needed not only to create harmonisation of concepts but also to give impetus to some areas, raise awareness about emerging issues and forewarn about upcoming dangers if actions are not initiated by countries well in time (Rehani et al. 2011). For example, the growing use of CT in some developed countries has alerted other countries that they will face the same situation in future years (Muhogora et al. 2009, 2010; Rehani et al. 2011).

After almost a decade now, the achievements of the IAP include harmonised training material (IAEA 2011a) developed in cooperation with WHO, PAHO, ILO, ISR, IOMP and ISRRT, guidance documents, a number of publications, a website on radiation protection of patients (http://rpop.iaea.org) and a series of actions in many countries that have shown positive impacts on patient protection (Rehani et al. 2011; Muhogora et al. 2008, 2009, 2010; Ciraj-Bjelac et al. 2011). The IAP approach is helping to reduce overlap and duplication of efforts. Recently, close collaboration with Image Gently Campaign and Society for Pediatric Radiology in the field of radiation protection in pediatric radiology has been established.

## 4 IAEA Actions in Radiation Dose Management in Computed Tomography

The actions include the following:

1. Coordinated research project (CRP) on dose reduction in CT while maintaining diagnostic confidence;
2. Assessment of doses in adult patients in a large number of developing countries and dose management actions;
3. Radiation protection of children undergoing CT examination in developing countries.

The IAEA has developed a specific approach and identified a number of issues pertaining to CT in developing countries. Some of these are:

(a) Is there a significant workload of procedures that involve relatively higher patient doses, such as CT?
(b) What is the workload of pediatric patients for CT?
(c) Is there an increase in CT examinations and, if so, at what rate?
(d) What are radiation doses to patients and how do they compare with international standards and with doses in developed countries?
(e) What can be done to improve the situation?
(f) Results of actions aimed at improvement of the situation (Rehani and Tsapaki 2011).

Based on these questions, a programme was developed in 2005, a framework for data collection was established in 2006 and the programme implemented in phases during 2006–2011. The results started coming in 2006 from some countries, whereas others who joined later have been submitting results in the following years.

The first strategy employed was to create a situation for increasing cooperation between regulatory authorities and hospitals. This required a shift in working style towards cooperation rather than enforcement. The second step was to create a work plan that can be implemented without dosimetry skills that was non-existent at the time. This step also filtered those participants who could not achieve cooperation. The third step was to impart patient dosimetry skills. This required the development of elaborate forms and instruction sheets for data collection. After providing these documents, mentoring was initially conducted through email correspondence from the IAEA headquarters, followed by the organisation of special training courses for hands-on training with compulsory presentation of data by each participant with discussion and feedback by experts. This also provided uniformity of data collection and presentation.

## 5 IAEA Efforts to Improve Justification

The IAEA has initiated activities in the field of justification of medical exposures, in particular dealing with the nature of justification and how to give effect to it in practice (Malone 2009). In order to review the arrangements to ensure effective justification of medical exposure in diagnostic imaging, the IAEA has developed the triple A campaign: Awareness (through effective communication about risk), Appropriateness (through up-to-date referral guidelines) and Audit (through clinical audit of justification) or AAA. The international campaign on AAA has included many international organisations (WHO, EC, ISR, American College of Radiology, Food and Drug Administration-FDA, PAHO) who have worked together with the IAEA in three different strands: practical application of tools for justification; regulatory issues and communication issues in justification.

A recent study on CT examinations in children was initiated by the IAEA with the aim to assess the level of appropriateness of CT in common examinations in 40 countries and frequency of pediatric CT as compared to adult. The study comprised results from 146 CT facilities at 126 hospitals in Europe, Africa and Asia (Vassileva et al. 2012a, b). According to this study, the lowest frequency in 2009 was in European facilities (4.3%) and over almost double in Asia (12.2%) and Africa (7.8%). Head CT was the most common CT examination in children, nearly 75%. While regulations in many countries assign the main responsibility to radiologists on deciding whether a radiological examination should be performed, radiologists alone were responsible for only 6.3% of situations. The study also highlighted that availability of written referral guidelines for imaging in hospitals is grossly inadequate as they were not available in almost half of the CT facilities. Justification criteria for CT examinations in children did not always follow guidelines set by agencies, in particular in patients with accidental head trauma, infants with congenital torticollis; children with possible ventriculo-peritoneal shunt malfunction and young children (<5 years old) with acute sinusitis. Non-availability of previous images and records on previously received patient doses in about one-third of situations has the potential for unnecessary examination and radiation dose.

The fact that this was a non-random sample of countries that were chosen because of their prior record of good progress on IAEA projects in the past is of concern. The progress made by these countries can be considered better than many others and thus one can only worry about the situation in other countries worldwide.

Not surprisingly, the study concluded that with increasing use of CT in children and lack of use of appropriateness criteria, there is a strong need to implement guidelines to avoid unnecessary radiation doses to children.

## 6 IAEA Optimisation Efforts

Many times radiation dose reduction is taken as an aim whereas actually dose reduction alone can lead to undesirable consequences. It is therefore desirable to have a clearer understanding of optimization. Optimization implies "the procedure or procedures used to make a system or design as effective or as functional as possible" or "making the best of anything". In medical imaging, one attempts to choose certain parameters to optimise, such as image quality and patient dose. However, if one increases image quality (which is desirable), one ends up increasing patient dose too (which is not desirable). For radiologists, image quality is the main focus. Similarly, physicists are concerned with radiation dose. Optimization, therefore, tends to imply the best image quality for a radiologist and the least radiation dose for a physicist (Rehani 2007).

Despite significant efforts and a large number of publications, CT has continued to pose a challenge in optimization. This happens because the rate at which technology has been progressing during the past decade has been faster than effective optimization in practice. In addition to what has been done by manufacturers, the important role is played by the user in day-to-day management of situations in clinical practice.

The IAEA initiated multiple optimization studies initially through a programme of Coordinated Research Projects (CRP) and subsequently through technical cooperation projects in developing countries. The CRP addressed wide aspects of optimization of radiological protection, including initial assessment of the situation of equipment, evaluation of image quality and patient dose followed by corrective actions through a Quality Control (QC) programme. A further objective was to promote awareness about practical implementation of QC protocols, image quality evaluation and to create a pool of expertise in each participating country (IAEA 2004). A subsequent CRP addressed the issue of optimization in CT in great detail. Increased utilization of CT and results of the previous project were motivation for this project. The work was undertaken in two phases using nine CT scanners in six centres worldwide (IAEA 2009b). In the first phase, protocols for patient dosimetry and image quality were established. Information was collected from 707 patients undergoing routine abdomen, chest or head CT examinations. In the second phase, similar information was collected on a smaller sample of patients with modified exposure protocols designed to achieve specific target noise levels according to weight of patients.

For abdominal CT analysis, the data showed a good correlation between image noise and patient weight. After normalization of the data, a simple linear relationship between image noise and patient weight was adopted. This relationship was used to calculate the dose adaptation necessary to achieve target noise levels for any size patient. Phase 2 showed that each centre was able to achieve the target noise values leading, in some cases, to significant decreases in patient doses. For chest CT, there was no correlation between image noise and patient weight. This was possible due to instabilities in the method of measuring image noise. It was felt appropriate to adopt a strategy, similar to that used for abdomen, to adapt noise based on patient weight. Measurements in phase 2 again showed that each center was able to achieve the target noise values. For abdominal CT, dose reduction varied from about 25–62%, while for chest CT, dose varied from 12 to 79% in individual cases. The correlation between noise and head size/diameter was low; thus, no attempt was made to reduce dose on this basis.

The work showed that there is scope to adapt patient image quality and dose. For all the countries involved in this work the average patient doses were below European Diagnostic Reference Levels (DRL) for CT of the abdomen and chest. For CT of the head, two countries had values well over the European DRL. The image noise was low in several cases, and it was still possible to reduce the patient dose even further. This finding indicated the need for population-specific diagnostic reference levels. In all cases, the dose reductions were achieved without reducing image quality below a level that was regarded as acceptable by the participating radiologists.

## 7 Dose Tracking Initiative

The alarming increase in the use of high radiation dose examinations such as CT made the IAEA propose the concept of cumulative record of patient dose, the so-called Smart Card/Smart Rad Track project (Rehani 2009; Holmberg et al. 2010). The project is aimed at: developing methodologies to track radiation history (the number of radiological procedures and/radiation dose as appropriate); helping countries to establish policies and mechanisms for tracking indices of radiation exposure for diagnostic examinations and interventional procedures involving ionizing radiation to individual patients; developing guidance where the number of procedures alone, rather than dose, are sufficient which, combined with generic radiation dose figures, can provide dose estimates; providing information to strengthen the basic tenets of radiation protection, namely justification and optimization; cooperating with bodies associated with manufacturers to aid in developing hardware and software for tracking of procedures and individual patients' radiation dose indices; promoting development of international standards for tracking radiological examinations and procedures across different countries; and making provisions in safety standards to require tracking of radiological examinations and procedures and to assess cumulative radiation dose to individual patients.

Typical options for dose tracking are: an electronic card that allows access to imaging data on servers, including radiation-exposure history, e-health systems with interoperability and capability to track records for radiological history of an individual patient, an electronic card that contains a patient's information, including radiation-exposure history, a web-based personal health record with methodology to help an individual track their radiological history, or a paper card containing radiological history. Different levels of records, depending on type of examination and age at exposure are proposed. For relatively low-dose examinations such as radiography, it might be more reasonable to track the number of examinations alone. With examinations associated with relatively high radiation doses, such as CT, interventional procedures, PET/CT and some of the nuclear medicine studies, dose per examination and number of examinations all require consideration. For individuals above the age of 50 years, having a record of the number of examinations might be sufficient, while for younger individuals, one should aim at recording either doses or factors that can give reasonable dose estimates (Rehani and Frush 2010).

In keeping with the spirit of international cooperation, the IAEA has involved a number of stakeholders in this initiative. Integrated Health Enterprises (IHE) connects healthcare professionals and industry to improve the way computer systems in healthcare share information. IHE promotes the coordinated use of established information standards such as DICOM and HL7 to address specific clinical needs in support of optimal patient care. The systems developed in accordance with IHE provide more effective communication with one another, thereby facilitating the tracking of individual patients. Medical imaging vendors are increasingly complying with IHE protocols. Another stakeholder group involved deals with Electronic Health Records (EHR). EHR is developing quickly in many countries, particularly in Europe. The IAEA is working to include the tracking of radiological procedures and dose information in the functional criteria of EHR (Holmberg et al. 2010).

The dose tracking activities made the IAEA the first United Nations organization to take a lead in this area, in a clear sign of its commitment to the radiation protection of patients with the hope that, despite increasing use of radiation which is for the benefit of patients, it will be possible to keep radiation risks to levels that are acceptable.

## 8 Networks of Medical Professionals on Radiation Protection

In 2010, the IAEA initiated the establishment of a network of medical professionals on radiation protection of children. This activity is based on the success of the cardiology network (IAEA 2011b) and the need for focus on radiation protection of children. Three networks have been established, one each in three regions namely Europe, Asia and Latin America. It consists of pediatric radiologists, medical physicists and radiographers from developing countries in these regions. Participants have been motivated in meetings and have started collecting data as per framework prepared. They are going to spearhead actions and provide feedback and have launched their newsletter (IAEA 2011c).

## 9 IAEA Dose Optimization Studies in Computed Tomography for Adults

A prospective multi-national study was launched by the IAEA in 2005 in developing countries from three different regions, Africa, Asia and Eastern Europe (Muhogora et al. 2009). The purpose was to survey frequency of CT examinations and dose levels to adult patients and to assess the potential for improvement in compliance with the 'as low as reasonably achievable' principle. Structured instructions and forms for data collection were provided to countries so that the results could be collected in a consistent and meaningful way for intercomparison. Data from 88 CT facilities in 18 countries was available. The dose assessment was performed in terms of weighted or volume computed tomography dose index ($CTDI_w$/$CTDI_{vol}$) and dose length product (DLP) for chest, chest (high resolution), lumbar spine, abdomen and pelvis CT examinations using standard methods (Muhogora et al. 2009). The radiologists were asked to subjectively assess the image quality of each CT image at their hospitals, where the concern was whether the images were used for diagnosis or not.

At a first glance, mean CTDI values were below European DRLs (EC 1999). However, wide variations up to a factor of 16 were observed largely due to the performance of CT equipment. Regarding DLP, 17% of cases were above DRLs. The $CTDI_w$ and DLP values for these countries are presented in Tables 1 and 2.

Large DLP variations were observed which were mainly due to differences in the CT performance characteristics and scanning parameters used such as pitch and scan lengths as well as varied patient characteristics. The most important finding of this study was the lack of adjusting CT exposure parameters to patient size. The studies of this kind serve to increase awareness about radiation dose in CT, orient staff towards dose management and build capability on radiation protection of patients in CT not only in participating centres but also in the country and region.

**Table 1** Mean $CTDI_w$ values for adult patients in different countries and regions (Muhogora et al. 2009)

| Country | Mean $CTDI_w$ (mGy) | | | | |
|---|---|---|---|---|---|
| | Chest | Chest HR | Lumbar spine | Abdomen | Pelvis |
| Algeria | 9.2 | 6.8 | 16.2 | 15.4 | 19.1 |
| Ghana | 17.1 | 17.2 | 20.4 | 20.4 | 20.4 |
| Kenya | 20 | – | – | 13 | 20 |
| Morocco | 10 | 25.8 | 11.9 | 11.9 | 10.6 |
| Sudan | 19.2 | 14.1 | – | 20.5 | 7.3 |
| Tanzania | 16.8 | 13.9 | 38.8 | 22.7 | 26 |
| Tunisia | 24.3 | – | – | – | 25.4 |
| Japan | 14 | 15 | 19.3 | 19.3 | 19.3 |
| Kuwait | 12 | 18.2 | – | 11.7 | – |
| Syria | 18.6 | 24.3 | – | 21.6 | 28.4 |
| Thailand | 15.3 | 14.4 | 19.5 | 18.5 | 16.8 |
| Bulgaria | 16.7 | 14.9 | 20.7 | 16.3 | 18.2 |
| Czech Republic | 21.3 | 16.9 | 23.9 | 18.4 | 20.3 |
| Bosnia & Herzegovina | 13.5 | 20.6 | 21.2 | 21.2 | 20.1 |
| Srpska B&H[a] | 6.9 | – | 22.8 | 10.2 | 8.3 |
| Estonia | 15.7 | – | – | 19 | 14.5 |
| FYROM | 11.4 | – | – | 13 | 11.4 |
| Malta | 11.5 | 10 | 15.4 | 14.8 | 21.8 |
| Serbia | 20.1 | – | 12.3 | 12.3 | 14.1 |
| Region | Mean $CTDI_w$ (mGy) | | | | |
| | Chest | Chest HR | Lumbar spine | Abdomen | Pelvis |
| Africa | 9.2–24.3 | 6.8–25.8 | 11.9–38.8 | 11.9–22.7 | 7.3–26 |
| Asia | 12–18.6 | 14.4–24.3 | 19.3–19.5 | 11.7–21.6 | 16.8–28.4 |
| Eastern Europe | 6.9–21.3 | 10–20.6 | 12.3–23.9 | 10.2–21.2 | 8.3–21.8 |

[a] Srpska B&H: Republic of Srpska

## 10 IAEA Dose Optimization Studies in Computed Tomography for Children

Another large scale international study was initiated with an aim to investigate the frequency of CT examinations for pediatric patients below 15 years of age in 128 CT facilities in 28 developing countries of Africa, Asia and Eastern Europe and to assess the magnitude of CT doses (Muhogora et al. 2010). In this study, radiation dose data were available from 101 CT facilities in 19 countries. The dose assessment was performed again in terms of weighted or volume computed tomography dose index ($CTDI_w$/$CTDI_{vol}$) and dose length product (DLP) for chest, chest HR (high resolution), lumbar spine, abdomen and pelvis CT examinations using standard methods. The $CTDI_w$ and DLP values for pediatric patients in three regions are presented in Tables 3 and 4.

The results showed that on average the frequency of pediatric CT examinations was 20, 16 and 5% of all CT examinations in participating centres in Africa, Asia and Eastern Europe, respectively. Eleven CT facilities in six countries were found to use adult CT exposure parameters for pediatric patients, thus indicating limited awareness and the need for optimization. The $CTDI_w$ variations ranged up to a factor of 55 (Africa), 16.3 (Asia) and 6.6 (Eastern Europe). The corresponding DLP values ranged by a factor of 10, 20 and 8 in three regions, respectively.

**Table 2** Mean DLP values for adult patients in different countries and regions (Muhogora et al. 2009)

| Country | Mean DLP (mGy·cm) | | | | |
|---|---|---|---|---|---|
| | Chest | Chest HR | Lumbar spine | Abdomen | Pelvis |
| Algeria | 347 | 194 | 646 | 554 | 604 |
| Ghana | 396 | 348 | 523 | 496 | 415 |
| Kenya | 933 | – | – | 1314 | 837 |
| Morocco | 256 | 121 | 341 | 341 | 271 |
| Sudan | 423 | 171 | – | 725 | 163 |
| Tanzania | 383 | 366 | 363 | 602 | 494 |
| Tunisia | 874 | – | – | – | 599 |
| Japan | 564 | 404 | 513 | 513 | 513 |
| Kuwait | 223 | 561 | – | 552 | – |
| Syria | 416 | 103 | – | 638 | 545 |
| Thailand | 301 | 99 | 720 | 574 | 390 |
| Bulgaria | 512 | – | – | 435 | 322 |
| Czech Republic | 341 | – | 507 | 444 | 466 |
| Bosnia & Herzegovina | 437 | 330 | 460 | 460 | 323 |
| Srpska B&H[a] | 246 | – | 541 | 448 | 231 |
| Estonia | 833 | – | – | 910 | 698 |
| FYROM | 342 | – | – | 526 | 416 |
| Malta | 296 | 117 | 289 | 480 | 268 |
| Serbia | 148 | – | 512 | 512 | 305 |
| Region | Mean DLP (mGy·cm) | | | | |
| | Chest | Chest HR | Lumbar spine | Abdomen | Pelvis |
| Africa | 256–933 | 121–366 | 341–646 | 341–1314 | 163–837 |
| Asia | 223–564 | 99–561 | 513–720 | 513–638 | 390–545 |
| Eastern Europe | 148–833 | 117–330 | 289–541 | 435–910 | 268–698 |

[a] Srpska B&H: Republic of Srpska

As far as pediatric CT procedures are concerned, the results of the IAEA survey revealed extremely large variations in the frequencies of pediatric CT examinations, which indicate variable approaches to justification of pediatric CT examinations (Muhogora et al. 2010). More specifically, the number of pediatric CT examinations is relatively higher in the majority of African countries compared with Asia and Eastern Europe. This may be due to the nonavailability of alternative imaging modalities such as magnetic resonance imaging, high-resolution ultrasound or even limited experience in justifying CT procedures. The CT exposure parameters that were reported during the study showed that in a number of centres, the exposure parameters used for pediatric patients were similar to those used for adults. This has enormous implications not only for each individual dose, but also in collective dose and the risk of lifetime radiation induced cancer. The study has indicated a stronger need in many developing countries to justify CT examinations in children and their optimization. Awareness, training and monitoring of radiation doses is needed as a way forward.

The presented initial results were motivation for deeper survey of practice in pediatric CT both in respect of utilization of CT in children and optimization of clinical protocols. Following creation of networks of specialists in different regions worldwide, initiated by the IAEA in 2010, first results of the study on appropriateness of CT in common examinations in 40 countries and frequency of pediatric CT as compared to adult, have already been presented

**Table 3** Mean $CTDI_w$ values for pediatric patients in different countries and regions (Muhogora et al. 2010)

| Country | Mean $CTDI_w$ (mGy) | | | | |
|---|---|---|---|---|---|
| | Chest | Chest HR | Lumbar spine | Abdomen | Pelvis |
| Algeria | 5.2 | 3.5 | 4.2 | 4.2 | 5.2 |
| Ghana | 11.9 | 11.9 | 12.8 | 13.8 | 16.3 |
| Morocco | 4 | 14 | 6.9 | 6.9 | 4.9 |
| Sudan | 17.1 | – | 30 | 30.3 | 4 |
| Tanzania | 14.2 | – | 14 | 13.1 | 11.7 |
| Kenya | – | – | – | – | – |
| Tunisia | 9.8 | – | – | 9 | 7.6 |
| Japan | 6.4 | 5.2 | 8.7 | 8.7 | 8.7 |
| Kuwait | 5.5 | 15.5 | – | 14.5 | – |
| Syria | 13.5 | 18.6 | – | 13.6 | 16.8 |
| Thailand | 15.9 | 9.9 | 18.5 | 11.6 | 17.8 |
| UAE | 10.5 | 14 | – | 20.4 | – |
| Czech Republic | 8.1 | – | 22.3 | 11.5 | 11.7 |
| Cyprus | 6.3 | – | 6.6 | 6.6 | 4.9 |
| Bosnia & Herzegovina | 7.2 | 6.5 | 7.5 | 7.5 | 14.2 |
| Srpska B&H[a] | 3.3 | – | 7.2 | 5.6 | 3.9 |
| Estonia | 5.2 | – | 11.9 | 3.5 | 5.7 |
| FYROM | 16.3 | – | – | 13.5 | 11.4 |
| Malta | 12 | – | – | 12 | – |
| Serbia | 11 | – | 11 | 13 | 13 |
| Region | Mean $CTDI_w$ (mGy) | | | | |
| | Chest | Chest HR | Lumbar spine | Abdomen | Pelvis |
| Africa | 4–17.1 | 3.5–14 | 4.1–14 | 4.2–20.1 | 4.9–17.1 |
| Asia | 5.5–15.9 | 5.2–18.6 | 8.7–18.5 | 8.7–20.4 | 8.7–17.8 |
| Eastern Europe | 3.3–16.3 | 6.5 | 7.1–22.3 | 3.5–13.5 | 3.9–14.2 |

[a] Srpska B&H: Republic of Srpska

(Vassileva et al. 2012a). The study comprised results from 146 CT facilities at 126 hospitals in Europe, Africa and Asia (Vassileva et al. 2012a). The first part consisted of surveys of frequency of pediatric CT examinations and appropriateness followed by procedures and protocols, and lastly on the impact of optimization. The results on assessment of technical aspects of performing CT examinations in children, including exposure parameters and dose values for children compared to adults, use of sedation, immobilization devices, need of parental support, and use of different dose reduction approaches, e.g. tube current modulation, shielding of sensitive organs, projection for scout image, etc. are already available (Vassileva et al. 2012b). The aim of this part was to survey practice in order to identify potential for optimization of CT procedures and dose reduction in children. Standard forms were answered by 140 participating facilities from 40 countries in Africa, Asia, Europe, and Latin America to survey important exposure parameters from routine scanning protocols, and resulting doses expressed either in weighted or volume CTDI. A questionnaire with 20 questions about the practice of performing CT examinations in children was answered by 141 radiographers/radiology technologists.

The survey demonstrated wide use of modern MDCT scanners with dose saving techniques and optimization approaches, as presented in Table 5. Dedicated scanning protocols for pediatric examinations were available in 94%, but indication-based

**Table 4** Mean DLP values for pediatric patients in different countries and regions (Muhogora et al. 2010)

| Country | Mean DLP (mGy·cm) | | | | |
|---|---|---|---|---|---|
| | Chest | Chest HR | Lumbar spine | Abdomen | Pelvis |
| Algeria | 169 | 79 | 121 | 121 | 105 |
| Ghana | 272 | 371 | 277 | 320 | 382 |
| Morocco | 103 | – | – | 124 | – |
| Sudan | 109 | 49 | 154 | 154 | 55 |
| Tanzania | 85 | 50 | – | 43 | 56 |
| Kenya | 144 | – | 252 | 187 | 50 |
| Tunisia | 190 | – | – | 311 | 138 |
| Japan | 134 | 157 | 150 | 150 | 150 |
| Kuwait | 159 | 145 | – | 821 | – |
| Syria | 166 | 64 | – | 220 | 176 |
| Thailand | 171 | 70 | 397 | 397 | 240 |
| UAE | 216 | 260 | – | 479 | – |
| Czech Republic | 110 | – | 131 | 131 | 88 |
| Cyprus | 76 | – | 127 | 115 | 268 |
| Bosnia & Herzegovina | 160 | 96 | 199 | 199 | 275 |
| Srpska B&H[a] | 190 | – | 133 | 235 | 82 |
| Estonia | 322 | 194 | 115 | 135 | – |
| FYROM | 326 | – | – | 613 | 487 |
| Malta | 138 | – | – | 154 | – |
| Serbia | 230 | – | 385 | 385 | 330 |
| Region | Mean DLP (mGy·cm) | | | | |
| | Chest | Chest HR | Lumbar spine | Abdomen | Pelvis |
| Africa | 85.5–272 | 49–371 | 121–277 | 43–320 | 50–382 |
| Asia | 134–216 | 64–260 | 150–397 | 150–821 | 150–240 |
| Eastern Europe | 76–326 | 96–194 | 115–385 | 115–613 | 82–487 |

[a] Srpska B&H: Republic of Srpska

protocols in only 58% of the CT facilities. In 50% of the facilities, protocols for some age groups were missing, or exposure parameters were not adapted to body size or patient age. Variations of CTDI values up to a factor of 100 were found for chest examination of children younger than 10 years. In 8% of the scanners, CTDI values for pediatric patients were 2–5 times higher than for adults in at least one age group and one examination. The third quartile values in this survey were comparable to the published DRL values for head examination, but higher for chest and abdomen examination. Bismuth shields for protection of sensitive organs were rarely used, but other approaches such as gantry tilting or patient head repositioning was applied by more than 75% of operators for CT of the head. This survey found that 60% of the operators used sedation in more than half of small children <5 years, and 49% declared parental support to be needed in more than 50% of small children, demonstrating the insufficient use of immobilization tools and means to improve child cooperation. Patient dose records were kept in 49% of the facilities. Medical physics support in optimization was available in only half of the facilities.

The study concluded that effective feedback, networking and training are important tools to improve practice and to increase awareness among medical specialists, to train people how to optimize protocols and to promote safer use of CT in children.

**Table 5** Summary of the answers of 141 radiographers to the questionnaire surveying practice (Vassileva et al. 2012b)

| | Total (141 answers) | Europe (60 answers) | Asia (63 answers) | Latin America (11 answers) | Africa (7 answers) |
|---|---|---|---|---|---|
| Dedicated scanning protocols for pediatric examinations available? | 130 Yes | 55 Yes | 59 Yes | 9 Yes | 5 Yes |
| | 8 No | 3 No | 4 No | 0 No | 1 No |
| | 3 Do not know | 2 Do not know | 0 Do not know | 0 Do not know | 1 Do not know |
| Indication based protocols available? | 83 Yes | 25 Yes | 46 Yes | 9 Yes | 3 Yes |
| | 57 No | 35 No | 16 No | 2 No | 4 No |
| | 1 Do not know | 0 Do not know | 1 Do not know | 0 Do not know | 0 Do not know |
| In which projection is scout image usually performed for pediatric patient? | 103 AP | 36 AP | 51 AP | 9 AP | 7 AP |
| | 12 PA | 4 PA | 8 PA | 2 No answer | – |
| | 6 Lat | 6 Lat | 1 AP/Lat | – | – |
| | 6 AP/Lat | 5 AP/Lat | 1 AP/PA | – | – |
| | 5 AP/PA | 4 AP/PA | 2 No answer | – | – |
| | 9 No answer | 5 No answer | – | – | – |
| Does typical scout image and CT scan of the pediatric abdomen extend to breast (B) or to diaphragm (D)? | 110 D | 46 D | 53 D | 6 D | 5 D |
| | 22 B | 11 B | 8 B | 1 B | 2 B |
| | 9 No answer | 3 No answer | 2 No answer | 4 No answer | – |
| Indicate the lowest point for a typical scout image and CT scan of the pelvis? | 128 to border of pubis symp | 56 to border of pubis symp | 58 to border of pubis symp | 8 to border of pubis symp | 6 to border of pubis symp |
| | 3 below symp | 2 below symp | 1 below symp | 1 No answer | 3 No answer |
| | 10 No answer | 2 No answer | 4 No answer | – | – |
| Pediatric head CT for trauma is usually performed in axial (A) or helical (H) mode? | 74 axial | 39 axial | 28 axial | 4 axial | 3 axial |
| | 63 helical | 18 helical | 34 helical | 7 helical | 4 helical |
| | 4 No answer | 3 No answer | 1 No answer | – | – |
| Do you use Automatic exposure control (AEC) for any body part protocol? | 104 Yes | 44 Yes | 50 Yes | 5 Yes | 5 Yes |
| | 26 No | 9 No | 10 No | 5 No | 2 No |
| | 11 Do not know | 7 Do not know | 3 Do not know | 1 Do not know | 0 Do not know |
| Bismuth breast shielding for pediatric patients available? | 16 Yes | 4 Yes | 12 Yes | 0 Yes | 0 Yes |
| | 121 No | 55 No | 50 No | 9 No | 7 No |
| | 4 Do not know | 1 Do not know | 1 Do not know | 2 Do not know | – |
| Bismuth eye shielding available? | 11 Yes | 1 Yes | 9 Yes | 1 Yes | 0 Yes |
| | 124 No | 56 No | 53 No | 8 No | 7 No |
| | 6 Do not know | 3 Do not know | 1 Do not know | 2 Do not know | 0 Do not know |
| Are any immobilization means available, e.g. swaddling clothes, straps, etc.? | 120 Yes | 54 Yes | 53 Yes | 7 Yes | 6 Yes |
| | 20 No | 6 No | 9 No | 4 No | 1 No |
| | 1 Do not know | – | 1 Do not know | – | – |

(continued)

**Table 5** (continued)

| | Total (141 answers) | Europe (60 answers) | Asia (63 answers) | Latin America (11 answers) | Africa (7 answers) |
|---|---|---|---|---|---|
| How often is sedation used for small children (<5 years old)? | 9 Hardly ever | 3 Hardly ever | 5 Hardly ever | 1 Hardly ever | 0 Hardly ever |
| | 44 in <50% | 20 in <50% | 20 in <50% | 6 in <50% | 0 in <50% |
| | 62 in >50% | 33 in >50% | 22 in >50% | 1 in >50% | 7 in >50% |
| | 17 Always | 2 Always | 15 Always | 2 Always | 0 Always |
| | 6 No answer | 2 No answer | 1 No answer | 1 Do not know | – |
| How often does CT examination of pediatric patient need supporter in the room? | 25 Hardly ever | 8 Hardly ever | 13 Hardly ever | 2 Hardly ever | 2 Hardly ever |
| | 48 in <50% | 20 in <50% | 25 in <50% | 3 in <50% | 0 in <50% |
| | 44 in >50% | 22 in >50% | 13 in >50% | 5 in >50% | 4 in >50% |
| | 24 Always | 10 Always | 12 Always | 1 Always | 1 Always |
| If support of pediatric patient is needed, who does this usually? | 120 parents | 53 parents | 56 parents | 5 parents | 6 parents |
| | 15 staff | 6 staff | 6 staff | 3 staff | 0 staff |
| | 6 No answer | 1 No answer | 1 No answer | 3 No answer | 1 No answer |
| If parents are in the room, do they wear protective aprons? | 131 Yes | 55 Yes | 60 Yes | 9 Yes | 7 Yes |
| | 7 No | 3 No | 3 No | 1 No | 0 No |
| | 2 Not always | 2 Not always | 0 Not always | 1 No answer | 0 Not always |
| | 1 No answer | – | – | – | – |
| If medical staff works in the room, do they have personal dosemeters? | 111 Yes | 42 Yes | 58 Yes | 7 Yes | 4 Yes |
| | 30 No | 18 No | 5 No | 4 No | 3 No |
| Do you keep records of patient doses? | 69 Yes | 33 Yes | 31 Yes | 4 Yes | 1 Yes |
| | 62 No | 20 No | 31 No | 5 No | 6 No |
| | 10 Do not know | 7 Do not know | 1 Do not know | 2 Do not know | 0 Do not know |
| Is a medical physicist available and participating in radiation protection optimization? | 71 Yes | 34 Yes | 32 Yes | 3 Yes | 2 Yes |
| | 68 No | 26 No | 31 No | 6 No | 5 No |
| | 2 Do not know | – | – | 2 Do not know | – |

## 11 Dose Management in Newer Imaging Technologies

It so happens that CT occupies a central stage in most newer imaging technologies, be it hybrid imaging such as PET/CT or SPECT/CT or the cone beam CT (Rehani 2010). Further newer applications of cardiac CT and CT colonography are emerging. In keeping with the intention to provide a systematic transfer of knowledge to the world on newer imaging technologies, the IAEA has provided specific information on radiation doses and dose management actions in PET/CT, cardiac CT and CT colonography through its website (IAEA 2011d, e, f). Further specific publications as Safety Reports for all these 3 areas have been released, PET/CT (IAEA 2008a), cardiac CT (IAEA 2008b) and CT colonography (IAEA 2008c). A training material on radiation protection in hybrid imaging as power point slides has been made available for free download (IAEA 2011g).

## 12 Conclusions

In the 1990s, there was a lack of information on patient doses in CT in most developing countries. Utilising whatever manpower was available in different countries, be it radiographers, radiologists, regulators, physicists working in universities, regulatory office or radiation protection centres in the absence of medical imaging physicists, preparing detailed guidelines and data collection forms, focussing training on acquiring dosimetry skills, developing a system of periodic report submission by countries, mentoring and motivating collaborations within each country are some of the actions that have been used by the IAEA. Currently more than 60 countries are actively involved in dose management actions. Nearly half of them have reached the stage of producing information that has been included in papers published in reputed journals, as stated earlier, and others are on the way to cross thresholds. Publications apart, learning achieved and skills developed in this process are valuable outcomes. The bottom-up approach, combined with the top-down approach used by the IAEA earlier for many years, has proved useful.

## References


Ciraj-Bjelac O, Beganovic A, Faj D et al (2011) Radiation protection of patients in diagnostic radiology: Status of practice in five Eastern-European countries, based on IAEA project. Eur J Radiol 79:e70–e77

EC (European Commission) (1999) European guidelines on quality criteria for computed tomography. EUR 16262 EN, Luxembourg

Holmberg O, Malone J, Rehani M et al (2010) Current issues and actions in radiation protection of patients. Eur J Radiol 76:15–19

IAEA (International Atomic Energy Agency) (1996) Food and Agriculture Organization of the United Nations, International Atomic Energy Agency, International Labour Organization, OECD Nuclear Energy Agency, Pan American Health Organization, World Health Organization. International basic safety standards for protection against ionizing radiation and for the safety of radiation sources. Safety series no. 115. IAEA, Vienna

IAEA (International Atomic Energy Agency) (2002a) Radiological protection for medical exposure to ionizing radiation. Safety guide no. RS-G-1.5. IAEA, Vienna

IAEA (International Atomic Energy Agency) (2002b) International action plan for the radiological protection of patients. IAEA, Vienna. http://www.iaea.org/About/Policy/GC/GC46/Documents/gc46-12.pdf. Accessed 14 Sept 2011

IAEA (International Atomic Energy Agency) (2004) Optimization of the radiological protection of patients undergoing radiography, fluoroscopy and computed tomography, IAEA-TECDOC-1423. IAEA, Vienna

IAEA (International Atomic Energy Agency) (2006) Applying radiation safety standards in diagnostic radiology and interventional procedures using X rays. Safety reports series no. 39. IAEA, Vienna

IAEA (International Atomic Energy Agency) (2007) Dosimetry in diagnostic radiology: An international code of practice. Technical report series no. 457. IAEA, Vienna

IAEA (International Atomic Energy Agency) (2008a) Radiation protection in newer medical imaging techniques: PET/CT. Safety reports series no. 58. IAEA, Vienna

IAEA (International Atomic Energy Agency) (2008b) Radiation protection in newer medical imaging techniques: cardiac CT. Safety reports series no. 60. IAEA, Vienna

IAEA (International Atomic Energy Agency) (2008c) Radiation protection in newer medical imaging techniques: CT colonography. Safety reports series no. 61. IAEA, Vienna

IAEA (International Atomic Energy Agency) (2009a) Establishing guidance levels in X ray guided medical interventional procedures: a pilot study. Safety reports series no. 59. IAEA, Vienna

AEA (International Atomic Energy Agency) (2009b) Dose reduction in CT while maintaining diagnostic confidence: a feasibility/demonstration study, TECDOC-1621. IAEA, Vienna

IAEA (International Atomic Energy Agency) (2010) Patient dose optimization in fluoroscopically guided interventional procedures, TECDOC-1641. IAEA, Vienna

IAEA (International Atomic Energy Agency) (2011a) https://rpop.iaea.org/RPOP/RPoP/Content/AdditionalResources/Training/index.htm Accessed 14 Sept 2011

IAEA (International Atomic Energy Agency) (2011b) https://rpop.iaea.org/RPOP/RPoP/Content/AdditionalResources/Training/2_TrainingEvents/asian-network.htm. Accessed 14 Sept 2011

IAEA (International Atomic Energy Agency) (2011c) https://rpop.iaea.org/RPOP/RPoP/Content/SpecialGroups/2_Children/children-network.htm. Accessed 14 Sept 2011

IAEA (International Atomic Energy Agency) (2011d) https://rpop.iaea.org/RPOP/RPoP/Content/InformationFor/HealthProfessionals/6_OtherClinicalSpecialities/PETCTscan.htm. Accessed 14 Sept 2011

IAEA (International Atomic Energy Agency) (2011e) https://rpop.iaea.org/RPOP/RPoP/Content/InformationFor/HealthProfessionals/1_Radiology/ComputedTomography/CardiacCT.htm. Accessed 14 Sept 2011

IAEA (International Atomic Energy Agency) (2011f) https://rpop.iaea.org/RPOP/RPoP/Content/InformationFor/HealthProfessionals/1_Radiology/ComputedTomography/CTColonography.htm. Accessed 14 Sept 2011

IAEA (International Atomic Energy Agency) (2011g) https://rpop.iaea.org/RPOP/RPoP/Content/AdditionalResources/Training/1_TrainingMaterial/PETCT.htm. Accessed 14 Sept 2011

Malone J (2009) Report of a consultation on justification of patient exposures in medical imaging. Radiat Prot Dosim 135:137–144

Muhogora W, Ahmed N, Almosabihi A et al (2008) Patient doses in radiographic examinations in 12 countries in Asia, Africa and Eastern Europe—initial results from IAEA projects. Am J Roentgenol 190:1453–1461

Muhogora W, Ahmed NA, Beganovic A et al (2009) Patient doses in CT Examinations in 18 countries: initial results from international atomic energy agency projects. Radiat Prot Dosim 136:118–126

Muhogora W, Ahmed NA, Beganovic A et al (2010) pediatric CT examinations in 19 developing countries: frequency and radiation dose. Radiat Prot Dosim 140:49–58

Rehani M (2007) Radiation dose optimization in biomedical imaging and intervention. Biomed Imaging Interv J 3:e50

Rehani M (2009) Smart protection. IAEA Bull 2009; 50. http://www.iaea.org/Publications/Magazines/Bulletin/Bull502/50205813137.html. Accessed 14 Sept 2011

Rehani M (2010) Radiation protection in newer imaging technologies. Radiat Prot Dosim 139:357–362

Rehani M, Frush D (2010) Tracking radiation exposure of patients. Lancet 4:754–755

Rehani M, Holmberg O, Ortiz Lopez P et al (2011) International action plan on the radiation protection of patients. Radiat Prot Dosim. doi:10.1093/rpd/ncr258

Rehani M, Tsapaki V (2011) Impact of the International Atomic Energy Agency (IAEA) actions on radiation protection of patients in many countries. Radiat Prot Dosim. doi:10.1093/rpd/ncr259

Tsapaki V, Ahmed NA, AlSuwaidi JS et al (2009) Radiation exposure to patients during interventional procedures in 20 countries: initial IAEA project results. Am J Roentgenol 193:559–569

Vassileva J, Rehani M, Al-Dhuhli H et al (2012a) IAEA survey of pediatric CT practice in 40 countries in Asia, Europe, Latin America and Africa: Part 1. Frequency and appropriateness. Am J Roentgenol (Accepted to appear in May 2012 issue)

Vassileva J, Rehani M, Al-Dhuhli H et al (2012b) IAEA survey of pediatric CT practice in 40 countries in Asia, Europe, Latin America, and Africa: Part 2. Procedures and protocols. J Am Coll Radiol (communicated)

# The Image Gently Campaign: Championing Radiation Protection for Children Through Awareness, Educational Resources and Advocacy

Marilyn J. Goske, Michael J. Callahan, Donald P. Frush, Sue C. Kaste, Gregory Morrison, and Keith J. Strauss

## Contents



M. J. Goske (✉) · K. J. Strauss
Department of Radiology,
Cincinnati Children's Hospital Medical Center,
MLC 5031, 3333 Burnet Ave, Cincinnati,
OH 45229-3039, USA
e-mail: Marilyn.Goske@cchmc.org

M. J. Callahan
Department of Radiology, Children's Hospital,
300 Longwood Ave, Boston,
MA 02115-5737, USA

D. P. Frush
Division of Pediatric Radiology,
Duke University Medical Center,
1905 McGovern Davison Childrens Health Center,
Durham, NC 27710-3808, USA

S. C. Kaste
Radiologic Science Division of Diagnostic Imaging,
St Jude Children's Research Hospital,
262 Danny Thomas Place, Memphis,
TN 38105-2794, USA

G. Morrison
American Society of Radiologic Technologists,
15000 Central Ave SE, Albuquerque,
NM 87123-3909, USA

**Abstract**

CT scans have been shown to improve pediatric patient care and because of its benefits, the use of this remarkable technology has grown worldwide. However, children are particularly vulnerable to potential effects from ionizing radiation due their small size, rapid cell division and longer lifetime to manifest changes. It is most important that radiologists ensure that every CT scan is justified by the

D. Tack et al. (eds.), *Radiation Dose from Multidetector CT*, Medical Radiology. Diagnostic Imaging,
DOI: 10.1007/174_2011_484, © Springer-Verlag Berlin Heidelberg 2012

medical indication, that alternative imaging such as ultrasound or magnetic resonance imaging cannot be substituted and that methods are used to "child-size" the technique for the scan. This chapter describes practical strategies to promote awareness, education and advocacy in radiation protection for children through "social marketing" used by the Alliance for Radiation Safety in Pediatric Imaging. The Alliance develops educational resources, including "universal protocols" and online modules for radiologists and radiologic technologists and parents. The chapter includes a discussion of the new Size Specific Dose Estimate (SSDE) and how it may be used for individual patient reports, approaches to optimize pediatric CT protocols in practice, particularly for oncology patients and finally postulates future trends in imaging and dose recording in children.

## 1 Image Gently: A Social Marketing Campaign in Pediatric CT Scanning

### 1.1 Introduction

In 2001, pediatric radiologists demonstrated that children were often receiving "adult doses" of medical radiation from CT scans (Paterson et al. 2001). Leaders in the medical community such as the Society for Pediatric Radiology and influential agencies including the National Council on Radiation Protection and Measurements, the United States Food and Drug Administration and the National Cancer Institute reminded medical practitioners that the benefits of CT must be weighed against any potential risk (Meinhold 1993; FDA Public Health Notification 2001; National Cancer Institute and the Society for Pediatric Radiology 2002).

The concept of "justification" and the need for individual protocols for every pediatric CT scan prior to the CT scan was emphasized. Conferences were held (Slovis 2002a, b; Linton and Mettler 2003). Yet, review of the medical literature suggests that widespread application of lower dose, size-based CT scans were challenging to implement in practice. There were several reasons for the situation:

1. Radiation risk estimates are controversial among radiology medical professionals making the basic premise of CT dose reduction problematic (Mezrich 2008)
2. CT images looked sharper and less "noisy" the higher the dose
3. CT technology was advancing rapidly, in some cases outstripping the education of the users of the technology
4. There was no simple method to record radiation dose for individual patients (Strauss et al. 2009)
5. Target doses or diagnostic reference levels for patients are poorly understood in the United States (Gray et al. 2005).

In 2007, the Society for Pediatric Radiology, the American Society for Radiologic Technologists, the American Association of Physicists in Medicine and the American College of Radiology formed the Alliance for Radiation Safety in Pediatric Imaging to address radiation protection through the *Image Gently*$^{sm}$ campaign (Goske et al. 2008). The mission of the group is summarized in this statement:

> The Alliance for Radiation Safety in Pediatric Imaging—the *Image Gently* Alliance—is a coalition of health care organizations dedicated to providing safe, high quality pediatric imaging worldwide. The primary objective of the Alliance is to raise awareness in the imaging community of the need to adjust radiation dose when imaging children. The ultimate goal of the Alliance is to change practice.

The Alliance has developed educational materials and advocated for radiation protection through the power of the Alliance that consists of over 64 medical societies and agencies. It uses "social marketing" defined as "the application of commercial marketing technologies to the analysis, planning, execution and evaluation of programs designed to influence the behavior of a target audience in order to improve their personal welfare and that of the society for which they are a part" (Andreasen 2006). The campaign uses the internal communication of its members, ads, posters and promotional items, a website (www.imagegently.org), social media as well as the usual scientific approaches such as journal articles and scientific conferences to convey its message. While actual estimates of radiation risk have been debated within the medical community, there are no direct data to support an increased stochastic risk of cancer associated with medical imaging. The best data are extrapolated from the Life Span Study of the survivors of the atomic bomb in Japan after World War II (Preston et al. 2004). This study demonstrated that the younger the child at the time of exposure, the greater the risk such that infants are at 15 times the risk compared to an adult. Girls are almost twice as radiosensitive as boys at all ages. After exposure, the potential for changes and possible cancer induction is greater in children as children are expected to have a longer lifetime to live. The risk while highly debated is unknown (Linet et al. 2009). As the risk is difficult to quantify or study, particularly as the excess cancer risk is layered above the baseline 22% incidence of fatal cancer in the United States population, the Alliance has taken the stance that it is imperative to act aggressively as if there may be a risk (Fahey et al. 2011). The Alliance has created educational and quality improvement materials to ensure that medical imaging professionals, referring physicians and parents are informed.

## 1.2 Educational Tools

The Alliance has been focused on educational materials for groups of medical professionals necessary to monitor, perform and interpret CT scans in children. This includes radiologists, radiologic technologists and medical imaging physicists. However, individuals with specific expertise in CT, let alone pediatric CT, may be scarce. While a full CT curriculum is available for radiologic technologist programs teaching post primary education in computed tomography, it was not until 2007 that the entry level curriculum for radiologic technologists contained an optional content area in CT. The *ACR Practice Guidelines for Performing and Interpreting Diagnostic Computed Tomography* requires that at a minimum a radiologic technologist performing CT be certified by American Registry of Radiologic Technologist and have documented training and experience in CT (Berland et al. 2011; American College of Radiology 2008). Data from the American Registry of Radiologic Technologists indicates that of those ARRT registrants indicating that their primary or secondary practice is CT, approximately 38% do not hold the post primary certification in CT. There are still eleven states in the United States where no certification is required for an individual prior to performance of a radiographic exam, let alone a CT scan. To date there are only three states that have licensure, certification or recognition standards for an individual who performs a CT.

The Image Gently campaign knows that medical professionals want to optimize CT scans for children and has worked to provide open-access online resources to aid in achieving this goal. Many of the materials included on the website may be used to respond to concerns raised in the Sentinal Event Alert on *Radiation Risks of Diagnostic Imaging* (The Joint Commission Sentinel Event 2011).

Key teaching points of the online modules include:

- *The number of CT scans in children has risen dramatically*. The number of CT scans in the United States has risen from 3 million in 1980 to 62 million in 2006 (IMV 2006) [This equals approximately one CT scan for every ten Americans! Approximately 4–7 million of these scans are performed annually in children (National Cancer Institute 2002)]. In a large insurance database covering over 350,000 children over a 3 year time period, almost 12% of children had a CT scan during that time (Dorfman et al. 2011). One study performed in a children's busy emergency room showed that some types of CT scans such as cervical spine CT after trauma and chest CT scans in young patients have risen from 366 to 435%, respectively, and that improved outcomes for pediatric patients who have not been well studied to date (Broder et al. 2007). It is also noted that approximately 90% of pediatric CT scans performed in the emergency room are performed by adult-focused hospitals (Larson et al. 2011). This last statistic is most important as it underscores the need for all radiologists and radiologic technologists to have in depth knowledge of radiation protection for children, as many of these studies are not performed at pediatric—focused hospitals.
- The *dose from a single CT scan is significantly higher than X-rays*. A single view chest X-ray yields an estimated effective dose of up to 0.01 mSv. Compare that with a routine chest CT of up to 3 mSv. A child could have *several hundred* single view chest X-rays before it would equal one chest CT. Compared to one day of background radiation for example, a single view chest X-ray is similar to one day of background radiation while an abdominal CT is similar to up to 20 months of background radiation (Bulas et al. 2009). This is why medical professionals are particularly concerned with lowering radiation dose associated with CT scans in children.
- *Increased radiosensitivity compared to adults as the relative absorption of the smaller body does not*

*attenuate the beam.* The dose at the midpoint of a patient's body is less than the dose at the surface (skin) of the patient. This occurs because the X-ray beam of the CT rotates around the patient's body and because the surface layers of patient tissue reduce the radiation in the X-ray beam. In the large adult, the multiple surface layers 'protect' the core tissues from radiation dose. Since children have less surface layers, their core doses are significantly greater than an adult when incorrect "adult-sized" techniques are used.

Modules also review medical physics as it relates to performance of CT and the changes that technical parameters, such as kVp and mAs have on pediatric patients. The modules also discuss the practical points when scanning the head, chest and abdomen in children and strategies to lower dose when scanning.

Another open source educational tool on the Image Gently website (www.imagegently.org) is a Practice Quality Improvement (PQI) project that may be used by radiologists who perform CT in children (Goske et al. 2010). It is approved by the American Board of Radiology for Maintenance of Certification credit when completed. In this PQI project, a radiologist reviews 25 CT scans performed in children in their practice in the past 6 months. The radiologist is asked to examine the entire process, from the information given on the request from the referring physician to justify the scan, to communicate with parents and caregivers and examining screening for pregnancy or allergies in children. The module provides feedback in the form of online surveys that allows the radiologist to estimate the performance of their practice to others who have taken the module. While not a scientific survey, it does give the radiologist using the module a sense of where their practice falls compares to others who have taken the module and also provides the radiologist with educational materials that can be used in their practice.

### 1.3 International Outreach

There is a strong need to emphasize radiation protection for children worldwide due to the increase in volume of medical imaging using ionizing radiation around the world. The United Nations Scientific Committee on the Effects of Atomic Radiation (UNSCEAR) reported a total number of 39 CT scans per thousand world populations that adds to the annual collective dose to the human population (UNSCEAR 2010). A recent report from the International Atomic Energy Agency indicated that "adult" technique is often used for pediatric CT scans. According to the same report, many countries lack medical physicists in hospitals and outpatient facilities. Lack of attention to dosimetry of both patients and staff was reported as a common problem. Older equipment, lack of dosimeters or skill to use them also contribute to the challenges in radiation protection of children on a global scale (Rehani and Tsapaki 2011).

The Alliance has worked with over 22 international groups including the International Atomic Energy Agency, The International Radiation Protection Association, The International Radiology Quality Network, The International Society of Radiology and the World Health Organization. These groups work together in an effort to raise awareness of the need for radiation protection using a consistent message and positive tone (Goske et al. 2011a, b). These worldwide partnerships take advantage of the strengths of each of the Alliance partners. There are many, active international groups, some with immense global reach that have considerable influence in promoting radiation protection for children. Each group has a unique perspective and target audience that provides complimentary strategies for outreach efforts to different audiences around the world. The Image Gently website contains translations of the parent brochures in more than 13 different languages.

## 2 Communicating with Parents and the Public About Pediatric CT

### 2.1 Why it is Important to Communicate with Parents About Radiation Risk

One of the most important goals in working with pediatric patients is communication about the medical imaging exam before, during and after the study is performed. This is part of the concept of health literacy. Health literacy is described as The degree to which individuals have the capacity to obtain process and understand basic health information and services needed to make appropriate decisions (Ratzan and Parker 2004). The goal is for parents to walk out of the radiology department after their child's imaging exam, having more information about their child's health and the reason for the performance of the exam than prior to the exam. This vision is part of the national imperative from the Institutes of Medicine's *Health Literacy: a Prescription to End Confusion*, a 2004 initiative that noted that the average literacy level in the United Stated is 8th grade with comprehension at 6th grade for many parents (Ratzan and Parker 2004). This document suggests that health information should be supplied to parents in a straightforward, concise manner with language, pictures and varied format that may be readily understood prior to the procedure. Radiation risk is but one part of that communication. It is interesting to note that when given the opportunity to learn about medical radiation, parents appreciated learning about the radiation risk prior to the procedures. In a study of 100 parents who were surveyed and given a pamphlet on medical imaging and CT, no parent refused a scan (Larson et al. 2007).

### 2.2 Controversies in the Discussion of Radiation Risk: Informed Decision versus Informed Consent

An area of controversy in medical communication is that of informed consent versus informed decision making. Informed consent is a legal document that signifies that the physician has "disclosed the relevant risks from a medical procedure and the patient has accepted those risks as possible outcomes" (Brink et al. 2011). Key components of informed consent according to the American Medical Association include: the nature and purpose of the proposed treatment or procedure, the risks and benefits of a proposed treatment or procedure, alternatives (regardless of their cost or the extent to which the treatment options are covered by health insurance), the risks and benefits of the alternative treatment or procedure, the risks and benefits of not receiving or undergoing a treatment or procedure. An alternate educational strategy called *informed decision making* is another option that seeks to provide more information to families and provides an opportunity for meaningful conversation in the context of the imaging study. Informed decision-making calls for "a meaningful dialogue between physician and patient instead of unidirectional, dutiful disclosure of alternatives, risks, and benefits by the physician" with informed consent (Braddock et al. 1999). Informed consent is challenging in the example of low-levels of ionizing radiation used in medical imaging as the benefits and risks are difficult to state clearly, are not unequivocal and easily measured (Cardinal and Gunderman 2011).

### 2.3 Image Gently Parent Pamphlets on Medical Imaging

The Image Gently campaign has developed pamphlets to communicate with parents in general medical imaging, CT, fluoroscopy used with interventional procedures, fluoroscopy in diagnostic imaging and nuclear medicine, Fig. 1. These are open source and may be downloaded for use in hospitals and clinics. The Image Gently website has a parent section with frequently asked questions. There is an imaging record card that encourages parents to record the name of their child's imaging test, the date and location of the exam. Similar to an immunization card, this card educates parents and may provide dates and location of critical comparison studies that may obviate repeat imaging, Fig. 2. The campaign has worked with the American Academy of Pediatrics to create a jointly sponsored parent pamphlet and resources for pediatricians through their on-line learning website, PediaLink.

## 3 Size Specific Radiation Dose Estimates

### 3.1 Introduction

CT scanners typically display two radiation dose indices: $CTDI_{vol}$ and DLP. Some CT manufacturers provide a dose report page that lists these doses. Alternatively, state-of-the-art CT scanners provide this information in a DICOM structured report that is stored in PACS. Unfortunately, $CTDI_{vol}$ is not an indication of patient dose (Shope et al. 1981; Strauss et al. 2009; Boone et al. 2011). It should not be recorded in the patient's medical record to represent the patient's dose. Pediatric radiologists have requested a method to estimate the patient dose from CT to pediatric patients (Berdon and Slovis 2002; Slovis 2002a, b). This section presents correction

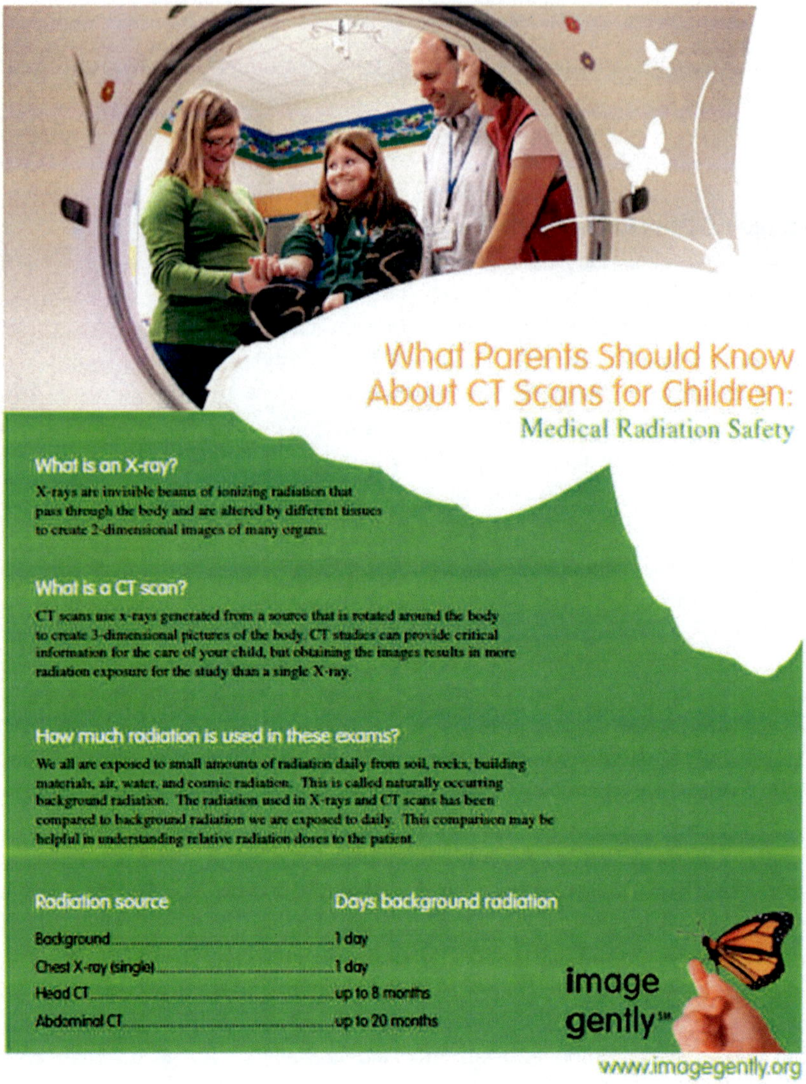


**Fig. 1** An Image Gently information pamphlet targeted to parents of children who will have a CT scans as part of their medical evaluation. Improving medical literacy for parents is one of the important goals of the Alliance for Radiation Safety in Pediatric Imaging. (Borrowed with permission. Alliance for Radiation Safety in Pediatric Imaging www.imagegently.org)

factors developed to better estimate the patient dose during a CT scan for patients of different body sizes, the Size Specific Dose Estimate. Radiologists can use these improved estimates of patient dose to better manage the radiation dose their patients receive and include the SSDE in the patient's radiology report.

## 3.2 Radiation Dose Indices Provided by CT Scanners

Radiation dose is the amount of energy transferred from X-rays passing through a medium to kinetic energy (energy of motion) of charged particles (electrons) within the medium divided by the mass of the medium that was irradiated by the X-rays (Bushberg et al. 2012). Most CT scanners electronically display two dose indices, $CTDI_{vol}$ and DLP. The $CTDI_{vol}$ is displayed in units of mGy for each completed scan. Each displayed $CTDI_{vol}$ has an associated DLP expressed in units of mGy-cm that takes into account the scan length along the z axis. For both indices, the 'medium' of the displayed doses is a cylindrical plastic phantom either 16 or 32 cm in diameter.

$CTDI_{vol}$ is based on radiation dose measurements completed by a qualified medical physicist using the phantoms and ionization chamber illustrated in Fig. 3.

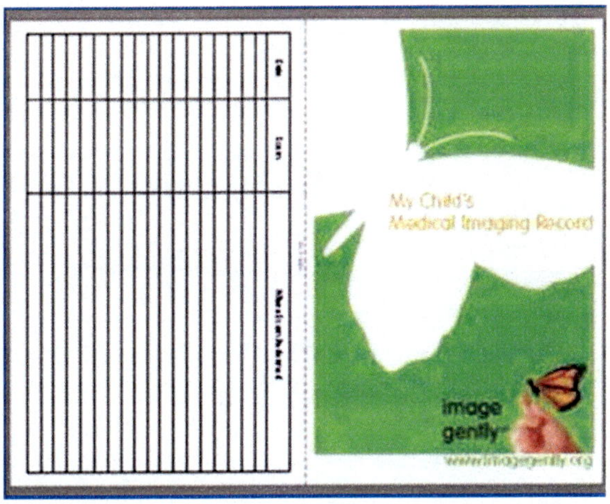


**Fig. 2** The Image Gently medical imaging record card provides parents with a simple method to track their child's imaging exams and includes the name of the study, date the exam was performed and location where the imaging study took place. (Borrowed with permission. The Alliance for Radiation Safety in Pediatric Imaging www.imagegently.org)

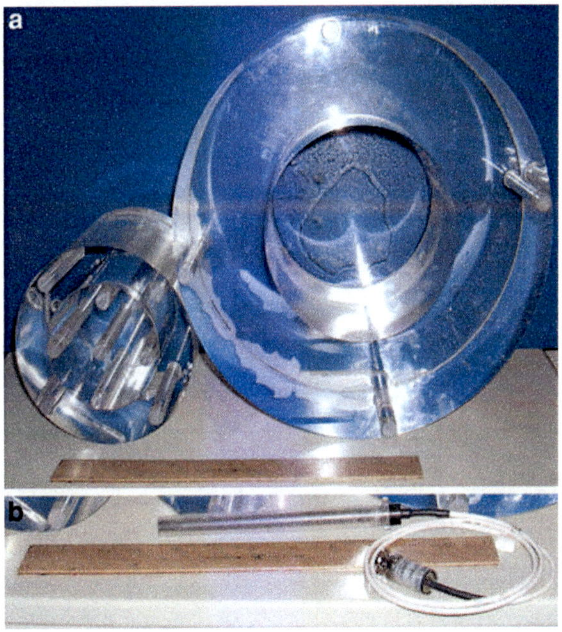


**Fig. 3** **a** Illustrates the two standard CTDI cylindrical plastic phantoms. The smaller cylinder on the *left*, sometimes called the 'adult head phantom', is 16 cm in diameter. This smaller cylinder is placed in the cylindrical cavity of the larger cylinder shown on the *right* to create a 32 cm, 'body' cylindrical phantom. **b** Illustrates the 100 mm long pencil ionization chamber used to measure CTDI doses by inserting it in the holes 1 cm below the surface and at the center of the cylindrical phantoms to make 'surface' and 'central' dose measurements. The ruler shown in both parts of this figure is a standard 12-inch ruler

Figure 4 illustrates the relative numerical values of measured dose in mGy that would be collected at each cylindrical hole with pencil chamber in Fig. 4 provided each phantom, 10, 16 and 32 cm, was centered in the gantry of the CT scanner. All of the scan parameters for measurements in Fig. 4, e.g., tube voltage, tube current, rotation time, pitch and bowtie filter are identical. The surface and central measurements for the 10 and 16 cm phantoms are approximately equal while the central measurement for the 32 cm phantom is approximately half of the surface measurement.

$CTDI_{vol}$ is defined as the single dose that best represents the distribution of doses delivered to the cross-sectional area of the phantom illustrated by each circle in Fig. 4. $CTDI_{vol}$ represents the radiation dose delivered to a *standard plastic phantom* from a specific model CT scanner using specified scan parameters. The listed $CTDI_{vol}$ values in Fig. 4 are *measured* values. $CTDI_{vol}$ provides a standardized method to estimate and compare the radiation output of different CT scanners to a standardized phantom. $CTDI_{vol}$ was defined to be a dose index of CT scanner radiation output, *not a patient dose index.*

The dose index, Dose Length Product (DLP), is the product of both the radiation dose to the selected CTDI phantom (represented by $CTDI_{vol}$) and the *length* of the phantom directly irradiated. The units of DLP are 'mGy-cm'. It is an indication of the total radiation energy transferred to the CTDI phantom. Since $CTDI_{vol}$ is not a patient dose index and DLP is estimated from $CTDI_{vol}$, *DLP does not represent a patient dose index.*

## 3.3 The Need for Patient Specific Dose Estimates Based on Size

Patients present a wide variation of path lengths for the x-rays to travel from the focal spot to the detector of the CT scanner. The neonate's shape is basically round and as small as 6 cm. As a patient grows, the path length can be greater than 40 cm (Kleinman et al. 2010). Age alone is not a good indicator of patient size. In a population of over 300 patients in New England, the abdomens of the largest 2 year-old patients equaled the size of the smallest 18 year-olds (Kleinman et al. 2010). Figure 4 illustrates that as patient size increases from 10 to 32 cm with the same

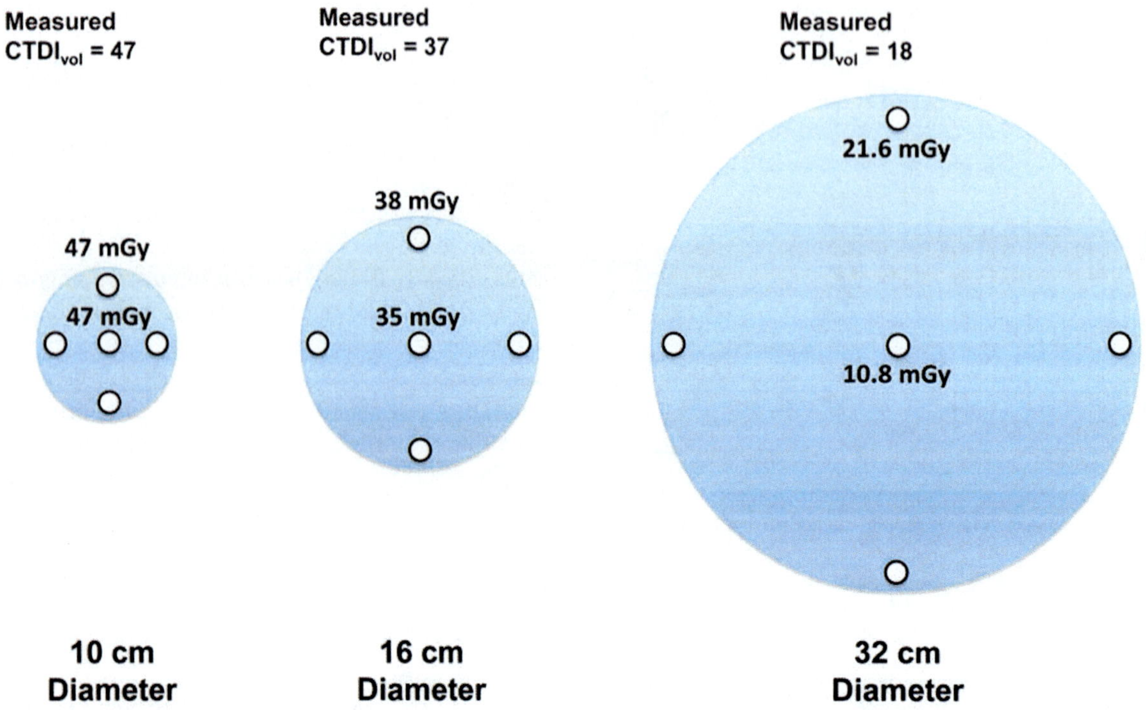


**Fig. 4** Labeled doses to 10, 16 and 32 cm cylindrical plastic phantoms at the surface and in the center of each phantom are actual measurements on a state-of-the-art CT scanner with 120 kVp, 200 mAs, pitch of 1, 1 cm fan beam width, and the same bowtie filter. All three phantoms were placed on gantry couch and centered within the CT gantry. The $CTDI_{vol}$ values are the measured values with the pencil ionization chamber shown in Fig. 3b

scan parameters, the measured $CTDI_{vol}$ decreases by approximately a factor of 2.6 (from 47 to 18 mGy).

While the *measured* dose index, $CTDI_{vol}$, is *very dependent* on phantom size when scan parameters for all three phantoms are identical as illustrated in the top row of data in Fig. 5 the *displayed* $CTDI_{vol}$ is *independent* of changes in patient size by definition. This displayed scan index accounts for the actual scan parameters used by the CT scanner, but the $CTDI_{vol}$, by definition, assumes the patient is either the 16 or 32 cm diameter cylindrical plastic. Therefore, the CTDI phantom is rarely a reasonable model for an individual patient with respect to attenuation; the patient's shape and clinical structures, e.g., bone and lung, change the dose distribution relative to that found in a cylindrical, homogeneous, plastic phantom.

The bottom rows of data in Fig. 5 illustrate the under or over estimate of the patient dose by the displayed $CTDI_{vol}$. If the 16 cm phantom is assumed, the scanner will display 37 mGy for $CTDI_{vol}$ for each of the three represented patient sizes (second row of data in Fig. 5); this over estimates the dose to adult patients and under estimates dose to infants. If the 32 cm phantom is assumed, the scanner displays 18 mGy for all patients (third row of data in figure); this *underestimates* the dose to all patients smaller than adults. The data presented in Fig. 5 demonstrates the need for the radiologist to know the phantom size associated with displayed $CTDI_{vol}$. *The displayed $CTDI_{vol}$ associated with the* 16 cm *CTDI phantom will be approximately twice the value of the displayed $CTDI_{vol}$ associated with the* 32 cm *CTDI phantom.* Without a straightforward method to assess pediatric patient dose (47 mGy) from the displayed $CTDI_{vol}$, the radiologist cannot assess their patient's risk from their CT radiation dose.

Since displayed $CTDI_{vol}$ assumes the use of either the 16 or 32 cm cylindrical plastic phantoms, one must know which phantom was selected by the scanner to estimate a more representative patient dose. Different manufactures use different criteria for selecting the CTDI phantom size. The manufacturer of the scanner should be consulted through their service representative to determine when the scanner uses each CTDI phantom size. If a newborn abdomen is scanned, the $CTDI_{vol}$ based on the 32 cm phantom

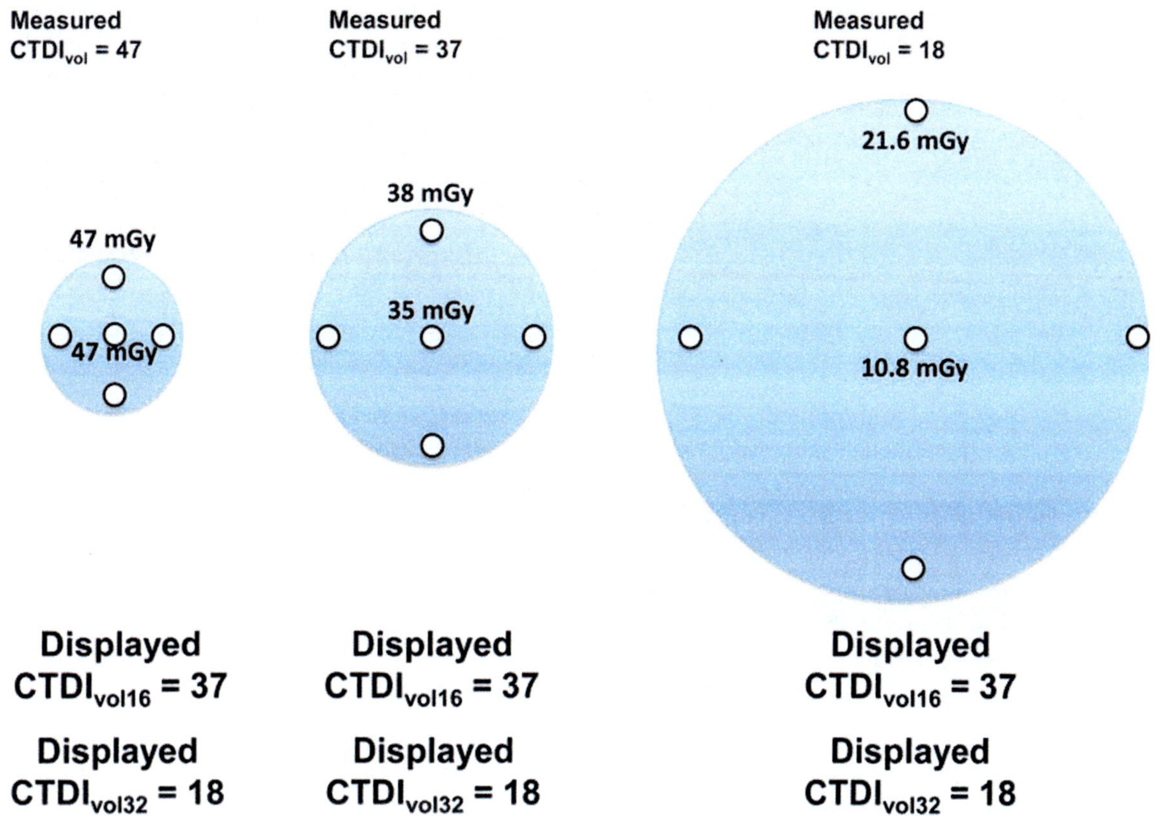


**Fig. 5** The measured $CTDI_{vol}$ dose values (pencil ionization chamber) for the representative patient size are listed at the top of the figure while the displayed $CTDI_{vol}$ values based on the 16 or 32 cm CTDI phantoms ($CTDI_{vol16}$ or $CTDI_{vol32}$) are listed below. While the measured $CTDI_{vol}$ is unique for each CTDI phantom, the displayed $CTDI_{vol}$, based on a given CTDI phantom, is independent of the representative patient size. When the displayed $CTDI_{vol}$ is based on the 32 cm CTDI phantom, the measured dose for all patient sizes smaller than 32 cm is underestimated by the displayed value. When the displayed $CTDI_{vol}$ is based on the 16 cm phantom, the measured doses for patient sizes that are smaller and larger than 16 cm are underestimated and overestimated by the displayed value, respectively

will be as little as 30% of the patient dose. If the $CTDI_{vol}$ is based on the 16 cm phantom, the $CTDI_{vol}$ will be approximately 80% of the newborn's dose.

## 3.4 The Science of Size Specific Dose Estimate

AAPM Report No. 204 (TG204), available on the AAPM website, entitled "Size-Specific Dose Estimates in Pediatric and Adult Body CT Examinations" was written to allow the estimation of patient dose from displayed $CTDI_{vol}$ by radiologic technologists or radiologists. These correction factors can be used to estimate patient dose for small as well as large patients. The scope is limited to correction factors associated with the variation in patient size for the trunk of the body (Boone et al. 2011). Data is not provided for head scans. The small scan variations in attenuation for pre- and post-contrast scans are ignored. The small doses associated with scan projection images at the beginning of the case are ignored. Additional errors in displayed $CTDI_{vol}$ due to the inability of these measurements to capture extended dose tails due to scatter in CT scans are not addressed (Dixon 2003, 2006; Boone 2007).

TG204 combines data from four different groups of investigators who independently studied the potential of size correction factors, see Fig. 6 (Boone et al. 2011). Two of these groups used Monte Carlo measurements, while the other two engaged in physical measurements on phantoms. Since $CTDI_{vol}$ is

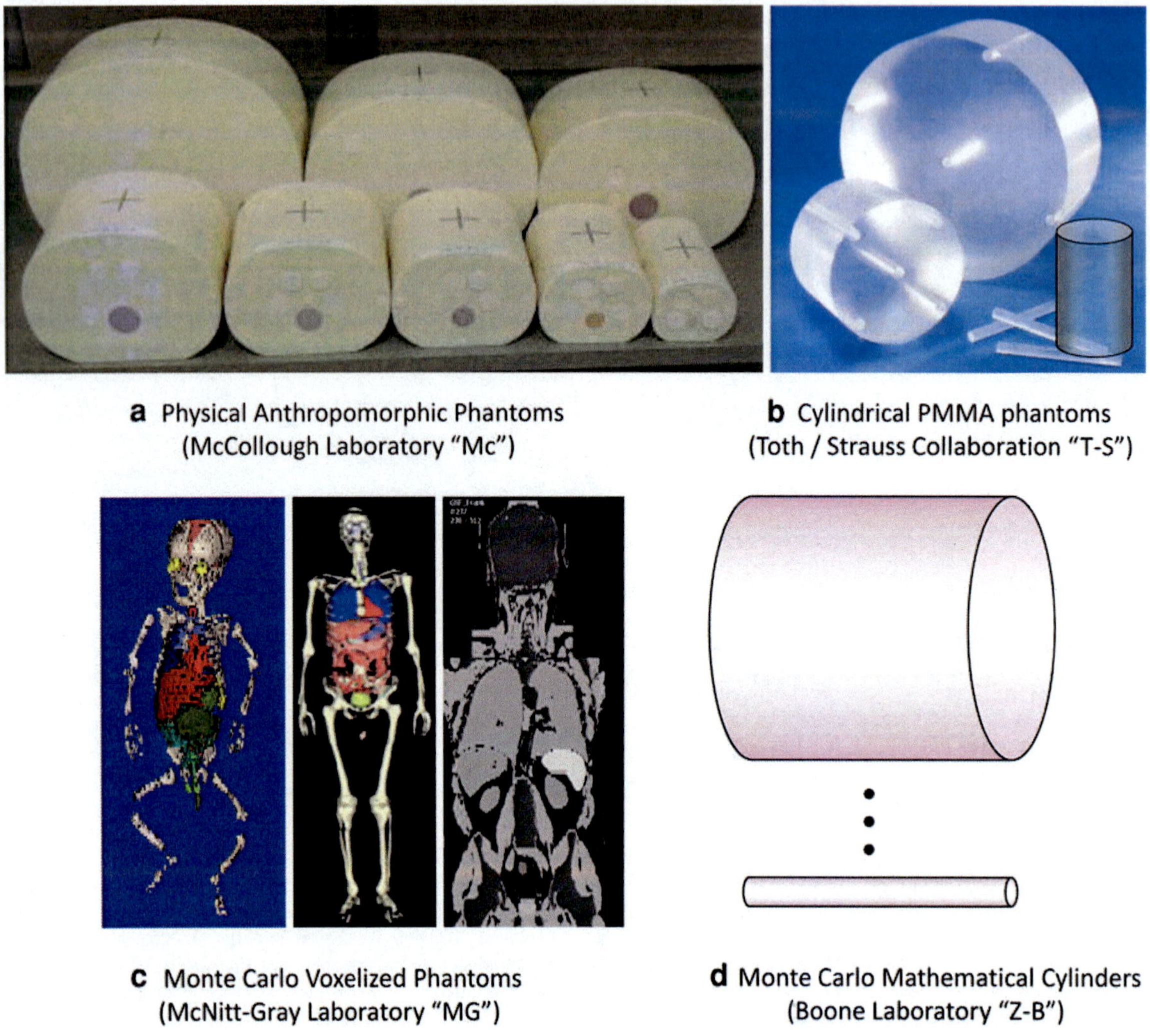


**Fig. 6** The various approaches used by the four independent research groups are illustrated. **a** Physical dose measurements were made using a series of eight anthropomorphic tissue equivalent phantoms. **b** The two existing PMMA phantoms in addition to a third 10 cm diameter phantom were used to make dose measurements on CT scanners from the four major manufacturers. **c** Monte Carlo dose calculations were made using a series of seven anthropomorphic mathematical phantoms, three of which are shown. **d** Monte Carlo calculations were made on a series of cylinders of different diameter and compositions. Borrowed with permission (Boone et al. 2011)

displayed immediately after acquisition of the scan projection image, the proposed correction factors can be used to estimate patient dose at the CT console prior to the actual CT scan that delivers the majority of the radiation dose (Boone et al. 2011).

Combined data from the four investigators is presented, normalized to the 32 cm CTDI phantom, Fig. 7, or to the 16 cm CTDI phantom, Fig. 8 for 120 kVp. The computer fit of the data assumes an exponential relationship ($Y = ae^{-bx}$) between the normalized dose coefficient and effective diameter (Boone et al. 2011). The normalized dose coefficient is the correction factor multiplied by $CTDI_{vol}$ that results in the Size-Specific Dose Estimate. The TG report develops the mathematical relationship between the equivalent diameter of Figs. 7 and 8 and the AP or LAT dimension of the patient. The dashed vertical lines correspond to the effective diameters of children of different ages. The report verifies that the mathematical fits in Figs. 7 and 8 for 120 kVp data are also reasonable fits for high voltage values that range from 80 to 140 kVp (Boone et al. 2011).

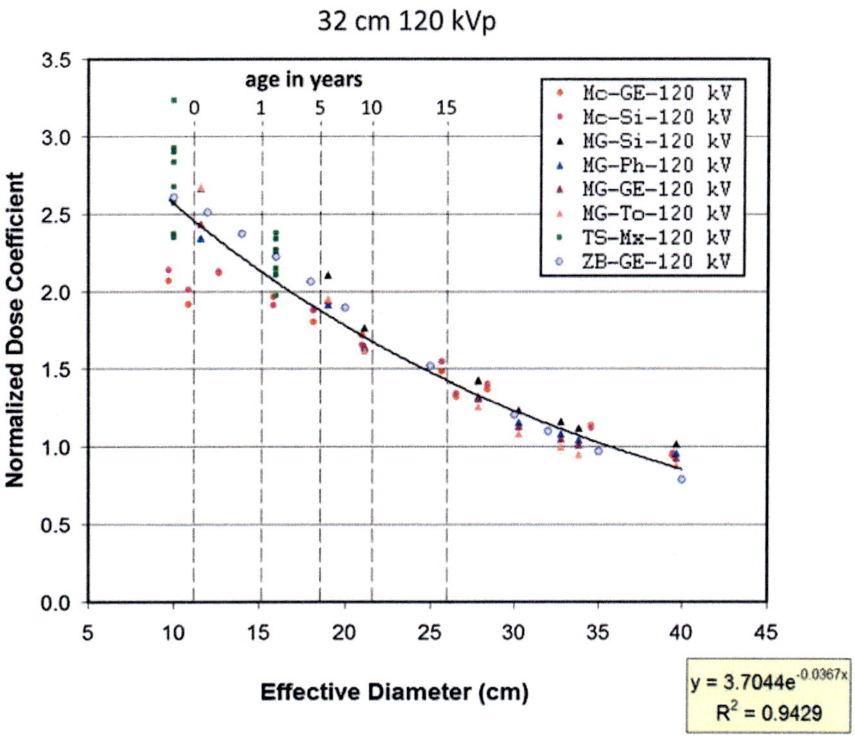


**Fig. 7** The normalized dose coefficient plotted as a function of effective diameter at 120 kVp for 32 cm CTDI phantom. The individual data points correspond to four independent research groups, as indicated in the key. (Mc = McCollough, MG = McNitt-Gray, TS = Toth/Strauss, ZB = Zhou/Boone). Scanners represented are also indicated in the key (GE = General Electric, Si = Siemens, Ph = Philips, To = Toshiba, Mx = Mixed Scanner manufacturers). Borrowed with permission (Boone et al. 2011)

The SSDE estimates the peak dose at the center of the scan length (in the z direction) of the irradiated patient. SSDE is an estimate of the radiation dose to the patient's tissues within the scan volume irradiated. Provided an organ is large compared to the transverse area of the scan and the organ completely lies within the scan length of the patient, SSDE may be a useful first approximation of organ dose, e.g., liver in an abdominal examination. SSDE cannot be substituted for $CTDI_{vol}$ in the calculation of DLP or the calculation of effective dose using published k-factors (Bongartz et al. 2004; Shrimpton et al. 2006). $CTDI_{vol}$ must be used for these latter two calculations.

The accuracy of SSDE is believed to be within 20% when the size of the CTDI phantom used by the scanner to display the $CTDI_{vol}$ is properly identified (Boone et al. 2011); a significant improvement over the errors illustrated in Fig. 5 for displayed $CTDI_{vol}$. Still, SSDE should be referred to as an estimate of patient dose. In addition, the user should use the appropriate number of significant figures when reporting SSDE. If the SSDE is greater than or equal to 5 mGy, only integer values should be expressed, for example 7 or 37 mGy and not 7.1 or 37.02. When the calculated SSDE is less than 5 mGy, one integer to the right of the decimal point is appropriate, for example 4.7 or 1.2 mGy (Boone et al. 2011).

## 3.5 Calculation of SSDE

Figure 9a, illustrates that the electronic distance-measuring tool on the scanner can be used to determine the lateral dimension (width) of the patient. In this example, the patient's body width measures 16.8 cm from the AP Projection Scan Image. The scanner displayed $CTDI_{vol}$ is 14.7 mGy based on the 16 cm CTDI phantom. Table 2B from TG204. illustrated in Fig. 9b assumes the 16 cm diameter CTDI phantom. One looks up a lateral dimension of 17 cm and obtains the correction factor of 1.08 (Boone et al. 2011). Thus, the SSDE for this patient is:

$$\text{SSDE} = 14.7\,\text{mGy} \times 1.08 = 16\,\text{mGy}$$

Assume after the scan you have the data illustrated in Fig. 10a (Boone et al. 2011). The displayed $CTDI_{vol}$ is 5.4 mGy based on the 32 cm CTDI phantom. One can electronically measure the PA dimension of 9.9 cm and a LAT dimension of

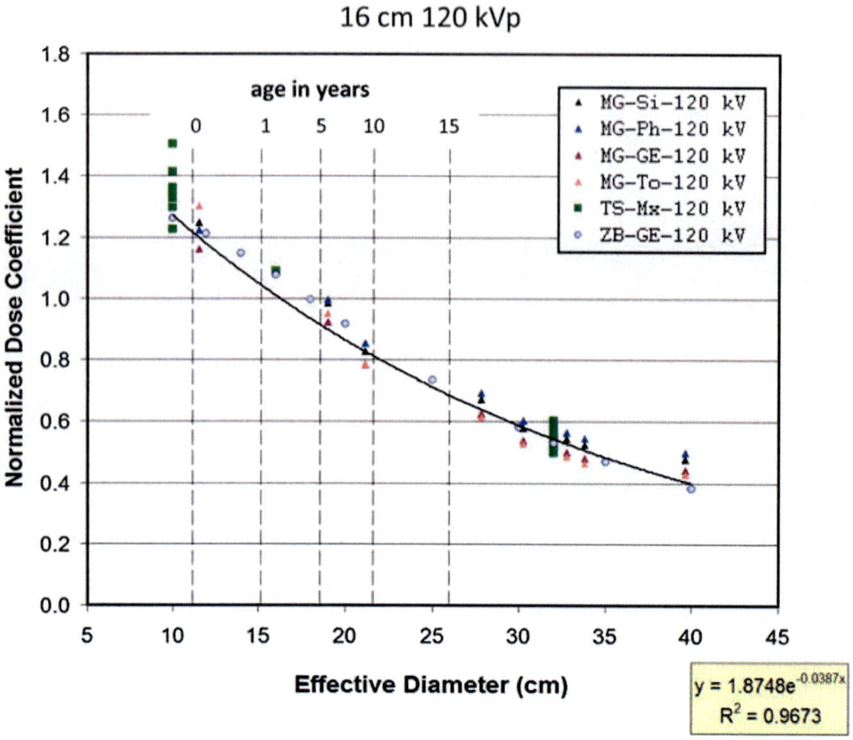


**Fig. 8** Same plot as Fig. 7, but now for the 16 cm CTDI phantom at 120 kV. The magnitude of the correction factors for pediatric doses is smaller than in Fig. 7. Borrowed with permission (Boone et al. 2011)

12.3 cm on the axial image of the patient. Thus, the PA plus LAT dimension is 22.2 cm. Table 1A from TG204 illustrated in Fig. 10b yields a correction factor of 2.50 for 22 cm (Boone et al. 2011). The SSDE for this patient is:

$$\mathrm{SSDE} = 5.4\,\mathrm{mGy} \times 2.5 = 13\,\mathrm{mGy}$$

If the CT scanner used the 16 cm CTDI phantom for the same patient and scan, the $\mathrm{CTDI}_{\mathrm{vol}}$ would be about 10.8 mGy. In this case one would obtain the correction factor from Table 2A in TG204 illustrated in Fig. 10c. A value of 22 cm yields a correction factor of 1.24. The SSDE for this patient is:

$$\mathrm{SSDE} = 10.8\,\mathrm{mGy} \times 1.24 = 13\,\mathrm{mGy}$$

Since the patient is unchanged, one would expect the same SSDE regardless of which CTDI phantom the CT scanner selected to estimate the $\mathrm{CTDI}_{\mathrm{vp}}$.

### 3.6 Clinical Application of SSDE

One may perform the SSDE calculation immediately after the scan projection images are produced or after the axial images are reformatted; the displayed $\mathrm{CTDI}_{\mathrm{vol}}$ should not change. If SSDE is estimated immediately after the scan projection images are completed and the calculated SSDE is significantly greater than the department's SSDE reference value for the particular CT study, the operator has the opportunity to appropriately adjust the scan parameters to obtain the correct patient dose prior to irradiating the patient.

As previously discussed in Sect. 3.4, in some clinical situations, SSDE may be a reasonable first approximation of the organ dose to relatively large organs completely contained within the scan volume. This information may assist the radiologist in estimating the risk associated with the CT examination.

Some departments currently elect or are mandated to include dose information in the dictated radiology report. Since $\mathrm{CTDI}_{\mathrm{vol}}$ or DLP dose indices provide only information about the amount of radiation used to perform the scan, these indices do not report an estimate of patient dose. A better solution is to report SSDE, the average radiation dose received by the patient's tissues in the scan volume when the thorax, abdomen and/or pelvis is imaged. The following is suggested language adapted from the information in TG204 (Boone et al. 2011).

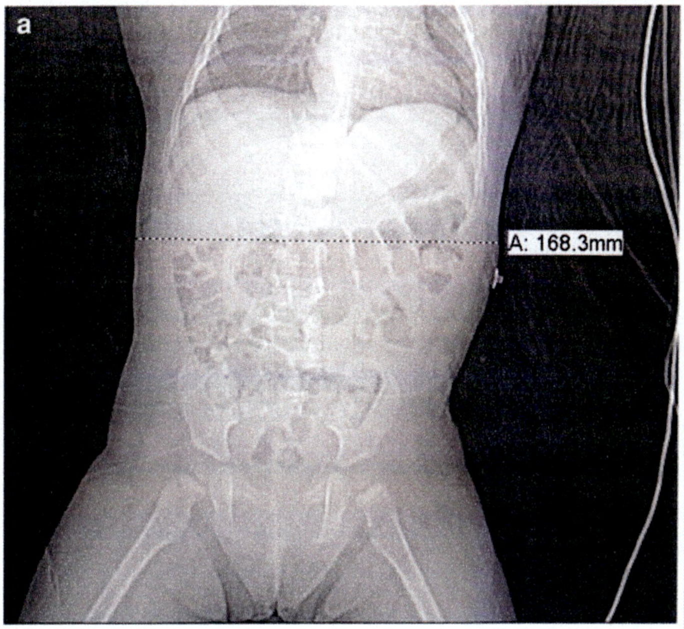


A
P
Scan

b

| Lateral Dim (cm) | Effective Dia (cm) | Correction Factor |
|---|---|---|
| 8 | 9.2 | 1.32 |
| 9 | 9.7 | 1.29 |
| 10 | 10.2 | 1.26 |
| 11 | 10.7 | 1.24 |
| 12 | 11.3 | 1.21 |
| 13 | 11.8 | 1.19 |
| 14 | 12.4 | 1.16 |
| 15 | 13.1 | 1.13 |
| 16 | 13.7 | 1.10 |
| 17 | 14.3 | 1.08 |
| 18 | 15.0 | 1.05 |
| 19 | 15.7 | 1.02 |
| 20 | 16.4 | 0.99 |
| 21 | 17.2 | 0.96 |
| 22 | 17.9 | 0.94 |
| 23 | 18.7 | 0.91 |
| 24 | 19.5 | 0.88 |
| 25 | 20.3 | 0.85 |
| 26 | 21.1 | 0.83 |
| 27 | 22.0 | 0.80 |
| 28 | 22.9 | 0.77 |
| 29 | 23.8 | 0.75 |
| 30 | 24.7 | 0.72 |
| 31 | 25.6 | 0.70 |
| 32 | 26.6 | 0.67 |

Table 2B from TG 204
16 cm CTDI phantom

**Fig. 9** **a** Is an AP scan projection performed prior to a CT scan in a child that demonstrates the method to electronically measure the lateral dimension of the patient prior to performance of a CT scan. In this patient the lateral dimension is 16.8 cm. **b** Illustrates Table 2B from the original AAPM Task group 204 document that lists the correction factor for the lateral dimension of the patient assuming the 16 cm CTDI phantom was used by the scanner to calculate and display $CTDI_{vol}$. The correction factor for a 17 cm lateral dimension is 1.08. Borrowed with permission (Boone et al. 2011)

The $CTDI_{vol}$ value reported on the scanner for the [32 or 16 cm] CTDI phantom was used with correction factors obtained from AAPM Report 204. The correction factor for this patient was based on the patient's lateral dimension [alternatively AP dimension, AP + LAT dimension, effective diameter, or age]. This method is thought to produce dose estimates with accuracy to within 20%. For this patient, the size-specific dose for this CT scan is ____ mGy.

It is imperative that language be adopted that clearly identifies how the dose estimate in the report was determined and that the correct phantom size and correction factors be used. Additional discussion concerning the application of SSDE pediatric dose estimates can be found elsewhere (Strauss and Goske 2011).

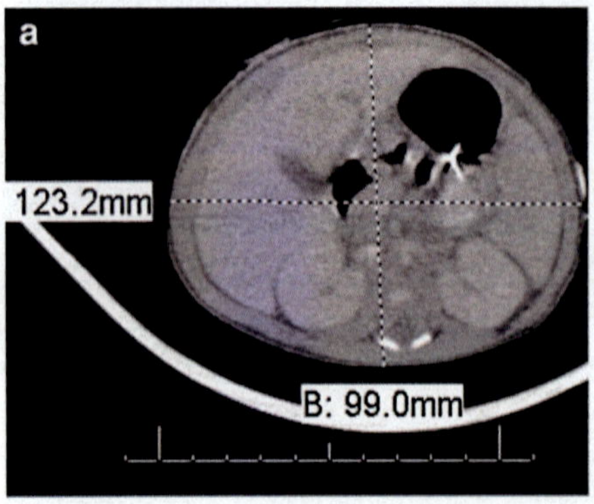


Axial Scan

b

| Lat + AP Dim (cm) | Effective Dia (cm) | Correction Factor |
|---|---|---|
| 16 | 7.7 | 2.79 |
| 17 | 8.2 | 2.74 |
| 18 | 8.7 | 2.69 |
| 19 | 9.2 | 2.64 |
| 20 | 9.7 | 2.59 |
| 21 | 10.2 | 2.55 |
| 22 | 10.7 | 2.50 |
| 23 | 11.2 | 2.46 |
| 24 | 11.7 | 2.41 |
| 25 | 12.2 | 2.37 |
| 26 | 12.7 | 2.32 |
| 27 | 13.2 | 2.28 |
| 28 | 13.7 | 2.24 |
| 29 | 14.2 | 2.20 |
| 30 | 14.7 | 2.16 |
| 31 | 15.2 | 2.12 |
| 32 | 15.7 | 2.08 |
| 33 | 16.2 | 2.05 |
| 34 | 16.7 | 2.01 |
| 35 | 17.2 | 1.97 |
| 36 | 17.6 | 1.94 |
| 37 | 18.1 | 1.90 |
| 38 | 18.6 | 1.87 |
| 39 | 19.1 | 1.83 |
| 40 | 19.6 | 1.80 |

Table 1A from TG 204
32 cm CTDI Phantom

| Lat + AP Dim (cm) | Effective Dia (cm) | Correction Factor |
|---|---|---|
| 16 | 7.7 | 1.39 |
| 17 | 8.2 | 1.36 |
| 18 | 8.7 | 1.34 |
| 19 | 9.2 | 1.31 |
| 20 | 9.7 | 1.29 |
| 21 | 10.2 | 1.26 |
| 22 | 10.7 | 1.24 |
| 23 | 11.2 | 1.22 |
| 24 | 11.7 | 1.19 |
| 25 | 12.2 | 1.17 |
| 26 | 12.7 | 1.15 |
| 27 | 13.2 | 1.13 |
| 28 | 13.7 | 1.10 |
| 29 | 14.2 | 1.08 |
| 30 | 14.7 | 1.06 |
| 31 | 15.2 | 1.04 |
| 32 | 15.7 | 1.02 |
| 33 | 16.2 | 1.00 |
| 34 | 16.7 | 0.98 |
| 35 | 17.2 | 0.97 |
| 36 | 17.6 | 0.95 |
| 37 | 18.1 | 0.93 |
| 38 | 18.6 | 0.91 |
| 39 | 19.1 | 0.89 |
| 40 | 19.6 | 0.88 |

Table 2A from TG 204
16 cm CTDI Phantom

**Fig. 10** **a** Is a single axial image from a pediatric CT scan that demonstrates the method to electronically measure the lateral or AP dimension of the patient: 12.3 or 9.9 cm, respectively. **b** Illustrates Table 1A from the original AAPM Taskgroup 204 document that lists the correction factor for the sum of the lateral and AP dimensions of the patient assuming the 32 cm CTDI phantom was used by the scanner to calculate and display $CTDI_{vol}$. The correction factor for a 22 cm summed dimension is 2.5. **c** illustrates Table 2A from the AAPM Taskgroup 204 original document which lists the correction factor for the sum of the lateral and AP dimensions of the patient, but assumes the 16 cm CTDI phantom was used by the scanner to calculate and display $CTDI_{vol}$. The correction factor for a 22 cm summed dimension is 1.24. Borrowed with permission (Boone et al. 2011)

## 4 Pediatric CT Protocols

### 4.1 Background

In 2001, a series of articles in the American Journal of Radiology changed the way Computed Tomography (CT) was performed and utilized in the pediatric population and changed perception of the potential age-adjusted risks for the development of radiation-induced cancer from doses similar to diagnostic CT studies (Brenner et al. 2001; Paterson et al. 2001; Donnelly et al. 2001). Over the past decade, both pediatric and adult radiologists have made a substantial effort to reduce CT doses in both adults and children while maintaining image quality, ensuring patient safety and adhering to the ALARA principle (Slovis 2002a, b). Developing effective pediatric CT protocols is a challenging and complex endeavor, and is fraught with many obstacles for the practicing radiologist and CT technologist. First and foremost is the challenge of appropriately adjusting patient dose to a widely variable ranges of patient size and body habitus. At the extreme ends of the spectrum, pediatric patients range from premature infants weighing just a few kilograms (path length of 4–6 cm of patient tissue X-rays travel through) to obese adolescent patients weighing as much as very large adult patients (path length of up to 40 cm). It is critical for the radiologist, radiologic technologist and qualified medical physicist work as a team to develop protocols that answer the clinical question while administering

| Abdomen Baseline: | kVp= | mA= | Time= sec | Pitch Abdomen= | Pitch Thorax= |
|---|---|---|---|---|---|
| PA Thickness (cm) | Approx Age | Abdomen | | Thorax | |
| | | mAs Reduction Factor (RF) | Estimated mAs = BL x RF *(fill in)* | mAs Reduction Factor (RF) | Estimated mAs = BL x RF *(fill in)* |
| 9 | newborn | 0.43 | | 0.42 | |
| 12 | 1 yr | 0.51 | | 0.49 | |
| 14 | 5 yr | 0.59 | | 0.57 | |
| 16 | 10 yr | 0.66 | | 0.64 | |
| 19 | 15 yr | 0.76 | | 0.73 | |
| 22 | small adult | 0.90 | | 0.82 | |
| 25 | med adult | Baseline (BL) | | 0.91 | |
| 31 | large adult | 1.27 | | 1.16 | |

**Fig. 11** This table lists a simple method to lower dose for pediatric patients using the Image Gently "universal protocols" available on the Image Gently website. This table assumes that the site is accredited and that the adult protocols fall within the ACR guidelines. Hospitals may use these protocols to work with their medical imaging physicist to lower dose further for pediatric patients as needed. Borrowed with permission (The Alliance for Radiation Safety in Pediatric Imaging www.imagegently.org)

the lowest possible radiation dose to the patient. This challenge is compounded by the fact that a steady evolution in scanner technology outpaces understanding of design of appropriate CT protocols (Frush 2009). Differences in CT design amongst the major CT vendors as well as differences in design within different models from the same vendor adds to the complexity of this issue.

In most situations, the benefit of a clinically indicated CT far outweighs the potential risks of the development of cancer later in life, but it cannot be understated that the best way to decrease risk from doses of ionizing radiation is to perform imaging studies that do not require their use such as ultrasound and magnetic resonance imaging, or not image the patient at all (Callahan 2011). If the clinical question can be effectively answered with ultrasound or MRI the need for a CT examination is eliminated.

## 4.2 Image Gently Universal Protocols

The Image Gently campaign and website were conceived by the Alliance for Radiation Safety in Pediatric Imaging in 2007. The Image Gently website (www.imagegently.org) contains a multitude of resources, including explicit guidelines for developing age and girth-based pediatric CT protocols (Fig. 11) (The Alliance for Radiation Safety in Pediatric Imaging 2008; Strauss 2008). The Image Gently pediatric protocols key off of the site's adult CT doses. This produces the relative level of quantum mottle in the pediatric images that are relatively independent of patient size and based on the basic level of quantum mottle that the radiologists have selected for their adult patients.

First, one must verify that the current adult CT techniques from the site do not result in radiation doses to the CTDI phantoms that exceed those recommended by the ACR (McCollough et al. 2006). A site radiologist or radiologic technologist should consult the qualified medical physicist who measured the radiation output from the site's CT scanners, and established $CTDI_{vol}$, for the site's baseline adult head and abdomen radiographic techniques (Strauss 2008). If the measured $CTDI_{vol}$ values are greater than the 75th percentile recommended by the ACR, the site should change their radiographic techniques to reduce their baseline dose values for their adult patients are below the 75th percentile. This basic first step insures that the selected baseline radiographic techniques are appropriate for the unique design of the site's CT scanner(s) and for the tolerance the site's radiologists have for quantum mottle in the CT images.

After establishing or verifying that the baseline radiographic techniques for adult heads or abdomens are reasonable, one can proceed to establish reasonable radiographic techniques for children. The conversion tables on the Image Gently website allow estimation of reduced mAs values (product of scanner's tube current and rotation time of the gantry) based upon patient age or PA thickness. These reduction factors result in radiation doses to pediatric patients that are equal or slightly less than the site's medium sized adult doses for the same CT examination. Reductions in the tube current or gantry rotation time (mAs) achieve the dose reduction from the Image Gently protocols; all other factors remain equal, including pitch, kVp, bow tie filter, etc. In certain clinical situations, and in certain patients, it may be prudent to adjust factors other than tube current in an attempt to reduce patient dose.

## 4.3 Strategies to Further Lower Dose

A significant change in CT practice is difficult to implement in most radiology practices. A reduction in CT dose for pediatric patients can be particularly challenging to implement, particularly in a primarily adult-based practice. In general, a reduction in patient dose for an individual CT examination results in an increase in quantum mottle, degrading image quality. However, a relatively significant amount of quantum mottle may be acceptable in some clinical situations. Image quality is a complex and subjective term; acceptable levels of quantum mottle vary among radiologists for the same examination, adding to the complexity of this issue.

Acceptable levels of quantum mottle vary for a wide range of diagnostic imaging tasks. Certain high contrast examinations of the chest, musculoskeletal system and select abdominal protocols such as the evaluation for renal stones can tolerate a relatively high level of quantum mottle. If a desired noise level is predefined by the user (Callahan 2011), CT scanners can use a multitude of technical factors including tube current, high voltage, pitch, slice thickness and automatic tube current modulation to deliver the minimum CT dose required to maintain the specified noise level and answer the clinical question at hand.

The advances in iterative reconstruction techniques offered by the CT manufacturers on their state-of-the-art CT scanners have been described by several authors in the chest (Singh et al. 2011; Prakash et al. 2010) and abdomen (Singh et al. 2010; Schindera et al. 2011). These studies demonstrate that iterative reconstruction significantly lowers quantum mottle and improves diagnostic image quality for certain clinical applications.

There are multiple steps that can be employed to decrease patient dose for individual CT studies in addition to the reduction of tube current as a function of reduced patient size by the radiologist, radiologic technologist and site's qualified medical physicist working as a team as discussed in Sect. 4.2. Many of these approaches have been summarized into ten steps published elsewhere (Strauss et al. 2010). The site's CT scanners should be accredited by the American College of Radiology to insure quality of every examination. The radiologists must be vigilant to insure the ordered CT examination is justified by clinical indication and alternative imaging strategies such as ultrasound or MRI are not appropriate substitutes. Only the indicated region of the patient's body should be scanned and scanned only once. Finally, a child friendly environment where the CT scanner is housed can reduce fear in the pediatric patient and encourage cooperation during the examination.

Obviously, all of the scan parameter choices provided by the CT scanner must be carefully considered when imaging children to properly manage the radiation dose; again summarized elsewhere (Strauss et al. 2010). The position of the stationary X-ray tube and the tube current used during the initial projection scan can significantly affect the radiation dose to critical organs such as the breast or gonads of the patient. The choice of axial or helical acquisition mode can alter both the patient dose and the image quality of the study. Reducing the detector size on the scanner in the z direction during scanning can significantly improve image quality. Most pediatric patients are imaged at a pitch of 1.3–1.4 in conjunction with a rapid gantry rotation time (<0.6 s) to minimize scan time and decrease patient motion (Strauss and Goske 2011). Certain musculoskeletal studies may benefit from a pitch of less than 1.0, which will theoretically result in improved bone detail as a result of tissue oversampling if all other factors are equal (Callahan 2011). Careful consideration is needed when choosing the manual or automatic exposure control (AEC) mode of the CT scanner. The AEC feature is designed to create images with the same quantum mottle regardless of the path length through the patient's body. While the design of some scanners allows straightforward application of AEC for both adult and pediatric patients, the design of the AEC is not intuitive on other scanners and can be difficult for the operator of the CT scanner to master when imaging pediatric patients (Strauss et al. 2010). The AEC mode of a site's CT scanner should not be used for pediatric imaging unless the site's qualified medical physicist has verified that the use of the AEC mode of the scanner results in reasonable pediatric patient doses.

Decreasing the high voltage (kVp) decreases the energy in each photon, which leads to a less penetrating beam, increased quantum mottle in the image, and less dose to the patient if no other scan parameters are adjusted (Strauss et al. 2010). In most situations, a lower kVp increases contrast in soft tissue organs and in CT angiography studies. The degree of change in radiation dose and quantum mottle caused by changes in high voltage may be reduced by changing the mAs in the opposite direction of the change in high voltage (Huda et al. 2008).

The choice of kVp should be made based on the need for subject contrast in the image (Huda et al. 2000; Huda 2002; Lucaya et al. 2000; Crawley et al. 2001). Soft tissue differentiation without the use of a contrast agent is typically improved by increases in the kVp with appropriate reductions in the mAs to result in reasonable patient doses; 120 kVp is reasonable for the majority of soft tissue imaging in children without intravenous or oral contrast. To improve contrast or to perform CT angiography, 100 kVp is reasonable for medium sized pediatric patients. Neonates to small pediatric patients may be imaged as low as 80 kVp. Some CT systems now also allow use of 70 kVp for scanning very small children. On many CT equipment, 80 kVp images at the maximum tube current of the CT scanner will not produce an adequate number of X-rays to avoid artifacts and maintain reasonable quantum mottle in the image for larger pediatric patients (Strauss and Goske 2011). Recently, at least one CT vendor has released software to enable automatic selection of appropriate kVp and consequent automatic adjustment of mAs based on patient size estimation and user-specified dose or image quality requirements.

How does one practically adjust patient dose for pediatric CT scanning with reduced high voltages? After reducing the high voltage as described above, the mAs is adjusted to either maintain radiation dose at its original level or reduce the radiation dose at the lower high voltage to maintain the contrast to noise ratio (CNR) in the original image. The first case is the simplest. First ensure that your current protocols at 120 kVp are adjusted appropriately for pediatric patients as described in Sect. 4.2. For a given size patient, dial your pediatric protocol with 120 kVp and reduced mAs into your scanner and note the displayed $CTDI_{vol}$. Dial in your reduced high voltage, either 80 or 100 kVp (depending on patient size), and increase the mAs until the displayed $CTDI_{vol}$ matches the original value (Strauss and Goske 2011).

In the second case, reduced high voltage and reduced dose, a reduction of kVp increases contrast in the image with a concurrent increase in noise. If the increase in noise is less than the increase in contrast, the contrast to noise ratio (CNR) and image quality will increase if the mAs is unchanged. For example, consider 80 vs 120 kVp imaging:

$$\begin{aligned}\text{CNR} &= \text{Contrast} / \text{Noise} = \text{Contrast increased } 70\% \\ &\quad / \text{Noise increased} < 70\%\end{aligned}$$

One is now able to reduce the mAs and patient dose until the quantum mottle in the image increases up to 70% with no reduction in CNR compared to the original image since the contrast in the image increased 70%. The degree to which the quantum mottle can be increased (dose reduced) is dependent on the imaging task and the size of the patient. A greater degree of dose reduction can be achieved with smaller sized patients (Strauss and Goske 2011).

Regardless of the strategy selected to reduce patient CT doses, one must increase the awareness and understanding of the CT radiation dose issues among radiologic technologists and radiologists to insure that adopted practices within the department are thoughtfully applied to all patients (Strauss et al. 2010). The wide range of patient sizes that are encountered in the clinical arena complicates this process. A color zone system has been used effectively to insure proper utilization of pediatric CT protocols based on a combination of clinical indication, prior CT history, and weight-adjusted protocols in an academic-based practice (Singh et al. 2009).

While weight-based and age-based protocols are commonly used to guide the use of variable CT techniques, a recent study showed that individual patient size does not correlate well with age (Kleinman et al. 2010). As a result, some institutions and the new American Association of Physicists in Medicine Task Group 204 previously discussed, use girth-based protocols as a more accurate assessment of patient size and body habitus.

## 5 Needs and Evolving Estimates of Radiation Dose and Risk for CT in Children

### 5.1 Introduction

Two of the principles of radiation protection are justification and optimization. Inherent in both of these is a firm understanding of both risk and benefit for CT in children. Some benefits of CT have been recently highlighted (Hricak et al. 2011), and are addressed in greater detail in other chapters. In addition, some of the current challenges and improvements with CT dose estimation in children are discussed elsewhere in this chapter. With growing awareness in both the medical community and public of CT radiation doses in children (Bogdanich 2009, 2010), and attendant cancer risks, imaging experts have a growing responsibility and accountability for continued refinements in the risk component of the risk benefit ratio, namely patient-specific dose assessment, and cumulative dose monitoring.

Several points are worth emphasizing as background for evolving needs in pediatric CT dose assessment. First, effective dose is a convenient, but ineffective in accurate and specific risk assessment (McCollough et al. 2010; Martin 2007). Furthermore, some uncertainty in dose and risk will remain. Fundamentally, the dose to the child from the CT scan will continue to be *estimation*, and the risk, if any, from low level radiation delivered by a pediatric CT examination will be debated. We must acknowledge the existence of conflicting data about potential benefits of low level radiation (Russo et al. 2011). There are assumptions using the linear no threshold (LNT) model (Little et al. 2009; Tubiana et al. 2009), as well as risk assignment through the most recent committee report on Biological Effects of Ionizing Radiation (BEIR VII). There are other nuances to risk assessment for pediatric CT including nonuniform exposures (e.g., at the periphery of the scan range where tissues and organs may be partially irradiated), and tissue inhomogeneity, such as variable contributions of fat in breast tissue or liver parenchyma (Samei et al. 2010).

**Current Pediatric CT Dose Estimations**

In clinical CT, effective dose is most often used as a dose metric. The unit for effective dose is the Sievert (Sv), and the effective doses for pediatric CT are in the millisieverts (mSv) range. The effective dose coverts a nonuniform radiation dose to a dose that is *effectively* an equivalent whole body dose. This is for a reference individual that is modeled by a reference phantom. Effective dose does not provide individual absorbed organ doses or organ risks and is not patient specific. For example, in a ten-year-old female, an effective dose of 10 mSv from an abdomen and pelvis CT has a lower potential (essentially zero) breast cancer risk than a chest CT with a 1.0 mSv effective dose, despite a 90% reduction in effective dose. The risk of breast cancer to a ten-year-old male will be lower that an identical 1.0 mSv examination in a ten-year-old girl.

With this understanding of some of the salient limitations of effective dose, how is effective dose currently estimated? Three methods to estimate effective dose from CT examinations are used. Doses can be estimated using mathematical, computer-based (Monte Carlo) modeling and geometric phantoms. Another method uses metal-oxide semiconductor field-effect transistor (MOSFET) dosimeters and anthropomorphic phantoms. The dose length product method, discussed in Sect. 3.2, is the third method (Strauss and Goske 2011). There are limitations with each of these (Frush 2011). Finally, there are resources that publish ranges of these doses, many of which are based on one or more of the three methods (or slight modifications) (Mettler et al. 2008), although information is limited in children. This absence of reference levels in the United States is one compelling reason in the push for CT dose registries in adults as well as children, such as the Quality Improvement Registry for CT Scans in Children (QuIRCC), discussed in more detail elsewhere in this chapter.

**Evolving Pediatric CT Dose Estimations**

Recent work, outlined in the American Association of Physicists in Medicine (AAPM) report (TG 204) (Boone et al. 2011) and based on refinements in dose estimation through scientific investigations by Boone, McCullough, McNitt Gray and Strauss, highlights the emerging recognition that dose estimations for pediatric (and adult CT) must go beyond contemporary effective dose determinations; sophisticated organ-based and even patient specific dose estimations are needed. This conceptual shift imparts an opportunity to include assignment of organ risk, that will be age and gender-based, and will likely be useful in the

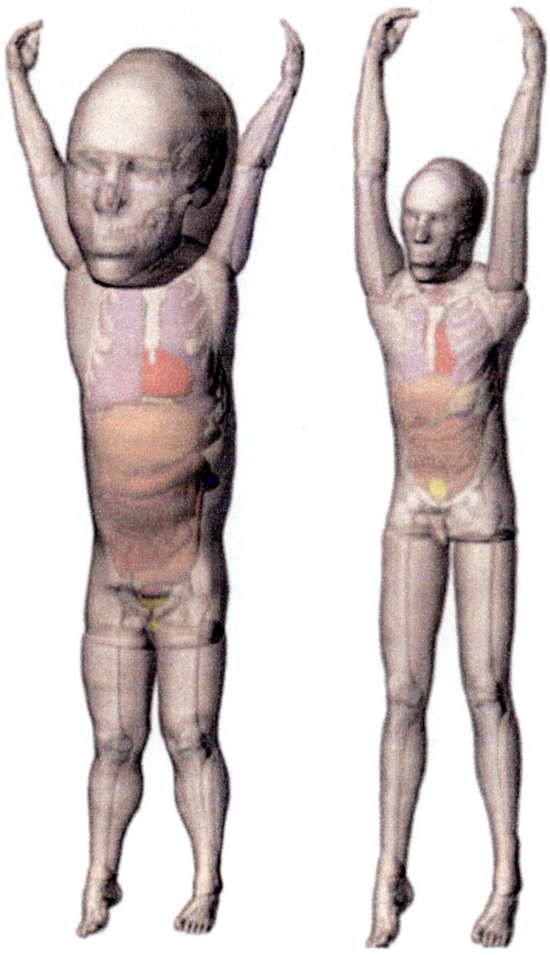

**Fig. 12** Computer models focused on the torso of the 5-week-old female (*left*) and 12-year-old male (*right*). To date the head, hands and feet have been scaled from adult data and not undergone age-specific modeling. Borrowed with permission (Li et al. 2011c)

growing cumulative dose mandate for medicine (The Joint Commission Sentinel Event 2011). While there are simultaneous and collaborative efforts in organ-based dose estimation, the following material will review one program's recent work (Li et al. 2011a, b, c, d, e, f).

It is important to emphasize that this paradigm is dependent on close collaboration within the imaging community, including medical physicists, technologist and imaging experts such as radiologists. The work consists of clinical pediatric CT data, geometric and mathematical modeling of this data (yielding a library of computer generated age-appropriate phantoms), validated Monte Carlo simulations for organ dose assignment for these phantoms, and translation of resultant organ doses to models of risk assessment. The product includes patient specific (age and gender based) organ dose, effective dose and (effective) risk indices and estimations.

The following are the steps for this paradigm. Images from essentially normal CT examination over a range of pediatric ages/sizes are de-identified. Organs that are completely within the scan range are individually and manually segmented (traced) and modeled. This is a very labor intensive process, but these contour data provide a bank of age/size-based organs that avoids the inaccuracies from other methods, such as geometrical models (e.g., cylinders, triangles, and rectangles) or scaling from adult organ data. Organs not fully covered in the scan range are modeled using existing data from full body computer models derived from visible human data with some other approximations. Based on these 3D organ determinations, full body gender-and age-specific computer phantoms are generated using non uniform rational B-spline—NURBS—methodology which accounts for complex surfaces and curves. This computer model is a hybrid between mathematical and geometrical models and results in a voxelized phantom, (Fig. 12) providing tremendous flexibility (i.e., individual voxel assessment) for organ dose determination. The phantom data is inputted into a Monte Carlo program for organ dose assignment. The Monte Carlo simulation has been validated in prior work with geometric phantoms on CT scanners across a range of protocols, consisting of different bow tie filters. Basically, knowing the parameters that contribute to the dose from a CT examination, such as kVp, mA, and pitch, organ dose can be determined for a broad range of clinical CT protocols in children from the computer phantom; this range comprises the clinical landscape for body CT protocols in children (Li et al 2011e) (Fig. 13). Finally, with these organ dose assessments, age and gender specific excess risks for cancer can be calculated from the models in the BEIR VII report (BEIR 2006). To date, the method described above has been used for assessment of organ doses and risks for pediatric chest and abdomen CT (Li et al. 2011b, d, f).

**Benefits of Patient-Specific CT Dose and Risk Assessment**

The imaging community has a responsibility for accurate dose assessment, practicing within reference

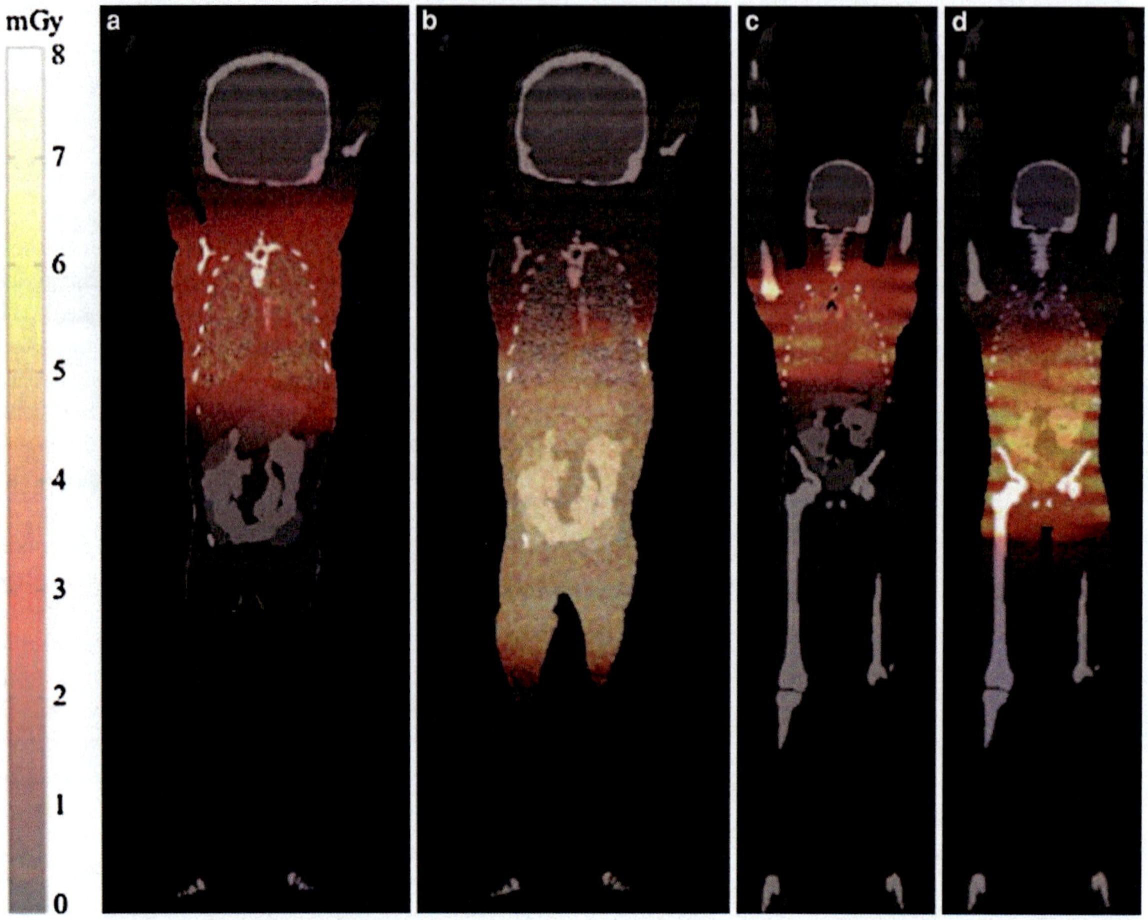


**Fig. 13** Modeled dose distributions from multidetector CT in the mid torso coronal plane in the same two pediatric voxelized phantoms from Fig. 1. **a** chest scan. **b** abdomen CT in the 5-year-old girl. **c** and **d** are the same regions for the 12-year-old. The gray scale organs are overlaid with a semitransparent colored dose distribution. Note the representation of the effect of the spiral course of the X-ray source. Borrowed with permission (Li et al. 2011c)

levels for radiation doses, and tracking radiation doses for individual patients. Current efforts with patient specific doses provide an opportunity for risk assignment, as discussed above. Whether or not this risk will find a place in patient records, through reports or be archived in other fashions such as PACS will require thoughtful discussion. Reporting of doses estimates for CT is on the horizon, required in California by July 2012 (Summary of the California Senate Bill 1237 2011), and as part of the Medicare Improvements for Patients and Providers Act (MIPPA) CT facility accreditation. The ACR is among accrediting organizations and requires submission threshold dose data for accreditation. The Food and Drug Administration and Medical Imaging and Technology Alliance (MITA) recently promoted mandates and developed guidelines for dose alerts on CT scanners (Hampton 2010; NEMA Standards Publication 2010). These and other actions underscore the growing need for dose accountability. With this accountability for dose, there is an implicit responsibility for the *significance* of this dose, primarily accurate and gender- and age-specific cancer risk in CT.

This improved dose information will be an important contribution for the development of dose registries, such as the ACR Dose Index Registry, and the ACR QuIRCC pediatric CT registry. Radiation dose reference levels are lacking for CT in the United States, and the growing body of registry data will help identify dose outliers (either over, or under dosing, the latter perhaps compromising image quality). Reference levels may help improve accreditation programs, fine tune equipment based dose alerts, function as benchmarks for practice and institution quality assessment and improvement (including protocol optimization), and serve as measures in practice quality improvement aspects of maintenance of certification, among others.

Cumulative dose archiving and tracking for patients, based on improved dose and risk assessments, can potentially help in decision making (or at least discussion of the risk and benefits with patients) at the point of care, and provide more accurate risk profiles for individuals, such as those undergoing multiple examinations. A summary of an international effort for cumulative dose tracking, including benefits (such as patient specific decision making for imaging, and guidance for CT protocol development and optimization) is being established by the International Atomic Energy Agency (Rehani and Frush 2010). The details of cumulative dose tracking will be dependent on resources of the health care system. To date, there is no existing national cumulative does tracking in the United States but the increasing presence of electronic medical records will be an important substrate for patient dose archiving and tracking. Institutional or other more local programs for patient dose tracking, initially based on frequency of CT examinations (Birnbaum 2008), are increasingly automated with technology such as optical character recognition (Li et al. 2011a, b, c, d, e, f). These and other efforts in improved dose and risk assessment for pediatric CT, together with advancements in technology and techniques, education and outcomes-based investigations, will contribute to the mandate for radiation protection of children during diagnostic imaging.

## 6 Challenges in Pediatric Oncologic Imaging

### 6.1 The Pediatric Oncology Population

Children treated for cancer represent a rapidly growing patient population for whom concern about exposures to ionizing radiation from medical imaging and their accumulative effects are rapidly being recognized. Currently, more than 12,000 children under the age of 20 years are diagnosed each year in the United States with cancer. With overall cure rates for all childhood cancers approximating 80% (Jemal et al. 2006), the number of cancer survivors in the United States has increased from 3 million to nearly 12 million over the past 40 years (Cancer Survivors 2011).

Childhood cancer patients and survivors may be at even greater risk from cumulative long-term effects of ionizing radiation exposure due to compounding of additional disease- and treatment-related exposures (e.g., chemotherapy, genetic sensitivity, radiation therapy). In addition, children treated for cancer are imaged considerably more frequently and many at younger ages than the general population, further contributing to radiation exposure burden. The results of treatment and associated exposures may contribute to development of second malignant neoplasms and secondary toxicities related to treatment (Armstrong et al. 2011); all necessitating repeated imaging. Thus, in caring for children and adolescents with cancer, the goals for patient and disease assessment must be considered as well as the need for clinical imaging such as would be seen in the general pediatric population.

In contrast with adults receiving cancer therapy, most of the pediatric cancer population undergoes protocol-based treatment. With this in mind, addressing scientific hypotheses with imaging must be considered when imaging childhood cancer patients as well as addressing potential clinical needs. The two need not necessarily conflict nor must they coincide with each other. To optimize patient care while minimizing imaging-associated toxicities, efforts should be made to limit unnecessary and oftentimes repeated imaging by obtaining and reviewing outside or referred studies prior to repeating on-site imaging, tailoring repeat studies to obtain information lacking on preceding examinations, using the lowest dose possible to obtain diagnostic quality studies, collaborating in the design of treatment protocols, serving as an imaging consultant to oncologists. As with general pediatric CT imaging, few instances exist when multi-phase CT imaging is justified for pediatric oncology patients. Diagnoses where multi-phase imaging may be considered include: differentiating hemangiomas from malignant hepatic tumors and preoperative surgical planning for such cases. In many cases, MR angiography can replace CT angiography.

Because exposures received in childhood and adolescence are cumulative, as discussed elsewhere in this chapter, any exposure to ionizing radiation whether it be directed by a scientific question, protocol requirement or clinical need must be considered on the basis of risk and benefit to the pediatric patient. Though children with cancer represent a small subset of the pediatric population, these children also participate in usual childhood activities such as playing and sports, acquire childhood infectious diseases and are typically cared for in local community hospitals for non-cancer related issues. Thus, limiting exposure to ionizing radiation is of paramount importance whenever imaging is indicated.

One subset of pediatric patients at particular risk for the development of radiation-induced malignant neoplasms, are those who possess a genetic sensitivity to the adverse effects to ionizing radiation. Such patients include those with ataxia telangiectasia, those with cellular blue nevus syndrome, those whose genetic heritage includes Li Fraumeni, Gardner's syndrome and other cancer-predisposition syndromes (Kleinerman 2009; Hall and Angèle 1999). In these subsets of patients, even limited radiation exposure may generate a malignant tumor; primary or secondary. Thus, in such cases, avoiding radiation by using ultrasound or MR instead of CT whenever possible is vitally important.

## 6.2 Oncologic Imaging

Oncologic medical imaging should be designed to answer the protocol question, provide detailed and complete staging information, effectively monitor disease response to therapy, and detect toxicities and complications (Kaste 2009, 2011) while subjecting the patient to the least exposure to ionizing radiation. Methods to ensure optimal imaging include standardization of imaging techniques to allow for accurate assessments of interval change in the extent and characteristics of the tumor. In the case of cross-sectional imaging, the type(s) and methods of contrast administration, anatomic sites imaged and exposure parameters should be consistent amongst examinations and adhere to protocol requirements. CT techniques exploiting inherent tissue contrast such as in the lungs for detection of pulmonary metastases and fungal lesions can conserve radiation exposure. However, detection of tiny lesions in liver, spleen and kidneys that may represent infectious microabscesses or metastatic deposits may require higher techniques than those recommended for abdominal imaging in trauma cases; a "miss" due to inability to detect tiny lesions on low dose studies may impact treatment and compromise patient outcomes.

## 6.3 Post Therapy Surveillance Monitoring

Few recent imaging studies have evaluated patient outcomes and the value of surveillance imaging in detecting disease relapse after completion of therapy. Of those available, most (with the exception of brain tumors) indicate little if any significant improvement in salvage rates between disease relapse detected by imaging and those detected by clinical history and examination (Kovanlikaya et al. 2003). Chong et al. 2010 found that the median 5 year cumulative estimate of radiation exposure from 690 medical imaging studies amongst a variety of pediatric cancers was 61 mSv (range, 10–642 mSv). Thirty-four percent of the studies performed were protocol driven; indications for the remaining studies were divided between clinical care and surveillance. These investigators found that the patients with highest exposures were those diagnosed with neuroblastoma (median, 214 mSv) and lymphoma (median, 61 mSV). Importantly, neuroblastoma is typically diagnosed in patients of very young ages (Chu et al. 2011; Lakhoo and Sowerbutts 2010; Maris 2010) when patients are most susceptible to the effects of ionizing radiation.

Investigation by Kan et al. (2011) found that inclusion of the pelvis CT among patients with Wilms tumor or hepatoblastoma failed to identify pelvic metastases that would alter treatment. Abdominopelvic CT has also been shown to be of limited value in initial or follow-up staging of patients with skeletal Ewing sarcoma, while contributing to increased radiation exposure, particularly when the primary site of disease is an extremity (Dobbs et al. 2010). Thus, routine off-therapy imaging needs further assessment with rigorous scientific study. Currently, except in the cases of brain tumors which are routinely evaluated with MR, routine off-therapy imaging should be subjected to outcome analysis to determine efficacy.

### 6.4 Future of Pediatric Oncologic Imaging

Imaging outcomes studies are critical to refining imaging follow-up, modality, frequency, sensitivity and specificity and must be undertaken in collaboration with pediatric oncologists, surgeons, and radiation oncologists. To be informative and limit potential toxicities from medical imaging, design of such studies must incorporate tumor- and patient-specific parameters such as

- Primary tumor type
  - Therapeutic response
  - Survival
  - Relapse risk and patterns
- Patient demographics
- Treatment toxicities
- Anticipated late effects

Tumor imaging must advance in concordance with evolving therapeutic research that focuses on molecularly targeted agents (Adamson 2009). The future role of CT and its function as a biomarker of oncologic disease will undoubtedly reflect such evolution of therapy.

As imaging technology advances, the value of incorporating new methods and replacing existing systems and techniques must be assessed. One example is demonstrated by the rapid incorporation of PET-CT into the clinical arena. PET-CT utilizes very low dose CT for attenuation correction and is oftentimes coupled with a higher dose CT of diagnostic quality. Thus, patients undergo two, though technically distinct CT studies, both of which contribute to radiation exposure. More recent PET-CT designs allow programing of variable CT techniques within the same study thereby obviating the need for separate CTs for attenuation correction and diagnosis; limiting radiation exposures. Cooperation between radiologists, nuclear medicine physicians, industry and oncologists will refine imaging while minimizing patient exposures to ionizing radiation.

In summary, pediatric patients diagnosed with a malignancy represent a growing and unique subset of the pediatric population. These patients undergo repeated imaging and thus accumulate considerable exposures to ionizing radiation. CT represents an important tool for diagnosing and assessing tumor response to therapy but its use also contributes to the growing exposure burden of these vulnerable patients. Refinement of CT techniques to optimize information obtained while limiting patient exposures is needed. Collaborative design of CT protocols to serve as a biomarker of disease and to serve a as a sensitive means of detecting infection and complications are important avenues to pursue.

## 7 Diagnostic Reference Levels

Diagnostic reference levels (DRL) are defined as target levels that can be used by hospitals, clinics, regions or nations "for identifying situations where the level of patient dose… is unusually high… if it is found that procedures are consistently causing the relevant diagnostic reference to be exceeded, there should be local review.. to determine whether the protection has been adequately optimized" (International Commission on Radiological Protection 1991). Typically DRL are defined for a specific exam and patient population and are not to be applied to an individual patient, but to populations of patients. In addition, as technology improves, it is assumed that DRL will change over time. Their purpose, as first defined by the International Commission on Radiologic Protection in 1991, was as a guidance tool (International Commission on Radiological Protection 1991). Gray emphasizes that DRL should not be used to define "good" or "bad" scan technique as individual patient protocols may require exceeding DRL for good clinical care and be justified based on the medical indication (Gray et al. 2005). DRL are most often based on 3rd quartile values of mean hospital doses as seen in national surveys. While groups such as the FDA and The Joint Commission have urged radiologists to monitor DRL for patients, their existence in the pediatric population is sorely lacking in the United States as noted above (U.S. Food and Drug Administration, White Paper 2010; The Joint Commission Sentinel Event 2011). While DRL are published in Europe in CT, they are only available for certain body parts, are based on age (a less optimal method than body size) and expressed in $CTDI_w$, making direct comparison across regions most challenging. The only United States pediatric DRL is that published by the American College of Radiology CT Accreditation program. For a CT scan of the abdomen for a 5 year old, using a 16 cm phantom as a reference standard, the target level is 20 mGy. This lack of

DRL for pediatric patients prompted action by the pediatric radiology community. Working with the American College of Radiology National Radiology Data Registries (NRDR), pediatric radiologists developed a prototype registry, the Quality Improvement Registry in CT Scans in Children (QUIRCC) (Goske et al. 2011a, b). This prototype registry has developed DRL from a six hospital consortium and has focused on CT of the abdomen and pelvis with IV contrast for study. Medical indication was for routine abdominal CT scan indications, most commonly CT scans of the abdomen for abdominal pain. Scan indication for other uses such as CT angiography or renal stone were excluded. While the registry is collecting exposure values of CTDI $_{vol}$ and DLP and pertinent technical values, the QuIRCC is using the new SSDE as discussed above to estimate patient radiation dose levels for patients of different body width. While still estimates, this is considered an advance over the use of exposure (CTDI $_{vol}$ or DLP) or effective dose as previously notes in the discussion in the section on SSDE.

## 7.1 Importance and the Future of Dose Index Registries

Dose Index Registries (DIR) such as the dose index registry developed by the American College of Radiology have the potential to rapidly acquire population data and provide feedback to radiology practices throughout the country. Though the use of automatic upload of de-identified data from CT scanners throughout the country, hospitals and institutions will be able to compare their practice with other practices and determine whether or not their scans fall within DRL as defined by the registry or other national organizations or agencies. The use of quality improvement methodology *will reduce variability of scan technique and potentially reduce or optimize radiation dose for children of the same body size for similar scan indications.* More importantly, the ability to define target reference levels based on body size and determine that the appropriate technique factors are being used for the specific medical indication (low versus higher resolution) *prior* to the scan being performed is the goal. Likely, in the not too distant future, determination of scan technique will be automated based on information gained from the scout view. The scanner will automatically assign specific scan parameters based on the protocols which have been determined from DRLs. Through these technical advances and the use of quality improvement methodology, practices may review and improve CT safety for pediatric patients undergoing CT.

## References


Adamson PC (2009) Imaging in early phase childhood cancer trials. Pediatr Radiol 39(Suppl 1):S38–S41

American College of Radiology (2008) New CT accreditation dose requirements effective. 1 Jan 2008. http://www.acr.org/accreditation/FeaturedCategories/ArticlesAnnouncements/NewDoseReq.aspx. Accessed 2 Oct 2011

Andreasen A (2006) The role of social marketing. In: Andreasen A (ed) Social marketing in the 21st century. Sage Publications, Thousand Oaks, pp 87–107

Armstrong GT, Liu W, Leisenring W, Yasui Y, Hammond S, Bhatia S, Neglia JP, Stovall M, Srivastava D, Robison LL (2011) Occurrence of multiple subsequent neoplasms in long-term survivors of childhood cancer: a report from the childhood cancer survivor study. J Clin Oncol 29: 3056–3064

BEIR (2006) Committee to assess health risks from exposure to low levels of ionizing radiation. Health risks from exposure to low levels of ionizing radiation: BEIR VII Phase II. National Academies Press, Washington, p 406

Berland LL et al (2011) American College of Radiology. ACR practice guidelines for performing and interpreting diagnostic computed tomography. http://www.acr.org/SecondaryMainMenuCategories/quality_safety/guidelines/dx/ct_performing_interpreting.aspx. Accessed 25 Sept 2011

Berdon WE, Slovis TL (2002) Where we are since ALARA and the series of articles on CT dose in children and risk of long-term cancers: what has changed? Pediatr Radiol 32:699. doi:10.1007/s00247-002-0794-4

Birnbaum S (2008) Radiation safety in the era of helical CT: a patient-based protection program currently in place in two community hospitals in New Hampshire. J Am Coll Radiol 5:714–718

Bogdanich W (2009) New York Times. Radiation overdoses point out dangers of CT scans. http://www.nytimes.com/2009/10/16/us/16radiation.html. Accessed 2 Oct 2011

Bogdanich W (2010) Radiation worries for children in dentists chair. New York Times. http://www.nytimes.com/2010/11/23/us/23scan.html. Accessed 2 Oct 2011

Bongartz G, Golding S, Jurik A, Leonardi M, van Meerten EvP, Geleijns J, Jessen KA, Panzer W, Shimpton PC, Tosi G (2004) European guidelines for multslice computed tomography. European Commission

Boone JM (2007) The trouble with CTD100. Med Phys 34(4): 1364–1371

Boone JM, Strauss KJ, Cody DD, McCollough CH, McNitt-Gray MF, Toth TL Goske MJ, Frush DP (2011) Size-specific dose estimates (SSDE) in pediatric and adult body CT examinations. AAPM Report No. 204 posted at http://www.aapm.org. ISBN: 978-1-936366-08-8, ISSN: 0271-7344. http://www.aapm.org/pubs/reports/RPT_204.pdf. Accessed 2 Oct 2011

Braddock CH 3rd, Edwards KA, Hasenberg NM et al (1999) Informed decision making in outpatient practice: time to get backto the basics. JAMA 282:2313–2320

Brenner DJ, Elliston CD, Hall EJ, Berdon WE (2001) Estimated risks of radiation-induced fatal cancer from pediatric CT. AJR 176(2):289–296

Brink JA, Goske MJ, Patti J (2011) Informed decision-making trumps informed consent for medical imaging with ionizing radiation. Radiology (in press)

Broder J, Fordham LA, Warshauer DM (2007) Increasing utilization of computed tomography in the pediatric emergency department, 2000–2006. Emerg Radiol 14(4): 227–232

Bulas D, Goske M, Applegate K, Wood N (2009) Image gently: improving health literacy for parents about CT scans for children. Pediatr Radiol 39:112–116

Bushberg JT, Seibert JA, Leidholdt EM, Boone JM (2012) The essential physics of medical imaging. Lippincott Williams and Wilkins, Philadelphia, p 1030

Callahan MJ (2011) CT Dose reduction in practice. Pediatric Radiol 41(Suppl 2):S488–S492. doi:10.1007/s00247-011-20990y

Cancer Survivors (2011) United States 2007 MMWR Morb Mortal Wkly Rep 60(9): 269–272

Cardinal JS, Gunderman RB, Tarver RD (2011) Informing patients about risks and benefits of radiology examinations: a review article. J Am Coll Radiol 8:402–408

Chong AL, Grant RM, Ahmed BA, Thomas KE, Connolly BL, Greenberg M (2010) Imaging in pediatric patients: time to think again about surveillance. Pediatr Blood Cancer 55: 407–413

Chu CM, Rasalkar DD, Hu YJ, Cheng FW, Li CK, Chu WC (2011) Clinical presentations and imaging findings of neuroblastoma beyond abdominal mass and a review of imaging algorithm. Br J Radiol 84(997):81–91

Computed tomography dose check (2010) NEMA Standards Publication XR 25-2010, pp 1–15

Crawley MT, Booth A, Wainwright A (2001) A practical approach to the first iteration in the optimization of radiation dose and image quality in CT: estimates of the collective dose savings achieved. Br J Radiol 74:607–614

Dixon RL (2003) A new look at CT dose measurement: beyond CTDI. Med Phys 30(6):1272–1280

Dixon RL (2006) Restructuring CT dosimetry: a realistic strategy for the future requiem for the pencil chamber. Med Phys 33(10):3973–3976

Dobbs MD, Lowas SR, Hernanz-Schulman M, Holt GE, Yu C, Kan JH (2010) Impact of abdominopelvic CT on Ewing sarcoma management. Acad Radiol 17:1288–1291

Donnelly LF, Emery KH, Brody AS, Laor T et al (2001) Minimizing radiation dose for pediatric body CT applications of single detector helical CT strategies at a large children's hospital. AJR 176(2):303–306

Dorfman AL, Fazel R, Einstein AJ et al (2011) Use of medical imaging procedures with ionizing radiation in children: a population-based study. Arch Pediatr Adolesc Med 165: 458–464

Fahey FH, Treves ST, Adelstein SJ (2011) Minimizing and communicating radiation risk in pediatric nuclear medicine. J Nucl Med 52:1240–1251

FDA (2001) Public health notification reducing radiation risk from computed tomography for pediatric and small adult patients. http://www.fda.gov/cdrh/safety/110201-ct.html. Accessed 21 Aug 2011

Frush DP (2009) Radiation, CT, and children: the simple answer is…it's complicated. Radiology 252:4–6

Frush DP (2011) CT dose and risk estimates in children. Pediatr Radiol 41(Suppl 2):483–487

Goske MJ, Applegate KE, Boylan J et al (2008) The image gently campaign: working together to change practice. AJR 190:273–274

Goske MJ, Phillips RR, Mandel K, McLinden D, Racadio J, Hall S (2010) A web-based practice quality improvement program in CT safety for children (Invited Paper). AJR 194(5):1177–1182

Goske MJ, Applegate KE, Butler PF, Frush DP, Morrison G, Strauss KJ (2011a) Image gently: partnerships to promote radiation protection for children worldwide. Pediatr Radiol 41(Suppl 1):S207–S209

Goske M, Strauss KJ, Coombs L et al (2011b) Quality improvement registry in CT scans in children (QuIRCC): use of a new pediatric CT dose estimate (CTPD) to develop diagnostic reference levels (DRL) for abdominal CT. Pediatric Radiol (abstract) 41(Suppl 1):250–311

Gray JE, Archer BJ, Butler PF, Hobbs BB et al (2005) Reference values for diagnostic radiology: application and impact. Radiology 235:354–358

Hall J, Angèle S (1999) Radiation, DNA damage and cancer. Mol Med Today 5:157–164

Hampton T (2010) Radiation oncology organization, FDA announce radiation safety initiatives. JAMA 303(13): 1239–1240

Hricak H, Brenner DJ, Adelstein SJ et al (2011) Managing radiation use in medical imaging: a multifaceted challenge. Radiology 258:889–905

Huda W (2002) Dose and image quality in CT. Pediatr Radiol 32:709–713

Huda W, Scalzetti EM, Levin G (2000) Technique factors and image quality as functions of patient weight at abdominal CT. Radiology 217(2):430–435

Huda W, Ogden KM, Khorasani MR (2008) Effect of dose metrics and radiation risk models when optimizing CT X-ray tube voltage. Phys Med Biol 53(17):4719–4732

IMV(2006) CT Marketing Summary Report. Des Plains, IL: IMV Medical Information Division

International Commission on Radiological Protection (1991) 1990 recommendations of the international commission on radiological protection. ICRP publication no. 60, Oxford

Jemal A, Siegel R, Ward E, Murray T, Xu J, Smigal C, Thun MJ (2006) Cancer statistics 2006. CA Cancer J Clin 56(2):106–130

Kan JH, Hwang M, Lowas SR, Hernanz-Schulman M (2011) Impact of pelvic CT on staging, surveillance, and survival of pediatric patients with Wilms tumor and hepatoblastoma. AJR Am J Roentgenol 196:W515–W518

Kaste SC (2009) Imaging challenges: a US perspective on controlling exposure to ionizing radiation in children with cancer. Pediatr Radiol 39(Suppl 1):S74–S79

Kaste SC (2011) Oncology protocols: how can we do better? Pediatr Radiol 41(Suppl 1):S166–S169

Kleinerman RA (2009) Radiation-sensitive genetically susceptible pediatric sub-populations. Pediatr Radiol 39(Suppl 1): S27–S31

Kleinman PL, Strauss KJ, Zurakowski D, Buckley KS, Taylor GA (2010) Patient size measured on CT images as a function of age at a tertiary care children's hospital. AJR Am J Roentgenol 194(6):1611–1619. doi:10.2214/AJR.09.3771

Kovanlikaya A, Karabay N, Cakmakci H, Uysal K, Olgun N, Ergör G (2003) Surveillance imaging and cost effectivity in pediatric brain tumors. Eur J Radiol 47(3):188–192

Lakhoo K, Sowerbutts H (2010) Neonatal tumours. Pediatr Surg Int 26:1159–1168

Larson DB, Rader SB, Forman HP et al (2007) Informing parents about CT radiation exposure: it's OK to tell them. AJR 189:271–275

Larson DB, Johnson LW, Schnell BM, Goske MJ, Salisbury SR, Forman HP (2011) Increasing utilization of CT in children visiting emergency departments in the United States, 1995–2007. Radiology 259(3):793–801

Li X, Da Zhang D, Liu B (2011a) Automated extraction of radiation dose information From CT dose report images. AJR 196:W781–W783

Li X, Samei E, Frush D et al (2011b) Patient-specific dose estimation for pediatric abdomen-pelvis CT. SPIE 7258: 725804-1725804-10

Li X, Samei E, Frush D et al (2011c) Patient-specific radiation dose and cancer risk estimation in CT: Part II. Applications to patients. Med Phys 38:408–419

Li X, Samei E, Frush D et al (2011d) Patient-specific dose estimation for pediatric chest CT. Med Phys 35:5821–5828

Li X, Samei E, Frush D et al (2011e) Patient-specific radiation dose and cancer risk estimation in CT: Part I. Development and validation of a Monte Carlo program. Med Phys 38: 397–407

Li X, Samei E, Frush D et al (2011f) Patient-specific radiation dose and cancer risk for pediatric chest CT. Radiology 259:862–874

Linet MS, Kim KP, Rajaraman P (2009) Children's exposure to diagnostic medical radiation and cancer risk: epidemiologic and dosimetric considerations. Pediatr Radiol 39(Suppl 1):S4

Linton OW, Mettler FA (2003) National conference on dose reduction in CT with an emphasis on pediatric patients. AJR 181:321–329

Little MP, Wakeford R, Tawn EJ, Bouffler SD, Gonzalez AB (2009) Risks associated with low doses and low dose rates of ionizing radiation: Why linearity may be (almost) the best we can do. Radiology 251:6–12

Lucaya J, Piqueras J, Garcia-Pena P, Enriquez G, Garcia-Macias M, Sotil J (2000) Low-dose high-resolution CT of the chest in children and young adults: dose, cooperation, artifact incidence, and image quality. AJR Am J Roentgenol 175:985–992

Maris JM (2010) Recent advances in neuroblastoma. N Engl J Med 362:2202–2211

Martin CJ (2007) Effective dose: How should it be applied to medical exposures?. Br J Radiol 80:639–647. Expand+ European Heart Journaleurheartj.oxfordjournals.org

McCollough C, Branham T, Herlihy V et al (2006) Radiation doses from the ACR CT accreditation program: review of data since program inception and proposals for new reference values and pass/fail limits. Presented at the RSNA 92nd scientific assembly

McCollough CH, Christner JA, Kofler JM (2010) How effective is effective dose as a predictor of radiation risk? AJR Am J Roentgenol 194:890–896

Meinhold CB (1993) Report No. 116-limitation of exposure to ionizing radiation. National council on radiation protection and measurements. http://www.ncrppublications.org/Reports/116. Accessed 21 Aug 2011

Mettler FA, Huda W, Yoshizumi TT et al (2008) Effective doses in radiology and diagnostic nuclear medicine: a catalogue. Radiology 248(1):254–256

Mezrich R (2008) Are CT scans carcinogenic? J Am Coll Radiol 5:691–693

National Cancer Institute (2002) Radiation risks and pediatric computed tomography (CT): a guide for health care providers. http://www.cancer.gov/cancertopics/causes/radiation-risks-pediatric-CT. Accessed 2 Oct 2011

Paterson A, Frush DP, Donnelly LF (2001) Helical CT of the body: are settings adjusted for pediatric patients. AJR Am J Roentgenol 176:297–301

Prakash P, Kalra MK, Ackman JB et al (2010) Diffuse lung disease: CT of the chest with adaptive statistical iterative reconstruction technique1. Radiology 256:261–269. doi: 10.1148/radiol.10091487

Preston DL, Pierce DA, Shimizu Y et al (2004) Effect of recent changes in atomic bomb survivor dosimetry on cancer mortality risk estimates. Radiat Res 162:377–389

Ratzan SC, Parker RM (2004) What is health literacy? In: Nielsen-Bohlman L, Panzer AM, Kindig DA (eds) Health literacy: a prescription to end confusion. Institute of Medicine of theNational Academies, p 32. http://www.nap.edu/openbook.php?record_id=10883&pa

Rehani M, Frush DP (2010) Tracking radiation exposure of patients. Lancet 376:754–755

Rehani MM, Tsapaki V (2011) Impact of the international atomic energy agency (IAEA) actions on radiation protection of patients in many countries. Radiation Protection Dosimetry, pp 1–4. doi:10.1093/rpd/ncr259

Russo GL, Tedesco I, Russo M et al (2011) Cellular adaptive response to chronic radiation exposure in interventional cardiologists. Eur Heart J, 23 Aug 2011. [Epub ahead of print]

Samei E, Li X, Chen B, Reiman B (2010) The myth of mean dose as a surrogate for radiation risk? Proc SPIE 7622:76220T

Schindera ST, Diedrichsen L, Muller HC et al (2011) Iterative reconstruction algorithm for abdominal multidetector CT at different tube voltages: assessment of diagnostic accuracy, image quality and radiation dose in a phantom study. Radiology 260:454–462. doi:10.1148/radiol.11102217

Shope TB, Gagne RM, Johnson GC (1981) A method for describing the doses delivered by transmission X-ray computed tomography. Med Phys 8(4):488–495

Shrimpton PC, Hillier MC, Lewis MA, Dunn M (2006) National survey of doses from CT in the UK: 2003. Br J Radiol 79:968–980

Singh S, Kalra MK, Moore MA et al (2009) Dose reduction and compliance with pediatric CT protocols adapted to patient size, clinical indication, and number of prior studies. Radiology 252(1):200–208

Singh S, Kalra MK, Hsieh J et al (2010) Abdominal CT: comparison of adaptive statistical iterative and filtered back projection reconstruction. Tech Radiol 257:373–383. doi: 10.1148/radiol.10092212

Singh S, Kalra MK, Gilman MD et al (2011) Adaptive statistical iterative reconstruction techniques for radiation dose reduction in chest CT: a pilot study. Radiology 259:565–573. doi:101148/radiol.11101450

Slovis TL (2002a) The ALARA concept in pediatric CT: myth or reality? Radiology 223:5–6

Slovis TL (2002b) ALARA Conference Proceedings. The ALARA concept in Pediatric CT-intelligent dose reduction. Pediatr Radiol 32:217–317

Strauss KJ (2008) Image gently universal protocols. http://www.pedrad.org/associations/5364/files/Protocols.pdf. Accessed 2 Oct 2011

Strauss KJ, Goske MJ (2011) Estimated pediatric radiation dose during CT. Pediatr Radiol 41(Suppl 2):472–482

Strauss KJ, Goske MJ, Frush DP, Butler PF, Morrison G (2009) Image gently vendor summit: working together for better estimates of pediatric radiation dose from CT. AJR Am J Roentgenol 192(5):1169–1175. doi:10.2214/AJR.08.2172

Strauss KJ, Goske MJ, Kaste SC et al (2010) Image gently: ten steps you can take to optimize image quality and lower CT dose for pediatric patients. AJR 194:868–873

Summary of the California Senate Bill 1237 (2011). http://www.leginfo.ca.gov/pub/09-10/bill/sen/sb_1201-1250/sb_1237_bill_20100929_chaptered.html. Last Accessed 9 Sep 2011

The Alliance for Radiation Safety in Pediatric Imaging (2008) The Image Gently website. www.imagegently.org. Accessed 2 Oct 2011

The Joint Commission Sentinel Event (2011) Alert Radiation risks of diagnostic imaging. Issue 47, pp 1–4. http://www.jointcommission.org/assets/1/18/SEA_471.PDF Accessed 2 Oct 2011

The National Cancer Institute and the Society for Pediatric Radiology (2002) updated 2008. Radiation and pediatric computed tomography: a guide for health care providers. http://www.cancer.gov/cancertopics/causes/radiation/radiation-risks-pediatric-CT. Accessed 2 Oct 2011

Tubiana M, Feinendegen LE, Yang C, Kaminski JM (2009) The linear no-threshold relationship is inconsistent with radiation biologic and experimental data. Radiology 251:13–22

UNSCEAR (United Nations Scientific Committee on the Effects of Atomic Radiation) (2011) Sources-report to the general assembly scientific annexes a. and b. 2008 Report, vol 1. UNSCEAR (2010)

U.S. Food and Drug Administration, White Paper (2010) Initiative to reduce unnecessary radiation exposure for medical imaging, 16 Feb 2010. http://www.fda.gov/Radiation-EmittingProducts/RadiationSafety/RadiationDoseReduction/ucm199904.htm. Accessed 9 Nov 2010

# CT Radiation Dose and Safety: Perspectives at the U.S. Food and Drug Administration

Stanley H. Stern, Sean Boyd, Kish Chakrabarti,
Iacovos S. Kyprianou, Thalia T. Mills,
and David C. Spelic

## Contents





S. H. Stern (✉) · S. Boyd · K. Chakrabarti ·
I. S. Kyprianou · T. T. Mills · D. C. Spelic
U.S. Department of Health and Human Services,
U.S. Food and Drug Administration,
Silver Spring, MD, USA
e-mail: Stanley.Stern@fda.hhs.gov

**Abstract**

With an emphasis on the regulatory framework, we describe three approaches that the U.S. Food and Drug Administration applies to promote dose control and radiation safety in X-ray computed tomography: (1) equipment radiation safety established through consensus standards and regulatory guidance, (2) clinical quality assurance promoted through collaboration with government agencies, industry groups, professional organizations and societies, and outreach to healthcare providers and consumers, and (3) surveillance and improved characterizations of dose and image quality enabled through research.

## 1 Introduction

Over the last few decades, FDA has been involved in efforts to determine essential elements for characterizing and controlling radiation dose in diagnostic radiography and fluoroscopy in general, and computed tomography (CT) in particular. Beginning about 30 years ago with a proposed rule[1] to establish federal regulation of the radiation safety of X-ray computed tomography equipment, the U.S. Food and Drug Administration (FDA) Center for Devices and Radiological Health (CDRH) adapted the computed

[1] Department of Health and Human Services, Food and Drug Administration (1980)

D. Tack et al. (eds.), *Radiation Dose from Multidetector CT*, Medical Radiology. Diagnostic Imaging,
DOI: 10.1007/174_2011_506, © Springer-Verlag Berlin Heidelberg 2012

tomography dose index (*CTDI*)[2] as a practical metric for characterizing the radiation output of CT scanners.[3] FDA also identified associated longitudinal dose profiles as graphical means to represent the spatial efficiency of dose disposition (see footnote 3). In its approach to regulation, FDA complemented such dose characterization with a few objectively measurable characteristics of image quality—the tomographic section sensitivity profile, the modulation transfer function, and image noise quantified by definition as the "standard deviation of the fluctuations in the CT number" of the reconstructed image.[4] All of these image-quality parameters are to be specified under the same conditions of scanner operation used for dose representation and reflective of the manufacturer's suggestions for typical values associated with CT of the adult head and body (see footnote 3). In a nutshell, for any particular model of CT scanner with its own dosing and imaging characteristics, the overarching intent was to provide users with *basic dose information* for that scanner. Such information is simply *indicative* of the magnitude of doses associated with CT procedures involving adult patients, and along with image-performance information, it is provided as a function of CT system operating conditions (see footnotes 1 and 3). The thinking was that this information enables users to "make appropriate choices" of operating conditions which assure that the corresponding doses result in clinically meaningful images (see footnotes 1 and 3). Although the FDA CT standard (see footnote 4) also mandated some equipment-performance features,[5] the focus of the regulation was on *disclosure requirements* under which manufacturers provide users with the specified, standardized dose-index and image-quality data as system-performance *information* (see footnote 3). In 1984, the rationale for limiting federal prescription of the number and kinds of equipment-performance features was a concern about "unduly constraining" CT as a "developing, dynamic technology" (see footnote 3). As it turned out, the final rule (see footnote 3) issued at that time has remained essentially unchanged[6] and has been ever since incarnated as the current federal radiation-safety standard (see footnote 4) covering CT scanners in the United States.

FDA reticence to impose regulatory constraints before CT equipment matured has proven to be prescient, as over these past 30 years CT technology advanced at a blistering pace: fast spiral (helical) scanning, automatic tube-current modulation, and cardiac-gated synchronization, development of shuttle-mode table movement to enable brain perfusion studies, extension of the simultaneous data-

---

[2] The "computed tomography dose index" (CTDI) is a metric of absorbed does in standardized dosimetry phantoms (or dose free-in-air) undergoing CT irradiation. See Shope et al. (1981)

[3] CTDI was adapted as a reference metric and was reflective of scanner operation, technology, and clinical applications circa 1980. Associated with CT dose are longitudinal "profiles" that accrue from scattered as well as primary radiation. As graphical plots of longitudinal dose in phantoms, dose profiles reveal the much longer extent of the dose spatial distribution compared to the nominal thickness associated with the tomographic section imaged. See the following notice of final rulemaking: Department of Health and Human Services, Food and Drug Administration, "Diagnostic X-ray Systems and Their Major Components; Amendments to Performance Standard," final rule amending 21 CFR 1020.30 and adding 1020.33, Federal Register Vol. 49, pp. 34698 ff., August 31, 1984.

[4] "Computed tomography (CT) equipment," title 21, part 1020, section 33, code of Federal Regulations (21 CFR 1020.33). http://edocket.access.gpo.gov/cfr_2011/aprqtr/pdf/21cfr1020.33.pdf; also see Guidance for Industry, FDA Staff, and Third Parties: Provision for Alternate Measure of the Computed Tomography Dose Index (CTDI) to Assure Compliance with the Dose Information Requirements of the Federal Performance Standard for Computed Tomography, U.S. Department of Health and Human Services, Food and Drug Administration, Center for Devices and Radiological Health, October 20, 2006. http://www.fda.gov/downloads/MedicalDevices/DeviceRegulationandGuidance/GuidanceDocuments/ucm094381.pdf.

[5] CT equipment features, as distinguished from user-directed *information* related to CT dose and imaging performance, that are required by the U.S. federal equipment-performance standard and that contribute significantly to radiation safety and imaging effectiveness include (1) pre-scanning visual indication of the scanner conditions of operation, (2) "timers" that automatically terminate X-ray exposure in the event of equipment failure affecting data collection and that could also be actuated at the operator's discretion to manually terminate exposure during scanning, (3) visual indication of the tomographic plane to facilitate appropriate alignment of a patient, (4) visual indication of X-ray activation and shutter status, and (5) a maximum tolerance of one millimeter in the deviation of the indicated scan increment from the actual scan increment.

[6] By and large, since 1984 the changes to the CT radiation-safety standard have been editorial rather than technical: See Federal Register, Vol. 49, pp. 37381 ff., September 24, 1984; Federal Register, Vol. 49, pp. 47388 ff., 4 December 1984; Federal Register Vol. 56, pp. 36098 ff., August 1, 1991; Federal Register, 67, No. (42), p. 9587, March 4, 2002; and Federal Register, Vol. 70, No. (111), p. 34042, June 10, 2005.

acquisition capability to 320 detector rows spanning a scanning range of 16 cm along the longitudinal axis swept out in a single rotation, incorporation of dual-source and dual-energy technology, development of flat-panel detectors and cone-beam technology, and development of novel, non-linear iterative reconstruction algorithms have led synergistically to expanded CT use in a broad range of clinical applications.[7] These advances contributed to increased CT utilization, and as of 2006 there were a total of 67 million sequences of CT scanning performed annually within the U.S.[8] The conduct of these CT scans resulted in a collective radiation dose that comprised 24% of the annual effective population dose (see footnote 8). The collective radiation dose from CT scanning represents approximately one-half of that from diagnostic imaging in general (see footnote 8). This large fraction is a particular concern, given that the effective dose from medical-imaging radiation per individual in the U.S. has increased six fold since the early 1980s (see footnote 8).

In response to technological advances during this period, and mindful of the tradeoff between the practicality of a dose-index measurement (implemented simply, for example, with an ionization chamber) versus fidelity in representation of actual patient dose and radiation risk, the medical physics community moved beyond the FDA regulatory definition of *CTDI*. *CTDI* has been adapted, corrected, converted, and appropriated for purposes ranging from more accurate characterization of patient dose in the development of diverse clinical protocols, to equipment quality control, to clinical quality assurance. For example, CT scanners eventually became capable of imaging tomographic sections along the longitudinal ($z$) axis of width $T$ that are significantly narrower ($T \leq 1$ mm) than the $T = 10$-mm section width that was typical of CT systems and practice in the 1980s. For $T = 10$ mm, the width-dependent limits of mathematical integration ($-7T$, $+7T$) defined for *CTDI* by FDA in 21 CFR 1020.33(b)(1) spanned a range corresponding to the 140-mm scanning length typically used in head exams and of the order of magnitude, albeit at the lower end, of scanning length used in body exams. However, for narrower section widths, say $T = 1$ mm, the narrower integration range ($-7$, $+ 7$ mm) is so much shorter than typical scanning lengths (head or body) that it limits the ability of *CTDI* to adequately account for contributions to dose from radiation scattered beyond those bounds.[9] In other words, as defined in 21 CFR 1020.33(b)(1), *CTDI* tends to significantly underestimate the accrual of dose for typical clinical scanning lengths as tomographic sections tend to widths smaller than 10 mm,[10] and *CTDI* therefore becomes less valid as a metric of a "reference" CT procedure characteristic of clinical practice. To rectify the accounting, $CTDI_{100}$ (and subsequently derived variants such as the weighted computed tomography dose index 100, abbreviated "$CTDI_w$," and later the volume weighted computed tomography dose index 100, abbreviated "$CTDI_{vol}$"), typically evaluated with a fixed-length (100 mm) "pencil" ionization chamber, were defined initially to serve as more practicably measurable dose indices (see footnote 10). For a reference scanning length of 100 mm, these $CTDI_{100}$-based indices initially provided relatively more realistic indications than that of the CFR-defined *CTDI* of the magnitude of dose accruing at the longitudinal mid-plane of a dosimetry phantom broadly representative of dose disposition in soft-tissue of adult patients with "typical" head or body dimensions.[11] "Dose-length product" (*DLP*),[12] a metric based on $CTDI_{100}$, was introduced as a dose-based indicator of radiation risk that could also be applied *grosso modo* to estimation (see footnote 12) of the ICRP parameter "effective dose" ($E$),[13] the whole-body equivalent-dose-index of

[7] An overview of technological advances in CT is provided by the book by Willi A. Kalendar, Computed Tomography: Fundamentals, System Technology, Image Quality, Applications, 3rd revised and enlarged edition, Publicis Corporate Publishing, Erlangen, Germany, 2011.

[8] NCRP Report No. 160 (2009)

[9] Guidance for Industry, FDA staff, and Third Parties: Provision for Alternate Measure of the Computed Tomography Dose Index (CTDI) to Assure Compliance with the Dose Information Requirements of the Federal Performance Standard for Computed Tomography, issued October 20, 2006, http://www.fda.gov/MedicalDevices/DeviceRegulationandGuidance/GuidanceDocuments/ucm094379.htm

[10] Leitz et al. (1995)

[11] Jessen et al. (1999)

[12] Shrimpton (2004)

[13] 2007 Recommendations of the International Commission on Radiological Protection, Annals of the ICRP Vol. 37, Nos. 2–4, pp. 1–332, Publication 103, Edited by J. Valentin, Elsevier, 2007.

population-averaged radiation detriment. Evolving extensions of the definition of $CTDI_{100}$, developed especially to accommodate novel modes of operation of CT scanners, have been standardized by the International Electrotechnical Commission (IEC),[14] have been adopted by CT manufacturers, and are mandated by various regulatory authorities for the assessment of diagnostic reference levels (*DRLs*).[15,16]

The proliferation of *CTDI*-based indices represents a technical struggle for CT metrics to keep pace with increasingly sophisticated CT scanner technologies and modes of equipment operation, with innovative clinical applications, and with the growing realization of the pertinence of individualized patient dosimetry. Especially since the development of wide-aperture, cone-beam CT scanners, the relevance of $CTDI_{100}$-based parameters as indicators of clinical dose in patients has been weakened; the shortcomings of these parameters has been cataloged extensively,[17] and even a new paradigm has been proposed for the evaluation of CT radiation dose.[18] One more manifestation of this technical struggle is the recent development of an algorithm to determine a patient-size-based "conversion factor" that could be applied to a $CTDI_{\mathrm{vol}}$ value to render it more realistically representative of the magnitude of soft-tissue dose associated with the individual habitus of any particular patient undergoing CT body scanning.[19] While each such variant of a dose-index is useful in its own terms, it is nevertheless true that to understand the radiation-related risk faced by an individual patient undergoing a CT procedure, no index is as meaningful as a comprehensive assessment of the individual organ doses. There simply is no avoiding the fact that risk attributable to radiation depends, among other factors, on the particular organ irradiated, on the sex of the patient, on the age of the patient, and on the magnitude of dose, all in a complex way[20] that cannot be faithfully represented by any single, average-value surrogate. In other words, accurate knowledge of organ dose is still a useful goal.

The range of clinical applications of CT and the frequent utilization of CT have come with increased radiation doses and associated cancer risks (see footnote 20), especially for pediatric patients,[21] and these trends have been followed for some time.[22,23] More recent developments have been the reports, beginning in September 2009, that FDA started to receive about acute radiation injuries—temporary epilation and erythema—associated with CT brain perfusion

---

[14] International Standard IEC 60601-2-44, Medical Electrical Equipment—part 2-44: Particular Requirements for the Safety of X-Ray Equipment for Computed Tomography—First Edition, October 1999; Second Edition, June 2001; Edition 2.1, November 2002; Edition 2.1 Corrigendum 1, April 2006; IEC 60601-2-44, Medical electrical equipment—part 2-44: Particular requirements for the basic safety and essential performance of X-ray equipment for computed tomography—Edition 3.0, February 2009; Edition 3.0 Corrigendum 1, May 2010, (International Electrotechnical Commission, Geneva, Switzerland)

[15] Annals of the ICRP Vol. 37, No. 6, publication 105: Radiological Protection in Medicine, edited by J. Valentin, Section 10 ("Diagnostic Reference Levels"), pp. 35–38 (summarizing pertinent sections of ICRP Publications 60, 73, and Supporting Guidance 2), published for the ICRP by Elsevier, December 2007; also see Diagnostic Reference Levels in Medical Imaging: Review and Additional Advice, web module produced by Committee 3 (Protection in Medicine) of the International Commission on Radiological Protection, 2002, http://www.icrp.org/docs/DRL_for_web.pdf

[16] For a brief overview of DRLs, see Matthews and Brennan (2009); for a particular example in CT, see Treier et al. (2010)

[17] For example, see Dixon (2003), (2006); Brenner (2005); Boone (2007)

[18] Comprehensive Methodology for the Evaluation of Radiation Dose in X-Ray Computed Tomography. A New Measurement Paradigm Based on a Unified Theory for Axial, Helical, Fan-Beam, and Cone-Beam Scanning with or Without Longitudinal Translation of the Patient Table, Report of AAPM Task Group 111: The Future of CT Dosimetry, American Association of Physicists in Medicine, February 2010, http://www.aapm.org/pubs/reports/RPT_111.pdf

[19] Size-Specific Dose Estimates (SSDE) in Pediatric and Adult Body CT Examinations, Report of AAPM Task Group 204 developed in collaboration with the International Commission on Radiation Units and Measurements (ICRU) and the Image Gently campaign of the Alliance for Radiation Safety in Pediatric Imaging, American Association of Physicists in Medicine 2011, http://www.aapm.org/pubs/reports/RPT_204.pdf

[20] Health Risks from Exposure to Low Levels of Ionizing Radiation (2006)

[21] FDA Public Health Notification: Reducing Radiation Risk from Computed Tomography for Pediatric and Small Adult Patients, November 2, 2001, http://www.fda.gov/MedicalDevices/Safety/AlertsandNotices/PublicHealthNotifications/ucm062185.htm

[22] Stern (2007)

[23] Spelic (2007)

procedures.[24] These reports crystallized FDA recognition of the importance of bolstering radiation safety through an *Initiative to Reduce Unnecessary Radiation Exposure from Medical Imaging*.[25,26]) Informed by two basic principles of radiation protection[27]—justification and optimization—the FDA/CDRH initiative reinforces a number of complementary approaches that taken together move beyond the current federal performance standard (see footnote 4) for CT equipment. These approaches broadly promote CT radiation safety and include

- CT equipment radiation safety established through consensus standards and regulatory guidance
- Clinical quality assurance promoted through collaboration with government agencies, industry groups, professional organizations and societies, and outreach to healthcare providers and consumers, and
- Surveillance and improved characterizations of dose and image quality enabled through research.

In this chapter we focus mostly on how CT radiation safety is facilitated in a regulatory framework.

[24] Safety Investigation of CT Brain Perfusion Scans: Initial Notification, October 8, 2009, http://www.fda.gov/MedicalDevices/Safety/AlertsandNotices/ucm193293.htm; Update, December 8, 2009, http://www.fda.gov/MedicalDevices/Safety/AlertsandNotices/ucm232560.htm; Update, November 9, 2010, http://www.fda.gov/MedicalDevices/Safety/AlertsandNotices/ucm185898.htm

[25] Initiative to Reduce Unnecessary Radiation Exposure from Medical Imaging, U.S. Food and Drug Administration, February 2010, (http://www.fda.gov/Radiation-EmittingProducts/RadiationSafety/RadiationDoseReduction/ucm199904.htm)

[26] White Paper: Initiative to Reduce Unnecessary Radiation Exposure from Medical Imaging, U.S. Food and Drug Administration, 16 Feb 2010, http://www.fda.gov/Radiation-EmittingProducts/RadiationSafety/RadiationDoseReduction/ucm199994.htm

[27] The principles of radiation protection—justification, optimization, and application of dose limits—are described in the Annals of the ICRP Vol. 37, Nos. 2–4, pp. 1–332, Publication 103: The 2007 Recommendations of the International Commission on Radiological Protection, edited by J. Valentin, published by Elsevier for the ICRP, April-June 2007. ICRP Publication 105 (Annals of the ICRP Vol. 37, No. 6, pp. 1–63, Radiological Protection in Medicine, edited by J. Valentin, published by Elsevier for the ICRP, December 2007) makes clear that "With regard to medical exposure of patients, it is not appropriate to apply dose limits or dose constraints, because such limits would often do more harm than good. Often, there are concurrent chronic, severe, or even life-threatening medical conditions that are more critical than the radiation exposure. The emphasis is then on justification of the medical procedures and on the optimisation of radiological protection."

## 2 CT Equipment: Overview of the US Regulatory Framework

FDA regulates manufacturers of CT devices through the Electronic Product Radiation Control (EPRC) and medical device provisions of the Federal Food, Drug, and Cosmetic Act.[28] FDA specifies requirements related to these provisions through prescription of "regulations" or "rules," which are mandatory, and it makes related recommendations through issuance of "guidance," which is not mandatory. For CT devices, FDA's regulatory authority applies to manufacturers and assemblers, not to facilities and users of the equipment. However, medical X-ray equipment users and facilities should report adverse events to the FDA. Other federal and state regulations may apply to CT facilities and users.

Manufacturers and assemblers of electronic radiation-emitting products sold in the United States are responsible for compliance with the radiological health regulations found in Title 21 of the *Code of Federal Regulations* (Subchapter J, *Radiological Health*).[29] In particular, CT manufacturers must comply with the performance standard for CT equipment (21 CFR 1020.33).

Medical X-ray equipment also must comply with medical device regulations found in Title 21 of the *Code of Federal Regulations* (Subchapter H, *Medical Devices*). Whereas the CT equipment-performance standard (21 CFR 1020.33) reflects very specific aspects of CT equipment design, operation, and user-directed information, the medical device regulations for the most part cover broadly applicable issues related to device pre-market clearance or approval and

[28] The Federal Food, Drug, and Cosmetic Act can be viewed at: http://www.fda.gov/RegulatoryInformation/Legislation/FederalFoodDrugandCosmeticActFDCAct/default.htm. Medical devices are covered under Chapter V (Drugs and Devices); radiation-emitting electronic products (including X-ray imaging devices such as CT) are covered under Chapter V, Subchapter C (Electronic Product Radiation Control).

[29] For an overview of the relevant laws and regulations applying to radiation control, see the FDA web page "Laws and Regulations (Radiation-Emitting Products)," http://www.fda.gov/Radiation-EmittingProducts/ElectronicProductRadiationControlProgram/LawsandRegulations/default.htm, updated November 14, 2011.

post-market compliance and surveillance.[30,31,32] Current FDA thinking on what a manufacturer needs to do to comply with the regulations for a specific device type is often reflected in FDA "guidance." "Guidance" refers to a formal regulatory document[33] that can address FDA staff, submitters of pre-market notifications (e.g., corporate sponsors, manufacturers, and assemblers), and the general public. Medical device manufacturers submit pre-market notifications to seek FDA *clearance* (for "class-II" devices[34]) or FDA *approval* (for "class-III" devices[35]) to market devices legally in the US.[36] "Guidance" describes FDA policies for regulated products. For devices, a guidance document can specify FDA recommendations covering safety and effectiveness with respect to device design, production, manufacturing, testing, labeling (including all manuals and documentation for users), as well as recommended limitations with respect to commercial promotion and marketing. "Guidance" can also describe FDA procedures for processing submissions of pre-market notifications, i.e., what the submitted material should contain, how it will be evaluated, what criteria are used for clearance and approval, and it can also specify policies of inspection and enforcement to ensure compliance with FDA decisions and regulations. FDA is currently drafting a guidance to apply to pre-market evaluation of CT systems.

A particular kind of guidance, deemed a "special control," is applicable to class-II devices (see footnote 34), i.e., devices for which general regulatory controls[37] are insufficient to provide reasonable assurance of safety and effectiveness. CT X-ray systems are currently classified as class-II devices. When guidance is designated as a "special control," the sponsor (e.g., medical device manufacturer) submitting a notification "must show that its device addresses the issues of safety and effectiveness identified in this guidance, either by meeting the recommendations of this guidance or by some other means that provides equivalent assurances of safety and effectiveness" in order to clear its medical device for marketing.[38] Special controls can be implemented through the promulgation of *new* federal performance standards, and special-controls guidance can incorporate particular equipment-feature recommendations or recommendations for compliance with consensus standards that FDA recognizes under the Food and Drug Modernization Act of 1997 (see footnote 34).

After a device is on the market and in use, prompt reporting of adverse events can help the FDA identify and better understand the risks associated with it. Any member of the public who suspects a problem with a CT device is encouraged to file a voluntary report through *MedWatch, the FDA Safety Information and Adverse Event Reporting Program.*[39] Device manufacturers and device user facilities, which include many health care facilities, must comply with the *Medical Device Reporting (MDR)* regulations (21 CFR

[30] For more information on the federal laws and regulations applying to medical devices, see the FDA web page "Device Advice: Comprehensive Regulatory Assistance," http://www.fda.gov/MedicalDevices/DeviceRegulationandGuidance/default.htm, updated October 17, 2011.

[31] For information on FDA's device premarket notification and premarket approval process, see the FDA webpage "How to Market Your Device," updated March 18, 2010, http://www.fda.gov/MedicalDevices/DeviceRegulationandGuidance/HowtoMarketYourDevice/default.htm

[32] Information about requirements for devices once they are on the market is available at the FDA web page "Postmarket Requirements (Devices)," http://www.fda.gov/MedicalDevices/DeviceRegulationandGuidance/PostmarketRequirements/default.htm, updated August 3, 2009.

[33] "What is a guidance document?" Title 21, part 10, section 115, paragraph (b) [21 CFR 10.115(b)], Code of Federal Regulations, edition of April 1, 2011

[34] "Medical Device Classification Procedures," Title 21, part 860, section 3, paragraph (c), sub-paragraph (2) [21 CFR 860.3(c)(2)], Code of Federal Regulations, edition of April 1, 2011.

[35] "Medical Device Classification Procedures," Title 21, part 860, section 3, paragraph (c), sub-paragraph (3) [21 CFR 860.3(c)(3)], Code of Federal Regulations, edition of April 1, 2011.

[36] For general information about medical device review, see the FDA web page "Device Advice: Comprehensive Regulatory Assistance," http://www.fda.gov/MedicalDevices/DeviceRegulationandGuidance/default.htm, updated October 17, 2011.

[37] "Medical Device Classification Procedures," Title 21, part 860, section 3, paragraph (c), sub-paragraph (1) [21 CFR 860.3(c)(1)], Code of Federal Regulations, edition of April 1, 2011.

[38] Department of Health and Human Services, Food and Drug Administration [Docket No. FDA-2011-N-0148] (2011)

[39] See the FDA web page MedWatch: The FDA Safety Information and Adverse Event Reporting Program, http://www.fda.gov/Safety/MedWatch/default.htm, updated November 17, 2011.

Part 803).[40] Health care personnel employed by facilities that are subject to FDA's user facility reporting requirements (see footnote 40) should follow the reporting procedures established by their facilities.

With the exception of the authority provided to FDA through the *Mammography Quality Standards Act (MQSA)* for broad regulation of mammography,[41] including setting requirements for facility accreditation and certification, setting standards for facility quality assurance, for quality control of equipment, and for personnel training and qualifications, FDA direct regulatory authority over imaging is otherwise limited to *manufacturers and equipment* and in some cases to the facility reporting requirements described in the preceding paragraph. States and other federal agencies regulate the *use* of CT equipment.

Facilities that seek reimbursement from the Centers for Medicare and Medicaid Services (CMS) must comply with relevant CMS regulations. Under the Medicare Improvements for Patients and Providers Act (MIPPA) of 2008,[42] by 2012 advanced diagnostic imaging facilities (performing CT, MRI, nuclear medicine) must be accredited by one of three accreditation organizations (the American College of Radiology,[43] The Intersocietal Accreditation Commission,[44] or The Joint Commission[45] recognized by CMS.[46] This requirement does not apply to hospitals, which have a separate set of guidelines.[47,48]

Individual states have regulations and guidelines applying to imaging facilities and personnel. The Conference of Radiation Control Program Directors (CRCPD) publishes *Suggested State Regulations for the Control of Radiation*,[49] which may be voluntarily adopted by states. A number of states are updating their regulations to improve radiation safety. In addition, professional organizations have published guidance to ensure that facilities and state inspectors have the information they need to follow these regulations. Examples of such efforts include training for state CT inspectors run jointly by the American Association of Physicists in Medicine (AAPM) and CRCPD[50] and recommendations of the California Clinical and Academic Medical Physicists (C-CAMP)[51] on how to implement the new California dose reporting law (SB 1237).[52]

---

40 For more information on adverse event reporting requirements, see the FDA webpage Reporting Adverse Events (Medical Devices), http://www.fda.gov/MedicalDevices/DeviceRegulationandGuidance/PostmarketRequirements/ReportingAdverseEvents/default.htm, updated June 18, 2009.

41 For information on MQSA, see the FDA web page Mammography Quality Standards Act and Program, http://www.fda.gov/Radiation-EmittingProducts/MammographyQualityStandardsActandProgram/default.htm, updated Novembr 8, 2011.

42 http://frwebgate.access.gpo.gov/cgi-bin/getdoc.cgi?dbname=110_cong_public_laws&docid=f:publ275.pdf

43 See The ACR Computed Tomography Accreditation Program web page, http://www.acr.org/accreditation/computed.aspx

44 See the Intersocietal Accreditation Commission for the Accreditation of Computed Tomography Laboratories web page, http://www.icactl.org/icactl/index.htm

45 See The Joint Commission web page on Seeking Imaging Center Accreditation, http://www.jointcommission.org/accreditation/ahc_seeking_imaging_centers.aspx

46 For more information on accreditation requirements under MIPPA, see the CMS web page Advanced Diagnostic Imaging Accreditation, https://www.cms.gov/MedicareProviderSupEnroll/03_AdvancedDiagnosticImagingAccreditation.asp, last modified September 26, 2011.

47 Information regarding CMS guidelines specific to radiological services in hospitals can be found in US Centers for Medicare & Medicaid Services, State Operations Manual 100–07, http://www.cms.gov/Manuals/IOM/itemdetail.asp?filterType=none&filterByDID=-99&sortByDID=1&sortOrder=ascending&itemID=CMS1201984&intNumPerPage=10, Appendix A—Survey Protocol, Regulations and Interpretive Guidelines for Hospitals. Rev 47 5 June 2009, http://cms.gov/manuals/Downloads/som107ap_a_hospitals.pdf, accessed through http://www.cms.gov/manuals/downloads/som107_Appendicestoc.pdf

48 A full list of CMS internet-only manuals which describe CMS policies and procedures are available here: https://www.cms.gov/Manuals/IOM/list.asp

49 The Suggested State Regulations for Control of Radiation are available on the Conference of Radiation Control Program Directors web page: http://www.crcpd.org/ssrcr.aspx

50 See slides from the Computed Tomography for State Inspectors and AAPM Training on Computed Tomography course (offered May 2011) on the CRCPD web page, http://www.crcpd.org/2011AnnualMeeting/Training/agenda_AAPM.aspx

51 Computed Tomography Dose Limit Reporting Guidelines for Section 3–115113; California Dose Reporting Law, Recommendations of the California Clinical and Academic Medical Physicists (C-CAMP), December 2010, http://www.aapm.org/government_affairs/documents/SB-1237Section3_v7.pdf

52 The California dose reporting law, as proposed in Senate Bill 1237, can be viewed at: http://www.leginfo.ca.gov/pub/09-10/bill/sen/sb_1201-1250/sb_1237_bill_20100929_chaptered.html

## 3 Consensus-Standard Safeguards of CT Radiation Safety

While the Electronic Product Radiation Control subchapter of the US Food, Drug, and Cosmetic Act requires FDA prescription of performance standards to protect public health and safety with respect to radiation-emitting products, it also authorizes FDA, in its establishment of a radiation-control program, to maintain liaison with a broad array of organizations interested in radiation control—including federal and state departments and agencies, professional societies, industry, trade, and labor associations.[53] In particular, since the year 2000, FDA has supported participation of its staff members as expert liaisons to the IEC maintenance team[54] MT 30 responsible for maintaining CT safety (see footnote 14), acceptance-test,[55] and constancy-test[56] standards developed on the basis of industry consensus. (In fact, FDA has been the only *governmental* public health agency of any country with staff as active, regularly participating members of MT 30.) At the national level, FDA has met regularly with the Medical Imaging Technology Alliance (MITA),[57] a trade organization and division of the National Electrical Manufacturers Association (NEMA),[58] to provide the MITA CT group with advice in its development of CT Dose-Check[59] (NEMA Standard XR 25–2010). FDA continues to have ongoing discussions with the MITA CT group about a number of issues and ways to improve CT radiation safety, including possible development of NEMA CT standards related to equipment access-control, equipment-usability features, automated estimation and recording of patient organ doses, and application of CT low-contrast detectability in order to evaluate algorithms and techniques related to dose reduction.

Under the Food and Drug Administration Modernization Act of 1997 (FDAMA), device standards published by any standards development organization (SDO) can be formally "recognized" by FDA. When manufacturers submit pre-market notifications to FDA for device clearance or approval, declarations of conformity to FDA-recognized standards obviate the need for manufacturers to provide data supporting the safety and effectiveness covered by the particular recognized standards to which the devices conform. Through FDAMA, FDA has formally recognized[60] several CT-related standards, including the IEC CT safety standard (see footnote 14), the IEC CT acceptance-test standard (see footnote 55), the IEC CT constancy-test standard (see footnote 56), and the NEMA CT dose-check standard (see footnote 59). The following sections detail how the CT safety standard and CT dose-check contribute to radiation safety.

### 3.1 International Electrotechnical Commission CT Safety Standard, IEC 60601-2-44

Although the US does not formally require manufacturer compliance with IEC CT standards, because many countries around the world do mandate such

[53] Laws and Regulations (Radiation-Emitting Products), FDA web page last updated January 21, 2010, http://www.fda.gov/Radiation-EmittingProducts/ElectronicProductRadiationControlProgram/LawsandRegulations/default.htm

[54] For a description of the current tasks and membership of the IEC maintenance team MT 30 responsible for CT, see http://www.iec.ch/dyn/www/f?p=103:14:0::::FSP_ORG_ID,FSP_LANG_ID:2530,25, accessed November 7, 2011.

[55] International Standard IEC 61223-3-5, Evaluation and routine testing in medical imaging departments—Part 3–5: Acceptance tests—Imaging performance of computed tomography X-ray equipment, Edition 1.0, August 2004, with corrigendum 1, March 2006, (International Electrotechnical Commission, Geneva, Switzerland).

[56] International Standard IEC 61223-2-6, Evaluation and routine testing in medical imaging departments—Part 2–6: Constancy tests—Imaging performance of computed tomography X-ray equipment, Edition 2.0, November 2006, (International Electrotechnical Commission, Geneva, Switzerland).

[57] http://www.medicalimaging.org/

[58] http://www.nema.org/

[59] NEMA Standards Publication XR 25-2010 Edition 1, Computed Tomography Dose Check, National Electrical Manufacturers Association, Arlington, Virginia, Oct 2010, http://www.nema.org/stds/xr25.cfm. NEMA XR 25-2010 Ed. 1 designates IEC 60601-2-44 Ed. 3 as a normative reference, i.e., it incorporates particular provisions of IEC 60601-2-44 Ed. 3 as its own.

[60] To search for consensus standard recognized by FDA, see the FDA web page Recognized Consensus Standards, http://www.accessdata.fda.gov/scripts/cdrh/cfdocs/cfStandards/search.cfm, updated March 18, 2011.

compliance,[61] manufacturers fabricate their systems to meet those standards. Moreover, if manufacturers declare their conformance to a voluntary, consensus standard and establish equipment-design specifications according to it, then according to US regulation they are obligated to assure that their scanners actually meet those specifications lest those scanners be deemed defective with regard to the emission of radiation.[62] Since for the most part the IEC CT safety standard (see footnote 14) (IEC 60601-2-44) harmonizes with the US mandatory performance standard (see footnote 4), i.e., IEC 60601-2-44 essentially incorporates all of the radiation-safety aspects of 21 CFR 1020.33 and indeed adds many more, IEC 60601-2-44 functions *de facto* as the vanguard for standardization of safety features of CT equipment marketed in the US. Furthermore, radiation safety is just one of the principal concerns of IEC 60601-2-44; the IEC CT safety standard also requires particular equipment features and user-directed information that preclude or mitigate other potential hazards affecting components and sub-systems involving electrical, mechanical, structural, excessive-temperature, controller- and instrument-inaccuracy, programmable-system, and electromagnetic-compatibility aspects of equipment operation. In other words, while 21 CFR 1020.33 basically remains dated to 1984 and limited to radiation safety, since 1999 the IEC CT safety standard (see footnote 14) has been updated through three editions—most recently in 2009—accommodating a rapidly evolving technology and effectively standardizing CT equipment safety in basically all of its aspects.

When IEC CT safety-standard (see footnote 14) features are applied by the user in collaboration with a medical physicist, they promote understanding and improve implementation of aspects of radiation safety well beyond those covered in the US federal performance standard covering CT (see footnotes 4, 5 and 6). The following examples indicate the broad domain of radiation hazards associated with CT equipment and the array of approaches to mitigate them. (Numbers in parentheses respectively identify the relevant subclauses of IEC 60601-2-44 Edition 3.0, February 2009.)

- *Information to preclude scanner operation causing detrimental tissue reactions associated with deterministic effects* (204.5.2.4.5): CT scanner documentation provides users with information about the particular conditions of operation that would yield a value of 1 Gy for the dose-index $CTDI_{100\ (\mathrm{peripheral})}$, a conservative lower bound to the threshold magnitude for skin injury.[63]
- *Advice about potential detrimental interaction of CT X-rays with electronically active medical devices* (203.5.2.4.101): Scanner documentation includes a cautionary statement regarding the potential malfunction—during CT X-ray irradiation—of active medical devices either implanted or worn on the body, such as neurostimulators, insulin infusion pumps, and pacemakers.[64] The cautionary statement directs the user to the manufacturer of the implanted or body-worn device for more information.
- *Limitation to the variability of radiation output* (203.6.3.2): For scanner operating conditions representative of typical clinical techniques, the amount of radiation output expressed as a single measurement of $CTDI_{\mathrm{free\ air}}$ is required to be within ±10% of the mean associated with a set of 10 measurements.
- *Confinement of extra-focal radiation* (203.8.4): X-ray source assemblies and radiation apertures limiting the spatial extent of the beam are required to be configured in a way that confines the extra-focal radiation (e.g., emanating from aperture edges rather than from the focal spot per se) to no more than 15 cm outside of the boundary of the largest selectable X-ray field projected onto a plane at a distance of 1 m from the focal spot and in a

[61] For example, see "Commission communication in the framework of the implementation of the Council Directive 93/42/EEC of 14 June 1993 concerning medical devices," Official Journal of the European Union, vol. 54, English edition, Notice no. 2011/C 242/02, pp. C 242/8—C 242/38, August 19, 2011, http://eur-lex.europa.eu/LexUriServ/LexUriServ.do?uri=OJ:C:2011:242:0008:0038:EN:PDF

[62] "Defect in an electronic product," title 21, part 1003, section 2 of the Code of Federal Regulations (21 CFR 1003.2). http://edocket.access.gpo.gov/cfr_2011/aprqtr/pdf/21cfr1003.2.pdf

[63] See the FDA web page, Radiation Dose Quality Assurance: Questions and Answers, last updated November 10, 2010, and references cited therein, http://www.fda.gov/Radiation-EmittingProducts/RadiationSafety/RadiationDoseReduction/ucm232550.htm

[64] FDA Preliminary Public Health Notification: Possible Malfunction of Electronic Medical Devices Caused by Computed Tomography (CT) Scanning, FDA web page last updated December 2, 2010, http://www.fda.gov/MedicalDevices/Safety/AlertsandNotices/PublicHealthNotifications/ucm061994.htm

direction parallel to the axis of rotation. For a representative distance ~57 cm between the X-ray focal spot and the scanner axis of rotation,[65] such extra-focal radiation would be limited in extent along the central axis, i.e., in a patient, to a distance of no more than approximately 8.6 cm for the largest X-ray field.

- *Protection against stray CT radiation* (203.13): Information for the user includes a 3-m × 3-m × 2-m map of values of air kerma per X-ray-tube current–time product (mAs) surrounding a 32-cm-diameter tissue-equivalent phantom irradiated under conditions of operation resulting in maximum stray-radiation values.
- *Control of radiation output* (203.106): Every CT scanner is required to have the capability of some kind of automatic exposure control (AEC) as a mode-of-operation alternative to manual selection of the conditions of operation. For most AEC modes, in setting a scanning sequence, a user would ideally select the highest tolerable amount of image noise acceptable for efficacious visualization of a region of interest. The AEC mode then automatically determines and—during scanning—dynamically adjusts the amount of incident X-ray flux needed to compensate for the variably attenuating anatomy so as to maintain the selected level of image noise, where image noise is quantified as the standard deviation of the fluctuation in the CT number of the reconstructed image. In principle, the resulting radiation dose corresponds to the (smallest) amount needed for optimal imaging as decided by the user according to the (largest) amount of image noise tolerable in achieving diagnostic efficacy. Among a variety of different modes exemplifying AEC operation, the amount of incident X-ray flux might be (1) kept constant for the entire sequence of scanning, or (2) adjusted as a function of projection angle about the $z$-axis (axis of rotation), or (3) adjusted as a function of position along the $z$-axis, or (4) adjusted as a function of position simultaneously *about* as well as *along* the $z$-axis, or (5) adjusted as a function of time, i.e., via electronic-gating triggers that synchronize and limit the duration of radiation to the clinically relevant phase of a rhythmic physiological process, for example, in cardiac, respiratory, or related procedures.[66]
- *Comprehensive specification of $CTDI_{\mathrm{free\ air}}$ as a basic metric of CT scanner radiation output* (203.109.2): In addition to the IEC CT safety standard provision (203.109.1) of head and body dosimetry-phantom values for $CTDI_{100}$, which is analogous to the requirement of 21 CFR 1020.33(c)(2), IEC 60601-2-44 Ed. 3 sub-clause 203.109.2 requires that scanner documentation provide users with a matrix of the values of $CTDI_{\mathrm{free\ air}}$ (measured at the scanner isocenter) and maximum deviations from those values at all selectable beam collimations and all kVp settings associated with typical conditions of operation for body scanning; at collimations and kVp settings associated with typical head scanning; and for each shaped or flat X-ray filter.
- *Dose profile depictions in phantoms and free-in-air* (203.110): While the US federal CT safety standard (see footnote 4) 21 CFR 1020.33(c)(2)(iv) as well as sub-clause 203.110 of the third edition of the international CT safety standard (see footnote 14) IEC 60601-2-44 both require the manufacturer to provide the user with a graphical depiction of the dose profile along the central axis of the head and the body dosimetry phantom, i.e., along the axis of rotation ($z$-axis), perpendicular to the tomographic plane, the IEC standard further stipulates that the range along $z$ extend to at least the full-width at one-tenth maximum of the dose profile. This stipulation ensures that the user will see the broad extent—far beyond the nominal width of the tomographic section(s) imaged—of scattered radiation along the axis of rotation. Furthermore, whereas there is no requirement in 21 CFR 1020.33(c)(2)(iv) for a graphical presentation of the dose profile free-in-air, there is such a requirement in sub-clause 203.110 of IEC 60601-2-44 Ed. 3. Free-in-air profiles contain basic dose spatial information reflecting X-ray focal-spot size, collimation, and the associated spatial distribution of the X-ray penumbra.[67]
- *Display and recording of $CTDI_{\mathrm{vol}}$ and DLP* (203.112): If one were to choose a provision of the IEC CT safety standard (see footnote 14) that

[65] Cf. Maier and Nagel (2002); Kalendar (2005)

[66] For a review of the optimal use of AEC in CT, see Gudjónsdóttir et al. (2010)

[67] Dixon et al. (2005); Dixon and Boone (2011)

promises to be the most powerful, helpful, and practical equipment feature facilitating clinical quality assurance of the safe use of radiation, it would be sub-clause 203.112. This sub-clause requires that *prior* to operator actuation of scaning, CT scanners automatically *display* values of the standardized dose indices $CTDI_{\mathrm{vol}}$ and *DLP* anticipated according to the preset conditions of scanner operation. Furthermore, it requires that *following* a sequence of scanning, CT scanners automatically (a) *display* the sequence-averaged, time-weighted mean values of those dose indices and (b) *record* those values (along with the associated dosimetry-phantom diameter—16 cm or 32 cm) in a DICOM-compliant CT dose structured report identifiable with each patient.[68] In other words, this requirement enables two aspects of safety and control that would otherwise be impractical: First, before the actuation of each programed sequence of scanning *for each individual patient examination*, the dose-index display feature allows the CT equipment operator to check the anticipated dose-index values that are displayed and verify that those values correspond to those expected for the particular scanning sequence set and patient habitus undergoing examination. If the dose-index values do not meet expectations, the scanner settings can be changed as appropriate without exposing the patient. Second, the automatically-generated dose-index and related scanner-setting data not only comprise one-time electronic dose records, respectively, associated with *each* of the individual patients, the data *for multiple patient examinations* can be compiled, sorted, and analyzed, for example, to (1) establish facility-based expectations (local "practice reference levels")[69] of dose-index values associated with particular clinical procedures and with categories of body habitus and age, (2) check practice trends versus time, versus operator or medical practitioner, and versus nationally-based *DRLs* (see footnotes 15 and 16), (3) track the multiple-examination dose histories of individual patients, (4) be uploaded to national dose registries for the analysis and development of *DRLs* (see footnotes 15 and 16).

- *Display and provision of information related to the dose-sparing efficiency of the irradiation geometry along the z-axis* (203.113): When multi-detector-row CT (MDCT) technology was introduced, collimation of the fan-beam width along the axis of rotation (*z*-axis) was automatically set wider than it had been for a single-row-detector scanner imaging a tomographic section of the same nominal width as that of the sum of the multiple-section widths imaged with a MDCT scanner. The wider collimation was warranted to avoid irradiation of the outer rows of the detector multiplex with X-ray flux of a variable and lower magnitude—associated with the beam penumbra—than that incident on the inner rows. The resulting widening has been characterized as "over-beaming" because it directly irradiates a broader region than that represented in the images.[70] Over-beaming tends to become especially significant for the imaging of a small number ($\leq 4$) of thin ($\leq 1$ mm) tomographic sections and less pronounced in imaging more sections.[71] Although focal-spot-tracking and dynamically-adaptive-collimation technology mitigate over-beaming, [72] over-beaming can still be significant for some irradiation configurations of current CT scanners. For that reason the IEC CT safety standard (see footnote 14) defines (201.3.213) an associated metric—the "geometric efficiency in the *z*-direction"—in terms of the integral of the free-in-air dose profile over the *data-acquisition range* along *z*, where this integral is expressed as a percentage of the total integral of the

[68] DICOM, a publicly available specification (http://medical.nema.org/), incorporates templates for automated transmission, storage, and retrieval of data, e.g., in the format of a "structured report" relevant to CT radiation dose and associated scanner parameter settings for each individual patient CT examination. The DICOM specification is normatively referenced in its entirety in the International Standards Organization (ISO) International Standard ISO 12052, Health informatics—Digital imaging and communication in medicine (DICOM) including workflow and data management, first edition, 2006, and ISO 12052 is a normative reference of the international CT safety standard, IEC 60601-2-44 Ed. 3.

[69] National Diagnostic Reference Level Fact Sheet, Australian Radiation Protection and Nuclear Safety Agency, June 2011, http://www.arpansa.gov.au/pubs/Services/NDRL/NDRLfactsheet.pdf

[70] Nagel (2002)

[71] McCollough and Zink (1999)

[72] Toth et al. (2000)

free-in-air dose profile over the *entire range* of $z$. In an idealized geometrical sense, i.e., ignoring the electronically passivated regions occupied by detector-row septa, this efficiency metric is inversely related to the relative amount of over-beaming.[73] Sub-clause 203.113 of IEC 60601-2-44 Ed. 3 requires scanners to display values of geometric efficiencies less than 70%, to warn operators when such values are displayed, and to require operator confirmation before proceeding to scan. Furthermore, a table of geometric efficiencies associated with all possible beam-collimation configurations, i.e., irrespective of the values of the efficiencies, is required to be provided to the user in the documentation accompanying the scanner.

The IEC CT safety standard (see footnote 14) undergoes review and revision on a regular cycle following IEC processes that are driven at the expert-group level in bi-annual meetings of the IEC CT group, MT 30 (see footnote 54). The following items represent some areas currently under active consideration for prospective inclusion in the IEC CT safety standard:

- Dose-check features
- Safety requirements for radiation-treatment planning
- Preview-image delineation of over-ranging in helical scans
- Regularization of the definition of $CTDI_{100}$ with respect to wide-collimation scanners
- Provision of dose profile and slice-sensitivity profile data in meaningfully informative graphical presentations updated to accommodate multislice scanners, and
- Standardization of the dosimetry-phantom diameter—applied as a basis for dose-index value display and recording—with respect to protocol type (head versus body) or sub population (adult versus pediatric).

## 3.2 National Electrical Manufacturers Association CT Dose-Check Standard, NEMA XR 25-2010

In the wake of reports of patient skin injuries from anomalously large doses of radiation associated with CT brain perfusion exams (see footnote 24), the MITA CT group—encouraged by FDA—stepped forward to fill an important niche in radiation safety by developing a CT *dose-check* standard (see footnote 59). The basic idea of CT dose-check is that if the expected magnitude of $CTDI_{vol}$ or $DLP$, each of which is estimated automatically by the CT unit *in advance* of a sequence of scanning, were to exceed a preset threshold, then the scanner would advise the operator of that possibility and would await confirmation or readjustment of scanner operational settings before proceeding to scan. The use of this feature is completely optional and configurable by the clinical facility: users can choose to preset dose-index thresholds to correspond to whatever magnitudes of dose they deem to be higher than they desire or expect for particular protocols, or they can choose not to use the feature at all. The AAPM, in collaboration with the American College of Radiology (ACR), the American Society of Radiologic Technologists (ASRT), the Medical Imaging and Technology Alliance (MITA), and FDA has developed recommendations on how to use the CT dose-check feature.[74]

*Dose-check* has a two-level architecture, where the two levels—*notifications* and *alerts*—are distinguished by different relationships to examination protocol elements and by different operational features: A dose *notification* would pop up automatically on the machine-user interface were the scanner-estimated dose-index to trip over a threshold preset at a value lower than that of a higher-level threshold that could activate a dose *alert*. To receive a dose *notification*, the user would need to preset threshold values for $CTDI_{vol}$ and/or $DLP$ in the scanner database for at least one of the "protocol elements" associated with the sequences of scanning comprising CT examinations. A "protocol element" is the set of equipment-operation parameters (e.g., X-ray tube voltage, current, rotation time, etc.) associated with a sequence of scanning; protocol elements and their associated scanning sequences may be grouped together and actuated automatically with a single press of a software button on the machine-user interface and with one or more activations of the "X-ray on" hardware

[73] Op. cit. footnote 18, AAPM report no. 111, p. 8.

[74] AAPM Recommendations Regarding Notification and Alert Values for CT Scanners: Guidelines for Use of the NEMA XR 25 CT Dose-Check Standard, AAPM Dose Check Guidelines version 1.0, 04/27/2011, http://www.aapm.org/pubs/CTProtocols/documents/NotificationLevelsStatement_2011-04-27.pdf

button (see footnote 59). For *each* protocol element configured with a notification threshold, before scanning, a dose-check-compliant CT scanner would automatically compare the estimated values of the dose indices against the respective pre-configured thresholds. If a pre-scanning estimate of the dose index were to exceed a notification threshold, the operator would be notified and could (a) reconfirm the selected machine settings, optionally enter a rationale for this decision, and proceed to scan or could (b) readjust the settings to reduce the estimated dose-index value below the threshold before proceeding to scan. For each sequence of scanning with a dose-index value exceeding a preset notification threshold, the system automatically establishes for the purpose of audit a record of the date, time, and unique identifier of the exam, the threshold value exceeded, the corresponding dose-index value tripping the notification, and any rationale provided for proceeding with scanning (see footnote 59).

Dose *alerts* are distinguished from dose *notifications* in several respects: Whereas a *notification* threshold is associated with only a single scanning sequence or single protocol element as one part of an examination, an *alert* threshold corresponds to a user-preset value of $CTDI_{vol}$ or of *DLP* associated with dose that is *cumulative* over the course of a complete examination comprised of multiple, different sequences of scanning, i.e., multiple protocol elements. In other words, to trigger an *alert*, for each successive scanning sequence (protocol element), the scanner tracks (1) the cumulative $CTDI_{vol}$ accruing at each position on the $z$-axis in the DICOM patient coordinate system and (2) the cumulative *DLP*. For each prospective scanning sequence of an exam, were a cumulative $CTDI_{vol}$ or *DLP* estimated by the scanner to exceed the *alert* threshold preset for that exam, the operator would receive an *alert* on the machine-user interface. Then, if an operator chooses not to readjust the settings to reduce the expected dose-index value below the threshold but instead elects to proceed with scanning, the operational process following an *alert* is subject to a greater degree of operator identification, action, and potential review than that following a *notification*: With an *alert*, the system would require the operator to enter his or her name, to reconfirm the selected protocol elements, possibly to enter a password (if the facility so configures the system), and, at the operator's discretion, to enter a brief "diagnostic reason" for proceeding with an examination where a cumulative dose-index would exceed the alert threshold. For purposes of review or audit, the system would then record the date and time, the operator's name, an identification number unique to the examination, the alert value(s) exceeded, the corresponding dose-index values that prompted the alert, and any explanation provided by the operator after receiving an alert (see footnote 59).

Facility setting of thresholds can be conceived to support distinct aspects of quality assurance (QA) in the use of radiation emitted by CT equipment in clinical examinations and procedures. In the most basic sense, threshold values would trigger a pause before scanning in any *individual* case in order to provide the operator with a "time out," i.e., a chance reconsider whether all operational parameters are indeed correctly set. If dose notification thresholds were preset to correspond to some high point, e.g., the 95 or 98th percentile of the dose-index distributions associated with various protocol scanning sequences, then the number of actual notifications and additional operator checking would be limited to those few cases that would represent true outliers in estimated dose, outliers warranting the extra steps needed to confirm the desirability of scanning as planned. This kind of high-percentile approach, as well as particular dose notification thresholds for several protocols, is reflected in recommendations of the American Association of Physicists in Medicine (see footnote 74). In a similar sense, i.e., to offer a pause before scanning, dose *alert* thresholds could be set conservatively to values of $CTDI_{vol} \sim 1{,}000$ mGy, the order of magnitude of a lower bound of approach to the regime associated with deterministic injury, e.g. skin injury.[75] In another sense, dose notification events automatically recorded and subsequently analyzed for thresholds preset to the 75 or 80th percentile of the dose-index distributions associated with various protocol scanning sequences and patient-size groups could possibly be used to reinforce operator and facility awareness and monitoring of *patterns* of dose emerging from many exams.

It is important to note that neither the notification nor alert threshold is intended to represent a dose "limit:" for any individual case, application of a dose that exceeds the preset notification or alert

[75] Balter et al. (2010)

threshold may be entirely warranted, as it depends on the patient habitus and clinical indication (see footnote 27).

Facility implementation of dose-check (see footnote 59) features would be just one component of CT QA. Among many other components, an ideal QA radiation-safety program would include (1) broadly-held cognizance amongst staff of the magnitudes of $CTDI_{vol}$ and *DLP* expected for particular CT protocols and sizes of patients, (2) operator accountability for selection and confirmation of equipment operating conditions for each individual patient examination, (3) periodic updating and follow-up on patterns of cases in which doses delivered exceed levels of concern, and (4) periodic adaptation of scanner operating conditions and development of protocols optimizing diagnostic efficacy with respect to dose, particularly for newly introduced clinical applications and technological advances in equipment features. Each such QA component should be carried out in a team approach, for example, by technologists and radiologists working together with medical physicists, and each component could be clinically validated by supervisory audits.

## 4 Prospective Safeguards in CT Equipment Design and Use to Improve Quality Assurance

In its *White Paper: Initiative to Reduce Unnecessary Radiation Exposure from Medical Imaging* (see footnote 26), FDA states that "FDA will issue targeted requirements for manufacturers of CT and fluoroscopic devices to incorporate important additional safeguards into the design of these machines, develop safer technologies, and provide additional training to support safe use by practitioners...." The following items represent particular access controls and equipment-usability features intended to improve CT system safety and quality assurance. They have been suggested as desiderata in discussions and presentations at meetings of CT stakeholders,[76] the public,[77] the IEC CT maintenance team, (see footnote 54) and the MITA (see footnote 57) CT group. While the items are under consideration, they might not necessarily be adapted as FDA policy via guidance or any other regulatory pathway, and they are presented here to stimulate thought and discussion:

- CT system interlock to preclude unauthorized CT scanner operation and to record operator identifier on image files and in the DICOM radiation dose structured report (see footnote 68).
- CT system interlock and record for audit to preclude unauthorized establishment or changes in user-defined scanning protocols.
- CT system interlock to preclude scanner operation without patient identification, except for emergency-use, service, engineering, and physics-test modes.
- Warnings and defaults to discourage user selection of an AEC mode in protocols for which the manufacturer recommends a manual mode (and vice versa).
- User-configurable display of interactive quality-assurance checklists.
- User-searchable information on dose reduction features integrated into the system-user interface.
- CT scanner capability for the user to enter patient anthropometric characteristics (e.g., gender, age, weight, height, circumference, etc.) that could be recorded by the scanner in the DICOM radiation dose structured report (see footnote 68).
- User-configurable capability to record the reconstruction algorithm on each image or dataset.
- Scanner capability to generate a detailed spreadsheet of protocols, manufacturer-recommended settings, user settings, and history of changes to settings.
- For each individual patient examination, CT scanner capability to automatically estimate and record in the DICOM radiation dose structured report (see footnote 68) values of organ doses and their uncertainties for each of the primary and remainder radiosensitive organs and tissues for which weighting factors are identified in the most recent recommendations of the International Commission on Radiological Protection (ICRP) (see footnote 13). The estimations should account for gender and for adult and pediatric X-ray attenuating patient habitus (i.e., body build specified in terms of anthropometric characteristics—such as weight, length, circumference, diameter, or, for pediatric patients, age related to size—that could be pertinent and useful in the estimation of organ doses).

---

[76] Stern (2009), (2010)

[77] See hyperlinks to transcripts of the Public Meeting: Device Improvements to Reduce Unnecessary Radiation Exposure from Medical Imaging, March 30–31, 2010, on the FDA web page http://www.fda.gov/MedicalDevices/NewsEvents/WorkshopsConferences/ucm201448.htm, last updated April 29, 2010.

## 5 Complementary Approaches to Promoting CT Radiation Safety Through Collaboration, Surveillance, and Research

The following summary of activities rounds out this chapter on FDA efforts to promote CT radiation safety.

### 5.1 Collaboration

As an advocate of quality assurance in CT, FDA has a broad range of formal and informal collaborative associations with government agencies, non-governmental standards development and radiation-protection organizations as well as with professional, industry, and trade groups. For example, in addition to work with the IEC and NEMA/MITA, FDA staff actively participates in standing work groups, research groups, or ad-hoc teams of the Center for Medicare and Medicaid Services (CMS), the National Institutes of Health (NIH) and its National Cancer Institute (NCI) Radiation Epidemiology Branch, the Department of Veterans Affairs, the National Institute of Standards and Technology (NIST), the National Naval Medical Center (NNMC), the CRCPD, the National Council on Radiation Protection and Measurements (NCRP), the AAPM, the Alliance for Radiation Safety in Pediatric Imaging (*Image Gently* campaign), and the *Image Wisely* collaborative initiative of the ACR, the Radiological Society of North America (RSNA), the ASRT, and the AAPM.

In particular, FDA has recommended that CMS integrate dose-management principles into its standards for CT personnel qualifications and facility quality assurance. In CMS guidelines for accreditation of free-standing advance diagnostic imaging facilities (those doing CT, nuclear medicine, magnetic resonance imaging) under the MIPPA (see footnote 41),[78] initial and continuing qualification of CT personnel could be made contingent on particular training requirements. Similar kinds of requirements could be included in CMS guidelines (see footnotes 47 and 48) related to participation of hospital radiologic services in CMS programs. Likewise, FDA has started to discuss with the CRCPD, the umbrella organization of US state radiation-control authorities, updates of its Suggested State Regulations for the Control of Radiation (SSRCR) (see footnote 49) covering CT. The SSRCR are templates frequently adapted—at times verbatim—by state governments to safeguard medical application of radiation, and they offer a potential regulatory pathway to require that the user community adopt desirable quality assurance practices and personnel-training criteria that are otherwise beyond the scope of current federal authority to mandate.

### 5.2 Surveillance

The Nationwide Evaluation of X-Ray Trends (NEXT)[79] is a surveillance program carried out cooperatively by the CRCPD and FDA. CT surveys of dose, techniques, and exam workloads are sampled typically from 200 to 300 randomly selected, voluntarily contributing facilities in approximately 30–40 participating states distributed across the United States. NEXT program CT surveys were done in 1990,[80] 2000–2001 (see footnotes 22 and 23), and 2005–2006 (see footnote 23);[81] results are being used to estimate diagnostic reference levels and also have been used to characterize X-ray trends in dose, e.g., in NCRP Report no. 160, *Ionizing Radiation Exposure of the Population of the United States* (2009) (see footnote 8). Figure 1 exemplifies some preliminary results from the 2005 to 2006 survey (see footnote 23), distributions of mAs (per rotation) applied by

[78] See Section 135 of U.S. Public Law 110–175, Medicare Improvements for Patients and Providers Act of 2008, http://frwebgate.access.gpo.gov/cgi-bin/getdoc.cgi?dbname=110_cong_public_laws&docid=f:publ275.pdf, July 15, 2008.

[79] Nationwide Evaluation of X-Ray Trends (NEXT), U.S. Food and Drug Administration web page, http://www.fda.gov/Radiation-EmittingProducts/RadiationSafety/Nationwide EvaluationofX-RayTrendsNEXT/default.htm, March 3, 2010; What is NEXT? Conference of Radiation Control Program Directors web page, http://www.crcpd.org/Pubs/NEXT.aspx, accessed September 28, 2011.

[80] Conway (1994)

[81] The data from the 2005–2006 NEXT survey of CT are currently undergoing final review and analysis. The original data set, neither edited, reviewed, nor analyzed, is currently available from hyperlinks to Excel files on the following FDA web page: Nationwide Evaluation of X-Ray Trends (NEXT) Computed Tomography Dataset, http://www.fda.gov/AboutFDA/CentersOffices/CDRH/CDRHTransparency/ucm202868.htm, last updated November 9, 2011.

**Fig. 1** (See footnote 23) Distributions of mAs applied by CT facilities for routine head exams in the US in 2005–06. *Bottom* and *top edges* of the *boxes* correspond respectively to the 25 and 75th percentiles, the *midline* to the median, the *diamond* to the mean, and the *whiskers* to the 5 and 95th percentiles. "Infant" refers to a patient who is 1-year old or younger, and "child" refers to a patient who is approximately 5- to 6-years old.[82]

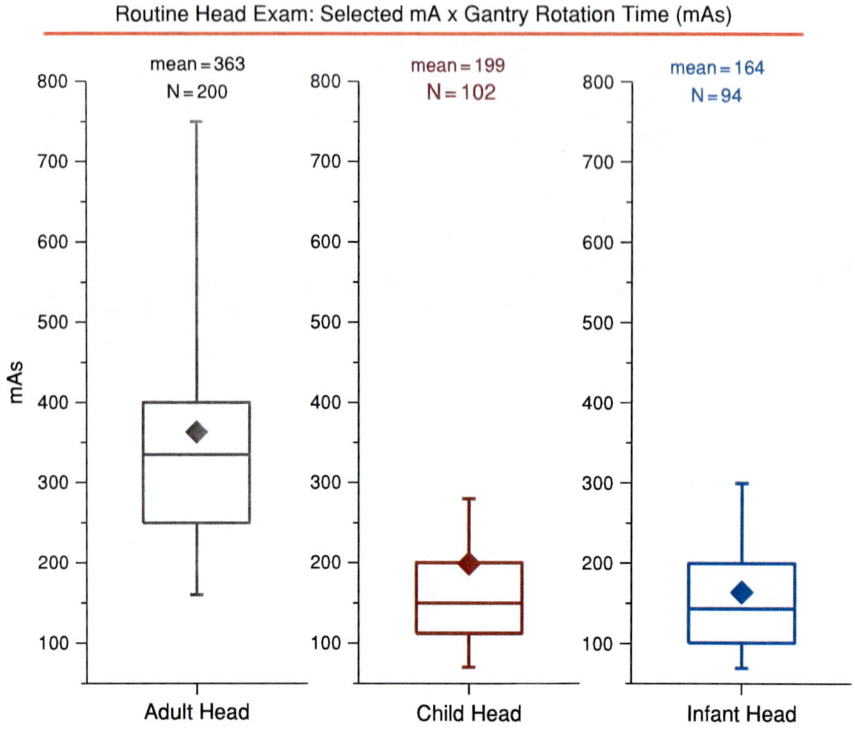


facilities for routine head exams in adult and pediatric patients.

### 5.3 Research

The FDA Center for Devices and Radiological Health has a vibrant research program in CT imaging and dosimetry. The bulk of this work is done under auspices and through collaborations of the Division of Imaging and Applied Mathematics (DIAM) of the CDRH Office of Science and Engineering Laboratories (OSEL), where research provides new and improved guidance for FDA evaluation of a wide variety of digital imaging devices including those of CT.[83,84] The following list of publication titles is a brief overview of the scope of recent CT work done by staff of the OSEL DIAM and their collaborators:

- Designing a phantom for dose evaluation in multislice CT[85]
- Accelerating Monte Carlo simulations of photon transport in a voxelized geometry using a massively parallel graphics processing unit[86]
- *PenMesh*—Monte Carlo radiation transport simulation in a triangle mesh geometry[87]
- Fast cardiac CT simulation using a graphics processing unit-accelerated Monte Carlo code[88]

82 Spelic et al. (2008)

83 FDA web page, laboratory of Imaging Physics, http://www.fda.gov/MedicalDevices/ScienceandResearch/ucm083231.htm, last updated May 21 2010; Laboratory of Image Analysis, http://www.fda.gov/MedicalDevices/ScienceandResearch/ucm083230.htm

84 FDA web page, FY 2010 OSEL Annual Report, http://www.fda.gov/AboutFDA/CentersOffices/OfficeofMedicalProductsandTobacco/CDRH/CDRHReports/ucm259763.htm, last updated November 9, 2011.

85 Abboud et al. (2010)

86 Badal and Badano ( 2009), (2011)

87 Badal et al. (2009)

88 Badal et al. (2010)

**Fig. 2** (See footnote 103) Head-phantom peak surface dose versus $CTDI_{\text{vol}}$ for four scanners. Note: nominal beam width at isocenter was 20 mm for the Philips, GE, Siemens scanners, and 40 mm for the Toshiba scanner

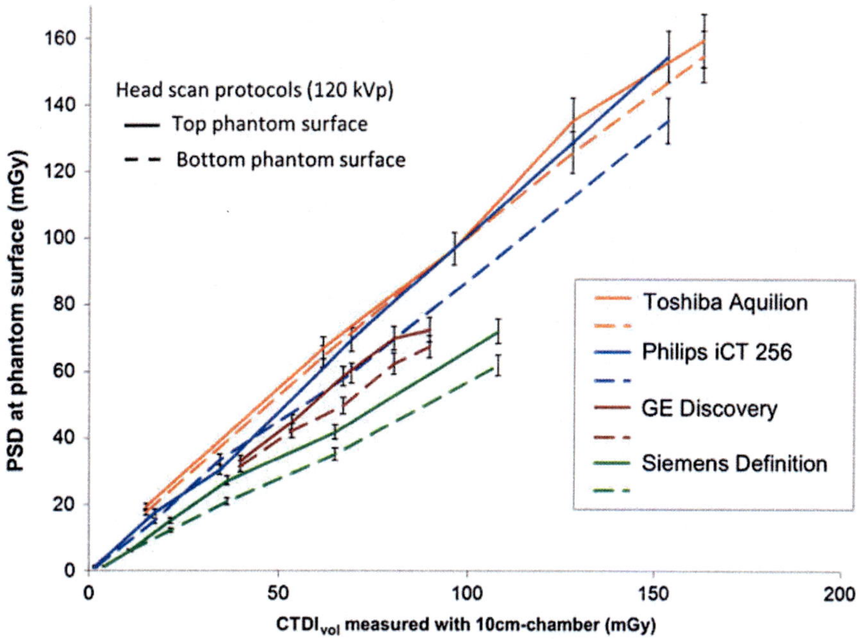


- Effect of oblique X-ray incidence in flat-panel computed tomography of the breast[89]
- A versatile laboratory platform for studying X-ray 3D breast imaging[90]
- A fast, angle-dependent, analytical model of CsI detector response for optimization of 3D X-ray breast imaging systems[91]
- A resource for the assessment of lung nodule size estimation methods: database of thoracic CT scans of an anthropomorphic phantom[92]
- Information-theoretic approach for analyzing bias and variance in lung nodule size estimation with CT: a phantom study[93]
- Computational high-resolution heart phantoms for medical imaging and dosimetry simulations[94]
- Improved computer-aided detection of small polyps in CT colonography using interpolation for curvature estimation[95]
- Distributed human intelligence for colonic polyp classification in computer-aided detection for CT colonography[96]
- CT colonography with computer-aided detection as a second reader: an observer performance study [97]
- Approximations of noise correlation in multi-slice helical CT scans: impact on lung nodule volume estimation.[98]

A recent investigation[99] of methods to estimate the modulation transfer function (MTF) and noise power spectrum (NPS) from measurements on a CT scanner has yielded interesting results that require further study and confirmation. Accounting for correlations in CT image noise, the method and its findings suggest that source-current-normalized magnitudes of signal-to-noise ratios (SNR) associated with various CT image-reconstruction kernels are significantly different from SNR evaluated under a presumption of uncorrelated noise. However, the assumptions and approximations underlying the method need to be better understood as well as validated. In this regard, the ongoing focus of FDA research on the evaluation of low-contrast detectability can inform and

[89] Badano et al. (2009)
[90] de las Heras et al. (2011)
[91] Freed et al. (2010)
[92] Gavrielides et al. (2010a)
[93] Gavrielides et al. (2010b)
[94] Gu et al. (2011)
[95] Liu et al. (2011)
[96] Nguyen et al. (2012)
[97] Petrick et al. (2008)
[98] Zeng et al. (2011)
[99] Brunner et al. (2011)

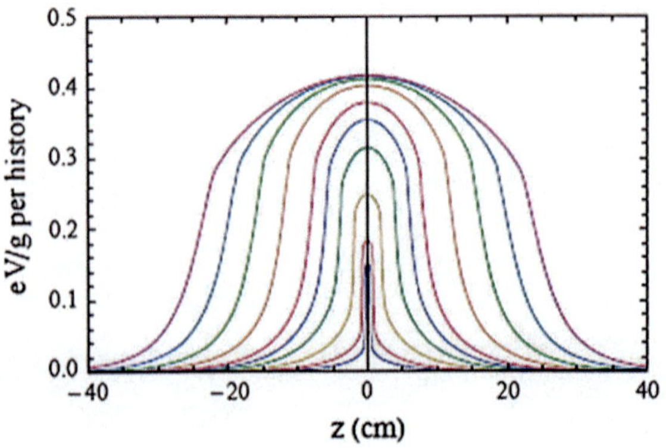


**Fig. 3** (See footnote 85) Calculated cross-sectional dose profiles in PMMA phantom, 32-cm diameter × 300-cm length, for beam widths from 1 to 60 cm

complement the development of metrics to characterize CT image-quality dependence on reconstruction algorithms and on techniques of dose reduction.

We close out this section with a few examples of CT dosimetry research projects at FDA and how they are promoted through a variety of FDA program sponsors:

- For a project to develop a handbook of organ doses associated with various CT examinations, the FDA *Commissioner's Fellowship Program*[100] supported research to establish CT scanner-independent estimates of organ dose in adult and pediatric patients.[101]
- The FDA *Critical Path Initiative*[102] supported work to determine organ doses experimentally in anthropomorphic phantoms and to characterize empirically the relationship between peak surface dose and the standardized dose-index $CTDI_{vol}$ (Fig. 2).[103]
- The FDA *Office of Women's Health*[104] supported Monte Carlo calculational dosimetry testing the design of phantoms for multi-slice CT (Fig. 3) (see footnote 85).

**Acknowledgment** At FDA, contributions to the advancement of radiation safety and effectiveness in CT depend on the efforts of many dedicated people in the CDRH Office of Communication, Education, and Radiation Programs; Office of Science and Engineering Laboratories; and Office of In Vitro Diagnostic Device Evaluation and Safety. We gratefully acknowledge their work.

## References

Abboud S, Badal A, Stern SH, Kyprianou IS (2010) Designing a phantom for dose evaluation in multi-slice CT. Proc SPIE 7622:762232

Badal A, Badano A (2009) Accelerating Monte Carlo simulations of photon transport in a voxelized geometry using a massively parallel graphics processing unit. Med Phys 36(11):4878

Badal A, Badano A (2011) Chapter 50, "Fast simulation of radiographic images using a monte carlo X-ray transport algorithm implemented in CUDA," in GPU computing gems: emerald edition, Wen-mei Hwu, Editor-in-Chief, Elsevier, Jan 2011. http://www.elsevier.com/wps/find/bookdescription.agents/724275/description#description

Badal A, Kypianou IS, Banh DP, Badano A, Sempau J (2009) penMesh—Monte Carlo radiation transport simulation in a triangle mesh geometry. IEEE Trans Med Imag 28(12):1894

Badal A, Kyprianou IS, Sharma D, Badano A (2010) Fast cardiac CT simulation using a graphics processing unit-accelerated Monte Carlo code. Proc SPIE 7622:762231

Badano A, Kyprianou IS, Freed M, Jennings RJ, Sempau J (2009) Effect of oblique X-ray incidence in flat-panel computed tomography of the breast. IEEE Trans Med Imag 28(5):696

Balter S, Hopewell JW, Miller DL, Wagner LK, Zelefsky MJ (2010) Fluoroscopically guided interventional procedures: a review of radiation effects on patients' skin and hair. Radiology 254(2):326–341

Boone JM (2007) The trouble with $CTDI_{100}$. Med Phys 34(4):1364–1371

Brenner DJ (2005) Is it time to retire the CTDI for CT quality assurance and dose optimization? Letter to the editor. Med Phys 32(10):3225–3226

Brunner CC, Renger B, Hoeschen C, Kyprianou IS (2011) Investigation of methods to estimate the MTF and NPS of CT towards creating an international standard. SPIE Medical Imaging 2011: Physics of Medical Imaging. Samei E, Pelc NJ (eds) 7961, 79613C Proceedings SPIE 2011

[100] FDA web page, Commissioner's Fellowship Program, http://www.fda.gov/AboutFDA/WorkingatFDA/FellowshipInternshipGraduateFacultyPrograms/CommissionersFellowshipProgram/default.htm, last updated October 28, 2011.

[101] Mills and Stern (2010).

[102] Critical Path Initiative, http://www.fda.gov/ScienceResearch/SpecialTopics/CriticalPathInitiative/default.htm, FDA web page last updated November 17, 2011.

[103] Fig. 2 is from the poster by de las Heras H, Minniti R, Wilson S, Skopec M, Stern S, Chakrabarti K (2011) "Peak skin dose and organ doses in CT examinations." 2011 joint AAPM/COMP Meeting Vancouver, 31 July-4 Aug 2011.

[104] Office of Women's Health, FDA web page, http://www.fda.gov/AboutFDA/CentersOffices/OC/OfficeofWomensHealth/default.htm, last updated March 15, 2011.

Conway BJ (1994) Nationwide evaluation of X-ray trends (NEXT) summary of 1990 computerized tomography survey and 1991 fluoroscopy survey, CRCPD publication 94–2. Conference of Radiation Control Program Directors, Inc., Frankfort, Kentucky

de las Heras H, Peng R, Zeng R, Freed M, O'Bryan E, Jennings RJ (2011) "A versatile laboratory platform for studying X-ray 3D breast imaging," Poster presentation at the IEEE Nuclear Science Symposium and Medical Imaging Conference, Valencia, Spain, 23–29 Oct 2011

Department of Health and Human Services, Food and Drug Administration (1980) Diagnostic X-ray systems and their major components; amendments to performance standard, proposed rule amending 21 CFR 1020.30 and adding 1020.33. Fed Regist 45(218):72204–72213 31 Oct 1980

Department of Health and Human Services, Food and Drug Administration [Docket No. FDA-2011-N-0148] (2011) Clarifying edits to existing special controls guidance documents; availability. Fed Reg 76(59):17135–17136, 28 Mar 2011

Dixon RL (2003) A new look at CT dose measurement: Beyond CTDI. Med Phys 30(6):1272–1280

Dixon RL (2006) Restructuring CT dosimetry—a realistic strategy for the future. Requiem for the pencil chamber. Med Phys 33(10):3973–3976

Dixon RL, Boone JM (2011) Analytical equations for CT dose profiles derived using a scatter kernel of Monte Carlo parentage with broad applicability to CT dosimetry problems. Med Phys 38(7):4251–4264

Dixon RL, Munley MT, Bayram E (2005) An improved analytical model for CT dose simulation with a new look at the theory of CT dose. Med Phys 32(12):3712–3728

Freed M, Park S, Badano A (2010) A fast, angle-dependent, analytical model of CsI detector response for optimization of 3D X-ray breast imaging systems. Med Phys 37(6):2593

Gavrielides MA, Kinnard LM, Myers KJ, Peregoy J, Pritchard WF, Zeng R, Esparza J, Karanian J, Petrick N (2010a) A resource for the assessment of lung nodule size estimation methods: database of thoracic CT scans of an anthropomorphic phantom. Opt Exp 18(14):15244

Gavrielides MA, Zeng R, Kinnard LM, Myers KJ, Petrick N (2010b) Information-theoretic approach for analyzing bias and variance in lung nodule size estimation with CT: a phantom study. IEEE Trans Med Imag 29(10):1795

Gu S, Gupta R, Kyprianou IS (2011) Computational high-resolution heart phantoms for medical imaging and dosimetry simulations. Phys Med Biol 56:5845

Gudjónsdóttir J, Ween B, Olsen DR (2010) Optimal use of AEC in CT: a literature review. Radiologic Technol 81(4):309–317

Health Risks from Exposure to Low Levels of Ionizing Radiation (2006) BEIR VII phase 2, National Research Council of the National Academies of Science and Engineering and the Institute of Medicine, The National Academies Press, Washington

Jessen KA, Shrimpton PC, Geleijns J, Panzer W, Tosi G (1999) Dosimetry for optimisation of patient protection in computed tomography. Appl Radiat Isot 50(1):165–172

Kalendar WA (2005) Computed tomography fundamentals, system technology, image quality, applications, 2nd revised edition, Publicis Corporate Publishing, Erlangen, Germany, p 42

Leitz W, Axelsson B, Szendrö G (1995) Computed tomography dose assessment: a practical approach. Radiat Prot Dosim 57:377–380

Liu J, Kabadi S, Van Uitert R, Petrick N, Deriche R, Summers RM (2011) Improved computer-aided detection of small polyps in CT colonography using interpolation for curvature estimation. Med Phys 38(7):4276–4284

Maier W, Nagel HD (2002) "Appendix," in radiation exposure in computed tomography, 4th revised and updated edition, edited by Nagel HD, CTB Publications, Hamburg, Germany, pp 71–74

Matthews K, Brennan PC (2009) The application of diagnostic reference levels: general principles and an Irish perspective. Radiography 15:171–178

McCollough CH, Zink FE (1999) Performance evaluation of a multi-slice CT system. Med Phys 26(11):2223–2230

Mills T, Stern S (2010) "Development of a handbook of radiation doses in organs of patients undergoing X-ray computed tomography (CT)," presentations at the 42nd national conference on radiation control, Newport, Rhode Island 18–22 Apr 2010, and at the 52nd Annual meeting of the American association of physicists in medicine, Philadelphia, Pennsylvania, 18–22 July 2010

Nagel HD (2002) "Aspects of dose for special technical features," in chapter 5 of radiation exposure in computed tomography, 4th revised and updated edition, edited by Nagel HD. CTB Pulications, Hamburg, Germany, pp 42–43

NCRP Report No. 160 (2009) Ionizing radiation exposure of the population of the United States, National Council on Radiation Protection and Measurements, Bethesda, Maryland

Nguyen TB, Wang S, Anugu V, Rose N, McKenna M, Petrick N, Burns JE, Summers RM (2012) Distributed human intelligence for colonic polyp classification in computer-aided detection for CT colonography. Radiology. doi: 10.1148/radiol.11110938, 24 Jan 2012

Petrick N, Haider M, Summers RM, Yeshwant S, Brown L, Iuliano EM, Louie A, Choi JR, Pickhardt PJ (2008) CT colonography with computer-aided detection as a second reader: an observer performance study. Radiology 246(1):148–156

Shope TB, Gagne RM, Johnson GC (1981) A method for describing the doses delivered by transmission X-ray computed tomography. Med Phys 8(4):488–495

Shrimpton PC (2004) Assessment of patient dose in CT, NRPB-PE/1/2004, national radiological protection board, Chilton, Didcot, Oxon, Mar 2004, and references cited therein

Spelic DC (2007) Nationwide Expansion of X-ray trends, CRCPD publication E-07-4. In: proceedings of the 39th national conference on radiation control, Conference of radiation control program directors, Inc., Frankfort, Kentucky, pp 98–100. http://www.crcpd.org/Pubs/07AMProceedingsWebVersion.pdf

Spelic DC, Stern SH, Kaczmarek RV (2008) Nationwide evaluation of X-ray trends (NEXT) protocol for 2005 survey of computed tomography, CRCPD publication E-08-2, conference of radiation control program directors, Inc., Frankfort, Kentucky, July 2008. http://www.crcpd.org/Pubs/NEXT_Protocols/NEXT-2005CT-Protocol.pdf

Stern SH (2007) Nationwide evaluation of X-ray trends (NEXT) tabulation and graphical summary of 2000 survey of computed tomography, CRCPD publication E-07-2, Conference of Radiation Control Program Directors, Inc., Frankfort, Kentucky. http://www.crcpd.org/Pubs/NEXT_docs/NEXT2000-CT.pdf

Stern SH (2009) "Improving quality assurance in CT," presentation at the Medical Imaging Technology Alliance (MITA) CT Stakeholders' Meeting at RSNA, Chicago, 30 Nov 2009

Stern SH (2010) "FDA dose-reduction initiative: progress," MITA CT Stakeholders' Meeting at RSNA, Chicago, 30 Nov 2010

Treier R, Aroua A, Verdun FR, Samara E, Stuessi A, Trueb PhR (2010) Patient doses in CT examinations in Switzerland: implementation of national diagnostic reference levels. Rad Prot Dosim 142(2–4):244–254

Toth TL, Bromberg NB, Pan TS, Rabe J, Woloschek SJ, Li J, Seidenschnur GE (2000) A dose reduction X-ray beam positioning system for high-speed multislice CT scanners. Med Phys 27(12):2659–2668

Zeng R, Petrick N, Gavrielides MA, Myers KJ (2011) Approximations of noise correlation in multi-slice helical CT scans: impact on lung nodule volume estimation. Phys Med Biol 56:6223

# ICRP's Role in Patient Dose Management in CT

Madan M. Rehani

## Contents



**Abstract**

The International Commission on Radiological Protection (ICRP) was established in 1928 and has been responsible for establishing principles and a system of radiological protection that is used world-wide. The main principles developed by the ICRP as applicable to patient protection are justification and optimisation of protection. ICRP has published two Annals on patient dose management in CT dealing with specific aspects of optimisation of protection in different clinical conditions besides guidelines on justification. Providing recommendations on dose management in clinical practice is another important aspect of the ICRP publications. In the ongoing effort to reach even more health professionals involved and make CT examinations safer, ICRP is planning to undertake actions on cone beam CT and hybrid systems.

**Abbreviations**

| | |
|---|---|
| AAPM | American association of physicists in medicine |
| AP | Anteroposterior |
| CTDI | CT dose index |
| $CTDI_{vol}$ | Volume weighted CT dose index |
| DLP | Dose-length product |
| DRL | Dose reference level |
| ICRP | International commission on radiological protection |
| IEC | International electrotechnical commission |
| MDCT | Multi detector CT |

M. M. Rehani (✉)
Secretary, Protection in Medicine Committee, International Commission on Radiological Protection (ICRP), Ottawa, ON, Canada
e-mail: madan.rehani@gmail.com

D. Tack et al. (eds.), *Radiation Dose from Multidetector CT*, Medical Radiology. Diagnostic Imaging,
DOI: 10.1007/174_2011_485, © Springer-Verlag Berlin Heidelberg 2012

| | |
|---|---|
| MRI | Magnetic resonance imaging |
| SSDE | size-specific dose estimates |

## 1 Introduction

The International Commission on Radiological Protection (ICRP) was established in 1928 and has been responsible for establishing principles and system of radiological protection that is used world-wide. ICRP is an independent, international organisation with more than 200 volunteer members from approximately 30 countries across six continents. These members represent leading scientists and policy makers in the field of radiological protection. ICRP is funded through a number of ongoing contributions from organisations with an interest in radiological protection.

Since 1928, ICRP has developed, maintained, and elaborated the International System of Radiological Protection used world-wide as the common basis for radiological protection standards, legislation, guidelines, programs, and practice. The system has been developed by ICRP based on (i) the current understanding of the science of radiation exposures and effects and (ii) value judgements. These value judgements take into account societal expectations, ethics, and experience gained in application of the system.

An understanding of the health effects of ionising radiation is central to the Commission's recommendations. There have been some controversies regarding radiation risks from one CT scan or several CT scans. The practical system of radiological protection recommended by the Commission continues to be based upon the assumption that at doses below approximately 100 mSv a given increment in dose will produce a directly proportionate increment in the probability of incurring cancer or heritable effects attributable to radiation. This dose-response model is generally known as 'linear-non-threshold' or LNT. The use of the LNT model is considered by the Commission to be the best practical approach to managing risk from radiation exposure and commensurate with the 'precautionary principle'. The Commission considers that the LNT model remains a prudent basis for radiological protection at low doses and low dose rates.

However, the Commission emphasizes that whilst the LNT model remains a scientifically plausible element in its practical system of radiological protection, biological/epidemiological information that would unambiguously verify the hypothesis that underpins the model is unlikely to be forthcoming. Because of this uncertainty on health effects at low doses, the Commission judges that it is not appropriate, for the purposes of public health planning, to calculate the hypothetical number of cases of cancer or heritable disease that might be associated with very small radiation doses received by large numbers of people over very long periods of time.

The probabilistic nature of stochastic effects and the properties of the LNT model make it impossible to derive a clear distinction between 'safe' and 'dangerous', and this creates some difficulties in explaining the control of radiation risks. The major policy implication of the LNT model is that some finite risk, however small, must be assumed and a level of protection established based on what is deemed acceptable.

This leads to the Commission's system of protection with its three fundamental principles of protection:

- Justification
- Optimisation of protection
- Application of dose limits (which is applicable for staff protection but not for patient protection).

Over the last decade, the Commission has published a number of documents that provided detailed advice related to radiological protection and safety in the medical applications of ionising radiation. CT is one such example in which two Annals have been published (ICRP 2001, 2007a).

These publications are written with the intent of communicating directly with the relevant medical practitioners, namely radiologists and supporting paramedical staff.

## 2 Justification of CT Examinations

Justification requires that the net benefit to be positive. Unlike occupational and public exposures, justification in medical practice lies more often with the profession than with the government or the competent regulatory authority. The responsibility for the justification of the use of a particular procedure falls on the relevant medical practitioners, who need to have special training in radiological protection.

According to principles established by the ICRP in its earlier publications and included in the latest recommendations (ICRP 2007b), the principle of justification applies at three levels in the use of radiation in medicine.

- At the first level, the use of radiation in medicine is accepted as doing more good than harm to the patient. In medicine, this level of justification is now taken for granted.
- At the second level, the justification is carried out by the health authority in conjunction with appropriate professional bodies for a given radiological procedure such as use of CT for colonography. The aim of the second level of justification is to judge whether the radiological procedure will usually improve the diagnosis or treatment or will provide necessary information about the exposed individuals.
- At the third level, it is a matter of applying justification to an individual patient (i.e., a particular CT examination should be judged to do more good than harm to an individual patient).

Justification in radiological protection of patients is different from justification of other radiation applications, in that generally the very same person enjoys the benefits and suffers the risks associated with a procedure (ICRP 2008). There may be other considerations: attendant occupational exposures could be correlated with patient doses or sometimes there can be a trade-off. Screening programmes may benefit the population rather than every screened person. Risks and benefits accrue to the same person. A very important aspect in daily medical practice is the fact that a method or procedure can be regarded as justified but this does not necessarily mean that its application to the particular patient being considered is justified and hence the need for a third level of justification is important.

According to ICRP Publication 87 (ICRP 2001), requests for a CT examination should be generated only by properly qualified medical or dental practitioners depending on the national educational and qualification system. Justification of CT is a shared responsibility between referring physician and radiologist. The radiologist should be appropriately trained and skilled in CT and radiation protection, and possess adequate knowledge concerning alternative techniques. Also to be considered in the justification process is the availability of resources and cost. The referring physician has responsibility for the justification of an examination in individual cases and obtaining the advice of a radiologist for any alternative examination that would provide the desired information. Justification of the CT study for a given indication and classification of the clinical indications into those requiring standard dose CT and those requiring only low dose CT is also a responsibility of the referring physician.

Clinical guidelines advising which examinations are appropriate and acceptable should be available to clinicians and radiologists. Ideally, these will be agreed at the national level, but where they are not, local guidelines are often developed within an institution. In CT, this requires consideration of whether the required information could be obtained by conventional radiography, ultrasound, or magnetic resonance imaging (MRI) without unduly hindering clinical management.

As in all X-ray procedures, CT examinations should not be repeated without clinical justification and should be limited to the area of pathology under request. Unjustifiable repetition of exposure may occur if the referring clinician or radiologist is unaware of the existence or results of previous examinations. The risk of repetitive examinations increases when patients are transferred between institutions. For this reason, a record of previous investigation should be available to all those generating or carrying out examination requests. The clinician who has knowledge that a previous examination exists has a responsibility to communicate this to the radiologist.

CT examinations for research purposes that do not have clinical justification at the level of immediate benefit to the person undergoing the examination should be subject to critical evaluation since the doses are significantly higher than doses in conventional radiography. Additional information on this is available in Publication 62 (ICRP 1993).

## 3 Optimisation of CT Examinations

Once referral for CT examination has been justified, the radiologist has primary responsibility to ensure that the examination is carried out conscientiously, effectively, and with good technique. This is usually described as the principle of optimisation. Within this process the radiologist and operator have considerable scope for limiting the radiation dose to the patient. The objective is to provide sufficient diagnostic information to influence the clinical management of the patient.

Clinical issues define the area to be examined and the extent of the examination required. However, even when these conditions are met, the radiologist has additional opportunity for limiting the radiation dose to the patient.

It is valuable to consider the role of contrast medium enhancement prior to commencing the examination. In some cases, a single examination following enhancement may be adequate for clinical purposes and initial unenhanced images may therefore be avoided. In multiphase enhancement studies, the examination should be limited to the number of phases which are clinically justified.

The basis for optimisation of protection of the patient in diagnostic procedures in the past has been that the source-related individual dose constraints are not relevant. Instead reference levels for a particular procedure, which apply to groups of similar patients rather than individuals, are used to ensure that doses do not deviate significantly from those achieved at peer departments for that procedure unless there is a known, relevant, and acceptable reason for the deviation. This has been based on the understanding that the same person gets the benefit and suffers the risk, and thus individual restrictions on patient dose could be counterproductive to the medical purpose of the procedure.

Radiologists should work closely with the medical physicists to ensure that proper protocols are used and the radiation dose that is applied is based on patient age, size, clinical indications, as well as the number of prior radiation-based examinations. Dose reference levels (DRLs) should be set in terms of the practical dose quantities used to monitor CT practice: volume weighted CT dose index ($CTDI_{vol}$, expressed in mGy) and dose-length product (DLP, expressed in mGy cm) are currently commonly displayed by CT scanners. These quantities are not patient doses (directly reflecting risk to individuals), but doses to standard phantoms. DRLs are used for characterising radiation exposure in CT for the purpose of comparison of practices. The standard CT dosimetry phantoms are acrylic cylinders with diameters of 16 cm (commonly referenced for head protocols) and 32 cm (commonly referenced for body protocols on adults). Under similar conditions of CT exposure, displayed values of $CTDI_{vol}$ or DLP referring to the smaller dosimetry phantom are about twice those referring to the larger phantom. In order to allow meaningful comparison of values of $CTDI_{vol}$ and DLP as part of the optimisation of patient protection, it is imperative to know the reference dosimetry phantom for each displayed dose. There is no merit in setting DRLs in terms of other derived dose quantities, such as an effective dose.

Whereas $CTDI_{vol}$ and DLP provide a general characterisation of the conditions of exposure in CT, American Association of Physicists in Medicine (AAPM) (2011) has suggested a complementary approach for monitoring doses to individual patient utilities. The concept of size-specific dose estimates (SSDE). Values of SSDE are derived from displayed values of $CTDI_{vol}$, though application of tabulated correction factors specific to patient age or effective diameter (determined from anteroposterior (AP) and lateral dimensions), in order to provide an estimate of the typical level of dose for an individual patient. In addition, the International Electrotechnical Commission (IEC) has proposed the use of dose notification and dose alert values of $CTDI_{vol}$ or DLP that can be set by CT centres to flag levels of potential concern for specific scan settings on the scanner. These dose values also represent a different concept to DRLs. AAPM (advice on website dated 27/04/11), for example, has recommended initial notification values for $CTDI_{vol}$ of 80 mGy (expressed in terms of the 16 cm dosimetry phantom) in relation to scans of the adult head and 50 mGy (32 cm dosimetry phantom) for scans on the adult torso.

## 4 Dose Management in Specific Clinical Practices

ICRP Publication 102 (ICRP 2007a) has a section that deals with specific conditions, namely chest CT, CT for coronary calcium quantification and non-invasive coronary angiography, CT colonography, CT for trauma, CT of the urinary tract, CT-guided interventions, CT in children, and CT of the pregnant patient. The summary points from that section are:

- Guidelines (selection criteria for CT examinations) are necessary so that inappropriate studies can be avoided. In addition, alternative non-radiation imaging techniques should be considered, when appropriate.

- Training of requesting physicians and CT staff can help in the management of scan indications, protocols, and patient dose.
- With the emergence of cardiac MDCT applications, many cardiologists have become users of MDCT scanners. The Commission recommends appropriate training in radiation protection for cardiologists.

## 5 Process for ICRP Publications

ICRP deliberates on topics on which it should provide guidance and publish documents. It creates a Task Group (TG) for each topic under the chairmanship of one of its members. Besides its Chair, the TG has full members and corresponding members suggested by the TG Chair. TG members may be from any country in the world but should have in the topic and be actively involved in the topic with skills to contribute towards sections of the report. For reports dealing with CT, TG members are typically medical physicists, radiologists, or engineers. TG members need to be approved by the relevant Committee and by the Main Commission (MC). The proposal for TG creation also recommends funds needed to hold TG meetings. Typically, one or two meetings may be held for completion of the document. The draft document created by the TG is reviewed by the concerned Committee(s) and, on approval, it is sent to the MC which provides feedback. The MC approves the document for placing on the ICRP website for public consultation. The TG Chair, with the help of TG members, addresses the comments and finalises the document which is again reviewed by the Committee(s) and MC before it is sent to the publisher for its publication as Annals of the ICRP.

The Scientific Secretary of the ICRP acts as Editor of the Annals of the ICRP. The Annals were listed in pubmed with editor as the author, but recently the ICRP decided to list TG members as authors in pubmed.

Occasionally, Working Parties (WP) are created to review topics which later are converted into TG(s).

The web address of the organisation is: http://www.icrp.org/

A list of ICRP publication is available at: http://www.icrp.org/publications.asp

Information about different Committees of the ICRP is available at: http://www.icrp.org/page.asp?id=3

Committee 3 deals with protection in medicine and information about the constitution of this Committee and all Task Groups is available at: http://www.icrp.org/icrp_group.asp?id=9

## References


American Association of Physicists in Medicine (2011) Size specific dose estimates (SSDE) in pediatric and adult body CT examinations. Report of AAPM Task Group 204

International Commission on Radiological Protection (1993) Radiological protection in biomedical research. ICRP Publication 62. Ann ICRP 22(3):1–70

International Commission on Radiological Protection (2001) Managing patient dose in computed tomography. ICRP Publication 87. Ann ICRP 30(4):1–45

International Commission on Radiological Protection (2007a) Managing patient dose in multi-detector computed tomography (MDCT). ICRP Publication 102. Ann ICRP 37(1): 1–79

International Commission on Radiological Protection (2007b) Recommendations of the ICRP. ICRP Publication 103. Ann ICRP 37(2-4):1–332

International Commission on Radiological Protection (2008) Radiological protection in medicine. ICRP Publication 105. Ann ICRP 37(6):1–63

# Software for Calculating Dose and Risk

Georg Stamm

## Contents



**Abstract**

Calculation or even rough estimation of patient dose and risk is a rather complicated and time-consuming process. Software tools may help to at least facilitate the calculations assuming some necessary simplifications. The different approaches from on-line tools and calculators for mobile devices for a quick mean dose display for selected regions up to examples for precise Monte-Carlo simulations for real scanner setups will be presented. As every patient has his own geometry and constitution it is nearly impossible to calculate individual dose values. To at least calculate data to compare the performance of different scanners or to benchmark own scan protocols a common used approach is using standard sized patient phantoms and databases matching the design and setup of different scanners. Due to rapidly evolving scanner technique with sophisticated methods of tube current modulations which cannot be covered by the dose calculators the use of some simplifications using mean conversion factors or mean values for the tube current are necessary to estimate a mean dose to the standard sized patient within a range of ±15%. This also holds for all calculations for specific organ dose values like uterus dose and eye-lens dose. Individual or personalized dose estimates will remain a task for future work.

G. Stamm (✉)
Medizinische Hochschule Hannover,
Institut für Diagnostische und Interventionelle Radiologie,
Carl-Neuberg-Str. 1, 30625 Hannover, Germany
e-mail: stamm.georg@mh-hannover.de

D. Tack et al. (eds.), *Radiation Dose from Multidetector CT*, Medical Radiology. Diagnostic Imaging,
DOI: 10.1007/174_2011_434, 

## 1 Introduction

Software for calculating dose from CT exams can be splitted into several groups:

(1) On-line dose calculators for a very short check of patient doses for selected regions.
(2) Rough dose estimates using conversion factors for the region of interest.
(3) More sophisticated approaches taking into account different scanner designs.
(4) Rather complicated methods using Monte-Carlo calculations to estimate dose to the (individual) patient.

## 2 On-line Dose Calculators

The easiest example for an on-line risk calculator helps to "determine the health risk associated with a radiation figure you encountered somewhere" (Radiation Dose to Risk Converter).

The sites XRayRisk or RADAR Medical Procedure Radiation Dose Calculator offer the possibility of estimating patient doses for commonly conducted examination using X-rays (either conventional or CT) and/or radioactive isotopes used in nuclear medicine procedures.

While the RADAR calculator allows only the display of mean dose values for listed exams (example: CT abdomen/pelvis—helical = 14 mSv) without the possibility of entering own dose values (e.g. dose-length-product DLP). The XRayRisk calculator either uses the same approach (example: CT abdomen/pelvis = 14 mSv) or an optional input of dose-length-product (example: CT abdomen/pelvis with 750 mGy * cm = 13.5 mSv).

The risk is presented either as excess/additional lifetime cancer risk or in terms of the natural background radiation.

The packages WAZA-ARI (Takahashi et al. 2011a, b) and the pediatric CT dose and risk estimator (Alessio and Phillips 2010) are already more sophisticated approaches but are limited either due to scanner models available or using simple conversion factors for the specified regions. But those two tools are very useful for a quick estimate and especially the paediatric CT dose and risk estimator shows the result as risk estimate in terms of natural background radiation, which is much more easier to explain to the patient than physical dose quantities. While dose calculators taking into account nearly all parameters of the examination often need the input and advice of medical physicist the on-line tools are very easy to use even for people with only basic skills in radiation physics.

## 3 Calculations Based on Conversion Factors

Rough dose estimates can be achieved by just multiplying recorded dose values with conversion factors. For conventional X-ray exams this can be done by multiplying the values from the measured dose-area-product (DAP) with corresponding conversion factors f (mSv/cGy * $cm^2$) for the relevant regions to estimate the effective dose for this exam (see e.g. Le Heron 1992; Bor et al. 2004). A similar approach can be done considering CT scans by using conversion factors f (mSv/mGy * cm) for the dose-length-product (DLP). Those conversion factors were first described in the European Guidelines on Quality Criteria for Computed Tomography (http://www.drs.dk/guidelines/ct/quality/) and modified in the 2004 CT Quality Criteria (Bongartz 2004).

Table 1 shows the corresponding values for some scan regions based on the EU values.

As an example on how to use these factors just record the dose-length-product of the CT series (usually displayed at the scanner console).

A DLP of 750 mGy * cm for one series in abdominal CT would result in an effective dose of 750 mGy * cm * 0.015 mSv/(mGy * cm) = 11.25 mSv.

This first approach was further adopted and improved by other authors to allow quick estimates of dose values in terms of effective dose. With the software tools OmnimAs and QuickDose the user selects the appropriate region and after the input of the values for the DLP the corresponding value for the effective dose will be displayed.

The main advantage of this approach is a fast result and no specific information on scanner design is necessary. On the other hand only rough dose estimates are possible as the conversion factors are only mean values for a whole body region of interest. Different setups for scanner design including (form)-filter and different focus-to-axis distance are not covered by

**Table 1** Conversion factors f [mSv/(mGy * cm)] for commonly used CT exams based on the values of the European Guidelines on Quality Criteria for CT

| Region | f according (Alessio and Phillips 2010; Bongartz et al. 2004) [mSv/(mGy * cm)] | Original EU values EU 16262 EN |
|---|---|---|
| Head/ Neck | 0.004 | n.a. |
| Head | 0.002 | 0.0023 |
| Neck | 0.005 | 0.0054 |
| Chest | 0.020 | 0.017 |
| Abdomen/ Pelvis | 0.015 | 0.015 |
| Pelvis | n.a. | 0.019 |
| Trunk | 0.017 | n.a. |

these dose calculations. Although there are already some efforts to publish specific conversion factors for children of different age (Shrimpton 2004) these values are up to now only included in one web-based calculation tool (Alessio and Phillips 2010).

## 4 Dose Calculators Using Different Scanner Design

Including different scanner design and hence a much more accurate approach has been done by several software products which are listed in the following Table 2.

**Table 2** Dose calculators taking into account different scanner designs and specific scan parameters

| Product | Platform | Remarks |
|---|---|---|
| P-Dose | Microsoft Windows® | Commercial, limited number of scanner data, only for adults |
| ImpactDose | Microsoft Windows® | Commercial, scanner data only for one vendor, only for adults |
| CTDosimetry | Microsoft Excel® | Spread sheet (freeware), data set (commercial), scanner data for different vendors available, only for adults |
| CT-Dose | Microsoft Windows® | Discontinued |
| CT-Expo | Microsoft Excel® | Spread sheet, shareware, scanner data for different vendors available, 3 age groups (adult, child, baby) |
| FetDose/OrgDose (Osei et al. 2003), (Osei and Barnett 2009) | Microsoft Windows® | Freeware, only limited data for scanners, only for adults |
| NCICT | Microsoft Windows® | Currently only available for beta tester |

Dose calculations with the above mentioned tools can be done nearly as quick as using only conversion factors and give a more precise result. On the other hand all calculations are based on a set of phantoms representing the standard patient. These phantoms are either hermaphrodite, gender specific like ADAM, EVA (Kramer et al. 1982) and may represent also different age groups like Child and Baby (Zankl et al. 1993). This means that dose calculations for individual patients are not possible. The calculated dose values in terms of either effective dose or organ doses have to taken as bench marks which may not proper represent the current situation for the individual patient. Different patient diameter and divergent location of relevant organs may cause different radiation absorption and hence lead to some discrepancy. But we can use the software packages as valuable tools to check compliance with the diagnostic reference dose levels (DRL) or to optimize the own scan protocols because the influence of every change in scan parameters on corresponding dose values can be directly recorded. Benchmarking the own scan protocols and monitoring the differences after the installation of a new scanner are possible as well. A further range of application is teaching students and radiographers the basics of radiation protection using the correct set of scan parameters.

Medical physicists are able to estimate dose for the uterus when a pregnant woman has been examined and the risk for the unborn child shall be evaluated with the above-mentioned constraints on reliable values for the individual patient.

The limitations for this approach are calculations or specific organ dose values. As these software tools do not take into account the tube current modulations correlated with the different approaches of automatic exposure control (AEC) in CT, all calculations are based on mean tube current values for the region of interest. As the real tube current values may be higher in regions with a high intrinsic absorption (e.g. pelvis) the estimated results for organs within this region (ovaries, kidney) may be too low. If a more precise estimate is necessary, the calculations should and can be done slice by slice using the real values for the tube current recorded in the DICOM metadata of every slice image.

## 5 Monte-Carlo Simulation

The most accurate and also most time consuming calculation can be done using Monte-Carlo simulation of radiation propagation in material. Several software packages are available, usually used for simulations in radiotherapy (EGSnrc package for the Monte Carlo simulation of coupled electron-photon transport; Geant4 Geometry and Tracking; MCNP General Monte Carlo N-Particle Transport Code or the eXtended version MCNPX). These packages allow the design of nearly every radiation field including the effects of filter material on the energy spectrum of the radiation. But the more possibilities exist for modelling the real situation the more complex is the whole simulation process. An exact and profound knowledge of radiation physics is necessary to properly setup the environment for the simulation.

But even if experts in medical physics and radiation physics are involved in the simulation process it is even impossible to get reliable data for some essential components. Material and shape of the form-filter used in modern CT devices are completely unknown to the public and kept secret by the manufacturers. Hence it is often impossible to launch a correct simulation because several important boundary conditions are unknown.

GMctdospp is an example for a software package where the EGSnrc code has been adapted to CT geometry and the energy spectrum of the corresponding X-rays. Some results for simulation of Cone-Beam-CT were published in (Voigt et al. 2010). Another commercial software package for simulating dose distributions in phantoms and patients is ImpactMC.

Some other publications deal with using voxel phantoms to do individual dose calculations (a wide range is covered in ImpactMC; Hunt et al. 2004; Petoussi-Henss et al. 2002; Zankl 2010; Zankl et al. 2000; Kramer et al. 2003, 2004). This approach needs a proper segmentation of the organs for a precise dose calculation. The segmentation process isn't as time consuming as some years ago, but we are far from having the segmentation results on the fly.

To at least partially overcome these difficulties other authors suggest the use of "phantom families" which take into account a matrix of different shape and weight of the patients (Cassola et al. 2011).

## 6 Dose Calculators for Mobile Devices and Other Software Packages

The current available software for mobile devices is also mainly based on conversion factors. QuickDose for Windows Mobile 6 Smartphone uses this feature for calculating dose values for CT exams and also includes the possibility of estimating dose values for the uterus of conventional X-ray and nuclear medicine exams. Another application is the CT Dose Calculator available for Android platforms.

Calculating dose values (effective dose and/or dose area product) for conventional X-ray exams can be done by the software packages PRDC dose (Kim et al. 2006), XL-Dose and RefDose (both discontinued), the freeware CALDose_X 4.1 and the commercial package PCXMC (current version 2.0). CALDose_X can now also be used on-line using already the mentioned phantom family and Monte-Carlo simulation with execution times of about 2 min. As contribution of conventional X-ray exams to collective dose has decreased during the last decades the importance for calculating corresponding dose values decreases as well. Dose evaluation are more and more focused on the (rapidly) increasing numbers of CT exams which have reached a contribution to collective dose in Germany of more than 50% (Annual Report of German National Radiation Protection Board 2008).

FetDose (Osei et al. 2003) and UterusDose, an Excel application based on the recommendations of the German Society of Medical Physicist (DGMP) and the German Röntgen Society (DRG), are special software tools which allow the estimation of dose to the unborn child in case of accidental exposition.

## 7 Conclusion

Regarding the rapidly evolving market for mobile solutions it will be just a question of time until other applications using modern web standards like HTML5 and/or JavaScript will provide functionalities in the range from using simple conversion factors up to including databases for different scanner design and ages for the patient under consideration. The Food and Drug Administration (FDA) has already recognized the great potential of mobile applications or "apps" and defined guidelines for the industry regarding mobile medical applications (FDA U.S. Food and Drug Administration, Draft Guidance for Industry and Food and Drug Administrative Staff—Mobile Medical Applications).

The rapid evolving techniques of the scanners and the new technical implementations of automatic exposure controls like mA-modulation, rolling collimator for reducing the over-ranging effect, rapid kV-switching or dual energy applications make it even more complicated to implement these new developments and features in the dose calculation software packages. Thus dose estimates using generic conversion factors with an uncertainty in the range of $\pm 15\%$ will always remain a quick and easy method to assess radiation exposure of CT exams. Online tools reading the scan parameters directly from the DICOM header of anonymized images could be used in future for optimization and benchmarking the own scan protocols.

For more individual dose calculations a quick (on-line) segmentation of the images is necessary to identify the position and extend of all critical organs and mapping the calculations based on the standard patient phantoms (or phantom family) to the real patient data.

## References

### On-line Calculators and Software Using Conversion Factors


Alessio AM, Phillips GS (2010) A pediatric CT dose and risk estimator. Pediatric Radiol 40:1816–1821. http://faculty.washington.edu/aalessio/doserisk2/

Bongartz G, Golding SJ, Jurik AG, Leonardi M, van Persijn van Meerten E, Rodríguez R, Schneider K, Calzado A, Geleijns J, Jessen KA, Panzer W, Shrimpton PC, Tosi G (2004) European guidelines for multislice computed tomography. Funded by the European commission. Contract number FIGM-CT2000-20078-CT-TIP, March 2004. http://www.msct.eu/CT_Quality_Criteria.htm

Bor D, Sancak T, Olgar T, Elcim Y, Adanali A, Sanlidilek U, Akyar S (2004) Comparison of effective doses obtained from dose-area product and air kerma measurements in interventional radiology. Br J Radiol 77:315–322

European Guidelines on Quality Criteria for Computed Tomography, EUR 16262 EN

Le Heron JC (1992) Estimation of effective dose to the patient during medical X-ray examinations from measurements of the dose-area product. Phys Med Biol 37:2117–2126

OmnimAs (Windows® platform). http://www.arwen.se/radiologi/omnimas_en/index.html

QuickDose (Windows Mobile 6 Smartphone® and Windows®) http://www.mh-hannover.de/1604.html

RADAR Medical Procedure Radiation Dose Calculator (http://www.doseinfo-radar.com/RADARDoseRiskCalc.html)

Radiation Dose to Risk Converter (http://www.wise-uranium.org/rdcri.html)

Shrimpton PC (2004) Assessment of patient dose in CT; NRPB-PE/1/2004. http://www.msct.eu/CT_Quality_Criteria.htm

Takahashi F et al (2011a) WAZA-ARI computational dosimetry system for X-ray CT examinations. I. Radiation transport calculation for organ and tissue doses evaluation using JM phantom. Radiat Prot Dosim 146:241–243

Takahashi F et al (2011b) WAZA-ARI computational dosimetry system for X-ray CT examinations II: development of web-based system. Radiat Prot Dosim 146:244–247

XRayRisk (http://www.xrayrisk.com/calculator/calculator.php)


### Software Packages Including Scanner Design Factors


CTDosimetry (IMPACTscan). http://www.impactscan.org/ctdosimetry.htm

CT-Expo (Demo version). http://www.mh-hannover.de/1604.html

ImpactDose. http://test.scanditronix-wellhoefer.com/Software-ImpactDose.1313+M52087573ab0.0.html?&cHash=5baba317bf

Kramer R, Zankl M, Williams G, Drexler G (1982) The calculation of dose from external photon exposures using reference human phantoms and Monte Carlo methods: part I. the male (Adam) and female (Eva) adult mathematical phantoms. GSF-Report S-885 (Neuherberg: GSF—National Research Center for Environment and Health)

Osei E, Barnett R (2009) Software for the estimation of organ equivalent and effective doses from diagnostic radiology procedures. J Radiol Prot 29:361–376

Osei E, Darko J, Faulkner K, Kotre C (2003) Software for the estimation of foetal radiation dose to patients and staff in diagnostic radiology. J Radiol Prot 23:183–194

P-Dose. http://www.qualitycontrol.org/index.php?page=modulo_p_dose_ct_en

Zankl M, Panzer W, Drexler G (1993) Tomographic anthropomorphic models, part II: organ doses from computed tomographic examinations in paediatric radiology. GSF-Report 30/93 (Neuherberg: GSF—National Research Center for Environment and Health)

## Software for Monte Carlo Simulation and Voxel Phantoms

Cassola VF, Milian FM, Kramer R, de Oliveira Lira CAB, Khoury HJ (2011) Standing adult human phantoms based on 10th, 50th and 90th mass and height percentiles of male and female Caucasian populations. Phys Med Biol 56:3749–3772

EGSnrc package for the Monte Carlo simulation of coupled electron-photon transport. http://irs.inms.nrc.ca/software/egsnrc/

Geant4 Geometry and Tracking. http://geant4.cern.ch/

GMctdospp. http://www.thm.de/imps/programme/95-gmctdospp

Hunt JG, Da Silva FCA, Mauricio LP, Dos Santos DS (2004) The validation of organ dose calculations using voxel phantoms and Monte Carlo methods applied to point and water immersion sources. Radiat Prot Dosim 108:85–89

ImpactMC. http://www.ct-imaging.de/en/dose-calculation.php

Kramer R, Vieira JW, Khoury HJ, Lima FRA, Fuelle D (2003) All about MAX: a male adult voxel phantom for Monte Carlo calculations in radiation protection dosimetry. Phys Med Biol 48:1239–1262

Kramer R, Khoury HJ, Vieira JW, Lima VJM, Lima FRA, Hoff G (2004) All about FAX: a Female Adult voxel phantom for Monte Carlo calculation in radiation protection dosimetry. Phys Med Biol 49:5203–5216

MCNP General Monte Carlo N-Particle Transport Code or the eXtended version MCNPX. http://mcnp-green.lanl.gov/ and http://mcnpx.lanl.gov/

Petoussi-Henss N, Zankl M, Fill U, Regulla D (2002) The GSF family of voxel phantoms. Phys Med Biol 47:89–106

Voigt JM, Wulff J, Danova D, Fiebich M (2010) Simulation der Dosisverteilung bei Cone-Beam-CT Untersuchungen mit GMctdospp 41. Jahrestagung der Deutschen Gesellschaft für Medizinische Physik – Tagungsband 2010 (in German). http://www.dgmp.de/oeffentlichkeitsarbeit/tagungsbaende/MedizinischePhysik2010.pdf

Zankl M (2010) The GSF voxel computational phantom family. In: George Xu X, Eckerman KF (eds) Handbook of anatomical models for radiation dosimetry, Chapter 3. Taylor & Francis, Boca Raton

Zankl M, Panzer W, Herrmann C (2000) Calculation of patient doses using a human voxel phantom of variable diameter. Radiat Prot Dosim 90:155–158

## Other Software Packages, Mainly for Conventional X-rays

Annual Report of the German Radiation Protection Board (Bundesamt für Strahlenschutz) 2008, 246. http://www.bfs.de/de/bfs/publikationen/berichte/jb/jb_ab_2003.html

CALDose_X 4.1. http://www.caldose.org/CaldoseEng1.aspx

CT Dose Calculator for Android. http://de.appbrain.com/app/ct-dose-calculator-free/com.whodunnit.medicalphysics.dosecalculatorfree

DGMP- and DRG-Report Nr. 7. http://www.dgmp.de/oeffentlichkeitsarbeit/papiere/Bericht7_Neuauflage2002.pdf

FDA U.S. Food and Drug Administration, Draft Guidance for Industry and Food and Drug Administrative Staff - Mobile Medical Applications. http://www.fda.gov/MedicalDevices/DeviceRegulationandGuidance/GuidanceDocuments/ucm263280.htm

Kim C-H, Cho SH, Xu XG (2006) PRDC - a software package for personnel radiation dose calculation. Radiat Prot Dosim 118:243–250

PCXMC Version 2.0. http://www.stuk.fi/sateilyn_kaytto/ohjelmat/PCXMC/en_GB/pcxmc/

UterusDose, Excel spreadsheet. http://www.mh-hannover.de/1604.html

# Image Wisely

James A. Brink and E. Stephen Amis

## Contents



**Abstract**

The American College of Radiology and the Radiological Society of North America formed the joint task force on adult radiation protection to address concerns about the surge of public exposure to ionizing radiation from medical imaging. The joint task force collaborated with the American Association of Physicists in Medicine and the American Society of Radiologic Technologists to create the Image Wisely campaign with the objective of lowering the amount of radiation used in medically necessary imaging studies and eliminating unnecessary procedures. Image Wisely offers resources and information to radiologists, medical physicists, other imaging practitioners, and patients.

J. A. Brink (✉)
Department of Diagnostic Radiology,
Yale University School of Medicine,
Tomkins East 2-230, 789 Howard Avenue,
New Haven, CT 06520-9128, USA
e-mail: james.brink@yale.edu

E. S. Amis
Department of Radiology,
Albert Einstein College of Medicine
and Montefiore Medical Center,
Department of Radiology, 111 E 210th St.,
Bronx, NY 10467-2401, USA

Since the discovery of the X-ray in 1895, imaging with ionizing radiation has revolutionized the practice of medicine. While many X-ray pioneers lost their digits, limbs, and lives to the harmful effects of the X-ray, much of the concern about potential harmful effects from medical radiation diminished to a low level in the several decades leading up to the turn of the century. In the last decade, largely due to evidence of carcinogenesis from low-level radiation experienced by survivors of the atomic bomb, imaging professionals, referring practitioners, patients, the public, and news media have mounted rising concerns about the potential carcinogenesis of medical imaging with ionizing radiation.

Radiologists have long been recognized as the purveyors of safe and effective use of ionizing radiation in medical imaging, and in the past several

D. Tack et al. (eds.), *Radiation Dose from Multidetector CT*, Medical Radiology. Diagnostic Imaging,
DOI: 10.1007/174_2011_504, © Springer-Verlag Berlin Heidelberg 2012 

years, radiologists have recognized the need to disseminate their knowledge broadly to the medical community, patients, and the public. Moreover, they have recognized the need for greater dissemination of best practices in dose optimization, monitoring, and control. As a result, in June 2009, the American College of Radiology (ACR) and the Radiological Society of North America (RSNA) established the Joint Task Force on Adult Radiation Protection (Brink and Amis 2010). The task force focused on medical imaging in adults as the Image Gently campaign had been established a few years earlier and was focused on pediatric imaging.

The Joint Task Force was charged to raise awareness of techniques to lower the amount of radiation used in adult medical imaging examinations to only that needed to acquire diagnostic medical images, and to heighten awareness of opportunities to reduce or eliminate unnecessary imaging examinations through adherence to best practice guidelines. Specifically, the task force was asked to consider a campaign to develop, catalog, and disseminate educational resources for imaging professionals, medical physicists, and imaging technologists who provide medical imaging services, and for referring physicians, patients, and the public who participate in medical imaging in one manner or another. Finally, the task force was charged to disseminate these educational resources using a wide array of electronic and print media. From its inception, the task force members also wished to institute initiatives through this campaign that would ensure adoption of best practices in dose optimization. Through social networking and marketing, the task force sought to involve other healthcare organizations, educational institutions, government agencies, and medical imaging equipment manufacturers in this initiative.

The task force first met in November 2009 and recommended a social marketing campaign targeted for adult medical imaging with ionizing radiation. The group quickly identified Image Wisely as an ideal name for this initiative, building in part on the successful moniker of the Image Gently campaign for pediatric imaging. A logo was developed (Fig. 1) composed of a wise owl with its tail in the shape of a 'W' to emphasize the 'wise' nature of our program's theme. With this logo, the task force hoped to establish a brand that would be instantly recognized when displayed in conjunction with educational materials and announcements of new opportunities for radiation dose monitoring and control in adult medical imaging. At its inaugural meeting, the task force also recognized the importance of widening the primary member institutions beyond the ACR and the RSNA to include medical physicists, as represented by the American Association of Physicists in Medicine (AAPM), and imaging technologists, as represented by the American Society of Radiologic Technologists (ASRT).

**Fig. 1** Image Wisely logo

While the Image Wisely campaign was inspired, in part, by the success of the Image Gently campaign for minimizing radiation exposure in children, the Image Wisely campaign for adults does not replicate the principles of Image Gently. This is due, in part, to differences in the sensitivity to ionizing radiation between the two populations. In children, the radiosensitivity of rapidly growing tissues in combination with their long life expectancy requires special considerations and precautions when imaging with ionizing radiation. Conversely, in adults, confounding variables such as advancing age and co-morbidities complicate assessment of the risks of medical imaging. Thus, the principles espoused in the Image Wisely campaign attempt to address these differences through its educational activities and programs about medical imaging in adults.

At its inception, Image Wisely campaign was planned to be executed in three distinct phases, ordered according to the magnitude of radiation exposure to the population in United States from medical imaging (NCRP 2009). The greatest population exposure from medical imaging comes from computed tomography, followed sequentially by nuclear medicine and radiography/fluoroscopy. In just one year after the task force was formed, Image Wisely launched a campaign targeting computed tomography at the annual meeting of the RSNA in November, 2010. In 2011, the second phase was launched targeting nuclear medicine, and in 2012, the third phase will be launched targeting radiography/fluoroscopy.

Many radiology organizations and professional societies have embarked on programs to educate imaging professionals, referring physicians, patients, and the public about the various issues associated with medical imaging with ionizing radiation. However, to date, there has not been an overarching educational program that organizes these collective educational offerings. The Image Wisely campaign seeks to answer that need by collecting and cataloging the best educational content and organizing it in a "tree of knowledge". This approach is the underpinning of the organizational structure for the Image Wisely website. Visitors to the website can approach a topic at a high-level and drill down with increasing levels of granularity through successive links on specific topics. Only the best educational content for a particular topic is included, and rather than simply providing links to the content, the website offers brief narratives that describe the content and put it into context. This format is replicated for the content targeting each group of imaging practitioners: imaging professionals, medical physicists, and imaging technologists. For referring physicians, the content is accessed through a "frequently asked questions" format. However, beneath each of these questions lies a hierarchical tree of knowledge similar to that described for the imaging practitioners.

Because imaging technology evolves rapidly, mechanisms for radiation protection, monitoring, and control change and evolve rapidly as well. And, because imaging technology is relatively complex, it is difficult for practitioners to keep pace with the latest innovations germane to their particular imaging equipment. Imaging equipment manufacturers often develop very different approaches to particular problems making it even more difficult for practitioners to be up-to-date with the latest advances specific to their imaging equipment. To help meet this need, the primary imaging equipment vendors have been solicited to provide micro-sites with the latest in user-specific technical innovations for radiation protection. These micro-sites are maintained by the vendors with links provided to the Image Wisely website. To date, the website content for imaging professionals, medical physicists, imaging technologists, and the vendor micro-sites are focused exclusively on computed tomography, whereas the content focused on referring physicians, patients, and the public is focused on medical imaging with ionizing radiation in general. With each successive phase of the Image Wisely implementation, additional sections of the website will be built out to accommodate the necessary content.

For patients and the public, many valuable resources have been developed that describe the benefits and risks of medical imaging with ionizing radiation in an easy-to-understand format. These include the radiology.info.org website that was developed jointly by the ACR and RSNA as well as the interactive radiation benefits-and-risks primer that was developed by the ACR. These resources allow patients and the public to understand the benefits of medical imaging while weighing them against the risks of ionizing radiation. Rather than re-inventing this educational content, the Image Wisely leadership decided that it was more than sufficient for patients and the public to get a good grasp of the issues related to ionizing radiation in medical imaging, and links to this content are provided to each of these resources. In addition, the ACR has developed video clips that address common questions for both adult and pediatric imaging with ionizing radiation. While these clips have appeared on television, links to this content are also provided through the Image Wisely website.

A key component of the Image Wisely campaign is the formal pledges taken by individuals among the targeted constituents, namely imaging professionals, medical physicists, and imaging technologists (Fig. 2). With launch of the Image Wisely program in 2010, a pledge specific to individual practitioners was made available, and within 1 year, over 10,000 individuals had committed to this pledge. However, from its inception, the Image Wisely leadership had intended to add higher levels of commitment for imaging facilities. Specifically, the Image Wisely leadership wished to go beyond simply adopting a pledge as proof that an individual imaging practitioner has embraced the Image Wisely principles and integrated them into his or her practice. In November 2011, at the start of the second year of the Image Wisely program, three additional pledges were made available: a pledge for imaging facilities, a pledge for referring physicians, and a pledge for professional associations (Figs. 3, 4, and 5, respectively). Imaging facilities offered the opportunity to achieve three levels of commitment. The first level of commitment involves pledging adherence to the principles of Image Wisely. For the second level of commitment, the imaging facility must participate in an accreditation program that focuses attention on radiation dose issues. And for the third level of commitment, the imaging facility must participate in a local, regional,

**Fig. 2** Image Wisely pledge for imaging professionals

**PLEDGE FOR IMAGING PROFESSIONALS**

Yes, I want to ***image wisely***.

I wish to optimize the use of radiation in imaging patients and thereby pledge:

1. to put my patient's safety, health and welfare first by optimizing imaging examinations to use only the radiation necessary to produce diagnostic quality images
2. to convey the principles of the Image Wisely Program to the imaging team in order to ensure that my facility optimizes its use of radiation when imaging patients
3. to communicate optimal patient imaging strategies to referring physicians, and to be available for consultation
4. to routinely review imaging protocols to ensure that the least radiation necessary to acquire a diagnostic quality image is used for each examination

or national dose index registry that allows benchmarking of radiation doses to population standards. For referring physicians, a simple form is provided to allow referring physicians the opportunity to pledge adherence to the principles of Image Wisely. For professional societies, rather than simply allowing them to join an alliance, the Image Wisely pledge allows them to make the commitment to promote the principles of Image Wisely among their members.

A new feature for the Image Wisely website that is presently under development is the radiation safety Case of the Fortnight. This feature will include a detailed case-based review of a key radiation safety principle in medical imaging. Patterned after the highly successful "Case in Point" popularized by the ACR, the radiation safety Case of the Fortnight promises to be a valuable addition to the educational offerings provided by Image Wisely with a blend of imaging physics and safety, a domain that is often neglected among continuing medical education offerings.

Marketing is a key component of campaigns such as Image Wisely and Image Gently, and the marketing departments of the ACR and the RSNA have done a tremendous job in getting the word out about these important initiatives. Banners, posters, and pins are among the many physical reminders that these organizations have developed to permeate the thoughts of the medical community with the principles of Image Wisely. Similarly, many multi-media marketing tools have been leveraged to promote the Image Wisely campaign. In addition, the marketing departments of the ACR and the RSNA have sought ways to integrate the principles of Image Wisely with those of Image Gently whenever possible. To this end, they have developed a joint poster for the 2011 annual meeting of the RSNA entitled "One-Size-Fits-All?", and effort to remind both adult and pediatric imaging practitioners of the importance of body habitus on parameter selection for medical imaging (Fig. 5).

With the launch of the second phase of Image Wisely targeting nuclear medicine, many of Image Wisely's achievements for computed tomography may translate to this arena, however some may not. While instrumentation greatly affects the radiation dose that may be achieved with each modality, important differences exist between CT and nuclear medicine, primarily related to the fact that CT is a transmission technology and nuclear medicine is an emission technology. In CT, X-rays are transmitted through the body from an X-ray source to an X-ray detector. Conversely, in nuclear medicine, radiation is emitted from radioactive tracers that are administered to the body. Thus, the educational content for nuclear medicine may differ in style and substance from that of CT. Representatives from the Society of Nuclear Medicine, the American Society of Nuclear Cardiology, the Society of Nuclear Medicine Technologists, as well as the four founding societies of Image Wisely met recently to plan the Image Wisely initiative for nuclear medicine. A "tree of knowledge" approach

**Fig. 3** Image Wisely pledge for imaging facilities

PLEDGE FOR FACILITIES

*Would your CT facility like to demonstrate its radiation safety awareness? You may do so by meeting one of the following* ***Image Wisely Levels of Commitment:***

**LEVEL 1** – Take the Image Wisely pledge

1. All imaging physicians interpreting CT exams and technologists performing CT scans must have an understanding of the radiation exposure involved in CT so as to be able to properly advise patients undergoing CT imaging.
2. CT doses should be optimized to the lowest levels required to produce images containing all necessary information for accurate interpretation (dose optimization).
3. The CT practice should comply with currently available recommendations for default CT dose protocols (AAPM, NCRP, ACR, etc.).
4. Whenever possible, automatic CT exposure control and other dose reduction methodologies (i.e. vendor supplied programs) should be employed to minimize patient exposure.
5. The CT practice should manually or electronically monitor CT dose indices for common examinations, compare these indices with established benchmarks, and evaluate outliers on a timely basis to prevent unnecessary exposure to patients or images with insufficient diagnostic information.
6. The practice should review the number of CT scans performed on patients with repetitive CT scans and notify the ordering physician when the total number of exams appear excessive relative to the expected clinical benefit.*
7. The radiology practice should be consultative in nature and provide ongoing education to referring practitioners on risks and benefits of CT imaging.

**Ideally, this process could be automated or semi-automated if ordering is via a suitable computerized physician order entry (CPOE) system. In the absence of a suitable CPOE system, this may be accomplished when the exam protocol is prescribed by the radiologist, or designated health care professional, for individual patients prior to their CT scans. This approach would not prevent placement of the order for CT, but should raise awareness of prior exposure, suggest consideration of the risk/benefit ratio, and reference the ACR Appropriateness Criteria for alternative imaging algorithms.*

**LEVEL 2** – Level 1 + Earn accreditation from an organization that directly evaluates the following radiation-related attributes:

- Radiation dose indices and compliance with accreditation pass/fail thresholds
- Clinical image quality (peer-reviewed by an external, qualified interpreting physician)
- Phantom image quality (peer-reviewed by an external, qualified medical physicist)
- Personnel (qualifications set by the accrediting organization)
- 

**LEVEL 3** – Level 2 + Participate in a dose index registry (*local or national*) that includes routine evaluation of procedures and dose indices

**Fig. 4** Image Wisely pledge for referring practitioners

**PLEDGE FOR REFERRING PRACTITIONERS**

I have reviewed the Image Wisely webpage for "Referring Practitioners" and pledge to the following:

1. I will educate myself regarding the relative radiation exposures for the various imaging exams which use ionizing radiation (plain x-rays, fluoroscopic studies, CT scans, and nuclear medicine studies). In my practice, I will balance the medical benefit to my patients for any of these imaging exams I order against any potential radiation risk associated with that exam.

2. I will consult, as needed, with professionals specializing in medical imaging (radiology, nuclear medicine, ultrasound, and magnetic resonance imaging) in order to choose the most appropriate imaging examinations for my patients.

**Fig. 5** Image Wisely pledge for professional associations

**PLEDGE FOR ASSOCIATIONS**

We will endorse and promote among our members the goals of Image Wisely to raise awareness throughout the medical community of opportunities to eliminate unnecessary imaging exams and to lower the amount of radiation used in necessary imaging exams to only that needed to capture optimal medical images.

was planned that will be focused on three broad areas: general nuclear medicine, PET/CT, and nuclear cardiology. Within general nuclear medicine and PET/CT, sub-sections will involve specific organ systems, radiopharmacy, and instrumentation. Within nuclear cardiology, sub-sections will address myocardial perfusion imaging with SPECT and PET/CT as well as gated blood pool imaging. With careful planning, the nuclear medicine initiative promises to be an important contribution to radiation protection for nuclear medicine imaging procedures.

In summary, the Image Wisely campaign has contributed greatly to radiation protection in adult medical imaging. Within the first year, over 10,000 individual practitioners pledged to adhere to the principles of Image Wisely. In the second year of the campaign, educational content is being developed for nuclear medicine, and additional pledges have been developed for imaging facilities, referring practitioners, and professional organizations. Imaging facilities have the opportunity to pledge at three levels of commitment. Beyond simply endorsing the principles of Image Wisely, facilities may embrace a second level of commitment involving accreditation by an organization that focuses on radiation protection, monitoring, and control. The third level of commitment involves participation in a dose index registry on either a local, regional, or national level. Referring physicians can pledge to commit to the principles of Image Wisely as can professional organizations. In this next year of the campaign, we hope to greatly widen the scope of education, commitment, and action regarding radiation protection, monitoring, and control in adult medical imaging.

## References

Brink JA, Amis ES (2010) Image Wisely: a campaign to increase awareness about adult radiation protection. Radiology 257:601–602

National Council on Radiation Protection and Measurements (2009) Ionizing radiation exposure of the population of the United States, NCRP Report No. 160, Bethesda

# Guidelines for Appropriate CT Imaging

Kristie M. Guite, J. Louis Hinshaw, Frank N. Ranallo, and Fred T. Lee

## Contents



**Abstract**

Computed Tomography (CT) is now used to diagnose or guide management of virtually every disease state. However, this increase in CT use is associated with a rapid increase in medical radiation exposure. In response, there has been increased emphasis on reducing the radiation exposure associated with CT. This includes both using alternate imaging modalities and optimizing the technical parameters of the CT scans that are performed. An insidious and often overlooked source of medical radiation exposure is multi-phasic examinations. Multiple CT phases (before and after contrast administration, delayed imaging, and venous and arterial phases among others) can be highly useful for certain specific clinical indications. However, when used incorrectly, multi-phase examinations multiply radiation dose for no benefit. In response to the need for guidelines for appropriate CT use, the American College of Radiology has created appropriateness criteria to provide guidance regarding the most efficacious use of multi-phase CT.

**Abbreviations**

| | |
|---|---|
| CT | Computed tomography |
| kVp | Kilovoltage |
| ma | Milliamperes |
| CTA | Computed tomography angiography |
| CTU | Computed tomography urography |
| MRI | Magnetic resonance imaging |
| ACR | American college of radiology |

K. M. Guite · J. L. Hinshaw (✉) · F. N. Ranallo · F. T. Lee
Departments of Radiology, University of Wisconsin, Mail Code 3252, 600 Highland Avenue, Madison, WI 53792, USA
e-mail: jhinshaw@uwhealth.org

F. N. Ranallo
Departments of Medical Physics, University of Wisconsin, Madison, WI, USA

D. Tack et al. (eds.), *Radiation Dose from Multidetector CT*, Medical Radiology. Diagnostic Imaging,
DOI: 10.1007/174_2011_528, 

## 1 Introduction

Computed Tomography (CT) was first introduced as a medical device in the 1970s, and has since become ubiquitous as an imaging tool. Recent technical advances including faster scan times, improved spatial resolution, and advanced multi-planar reconstruction techniques have allowed CT to be used for virtually every anatomic abnormality. Approximately 3 million scans were performed annually in the United States in 1980, but by 2008 that number had grown to 67 million and continues to rise (Gazelle et al. 2007). Over two-thirds of all medical radiation is attributable to CT, with 75% of CT scans being performed in the hospital setting. Approximately 40% of CT scans performed of the head/neck/spine, 10% of the chest, 47% of the abdomen/pelvis, and the remainder of the extremities or as a procedural tool (Brenner and Hall 2007; Mettler et al. 2000; Brix et al. 2009).

Along with the increased number of scans, an increasing awareness of medical radiation has permeated the popular and scientific press resulting in an emphasis by many organizations on reducing overall medical radiation exposure. The significance of the increased radiation exposure to the population caused by CT remains unclear. High levels of ionizing radiation exposure are known to increase cancer risk (Pierce and Preston 2000; Pierce et al. 1950; Muirhead 2003) but the data for lower doses of radiation, like those seen during medical imaging (including CT), is less clear and remains controversial (Mezerich 2008; Cardis et al. 2005; Little et al. 2009). Therefore, in the absence of clarity on this topic, the American College of Radiology (ACR), Health Physics Society (HPS), and other interested organizations have adopted the principles of *As Low As Reasonably Achievable (ALARA)*, *Image Gently* in pediatrics and *Image Wisely* in adults. The common theme of all of these statements is that physicians should limit radiation exposure to only what is medically necessary (Committee on the Biological Effects of Ionizing Radiation 1990; ICRP 1991).

Most strategies to reduce radiation associated with CT have focused on vetting CT as the appropriate diagnostic test, limiting the examination to the anatomic area in question, and optimizing scanning parameters (such as kVp and mA) (Tack et al. 2003; Paterson et al. 2001; Greess et al. 2002). Particularly in pediatrics, the *Image Gently* campaign has placed a large amount of emphasis on reducing radiation exposure through the preferential use of other imaging modalities instead of CT. If CT is felt to be necessary, applying optimized technical parameters and limiting the scan area can substantially reduce radiation exposure and result in dose reductions as high as 65% (ICRP 19901991; Greess et al. 2002). These important techniques are described in other chapters of this book and are not our focus. Rather, we will concentrate on an important, but potentially overlooked source of unnecessary medically radiation, namely, the use of multi-phase examinations when a single or lesser number of phases would suffice (Guite et al. 2011).

## 2 Potential CT Phases

The different phases that are possible with state-of-the-art CT scanners are myriad and include scanning before and after contrast administration, delayed imaging, venous and arterial phases, and several others (Table 1). These phases are performed for a variety of indications and may be useful in identifying specific patterns of contrast enhancement, or evolution of findings over time, which can dramatically aid in diagnosis. However, these additional phases are only necessary in very specific clinical scenarios, and need to be used judiciously as each phase will result in an additional CT scan of the area in question. When multi-phase examinations are performed with the same technical parameters as the original phase, the radiation dose is multiplied by the number of phases. Therefore, it is important that the scans are clinically indicated and relevant.

## 3 Use of Multiphasic CT

Multi-phase CT examinations are extremely useful in a subset of patients. The temptation in a busy practice is to perform CT with a "one size fits all" approach, so as to not miss the opportunity to characterize a potential finding. This approach requires the use of multi-phase scans to cover all potential scenarios, but since most patients do not benefit from additional phases, this practice results in unnecessary radiation for the majority of patients. The dose-multiplication

**Table 1** Common indications for multiphase CT

| Potential CT phases | Reason |
|---|---|
| Non-contrast | Identify calcifications |
| Contrast enhanced | Evaluate for soft tissue abnormalities and patterns of enhancement |
| Angiography | Evaluate vascular anatomy |
| Arterial phase imaging | Identify hypervascular processes |
| Portal venous phase imaging | Most routine imaging is performed with this phase |
| Delayed | Timing depends on indication. Can be used to characterize cholangiocarcinoma, adrenal adenomas, renal and urothelial masses, or for the evaluation of trauma patients |
| *Renal* | |
| Corticomedullary phase | Identification of renal cortical abnormalities |
| Nephrogenic phase | Characterization and improved visualization of renal masses |
| Excretory phase | Evaluate the renal collecting system |

effect of these unnecessary phases can be dramatically reduced or eliminated with individual tailoring of CT examinations to the specific clinical scenario (Guite et al. 2011). In an attempt to address this issue, the ACR has developed evidence and expert opinion-based appropriateness criteria matching scanning protocols with specific phase selections for various clinical conditions, and these will be the focus of our subsequent discussion (Criteria 2008).

There are individual ACR appropriateness criteria for the most common indications for diagnostic radiology, interventional radiology, and radiation oncology. For each indication in the appropriateness criteria, the varying imaging modalities are ranked, separating out the phases in CT, with one being the least appropriate study for the given indication and nine being the most appropriate. More specifically, the rating scale is as follows: usually not appropriate studies are given scores of 1–3, studies that may be appropriate are given scores of 4–6, and the studies that are usually appropriate are given scores of 7–9. Similarly, the Royal College of Radiology has also developed guidelines for the same purpose and these guidelines have many similarities to, but are not identical to the ACR guidelines (Royal College of Radiologists 2007). For the purposes of this discussion, we will attempt to describe relatively universally accepted utilization patterns for CT phases and while these recommendations are primarily based upon the ACR guidelines, we also recommend that you become familiar with the guidelines in use in the region in which you practice.

The majority of CT imaging in the head, chest, and extremities are performed with single-phase imaging and will not be specifically addressed. However, abdominal imaging is associated with many potential uses for multiple-phase imaging and will be discussed in detail. The majority of abdominal and pelvic CT's can be performed using a single-phase, but the evaluation of some tumor types (hepatic/pancreatic/renal), the urinary collecting system, and trauma patients among others, may be best evaluated with multiple phases.

## 4 Indications for CT by Phase

In discussing the numerous phases and indications for CT, it should be noted that best patient care requires individualized CT protocols based upon each patient's specific symptoms, pathology, and underlying comorbidities. Although labor intensive, this provides the highest likelihood of an accurate diagnosis with the lowest necessary radiation dose. The following discussion will provide a basic outline of current best practice, but for a more complete list of guidelines, the ACR appropriateness criteria can be found on the ACR website (http://www.acr.org/ac).

## 5 Unenhanced CT

Non-contrast CT scans (Fig. 1) are of limited use for the differentiation of soft tissue structures. However, various materials such as blood, calcium (renal stones, vascular

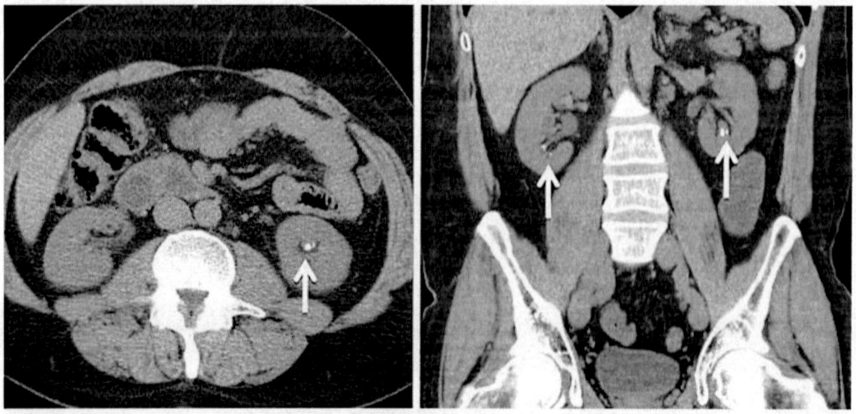

**Fig. 1** Non-contrast CT demonstrating multiple bilateral renal calculi (*arrows*); axial *left*, coronal reformat on *right*

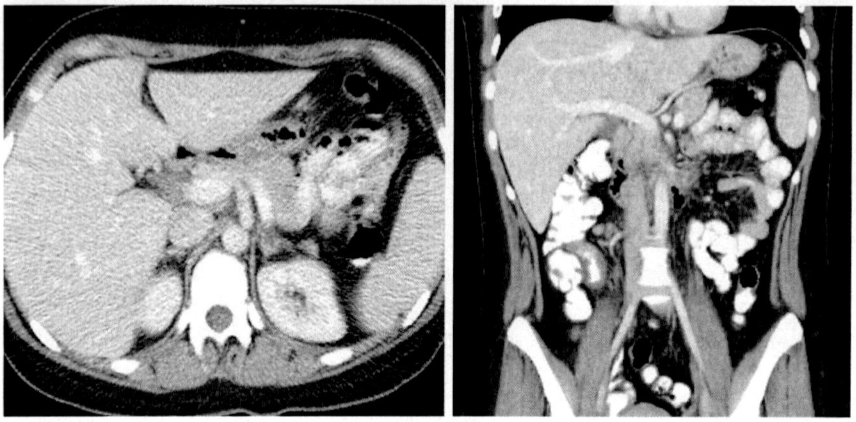

**Fig. 2** Contrast enhanced CT demonstrating parenchymal enhancement of the intra-abdominal organs (axial *left*, coronal reformat *right*)

atherosclerosis), bone, pancreas, and pulmonary parenchyma are highly visible and can be assessed with non-contrast CT. For example, non-contrast CT of the brain is typically performed as an initial screen in stroke, in altered mental status/dementia, trauma, and follow-up examinations. In the chest, pulmonary parenchyma is well visualized due to the high intrinsic contrast with aerated lung. Thus, pulmonary nodules are best evaluated with non-contrast CT imaging. In the abdomen and pelvis, there are several indications for non-contrast imaging such as the evaluation of renal calculi, some cases of bleeding, evaluation of various vascular abnormalities (including aneurysm and dissection), prerenal transplantation, and evaluation of the pancreas (in combination with contrast phases). Lastly, in the extremities, non-contrast CT scans are used in the evaluation for fractures and surgical planning, sometimes with 3D reconstructions.

## 6 Contrast Enhanced

Intravenous enhanced contrast enhanced CT examinations are acquired at a specific time after intravenous contrast injection (timing is dependent on the phase of contrast enhancement needed and organ system being evaluated). The timing is chosen to ensure contrast distribution within the solid organ parenchyma in question (Fig. 2). Single-phase contrast enhanced imaging of the abdomen is most commonly performed utilizing a single phase with opacification of the portal vein and solid abdominal organs. These scans are used in the evaluation of nonspecific abdominal pain, hernia, infection, masses (in any location with a few exceptions such as hypervascular tumors, renal, hepatic, and others), and in most follow-up examinations.

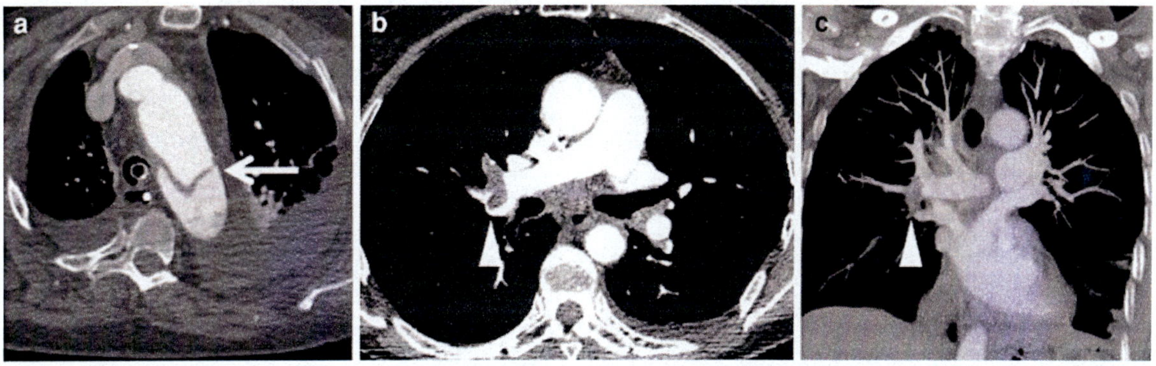


**Fig. 3** **a** CT angiography of the thoracic aorta which demonstrates a dissection (*arrow*) along the aortic arch/descending aorta. **b** CT angiography of the pulmonary arteries in evaluation of pulmonary embolus which demonstrates a large pulmonary embolus in the right main pulmonary artery (*arrowheads*). **c** Coronal reformation of the PE study in b

## 7 Arterial Phase

Arterial phase imaging is timed to correspond to the peak concentration of contrast material in the arteries or highly vascular tumors (approximately 15–35 s after the injection of intravenous contrast) and are generally divided into early (arteries) and late (hypervascular tumors) arterial phases. Arterial phase imaging is frequently used in conjunction with other phases to obtain complete information. Indications for arterial phase imaging include: evaluation of aneurysms or dissections (cerebral, aortic, etc.), hepatic, splanchnic or renal arterial anatomy, arterial imaging in liver or kidney transplantation, and the evaluation of specific tumors including hepatic, renal, and pancreatic neoplasms. Of note, hepatic masses are typically evaluated with both arterial- and venous-phase CT scans (biphasic imaging). Renal masses will be discussed under the renal imaging section. Single arterial phase imaging is often used in the evaluation of trauma patients, and in the evaluation for pulmonary emboli.

## 8 CT Angiography

CT angiography (CTA) is highly effective for evaluation of the arterial system, and has largely replaced conventional angiography due to the lower risk profile. Images are acquired after a rapid bolus of intravenous contrast material (3–7 cc/s) during the arterial phase (15–35 s after injection) when the concentration of contrast material in the arterial system is high (Figs. 3a–c. Images are usually acquired using narrow collimation (<1 mm) and can be retrospectively reconstructed using dedicated three-dimensional workstations and software. CTA is commonly used in the evaluation of pulmonary emboli, aneurysms, vascular malformations, dissection, and ischemia. CTA can also be used to evaluate for bleeding sources, and in the evaluation of the extremity vasculature.

## 9 Portal Venous Phase

Portal venous phase imaging (Fig. 4b) can be used alone (as this is typically the phase performed for a single contrast enhanced CT) or in combination with other phases in the evaluation for hepatic pathology. CT images are acquired after the injection of intravenous contrast when the portal vein is opacified (60–90 s after injection) to specifically evaluate enhancement of the hepatic parenchyma. Portal venous phase images are occasionally used in conjunction with other phases, such as the late arterial phase, to specifically evaluate contrast enhancement and washout patterns of hepatic tumors. Additionally, this phase can also be used for evaluation of the biliary tract, and for the evaluation of small bowel and mesentery and can be part of a CT enterography examination.

## 10 Delayed Phase

Delayed phase imaging (Fig. 5) encompasses scanning at a variety of different times following contrast administration, and depends on the pathology in

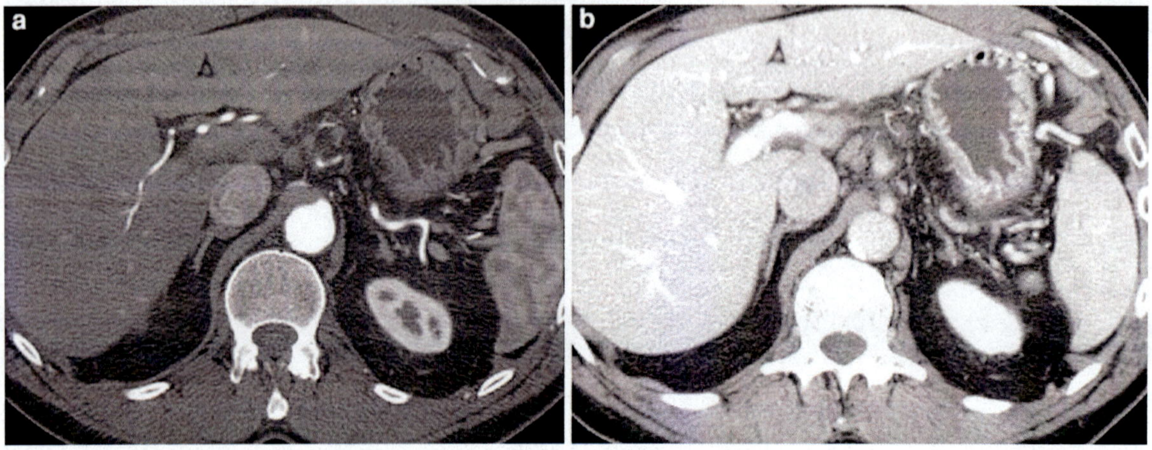


**Fig. 4** Biphasic liver CT. This includes an hepatic (late) arterial phase (**a**) where the aorta, hepatic artery, and splenic artery are opacified with contrast; however, the portal vein and other venous structures are not. This phase is used to look for arterially enhancing lesions or arterial anatomy. A portal venous phase (**b**) is also performed. In this phase, the portal vein is opacified and the solid organ parenchyma is enhancing which can be used to evaluate for patterns of contrast enhancement/washout

question. The most common indications for delayed phase imaging are evaluation of the kidneys, collecting system (ureters and bladder), and specific kidney, liver, and adrenal tumors (Boland et al. 1997; Lacomis et al. 1997). In addition, delayed phase images can also be used in the evaluation of active vascular extravasation in trauma patients. Typical delayed imaging times range from a few minutes to up to 15 min or sometimes even longer. For the evaluation for adrenal adenomas or cholangiocarcinoma, a delayed scan 10–15 min following contrast administration can be performed.

## 11 Renal Imaging

Detection and characterization of renal parenchymal masses is a frequent indication for CT. An initial non-contrast CT is important for detecting calcium or fat in a lesion, and to provide baseline attenuation of any renal masses. After the injection of intravenous contrast, a corticomedullary phase is obtained at approximately 70 s. The corticomedullary phase is characterized predominantly by enhancement of the renal cortex as well as the renal vasculature. This phase is valuable in the evaluation of benign renal variants, lymphadenopathy, and vasculature. There is minimal enhancement of the medulla and collecting system in this phase of imaging. The parenchymal phase is obtained approximately 100–200 s after the injection of contrast material. Parenchymal phase imaging demonstrates continued enhancement of the cortex, enhancement of the medulla, and various levels of contrast material in the collecting system. The parenchymal phase is highly important for the detection and characterization of renal masses, parenchymal abnormalities, and the renal collecting system (Szolar et al. 1997) (Figs. 6, 7).

## 12 CT Urography

CT urography (CTU) is commonly used in the evaluation of hematuria, and specifically tailored to image the renal collecting system, ureters, and bladder in addition to the renal parenchyma. Initial imaging includes a non-contrast phase to detect renal calculi as a source of hematuria. Note that dual energy CT may eventually allow the non-contrast phase to be eliminated. Contrast enhancement techniques for CTU vary from institution to institution. A common technique used at our institution and others is a double bolus, single-phase imaging algorithm. This technique is a hybrid contrast injection strategy that results in opacification of both the renal parenchyma (parenchymal phase) and the collecting system, ureters, and bladder (excretory phase). At our institution, a small contrast bolus is administered initially, followed 10 min later with a larger bolus that is

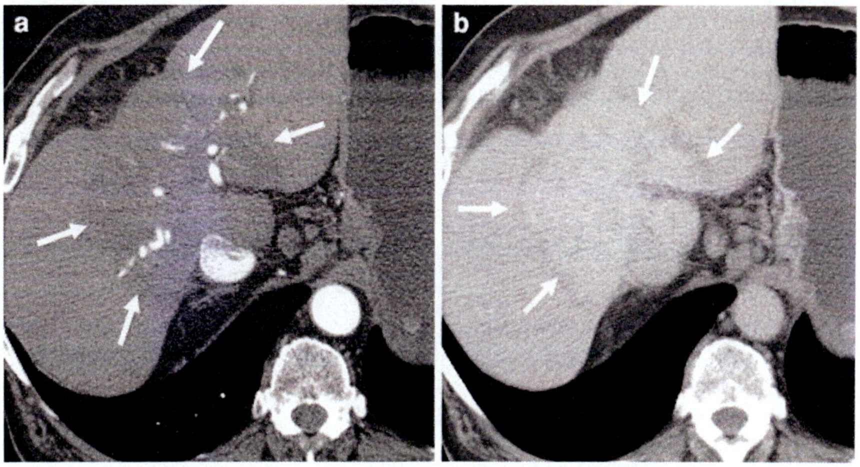


**Fig. 5** **a** Portal venous phase abdominal CT demonstrates a low attenuation mass (*arrows*) in the liver. **b** 15 minute delayed image demonstrates delayed enhancement of the liver mass (*arrows*) characteristic of cholangiocarcinoma

imaged in the corticomedullary phase. This ensures that contrast is being excreted by the kidneys and thus the collecting system is opacificed (excretory phase) from the initial injection, and that the renal parenchyma is enhancing as well from the second injection (parenchymal phase). At the conclusion of our urography protocol, we also perform a scout image in the supine and prone position to allow a global evaluation of the collecting system. Excretory phase imaging allows for not only evaluation of the ureteral lumen, but also periureteral abnormalities including external masses and lymphadenopathy (Caoili et al. 2003).

## 13 Incidental Findings

Incidental findings are noted in approximately 5–16% of patients scanned for an unrelated clinical indication (Pickhardt et al. 2008; Hassan et al. 2008). Complete characterization of incidental findings may require further scanning phases such as arterial phase (certain liver tumors) or delayed images (adrenal lesions). However, it is not acceptable practice to anticipate the possibility of incidental lesions and prospectively add additional phases to routine protocols. Unfortunately, several recent surveys demonstrated that this practice is more common than might be anticipated, and contributes to unnecessary medical radiation exposure to a large population of patients (Guite et al. 2011). Even more egregious is the fact that many of these findings could potentially be even more accurately evaluated with other non-radiation imaging modalities such as MRI or ultrasound.

Although the management of incidental findings is not the focus of this chapter, some of these findings will require further workup and this will be briefly addressed. Management of incidental findings has been controversial because they are relatively common, particularly in older populations and additional studies, particularly CT scans may be required for further characterization of what is frequently a benign finding. In an effort to provide guidance on which incidental findings should be appropriately further evaluated and what the appropriate imaging modality should be, the ACR published a white paper on management of incidental findings found on CT of the abdomen in 2010 (Berland et al. 2010).

## 14 Integrated Decision Support

Computerized order entry as part of an electronic medical record has streamlined the ordering process for all tests, including imaging. At least some of the exponential increase in the use of CT is related to the ease with which an order can be placed and executed. There is an associated need for decision support systems to aid clinicians in ordering imaging studies in an evidence-based manner. Several software programs have been developed for this purpose and are under investigation (Sistrom et al. 2009; Rosenthal et al. 2006). These programs are designed to help clinicians by determining what, if any, imaging modality is most appropriate based upon a given clinical scenario. Based upon the recommendations, clinicians may choose to change the study to

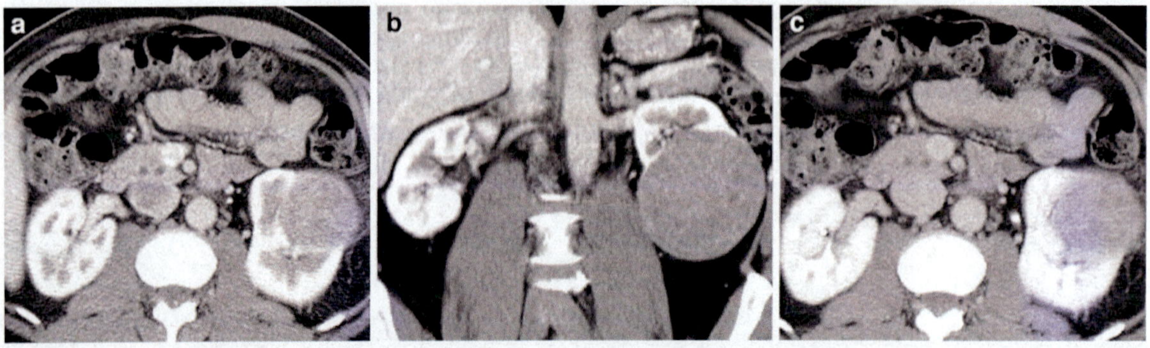

**Fig. 6** Corticomedullary phase (axial—**a**) demonstrates peripheral enhancement of the renal cortex with minimal opacification of the renal medulla. There is a large renal cell carcinoma in the *right* kidney which can be differentiated from the normal renal parenchyma by the heterogeneous and differential enhancement. The renal artery and vein are opacified in this phase as well. The collecting system is not opacified (coronal reformat—**b**). In the parenchmyal phase the renal cortex and the medulla are enhancing. The renal cell carcinoma in the *left* kidney is not as well defined when compared to the corticomedullary phase images, but is actually slightly more conspicuous. There is some contrast noted within the collecting system during this phase (**c**)

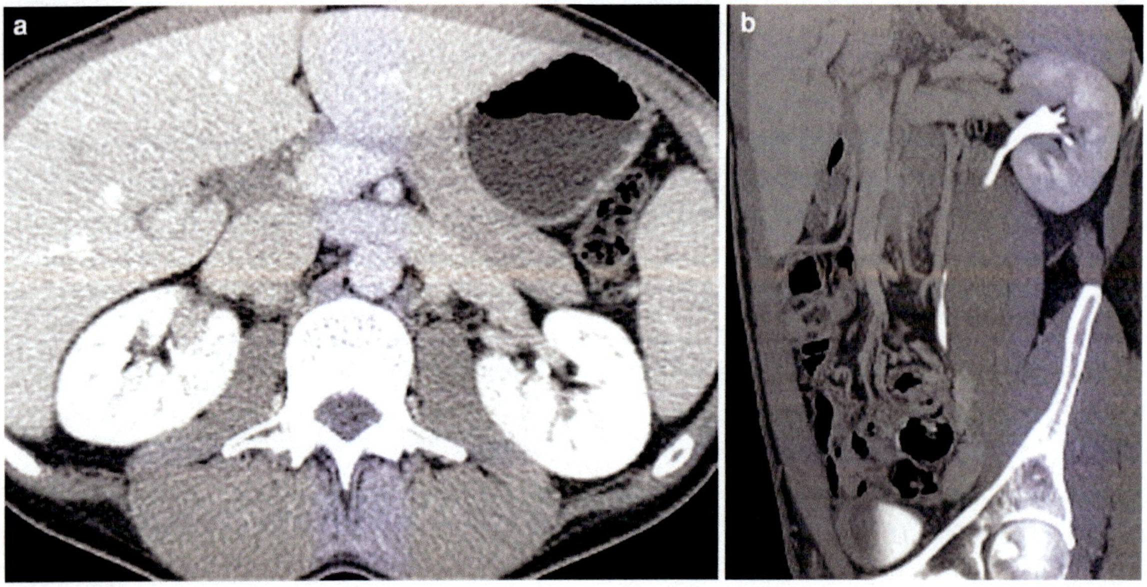

**Fig. 7** **a** This renal parenchymal phase again demonstrates enhancement of the renal cortex and medulla but no contrast within the collecting system. **b** With the double bolus technique of CT Urography, there is enhancement of the renal parenchyma and contrast within the renal calyces, renal pelvis, and ureter allowing evaluation of both

a more appropriate one, or they may choose to override the recommendation if they still feel that the original study is more appropriate. Interestingly, studies have shown that even with these systems in place, only 0.2% of providers change their initial order to the recommended study and when there is a duplicate study within one month, only 0.5% of requests were altered to reflect that fact (Bowen et al. 2011). This suggests that these systems may only have a small impact on ordering habits, but despite these findings, integrated decision support software has been shown to be successful in reducing the growth rate of CT use in the outpatient setting (Sistrom et al. 2009).

## 15 Conclusion

Multi-phase CT examinations are very important for the detection and characterization of certain clinical conditions, but should not be generalized for every patient undergoing CT of the abdomen and pelvis. A recent survey demonstrated that many physicians are routinely performing multi-phase CT for the majority of patients in an attempt to prospectively characterize potential lesions detected during the scan. However, unindicated multi-phase CT examinations are an important source of medical radiation that does not contribute to the care of patients. Adherence to published standards such as the ACR Appropriateness Criteria can both decrease medical radiation and optimize imaging for the specific clinical indication.

## References

ACR Appropriateness Criteria (2008) http://acr.org/acr

Berland LL, Silverman SG, Gore RM, Mayo-Smith WW, Megibow AJ, Yee J, Brink JA, Baker ME, Federle MP, Foley WD, Francis IR, Herts BR, Israel GM, Krinsky G, Platt JF, Shuman WP, Taylor AJ (2010) Managing incidental findings on abdominal CT: white paper of the ACR incidental findings committee. J Am Coll Radiol 7:754–773

Boland GW, Hahn PF, Pena C, Mueller PR (1997) Adrenal masses: characterization with delayed contrast-enhanced CT. Radiology 202:693–696

Bowen S, Johnson K, Reed MH, Zhang L, Curry L (2011) The effect of incorporating guidelines into a computerized, order entry system for diagnostic imaging. J Am Coll Radiol 8:251–258

Brenner DJ, Hall EJ (2007) Computed tomography—an increasing source of radiation exposure. NEJM 357: 2277–2284

Brix G, Nissen-Meyer S, Lechel U et al (2009) Radiation exposures of cancer patients from medical X-rays: how relevant are they for individual patients and population exposure? Eur J Radiol 72(2):342–347

Caoili EM, Inampudi P, Cohan RH et al (2003) MDCTU of upper tract uroepithelial malignancy. Am J Roentgenol 180:71

Cardis E, Vrijheid M, Blettner M et al (2005) Risk of cancer after low doses of ionizing radiation: retrospective cohort study in 15 countries. BMJ 331–377

Committee on the Biological Effects of Ionizing Radiation (1990) Health effects of exposure to low levels of ionizing radiation. National academy Press, Washington

Gazelle SG, Halpern EF et al (2007) Utilization of diagnostic medical imaging: comparison of radiologist referral versus same-specialty referral. Radiology 245(2):517–522

Greess H, Nomayr A, Wolf H, Baum U et al (2002) Dose reduction in CT examinations of children by an attenuation-based on-line modulation of tube current (CARE dose). Eur Radiol 12:1571–1576

Guite KM, Hinshaw JL, Ranallo FN, Lindstrom MJ, Lee FT (2011) Ionizing radiation in abdominal computed tomography: unindicated muliphase scans are an important source of medically unnecessary exposure. J Am Coll Radiol 8:756–761

Hassan C, Pickhardt PJ, Laghi A et al (2008) Computed tomographic colonography to screen for colorectal cancer, extracolonic cancer, and aortic aneurysm: model simulation with cost-effectiveness analysis. Arch Intern Med 168:696–705

ICRP (1991) 1990 Recommendations of the international commission on radiological protection. ICRP publication no 60. Pergamon, Oxford

Lacomis JM, Baron RL, Oliver JH 3rd, Nalesnik MA, Federle MP (1997) Cholangiocarcinoma: delayed CT contrast enhancement patterns 203(1):98–104

Little MP, Wakeford R, Tawn JE, Bouffler SD, Berrington de Gonzalez A (2009) Risks associated with low doses and low dose rates of ionizing radiation: why linearity may be (almost) the best we can do. Radiology 251(1):6–12

Mettler FA Jr, Wiest PW, Locken JA, Kelsey CA (2000) CT scanning: pattern of use and dose. J Radiol Prot 204:353–359

Mezerich R (2008) Are CT scans carcinogenic? Am Coll Radiol 5:691–693

Muirhead CR (2003) Studies on the Hiroshima and Nagasaki Survivors, and their use in estimating radiation risks. Radiat Prot Dosim 104:331–335

Paterson A, Frush D, Donnelly LF (2001) Helical CT of the body: are settings adjusted for pediatric patients? Am J Radiol 176:297–301

Pickhardt PJ, Hanson ME, Vanness DJ et al (2008) Unsuspected extracolonic findings at screening CT colonography: clinical and economic impact. Radiology 249:151–159

Pierce DA, Preston DL (2000) Radiation-related cancer risks at low doses among atomic bomb survivors. Radiat Res 154:178–186

Pierce DA, Shimizu Y, Preston DL, Vaeth M, Mabuchi K (1996) Studies of the mortality of atomic bomb survivors. Report 12, Part I. Cancer-1950–1990. Radiat Res 146:1–27

Rosenthal DI, Weilburg JB, Schultz T et al (2006) Radiology order entry with decision support: initial clinical experience. J Am Coll Radiol 3:799–806

Royal College of Radiologists (2007) Making the best use of clinical radiology services: referral guidelines, 6th edn. Royal College of Radiologists, London

Sistrom CL, Dang PA, Weilburg JB, Dreyer KJ, Rosenthal DI, Thrall JH (2009) Effect of computerized order entry with integrated decision support on the growth of outpatient procedure volumes: sever year time series analysis. Radiology 251(1):147–155

Szolar DH, Kammerhuber F, Altzieber S et al (1997) Multiphasic helical CT of the kidney: increased conspicuity for detection and characterization of small (<3 cm) renal masses. Radiology 201:211–217

Tack D, De Maertelaer V, Gevenois PA (2003) Dose reduction in multidetector ct using attenuation-based online tube current modulation. Am J Roentgenol 181:331–334

# Part VI

# Vendor Perspective on CT Radiation Dose

# Practical Approaches to Dose Reduction: GE Perspective

Roy A. Nilsen

## Contents




**Abstract**

This chapter will cover the GE perspective on controlling CT dose through system design features in both hardware and software. We will show how GE scanners have been designed to optimize the dose delivered while achieving the image quality required for the clinical task.


## 1 Optimizing Image Quality and Dose Through Software Features

### 1.1 Adaptive Filtration

Techniques exist to reduce noise (pixel standard deviation) in CT through the choice of reconstruction kernel and image space smoothing. These basic techniques can come with a significant trade off in image resolution for noise reduction. To address this, GE Healthcare has developed a suite of advanced adaptive image filters. These filters recognize the features in the image and modify their processing to give significant noise reduction while minimizing the effect on resolution. Small regions of voxels are examined to determine the presence and orientation of image features. The image smoothing is then adjusted to retain, or possibly enhance, the features while still achieving the desired noise reduction. Conversely, uniform smoothing can be applied in regions without image features.

Some examples of this type of feature in current GE Healthcare systems are:


R. A. Nilsen (✉)
GE Healthcare, Waukesha, WI, USA
e-mail: Roy.Nilsen@med.ge.com



D. Tack et al. (eds.), *Radiation Dose from Multidetector CT*, Medical Radiology. Diagnostic Imaging,
DOI: 10.1007/174_2011_486,

1. ECG-Gated Cardiac—A suite of specific filters have been developed to deal with the specific challenges and features of cardiac imaging. Half-scan reconstruction and the lower mA present outside of the targeted heart phase lead to potentially higher noise in this class of clinical procedure. Three cardiac imaging adaptive filters are provided to reduce noise while maintaining heart anatomy-specific edges in cardiac imaging modes for all patient sizes including obese. Reductions in dose of upto 10–30% have been demonstrated by leveraging these adaptive filtration techniques.
2. Neuro—A suite of three-dimensional filters tuned for the challenges and characteristics of neuro imaging have been developed. The specific issues inherent in brain imaging have been addressed to allow for additional noise reduction. These filters are user selectable in head protocols to allow for improvement in image quality or dose reduction.

Filtration can also take place in the projection data before image reconstruction. By examining the signal levels and characteristics of each view, filtration is appropriately applied in each case. This is especially important in areas of large, asymmetric anatomy where there is high electronic noise in low signal rays relative to quantum noise due to the interaction of radiation with matter. The adaptive low signal processing adjusts its strength to the quality of the signal for each view and ray. Dramatic differences in the signal quality and noise statics across the views used to reconstruct an image can lead to significant streaking artifacts.

Use of these filtration techniques allow our customers to push the scanning techniques to their lower limit, while retaining sufficient diagnostic image quality.

## 1.2 Statistical Iterative Reconstruction Algorithms

Among such techniques as optimizing scan protocols, filtering and modulating the X-ray beam around the patient, or minimizing the range of exposure, the image reconstruction itself is an area often overlooked. Indeed, the same analytical Filtered Back-Projection (FBP) algorithm has been used as the foundation of commercially available CT reconstruction techniques since the 1970s. Its well-known advantages are speed and a simple closed-form solution available from a single pass over the acquired data. It is still widely used today and considered acceptable for clinical diagnosis, but it does not provide optimal results for depiction of the patient (Thibault 2010).

This is apparent in the inherent level of artifacts and noise in FBP images. In fact, FBP fails to account for a fundamental component of data acquisition: it simply ignores that the projection data are corrupted by quantum noise and electronic noise during acquisition.

Instead, it may propagate and sometimes amplify noise into patient images, creating streaks, artifacts, and potentially hiding pathology, and valuable diagnostic information. This makes low dose imaging with standard reconstruction techniques a significant challenge for radiologists and technologists.

Rather than building upon FBP and its limitations, GE Healthcare has invested many years of research into building from the ground a powerful class of new reconstruction algorithms, which are designed to explicitly include the description of data statistics into the reconstruction. With ASiR™, commercially available since 2008 (auntminnie.com 2009; diagnosticimaging.com 2009), and now with Veo™*, the world's first Model-Based Iterative Reconstruction (MBIR) product (Budovec et al. 2008), GE Healthcare makes it possible to generate low dose CT images that may reveal pathology previously hidden in noise, all without sacrificing detail in the usual manner of classical analytical techniques. Advanced statistical algorithms can extract more information from the same CT data that would normally yield poor results using FBP-based approaches, allowing radiologists greater confidence in their diagnosis from images with improved image quality at lower dose (Fig. 1).

### 1.2.1 Veo™: The Model-Based Paradigm

The key to such algorithms lies in the ability to accurately model the interactions of radiation with matter as X-rays are produced in the tube, attenuated through the CT system and the patient, measured at the detector, and transformed into digital signal (Thibault 2010).

The fundamental concept is that a physically realistic algorithm will achieve reconstruction results significantly better than a technique that assumes the

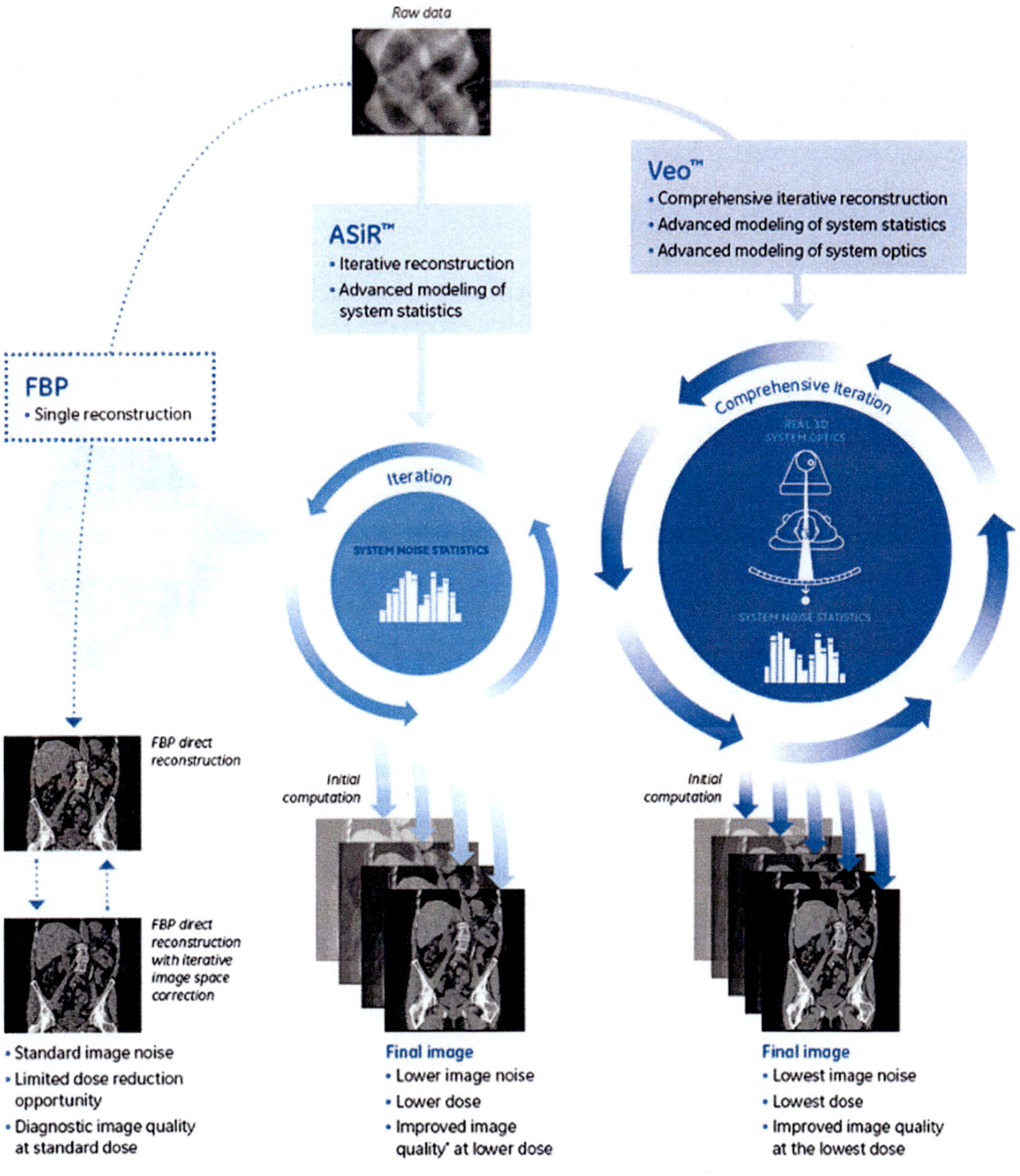


**Fig. 1** Comparison of the reconstruction flows of FBP, ASiR$^{TM}$, and Veo$^{TM}$ ("Veo$^{TM}$ CT model-based iterative reconstruction" by Jean-Baptiste Thibault PhD, © 2010 General Electric Company)

signal is perfect like FBP because it describes more accurately the real data acquisition process.

The problem of CT reconstruction is turned into that of estimating the image that represents the projection data under a statistical metric based on the physics of data acquisition and desired image properties.

Individual models for measured noise statistics, system optics, radiation and detection physics, medical image characteristics, etc., can be developed independently with as few approximations as possible to provide a faithful representation of the actual scanning process. The collection of all these models is

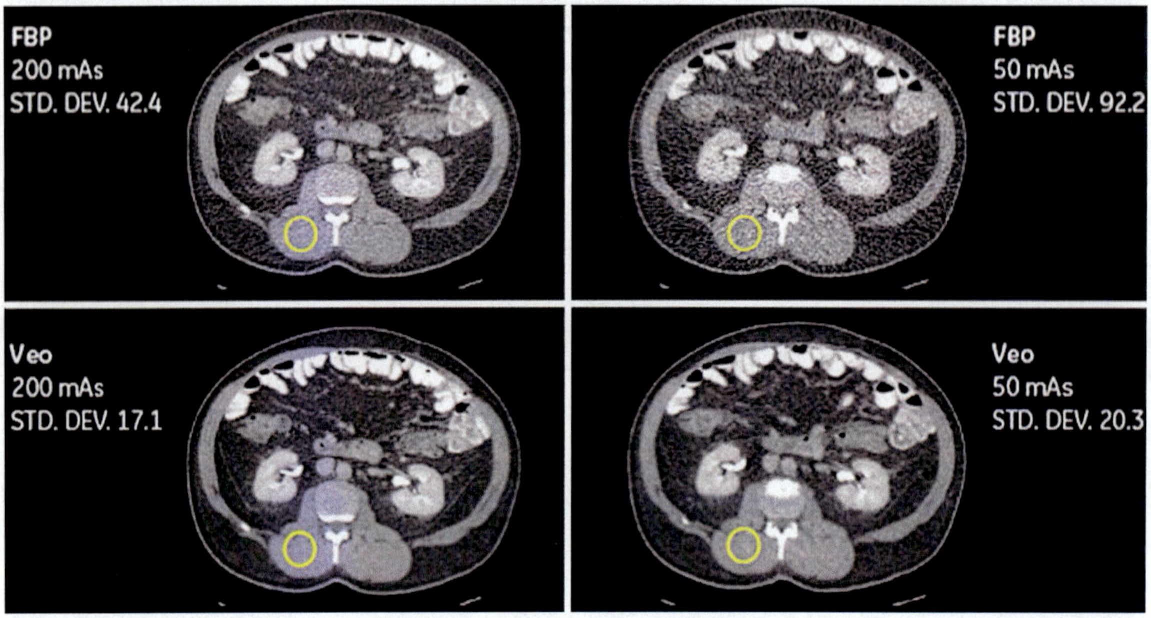


**Fig. 2** Illustration of image quality in low-dose abdominal CT scanning at two different dose levels of 200 and 50 mAs, respective, from a multi-dose prospective study conducted at Massachusetts General Hospital (images courtesy of Dr. Kalra, MD)

fed into a mathematical formulation to describe the reconstructed image in a manner representative of the way the corresponding projection data was acquired. The resulting function is optimized to find the best possible match between the reconstructed image and the acquired projection data given the knowledge of the CT system operation. This model-based approach originates from the inverse problem of predicting what projection data should be given to the scanned object. It compares the projection data synthesized from the combined model to the real data in order to minimize discrepancies while disallowing the propagation of noise into the image and enforcing desirable constraints for a medical image.

To further assess possible clinical impact, a prospective pilot study was led by Dr. Mannudeep Kalra, Professor of Radiology at the Massachusetts General Hospital, to compare objective noise between FBP and MBIR in low-dose abdominal CT examinations acquired at multiple dose levels on large patients (Singh et al. 2009).

Figure 2 illustrates some reconstructed images of 0.625 mm thickness at 200 and 50 mAs. While noise (pixel standard deviation) was found to increase markedly in standard FBP images, no significant difference was observed in the MBIR images: model-based reconstruction does not trade off higher noise for improved resolution in the usual manner of FBP. No significant artifacts were seen either. Although signal degradation is significant at the low end of the dose range, the impact on texture in the MBIR images did not diminish clinical relevance. This analysis suggests that model-based reconstruction may allow significant dose reduction for abdominal CT scanning without affecting noise or artifacts, or may offer higher image quality without compromise at the same dose.

These results illustrate how statistical reconstruction offers expanded options for patient management compared to standard reconstruction: with a model-based approach such as Veo, radiologists can use the improved resolution versus noise trade off to enhance image quality from a standard acquisition protocol, or they can image patients at significantly lower dose without sacrificing quality. A balance may also be chosen to achieve dose reduction together with improving image quality relative to today's standards.

### 1.2.2 Adaptive Statistical Iterative Reconstruction (ASiR$^{TM}$)

Adaptive Statistical Iterative Reconstruction (ASiR) is a reconstruction technique that may enable reduction in image pixel standard deviation. The ASiR

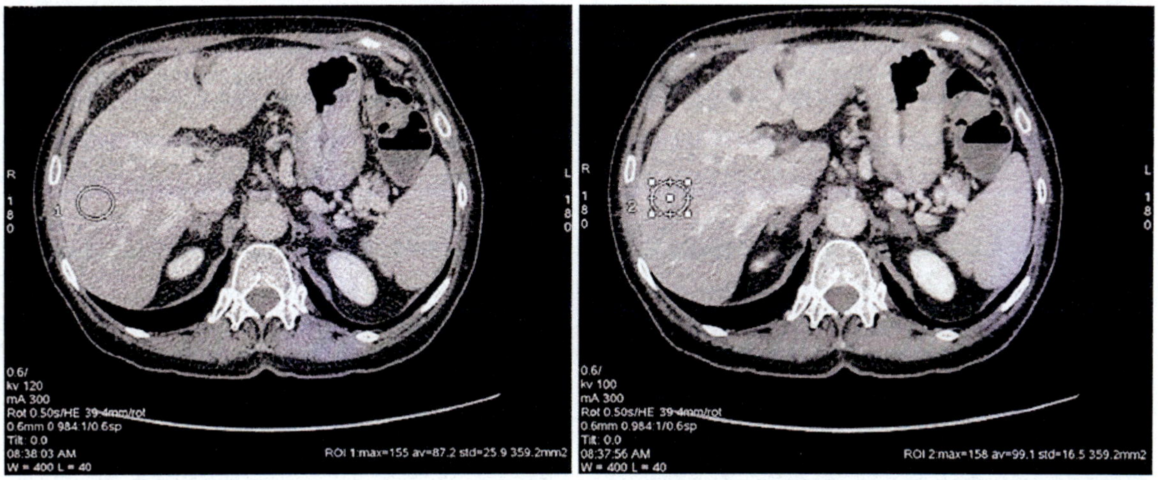


**Fig. 3** ASiR image on right demonstrating noise suppression combined with low contrast detectability increase. "ASiR", GE Healthcare online information (http://www.gehealthcare.com/usen/ct/products/asir.html)

reconstruction algorithm may allow for reduced mA in the acquisition of diagnostic images, thereby reducing the dose required. ASiR may also enable improvement in low contrast detectability.

#### 1.2.2.1 Theory

ASiR studies how noise propagates through the reconstruction steps to feed this model back into the loop and iteratively reduce noise in the reconstructed image without affecting other properties such as detail. To keep complexity down to a minimum and facilitate fast convergence, ASiR uses the same idealized system optics representation as FBP and results in similar data utilization per image.

MBIR, on the other hand, directly weighs each individual data point to give noisy projections lower influence on the final result than less noisy projections, which eliminates correlated noise and streaks arising from non-circular objects. The metric applied to the discrepancy between each measured projection point and the estimated image is weighted by this factor to minimize the noise content in the reconstructed image (Thibault 2010).

#### 1.2.2.2 Features

ASiR reconstruction is available in two modes:

- Slice Mode ASiR
- Volume Mode ASiR

The two modes are user selectable for thin slice acquisitions, but the slice mode is available for all slice thickness settings.

In addition to providing a selection of the mode of ASiR reconstruction, the scanner allows the user to select levels of ASiR settings from 0 to 100% in 10% increments. These "levels" or "blend levels" provide a varying degree of noise (pixel standard deviation) removal from the images. In order to enable the user to select the right level of ASiR, an ASiR review tool is provided that allows the user to change the settings and review the images for each protocol.

Volume mode is applied to 0.625 mm slice thickness and slice mode is applied to 1.25, 2.5, and 5 mm slice thicknesses (GE Healthcare System Documentation 2011; Fig. 3).

## 1.3 Pediatric Protocol Selection Through Color-Coding for Kids

For over 20 years, the Broselow–Luten system has been used in emergency departments (ED) to facilitate care and reduce medical errors. The system categorizes children into one of eight color zones based on their weight and size. With these color-coded categories, clinicians can determine a safe medication dose and utilize appropriately sized equipment (GE Healthcare CT Publication 2007).

Radiation and contrast dose remain a primary concern when conducting CT scans of pediatric patients. To address this, Donald P. Frush, M.D., Chief of Pediatric Radiology at Duke Children's Hospital and Health Center (CHC), developed the

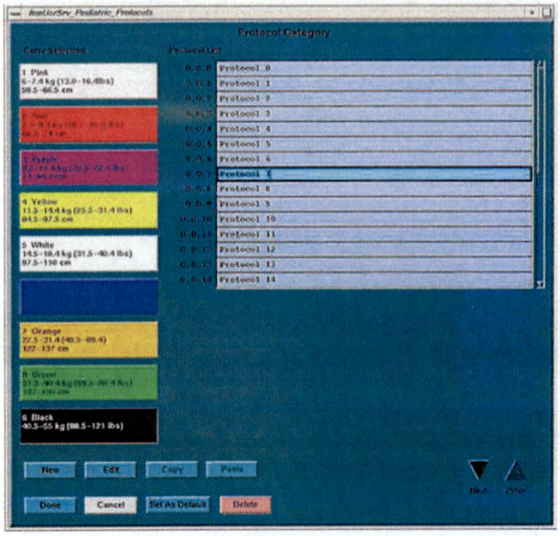


**Fig. 4** Length and weight based color-coding for kids protocol identification speeds selection and reduces error in pediatric protocol selection ("FeatherLight, Technology for Dose Optimization" © 2008, GE Healthcare)

Broselow–Luten color-coding protocols for use with GE's LightSpeed® scanners, and are also available on the BrightSpeed product line. In 2001, GE became the first CT manufacturer to introduce preloaded pediatric protocols based on the child's color classification.

"By implementing color-coding for kids, GE seized a major leadership role to lower dose in children and help improve the way physicians scan children with CT," said Dr. Frush.

His research with CT examinations revealed the system helps medical professionals provide more expedient and standardized care while maintaining clinical confidence.

Use of GE's color-coding for kids CT protocols has also helped facilities conform to the standard radiation safety principle, As Low As Reasonably Achievable (ALARA), as well as the FDA's public health notification of 2001 that emphasized the importance of adjusting CT scanner parameters according to the patient's size and weight.

Today, color-coding for kids on GE's LightSpeed® VCT is routine at Duke's CHC. Children are first classified according to the Broselow–Luten system, for example, a 35-pound child would be classified as "white." With the "white" color classification, a nurse can use the system as a guide to administer the appropriate color-coded "white" dose of contrast and the technologist selects the "white" protocol on the CT Scanner.

Dr. Frush's experience with color-coding for kids on the LightSpeed VCT has made a significant impact. "Many of the questions regarding radiation dose are addressed by this method. Plus, our technologists overwhelmingly prefer this method as it helps simplify protocol selection and performance" (Fig. 4).

## 1.4 Dose Display and Reporting

The standard CT dose values of $CTDI_{vol}$, DLP and CTDI phantom size are reported by GE Healthcare CT scanners. This information is shown before the scan to be evaluated by the operator and reported after the scan. The post-scan reports take two forms: a text page breakdown by scan groups and the DICOM Radiation Dose Structured Report (RDSR). Production of the RDSR allows GE Healthcare CT scanners to be compliant with the IHE-Radiation Exposure Monitoring (IHE-REM) standard. The RDSR allows for electronic tracking, analysis, and recording of CT Dose information.

## 1.5 Dose Check

The dose check feature intends to notify and alert the operating personnel, generally technologists that prepare and set the scan parameters, prior to starting a scan, whether the estimated dose index is above the value defined and set by the operating group, practice, or institution to warrant notification to the operator. The dose check feature is designed to comply with the NEMA XR-25 standard (GE Healthcare CT Publication 2011).

Dose check is designed to be a tool that enables users to be more aware of the associated dose index of the scan they are prescribing, and provides a "Notification" upon confirming the scan or saving the protocol if that dose index is above the institution's established range for the protocol element. This notification level is intended to be set at a level that would be considered above "routine" or "normally expected" dose, but not at such a high level as to pose a significant risk to the patient. In fact, depending on patient size or imaging need it may be appropriate to

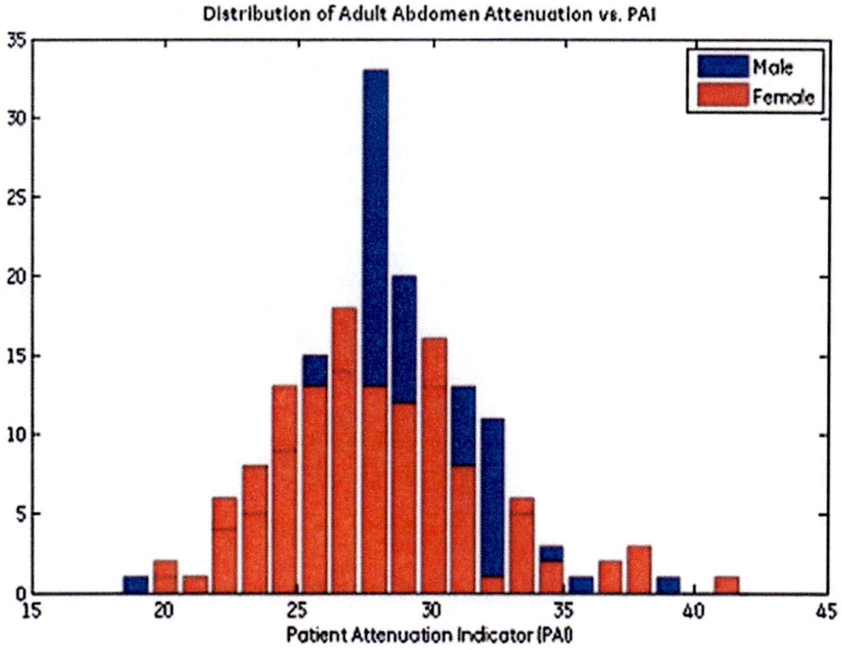


**Fig. 5** Adult abdominal patient distribution in terms of average patient attenuation ("Discovery™ CT750 HD Technical Reference Manual", © 2011 General Electric Company)

scan at a value above the Notification Value in order to achieve the diagnostic intent of the exam.

Notification values are not necessarily the same as published "Diagnostic Reference Values" (DRLs); however, these may be consulted as a guide in helping to determine the appropriate notification value for your site and patient population. Because routine scanning involves a range of applicable techniques due to patient sizes and imaging needs, another consideration on where to set the notification level will be the frequency in which your practice would want it posted. GE encourages sites' to establish appropriate notification values for pediatric scanning. The dose check feature also provides an "Alert" upon confirming when the dose exceeds a value determined by the institution that represents a value above which the accumulated dose index value would be well above the institution's established range for the examination, potentially excessive, that warrants more stringent review and consideration before proceeding.

## 1.6 System Software for X-Ray Exposure Control

A key step in performing a high quality diagnostic imaging examination is matching the scan technique to the clinical need and patient size. GE Healthcare has developed AutomA to assist in this process. AutomA is a powerful tool, but it is critical that healthcare professionals continue to use their judgment when deciding whether and precisely how, to employ CT scanning techniques.

### 1.6.1 AutomA

#### 1.6.1.1 Background

A significant factor in the quality of a CT image is the amount of X-ray quantum noise contained in the scan data used to reconstruct the image. Most technologists know how the choices of X-ray scan technique factors affect image noise. That is, noise decreases with the inverse square root of the mAs and slice thickness. Noise also decreases approximately inversely with kVp. For example, increasing the mA from 50 to 200 (a factor of 4) will decrease quantum noise by a factor of 2 (the square root of 4). Quantum noise also increases with increasing helical pitch; however, the exact relationship is dependent on the details of the helical reconstruction process (GE Healthcare System Documentation 2011).

The most significant factor that influences the quantum noise in the scan data is the X-ray attenuation of the patient section being scanned. The X-ray attenuation is related to the size and tissue composition of the patient section. Figure 5 shows a

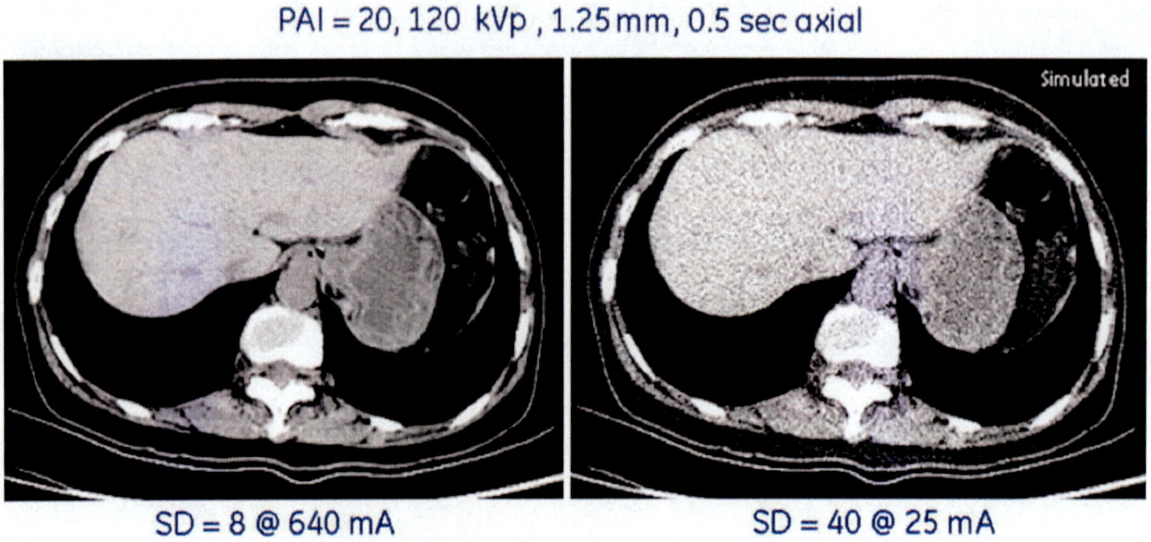


**Fig. 6** Example small patient (PAI = 20) with factor of five noise increase (simulated) ("Discovery™ CT750 HD Technical Reference Manual", © 2011 General Electric Company)

distribution of patient attenuation area values (PAA) for adult abdominal images that ranges from 19–41 with a mean of 27.6 (for this patient sample set). The patient attenuation area (also called the Patient Attenuation Indicator, PAI) (Toth et al. 2006) is computed for the patient section as the square root of the product of the sum of raw pixel attenuation values times the pixel area.

For a given fixed scan technique, the quantum noise varies by about a factor of 5 from the smallest to the largest patients attenuation (PAI range of 17– 41). Figure 6 shows an example of a five times noise increase simulated for a small patient (20 PAI). With a fixed mA scan protocol, the technologist must select the mA using a qualitative estimate of the patient attenuation. This is may be accomplished using patients weight, diameter measurements, body mass index, or just as a qualitative visual classification. Because these methods provide very rough X-ray attenuation estimates and do not account for attenuation changes within the patient region being scanned, the technologist must use a high enough technique margin to avoid the possibility of compromising the diagnostic quality of the images with too much noise. Since dose is inversely related to the square of the noise, many patients are likely to be receiving more dose than necessary for the required diagnostic quality using such manual methods. Automatic tube current modulation: AutomA is an automatic tube current modulation feature that can make necessary mA adjustments more accurately than those estimated for the patient by the user and thereby can obtain a more consistent desired image noise in spite of the wide range of patients. Since image noise variability is substantially reduced, a significant overall patient dose reduction is possible with proper scan parameter selection.

AutomA (Z-axis modulation) adjusts the tube current to maintain a user selected quantum noise level in the image data. It regulates the noise in the final image to a level desired by the user. AutomA is the CT equivalent of the auto exposure control systems employed for many years in conventional X-ray systems. The goal of AutomA is to make all images contain similar X-ray quantum noise independent of patient size and anatomy. The AutomA tube current modulation is determined from the attenuation and shape of scout scan projections of the patient just prior to CT examination sequence.

SmartmA (angular or xy modulation) has a different objective than Z-modulation. It adjusts the tube current to minimize X-rays over angles that have less importance in reducing the overall image noise content. In anatomy that is highly asymmetric, such as the shoulders, X-rays are significantly less attenuated in antero-posterior (AP) direction than in the lateral

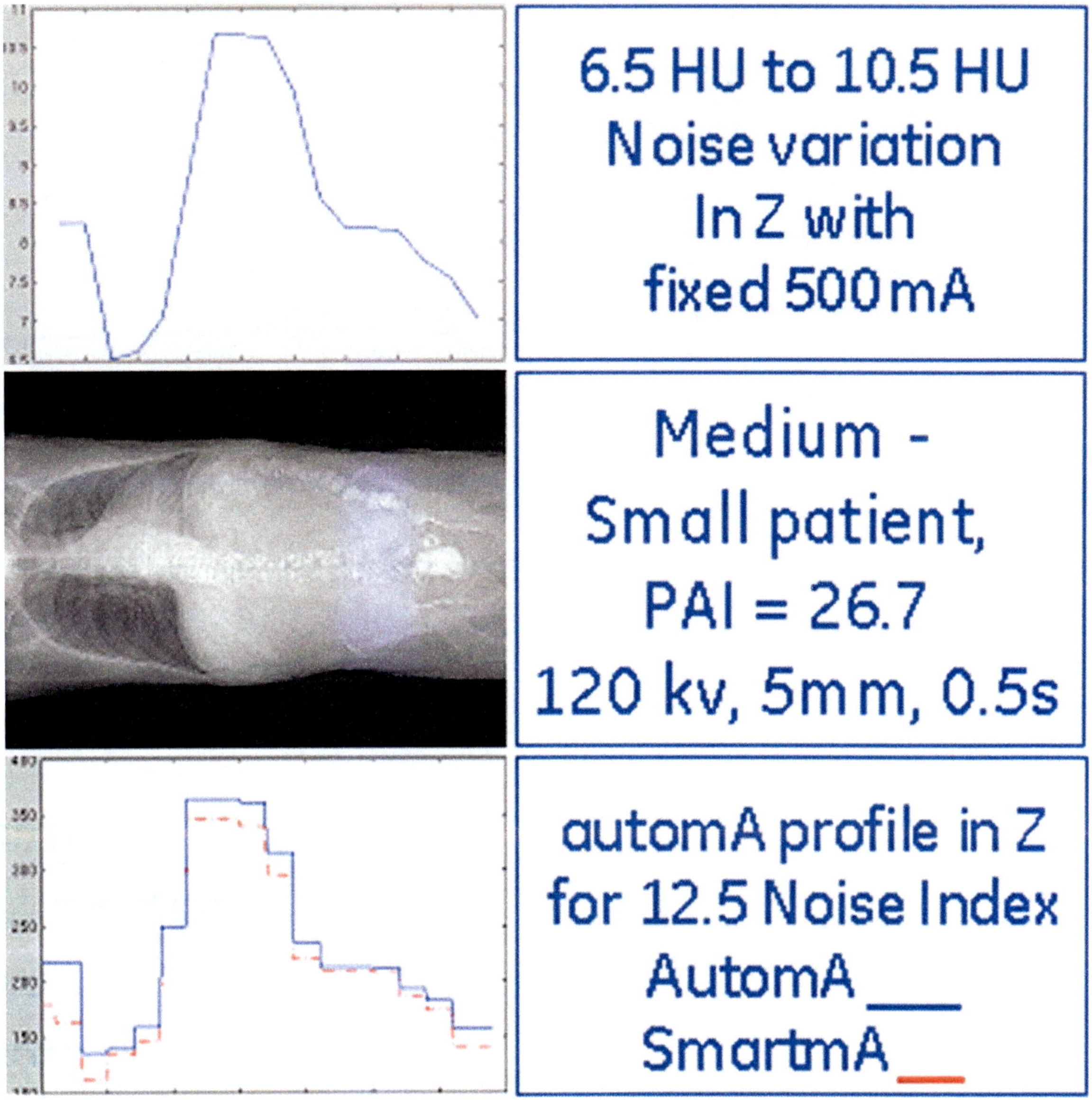


**Fig. 7** Example noise variation with fixed mA and mA variation with AutomA with a Noise Index setting ("Discovery™ CT750 HD Technical Reference Manual", © 2011 General Electric Company)

direction. Thus, the overwhelming abundance of AP X-rays can be substantially reduced without a significant effect on overall image noise. Angular modulation was first introduced in GE single slice scanners in 1994 (Kopka and Funke 1995; Jacobson et al 1996).

#### 1.6.1.2 AutomA Theory

AutomA is an automatic exposure control system that employs Z-axis tube current modulation and is available on GE multislice scanners. A noise index parameter allows the user to select the amount of X-ray noise that will be present in the reconstructed images. Using a single patient scout exposure, the CT system computes the required mA to be used based on the selected Noise Index setting. The Noise Index value will approximately equal the standard deviation in the central region of the image when a uniform phantom (with the patient's attenuation characteristics) is scanned and reconstructed using the standard reconstruction algorithm (Fig. 7).

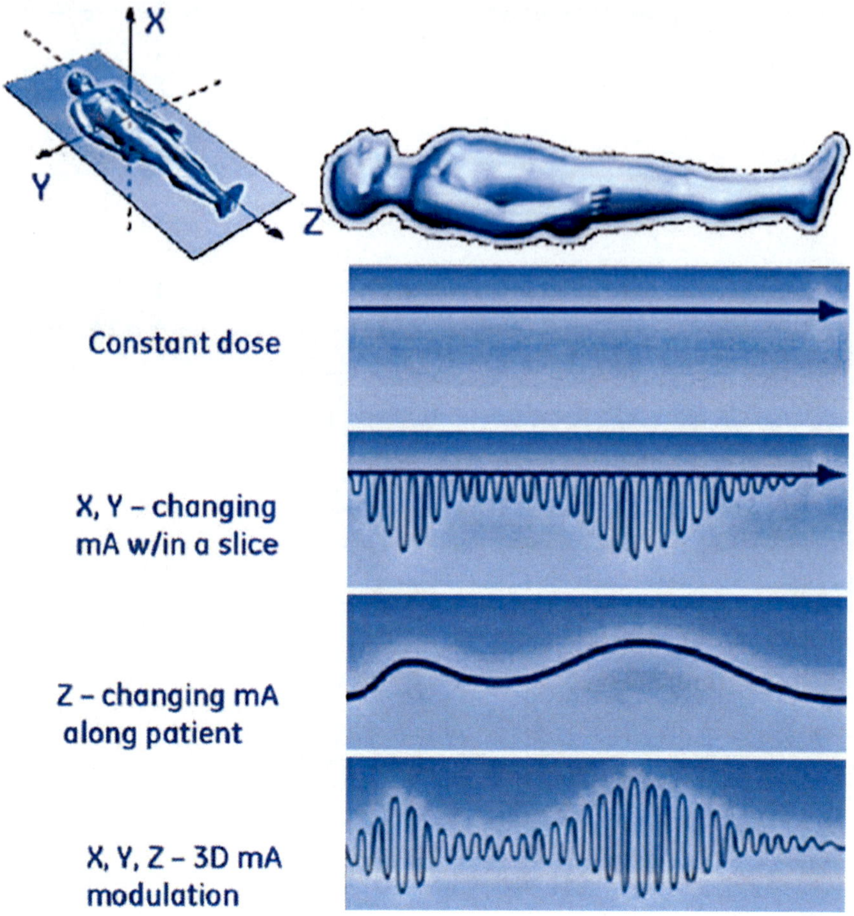


**Fig. 8** GE Healthcare's "Auto mA" and "Smart mA" techniques for mA modulation. GE Healthcare online training, AutomA/SmartmA Theory" (http://www.gehealthcare.com/usen/education/tip_app/docs/AutomA-SmartmA%20Theory.pdf)

The system determines the tube current using the patient's scout projection data and a set of empirically determined noise prediction coefficients for a reference technique. The reference technique is the selected kVp, and an arbitrary 2.5 mm slice at 100 mAs for an axial reconstruction using the standard reconstruction algorithm. The scout projections contain density, size and shape information about the patient. The total projection attenuation (projection area) contains the patient density and size information and the amplitude and width of the projection contains the patient shape information. These patient characteristics determine how much X-ray will reach the detector for a specified technique and hence predict the image standard deviation due to X-ray noise for the standard reconstruction algorithm.

To predict the image noise at a given z position for the reference technique, the projection area and oval ratio are obtained from the patient's scout. The oval ratio is an estimate of the patient asymmetry that is determined from the amplitude and width of the projection data.

The expected X-ray noise for the reference technique (reference noise) is then calculated as a function of the projection area and oval ratio from the scout using polynomial coefficients that were determined by a least squares fit of the noise measurements from a set of phantoms representing a clinical range of patient sizes and shapes. Knowing the reference noise and the difference between the reference technique and the selected prescribed technique, the mA required to obtain the prescribed Noise Index is calculated using well-known X-ray physics equations. That is, the noise is inversely related to the square root of the number of photons and the number of photons is proportional to the slice thickness, slice acquisition time, and mA. In the GE AutomA design, an adjustment factor for helical pitches is also incorporated in the calculation to account for noise differences that scale between helical selections and the axial reference technique (Fig. 8).

AutomA provides a framework to adapt the scanning technique to each patient based on the user input of Noise Index and mA limits. A key point to remember is that any automatic exposure control system must be well understood and used properly in order to achieve the benefits which the system is designed to deliver. Improper use can lead to several unintended consequences, including higher doses than warranted or expected, poor image quality, the need to re-scan, or other issues with the quality of the diagnostic examination.

## 1.7 Cardiac Imaging

Cardiac CT Angiography (CTA) is an area requiring special consideration for dose reduction. Retrospectively gated studies can result in in-effective dose utilization. The use of only the portion of the data pertaining to the phases of interest, combined with the required low pitch can leave a significant portion of the scan data unused. Prospectively integrating the ECG signal in the scan acquisition enables multiple avenues for dose optimization.GE Healthcare has implemented two techniques for minimizing the X-ray exposure outside of the heart phase(s) of interest.

### 1.7.1 Electrocardiograph Tube Current Modulation

Modulating tube current based on an electrocardiograph (ECG) signal is a technical innovation that significantly reduces radiation dose to cardiac patients. The concept is based on the fundamental principles of cardiac CT imaging (GE Healthcare System Documentation 2011).

#### 1.7.1.1 ECG-Modulated mA Theory

The motion of the heart has always been challenging for diagnostic imaging of the heart and surrounding areas. Motion can cause blurring and mis-registration of artifacts in images. Cardiac CT acquires images when the heart motion is minimal. The motion is generally least near the end of the diastolic phase of the cardiac cycle. The motion is generally greatest during the systolic phase of the cardiac cycle, in which the heart is contracting. The ECG-modulation feature takes advantage of this fact, and only provides full tube current to the patient during the diastolic period of the cardiac cycle, which is most likely to produce the best image quality. The tube current is modulated to a lower mA setting during systole to decrease the dose to the patient.

ECG-modulated mA applies to cardiac helical scans only. Cardiac helical acquisitions utilize retrospectively gated reconstructions. Without ECG-modulation, radiation is on for the entire length of the scan and images can be created at any phase of the cardiac cycle. ECG electrodes are connected to the patient prior to the scan and an ECG monitor stores the ECG data during the scan. The scanner measures one full heart period as the time from one QRS complex to the next.

The QRS complex is the portion of the ECG waveform corresponding to ventricular depolarization signaling contractions. A particular time period in the cardiac cycle is prescribed in terms of a percent phase of the heart period. With the ECG gating information and acquisition data from the entire scan, the image reconstruction software can retrospectively create images centered on any phase in the cardiac cycle. For most patients, 75% is considered to be the best phase for imaging of the coronary arteries.

The ECG-modulated mA feature requires the user to input the maximum and minimum tube current values and the start and end cardiac phase for the tube to be at maximum current for each cycle. Minimum tube current can be no less than 20% of the maximum. Twenty percent of the peak mA may yield adequate image quality at systole to assess cardiac function from images generated outside of the maximum mA phases. Start and end phases can be prescribed from 0 to 99% of the cardiac cycle. The scan will start off at the maximum tube current. The algorithm uses a moving average of the heart periods to predict when the next QRS complex will occur. Once the initial average is set, the system will start modulating the tube current. To guarantee the tube current is at the minimum and maximum values when it should be, the system must take into account the time required for the generator to ramp the tube up to maximum current and down to minimum current.

In the event that the patient should experience a preventricular contraction (PVC) or a missed beat, there is the possibility that the images at full mA could become shifted from the prescribed phases. The system has special checks in place for these abnormal

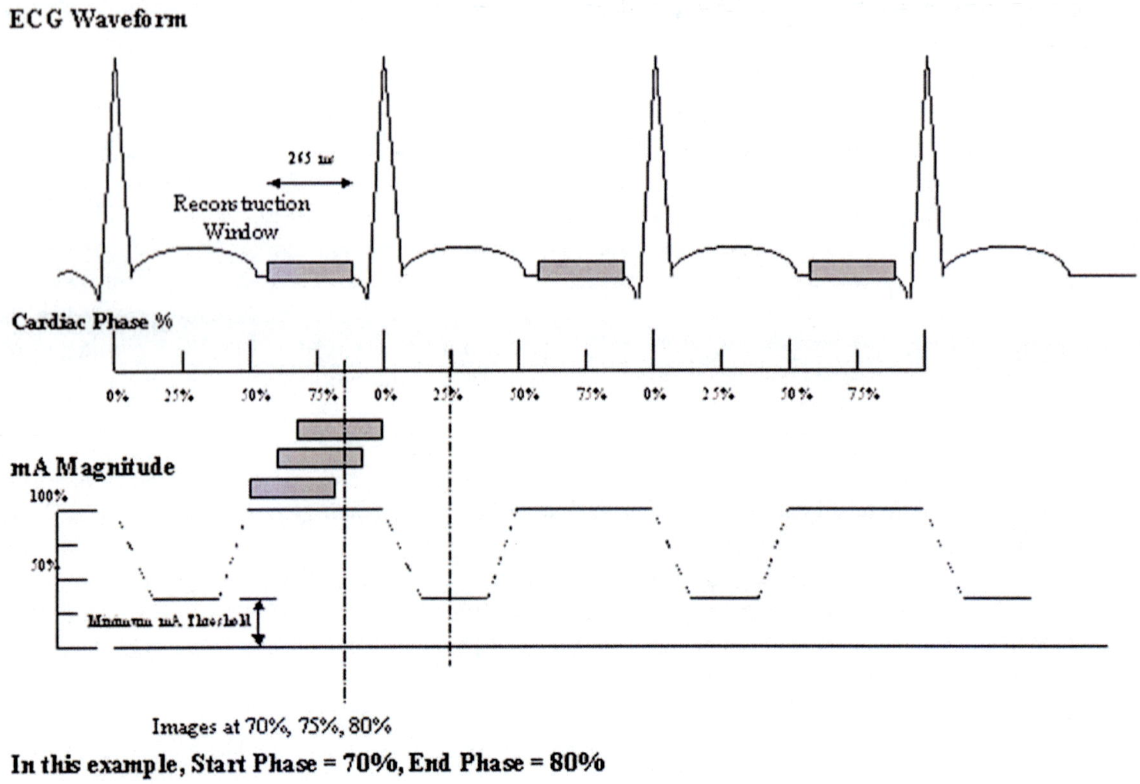


**Fig. 9** ECG based mA modulation for Cardiac helical ("Discovery™ CT750 HD Technical Reference Manual", © 2011 General Electric Company)

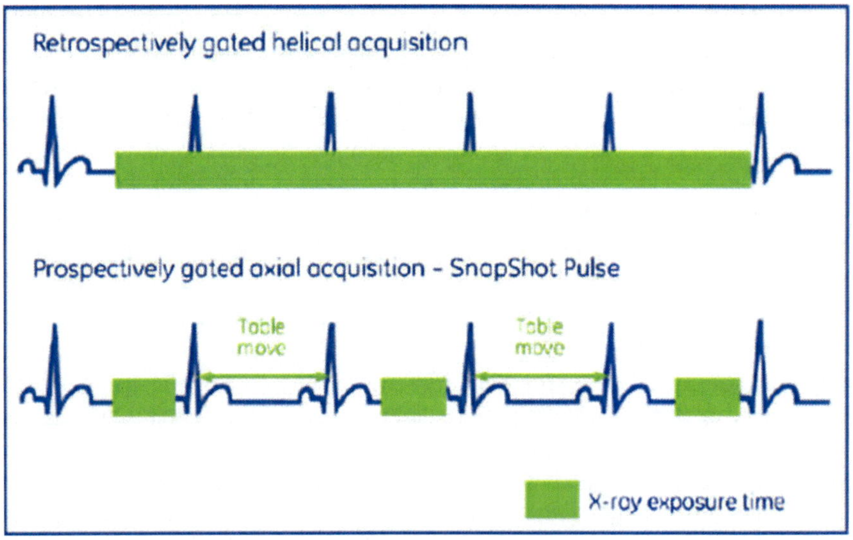


**Fig. 10** SnapShot Pulse™ method of cardiac scanning only turns X-ray on at the locations and heart phases required ("SnapShot Pulse: low dose cardiac imaging" © 2006 General Electric Company)

heart beat situations and will immediately ramp the tube up to full current in order to minimize the number of noisy images that can occur during these abnormal cycles. Once the heart has settled into a normal rhythm again, the system will resume modulation (Fig. 9).

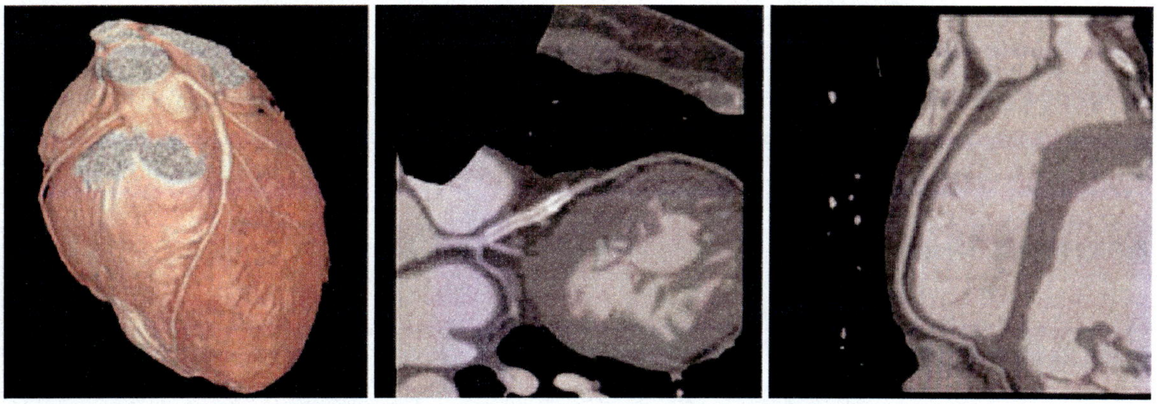

**Fig. 11** Examples of SnapShot Pulse$^{TM}$ cardiac images ("Snap Shot Pulse: low dose cardiac imaging" © 2006 General Electric Company)

#### 1.7.1.2 Prospective Cardiac Gating, SnapShot Pulse

Cardiac cine acquisition for cardiac imaging is available in conjunction with CardIQ SnapShot Pulse and prospective cardiac gating. In this step and shoot cine scanning mode, the heart rate is monitored during the scan and the R-Peak triggers the acquisition of data for that location. The table moves to the next location and waits for the next R-Peak to trigger acquisition of data for the phase specified. SnapShot Pulse is a lower dose mode compared to cardiac helical modes. A padding value allows for flexibility of neighboring phase locations to accommodate small fluctuations in heart rate (a few BPM or less). However, a stable heart rate of 65 BPM or less is recommended for SnapShot Pulse (Figs. 10, 11).

## 2 Optimizing Image Quality and Dose Through Hardware Features

### 2.1 Reduction of Off-Focal Radiation

X-rays generated by electrons striking the anode outside of the focal spot contribute only to artifact and additional dose. The primary source of this effect is back-scattered electrons randomly re-striking the anode after their initial collision. Artifacts appear near sharp anatomical structures and as additional image noise. An electron collection ring is designed into GE Healthcare X-ray tubes to remove these backscattered electrons. The net effect of this design is high image quality and up to 5% dose reduction.

### 2.2 X-Ray Beam Quality

X-ray Beam Quality encompasses multiple facets in the context of a CT scanner. The spectrum or "hardness" affects the level of contrast seen in human tissue and the ability to penetrate large or dense anatomy. Low energy X-rays provide more tissue contrast, but in cases of large anatomy they will be fully absorbed and only contribute to patient dose. The "shape" of the filter matches the X-ray intensity level across the beam to the attenuation level across the patient. This is especially import near the surface of the patient. Selecting the optimal beam hardness and shape for the particular clinical task and patient habitus is key to optimizie the dose and image quality of any CT procedure. By assigning clinically relevant names to the scan field of view (SFOV) selections, GE Healthcare MDCT scanners facilitate this matching for the operator. Two or three bowtie filter sizes and two hardness levels are provided to give flexibility in matching the clinical scenario. The small and medium filters preserve the softness of the beam and are tuned for anatomy of less than 30 cm. These qualities are appropriate for head or pediatric scanning. The filter size can also be set according to the region of interest. For instance in cardiac scanning, the heart will fit into the field of view of the small and medium filters. Use of a smaller filter can bring a dose reduction and image quality improvement for these

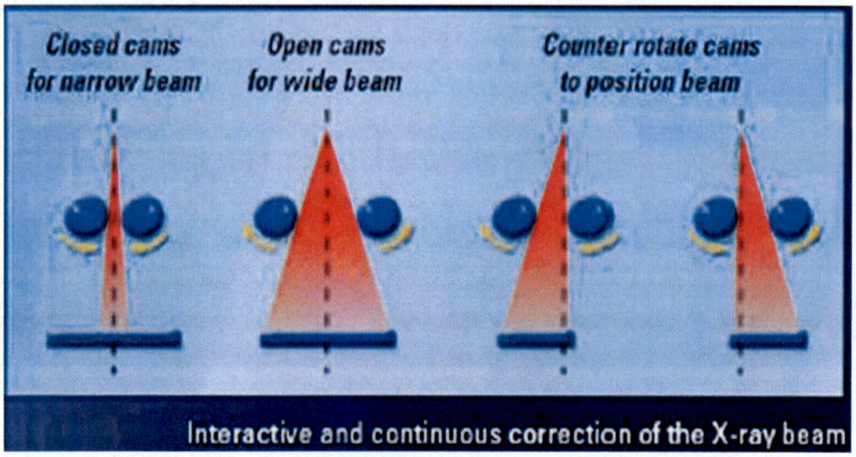


**Fig. 12** "Focal spot tracking" updates the position of both edges of the beam in real-time to maintain the narrowest beam possible ("FeatherLight, Technology for Dose Optimization" © 2008, General Electric Company)

cases. The large filter is designed for larger anatomy by providing a harder beam and wider X-ray field. The low energy X-rays would be absorbed by large patients, therefore removing them in filter has no impact on image quality. Uniform image quality across the full scan field of view is delivered by the increased X-ray intensity width. Shaped filters can provide a surface dose reduction of up to 50% as compared to a uniform X-ray field.

### 2.3 Beam Tracking and Focal Spot Size to Optimize Z-Axis Dose Efficiency

Ideally all rows of an MDCT scanner would receive uniform X-ray intensity. The inherent nonuniformity of a collimated X-ray beam must be considered in a system design. The central region of the beam (umbra) will be uniform, but there will be regions on the edges of diminishing intensity (penumbra). The penumbra is not of sufficient quality for imaging and only contributes to patient dose. The size of the focal spot is a key determining factor in the amount of penumbra. The size of the penumbra region can differ by 50% from large to small sizes. By automatically determining the spot size based on tube current levels, GE Healthcare CT scanners only use the large when required. One option to ensure that the active area of the detector sees a uniform X-ray field is to open the source collimator wide enough to have an umbra region that covers not only the active z-range of the detector, but also has margin to cover the thermal and mechanical motion inherent in the focal spot. This would result in an umbra region significantly larger than required and the X-ray falling outside the active detector region contributes only to patient dose. GE Healthcare has chosen a different approach for their MDCT scanners. A closed loop tracking system monitors the position of the X-ray beam edges on the detector (Fig. 12). Each beam edge is independently measured and adjusted to keep the beam width in tight to the active detector region every few milliseconds.

### 2.4 Dynamic Z-Axis Tracking

Helical scanning brings many clinical benefits, but it brings along over ranging acquisition to complete the sampling required for image reconstruction. Even with highly efficient image reconstruction algorithms, some of the outer row data is not required at the ends of the scan range. The independent beam edge control provided for beam tracking is perfectly suited to deal with this. GE Healthcare has developed a Dynamic Z-Axis Tracking mode that independently adjusts the beam edges at the start and end of a helical acquisition. The trailing edge is brought in at the start and opened as the scan progresses. The leading edge is brought in as the acquisition completes. This feature is available on particular GE Healthcare CT MDCT scanners and is automatically enabled for the scanning scenarios that can leverage it.

### 2.5 System Design for Data Acquisition

Multiple design factors play a role in the robustness of the Data Acquisition System (DAS), especially in situations of low X-ray flux at the detector such as large patients, highly attenuating anatomy or low dose scanning techniques. Electronic systems have an inherent level of noise. If the signal levels to be measured are of the same magnitude as the noise, severe imaging artifacts will appear. GE Healthcare MDCT scanners address this issue with multiple design aspects:

(i) *HiLight*$_{TM}$ or *Gemstone*$_{TM}$ scintillator materials bring 98% X-ray detection efficiency and very high light signal output.
(ii) A type of photodiode that can be mated to the scintillator without electrical connections interfering with the light transfer is used. These backlit photodiodes engage 100% of their active area to collect light from the scintillator, even in very high resolution systems.
(iii) Collapsing the electronics into smaller packages through higher levels of integration has increased immunity to electrical interference and inherent capacitance.

All of these design features come together to give the DAS superior performance in low signal situations allowing for low technique scanning without artifact.

## 3 Summary

GE Healthcare has developed a rich toolbox of features to optimize dose for many different clinical needs. Understanding how and when to use all the capabilities of your specific CT are key to getting the required image quality at the lowest possible dose for each clinical need.

## References

ASiR reconstruction sharpens images, slices abdominal CT dose, auntminnie.com. Accessed 21 May 2009

Budovec J et al (2008) Iterative reconstruction algorithm for multi detector computed tomography decreases image noise and improves image quality. In: Proceedings of SCBT-MR conference, 2 April 2008

Estimated radiation dose of coronary CT angiography using adaptive statistical iterative reconstruction (ERASIR 1) study, diagnosticimaging.com. Accessed 2 December 2009

GE Healthcare CT Publication (2007) Color-coded CT protocols help reduce dose for pediatrics. ©2007 General Electric Company

GE Healthcare System Documentation (2011) Discovery™ CT750 HD technical reference manual, ©2011 General Electric Company

GE Healthcare CT publication (2011) Dose check quick guide, ©2011 General Electric Company

Jacobson DR, Foley WD, Metz S, Peterswen AL (1996) Variable milliampere CT: effect on noise and low contrast detectability. Radiology 326:210

Kopka L, Funke M (1995) Automatically adapted CT tube current: dose reduction and image quality in phantom and patient studies. Radiology 197:292

Singh S et al (2009) Noise and attenuation characteristics of ultra low-dose abdominal CT reconstructed with model-based iterative reconstruction: a prospective pilot study. In: Proceedings of the RSNA meeting, 3 December 2009

Thibault J-B (2010) GE Healthcare white paper, Veo™ CT model-based iterative reconstruction, ©2010 General Electric Company

Toth T, Ge Z, Daley M (2006) The influence of bowtie filter selection, patient size and patient centering on CT dose and image quality. In: Poster SU-FF-I42, 2006AAPM conference (MedPhy, vol 33, No.6)

## Additional Information

## ASiR™ Sources

Singh S, Kalra MK, Gilman MD, Hsieh J, Pien HH, Digumarthy SR, Shepard JO (2011) Adaptive statistical iterative reconstruction technique for radiation dose reduction in chest CT: a pilot study. Radiology 259:566–573

Singh S, Kalra MK, Hsieh J, Licato PE, Do S, Pien HH, Blake MA (2010) Comparison of adaptive statistical iterative and filtered back projection reconstruction techniques. Radiology 257:373–383

Prakash P, Kalra MK, Ackman JB, Digumarthy SR, Hsieh J, Do S, Shepard JA, Gilman MD (2010a) Diffuse lung disease: CT of the chest with adaptive statistical iterative reconstruction technique. Radiology 256(1):261–269

Leipsic J, Labounty TM, Heilbron B, Min JK, Mancini GB, Lin FY, Taylor C, Dunning A, Earls JP (2010a) Adaptive statistical iterative reconstruction: assessment of image noise and image quality in coronary CT angiography. Am J Roentgenol 195(3):649–654

Sagara Y, Hara AK, Pavlicek W, Silva AC, Paden RG, Wu Q (2010) Abdominal CT: comparison of low-dose CT with adaptive statistical iterative reconstruction and routine-dose CT with filtered back projection in 53 patients. Am J Roentgenol 195(3):713–719

Prakash P, Kalra MK, Kambadakone AK, Pien H, Hsieh J, Blake MA, Sahani DV (2010b) Reducing abdominal CT radiation dose with adaptive statistical iterative reconstruction technique. Invest Radiol 45(4):202–210

Leipsic J, Labounty TM, Heilbron B, Min JK, Mancini GB, Lin FY, Taylor C, Dunning A, Earls JP (2010b) Estimated radiation dose reduction using adaptive statistical iterative reconstruction in coronary CT angiography: the ERASIR study. AJR Am J Roentgenol 195(3):655–660

Fleischmann D, Boas FE (2011) Computed tomography—old ideas and new technology. Eur Radiol 21(3):510–517. doi:10.1007/s00330-011-2056-z

## Veo™ Sources

Budovec J, Foley D et al (2008) Iterative reconstruction algorithm for multi detector computed tomography decreases image noise and improves image quality. In: Proceedings of SCBT-MR conference, 2 April 2008

Singh S, Kalra MK, Licato P, Thibault JB (2009) Noise and attenuation characteristics of ultra-low dose abdominal CT reconstructed with model based iterative reconstruction: a prospective pilot studym, RSNA 09

Kinahan P (2010) Impact of model-based iterative reconstruction on image quality and radiation dose. ISCT, San Francisco, CA, 18 May 2010

Nelson RC (2010) The trade-off between adaptive statistical iterative reconstruction (ASIR) and model based iterative reconstruction (MBIR). ISCT, San Francisco, 18 May

Nelson RC (2011) Use of iterative reconstruction for low radiation dose imaging in clinical practice. ISCT, San Francisco, 13–16 June

Shuman W (2011) Model-based iterative reconstruction (MBIR), ASiR and FBP of the liver: impact on image noise, lesion detection, and image quality. ISCT, San Francisco, 13–16 June

Yadava G, Kulkarni S, Colon ZR, Thibault J (2010) Dose reduction and image quality benefits using model based iterative reconstruction (MBIR) technique for computed tomography. Med Phys 37:3372

## General Sources

Toth TL, Bromberg B, Pan T-S, Rabe J, Steven JW, Li J, Seidenschnur GE (2000) A dose reduction X-ray beam positioning system for high-speed multislice CT scanners. Med Phys 27(12):2659–2668

Kalra MK, Maher MM, Toth TL, Schmidt B, Westerman BL, Morgan HT, Saini S (2004) Techniques and applications of automatic tube current modulation for CT. Radiology 233(3): 649–657

Jiang H, Londt J, Vass M, Li J, Tang X, Okerlund D (2006) Step-and-shoot data acquisition and reconstruction for cardiac X-ray computed tomography. Med Phys 33(11): 4236–4248

James PE, Berman EL, Urban BA, Curry CA, Lane JL, Jennings RS, McCulloch CC, Hsieh J, Londt JH (2008) Prospectively gated transverse coronary CT angiography versus retrospectively gated helical technique: improved image quality and reduced radiation dose. Radiology 246(3):742–753

Husmann L, Valenta I, Gaemperli O, Adda O, Treyer V, Christophe AW, Veit-Haibach P, Tatsugami F, von Schulthess GK, Kaufmann PA (2008) Feasibility of low-dose coronary CT angiography: first experience with prospective ECG-gating. Eur Heart J 29(2):191–197

# Dose Reduction in Computed Tomography Siemens Perspective

Christianne Leidecker and Bernhard Schmidt

## Contents



C. Leidecker (✉) · B. Schmidt
Siemens Medical Solutions, Erlangen, Germany
e-mail: Christianne.Leidecker@siemens.com

**Abstract**

With CT being the imaging modality of choice in many situations, dose reduction is of concern for both manufacturers and users. To reduce the dose for an individual exam, the first and foremost principle to adhere to is ALARA (As Low As Reasonably Achievable), i.e., to use the lowest possible dose to obtain the required diagnostic quality images. Besides adjusting the techniques to the diagnostic question, it is vital to know and understand dose reduction techniques available on the CT system. Whereas the availability of individual techniques typically depends on the model type as well as the installed scanner software, this chapter gives an overview of technologies and algorithms available on Siemens systems to reduce the absorbed dose to a minimum.

## 1 Real-Time Anatomic Exposure Control: CARE Dose4D™

Probably the most powerful lever to optimize radiation dose in CT is through adaptation of the scan parameters to the anatomy of the individual patient. Centering the patient correctly, using the right protocols and adjusting the X-ray tube output to the patient's size and shape help to minimize radiation exposure. In clinical routine, however, this may be time consuming and rather challenging; for example, users may not be aware that a decrease in the patient's diameter by only 4 cm allows reducing the tube output by a factor of two while still maintaining adequate image quality. Another disadvantage of scanning

D. Tack et al. (eds.), *Radiation Dose from Multidetector CT*, Medical Radiology. Diagnostic Imaging,
DOI: 10.1007/174_2012_571, © Springer-Verlag Berlin Heidelberg 2012

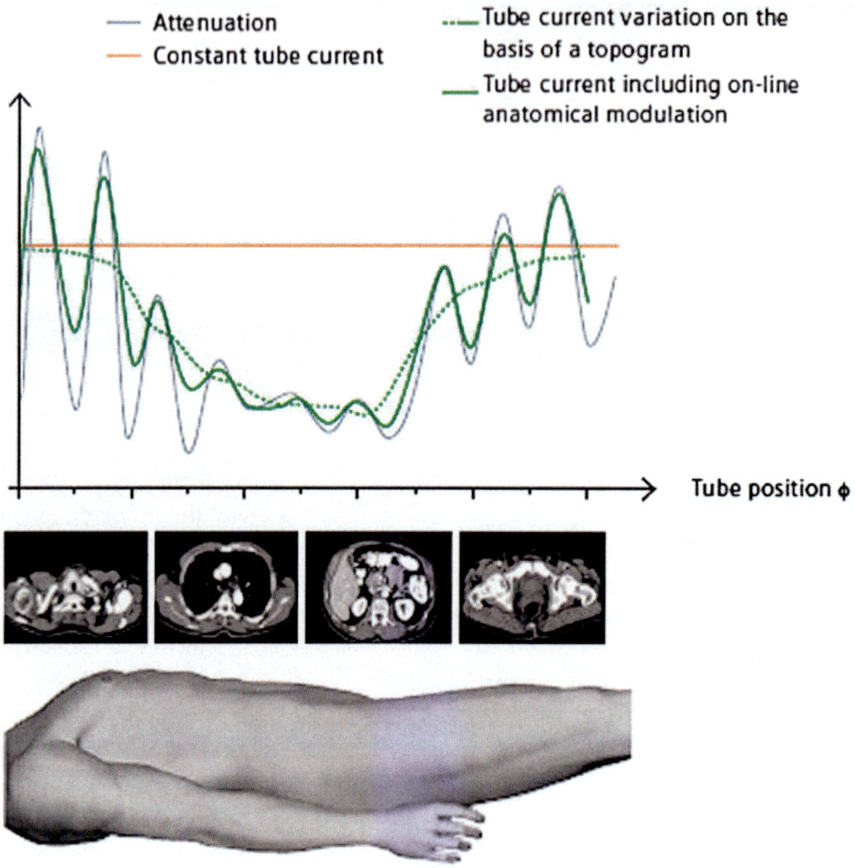


**Fig. 1** Working principle of CARE Dose4D. With constant tube current, regions in the shoulder and the pelvis would be under-dosed, while the thorax and abdomen would be significantly over-dosed. On-line anatomical dose modulation efficiently adapts the tube current and hence the radiation dose to the patient's attenuation

patients with a constant tube current is that it leads to noisy images in areas of high attenuation and over-dosing in areas of lower attenuation of a given patient. In addition, young or slim patients might receive much more dose than required to get a desired image quality, while image quality of obese patients might be compromised.

Hence, an automatic adaptation of scan parameters to the patient's anatomy is highly desirable. In all modern Siemens CT scanners, control mechanisms are available that automatically adjust the radiation dose level to the patient's anatomy—similar to a highly sophisticated camera's automatic exposure mode. Siemens CARE Dose4D (see Figs. 1 and 2) automatically adapts radiation dose to the size and shape of the patient, achieving optimal tube current modulation in two ways (Kalra et al. 2004a, b; Greess et al. 2002; Rizzo et al. 2006; Mulkens et al. 2005; Graser et al. 2006). First, tube current is varied on the basis of a single topogram (either lateral or AP/PA), by comparing the actual patient to a "standard-sized" patient using sophisticated algorithms. As might be expected, tube current is increased for larger patients and reduced for smaller patients. Differences in attenuation in distinct body regions are taken into account. For example, in an adult patient, a high tube output might be needed in the shoulder region, whereas it can be considerably lowered in the thorax. Tube output increases again in the abdomen and slightly further in the pelvis.

Second, adaptation is not only done along the patient's length axis, but also in the scan plane as the scan progresses to account for changes in attenuation within one tube rotation. This is particularly important for efficiently reducing dose in the shoulder and pelvic region, where the lateral attenuation is much higher than the anterior–posterior attenuation.

As mentioned above, the dose is adapted by comparing the actual patient to a "standard-sized" patient—roughly speaking. Hence, the user has to specify the image quality he would expect in this "reference" patient. In Siemens terminology, this

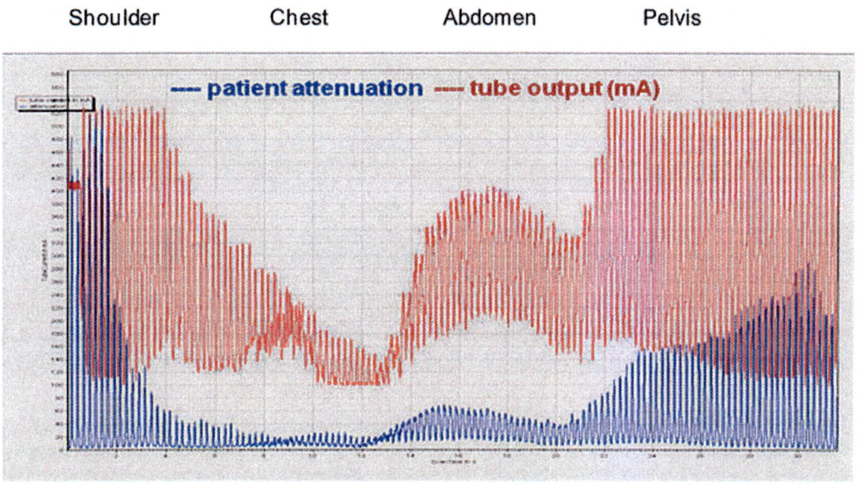


**Fig. 2** CARE Dose4D for a scan from the shoulders to the pelvis. The real-time anatomic exposure control (CARE Dose4D) and on-the-fly compensation of attenuation differences of different body parts are shown as the CT scan progresses

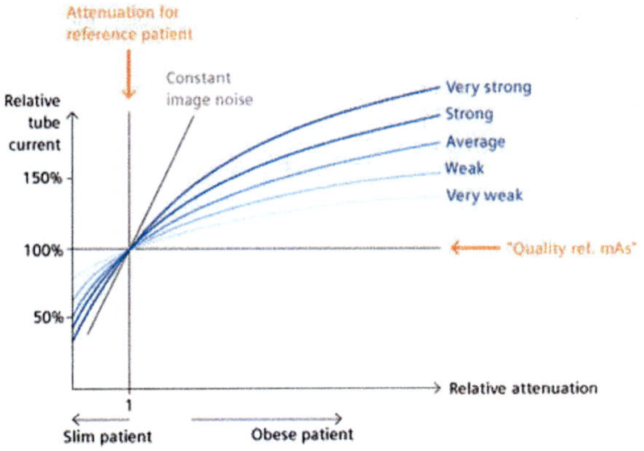


**Fig. 3** Different settings for modulation strength. Depending on the user preferences, a fine tuning of the strength of the attenuation-based mAs-adaptation for is possible

value is called the "Quality reference mAs" and is defined for a value one would use for a standard-sized adult patient weighing 75 kg. This value should be defined according to the clinical question and can be stored in the corresponding reference protocols. For an actual patient, in areas of higher attenuation the mAs-value will be higher that the reference, whereas in low attenuation areas mAs-values will be reduced compared to the reference.

Clinical experience has shown that the relationship between optimal tube current and patient attenuation is not linear. Larger patients clearly need a higher dose than average-sized patients and smaller patients need a lower dose than average-sized patients. During real-time dose modulation, CARE Dose4D adjustments follow a user configurable curve to best fit clinical needs. Up to five different configurations are available (see Fig. 3) and while radiation dose reduction or increase might be less than expected for smaller patients and larger patients, respectively, it allows maintaining good diagnostic image quality while achieving an optimal radiation dose.

## 2 Automated Dose-Optimized Selection of the X-ray Tube Voltage: CARE kV™

Conventional dose modulation approaches available, since the mid-1990s, control only the X-ray tube current while the X-ray tube voltage (the kV-setting) is left untouched. Yet there is untapped potential for dose reduction by adapting the radiation energy to the diagnostic task, such that an optimized contrast-to-noise ratio is achieved.

The quality of CT images is mainly characterized by three parameters: contrast, noise, and resolution/ sharpness. Improving all or any of these parameters will render a better image and enable the physician to make a more precise diagnosis. For example, if the contrast is high and the noise is low, the image quality improves. While image sharpness is independent of the radiation energy, noise, and contrast in the image do depend on the radiation energy and thus can be optimized with respect to the lowest possible dose without compromising the quality of the image. It is well known that the radiation energy can be modulated by changing the tube voltage.

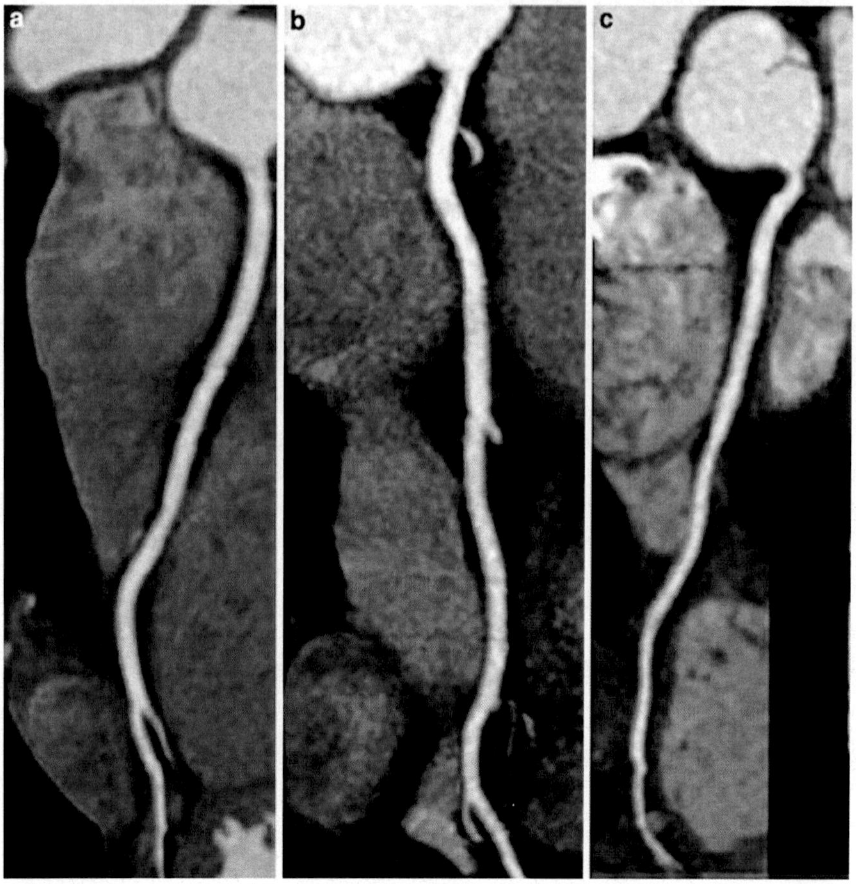


**Fig. 4** Three CT angiographies with three different current and voltage settings. Note that the mean contrast aorta is highest with the lowest CTDIvol of 21.2 mGy. **a** 120 kV 330 mAs, CTDIvol = 43.1 mGy, Mean contrast aorta: 322 HU. **b** 100 kV 330 mAs, CTDIvol = 31.8 mGy, Mean contrast aorta: 561 HU. **c** 100 kV 230 mAs, CTDIvol = 21.2 mGy, Mean contrast aorta: 559 HU

To maintain the same image quality, the contrast-to-noise ratio (CNR) has to be constant. Typically, an iodine contrast agent is administered to improve the visibility of organ structures in CT images (particularly in CT angiography examinations). This improves the contrast, thus allowing higher levels of noise without losing image quality. The contrast is best if the energy of the X-rays is low, since the low energetic X-rays are better absorbed by iodine than the surrounding tissue. However, in order to maintain constant CNR, the tube current usually requires adjustment. Nevertheless, for a constant CNR in CT angiographic studies, the radiation dose can be significantly reduced by choosing 80 or 100 kV tube voltages instead of 120 kV (see Fig. 4).

For larger patients though, who have a higher X-ray attenuation, the output of the X-ray tube at lower kV-settings may not be sufficient to produce the required contrast-to-noise ratios. For these patients, higher X-ray tube voltages will have to be selected, despite reduced iodine contrasts.

In a busy environment, a technician often has insufficient time to measure the attenuation of each patient. Automatic tools that define the optimal combination of voltage and current for each patient according to the patient's topogram are necessary. CARE kV is a fully automated feature that adjusts the tube voltage tailored to the individual patient, the system capabilities and the clinical task. In combination with CARE Dose4D, it allows the patient-specific adaptation of both dose relevant parameters, tube current and tube voltage.

When using CARE kV, a "Reference kV"-value has to be defined for each protocol, similar to CARE Dose4D. The "Reference kV" refers to a standard patient, weighing 75 kg. Additionally, one has to specify the exam type (e.g. CT Angiography, non-contrast exam, etc.) for which the CNR has to be

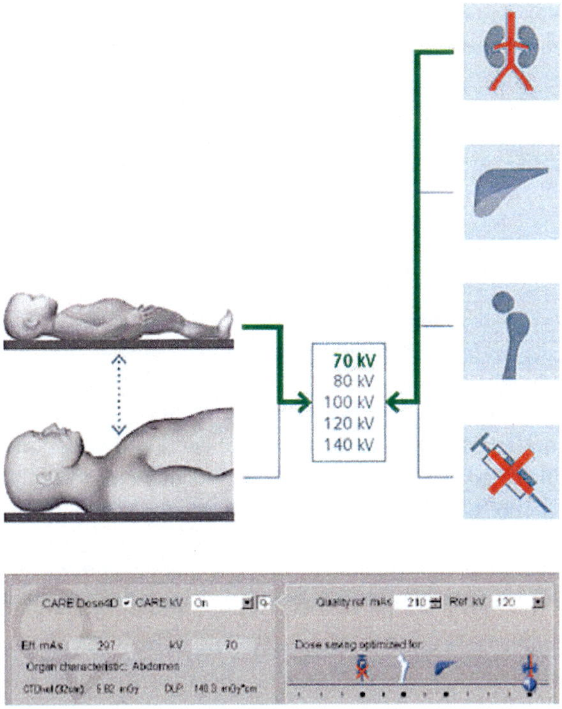


**Fig. 5** With CARE Child, low dose 70 kV scan modes with dedicated modulation for children are available

maintained. Last but not least, it is important to note that lowest kV-setting does not necessarily mean lowest dose. Depending on the individual patient and exam type, a higher kV-setting will achieve the specified image quality at a lower dose.

## 3 Low kV Scanning (70 kV): CARE Child™

When imaging pediatric patients, special attention is needed on the one hand to meet the image quality requirements and on the other hand, to ensure lowest dose given that children are more sensitive to radiation than adults. As a consequence, the ALARA principle (As Low As Reasonably Achievable) is of particular importance in pediatrics. It calls for always selecting the dose that is as low as possible, yet sufficient for a reliable diagnosis.

Studies investigating the potential for dose reduction by adapting the tube voltage have shown that in particular in the case of CT angiography studies and generally contrast enhanced CT scans lower kV-settings allowed for a substantial reduction in dose. In fact, the smaller the patient, the higher was the benefit of using lower kV-settings. While voltages commonly available on today's CT systems lie between 80 and 140 kV, Siemens offer the additional low kV-setting of 70 kV with CARE Child. Dedicated tube technology enables CT scanning at such low kV-settings. Initial studies have shown that for example in the case of CTA examination an additional reduction of 30% in dose is possible by using 70 kV instead of 80 kV (Schmidt et al. 2010) (Fig. 5).

Last but not least, with the introduction of high pitch scanning on Dual Source CT scanners, the achieved scan speeds allow even uncooperative children to be examined without sedation, reducing stress for the patient and saving time and money. Typical dose values of below 0.5 mSv in pediatric applications can be achieved with full diagnostic image quality.

## 4 Organ-Based Dose Modulation X-CARE™

With the most recent edition of the ICRP (recommendations of the International Commission on Radiological Protection of 2007, ICRP 103), tissue weighting factors which are used to calculate effective dose values, have been changed. In particular, the tissue weighting factor for the female breast tissue has been increased, indicating that it is more radiation sensitive than previously assumed. In any CT examination of the thorax, the breast—even without being the primary body part of interest—is irradiated and should therefore be especially protected. In current clinical practice, a common approach to protect the female breast is by the use of so-called breast shields made out of e.g. bismuth. While they allow for a reduction in dose to the breast tissue, they typically also lead to a drop in image quality through increased image noise and local artifacts. An alternative approach without the negative impact on image quality is the modulation of the tube current in such a way that the radiation intensity is reduced when the patient is irradiated from the front as shown in Fig. 6, thus reducing the absorbed dose in areas with particularly sensitive tissue.

Siemens X-CARE, an organ-based dose modulation mode, can selectively limit the radiation exposure of sensitive organs. With this method, the radiation exposure of sensitive tissue (such as the breast or the eyes) is reduced by 30–40%, while image noise and

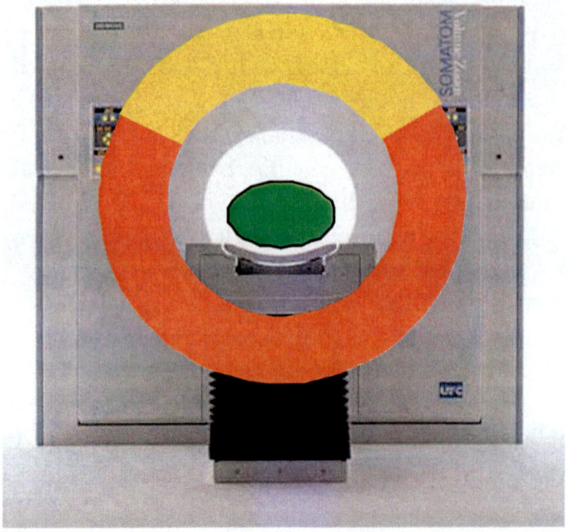

**Fig. 6** Scheme of the X-CARE principle. Tube current is reduced substantially in the anterior part of the patient and slightly increases in the back of the patient

detailed visualization remain unaffected as shown in Fig. 7.

## 5 Asymmetric Collimator Control: Adaptive Dose Shield

In spiral CT, it is necessary to do an extra half-rotation of the gantry before and after the planned scan length, due to data interpolation requirements. With today's multislice CT scanners, it is routing to fully irradiate the detector throughout these half-rotations, even though only part of the acquired data is necessary for image reconstruction. This problem is typical for spiral CT and commonly referred to as "over-ranging". In the case of conventional collimators that are moving synchronous together therefore, the patient is unnecessarily irradiated at the beginning and end of the scanned area (Fig. 8). The contribution of this wasted dose increases for wider detectors, which are used lately in modern CT systems.

The above mentioned waste of dose can be limited by using a pre-patient collimator with an asymmetric opening and closing to prevent over-ranging at the beginning and at the end of a spiral CT scan as shown in Fig. 9.

Thus, dose can be significantly reduced, depending on the scanned range, without affecting image quality as has been shown in Scientific Poster Session, Physics and basic Science; LL-PH2102-B04; Dose Reduction in Spiral CT Using Dynamically Adjustable Z-axis Beam Collimation; RSNA 2008.

## 6 Iterative Reconstruction Algorithms: IRIS and SAFIRE™

Today, image reconstruction in CT is based on conventional filtered back projection methods in which the spatial resolution is directly correlated with increased image noise. Thus, conventional methods are limited by this trade-off: higher spatial resolution is always accompanied by higher image noise. Iterative reconstruction approaches enable a decoupling of spatial resolution and image noise. Spatial resolution is thus enhanced in areas with high contrast and image noise in low contrast areas is reduced therefore enabling the user to perform CT scans with a lower absorbed dose.

As a general rule, iterative reconstruction algorithms include a correction loop in the image reconstruction process. Once an image has been reconstructed from the measured projections, a ray-tracing of the image is performed to calculate new projections that exactly represent the reconstructed image. This step, called reprojection, simulates the CT measurement process, but with the image as the "measured object". If the original image reconstruction were perfect, measured, and calculated projections would be identical. In reality they are not and the deviation is used to reconstruct a correction image and to update the original image.

Then the loop starts again. The images are improved step by step, and a significant noise reduction can be obtained by carefully modeling the data acquisition system of the CT scanner and its physical properties in the reprojection algorithm. This method is known as "model-based iterative reconstruction". The drawback of this approach is that the exact modeling of the scanner during reprojection requires high computer processing power, therefore significant hardware capacity is needed to avoid long image reconstruction times.

Simplified approaches with less computer complexity and faster reconstruction are possible with less accurate reprojection and calculation of the

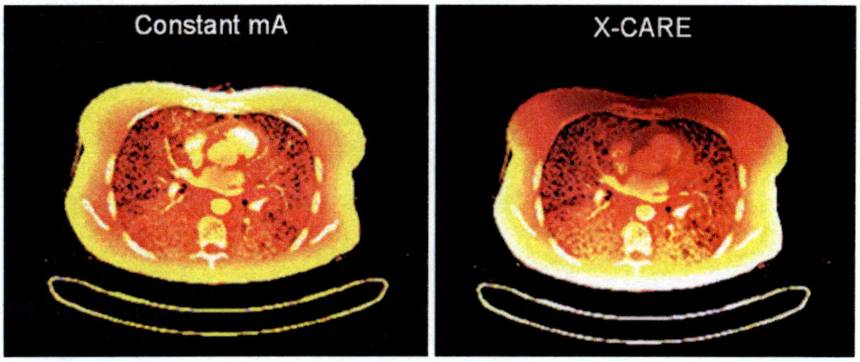


**Fig. 7** Radiation doses without X-CARE and with X-CARE. *Darker areas* indicate lower absorbed dose

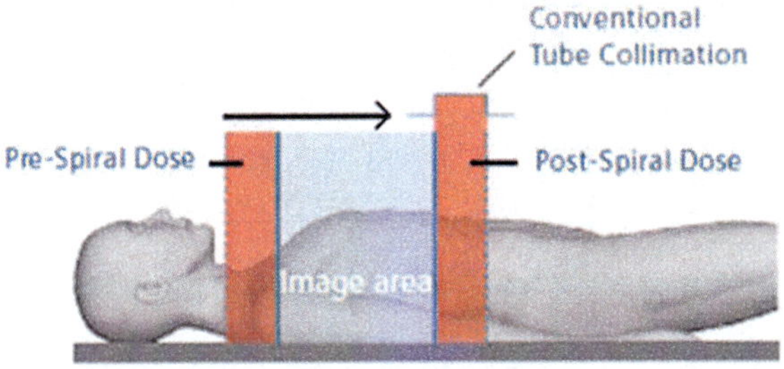


**Fig. 8** Conventional collimators moving together. The areas marked in *red* are out of the necessary scan range but still irradiated with full power

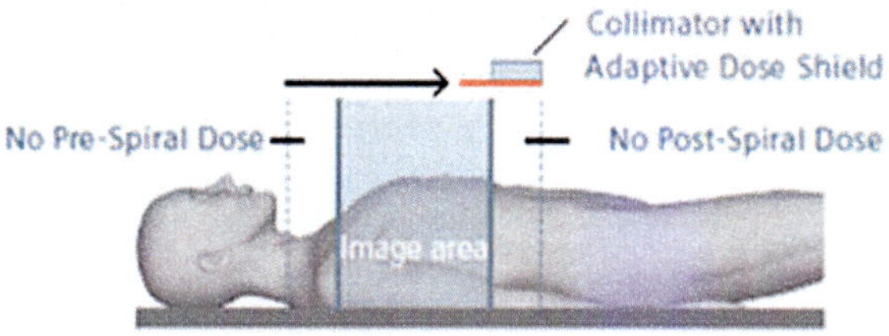


**Fig. 9** Adaptive Dose Shield. When the CT scan starts, the collimator opens asymmetrically. In the center of the scan range, the collimator is fully open to match the selected beam width. At the end of the scan range the collimator again closes asymmetrically, thereby limiting unnecessary exposure

correction image. Often, only the statistical noise of the data is taken into account in a simplified way. This may result in strange, unfamiliar noise textures and a plastic-like look of the images. This method is known as "statistical iterative reconstruction". See Fig. 10.

Yet another alternate implementation which accelerates the image reconstruction without loss in the image quality has been developed and implemented by Siemens. Iterative reconstruction in image space (IRIS) offers both a significant image noise reduction corresponding to up to 60% potential dose reduction and fast reconstruction times for routine clinical use. In addition, the noise texture of the images is similar to standard well established convolution kernels. With the IRIS method, a master reconstruction is performed that optimally utilizes all measured data and provides all available detail information but with increased noise in the so-called master image.

Within the IRIS iterative loop, this master image is "cleaned up" step by step, enhancing object contrasts and reducing image noise in each iteration, see Fig. 10b.

The traditional reprojection is not necessary, therefore the time consuming calculation of the deviations from the original raw data is avoided and allows fast reconstruction times.

Further developing on this method, Siemens introduced Sinogram Affirmed Iterative Reconstruction (SAFIRE) as the newest generation of iterative reconstruction algorithms. SAFIRE is a raw data and model-based iterative reconstruction algorithm which enables CT dose reduction of up to 60% (Winklehner et al. 2011; Moscariello et al. 2011). It builds on an improved regularization technique compared to IRIS, used to reduce the noise in the data. Additionally, the use of projection raw data during the iterative image improvement process enables a reduction of subtle image artifacts and therefore a further improvement in general image quality. The actual number of applied raw data loops depends on the expected artifact level in the images, Fig. 11.

With SAFIRE, pixel noise, low contrast detectability and high contrast resolution in images are maintained while radiation dose is reduced. Figure 12 shows an example of a standard FBP reconstruction and the reconstruction of the same data with SAFIRE.

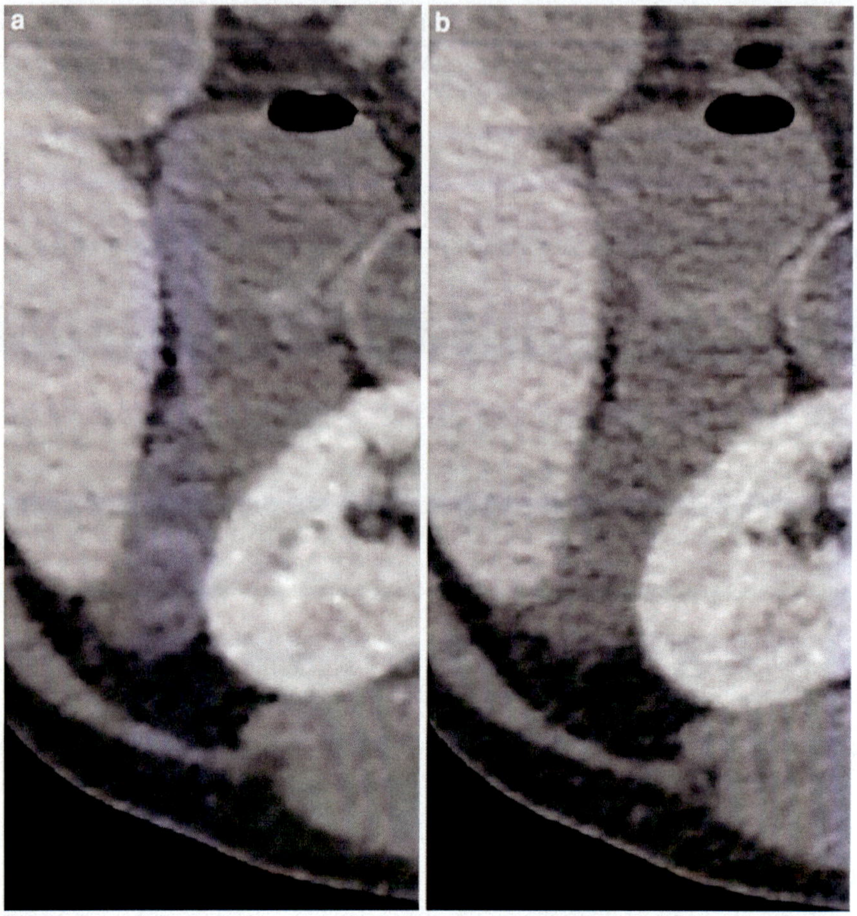

**Fig. 10** **a** Example of a simplified approach with less computer complexity and faster reconstruction with statistical iterative reconstruction. **b** Example of a iterative reconstruction with IRIS: 50% dose reduction

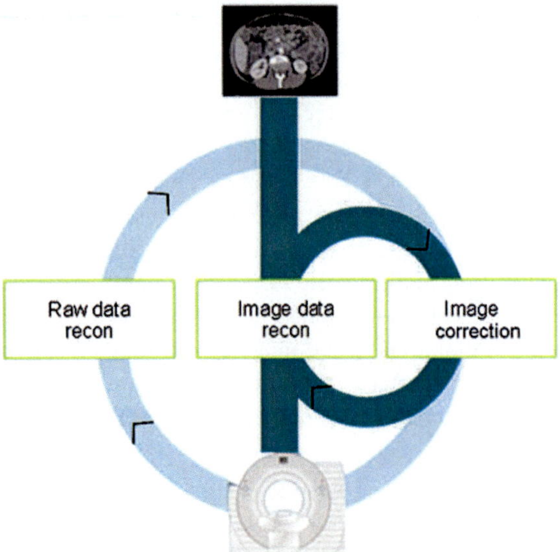


**Fig. 11** Principle of SAFIRE: Combination of a raw data and model-based iterative reconstruction algorithm with an iterative image based loop

# 7 Dose Reduction Techniques for Specific Applications

## 7.1 Dose Neutral Dual Energy Scanning with Selective Photon Shield

Dual Energy CT is an evolving technology in today's CT landscape. It has the potential to offer additional information that is not available in single energy scans. However, maintaining the dose levels that are used in single energy scans is of equal importance. The Siemens realization of Dual Energy scanning in a Dual Source CT scanner allows exploring the full potential of dose reduction technologies such as e.g. CARE Dose4D and Adaptive Dose Shield used in single energy scanning and, in addition to, dedicated technologies for dose reduction in Dual Energy scanning.

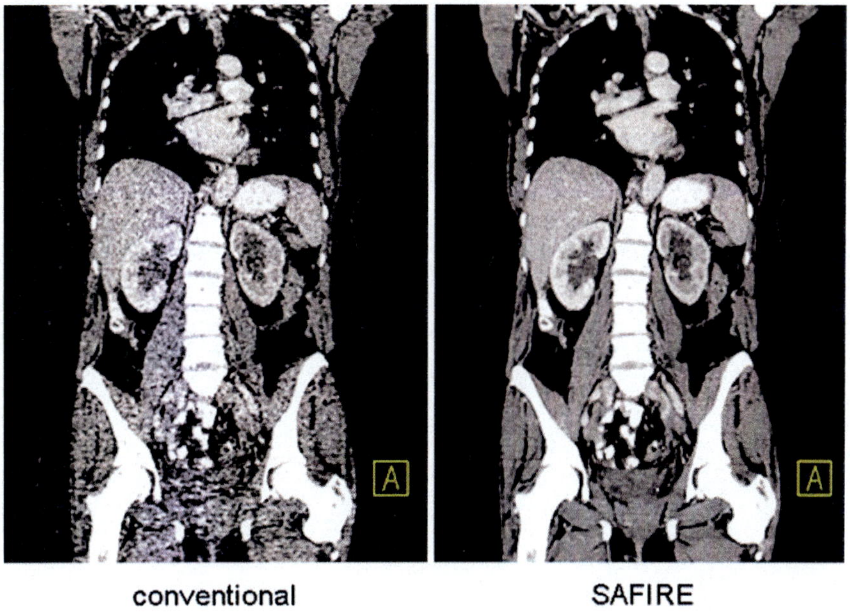


**Fig. 12** Example of a conventional reconstruction (*left*) and the reconstruction of the same data with SAFIRE (*right*)

With the introduction of the second generation of Dual Source CT scanners, Siemens added an important new feature to the SOMATOM Definition Flash. The Selective Photon Shield allows dedicated filtration of the high energy spectrum, removing low energy photons, see Fig. 13. This improves separation of the low and high energy images and, therefore, improves material differentiation by about 80%. In addition, the photon filter helps reducing image noise and eliminates the dose penalty of typically 10–20% for first generation Dual Source CT scanners in most types of Dual Energy studies.

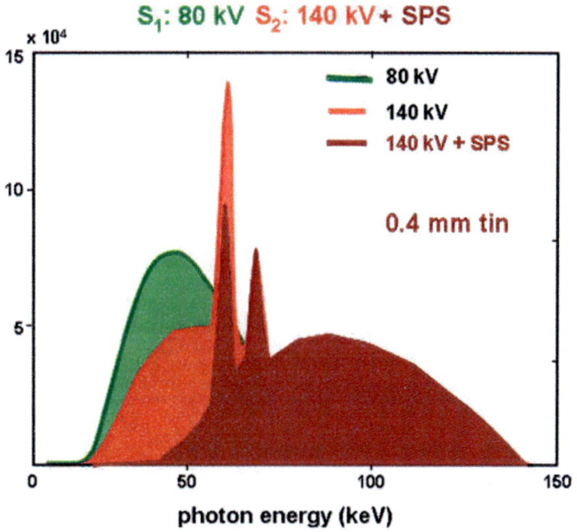


**Fig. 13** Typical spectra used in CT do considerably overlap (shown for typical energies of 80 and 140 kV, respectively). With the Selective Photon Shield, dedicated filtration of the high energy spectrum is performed, substantially removing the overlap

## 7.2 Dose Reduction in Cardiac CT

While already introduced in the mid-1980s, it was mainly due to technological advances in the last decade that imaging of the heart with CT has become a reliable technique. However, the demands on image quality—high temporal resolution to avoid image distortion by cardiac motion as well as sub-millimeter spatial resolution for adequate visualization of the heart's small anatomical structures—require scan data acquisition to be controlled by the patient's electrocardiogram (ECG) and resulted in relatively high exposure. Hence, radiation exposure of coronary CT angiography has been a concern and efforts have been undertaken to provide additional techniques for dose reduction in gated CT acquisitions.

Typically, modern CT scanners will offer various acquisition techniques together with dedicated means of reducing exposure during gated CT acquisitions. With the introduction of dual source CT systems, the methods available with Siemens technology are

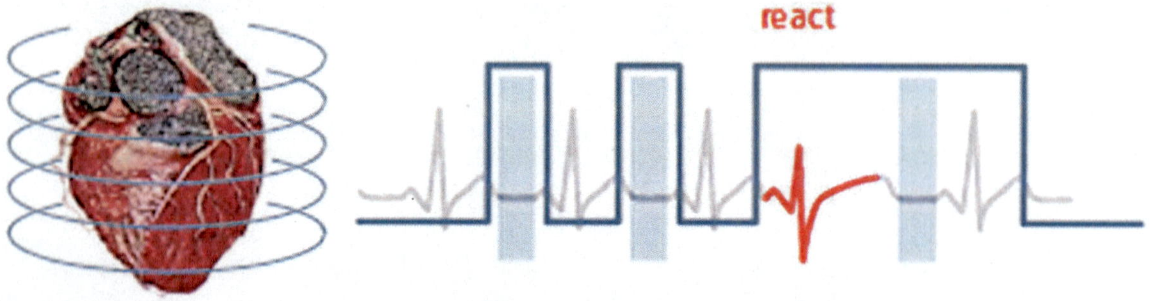


**Fig. 14** The CT generates images only during a predefined phase of the heart beat. During this phase, the current (*solid line*) is 100% of the necessary level to achieve the specified image quality and is reduced outside this phase to 20 or even 4%. Advanced algorithms additionally allow to flexibly react to arrhythmia occurring during the scan

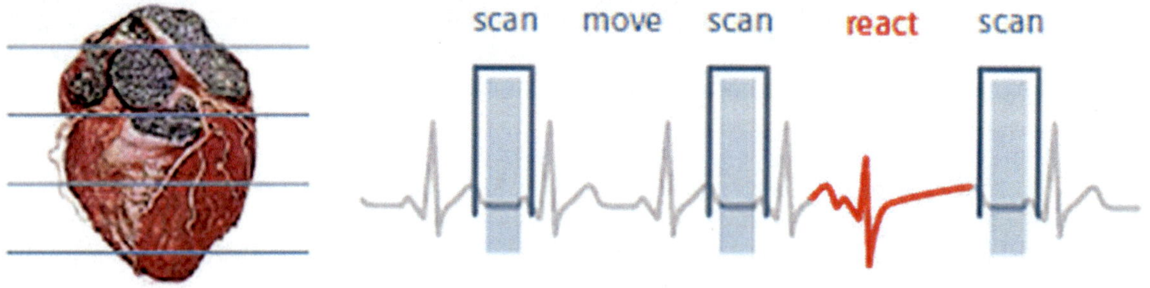


**Fig. 15** Each slice of the heart is scanned during the same ECG phase. With this method, substantial dose reductions with no image quality loss are possible

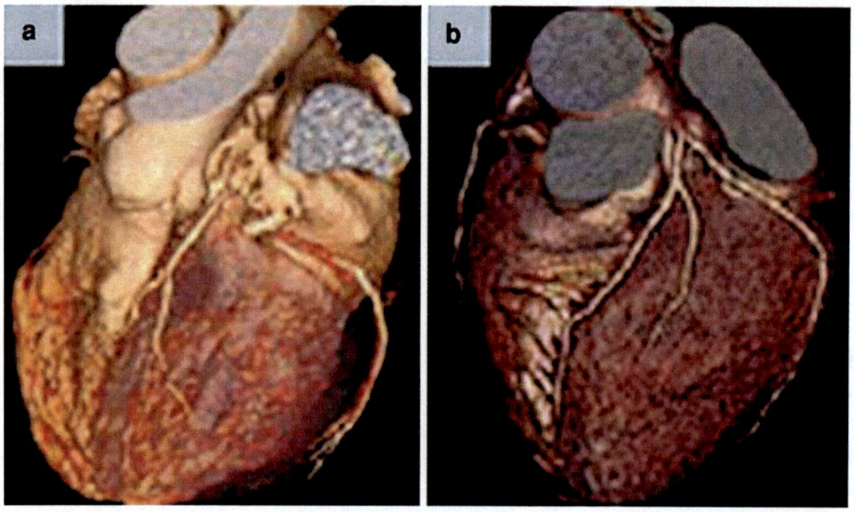


**Fig. 16** The Adaptive ECG-Pulsing spiral CT scan (**a**) with a 4–8 mSv dose and the Adaptive Cardio Sequence scan (**b**) with a 1–3 mSv dose

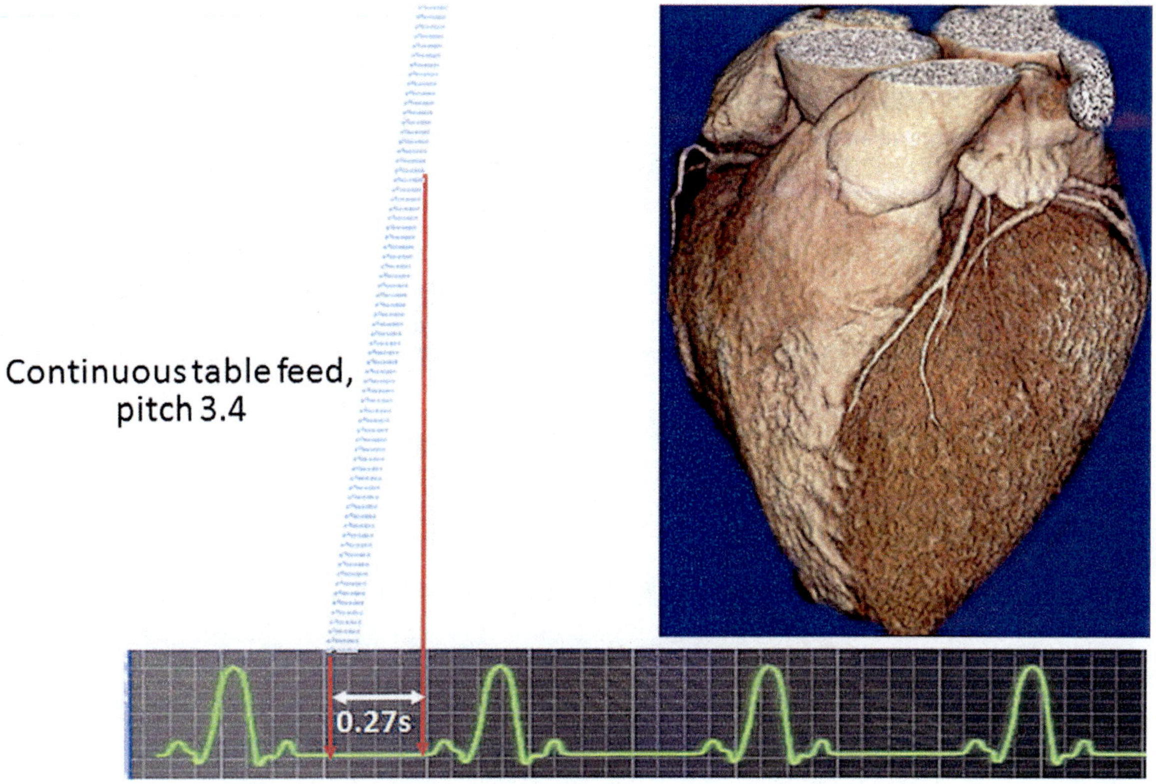


**Fig. 17** Principle of ECG-triggered DSCT spiral scan data acquisition and image reconstruction at very high pitch. The patient table reaches a preselected z-position (e.g., the apex of the heart) at a preselected cardiac phase after acceleration to maximum table speed. Data acquisition begins at this preselected z-position. Because of the rapid movement of the table, the entire heart can be scanned in a fraction of a heartbeat. The total scan time is typically 0.25–0.2 s. The scan data for images at adjacent z-positions (indicated by *short horizontal lines*) are acquired at slightly different phases from the cardiac cycle. Each of the images is reconstructed using data of a quarter rotation per X-ray tube, resulting in a temporal resolution of 75 ms per image

- ECG-controlled dose modulation for cardiac spiral CT—Adaptive ECG-Pulsing
- ECG-triggered sequential CT—Adaptive Cardio Sequence
- ECG-triggered Dual Source spiral CT using very high pitch values—Flash Spiral.

### 7.2.1 ECG-Controlled Dose Modulation for Cardiac Spiral CT: Adaptive ECG-Pulsing

In this acquisition mode data is acquired continuously over multiple heart phases while the patient table moves at low pitch values. Thus, it typically provides the ability to retrospectively select the phase of the cardiac cycle during which images are reconstructed, thus maximizing image quality. To reduce dose, Adaptive ECG-Pulsing should be used. With this method, the radiation dose is modulated during the complete spiral CT scan: the tube current is maintained at 100% of the desired level only during a predefined phase of interest of the heart cycle. During the rest of the time the current is reduced to 20% or even down to 4% (a feature called MinDose), thus reducing the mean absorbed dose by up to 30–50%, see Fig. 14. This method is based on the continuous monitoring of the ECG and an algorithm that predicts when the desired ECG phase will start, and it is reliable for high and/or irregular heart rates.

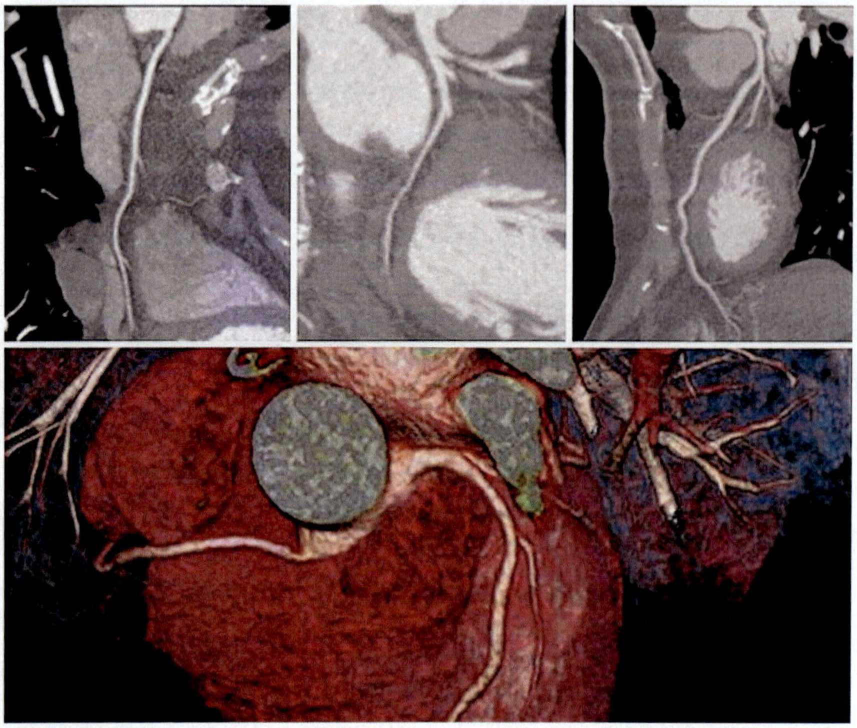

**Fig. 18** The images reconstructed in this modus with an acquisition time of 280 ms, a temporal resolution 75 ms, 80 kV, and 0.4 mSv

### 7.2.2 ECG-Triggered Sequential CT: Adaptive Cardio Sequence

Dubbed as ''step-and-shoot'' mode, this acquisition mode allows substantial dose reductions down to the range of 1.2–4.3 mSv. The trade-off is the somewhat reduced ability of selecting the heart phase for reconstruction.

Prospective ECG-triggering combined with "step-and-shoot" acquisition of axial slices is a very dose-efficient way of ECG-synchronized scanning because only the very minimum of scan data needed for image reconstruction is acquired during the previously selected heart phase, see Fig. 15. The patient's ECG signal is monitored during examination, and axial scans are started with a predefined temporal offset relative to the R-waves. With conventional approaches, the method reaches its limitations with patients with severe arrhythmia, since ECG-triggered axial scanning depends on a reliable prediction of the patient's next cardiac cycle by using the mean length of the preceding cardiac cycles.

With Adaptive Cardio Sequence, a more refined analysis of the patient's ECG is performed. Irregularities are reliably detected, and in case of an ectopic beat, the scan can be either skipped if the ectopic beat happens earlier than the predicted scan start, thus saving unnecessary dose, or repeated at the same position (Fig. 16).

### 7.2.3 ECG-Triggered Dual Source Spiral CT Using Very High Pitch Values: Flash Spiral

With the introduction of Dual Source CT (DSCT), a new way of scanning the heart within one heartbeat arose. The pitch limitation for gapless volume coverage of a single source CT being overcome, pitch values of up to 3.4 in combination with detector coverage of 38.4 mm and 0.28 s gantry rotation time allow for scanning of the heart within approximately 0.27 s with a temporal resolution of 75 ms (Figs. 17 and 18).

## 8 Summary and Conclusion

Dose reduction in CT is an important consideration in today's clinical practice. It is therefore vital to know the technical possibilities a CT system offers to ensure a minimal radiation dose applied with the best possible outcomes for diagnosis.

An equally important part is the assessment and management of patient dose and has become one of the most frequently discussed topics in CT imaging. On Siemens CT scanners, the reporting of established dose parameters like CTDI and DLP has been implemented since 1990. For each exam, the information is available in the Patient Protocol after the scan, and can be viewed and archived as a DICOM image. More recently, new standards in dose reporting have been established (DICOM Dose Structured Reports—DICOM Dose SR) and implemented by Siemens.

Last but not least, education and training are equally important pillars in this area. Only then one can take advantage of all existing dose reduction technologies to their fullest extent.

## References

Graser A et al (2006) Am J Roentgenol 187:695–701
Greess H et al (2002) Eur Radiol 12:1571–1576
Kalra MK et al (2004a) Radiology 230:619–628
Kalra MK et al (2004b) Radiology 233:649–657
Moscariello M et al (2011) Eur Radiol
Mulkens TH et al (2005) Radiology 237:213–223
Rizzo S et al (2006) AJR Am J Roentgenol 186:673–679
Schmidt M et al (2010) Radiology Proc
Winklehner M et al (2011) Eur Radiol

# CT Radiation Dose: Philips Perspective

Alain Vlassenbroek, Dhruv Mehta, and Jeffrey Yanof

## Contents




**Abstract**

Fulfilling the demand for effective diagnostic and therapeutic information has led to a steady increase in the use of computed tomography (CT). With this trend, CT departments strive to scan with the "As Low As Reasonably Achievable" (ALARA) principle; however, its practice varies significantly among sites and scanners servicing an ever-widening range of clinical indications and patient populations. Philips strategies for simplifying CT dose management are described. Multiple components of the Philips CT imaging chain have been designed to increase volume imaging speed, dose efficiency, and image quality, thereby enabling opportunities for lower dose scan protocols and helping to achieve doses ALARA. In addition, nine seamlessly integrated protocol-driven and patient-adaptive technologies including DoseRight Automatic Current Selection, DoseRight dose modulation, DoseRight Cardiac, Step & Shoot, IntelliBeam Filters, SmartShape Wedge (bowtie) Filters, Eclipse DoseRight collimator, and iDose$^4$ Iterative Reconstruction Technique are described. These combined technologies automatically use the quantity and quality of radiation where and when needed, leading to image quality improvements and dose reductions. Combining Philips' dose optimized CT imaging chain with automatic dose optimization tools begins a new era where expanding multi-detector CT will be fueled not only by increasing clinical benefits, but also by easily lowering dose to levels not previously possible for broader patient populations.



A. Vlassenbroek (✉)
Philips Healthcare, Rue des Deux Gares 80, 1070, Brussels, Belgium
e-mail: alain.vlassenbroek@philips.com

D. Mehta · J. Yanof
Philips Healthcare, Miner Road 595, Cleveland, OH, USA


D. Tack et al. (eds.), *Radiation Dose from Multidetector CT*, Medical Radiology. Diagnostic Imaging,
DOI: 10.1007/174_2012_544, © Springer-Verlag Berlin Heidelberg 2012

## 1 Introduction

During the last decade, technological advances have markedly enhanced and expanded the range of clinical applications of computed tomography (CT) (Boll et al. 2006). Consequently, physicians have ranked CT atop the list of innovations that have improved patient care (Fuchs and Sox 2001). While the benefits of CT have been very well documented, increasing radiation doses to the population drew attention to the need for reducing radiation exposure from CT (Mettler et al. (2000); Brenner and Hall 2007). In response, the radiology community has worked to adhere to As Low As Reasonably Achievable (ALARA) principles in CT imaging (FDA 2001; Frush et al. 2003; Golding and Shrimpton 2002; Kalra et al. 2004). While meeting diagnostic and therapeutic imaging objectives, most CT departments and centers strive to routinely scan with patient radiation doses ALARA. However, techniques for practicing ALARA can vary significantly by clinical indication and patient population (Frush et al. 2002; Technical report 2007). Surveys have shown significant variations between sites and scanners including wide ranges of radiation dose for the same scan indication (Frush et al. 2002), utilization of adult scan protocols for pediatrics (Goske et al. 2008a), and opportunities to increase awareness of CT dose estimates (Lee et al. 2004; Technical report 2007).

Dose management is simplified with Philips Healthcare's DoseWise philosophy (Morgan 2002) and the advances embodied in modern Philips MDCT scanners. Multiple components of the imaging chain—from the tube to the detectors to the reconstruction of the final CT images—have been enhanced to increase volume imaging speed, dose efficiency, and image quality (Sect. 2), integrated with new dose optimization (Sect. 3) and reporting tools (Sect. 4), thereby enabling opportunities for lower dose scan protocols. The dose optimization tools are integrated with each stage to automatically control the quantity and quality of radiation where and when needed and help to simplify dose management for routine CT scanning. The resulting image quality and dose efficiency improvements help to meet the imaging objectives with doses ALARA.

## 2 Essence Technology: Improved Image Quality and Dose Efficiency

A high-performing volumetric CT imaging chain with inherent image quality (IQ) and dose efficiency can enable the optimization and routine use of lower dose scan protocols. Philips' iCT 256-slice scanner is based on a highly scalable platform, referred to as Essence technology, that provides a new standard of fast volumetric imaging performance with inherent IQ and dose efficiency, including:

- *Wider detector coverage.* The iCT's NanoPanel$^{3D}$ detector reduces overbeaming by increasing z-axis dose efficiency to 96.4% at 8 cm from 93.0% at 4 cm coverage, as shown in Fig. 1. (Philips Healthcare 2009)
- *ClearRay 2D anti-scatter collimation (ASC).* Scattered radiation primarily originates from the scanned object and adds to the primary transmitted X-ray intensity which we measure at CT. This deviation from the true attenuation measurements can result in artifacts, inaccuracy in reconstructed CT attenuation (HU) measurements, and degradation of low contrast resolution within an image. The increasing z-axis coverage in latest generation of MDCT scanners requires larger cone angles for X-rays to ensure an increased field of view. This increasing cone angle increases the scatter radiation along the z-axis. Scattering is the dominant, most probable, way that diagnostic X-rays interact with human tissue. Scatter radiation is one of the primary contributors to image quality degradation when it reaches the detector. This amount of scattered radiation that reaches detectors grows with increasing z-axis scanner coverage (Engel et al. 2008). As the amount of scattered radiation has been growing continuously, the scatter rejection technology (1-dimensional anti-scatter grids) has barely undergone any improvements in the wide area MDCT scanners. Starting from 64-slice scanners, this scatter radiation results in large scale inhomogeneities in CT attenuation (HU) values as well as dark streaks between strongly absorbing objects (Joseph and Spital 1982) in an image. In the iCT, the NanoPanel$^{3D}$ detector is spherically shaped so its ClearRay 2D anti-scatter grids (Fig. 2a) can be focused for true 3D cone beam geometry.

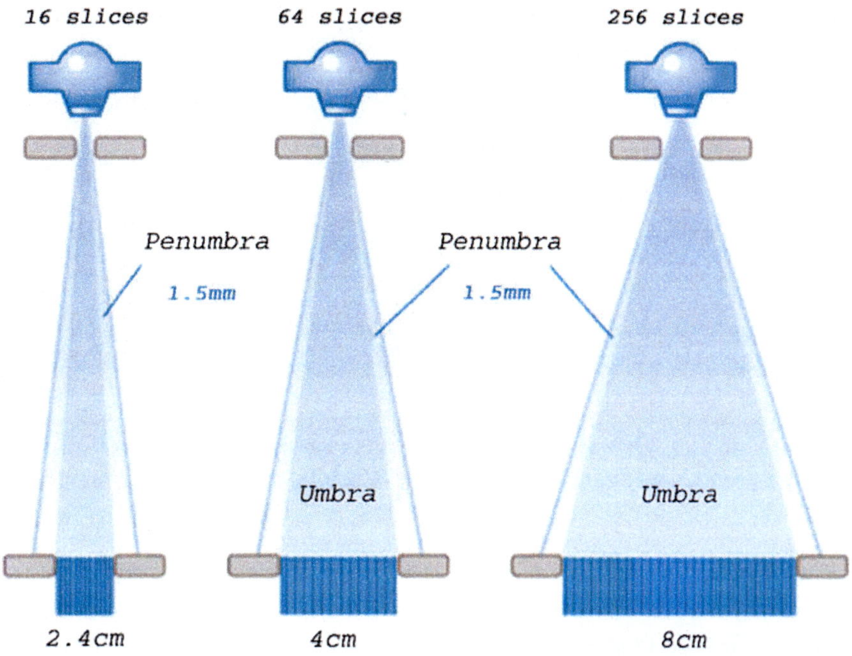


**Fig. 1** Larger detector coverage provides more dose efficiency since overbeaming is reduced. The Z-axis dose efficiency with 8 cm coverage is 3.4 and 7.5% higher than with 4 and 2.4 cm of coverage, respectively. "CT radiation dose: Philips Perspective", by Alain Vlassenbroek: *"Published with kind permission of © A. Vlassenbroek, 2012. All Rights Reserved"*

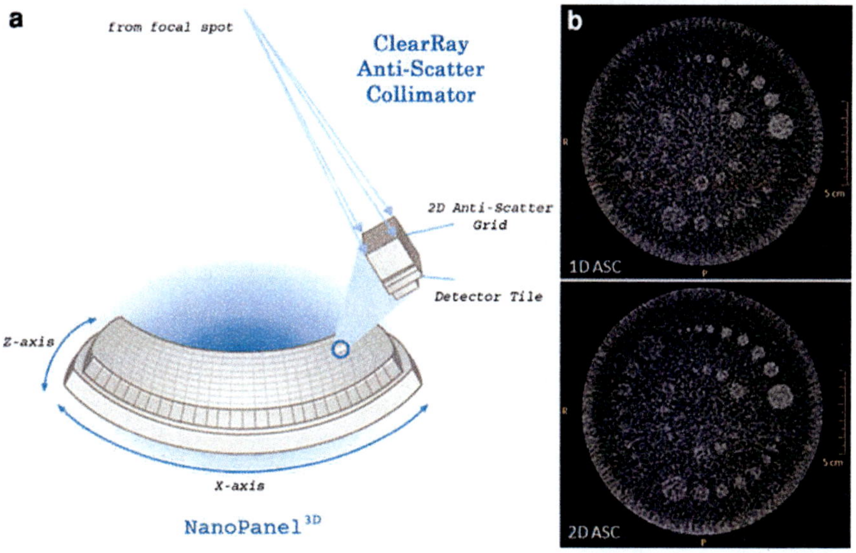


**Fig. 2** **a** ClearRay 2D anti-scatter collimators (ASC) integrated on NanoPanel$^{3D}$ detector tiles decrease volume scatter more effectively than the 1D ASC. **b** Scans of a Catphan phantom at the same dose show improved low contrast with the 1D ASC (lower) compared with the 1D ASC (upper). "CT radiation dose: Philips Perspective", by Alain Vlassenbroek: *"Published with kind permission of © A. Vlassenbroek, 2012. All Rights Reserved"*

The resulting scatter reduction can improve low contrast resolution and uniformity by reducing the scatter-to-primary ratio (SPR) to 6% from 18% for the 1D ASC (Vogtmeier et al. 2008). Scans of a Catphan phantom (The Phantom Laboratory, NY, USA) at the same dose show improved low contrast with the 2D ASC compared with the 1D ASC (Fig. 2b) using the same scan protocol.

- *Fast rotation speed.* The new AirGlide gantry uses a frictionless system—as an alternative to ball bearings—that enables rotation speeds of 0.27 s resulting in a substantial improvement in temporal resolution. This speed helps minimize motion artifacts for challenging examinations such as Step & Shoot Cardiac imaging with higher heart rates or when scanning restless children.

These dose efficiency and IQ improvements, such as a reduction in scatter and motion artifact, and others from Essence technology, can provide opportunities to meet imaging objectives with scan protocols adapted

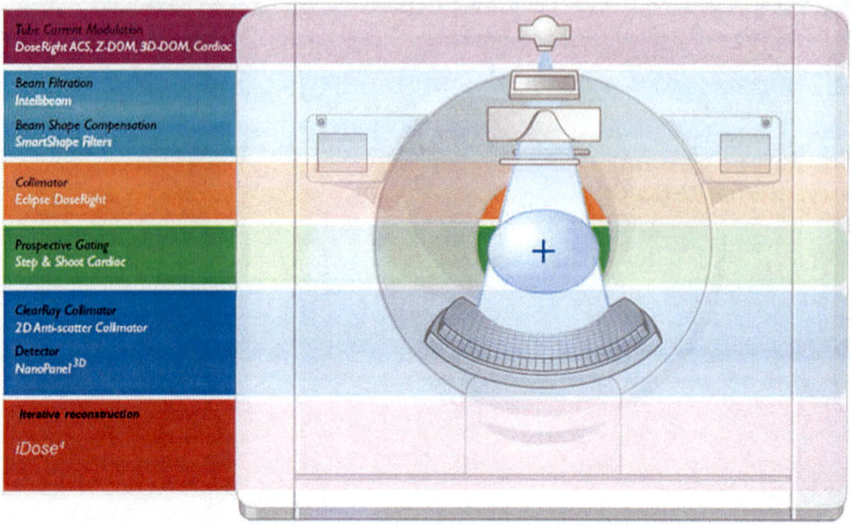


**Fig. 3** The iCT platform has a complete set of advanced dose optimization tools integrated in each stage of the imaging chain and which control the *quantity* and *quality* of exposure *where* and *when* needed. "CT radiation dose: Philips Perspective", by Alain Vlassenbroek: *"Published with kind permission of © A. Vlassenbroek, 2012. All Rights Reserved"*

for doses ALARA. Advances in Essence technology—integrated with dose optimization tools described in the Sect. 3—show that dose and image quality do not need to be difficult trade-offs.

## 3 Improved Image Quality and Dose Optimization Technologies

To further simplify dose management, the iCT platform has a complete set of advanced image quality and dose optimization tools seamlessly integrated with Essence technology. These tools optimize image quality and control the quantity and quality of exposure where and when needed as summarized in the stages of the imaging chain (Fig. 3). Tube current modulation techniques (DoseRight ACS, Z-DOM, 3D-DOM, Cardiac), advanced gating techniques (Step & Shoot Cardiac and Complete), beam shaping (SmartShape) and quality filters (IntelliBeam), the helical end-effect collimation (Eclipse DoseRight Collimator), and iterative reconstruction technique (iDose$^4$) are described below in sequence from X-ray source to final reconstructed images.

Special pediatric dose saving techniques are then described to show how dose optimization tools are used in concert along with age- and weight-based tube current reduction factors.

The integrated set of dose optimization tools is patient-adaptive and protocol-driven to automatically deploy the optimum component configurations for each scan. A number of dose optimization techniques, such as the SmartShape wedge (bowtie) filters, are designed to optimize both dose and image quality, while others, such as the Eclipse DoseRight collimator, lower exposure without affecting IQ (Philips Healthcare 2009).

### 3.1 DoseRight Automatic Current Selection

If scan parameters were not adapted for the size of the scan region, larger (smaller) patients would receive less (more) dose per kilogram. This is because for a given projection, the center and peripheral region nearest the detector would typically have lower (higher) beam intensity for a larger (smaller) patient due to attenuation along a larger (smaller) diameter. The summative effect with each tube rotation would result in higher (lower) average noise levels for larger (smaller) patients.

DoseRight ACS automatically suggests tube current settings according to the maximum estimated patient size in the scan region. A default "reference" tube current corresponding to an average patient size is defined for each scan protocol and can be modified by the user. This reference size is defined for each scan type and age group. For example, the reference size for the scan type "body" is 33 cm for an adult, 20 cm for a child, and 16 cm for an infant.

When planning an examination, the patient's maximum diameter is estimated from the "surview"

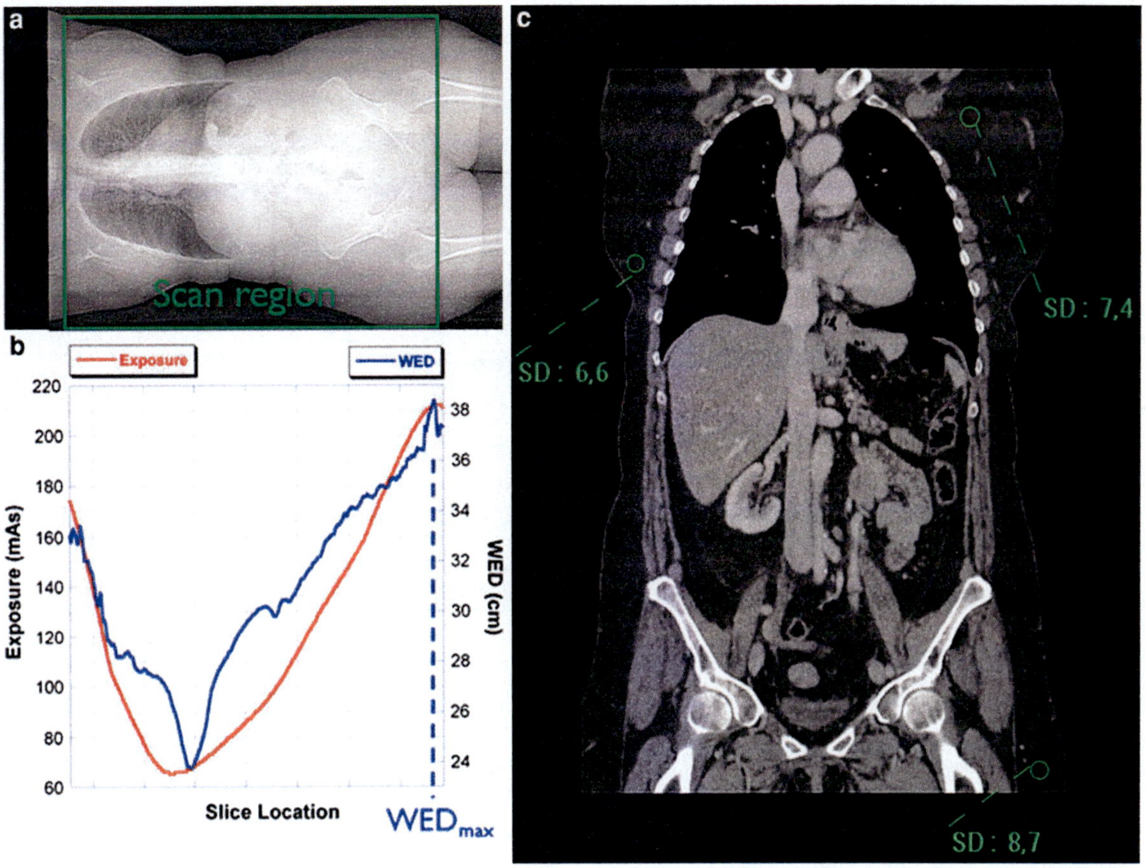


**Fig. 4** **a** Surview image and definition of the scan region. **b** The Water Equivalent Diameter WED(z) along the table direction is measured from the Surview image. $WED_{max}$ is compared to the reference diameter to scale the X-ray exposure. In this example, DoseRight ACS recommends an exposure of 210 mAs for $WED_{max}$ = 38 cm. WED(z) profile is used to modulate the exposure (mAs) for each table position with DoseRight Z-DOM. **c** Coronal reformat of the reconstructed axial images shows that DoseRight Z-DOM does not adapt the tube current to maintain a constant noise level for every patient size but gives a lower noise level for smaller attenuating sizes. The noise measured as the standard deviation (SD) of the pixel value (HU) is lower in the thorax (SD = 6.6 HU; WED ~ 24 cm) compared to the shoulder (SD = 7.4 HU; WED ~ 32 cm) and the pelvis region (SD = 7.4 HU; WED ~ 38 cm). "CT radiation dose: Philips Perspective", by Alain Vlassenbroek: *"Published with kind permission of © A. Vlassenbroek, 2012. All Rights Reserved"*

(Fig. 4a). This maximum diameter is expressed as a "water equivalent diameter" ($WED_{max}$) which corresponds to the diameter of a cylindrical water phantom with the same total attenuation. The patient diameter WED(z) is actually measured from the surview for every position along the craniocaudal (z) axis and DoseRight ACS uses the maximum value $WED_{max}$ of WED(z) and compares it to the reference diameter to scale the reference tube current to control the dose and noise level by suggesting a higher or lower value for larger or smaller diameters, respectively (Fig. 4b). Note that DoseRight ACS does not adapt the tube current to maintain a constant noise level for every patient size but keeps a lower noise level for smaller patient size (including pediatric patients) (see Fig. 4c). This is in agreement with the observation noted by McCollough et al., "Radiologists most strongly prefer less image noise on images obtained in small patients and/or children, probably because most small patients/children do not have the fat planes between tissues and organs that are typical in larger adults and that enhance contrast and tissue differentiation. In addition, because the details of interest are smaller in small patients/children, higher contrast-to-noise ratios (CNR) are required" (McCollough et al. 2006; Wilting et al. 2001).

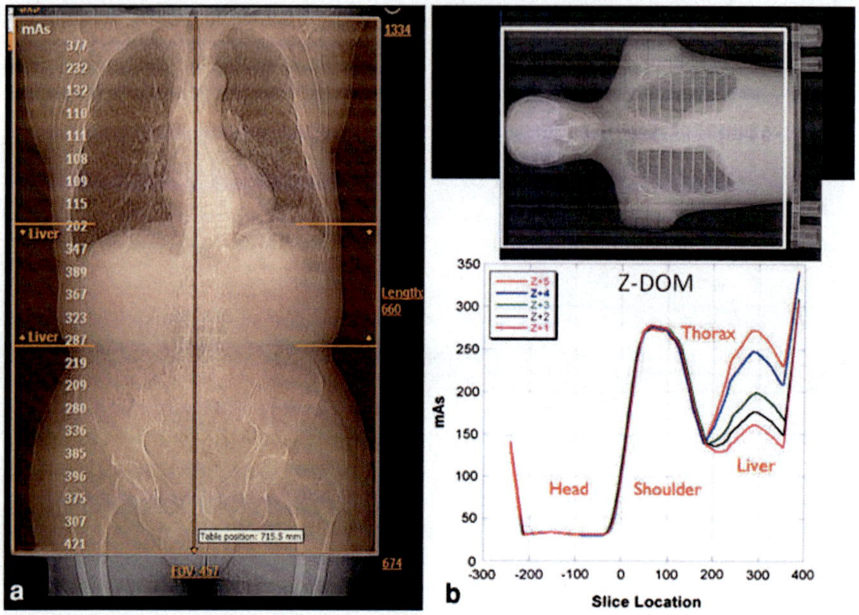


**Fig. 5** **a** Surview image demonstrating the liver detection algorithm in a CAP examination. The DoseRight Z-DOM exposure profile (mAs) is displayed on the image. **b** CAP protocol applied to a RANDO phantom and the corresponding mAs profiles corresponding to five different strenghts of the "liver image quality boosting" parameter in the scan protocol. "CT radiation dose: Philips Perspective", by Alain Vlassenbroek: *"Published with kind permission of © A. Vlassenbroek, 2012. All Rights Reserved"*

### 3.2 DoseRight Z-axis Dose Modulation

Average X-ray attenuation can vary significantly along the craniocaudal (z) axis as can be seen on Fig. 4b. For example, the chest has a much lower average attenuation than the abdomen due to air in the lungs and will require a much lower tube current to achieve the desired image quality. As mentioned in Sect. 3.1, WED(z) is measured from the surview for every position along the craniocaudal (z) axis in the scan region. This z-profile can be used to modulate the tube current for each table position. The maximum, average, and minimal tube current levels for Z-DOM are displayed when planning the scan, and the percentage dose reduction is displayed with the reconstructed images. Note that DoseRight ACS and Z-DOM can be switched on separately or used in combination.

Phantom measurements performed on a RANDO phantom (Fluke Biomedical, WA, USA) show that the absorbed organ dose is reduced by 23% in the Thyroid, 19% in the Breast, and 26% in the eyes when Z-DOM is used compared to measurements performed without Z-DOM (Lee et al. 2010). Other unpublished data show that, in multi-region examinations such as chest-abdomen-pelvis (CAP) or head-neck scan protocols, DoseRight Z-DOM has been seen clinically to lower patient dose by about 20–40%.

For scans where the brain or the liver are included in multi-region examinations and where low contrast detectability is of primary importance (e.g., oncology scans), a low dose acquisition with Z-DOM may deliver insufficient image quality. Brain and liver require excellent low contrast detectability and an image quality above what is expected for other organs like the pelvis or the thorax. A solution consists of increasing the DoseRight ACS-recommended tube current. However, doing this results in a global shift of the tube current profile for the whole region to larger values which results in an inadequate dose delivered to the shoulder-thorax and pelvis regions. To solve this issue, Philips has introduced neck- and liver detection algorithms that enable increasing the tube current in the brain and liver area only. This improves the corresponding image quality and low contrast detectability for these organs. Figure 5a shows a surview image demonstrating the liver detection algorithm for a patient referred to CT for a CAP scan in an oncology follow-up examination. Also shown on Fig. 5a is the corresponding mAs modulation profile displayed on the surview image. Figure 5b shows a similar CAP protocol applied to a RANDO phantom together with a plot of the mAs profiles corresponding to five different strenghts of the "liver image quality boosting" parameter in the scan protocol (scale 1–5).

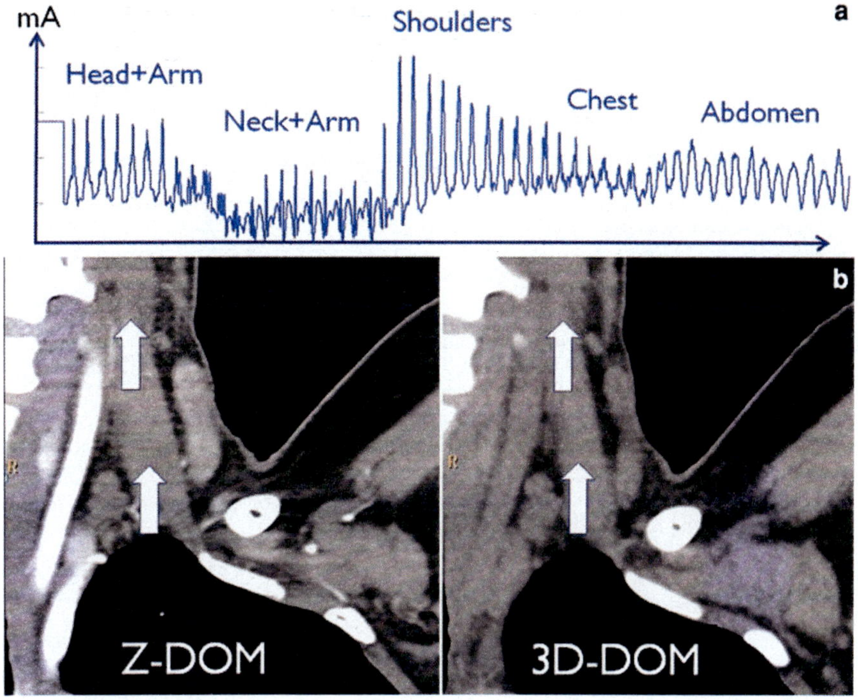


**Fig. 6** **a** DoseRight 3D-DOM applies an angular modulation of the tube current around the DoseRight Z-DOM modulation profile during the tube rotation according to changes in patient shape eccentricity. For each rotation, projections are processed to determine the maximum and minimum patient diameter. **b** Improvement of image quality with DoseRight 3D-DOM against DoseRight Z-DOM is due to a more homogeneous distribution of X-ray photons on the detectors during each rotation leading due a reduction of the streak noise in the reconstructed images as pointed out by the *arrows*. "CT radiation dose: Philips Perspective", by Alain Vlassenbroek: "*Published with kind permission of © A. Vlassenbroek, 2012. All Rights Reserved*"

## 3.3 DoseRight 3D Dose Modulation

The X-ray attenuation of the patient can also vary with tube rotation angle. For example, the shoulder region can have a higher attenuation lateraly than anteroposteriorly. DoseRight 3D-DOM applies an angular modulation of the tube current around the DoseRight Z-DOM modulation profile during the tube rotation according to changes in patient shape (eccentricity). For each rotation, projections are processed to determine the maximum and minimum patient diameter (see Fig. 6a). The tube current for the next rotation is then modulated between these limits. Improvement of image quality with DoseRight 3D-DOM above Z-DOM is due to a more homogeneous distribution of X-ray photons on the detectors during each rotation, thus leading to a reduction of the streak noise in the reconstructed images (see Fig. 6b).

## 3.4 DoseRight Cardiac: Dose Modulation for Retrospectively-Gated Helical Scans

In helical cardiac scans, radiation dose reduction can be achieved by prospectively modulating the tube current using the ECG information. The tube current can be kept at the nominal level (100%) during the targeted cardiac phase of interest and can be reduced to 20% during all other phases of the cardiac cycle (see Fig. 7a). Using this approach, dose savings of up to 45% can be achieved without compromising the image quality in the cardiac phase of interest, depending on the heart rate during the acquisition (Hesse et al. 2006).

## 3.5 Step & Shoot Cardiac and Complete: Prospective Gating

Imaging an organ over multiple physiological phases (e.g., over the cardiac cycle) can provide both anatomical and functional information (see Sect. 3.4); however, for many indications it is only necessary to image—and expose—a single phase. With the Step & Shoot Cardiac and Complete techniques, the tube current can be prospectively modulated to image only a desired phase in an axial scanning mode, thus enabling prospectively gated axial cardiac scanning during the "quiet" phase of the cardiac cycle. Step & Shoot Cardiac scans can result in a dose savings of up to 80% compared with a retrospectively-gated helical technique, while maintaining optimum image quality (see Fig. 7b). Furthermore, larger detector width can

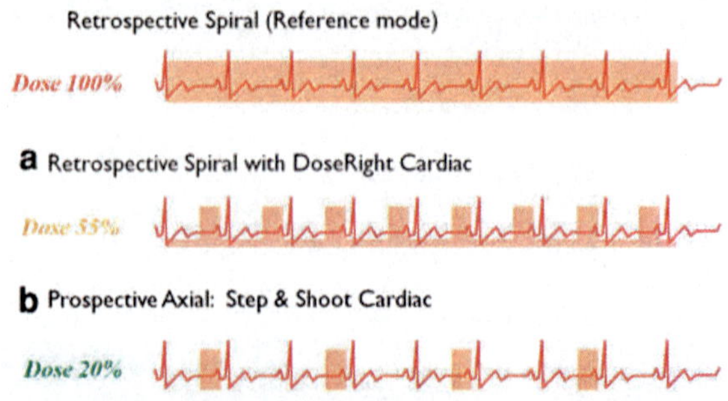


**Fig. 7** **a** With retrospective gating during spiral scanning, the tube current can be kept at the nominal level (100%) during the targeted cardiac phase of interest (in this example, the diastolic phase) and can be reduced to 20% during all other phases of the cardiac cycle. Using this approach, dose savings of up to 45% can be achieved without compromising the image quality in the cardiac phase of interest, depending on the heart rate during the acquisition. **b** With prospective gating, the tube current can be prospectively modulated to image only the desired cardiac phase in an axial scanning mode. Step & Shoot Cardiac or Complete scans can result in a dose savings of up to 80% compared with a retrospectively-gated reference helical technique. "CT radiation dose: Philips Perspective", by Alain Vlassenbroek: *"Published with kind permission of © A. Vlassenbroek, 2012. All Rights Reserved"*

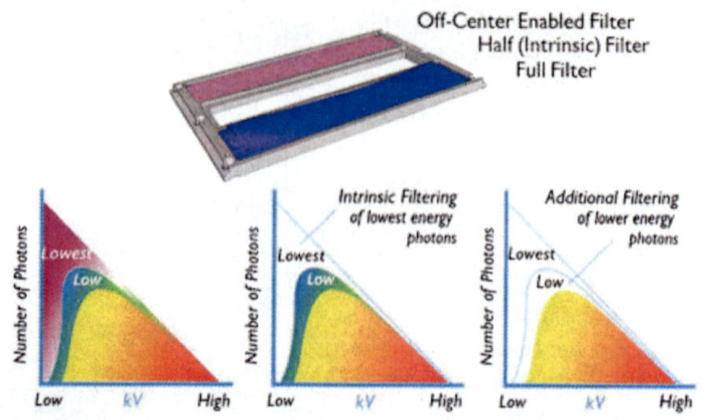


**Fig. 8** The low energy content (softness) of X-ray spectrum can affect dose and image quality and can be controlled with the IntelliBeam filters. The filter selection is automatically configured with the scan protocol. "CT radiation dose: Philips Perspective", by Alain Vlassenbroek: *"Published with kind permission of © A. Vlassenbroek, 2012. All Rights Reserved"*

be further leveraged by increasing the axial shot coverage for decreasing field of view. This enables larger step lengths with minimum cone beam overlap.

### 3.6 IntelliBeam Filters

For a selected peak kilo-voltage setting (80, 100, 120, and 140 kVp), the low energy content (softness) of X-ray spectrum can affect dose and image quality: a beam that is too "soft" can increase skin dose and a beam that is too "hard" (higher "quality") can decrease contrast detail. On the iCT, the beam's hardness (quality) can be controlled with selectable IntelliBeam filters (see filter tray on Fig. 8). The filter selection is configured with scan protocols, and is used automatically in combination with SmartShape wedges (see Table 1 and Fig. 9) and the X-ray tube's intrinsic filtration to optimize both low contrast resolution and dose.

The filters are designated "full", "half", and "off-center enabled".[1] The full IntelliBeam filter used with all adult head and body protocols reduces dose by about 30% at 120 kVp and 46% at 80 kVp relative to half filter. The half filter is used with infant scan protocols to enhance low contrast resolution. This helps manage dose in combination with the small wedge and intrinsic filtration (as shown in Table 1).

### 3.7 SmartShape Wedge (Bowtie) Filters

Wedges, also known as bowtie filters, can increase both dose efficiency and image quality. This double advantage is achieved by filtering the beam's intensity according to the patient's shape. Each wedge provides more filtering from medial—where the patient thickness is greatest—to lateral, thereby facilitating a uniform dose and noise distribution as the tube rotates. Three SmartShape wedges are provided: (a) small: infants 0–8 months, (b) medium: cardiac, and (c) large: adult head and body (see Fig. 9a).

A medium size phantom is used in Fig. 9b to illustrate the importance of wedge. It shows a green shaded beam intensity in the center region for all three wedge sizes. When a large (small) wedge is used on the medium phantom, as shown on the right (left), the wedge's peripheral attenuation thickness is too small (large), the peripheral beam intensity is too high (low), resulting in a higher (lower) peripheral dose. When appropriately sized, the wedge's curvature facilitates a uniform exit beam intensity and image quality throughout the scanned region. They are used in

[1] A special trauma scan protocol uses a 1.2 mm aluminum filter without a wedge filter. This protocol is useful when patient centering is either not possible or not a priority.

**Table 1** The IntelliBeam filter selection is configured with the scan protocols, and is used automatically in combination with SmartShape wedges (see Fig. 9) and the X-ray tube's intrinsic filtration to optimize both low contrast resolution and dose

| Default scan protocol | Tray position | HVL[d] (mm AI equiv) | Wedge |
|---|---|---|---|
| Adult head and body | Full | 8.7 | Large |
| Cardiac | Full | 8.7 | Medium |
| Infant | Half | 7.4 | Small |
| Trauma | Off-center | 7.8 | Open |

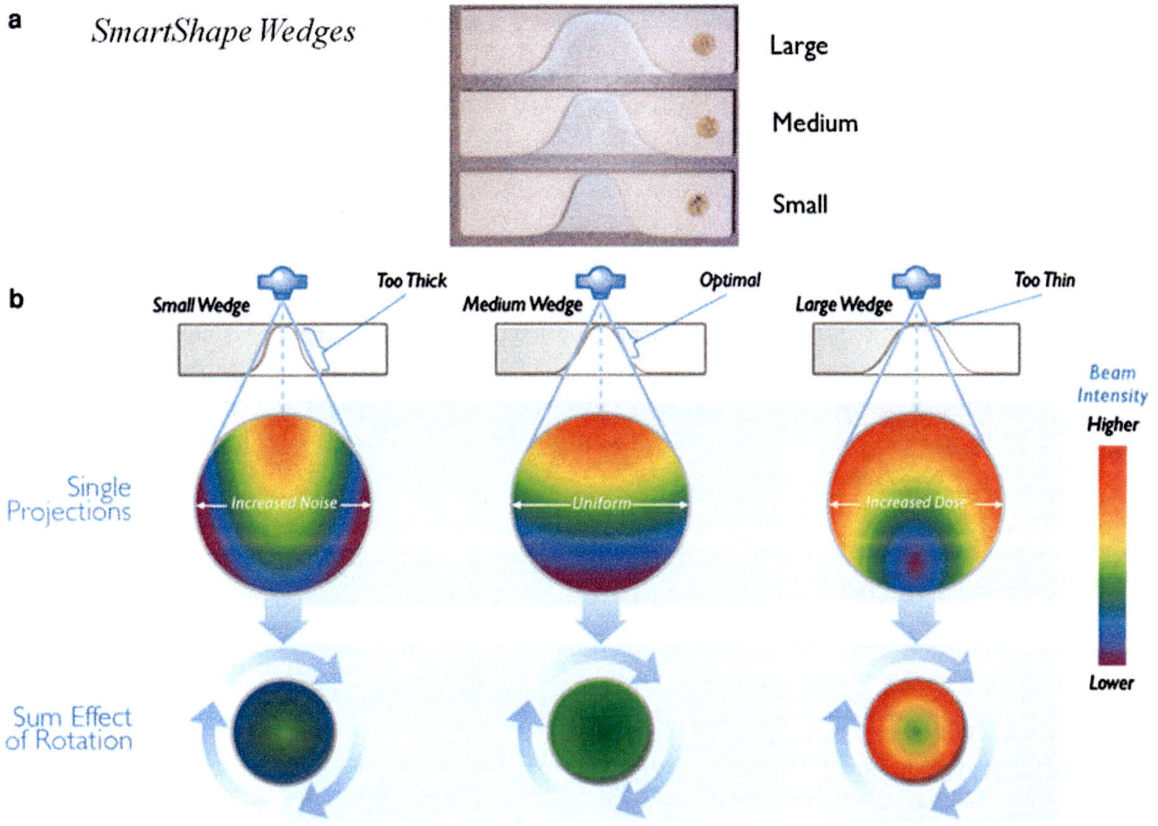


**Fig. 9** **a** Three SmartShape wedges are provided: (a) small: infants 0-18 months, (b) medium: cardiac, and (c) large: adult head and body. **b** A medium size phantom is used to illustrate the importance of wedge. It shows a green shaded beam intensity in the center region for all three wedge sizes. When a large (*small*) wedge is used on the medium phantom, as shown on the right (*left*), the wedge's peripheral attenuation thickness is too small (*large*), the peripheral beam intensity is too high (low), resulting in a higher (*lower*) peripheral dose. When appropriately sized, the wedge's curvature facilitates a uniform exit beam intensity and image quality throughout the scanned region. "CT radiation dose: Philips Perspective", by Alain Vlassenbroek: *"Published with kind permission of © A. Vlassenbroek, 2012. All Rights Reserved"*

conjunction with the IntelliBeam filters, and are automatically selected based on the protocol being used.

*Infant wedge.* $CTDI_{(vol)}$ is reduced by approximately 14 and 22% as measured with the standard FDA head (16 cm) and body (32 cm) phantoms, respectively, compared with the large wedge. A dose savings of 10–14% can therefore be estimated for properly centered infant body examinations since the head phantom better approximates infant body size (less than 18 months).

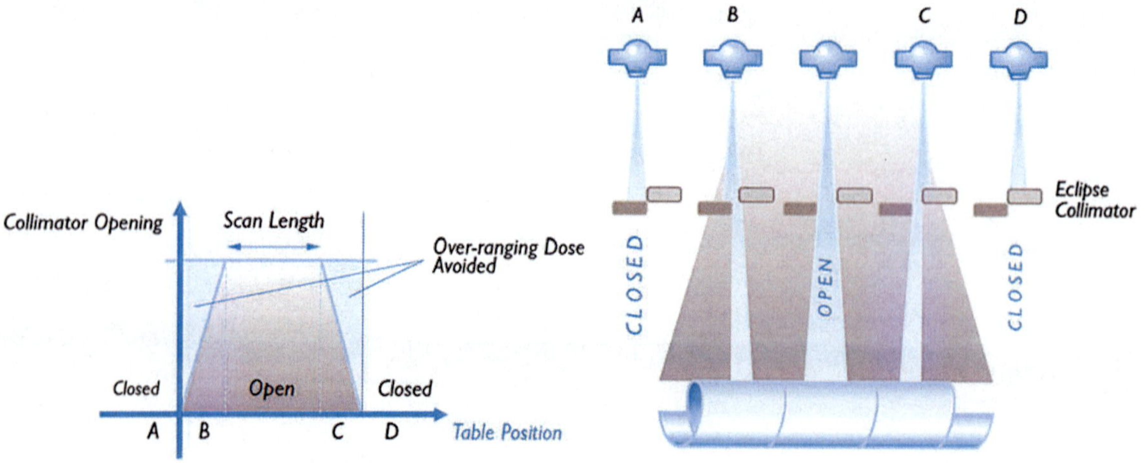


**Fig. 10** The Eclipse collimator automatically opens at the beginning and closes at the end of helical acquisitions. This dynamic collimator reduces unnecessary exposure without affecting image quality. DLP is reduced by one-half rotation at the start and by one-half rotation at the end of the helix (shown as regions a–b and c–d). "CT radiation dose: Philips Perspective", by Alain Vlassenbroek: *"Published with kind permission of © A. Vlassenbroek, 2012. All Rights Reserved"*

**Table 2** The Eclipse DoseRight Collimator reduces unnecessary exposure during spiral scanning without affecting image quality. Dose reduction is proportionally higher in scans with wider collimation, larger pitch, and shorter scan lengths such as those used in cardiac, pediatric, and brain exams

| | Typical scan length (cm) | Dose savings on DLP |
|---|---|---|
| Pediatric chest | 8 | 33% |
| Abdomen | 32 | 17% |
| Head/Brain | 16 | 25% |

*Cardiac wedge.* Body $CTDI_{(vol)}$ and $CTDI_{(peripheral)}$ is reduced by approximately 11 and 13%, respectively, relative to the large wedge. These results can be used to estimate a lung dose savings of 11–13% for properly centered cardiac examinations.

## 3.8 Eclipse DoseRight Collimator

Unnecessary, wasted exposure that does not contribute to imaging can occur at the beginning and end of helical scans. The Eclipse DoseRight Collimator—a component of the iCT imaging chain that complements wide detector coverage—automatically opens at the beginning and closes at the end of helical acquisitions as shown in Fig. 10. This dynamic collimator reduces unnecessary exposure without affecting image quality. DLP[2] is reduced by one-half rotation at the start and by one-half rotation at the end of the helix (shown as regions a–b and c–d, see Fig. 10). Therefore, dose reduction is proportionally higher with wider collimation, when using a larger pitch, and for shorter scan lengths (see Table 2). The combination of wider detector coverage and dynamic collimation reduces both "over-beaming" and "over-ranging" (Goske et al. 2008b). Dose reductions can be considerable, especially with short length helical scans, such as those used in cardiac, pediatric, and brain exams.

## 3.9 iDose$^4$ Iterative Reconstruction Technique

Filtered back projection (FBP) has been the industry standard for CT image reconstruction for decades (Radon 1917). While it is a very fast and fairly robust method, FBP is a sub-optimal algorithm choice for poorly sampled data or for cases where noise overwhelms the image signal. Such situations may occur in low dose or tube-power–limited acquisitions (e.g., scans of morbidly obese individuals). Noise in CT projection data is dominated by photon count statistics.

[2] Dose-length product = irradiated scan length * CTDI.

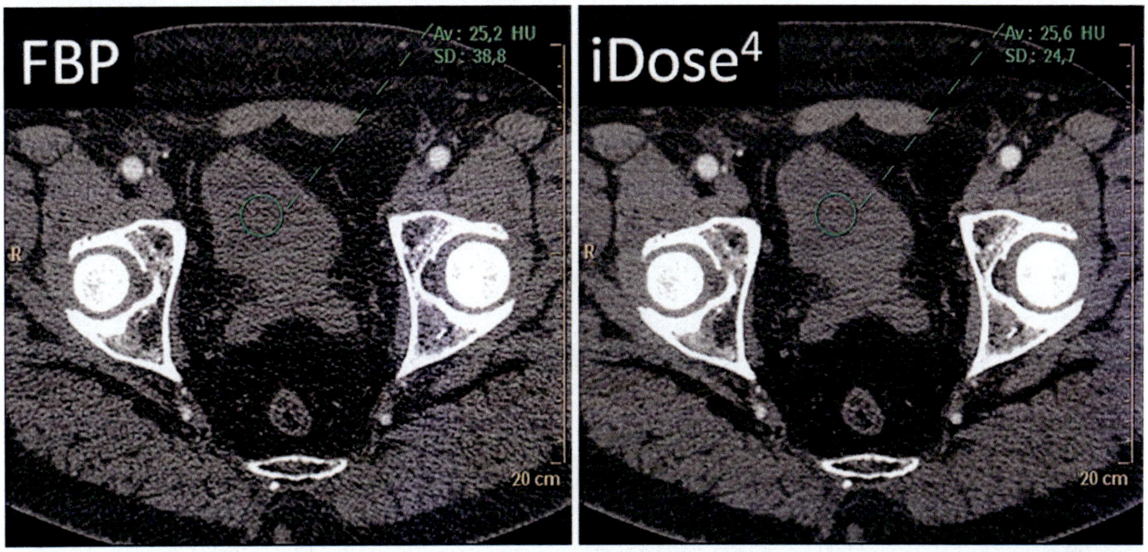


**Fig. 11** Image quality improvement with iDose$^4$ reconstruction compared to conventional filtered back projection reconstruction with the same scan. With FBP, the standard deviation of the pixel value (noise) measured on the image (SD = 38.8 HU) is 57% larger compared to the same measurement performed on the image reconstructed with iDose$^4$ (SD = 24.7 HU). A similar image quality improvement could only be achieved with FBP by increasing the patient dose by a factor 2.47. "CT radiation dose: Philips Perspective", by Alain Vlassenbroek: *"Published with kind permission of © A. Vlassenbroek, 2012. All Rights Reserved"*

As the dose is lowered, the variance in the photon count statistics increases disproportionately (Whiting et al. 2006). When these very high levels of noise are propagated through the reconstruction algorithm, the result is an image with significant artifacts and high quantum mottle noise. Over time, incremental enhancements were made to FBP to overcome some of its limitations. These improvements continued until recently, when a completely different approach to image reconstruction was explored through the clinical implementation of iterative reconstruction (IR) techniques. IR techniques attempt to formulate image reconstruction as an optimization problem (i.e., IR attempts to find the image that is the "best fit" to the acquired data). The noisiest measurements are given low weight in the iterative process; therefore, they contribute very little to the final image. Hence, IR techniques treat noise properly at very low signal levels, and consequently reduce the noise and artifacts present in the resulting reconstructed image. This results in an overall improvement of image quality at any given dose. With IR techniques, the noise can be controlled for high spatial resolution reconstructions; hence providing high-quality, low contrast, and spatial resolution within the same image. While IR techniques have been used for many years in PET and SPECT imaging, the sampling density and the data set sizes in CT have historically caused IR techniques to perform extremely slowly when compared to FBP. However, recent innovations in hardware design and algorithm optimizations have permitted the clinical use of an IR technique in CT.

iDose$^4$, a 4th generation reconstruction technique, is the latest addition to Philips' scanners that has been integrated with Essence technology and that provides significant improvements in image quality as well as noise reduction (Philips Healthcare 2011).

iDose$^4$ provides an innovative solution in which iterative processing is performed in both the projection and image domains. The reconstruction algorithm starts first with projection data where it identifies and corrects the noisiest CT measurements—those with very poor signal to noise ratio, or very low photon counts. Each projection is examined for points that have likely resulted from very noisy measurements using a model that includes the true photons statistics. Through an iterative diffusion process, the noisy data is penalized and edges are preserved. This process ensures that the gradients of underlying structures are retained, thus preserving spatial resolution while allowing a significant noise

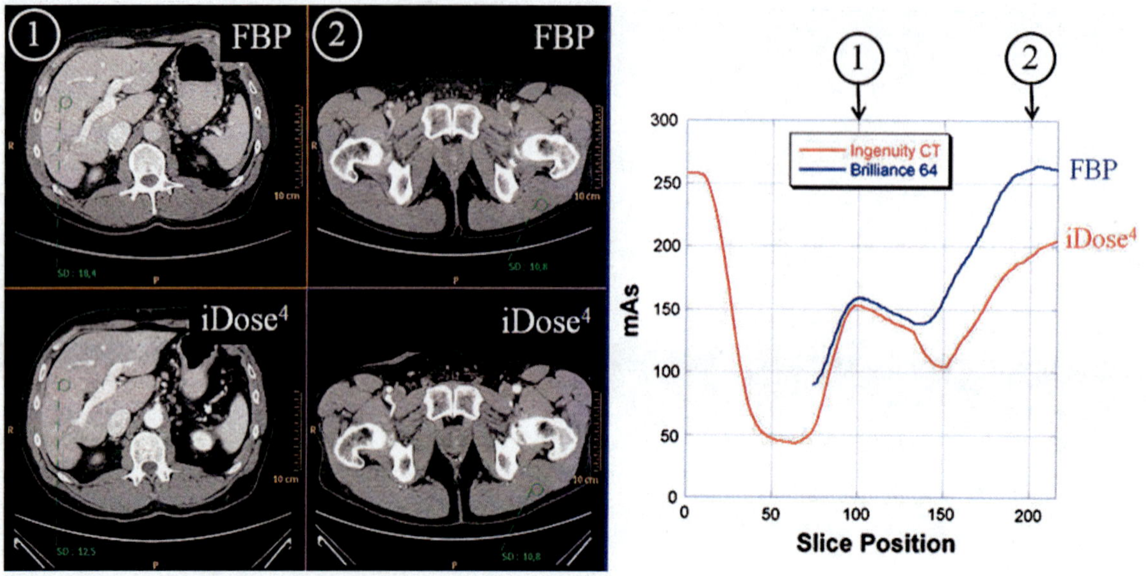


**Fig. 12** *Left upper raw* Acquisition performed on the Brilliance 64-Channel scanner and reconstructed with FBP. The aquisition was performed with DoseRight Z-DOM without liver image quality boosting (see Sect. 3.2). In the liver parenchyma, we measure the noise as SD = 18.4 HU at an exposure = 159 mAs. In the pelvis, we measure SD = 10.8 HU at an exposure = 261 mAs. *Left lower raw* Acquisition performed on the Ingenuity CT scanner and reconstructed with iDose$^4$ on the same patient at a later date for an oncology follow-up. The acquisition was performed with DoseRight Z-DOM with liver image quality boosting. All other acquisition parameters were identical compared to the acquisition performed on the Brilliance 64-Channel scanner. In the liver parenchyma, we measure the noise as SD = 12.5 HU at an exposure = 152 mAs. In the pelvis, we measure SD = 10.8 HU at an exposure = 191 mAs. *Right*: shows the respective DoseRight Z-DOM modulation profiles of the acquisitions performed on the Brilliance 64-Channel scanner (*in blue*) and on the Ingenuity CT (*in red*). We note the increased exposure values of the DoseRight Z-DOM profile in the liver region on the Ingenuity CT due to the liver IQ boosted modulation. As can be seen in the pelvis region (*position 2*), the iDose$^4$ reconstruction on the Ingenuity CT leads to a similar image quality as compared to FBP reconstruction on the Brilliance 64-Channel scanner. However, on the liver region (*position 1*) where low contrast is of primary importance for oncology patients, similar patient dose is delivered but a huge image quality improvement is obtained on the Ingenuity CT due to the iDose$^4$ reconstruction. "CT radiation dose: Philips Perspective", by Alain Vlassenbroek: *"Published with kind permission of © A. Vlassenbroek, 2012. All Rights Reserved"*

reduction. In doing so, this process prevents the primary cause of low signal streaks. Also, since the corrections are performed on the acquisition data (unlogged projections); this method successfully prevents bias error. The noise that remains after this stage of the algorithm is propagated to the image space; however, the propagated noise is now highly localized and can be effectively removed to support the desired level of image noise. The next major component of the iDose$^4$ algorithm deals with subtraction of the image noise while preserving the underlying edges associated with true anatomy or pathology. This subtraction begins with an estimate of the noise distribution in the image volume. This estimate is used to reduce the noise while preserving the true structure. This estimate also allows the preservation of the image noise power-spectrum characteristic of a lower noise acquisition and FBP reconstruction. Following this, a selector chooses among noiseless structural models, and the model that best fits the local topology of the image volume is chosen. Once the best model is chosen, it is used to reduce the noise in the image volume. To ensure uniform noise removal at all frequencies, multifrequency noise removal is performed.

Evidence from phantom tests and rigorous clinical evaluations with global clinical collaborators demonstrate the potential of iDose$^4$ to improve image quality and/or lower image noise levels beyond those previously achievable with conventional, routine acquisitions, filtered back projection reconstructions (see Fig. 11). Also demonstrated is the benefits of this 4th generation reconstruction technique in preventing photon-starvation artifacts (streaks, bias) prior to image

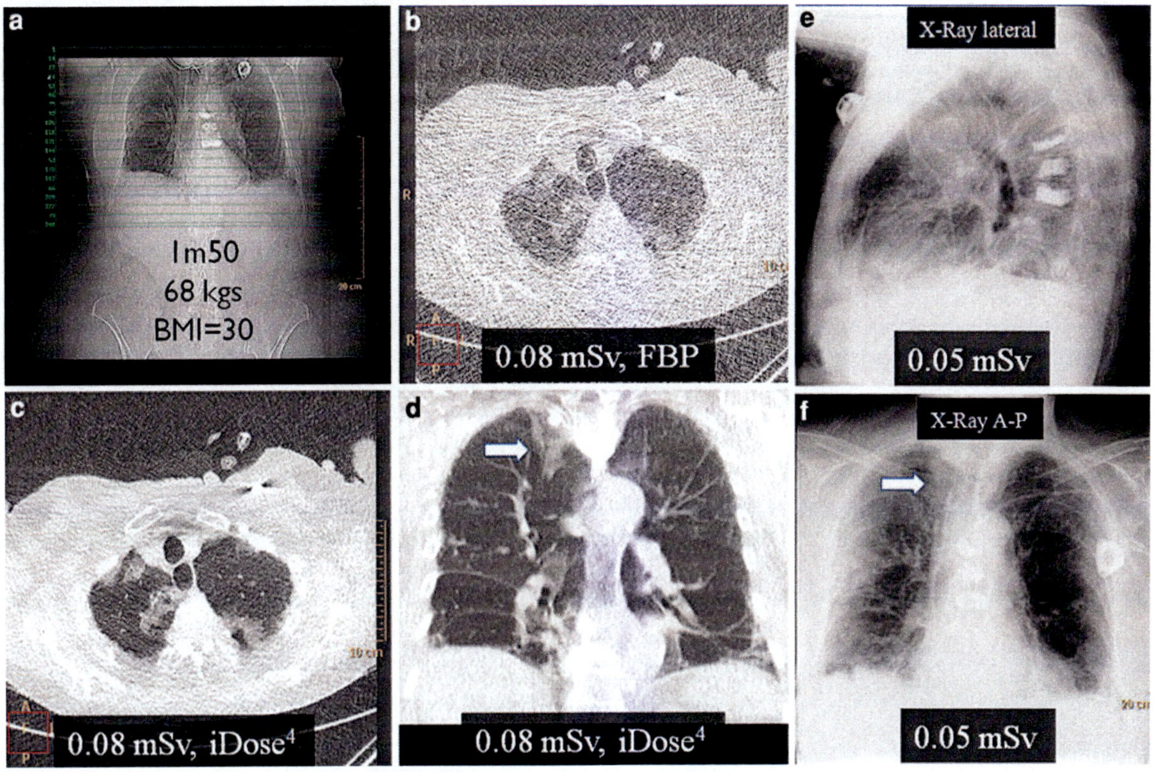


**Fig. 13** Comparison between ultra low dose chest MDCT and Chest X-Ray. **a** Surview image used to plan an ultra low dose MDCT scan (80 kVp/10 mAs, DLP = 5.8 mGy.cm, effective dose = 0.08 mSv) performed on a patient with breast cancer (1m50, 68 kg, bmi = 30). The MDCT axial images were reconstructed with **b** FBP and **c** iDose$^4$ reconstruction algorithms. Images reconstructed with FBP cannot be assessed because of the large amount of noise in the images. However, the images reconstructed with iDose$^4$ can be assessed to provide comprehensive diagnostic information and visualize opacities in the upper part of the lung. **d** A coronal reformat of the ultra low dose images reconstructed with iDose$^4$ enables a better 3D visualization of the abnormal structures (*white arrow*) as compared to the 2D views **e** and **f** of the chest X-Ray for a similar total patient dose (X-ray effective dose ~0.05 mSv per view). "CT radiation dose: Philips Perspective", by Alain Vlassenbroek: *"Published with kind permission of © A. Vlassenbroek, 2012. All Rights Reserved"*

creation and in maintaining image texture to overcome the artificial or "plastic" look of images that have been frequently reported when using previous-generation iterative reconstruction techniques. iDose$^4$ can be used in conjunction with all other dose optimization tools previously described (see example on Fig. 12).

From the workflow perspective, iDose$^4$ reconstruction is triggered by changing the reconstruction type from "standard" (FBP) to "iDose". iDose$^4$ reconstruction can be either selected prospectively (before the scan) or performed retrospectively on datasets for which the projection (raw) data is still available on the scanner. Scan protocols may utilize iDose$^4$ by default. An additional parameter—iDose$^4$ level (scale: 1–7) is used to define the strength of the iterative reconstruction technique in reducing image quantum mottle noise (range 11–55% noise reduction relative to a corresponding FBP reconstruction). The chosen level does not affect the reconstruction time (up to 20 images per second) and can be defined independent of the radiation dose with which an acquisition is performed.

With these techniques, an array of new CT applications may emerge, where a comprehensive diagnostic is enabled by noise reduction (see example on Fig. 13).

## 3.10 Pediatric Scan Protocols

Without adjusting scan parameters, smaller patients—particularly children—could receive a higher and

**Chest / Abdomen / Pelvis (CAP) – Weight Specific Protocols**

| Patient weight | Relative mAs or $CTDI_{vol}$ dose |
|---|---|
| Newborn to 10 kgm | 0.2-0.4 |
| 10 to 30 kgm | 0.6 |
| 30 to 50 kgm | 0.8 |
| 50 to 70 kgm | 0.9 |
| 70 to 90 kgm (ave. adult) | 1.0 |
| Above 90 kgm (large adult) | 1.4 |

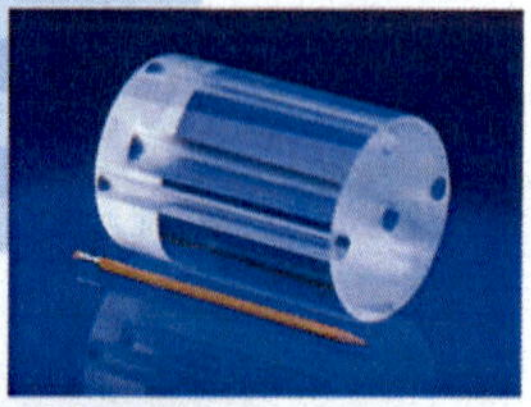

**Routine Brain – Age Specific Protocols**

| Patient age | Relative mAs or $CTDI_{vol}$ dose |
|---|---|
| Infant (up to 12 months) | 0.4 |
| Child (1 to 6 yrs) | 0.7 |
| Teen (7 yrs to 18 yrs) or average adult head | 0.9 |

**Fig. 14** Special scan protocols have been developed to lower dose for pediatric and infant CT examinations according to age (for head scans) and weight (for body scans). The protocols were developed with custom-made phantoms, such as the 10 cm phantom displayed on the right. "CT radiation dose: Philips Perspective", by Alain Vlassenbroek: *"Published with kind permission of © A. Vlassenbroek, 2012. All Rights Reserved"*

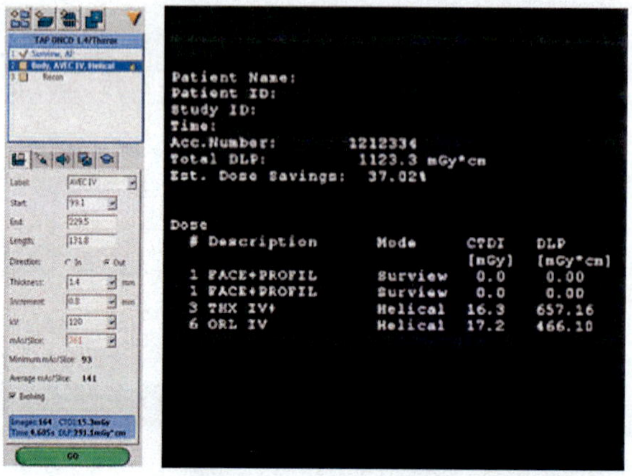


**Fig. 15** Dose estimates are displayed on the operator's console for all scan protocols prior to and throughout the examination. Also, a dose report is included as a DICOM secondary capture with the reconstructed data set, including the percentage dose savings from dose reduction tools, such as DoseRight z-axis dose modulation (Z-DOM). "CT radiation dose: Philips Perspective", by Alain Vlassenbroek: *"Published with kind permission of © A. Vlassenbroek, 2012. All Rights Reserved"*

unnecessary dose due to reduced beam attenuation as discussed above. Special scan protocols have been developed to lower dose for pediatric and infant CT examinations according to age (for head scans) and weight (for body scans), as shown in Fig. 14. The protocols were developed with custom-made phantoms, such as the 10 cm phantom on the right of Fig. 14, to prevent the underestimation of absorbed dose for smaller patients (Karabulut and Ariyürek 2006), as is the case when using FDA-standard 32 (body) and 16 cm adult (head) phantoms. The tube current reduction factors shown suggest mAs settings relative to ALARA-optimized adult protocols, and they can be further adapted according to the clinical indication, imaging objective, and physician preferences.

These pediatric protocols are used in combination with dose reducing tools, such as the infant SmartShape wedge filter and the Eclipse DoseRight Collimator, to provide multiple advantages and a comprehensive solution for pediatric dose management.

## 4 Dose Reporting

Advances in Philips' CT platforms also include intuitive reporting and recording of estimated dose, dose reduction, and dose efficiency. This feedback enables intra- and inter-scan assessments and comparisons of estimated dose levels. It can also be used in conjunction with image quality reviews to optimize scan protocols.

Dose estimates are displayed on the operator's console for all scan protocols prior to and throughout the examination (Fig. 15). Average volume dose index ($CTDI_{vol}$), dose-length product (DLP), and geometric dose efficiency are automatically updated as the operator plans the scan. If the planned $CTDI_{vol}$ exceeds the maximum allowed dose, a dose alert is generated to inform the technologist. Also, a dose report is included as a DICOM secondary capture with the reconstructed data set (Fig. 15). It includes the percentage dose savings from dose optimization tools, such as z-axis dose modulation (Z-DOM).

## 5 Summary

The advances of Philips' CT platforms were designed to increase dose efficiency and optimize image quality, thereby helping to achieve doses ALARA for ever-widening patient populations. This was achieved through Essence technology and by integrating dose optimization technologies in each stage of the imaging chain. These advances simplify the delivery of the right quantity and quality of exposure when and where needed for routine as well as challenging examinations.

The DoseWise philosophy also includes ongoing investments in innovative research and development and clinical collaboration. Further dose reductions will be achieved: X-ray beams will be dynamically shaped, filtered, modulated, and localized according to the reason for scanning and the tissue to be scanned. Dose estimates will be reported and recorded more accurately, taking into account patient size, shape, and tissue sensitivity. An array of new low dose CT applications will emerge such as those low enough to replace the radiograph. New partnerships and alliances will be forged to update ALARA practice standards, including education and reporting, and to provide a forum for sharing low dose scan protocols and techniques.

Together in clinical partnership, the modern Philips MDCT platforms and the DoseWise strategies embolden a vision of a new era of expanding MDCT use, fueled by increasing clinical benefits and decreasing doses. This vision shows the way to routine detection of disease before the onset of symptoms and provides timely information to improve treatment decisions, leading to better patient care.

**Acknowledgments** We would like to thank our colleague Mark Olszewski, from Philips HealthCare CT Product Management, for taking the time to assess this manuscript. His comments were greatly appreciated. We also would like to thank our colleagues Efrat Shefer and Leon de Vries, from Philips CT Clinical Science for their careful reading and corrections to this chapter. All clinical images presented in this chapter are courtesy of Professor E. Coche, from the Cliniques Universitaires Saint-Luc (UCL) at Brussels in Belgium.

## References

Boll DT, Hoffmann MH, Huber N, Bossert AS, Aschoff AJ, Fleiter TR (2006) Spectral coronary multidetector computed tomography angiography: dual benefit by facilitating plaque characterization and enhancing lumen depiction. J Comput Assist Tomogr 30(5):804–811

Brenner DJ, Hall EJ (2007) Computed tomography: an increasing source of radiation exposure. N Engl J Med 357: 2277–2284

Engel KJ, Herrmann C, Zeitler G (2008) X-ray scattering in single and dual-source CT. Med Phys 35(1):318–332

FDA Public Health Notification: Reducing radiation risk from computed tomography for pediatric and small adult patients. November 2001; Available at http://www.fda.gov/MedicalDevices/Safety/AlertsandNotices/PublicHealthNotifications/ucm062185.htm

Frush DP, Slack CC, Hollingsworth CL, Bisset GS, Donnelly LF, Hsieh J, Lavin-Wensell T, Mayo JR (2002) Computer-Simulated radiation dose reduction for abdominal multidetector CT of pediatric patients. AJR 179:1107–1113

Frush DP, Donnelly LF, Rosen NS (2003) Computed tomography and radiation risks: what pediatric health care providers should know. Pediatrics 112(4):951–957

Fuchs VR, Sox HC Jr (2001) Physicians' views of the relative importance of thirty medical innovations. Health Aff 20(5): 30–42

Golding SJ, Shrimpton PC (2002) Commentary. Radiation dose in CT: are we meeting the challenge? Br J Radiol 75(889): 1–4

Goske MJ, Applegate KE, Boylan J, Butler PF, Callahan MJ, Coley BD, Farley S, Frush DP, Hernanz-Schulman M, Jaramillo D, Johnson ND, Kaste SC, Morrison G, Strauss KJ, Tuggle N (2008a) The image gently campaign: working together to change practice. AJR Am J Roentgenol 190(2): 273–274

Goske MJ, Applegate KE, Boylan J, Butler PF, Callahan MJ, Coley BD, Farley S, Frush DP, Hernanz-Schulman M, Jaramillo D, Johnson ND, Kaste SC, Morrison G, Strauss KJ, Tuggle N (2008b) The image gently campaign: increasing CT radiation dose awareness through a national education and awareness program. Pediatr Radiol 38(3): 265–269

Hesse B, Murphy RT, Sigurdsson G et al (2006) Use of tissue doppler imaging to guide tube current modulation in cardiac multidetector computed tomographic angiography. AJC 98(5):603–607

Joseph PM, Spital RD (1982) The effects of scatter in X-ray computed tomography. Med Phys 9(4):464–472

Kalra MK, Maher MM, Toth TL et al (2004) Strategies for CT radiation dose optimization. Radiology 230(3):619–628

Karabulut N, Arıyürek M (2006) Low dose CT: practices and strategies of radiologists in university hospitals. Diagn Interv Radiol 12(1):3–8

Lee CL, Haims AH, Monico EP, Brink JA, Forman HP (2004) Diagnostic CT scans: assessment of patient, physician, and radiologist awareness of radiation dose and possible risks. Radiol 231:393–398

Lee K, Lee W, Lee J, Lee B, Oh G (2010) Dose reduction and image quality assessment in MDCT using AEC (D-DOm and Z-Dom) and in-plane bismuth shielding. Radiat Prot Dosimetry 141(2):162–167

McCollough CH, Bruesewitz MR, Kofler JM (2006) CT dose reduction and dose management tools: overview of available options. Radiographics 26:503–512

Mettler FA, Wiest PW, Locken JA, Kelsey CA (2000) CT scanning patterns of use and dose. J Radiol Prot 20:353–359

Morgan HT (2002) Image quality improvement and dose reduction in CT pediatric imaging. Medica Mundi 46(3): 16–21

Philips Healthcare (2009) The Brilliance iCT and DoseWise strategies, White Paper

Philips Healthcare (2011) iDose$^4$ iterative reconstruction technique, White Paper

Radon J (1917) Über die Bestimmung von Funktionen durch Ihre Integralwerte längs gewisser Mannigfaltigkeiten. Berichte über die Verhandlungen der Sächsische Akademie der Wissenschaften (Reports on the proceedings of the Saxony Academy of Science) 69:262–277

Technical report (2007) CT Market Summary Report, INV 2007, IMV Medical Information Division, Des Plaines, IL

Vogtmeier G, Dorscheid R, Engle K, Lutha R, Mattson R, Harwood B, Appleby M, Randolph B, Klinger J (2008) Two dimensional anti-scattergrid for computed tomography detectors. Proc SPIE 6913:691359-1–11

Whiting BR, Massoumzadeh P, Earl OA, O'Sullivan JA, Snyder DL, Williamson JF (2006) Properties of preprocessed sinogram data in X-ray computed tomography. Med Phys 33(9):3290–3303


Whiting BR, Massoumzadeh P, Earl OA, O'Sullivan JA, Snyder DL, Williamson JF (2006) Properties of preprocessed sinogram data in X-ray computed tomography. Med Phys 33(9):3290–3303


Wilting JE, Zwartkruis A, van Leeuwen MS, Timmer J, Kamphuis AG, Feldberg M (2001) A rational approach to dose reduction in CT: individualized scan protocols. Eur Radiol 11:2627–2632

# Practical Approaches to Dose Reduction: Toshiba Perspective

Jacob Geleijns and R. Irwan

## Contents




J. Geleijns (✉)
Radiology Department, Leiden University Medical Center, Albinusdreef 2, 2333 ZA, Leiden, The Netherlands
e-mail: J.Geleijns@lumc.nl

R. Irwan
CT Business Unit, Toshiba Medical Systems Europe, Zoetermeer, The Netherlands



**Abstract**

Since its inception, computed tomography (CT) has advanced medicine and became an invaluable diagnostic tool. Technological advances in CT have expanded its clinical capabilities leading to a substantial increase in CT utilization. The large number of patients and diagnostic tasks in CT imaging warrants methods for ensuring that every individual patient receives the best diagnostic image quality at the lowest possible dose. A busy clinical practice will interact with a wide range of patients varying in age and body habits, each requiring a personalized CT examination. The optimized image quality for a clinical exam will depend on the diagnostic task and the size and shape of the patient being imaged. Toshiba has designed its Aquilion line of CT scanners to yield high image quality with minimal radiation dose for all patients. From the dual-supported anode X-ray tube, to the efficient detector system and low-noise data acquisition system (DAS), to the dose-saving SURE Exposure 3D tube current modulation software, to advanced, adaptive and iterative reconstruction, and noise reduction algorithms, the range of Aquilion CT systems is designed to deliver optimal image quality at the lowest possible dose.


## 1 Detector Efficiency

No single hardware aspect of a scanner has more influence on dose than the efficiency of the detection system. The detector's ability to catch the X-ray,

D. Tack et al. (eds.), *Radiation Dose from Multidetector CT*, Medical Radiology. Diagnostic Imaging,
DOI: 10.1007/174_2011_501, © Springer-Verlag Berlin Heidelberg 2012

convert it to light, transmit that light, and convert it to an electrical signal with minimal loss defines the overall efficiency of the detector. More efficient detectors result in lower patient dose for a given level of image quality. In order to create the highly efficient scintillator detector material, Toshiba developed a new method of sintering the Gadolinium Oxysulfide (GOS) ceramic. With this new method, only Praseodymium is added to the base ceramic which keeps the light output high and allows the material to be accurately machined to 0.5 mm slices with clean, sharp edges. Toshiba's detector system, based on this scintillator, is the only detector system that achieves 0.5 mm slice thickness for their entire range of scanners, from the 4 detector row scanner all the way up to the 320 detector row scanner. The detector's low afterglow and fast decay times allow fast scanning and rotation times, avoidance of image artifacts, while its high light output contributes to good sensitivity and low contrast detectability. The scintillator is over 99% absorption efficient and optically transparent with a high light output, for example 2.3 times that of cadmium tungstate ($CdWO_4$). It is characterized by fast decay times and low afterglow properties that allow for high quality scanning at rotation times down to 0.35 s per rotation and below. Combined with precise and highly shielded electronics to ensure the best possible recording of the signal, the detector ensures optimal recording of the signal, even in case of low-dose acquisitions.

## 2 Tube Filtration

X-rays, upon leaving the tube, have a spectrum of energies that range from very low up to a maximum energy which is equal to the tube voltage. Low energy X-ray photons do not penetrate through the body as well as higher energy ones. In fact, the lowest energy photons will not pass through the body at all. Since image formation relies upon photons getting through the body and being picked up by the detectors, these lowest energy photons only contribute to patient dose. Therefore, all CT scanners add a certain amount of filtration to block the low energy X-rays. There is, however, a trade off involved when choosing the amount of filtration: in the process of removing low energy X-rays, some desirable, medium- and high-energy X-rays will be removed as well, thus decreasing the overall output of the tube. This means that higher tube currents are needed to realize a given image noise level. Furthermore, it is the medium energy X-rays that provide the best soft tissue contrast. Thus, heavier filtering will compromise the system's low contrast detectability. Therefore, a CT system needs enough filtration to block the lowest energy photons but not so much as to lose the ability to optimally distinguish low-contrast anatomy.

## 3 Scan Geometry

It is the ratio of the scanner's focus to isocenter and focus to detector distances that determines the geometry's role in patient exposure, mainly with regard to skin dose. There is skin dose reduction with a longer geometry since the patient is further away from the X-ray tube during scanning. Reduction of skin dose is particularly relevant in CT fluoroscopy and dynamic CT studies, where cumulative skin dose may become relatively high. Furthermore, longer geometries are more resistant to scatter, and thus contribute to better image quality, since there is a higher probability that a scattered photon will miss the detector entirely (Joemai et al. 2009).

## 4 X-ray Tube

Toshiba's X-ray tube has a feature to collect off-focal electrons and prevent them from producing X-rays. If these electrons are not captured, they can lead to artifacts and image quality degradation as well as unnecessary patient dose. By fitting a positively charged grid near the electrically grounded anode, any secondary, off-focal electrons are captured and removed from the system. In this way, the X-ray tube provides optimum image quality with a minimum of radiation dose to the patient.

## 5 Active Collimation

In helical scanning, exposure is needed before the start and after the end of the planned scan range in order to reconstruct images at these positions (Van der Molen and Geleijns 2007). This overranging requires at least one extra rotation, although

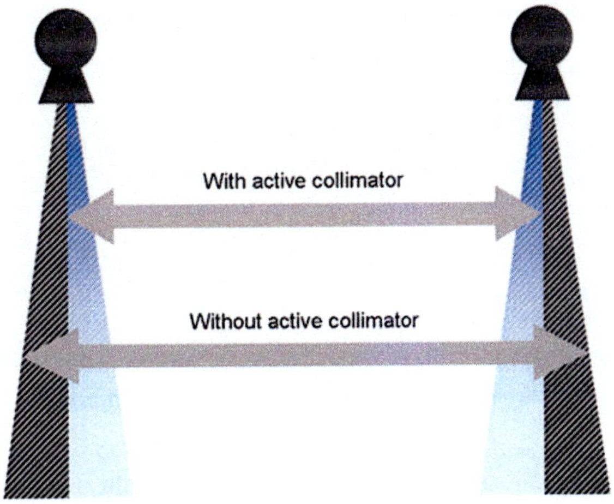


**Fig. 1** Active collimator diagram demonstrating elimination of the unnecessary radiation exposure at the beginning and end of the scan (*dark, dashed* areas), the active collimator reduces the exposed range considerably

only a small portion of this data is utilized. Active collimation synchronizes the width of the X-ray beam at the ends of the scan range to the clinically useful area needed for image reconstruction. By eliminating exposure that is not used for diagnosis, patient dose can be reduced. The collimator automatically opens at the start of the scan and closes at the end of the scan to keep the exposed area as short as possible, as illustrated in Fig. 1.

## 6 SURE Exposure 3D, Technique

The ultimate goal of CT technology is to create the best diagnostic image quality while minimizing radiation dose to the patient. Individual patients undergoing CT imaging have different needs depending on their size and shape and depending on the diagnostic task. Thus, it is essential that tools are being used to tailor each scan for the individual patient to ensure excellent image quality while maintaining the lowest possible radiation dose.

Analogous to automatic exposure control in X-ray imaging, in CT technologies such as SURE Exposure are used for managing dose on a patient-specific basis. SURE Exposure is a suite of dose reduction applications that integrate acquisition and reconstruction parameters with advanced dose reduction algorithms (Van der Molen et al. 2011).

Since the human body is not perfectly round and uniform in size and density, during a CT scan a varying tube current is required to achieve the same image quality in different parts of the body. For example, during a typical lung scan, the first part of the acquisition must penetrate the bony shoulder area, while the middle part is largely low-attenuating air, and the end has to penetrate the liver and diaphragm. In this example, a higher tube current is needed through the shoulders, a smaller amount through the lungs, and an amount somewhere in between for the abdomen. Furthermore, patients are not all the same size. A sumo wrestler would clearly require a higher tube current to achieve a given image quality level than would a ballerina. In addition because patients are shaped in an elliptical fashion, more tube current is typically needed when X-rays are passing laterally through the body than when they are passing anterior-posterior.

Toshiba's SURE Exposure 3D software automatically adjusts the mAs rapidly during the scan to adapt to and compensate for all of these changes in attenuation level. To accomplish this, SURE Exposure determines the relative attenuation of a patient from either a single or dual scanogram, and converts this information into a "water equivalent thickness". The user-chosen image quality level is then used to calculate the amount of tube current needed to achieve the desired image quality. If a single scanogram is used, SURE Exposure will modulate longitudinally along the length of the patient in the z-direction. If a dual scanogram is used, SURE Exposure will modulate in all three dimensions as the tube rotates and traverses the patient (Fig. 2).

Therefore, as the scan moves from the shoulders to the lung, the mAs goes down, and as the tube rotates around the patient, less tube current is used anterior-posterior than laterally. In addition, SURE Exposure adjusts the tube current appropriately for the selected acquisition and reconstruction parameters, and dose reduction algorithms. SURE Exposure tube current modulation has the ability to reduce patient dose while maintaining optimized image quality. For the same image quality level, compared to non-modulated scanning, SURE Exposure 3D can reduce the dose by up to 40%.

The unique nature of coronary imaging gives another opportunity for dose saving (Seguchi et al. 2010). With low and steady heart rates, the optimum phase for reconstruction is typically between 65 and 80% R–R. Since the data in the rest of the cardiac cycle

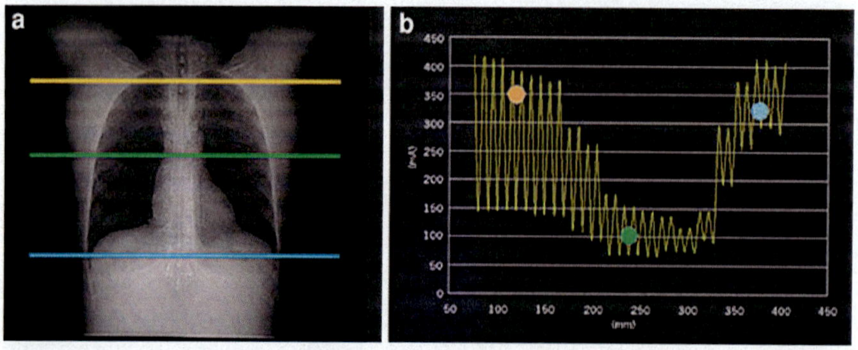


**Fig. 2** Three-dimensional exposure control by modulation of the tube current. The tube current is higher at the level of the shoulders and the upper abdomen, and lower at the level of the lungs. Periodic tube current modulation compensates for differences in the attenuation in the lateral and frontal directions

is used only for examining the bulk ventricular function, a much lower tube current may be used. SURE Exposure 3D with ECG dose modulation allows the tube current to be significantly reduced during the systolic phases of the cardiac cycle, enabling a reduction in patient dose of as much as 50%.

## 7 SURE Exposure 3D, Image Quality

The appropriate image quality for each diagnostic task is determined by the physician. SURE Exposure then modulates tube current to achieve the lowest possible dose for that desired image quality. The image quality level can be automatically set by the protocol selected for the clinical examination. Three or more global image quality settings are available for each scan region. For example, an adult abdomen protocol has the global settings: High Quality, Standard, and Low Dose. The global settings are specific to the image quality requirements of the body region being imaged (adult head, adult body, pediatric head, or pediatric body). Each image quality setting is defined by a target standard deviation of noise. The range of tube current values used for each image quality setting is limited by an adjustable minimum and maximum tube current.

The automated image quality settings operate on a global level, are tailored for the body region, and are available from any protocol. SURE Exposure is fully customizable and any adjustments can be made to the default image quality levels. Some users may also prefer to generate additional global settings. A good example of this is the addition of an Ultra Low Dose image quality setting which may be used for protocols that tolerate higher noise levels such as follow-up examinations.

Protocol-specific image quality settings can be used for examinations that have specific image quality or dose requirements. For example, a group of patients may require chest CT studies for the purpose of lung volume measurements. Since the images will not require as high of image quality as required for conventional chest CT, the protocol for these volume scans can achieve maximum dose savings by allowing a higher noise level than in a standard chest protocol. This customized protocol can then be saved and used for all lung volume measurement examinations. Protocol-specific image quality settings can also be useful for sites involved in clinical trials with protocols that require specific tube current limits and noise levels. Creating automatic image quality settings for such specific protocols helps avoid operator error and accelerates workflow. SURE Exposure can also be adjusted for individual patient examinations. To adjust the image quality settings for an individual patient, the CT operator selects a desired standard deviation noise level and/or a minimum and maximum tube current. This type of individualized image quality adjustment may be necessary in patient-specific situations, which may be warranted for a patient with a known pregnancy, or an inherently radiosensitive patient (i.e., ataxia-telangiectasia patients).

SURE Exposure incorporates acquisition and reconstruction parameters, and is not just a stand-alone tube current modulation algorithm. One of the unique benefits of SURE Exposure is its ability to achieve excellent image quality by incorporating the acquisition and reconstruction parameters. Since acquisition and reconstruction parameters can have substantial effects on image noise, the tube current must be appropriately adjusted. SURE Exposure helps to ensure optimized image quality by tailoring not only to patient size and shape, but also to the imaging parameters selected for each imaging task.

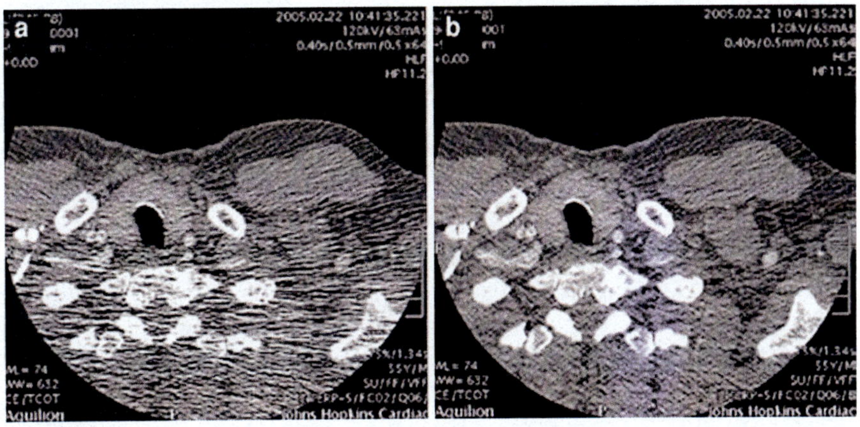


**Fig. 3** Effect of Boost3D on streaks from low photon count; image with typical streaks through the shoulder region (*left*), and image from the same dataset but reconstructed with Boost3D (*right*). (Courtesy of Johns Hopkins)

The primary acquisition parameters affecting image noise, in addition to tube current, are pitch, rotation time, and tube voltage. In helical scanning, higher pitch values (or faster table travel) can not only reduce scan time but can also affect image noise. SURE Exposure counteracts this effect by adjusting the tube current to achieve optimized image quality regardless of the selected pitch value. Likewise, SURE Exposure adjusts tube current to account for faster rotation times or lower tube voltage. By automatically adjusting to these acquisition parameters, SURE Exposure helps ensure that the target image quality is obtained at the lowest possible dose.

The parameters used to reconstruct an image can also have an effect on image noise. SURE Exposure accounts for reconstruction parameters selected for the initial reconstruction to adjust for these effects. For example, smoother reconstruction kernels will decrease image noise. SURE Exposure recognizes the selection of a smooth kernel and reduce the tube current to achieve the lowest possible dose for that scan while achieving the target image quality. SURE Exposure also recognizes the selection of reconstructed slice width and automatically adjusts to ensure high quality images.

An "Easy Mode" is also available, which offers users the option to automatically set SURE Exposure settings according to the reconstruction parameters most used for viewing each task-specific protocol.

## 8 Boost3D

Even with an optimized detector system and tube current modulation, highly attenuating anatomy such as the shoulders and pelvis as well as metal implants in the body can severely reduce the number of photons reaching the detectors. This localized reduction in photon count can lead to degradation in image quality in the form of excess noise and streak artifacts. Conventionally, these highly attenuating areas are imaged using increased tube current and tube voltage to overcome the low photon count. However, since increasing the imaging technique results in higher patient dose, Toshiba developed an adaptive, three-dimensional algorithm that preferentially corrects the raw data in areas with low photon count. This algorithm, known as Boost3D, seeks out portions of the raw-projection data where there is a disproportionate loss in X-ray signal and applies the three-dimensional filter locally to reduce the image noise and streak artifacts. In areas of normal signal, no correction is applied and the native image quality is preserved. Such local, or adaptive, techniques produce the optimum results because the filter is applied only where it is needed. Since this algorithm removes streak artifacts caused by photon

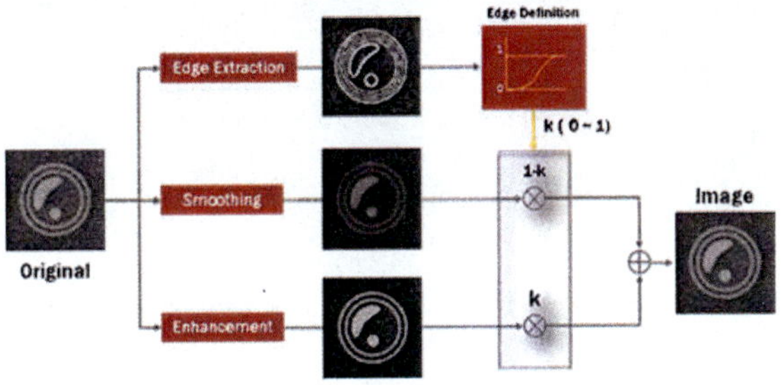


**Fig. 4** Quantum denoising software (QDS) reduces noise by adaptively targeting quantum noise in the reconstructed image. QDS applies a combination of smoothing and enhancing filters to an image, reducing quantum noise while maintaining spatial resolution and image texture. QDS is integrated into the imaging chain to automatically maximize dose savings and image quality without any guesswork on part of the user

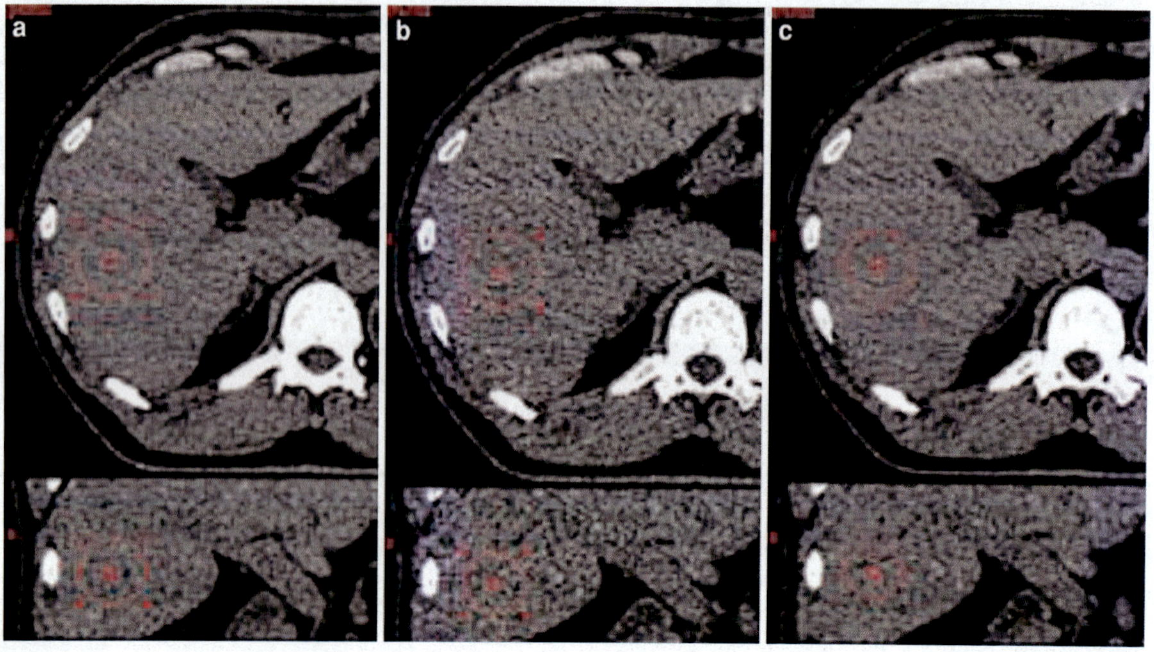


**Fig. 5** Effect of Quantum Denoising Software on a liver scan. **a** shows a scan at standard X-ray exposure and noise level. **b** shows a scan at 45% lower mAs. The noise value is increased. **c** shows the lower mAs scan with QDS. The noise is the same as the standard exposure, but with significantly less dose

starvation, it can either be applied to enhance images using conventional tube current settings, or to allow low-dose imaging with acceptable image quality by reducing the scan technique and, thereby, the patient dose. Figure 3 demonstrates images through the shoulder in a cardiac bypass patient using a relatively low scan technique. The images exhibit typical structured noise and streak artifacts resulting from the low photon count. However, when Boost3D is applied, Fig. 3 shows the resulting image quality: the image noise is greatly reduced and the streak artifacts disappear. By reducing the noise and mitigating the effects of low-dose scanning, adaptive techniques such as Boost3D are key developments in low dose CT imaging. Boost3D is easily selectable in any given protocol, making it convenient and simple to use.

## 9 Quantum Denoising Software

One method of improving image quality is through noise reduction. Image noise competes with signal, i.e. the representation of the anatomical object, and therefore the greater the amount of noise, the harder it becomes to visualize an object. Historically, obtaining the desired noise level for a task has been achieved by adjusting the tube voltage and tube current. However, increasing these settings increases radiation dose to the patient and requires more powerful generators. An alternative to increasing protocol settings is to reduce noise through image processing tools designed to reduce noise while preserving signal. Such tools allow the user to either improve image quality at a given dose without raising the tube current or to maintain image quality while decreasing tube current and patient dose. Quantum denoising software (QDS) was introduced in 2004 and has been routinely employed in routine clinical examinations and resulted in a dose reduction of up to 50%. Until the emergence of iterative reconstruction algorithms, QDS was offering unique and robust noise reduction that contributed to reducing patient dose. Beyond optimized scanning techniques and streak removal, with QDS it is possible to minimize the overall noise left in the reconstructed image. QDS is an adaptive noise reduction filter that works on reconstructed image data by preferentially smoothing areas of uniform density while preserving the edge information of the image. The algorithm uses locally sampled edge information within the image to blend together variable strength smoothing and sharpening filters. In areas of uniform density with few edges, the algorithm smoothes the image and reduces the noise; in areas with edges, such as near tissue boundaries and other complex structures, the algorithm enhances the image (Fig. 4).

QDS works in both two and three dimensions and can drastically reduce image noise, allowing a corresponding saving of patient dose. Figure 5 illustrates the substantial dose saving possible with QDS. Figure 5a shows the relative noise in the liver of a patient using a standard scan technique. Figure 5b demonstrates the increase in image noise as the tube current is reduced by 45%. Finally, Fig. 5c highlights the ability of the QDS to reduce the noise in the liver to a level similar to that of the original, higher dose image. QDS works in conjunction with the SURE Exposure 3D software to adjust the tube current based on the expected noise reduction from the adaptive filter.

## 10 Adaptive Iterative Dose Reduction 3D

AIDR 3D is the abbreviation of Adaptive Iterative Dose Reduction 3D and is the most recent algorithm for noise reduction. AIDR 3D has been specially designed to work iteratively in both the three dimensional reconstruction data and raw data domains. The collective AIDR 3D process results in robust noise reduction, which is essential for achieving ultra low dose examinations in routine clinical CT imaging. AIDR 3D can be routinely applied to all clinical acquisition modes and is able to remove up to 50% of image noise, while maintaining image quality, and resulting in dose reduction of up to 75% (Fig. 6).

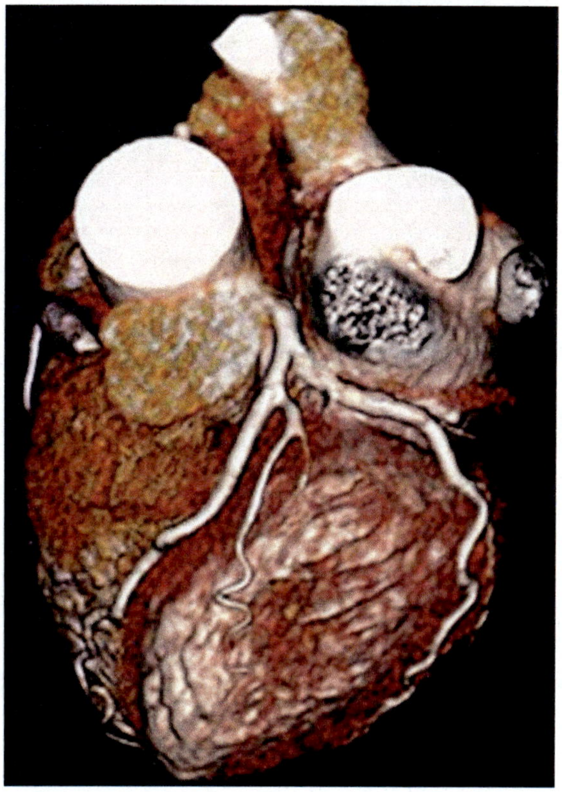

**Fig. 6** Volume rendered 3D cardiac CTA acquired on Aquilion ONE using AIDR software. This examination was acquired in a single heartbeat with 0.9 mSv of effective radiation dose. (Courtesy of Monash Medical Center)

Integration of dose reduction technologies is essential for optimal dose management. Therefore, AIDR 3D has been integrated with SURE Exposure 3D, Toshiba's automatic tube current modulation software. SURE Exposure 3D modulates the exposure for each patient, based on a preset, target level of image quality. When combined with AIDR 3D, reduced X-ray the optimal exposure setting are automatically calculated before the scan, while maintaining the preprogramed image quality. This combination provides a good solution for robust dose management.

SURE Exposure 3D is fully integrated into the imaging chain, including AIDR 3D, and can therefore calculate the minimum radiation exposure required for each examination in every patient. With the inclusion of AIDR 3D in the scan protocol, the calculated exposure can be reduced by up to 75% when compared to a scan performed with traditional filtered back projection (FBP) reconstruction. The AIDR 3D algorithm is designed to work in both the raw data and reconstruction domains (Fig. 7). In a low dose scan, the number of X-ray photons reaching the detector becomes very small and electronic noise in the Data Acquisition Systems (DAS) might become dominant which will degrade image quality. To avoid this, AIDR 3D processing uses a scanner model and a statistical noise model considering both photon and electronic noise to eliminate noise due to photon starvation in the projection data.

The statistical and scanner models are used together to achieve electronic noise reduction in the raw data domain. The models analyze the physical properties of the CT system at the time of the acquisition, and characterize both electronic and quantum noise patterns in the raw data domain. The projection noise estimation

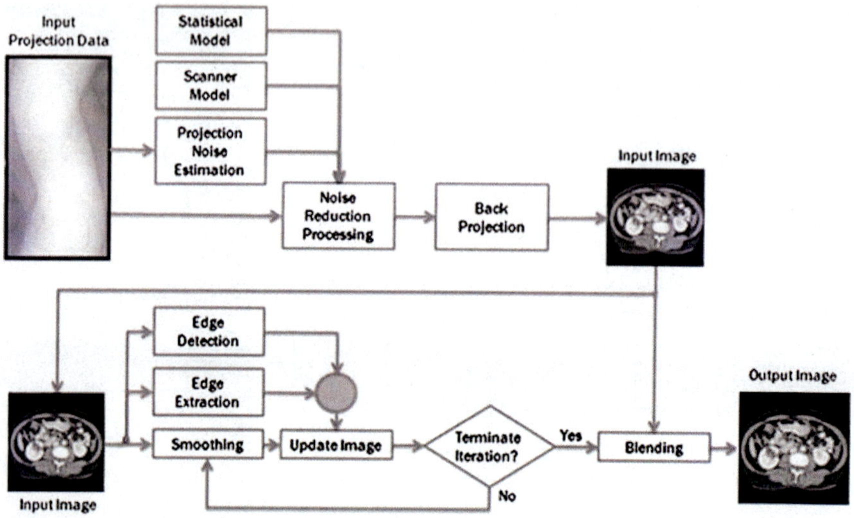


**Fig. 7** AIDR 3D is an advanced iterative reconstruction algorithm that reduces noise both in the raw data domain and also in the reconstruction process in three-dimensions

takes care of noise and artifacts reduction. An initial image (filtered backprojection) is used as an input image in every iteration to be compared with the output image. A sophisticated iterative technique is then performed to optimize reconstructions for the particular body region being scanned by detecting and preserving sharp details and smoothing the image at the same time. Finally, a weighted blending is applied to the original reconstruction and the output of this iterative process to maintain the noise granularity. The complete AIDR 3D reconstruction therefore increases the SNR while improving the spatial resolution and produces images which look natural. With AIDR 3D, image noise can be reduced while spatial resolution and structural edges are preserved or even improved.

Figure 8 shows the effect of AIDR 3D (right) compared to conventional filtered backprojection (left) for a low dose scan of an anthropomorphic phantom. The improvement in image quality is clearly noticeable. Especially the small details in the pulmonary branches can be clearly seen. The dose length product (DLP) is 6.43 mGy cm which is equivalent to 0.09 mSv (tube voltage 120, tube current 10, rotation time 0.35 s)

## 11 Clinical Cases

### 11.1 Cardiac

A 75-year-old female with a body mass index (BMI) of 20 was scanned with a prospectively gated volume acquisition with the Aquilion ONE CT scanner (scan time 0.35 s; 80 kV). SURE Exposure 3D and AIDR 3D, the scan resulted in a DLP of 29 mGy cm which is equivalent to an effective dose of 0.4 mSv ($k$–factor = 0.014 mGy cm/mSv). Images reconstructed with FBP or AIDR 3D are presented in Fig. 9. More on cardiac CT with Toshiba scanners in papers by Geleijns et al. (2011); George et al. (2011), and Joemai et al. (2008a, b).

### 11.2 Pediatric

Radiation protection in pediatric imaging is a major concern because children are particularly sensitive to radiation. With the Aquilion ONE scanner, dose savings of 20–40% have been reported (Kroft et al. 2010). Furthermore, with 16 cm longitudinal coverage and an acquisition time of 0.35 s, the use of sedation can often be avoided. AIDR 3D can reduce the dose even further for example for a one-day-old baby with a congenital heart defect. Figure 10 shows the clinical images demonstrating narrowing of pulmonary trunk while there is no compression of the airways (80 kVp, 100 mA, 0.35 s, and 8 cm scan range, DLP of 6.8 mGy cm, 0.27 mSv effective dose). More on pediatric CT in the paper by Kroft et al. (2010).

### 11.3 Dual Energy

Dual energy is another clinical applications, where AIDR 3D can be applied to in order to achieve dose

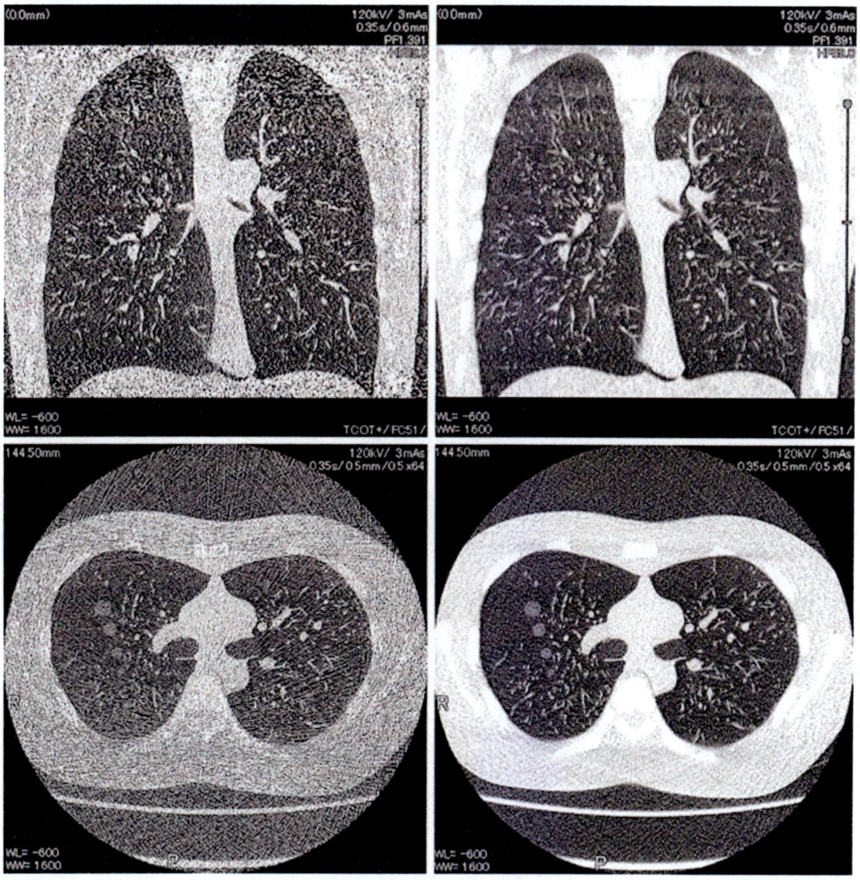


**Fig. 8** Images obtained with FBP reconstruction (*left*), and AIDR 3D reconstruction (*right*) of a Thorax scan of an anthropomorphic phantom. The effective dose is 0.09 mSv ($k$–factor = 0.014 mGy cm/mSv). (Courtesy of Keio University Hospital)

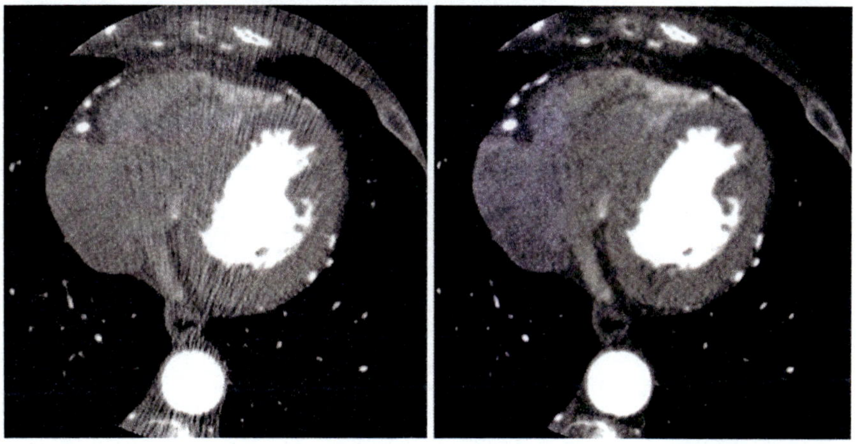

**Fig. 9** Cardiac CTA: FBP reconstruction (*left*) and AIDR 3D reconstruction (*right*) (DLP of 29 mGy cm and an effective dose of 0.4 mSv). (Courtesy of Monash Medical Center)

reduction. For example, standard abdominal pelvic CT scanning protocols can be converted to dual energy protocols by maintaining the same cumulative DLP. Tube currents for each energy arc chosen so that the image noise of both images is matched. Figure 11 shows coronal and axial images of a patient with renal colic with a total effective dose of just 2.2 mSv. Images without AIDR 3D (left) and with AIDR 3D (right), images reconstructed using AIDR 3D demonstrate substantial noise reduction compared to images without AIDR.

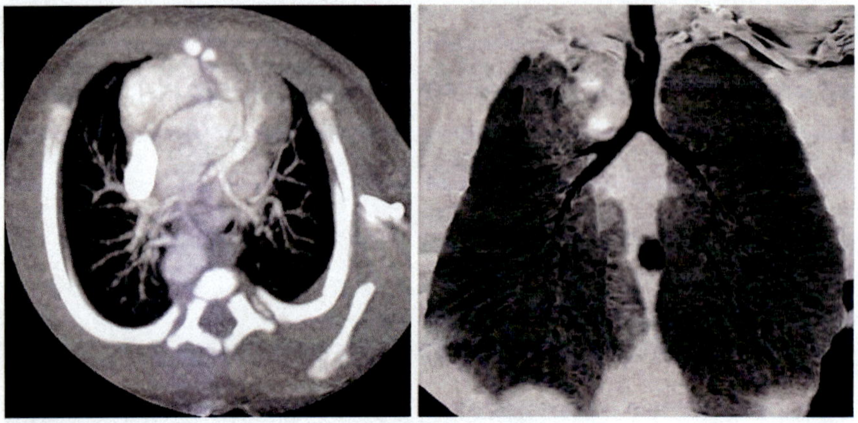

**Fig. 10** One day old baby with Tetralogy of Fallot. In 0.35 s the infant was scanned with the Aquilion ONE scanner and images were reconstructed with AIDR 3D (DLP of 6.8 mGy cm, equivalent of 0.27 mSv). (Courtesy of Monash Medical Center)

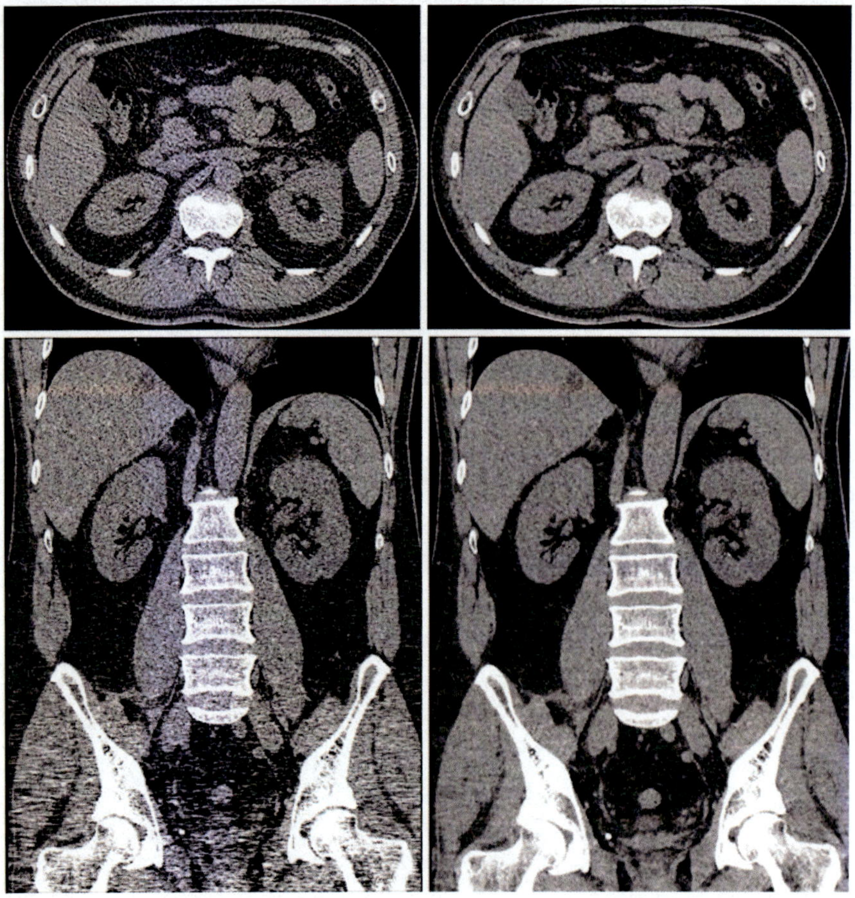

**Fig. 11** Dual Energy coronal and axial images of patient with renal colic: without AIDR 3D (*left*), and with AIDR 3D (*right*). The total effective dose is 2.2 mSv. (Courtesy of CHU Nancy)

## 11.4 Body Perfusion

Renal cell carcinoma (RCC) is the most common renal neoplasm. While ultrasound and MRI have been used to diagnose this disease, body perfusion with CT is becoming an interesting alternative as it produces fast and accurate diagnostic results and allows evaluation of malignant or benign renal masses. Figure 12 demonstrates a clinical application of AIDR 3D for low dose kidney perfusion.

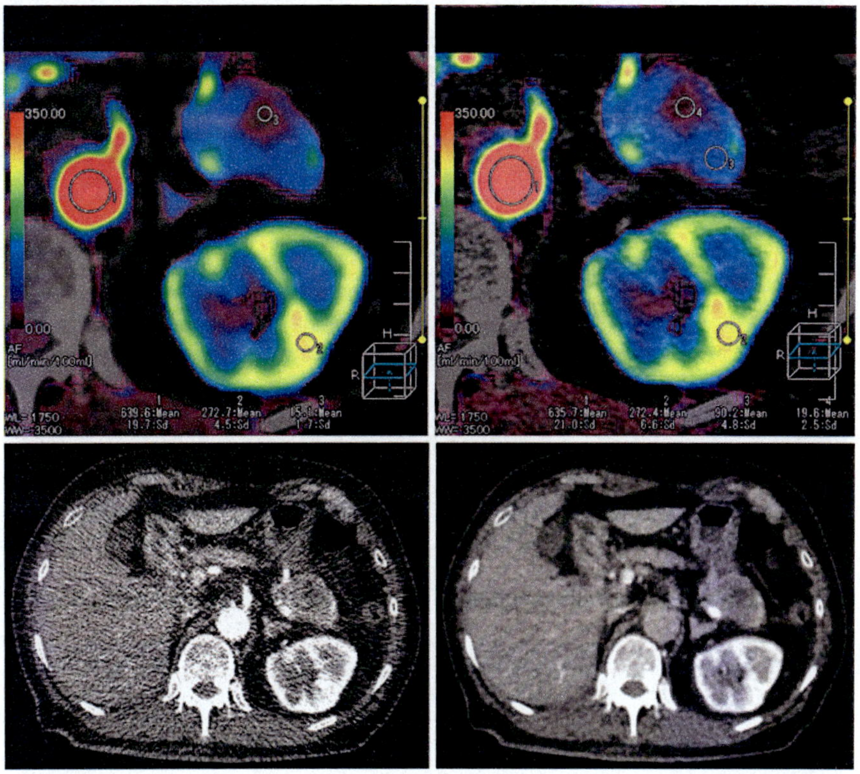


**Fig. 12** AIDR 3D (*right*) was applied to a low dose kidney perfusion protocol: 100 kV, 25 mAs, 16 cm z-coverage, producing an effective dose of 9 mSv (*k*–factor = 0.015 mGy cm/mSv). (Courtesy of Keio University Hospital)

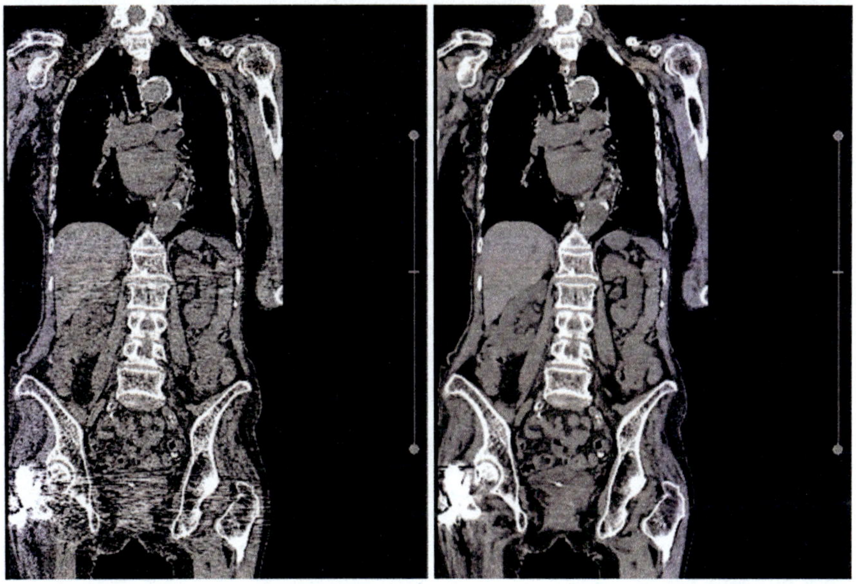

**Fig. 13** FBP reconstruction (*left*) and AIDR 3D (*right*) reconstruction of a trauma patient. The total scan range was 65 cm, and scan time was 4 s. The difference in reconstruction time between FBP and AIDR 3D was smaller than 10%. (Courtesy of Fujita Health University Hospital)

With a longitudinal coverage of 16 cm (Toshiba Aquilion ONE), body perfusion guarantees temporal (phase) uniformity across the entire volume. An image registration algorithm was applied to make sure that the mismatch due to the motion from respiration is eliminated. Using a low dose protocol of 100 kV, 25 mAs for each volume, and a full longitudinal coverage of 16 cm, renal masses can be detected with a total effective dose of below 10 mSv.

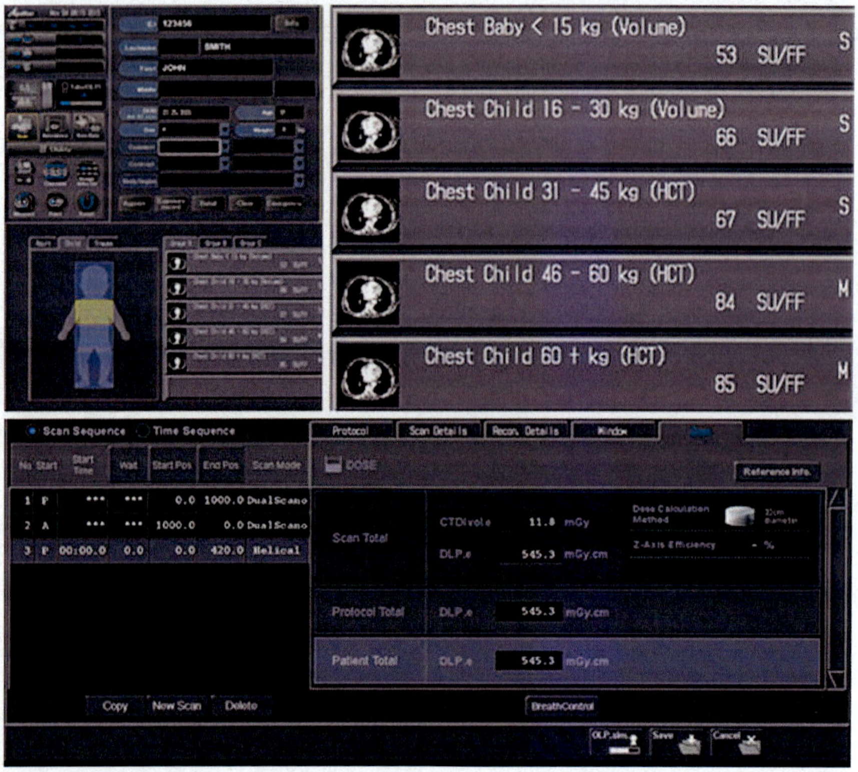


**Fig. 14** Some screenshots from the user interface. The patient is registered from Modality Worklist (*above*, *left*), and there is an automatic selection of age-based protocols. Weight-based exam plans are available for pediatric applications (*above*, *right*). Detailed information about patient dose is available at all stages of the CT examination (*below*)

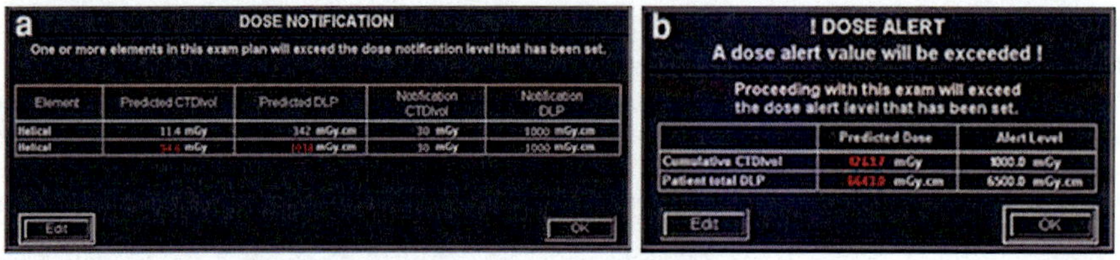


**Fig. 15** Screens corresponding to the Dose Notification (*above*) and the Dose Alert, (*below*) both are part of the "Dose Check" safeguard

## 11.5 Trauma

Fast acquisition and reconstruction is very important in the emergency department, the increase in reconstruction time with AIDR 3D is below 10% depending on anatomical regions being scanned. Figure 13 illustrates an example of whole body (thorax, abdomen, and pelvis) of a trauma patient (helical acquisition, 80 × 0.5 mm, pitch factor of 1.4, and rotation time of 0.35 s).

### 11.5.1 User Interface

A good user interface is essential for achieving optimal and consistent use of a CT scanner. The Toshiba user interface is intuitive, and efficient, some screenshots are presented in Fig. 14. The selection of the CT study starts with pictograms (to select adult or pediatric, and for selection of the body part), and after that a specific protocol can be selected. There is always information available with regard to patient dose.

Toshiba supports international initiatives on patient safety, it implemented the Dose Notification Feature and the Dose Alert Feature, both are part of the "Dose Check" safeguard. Figure 15 shows the corresponding screens.

## References

Geleijns J, Joemai RM, Dewey M, de Roos A, Zankl M, Cantera AC, Artells MS (2011) Radiation exposure to patients in a multicenter coronary angiography trial (CORE 64). Am J Roentgenol 196(5):1126–1132

George RT, Arbab-Zadeh A, Cerci RJ, Vavere AL, Kitagawa K, Dewey M, Rochitte CE, Arai AE, Paul N, Rybicki FJ, Lardo AC, Clouse ME, Lima JA (2011) Diagnostic performance of combined noninvasive coronary angiography and myocardial perfusion imaging using 320-MDCT: the CT angiography and perfusion methods of the CORE320 multicenter multinational diagnostic study. Am J Roentgenol 197(4):829–837

Joemai RM, Geleijns J, Veldkamp WJ, Kroft LJ (2008a) Clinical evaluation of 64-slice CT assessment of global left ventricular function using automated cardiac phase selection. Circ J 72(4):641–646

Joemai RM, Geleijns J, Veldkamp WJ, de Roos A, Kroft LJ (2008b) Automated cardiac phase selection with 64-MDCT coronary angiography. Am J Roentgenol 191(6):1690–1697

Joemai RM, Zweers D, Obermann WR, Geleijns J (2009) Assessment of patient and occupational dose in established and new applications of MDCT fluoroscopy. Am J Roentgenol 192(4):881–886

Kroft LJ, Roelofs JJ, Geleijns J (2010) Scan time and patient dose for thoracic imaging in neonates and small children using axial volumetric 320-detector row CT compared to helical 64-, 32-, and 16-detector row CT acquisitions. Pediatr Radiol 40(3):294–300

Seguchi S, Aoyama T, Koyama S, Fujii K, Yamauchi-Kawaura C (2010) Patient radiation dose in prospectively gated axial CT coronary angiography and retrospectively gated helical technique with a 320-detector row CT scanner. Med Phys 37(11):5579–5585

Van der Molen AJ, Geleijns J (2007) Overranging in multisection CT: quantification and relative contribution to dose–comparison of four 16-section CT scanners. Radiology 242(1):208–216

Van der Molen AJ, Joemai RM, Geleijns J (2011) Performance of longitudinal and volumetric tube current modulation in a 64-slice CT with different choices of acquisition and reconstruction parameters. Phys Med (in press)

# Index




DOI: 10.1007/978-3-642-24535-0, © Springer-Verlag Berlin Heidelberg 2012